RXPREP COURSE BOOK
2015 EDITION

KAREN SHAPIRO, PHARMD, BCPS

SHERRY A. BROWN, PHARMD, MBA, BCPS

With Stephanie D. Garrett, PharmD, BCPS

CONTRIBUTORS

AMINE ALE-ALI
PHARMD, BCOP

PAUL BERINGER
PHARMD

HEATHER R. BREAM-ROUWENHORST
PHARMD, BCPS

KATIE E. CARDONE
PHARMD, BCACP, FNKF, FASN

GEORGE DEMAAGD
PHARMD, BCPS

PAULINA DEMING
PHARMD, PHC

CATRINA DERDERIAN
BS, PHARMD

JEFFREY FUDIN
BS, PHARMD, FCCP

MUOI GI
PHARMD, BCPS, BCOP

JEFF GOAD
PHARMD, MPH, FAPHA, FCPHA, FCSHP

SUSAN E. GORMAN
PHARMD, MS, DABAT, FAACT

ERIC GUPTA
PHARMD, FNLA, BCPS, CLS

BRETT HEINTZ
PHARMD, BCPS-ID, AAHIVE

JAN D. HIRSCH
BSPHARM, PHD

DOUG HUMBER
PHARMD

KIM JONES
PHARMD, BCPS

JEFF LEE
PHARMD, FCCP

KELVIN LI
RPH

JOSEPH D. MA
PHARMD

JOEL C. MARRS
PHARMD, FCCP, FNLA, BCPS-AQ CARDIOLOGY, BCACP, CLS

CRAIG MARTIN
PHARMD, BCPS

JESS MARTINEZ
PHARMD

CYNTHIA L. MORRIS-KUKOSKI
PHARMD, DABAT, FAACT

TIEN NG
PHARMD, FCCP, BCPS (AQ-C)

NANCY N. NGUYEN
PHARMD, BCPS, AAHIVP

NATHAN PAINTER
PHARMD, CDE

ALLISON PROVINE
PHARMD, BCPS

RENU F. SINGH
PHARMD, BCACP, CDE

KIMBERLY B. TALLIAN
PHARMD, BCPP, FASHP, FCCP, FCSHP

STACY A. VOILS
PHARMD, MSC, BCPS

ROBIN WACKERNAH
PHARMD, BCPP

D. RAYMOND WEBER
PHARMD, BSPHARM, BCOP, BCPS, RPH

Cover design by Creativeshoebox.com

Book design by Media Arts International

Graphics by Zoe Gallagher & Media Arts International

Proofing Assistance from Pauline Park, PharmD & Pamela Tu, PharmD

TABLE OF CONTENTS

EXAM OVERVIEW

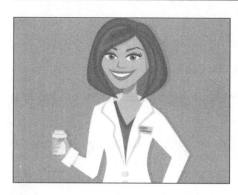

INTRODUCTION
This section includes four topics:

- NAPLEX® Overview
- Test Taking Tips
- How to Use this Book
- CPJE Pointers – for CA exam takers

NAPLEX® OVERVIEW

The NAPLEX® exam blueprint (outline) is available on the board's website at www.nabp.net. Please review the complete blueprint on the website. The blueprint is expected to change in November 2015. This is the summary of the 2014 blueprint, that will be in effect for most of 2015. The exam has three sections. Each section requires a passing score.

The first section is "Safe and Effective" use and is the majority of the exam (56%).

- These are largely asked in a patient-case format. You will need to identify aberrant labs, medical histories, medication use history – and recognize appropriate or inappropriate treatments.

- This section includes expected dosing options, regimens, and formulations. Pharmacoeconomic factors may be important: if a patient cannot afford a drug and a less-expensive, but valid option is available, the pharmacist should recommend the preferable drug. This is an important area for pharmacists; manufacturers can entice clinicians to use their new, expensive drugs – but part of a pharmacist's job is to review study data in order to protect the patient and help control costs.

- The ability to monitor patient outcomes is assessed, such as the patient's response to treatment and the drug's effect on renal or liver function. This requires selecting correct monitoring tests. Improving medication adherence and recommending better treatment options are tested on as well.

The second section is safe and accurate preparation and dispensing of medications (33%).

■ This includes calculations, including nutritional requirements and basic <u>PN calculations</u>. Flow rates for drugs administered by IV infusion <u>are essential</u>, along with drug concentrations, and the other general calculations in the section. Poor math skills will result in an unacceptable grade on the exam. A math mistake in pharmacy is a dosing mistake. Accuracy in calculations is an important skill to demonstrate on the exam.

■ Trade/generics are tested, along with common dosage forms. Be able to use PK parameters and quality assurance information to identify appropriate interchange and information regarding storage, packaging, handling, administration, and medication disposal.

The third section requires assessment, recommendations, and providing health care information to promote public health (11%).

■ Know the drug reference sources, how to administer and counsel on emergency care and vaccinations, and be able to make recommendations regarding common dietary supplements.

■ Be able to read simple study summaries and interpret the data.

■ Review self-care products and durable medical equipment, and self-monitoring of health status by the patient.

NAPLEX® is a computer-adaptive exam that consists of 185 multiple-choice questions. Of these, 150 questions are used to calculate the test score.

■ The majority of the questions are asked in a scenario-based format (such as patient profiles with accompanying questions). There are also stand alone questions.

■ The total test time is 4.25 hours, which includes an optional 10-minute break after approximately 2 hours. Any other breaks that are needed will be subtracted from the total testing time.

■ On the day of the exam, arrive 30 minutes prior to your appointment to get signed in (fingerprints will be taken, you will need 2 forms of ID, and do not bring prohibited items into the exam room). Acceptable forms of ID and the list of prohibited items is in the exam registration booklet.

■ If you arrive 30 minutes or later than your scheduled appointment, and are refused admission to sit for the exam, you will be required to forfeit your appointment.

■ A computer-adaptive exam assesses the answer to a given question in order to determine the level of difficulty to be selected for the following question. If you answer a question correctly, the computer will select a more difficult question from the test pool in an appropriate content area. If you answer a question incorrectly, an easier question will be selected by the computer. If you miss a calculation you are likely to get another similar item worth less and you may not accumulate enough points to pass.

■ All questions must be answered in the order in which they are presented. It is not possible to skip questions, or to go back at a later time.

- If you have not recently finished a year or more of clinical rotations in school or are coming from practice in a hospital setting please review the Lab Values and Patient Charts chapter which discusses how to <u>interpret charts</u> (medical records); this is required in order to answer questions. The two types of common case formats are in this text at the end of most of the clinical chapters. Interpreting medical records requires an understanding of <u>lab values</u> (what the value is used for and the interpretation of common measurements).

- The Pearson VUE testing center console uses an <u>on-screen calculator</u> which looks similar to the Texas Instruments TI-30XS Multiview or another similar hand-held. The on-screen calculator can be opened in a pop-up window during the exam at any time. Some of the calculations require functions on the on-screen calculator. You can do multiple-step problems; do not round until the last step or the answer could be wrong. A candidate requesting a handheld calculator will be supplied a five function calculator by Pearson VUE. If requested, this should be used only for simple math.

TEST TAKING TIPS

- Study the top selling drugs (group them together; you'll see all the statins are there, many ACE Is, etc) – and focus on the doses for the common agents. We have bolded most of them in this text. The RxPrep test bank can be used to check your retention of all the top sellers (and the essential others).

- When reading the case, you may wish to note allergies, abnormal labs and major enzyme inducers/inhibitors. They are there for a reason. You will have a dry erase board – you can quickly jot these things down – so they are in your mind when looking at the questions. Although time is limited it is easy to get cases confused after an hour or more of testing.

- Counseling is key; pharmacists must be able to make sure that patients use their drugs safely. In this text, counseling for key drugs is presented after the drug tables in each chapter. It is essential to be able to counsel on formulations that come in novel delivery vehicles, such as dry powder inhalers, self-injectables, patches and other formulations. These are each demonstrated in the videos, and are tested in the correlating test bank section. A patient can often figure out how to swallow a compressed tablet (with a glass of water), but will not be able to figure out how to self-administer an enoxaparin injection or how to use a dry-powder inhaler. Increasingly, drugs are being given in alternative formulations.

- Conditions for which "lifestyle" is essential (heart failure, diabetes) will require that you know how to counsel on healthy-living and disease-monitoring.

- <u>Pharmacoeconomics</u> (with the necessary <u>biostatistic</u> equations) is a required competency; this area, similar to calculations, must be known well prior to sitting for licensure. <u>Pharmacokinetic calculations have become more complex</u>. The calculations in this area can be mastered through repetition; you must do the math repeatedly until you can do the math in all the sections <u>with decent speed</u>, and <u>with accuracy</u>. If you cannot manage to make this happen, please consider getting help with the RxPrep Online Course. The instructors explain each calculation in the simplest manner, step by step. The course also includes our assistance, as-needed.

- Dosing? What is important to know? Trade/generics? Use the underlining (for key information) and bolding (for key drugs) that is present throughout this text as our "best guess" on material that should be known prior to testing. Use your own judgement as well. When we decide, for example, that a dose is important, it is because our team here agrees that the drug is used commonly or is particularly toxic, and an unsafe dosing level would be <u>dangerous</u>. For example, if a patient begins a dopamine agonist at too high a dose the patient could get hurt, or could cause hurt to others. Dopamine agonists cause excessive sedation, with onset that can be sudden. They must be started low and titrated carefully.

- It is advisable to start with the beginning chapters in this text which represent the "foundation" material; the math should be done at the beginning of study, throughout, and before testing. Other foundation topics (such as drug interactions) will help make the clinical chapters easier to manage. For example, if you are familiar with the big inducers or big inhibitors you will have familiarity when reviewing them in the specific topic chapters in which they are used. It will make the process go smoother if the study is done in a logical fashion.

HOW TO USE THIS BOOK

This book is designed as a companion to our live or online courses. You can register for a review program at www.rxprep.com. Select the online course without the text if you have the current version; this reduces the course cost by the price of the text and prevents another text from being sent.

If you are using the book as a stand-alone, here are some pointers:

- If an item is bolded it is a key drug and if it is underlined it is essential information.

- Not all essential information is designated. Use the top seller list as a guide to must-know drugs. You will be tested on drugs that are not top sellers, but have safety considerations. Hospital drugs that are essential are noted in the text.

- This book is complete; you do not need to have a myriad of additional resources. If you are testing through most of 2015, this book is sufficient. However, if it is towards the latter part of the year, you should check for key updates. We often post these as they come along on our Facebook page. Only reputable resources should be used.

- At the end of many of the core chapters are patient cases with practice questions. These are designed to be somewhat similar to NAPLEX® style cases – either in a written format, or the profile you might see on a pharmacy computer. The cases are designed to review key drug points and should not be missed. They do not overlap with the test bank questions.

- The questions in the RxPrep test banks match to the chapters in this text. The questions are designed to test the most basic drug competency knowledge. The knowledge in these questions, including calculations, should be at 100%. If you get something wrong do not skip it! Follow the instructions on "how to pass the exam the first time" that is under the "Announcements" section on your student Dashboard when logged into your account on the RxPrep website. You can access the announcements with the test bank or with the online course. Adult learners do not learn well passively by sitting in front of a text or computer screen; this announcement includes our best experience on how an adult learner can learn all this information, including how to remember oddball drug names (such as *Argatroban* and *Ivacaftor)*. It is possible. The exam is not complex; rather, there is much information to pack inside your brain, and the math must be done with good speed and accuracy.

CPJE POINTERS – FOR CA EXAM TAKERS

This text includes the topics that <u>overlap</u> with the CPJE (Medication Safety, ID, Immunizations, HIV, others). The clinical topics <u>not covered on that NAPLEX</u> that <u>are tested in the CPJE</u> are included in the separate CPJE course (NPSGs, therapeutic interchange, formulary, others). The California <u>law is covered completely</u>. The CPJE course is available at www.rxprep.com. We recommend, in addition, reading through Fred Weissman's book on California community law; this is a standard resource in California for community pharmacy law.

Best wishes for your exam preparation.

2

CALCULATIONS

ABBREVIATIONS USED IN PRESCRIPTIONS

ABBREVIATION	MEANING	ABBREVIATION	MEANING
ss	one-half	mL	milliliter
ac	before meals	NTE	not to exceed
pc	after meals	MDI	metered-dose inhaler
gtt, gtts	drop, drops	q	every
au	each ear *auris*	qd	every day
as *sinistra*	left ear	qod	every other day
ad *dextra*	right ear	PO	by mouth or orally
ATC	around the clock	NPO	nothing by mouth
hs	at bedtime	IV	intravenous
bid	twice a day	IVP	intravenous push
tid	three times a day	IVPB	intravenous piggy back
qid	four times a day	ID	intradermal
biw	two times a week	IM	intramuscular
tiw	three times a week	subc, subq, SC, SQ	subcutaneous
os	left eye *oculus*	ung	ointment
od	right eye	top	topically
ou	each eye	WA	while awake
qs	sufficient quantity	prn	as needed
qs ad	a sufficient quantity to make	stat	immediately
NR	no refills	SL	sublingual
c or w/	with	sup or supp	suppository
s or w/o	without	PR	per rectum
inj	injection	BM	bowel movement
X	times	N/V or N & V	nausea and vomiting

Not all of the above are considered safe abbreviations; all are used outpatient. In hospital settings use abbreviations included on the approved abbreviation list.

EQUIVALENT MEASUREMENTS

MEASUREMENT	EQUIVALENT
tsp (t)	5 mL
tbsp (T)	15 mL
1 fl oz	30 mL (approx.); 29.6 mL (actual)
1 cup	8 oz
1 pint (16 oz)	473 mL
1 quart	2 pints; 946 mL
1 gallon	4 quarts; 3,785 mL

MEASUREMENT	EQUIVALENT
1 kg	2.2 pounds
1 oz	28.4 g
1 pound	454 g
1 in	2.54 cm
1 grain (gr)	65 mg (approx); 64.8 mg (actual)
% (w/v)	g/100 mL
% (v/v)	mL/100 mL
% (w/w)	g/100 g

METRIC CONVERSIONS

PREFIX	DEFINITION
kilo	1,000 (one thousand), as in kg
deci	1/10 (one-tenth), as in dL
milli	1/1,000 (one-thousandth), as in mL
micro	1/1,000,000 (one-millionth), as in mcg
nano	1/1,000,000,000 (one-billionth), as in ng

LABELING INSTRUCTIONS

- Begin with an instructive word (such as: Take, Place, Unwrap, Insert, Inhale).
- Follow with the quantity and dosage form (such as: 1 capsule).
- Follow by the location (such as: by mouth, rectally, vaginally, under tongue).
- Follow with the frequency (such as: daily, twice daily, at meals and bedtime).
- Finish with any noted instructions (such as: for pain, for cholesterol, on an empty stomach).

CPJE Students Only

Note in California, the 2011 new prescription label requirements include changes to the label layout such as 16 phrases of directions for use. In most cases, these phrases should be used on the prescription label. Please refer to *A Guide To California Community Pharmacy Law*, by Fred G. Weissman, PharmD, J.D. or, the law statement on the board's website or RxPrep's CPJE Course, which covers legal requirements and several items not covered in this book (including NPSG's, ADC requirements, P&T and Formulary, and Therapeutic Interchange).

Labeling Prescriptions

1. **Choose the correct wording for the prescription label:**

   a. Take 1-2 tablets by mouth every 4-6 hours as-needed for pain for 2 days. Do not exceed 6 tablets per day.

   b. Take up to 2 tablets by mouth every 4-6 hours as-needed for pain. Do not exceed 6 tablets per day.

   c. Take 1-2 tablets by mouth every 4-6 hours as-needed for pain. NTE 6 tablets per day.

   d. Take 1-2 tablets by mouth every 4-6 hours for pain. Do not exceed 6 tablets per day.

   State of California
   PRESCRIPTION BLANK

   Joe Jackson, MD
   927 Deep Valley Drive
   Los Angeles, California
   Phone (310) 555-3333

   DEA#FJ3829150
   BATCH# HTS5058903765

   CA LIC#568596

   0200

   Name _Edward Richards_   D.O.B. _May 15, 1949_

   Address _177 Green Street_   Date _November 29, 2013_

   Touch Rx symbol, color will disappear then reappear.

   Rx **Vicodin 5/325 mg #12**

   Sig: i-ii tabs PO q 4-6 hrs prn pain X 2 days. NTE 6/d.

   Qty/Units
   ☑ 1-24 / _12_
   ☐ 25-49 / ____
   ☐ 50-74 / ____
   ☐ 75-100 / ____
   ☐ 101-150 / ____
   ☐ 151 and over / ____

   SUBSTITUTION PERMISSABLE _____   DO NOT SUBSTITUTE _____

   DO NOT REFILL ____   REFILL ____ TIMES   SIGNATURE OF PRESCRIBER

   Prescription is void if more than one controlled substance is written per blank.
   Security Features. Details on Back

   e. Take 1-2 tablets by mouth up to 6 times daily as-needed for pain for 2 days. Do not exceed 6 tablets per day.

The correct answer is (A). Generally, the acetaminophen component has the higher risk of toxicity (liver toxicity).

2. **Choose the correct wording for the prescription label:**

   a. Take 1 capsule by mouth every six hours.

   b. Take 1 capsule by mouth four times daily: take 1 on an empty stomach and take 1 at bedtime.

   c. Take 1 capsule by mouth four times daily: take 1 after meals and take 1 at bedtime.

   d. Take 1 capsule by mouth four times daily: take 1 with meals and take 1 at bedtime.

   JOE JACKSON, MD
   927 DEEP VALLEY DRIVE
   LOS ANGELES, CALIFORNIA

   PHONE (310) 555-3333   DEA No. FJ3829150

   NAME _Melissa Atkins_   DATE _October 29, 2013_

   ADDRESS _18469 Lotus Circle_   AGE _57_

   Rx

   Keflex 500 mg PO QID: ac and hs. #28

   ☐ LABEL

   REFILL __0__ TIMES

   _____ , M.D.   _____ , M.D.

   DO NOT SUBSTITUTE   SUBSTITUTION PERMISSIBLE

   e. Take 1 capsule by mouth four times daily: take 1 before meals and take 1 at bedtime.

The correct answer is (E). The patient should be counseled to finish all of the medication even if they start to feel better. Cephalexin *(Keflex)* comes as tablets, capsules and powder for suspension.

3. A pharmacist receives a prescription for "APAP 5 gr supp #6 1 PR prn temperature > 102 degrees". Choose the correct wording for the prescription label:

  a. Insert 1 suppository as needed when temperature is greater than 102 degrees.

  b. Unwrap and insert 1 suppository rectally as needed for a temperature greater than 102°.

  c. Take 500 mg of APAP suspension as needed 6 times per day for a temperature greater than 102°.

  d. Take 6 suppositories vaginally as needed for a temperature greater than 102°.

  e. Insert 500 mg of APAP into the rectum as needed for a fever greater than 102°.

The correct answer is (B). It is important to tell patients exactly how to take a medication. Five grains is 325 milligrams (65 mg/gr x 5 gr).

---

4. A pharmacist receives a prescription for "*Vigamox* 0.5% #3 1 gtt tid ou x 5d". Choose the correct wording for the prescription label:

(handwritten: moxifloxacin)

  a. Insert 3 mL into the right eye three times daily for 5 days.

  b. Insert 1 drop into the right eye three times daily for 3 days.

  c. Instill 1 drop into both eyes three times a day for 5 days.

  d. Instill 3 drops into the right eye three times a day for 5 days.

  e. Instill 3 drops into both eyes three times a day for 5 days.

The correct answer is (C). It is important to properly counsel patients on the correct technique for instilling eye drops. Refer to the Ophthalmics chapter.

Calculating the Correct Dose and/or Amount for a Prescription

Instructions to perform with each calculation problem in order to increase accuracy:

- Check your math. Time permitting, double-check the calculations. It is very easy to make mistakes that you will catch when repeating the calculations.

- If you are using proportions to solve the problem, place your answer directly back into the equation as another accuracy check. For example:

$$\frac{5\text{ g}}{100\text{ g}} = \frac{X\text{ g}}{1{,}000\text{ g}} \quad X = 50\text{ g}$$

Check: 5/100 = 0.05; 50/1,000 = 0.05

- When setting up proportions, make sure the units (including route and drug if applicable) in the numerators match, and the units (route and drug) in the denominators match as well.

- Read the question again after solving the problem to be certain you have answered with the correct units (g or mg, mEq, mL or L, etc.) and have rounded your answer as specified in the question. If rounding is required, look at the number to the right of the one you are rounding to; for example, if rounding to the nearest whole number look at the tenths column. If the number to the right is 0 to 4, round down. If it is 5 to 9, round up. For example, 31.27 rounded to the nearest whole number is 31, and 31.635 rounded to the nearest whole number is 32. Round only at the end of the equation, not at each step.

- <u>Make sure you are answering the question</u>. The next problem illustrates that the problem may have more than one step, and you want to be careful to get to the right step to get to the requested response.

- The math in this section, and on the exam, is not complex. Most formulas are not provided. How do you get to the point where you can do the math easily and accurately, in a timely fashion: by repetition. Do the math over and over until you are doing the problems easily. The problems shown here are repeated, with different numbers, in the RxPrep test bank which can be used for knowledge assessment. Your math ability should be at 100% prior to testing; math mistakes are not acceptable in this profession; a math mistake is a dosing mistake.

5. In the prescription to the right, the pharmacist dispensed 3 oz to Ms. Brooks. How many days of therapy will Ms. Brooks be short? Round to the nearest whole number. Use 30 mL for 1 fluid ounce.

disp 90 ml
needs 100 ml

    a. 10 mL
    b. 90 mL
    c. 1 day
    d. 3 days
    e. 9 days

The correct answer is (C). Use caution with calculations where a step of the answer (but not the final step) will be a selection. Always go back and read the question prior to selecting your response.

- 5 mL (per dose) x 2 times/day x 10 days = 100 mL needed

- Quantity dispensed: 3 oz x 30 mL/oz = 90 mL dispensed

- Difference: Quantity needed – Quantity dispensed = 100 mL – 90 mL = 10 mL

Gene Tran, MD 5445 Grand Ave. Fallbrook, California Phone (760) 555-2112	**005–1015** CA LIC. #A19666 D.E.A. #SK456789

Name   *Angelina Brooks*   Date   *January 22, 2014*

Address   *33 Walden Rd. N Falls*   D.O.B.   *May 5, 1951*

℞

    TMP/SMX 40-200 mg/5 mL
    Sig: 1 tsp PO BID x 10 days, until all taken.

    5 ml x 2 = 10 ml/ day
                 x 10 days
                 = 100 ml

❏ Do Not Substitute   Refill _____ Times

Quantity	**Units**
❏ 1-24	_____
❏ 25-49	_____
❏ 50-74	_____
❏ 75-100	_____
❏ 101-150	_____
❏ 151 and over	_____

                               Physician Signature

Prescription is void if more than one controlled substance is written per blank.

- Each tsp (t) is 5 mL. She needs 2 tsp (t) daily, which is 10 mL. She is 1 day short for her course of therapy.

$$\begin{array}{r} 120 \\ -70 \\ \hline 50\ \text{ml} \end{array}$$

$$\frac{50\ \text{ml}}{120\ \text{ml}} = \frac{x}{5\ \text{ml}} \Rightarrow x = 2.$$

6. How many milliliters (mL) of *Mylanta* suspension are contained in each dose of the prescription below? Round to the nearest whole number.

PRESCRIPTION	QUANTITY
Belladonna Tincture	10 mL
Phenobarbital	60 mL
Mylanta susp. qs. ad	120 mL
Sig. 5 mL BID	

The total prescription is 120 mL; 10 mL belladonna, 60 mL of phenobarbital, and that leaves 50 mL left for the *Mylanta*.

$$\frac{50\ \text{mL } Mylanta}{120\ \text{mL total Rx}} = \frac{X\ \text{mL } Mylanta}{5\ \text{mL total Rx dose}} \qquad X = 2.08,\ \text{or 2 mL } Mylanta/\text{dose}$$

After solving the problem, read the question again to be certain you have answered the question with the correct units (mL of *Mylanta* per dose).

---

7. You have tablets that contain 0.25 mg of levothyroxine per tablet. You are crushing the tablets and mixing with glycerol and water for a 36 pound child. How many levothyroxine tablets will be needed to compound the following prescription?

PRESCRIPTION	QUANTITY
Levothyroxine Liq.	0.1 mg/mL
Disp.	60 mL
Sig. 0.01 mg per kg PO BID	

$$60\ \text{mL total Rx} \quad X \quad \frac{0.1\ \text{mg levo}}{\text{mL}} = 6\ \text{mg of levothyroxine needed}$$

$$\frac{0.1\ \text{mg}}{\text{ml}} = \frac{x}{60\ \text{ml}} \Rightarrow x = 6\ \text{mg}$$

$$6\ \text{mg levo} \quad X \quad \frac{1\ \text{tab}}{0.25\ \text{mg levo}} = 24\ \text{tabs of levothyroxine needed}$$

$$\frac{6\ \text{mg}}{\frac{0.25\ \text{mg}}{\text{tab}}} = 24\ \text{tabs}$$

Or, solving by dimensional analysis:

$$\frac{1\ \text{tab levo}}{0.25\ \text{mg levo}} \quad X \quad \frac{0.1\ \text{mg levo}}{\text{mL}} \quad X \quad 60\ \text{mL total Rx} = 24\ \text{tabs of levothyroxine needed}$$

After solving the problem, read the question again to be certain you have answered the question with the correct units (tablets).

8. A pharmacist will prepare an *Amoxil* suspension to provide a 1600 mg dose for a child with an otitis media infection, to be divided BID. To prepare an *Amoxil* suspension containing 200 mg/5 mL the pharmacist should add 76 mL of water to the powder for a final volume of 100 mL. The pharmacist will add approximately 1/3 of the water first, shake vigorously, add the remaining water, and shake again to form the suspension. The pharmacist mistakenly adds too much water and finds she has a final volume of 110 mL. There are no other bottles of *Amoxil* on the shelf and he will dispense the bottle with the extra water added. How many mL does the patient need to receive the correct dose? Provide the mL for a single dose, rounded to the nearest mL.

$$\frac{200 \text{ mg}}{5 \text{ mL}} = \frac{X \text{ mg}}{100 \text{ mL}} \qquad X = 4{,}000 \text{ mg}$$

$$\frac{4{,}000 \text{ mg}}{110 \text{ mL}} = \frac{800 \text{ mg}}{X \text{ mL}} \qquad X = 22 \text{ mL}$$

Handwritten:
1600 mg BID = 800 $\frac{mg}{dose}$

$\frac{200 \text{ mg}}{5 \text{ ml}} \cdot 100 \text{ ml} = 4000 \text{ mg}$

$\frac{4000 \text{ mg}}{110 \text{ ml}} = \frac{800 \text{ mg}}{x \text{ ml}} \Rightarrow x = 22 \text{ ml}$

9. How many milligrams of codeine will be contained in each capsule?

PRESCRIPTION	QUANTITY
Codeine Sulfate	0.6 g
Guaifenesin	1.2 g
Caffeine	0.15 g
M. ft. caps. no. 24	
Sig. One capsule TID prn cough	

Begin by converting to the unit requested in the answer (mg).

Handwritten: 0.6 g = 600 mg

$\frac{600 \text{ mg}}{24} = 25 \text{ mg per cap}$

$$0.6 \text{ g Codeine} \times \frac{1{,}000 \text{ mg}}{1 \text{ g}} = 600 \text{ mg of codeine for the total prescription}$$

The prescription order is for 24 capsules.

$$\frac{600 \text{ mg codeine total}}{24 \text{ caps}} = 25 \text{ mg of codeine/capsule}$$

After solving the problem, read the question again to be certain you have answered the question with the correct units (mg of codeine per capsule).

10. A physician writes an order for aminophylline 500 mg IV, dosed at 0.5 mg per kg per hour for a patient weighing 165 pounds. There is only theophylline in stock. How many milligrams (mg) of theophylline will the patient receive per hour? Round to the nearest whole number.

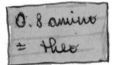
Handwritten note: 0.8 amino ≒ theo

$$\frac{0.5 \text{ mg Amino}}{\text{kg/hr}} \times \frac{1 \text{ kg}}{2.2 \text{ pounds}} \times 165 \text{ pounds} = 37.5 \text{ mg/hr aminophylline}$$

To get the theophylline dose, multiply by 0.8. Therefore, 37.5 mg/hr aminophylline x 0.8 = 30 mg/hr of theophylline. You must know how to convert between aminophylline and theophylline.

Handwritten:
$\frac{0.5 \text{ mg}}{kg \, hr} \cdot \frac{165}{2.2} kg = 37.5 \frac{mg}{hr}$

0.8 × amino = theo
0.8 · 37.5 = 30 mg/hr

■ Aminophylline to theophylline; multiply by 0.8

■ Theophylline to aminophylline; divide by 0.8

After solving the problem, read the question again to be certain you have answered the question with the correct units (mg per hour of theophylline).

---

11. How many grains of aspirin will be contained in each capsule? Round to the nearest tenth.

PRESCRIPTION	QUANTITY
Aspirin	6 g
Phenacetin	3.2 g
Caffeine	0.48 g
M. ft. no. 20 caps	
Sig. One capsule Q6H prn pain	

$$6 \text{ g ASA} \times \frac{1{,}000 \text{ mg}}{1 \text{ g}} \times \frac{1 \text{ gr}}{65 \text{ mg}} = 92.3 \text{ grains}$$

(handwritten) $\dfrac{6 g}{20} = 0.3 \ g/cap$

We have 92.3 grains per 20 capsules.

$$\frac{92.3 \text{ gr}}{20 \text{ capsules}} = 4.6 \text{ grains/capsule}$$

(handwritten)
1 gr = 65 mg
4.6 gr ? = 300 mg

After solving the problem, read the question again to be certain you have answered the question with the correct units (grains per capsule).

---

12. A 45 milliliter nasal spray delivers 20 sprays per milliliter of solution. Each spray contains 1.5 mg of active drug. How many milligrams of drug are contained in the 45 mL package?

First, add up the amount of drug per mL.

$$\frac{1.5 \text{ mg drug}}{\text{spray}} \times \frac{20 \text{ sprays}}{\text{mL}} = 30 \text{ mg/mL}$$

(handwritten) $\dfrac{20 \text{ sprays}}{ml} \cdot \dfrac{1.5 mg}{spray} = 30 \ mg/ml$

Then solve for milligrams of drug in 45 mL.

$$\frac{30 \text{ mg}}{\text{mL}} = \frac{X \text{ mg}}{45 \text{ mL}} \quad X = 1{,}350 \text{ mg}$$

(handwritten) $\dfrac{30 mg}{ml} \cdot 45 \ ml = 1350 \ mg$

---

13. A metered dose inhaler provides 90 micrograms of albuterol sulfate with each inhalation. The canister provides 200 inhalations. If the patient uses the entire canister, how many total milligrams will the patient have received?

$$200 \text{ inhalations} \times \frac{90 \text{ mcg}}{\text{inhalation}} = 18{,}000 \text{ mcg}$$

$$18{,}000 \text{ mcg} \times \frac{1 \text{ mg}}{1{,}000 \text{ mcg}} = 18 \text{ mg}$$

(handwritten)
$\dfrac{90 \ ug}{inh} \cdot 200 \ inh = 18\,000 \ ug$
$= 18 \ mg$

Proportions

A proportion represents the equality of two ratios. Given any three values of a proportion, it is easy to calculate the fourth. Remember to keep the same units (route, drug, etc.) in the numerator and the same units (route, drug, etc.) in the denominator.

$$\frac{a}{b} = \frac{c}{d}$$

[handwritten: 50 mg]

14. If one 10 mL vial contains 0.05 g of diltiazem, how many milliliters should be administered to provide a 25 mg dose of diltiazem?

First, convert grams to milligrams. Usually, it is best practice to convert to the units required in the answer when you begin the problem.

0.05 gram of diltiazem x $\dfrac{1,000 \text{ mg}}{1 \text{ g}}$ = 50 mg

[handwritten: 10 ml = 50 mg / x = 25 mg / 5 ml]

Use proportions to calculate the number of mL for a 25 mg dose.

$\dfrac{50 \text{ mg}}{10 \text{ mL}} = \dfrac{25 \text{ mg}}{X \text{ mL}}$ X = 5 mL dose

---

[handwritten left margin: 1 pint = 473 ml]

15. If phenobarbital elixir contains 18.2 mg of phenobarbital per 5 mL, how many grams of phenobarbital would be used in preparing a pint of the elixir? Round to the nearest hundredth.

First, convert milligrams to grams.

18.2 mg x $\dfrac{1 \text{ g}}{1,000 \text{ mg}}$ = 0.0182 g

[handwritten: 18.2 mg = 5 ml / x = 473 ml / 1.72 g]

Use proportions to calculate the amount of grams needed for 1 pint.

$\dfrac{0.0182 \text{ g}}{5 \text{ mL}} = \dfrac{X \text{ g}}{473 \text{ mL}}$ X = 1.72 g

---

16. Digoxin injection is supplied in ampules of 500 mcg per 2 mL. How many milliliters must a nurse administer to provide a dose of 0.2 mg? Round to the nearest tenth.

First, convert 500 mcg to mg.

500 mcg x $\dfrac{1 \text{ mg}}{1,000 \text{ mcg}}$ = 0.5 mg

[handwritten: 0.2 mg = 200 ug / $\frac{500 \text{ ug}}{2 \text{ ml}} = \frac{200 \text{ ug}}{x}$ / 0.8 ml]

$\dfrac{0.5 \text{ mg}}{2 \text{ mL}} = \dfrac{0.2 \text{ mg}}{X \text{ mL}}$ X = 0.8 mL

---

17. If 200 capsules contain 500 mg of an active ingredient, how many milligrams of the active ingredient will 76 capsules contain?

$\dfrac{200 \text{ caps}}{500 \text{ mg}} = \dfrac{76 \text{ caps}}{X \text{ mg}}$ X = 190 mg

[handwritten: 200 caps = 500 mg / 76 = x / 190 mg]

18. A penicillin V 250 mg tablet equals 400,000 units of penicillin activity. A patient is taking penicillin V 500 mg tablets QID for 7 days. How much penicillin activity, in units, will this patient receive in the total prescription?

If 250 mg contains 400,000 units, then 500 mg contains 800,000 units. The patient is taking 4 tablets daily, for 7 days (or 28 total tablets), at 800,000 units each.

$$\frac{800,000 \text{ units}}{1 \text{ tab}} = \frac{X \text{ units}}{28 \text{ tabs}} \quad X = 22,400,000 \text{ units}$$

[handwritten: 250 mg = 400 000 units; 500 mg × 4 × 7 = ?; 22,400,000]

19. A cough syrup contains 4 g of brompheniramine maleate per liter. How many milligrams are contained in a teaspoonful dose of the elixir?

First, convert grams to milligrams.

$$4 \text{ g} \times \frac{X \text{ mg}}{1 \text{ g}} = 4,000 \text{ mg per 1 liter}$$

[handwritten: 4 000 mg = 1000 ml; 20 mg ? = 5 ml]

- 1 L = 1,000 mL

- 1 teaspoonful = 5 mL

Next, solve using proportions.

$$\frac{4,000 \text{ mg}}{1,000 \text{ mL}} = \frac{X \text{ mg}}{5 \text{ mL}} \quad X = 20 \text{ mg}$$

20. A patient is to receive acyclovir 5 mg/kg every 8 hours for an acute outbreak of herpes zoster. What daily dose, in milligrams, should a 110 pound female receive?

Begin by converting the patient's weight in pounds (lbs) to kilograms (kg).

- 2.2 pounds = 1 kg

$$110 \text{ pounds} \times \frac{1 \text{ kg}}{2.2 \text{ pounds}} = 50 \text{ kg}$$

[handwritten: $\frac{5 \text{ mg}}{kg} \cdot \frac{110}{2.2} kg = 250 \text{ mg}$; ↓; × 3; = 750 mg]

$$\frac{5 \text{ mg}}{1 \text{ kg}} = \frac{X \text{ mg}}{50 \text{ kg}} \quad X = 250 \text{ mg/dose} \times 3 \text{ doses/day} = 750 \text{ mg/day}$$

21. MH is a 72 year old male patient hospitalized with decompensated heart failure and fever. Cultures are positive for aspergillosis. MH weighs 110 kg and will receive 0.25 mg/kg per day amphotericin B (reconstituted and diluted to 0.1 mg/mL) by IV infusion. What volume of solution, in milliliters, is required to deliver the daily dose?

Begin by calculating the total daily dose (mg) for this patient.

$$\frac{0.25 \text{ mg}}{1 \text{ kg}} = \frac{X \text{ mg}}{110 \text{ kg}} \quad X = 27.5 \text{ mg daily}$$

Calculate the volume of reconstituted amphotericin B solution needed per day.

[handwritten: $110 \text{ kg} \cdot 0.25 \frac{mg}{kg} = 27.5 \text{ mg}$; $\frac{0.1 \text{ mg}}{ml} = \frac{27.5 \text{ mg}}{x} \Rightarrow 275 \text{ ml}$]

$$\frac{27.5 \text{ mg}}{X \text{ mL}} = \frac{0.1 \text{ mg}}{1 \text{ mL}} \qquad X = 275 \text{ mL}$$

---

22. An elixir of ferrous sulfate contains 220 milligrams of ferrous sulfate in each 5 milliliters. If each milligram of ferrous sulfate contains the equivalent of 0.2 milligrams of elemental iron, how many milligrams of elemental iron would be in each 5 milliliters of elixir?

Ferrous sulfate ($FeSO_4$) contains 20% elemental iron (Fe); this is given in the problem which states that 1 milligram has 0.2 milligrams of elemental iron, which is 20%.

$$\frac{0.2 \text{ mg Fe}}{1 \text{ mg FeSO}_4} = \frac{X \text{ mg Fe}}{220 \text{ mg FeSO}_4} \qquad X = 44 \text{ mg Fe}$$

(handwritten) 1 mg = 0.2 mg Fe
220 mg = ? 44 mg Fe

---

23. A 10 gram packet of potassium chloride provides 20 mEq of potassium and 4 mEq of chloride. How many grams of powder would provide 8 mEq of potassium?

$$\frac{10 \text{ g}}{20 \text{ mEq K}^+} = \frac{X \text{ g}}{8 \text{ mEq K}^+} \qquad X = 4 \text{ g}$$

(handwritten) 10 g = 20 mEq K = 4 mEq Cl
4 g ? = 8 mEq K

✳ **24. Oral potassium chloride 20% solution contains 40 mEq of potassium per 15 milliliters of solution. A patient needs 25 mEq of potassium daily. What is the amount, in milliliters, of 20% potassium chloride that the patient should take? Round to the nearest tenth.**

$$\frac{40 \text{ mEq K}^+}{15 \text{ mL}} = \frac{25 \text{ mEq K}^+}{X \text{ mL}} \qquad X = 9.375, \text{ or } 9.4 \text{ mL}$$

(handwritten) $\frac{40 \text{ mEq}}{15 \text{ ml}} = \frac{25 \text{ mEq}}{x}$ 9.4 ml

Percentage Strength

A percentage is a number or ratio as a fraction of 100. Expressions of concentration describe the amount of solute that will be contained in the total preparation. The percentage concentrations are defined as follows:

- Percent weight-in-volume (% w/v) is expressed as g/100 mL (a solid mixed into a liquid)

- Percent volume-in-volume (% v/v) is expressed as mL/100 mL (a liquid mixed into a liquid)

- Percent weight-in-weight (% w/w) is expressed as g/100 g (a solid mixed into a solid)

25. How many grams of NaCl are in 1 liter of normal saline (NS)?

Normal saline (NS) is 0.9% (w/v) NaCl solution

Remember (w/v) is always expressed as grams per 100 mL, therefore, NS contains 0.9 g NaCl per 100 mL of solution.

$$\frac{0.9 \text{ g}}{100 \text{ mL}} = \frac{X \text{ g}}{1,000 \text{ mL}} \qquad X = 9 \text{ g}$$

(handwritten) $\frac{0.9 \text{ g}}{100 \text{ ml}} = \frac{x}{1000 \text{ ml}} \Rightarrow x = 9 \text{ g}$

---

26. How many grams of NaCl are in 500 mL of ½ NS? Round to the nearest hundredth.

NS is 0.9 g/100 mL; ½ NS is 0.45 g/100 mL.

(handwritten) $\frac{0.45 \text{ g}}{100 \text{ ml}} = \frac{x}{500 \text{ ml}}$

$\Rightarrow 2.25 \text{ g}$

$$\frac{0.45\ g}{100\ mL} = \frac{X\ g}{500\ mL} \qquad X = 2.25\ g$$

---

27. How many grams of dextrose 5% are in 250 mL of D5W? Round to the nearest tenth.

$$\frac{5\ g}{100\ mL} = \frac{X\ g}{250\ mL} \qquad X = 12.5\ g$$

$$\frac{5g}{100\ ml} \cdot 250\ ml = 12.5\ g$$

---

28. How many milligrams of triamcinolone should be used in preparing the following prescription? Round to the nearest whole number.

PRESCRIPTION	QUANTITY
Triamcinolone (w/v)	5%
Glycerin qs	60 mL
Sig. Two drops in right ear	

$$\frac{5\ g}{100\ mL} = \frac{X\ g}{60\ mL} \qquad X = 3\ g,\ or\ 3{,}000\ mg$$

$$\frac{5g}{100\ ml} = \frac{x}{60\ ml} \Rightarrow x = 3000\ mg$$

---

29. A prescription reads as follows: Prepare a 3% w/w coal tar preparation qs with petrolatum to 150 g. How much petrolatum, in grams, will be needed to make the prescription? Round to the nearest tenth.

$$\frac{3\ g}{100\ g} = \frac{X\ g}{150\ g} \qquad X = 4.5\ g$$

150 g (total weight) – 4.5 g (active ingredient) = 145.5 g petrolatum

$$\frac{3g}{100\ g} \cdot 150g = 4.5\ g\ coal\ tar$$

$$\begin{array}{r} 150\ g \\ -\ \ 4.5\ g \\ \hline 145.5\ g\ petro \end{array}$$

---

30. JL has mucositis secondary to methotrexate chemotherapy. The physician has ordered lidocaine HCl 2% w/v solution; qs with pure water to 120 mL. How much lidocaine, in grams, is required to make the prescription? Round to the nearest tenth.

$$\frac{2\ g}{100\ mL} = \frac{X\ g}{120\ mL} = X = 2.4\ g$$

$$\frac{2g}{100\ ml} \cdot 120\ ml = 2.4\ g$$

Compounding steps for this problem:

Weigh the drug (2.4 g), place in a beaker, add water to the 120 mL line, stir, and place into a container labeled: Lidocaine 2% solution, 120 mL, with additional labeling as required.

Common steps for compounding an ointment or cream:

- Weigh or measure the active ingredient/s.

- If you are using a dry powder or granules, you will need to triturate with the pestle to reduce the particle size.

- Levigate on an ointment slab with a metal spatula (unless you are mixing metal ions, then use a plastic spatula).

- Package into a tube or jar. See further discussion in the Compounding chapter.

---

31. SS is a 79 year old female with dry mouth and dry eyes from Sjögren's syndrome. She is picking up the prescription below. What is the maximum milligrams of pilocarpine she will receive per day?

PRESCRIPTION	QUANTITY
Pilocarpine	1% (w/v)
Sodium Chloride qs ad	15 mL
Sig: 2 gtts (0.1 mL) po TID prn up to 5 days for dry mouth	

First, calculate the amount of pilocarpine in the prescription.

$$\frac{1\ g}{100\ mL} = \frac{X\ g}{15\ mL} \quad X = 0.15\ g$$

(handwritten: 0.1 ml × 3 = 0.3 ml/day)

(handwritten: $\frac{1g}{100\ ml}$ · 0.3 ml = 3 mg)

Then, convert to mg since the problem wants the answer in mg.

$$0.15\ g \quad \times \quad \frac{1{,}000\ mg}{1\ g} \quad = \quad 150\ mg\ of\ pilocarpine$$

The patient will receive up to 3 doses per day (0.1 mL x 3 = 0.3 mL). Calculate the amount of pilocarpine in 0.3 mL.

$$\frac{150\ mg\ pilocarpine}{15\ mL} = \frac{X\ mg}{0.3\ mL} \quad X = 3\ mg\ pilocarpine$$

---

32. If 1,250 g of a mixture contains 80 g of drug, what is the percentage strength (w/w) of the mixture? Round to the nearest tenth.

$$\frac{80\ g}{1{,}250\ g} = \frac{X\ g}{100\ g} \quad X = 6.4\ g,\ which\ is\ 6.4\%$$

(handwritten: $\frac{80\ g}{1250\ g}$ · 100% = 6.4%)

---

33. A mouth rinse contains 1/12% (w/v) of chlorhexidine gluconate. How many grams of chlorhexidine gluconate should be used to prepare 18 liters of mouth rinse? Round to the nearest whole number.

- 1/12% = 0.083 g per 100 mL (w/v)

- 18 L x 1,000 mL/L = 18,000 mL

$$\frac{0.083\ g}{100\ mL} = \frac{X\ g}{18{,}000\ mL} \quad X = 14.94,\ or\ 15\ g$$

(handwritten: $\frac{1/12\ g}{100\ ml} = \frac{X}{18\ 000\ ml}$ → x = 15 g)

---

34. If 12 grams of lanolin are combined with 2 grams of white wax and 36 grams of petrolatum to make an ointment, what is the percentage strength (w/w) of lanolin in the ointment?

$$\frac{12\ g\ lanolin}{50\ grams\ ointment} = \frac{X\ g}{100\ grams} \quad X = 24\%\ w/w$$

(handwritten: 12 g lan / 2 g ww / 36 g pet)

(handwritten: $\frac{12\ g}{50\ g}$ · 100% = 24%)

35. A pharmacist dissolves 6 tablets. Each tablet contains 250 mg of metronidazole. The pharmacist will put the drug into a liquid base to prepare 60 mL of a topical solution. What is the percentage strength (w/v) of metronidazole in the prescription? Round to the nearest tenth.

6 tablets x $\dfrac{250 \text{ mg}}{1 \text{ tab}}$ = 1,500 mg, or 1.5 g

$\dfrac{1.5 \text{ g}}{60 \text{ mL}} = \dfrac{X \text{ g}}{100 \text{ mL}}$ X = 2.5 g, which is 2.5% w/v

6 · 250 mg = 1500 mg = 1.5 g

$\dfrac{1.5 \text{ g}}{60 \text{ mL}} \cdot 100\% = 2.5\%$

---

36. A pharmacist adds 5.3 grams of hydrocortisone to 150 grams of a 2.5% hydrocortisone ointment. What is the percentage (w/w) of hydrocortisone in the finished product? Round to the nearest whole number.

First, determine the amount of hydrocortisone (HC) in the current product.

$\dfrac{2.5 \text{ g HC}}{100 \text{ g}} = \dfrac{X \text{ g HC}}{150 \text{ g}}$ X = 3.75 g HC

$150 \text{ g} \cdot \dfrac{2.5 \text{ g}}{100 \text{ g}} = 3.75 \text{ g}$

$\begin{array}{r} 3.75 \text{ g} \\ + \ 5.3 \text{ g} \\ \hline 9.05 \text{ g} \end{array}$

$\dfrac{9.05 \text{ g}}{155.3 \text{ g}} \times 100\% = 6\%$

Next, add this amount (3.75 g) to the amount of hydrocortisone being added (5.3 g): 3.75 g + 5.3 g = 9.05 g.

Then, find the percent concentration of the total product (5.3 g + 150 g = 155.3 g).

$\dfrac{9.05 \text{ g}}{155.3 \text{ g}} = \dfrac{X}{100 \text{ g}}$ X = 5.82743, or 6%

---

37. How many milliliters of hydrocortisone liquid (40 mg/mL) will be needed to prepare 30 grams of a 0.25% cream (w/w)? Round to the nearest hundredth.

First, calculate the amount of hydrocortisone in the current product.

$\dfrac{0.25 \text{ g}}{100 \text{ g}} = \dfrac{X \text{ g}}{30 \text{ g}}$ X = 0.075 g or 75 mg

$30 \text{ g} \cdot \dfrac{0.25 \text{ g}}{100 \text{ g}} = 0.075 \text{ g}$

Then, solve for mL of hydrocortisone liquid needed.

$\dfrac{40 \text{ mg}}{\text{mL}} = \dfrac{75 \text{ mg}}{X \text{ mL}}$ X = 1.875 mL, rounded to 1.88 mL

$\dfrac{40 \text{ mg}}{\text{mL}} = \dfrac{75 \text{ mg}}{X}$

$\Rightarrow x = 1.88 \text{ mL}$

After solving the problem, read the question again to be certain you have answered the question with the correct units (mL).

✱ **38. What is the percentage strength of imiquimod in the following prescription? Round to the nearest hundredth.**

PRESCRIPTION	QUANTITY
Imiquimod 5% cream	15 g
Xylocaine	20 g
Hydrophilic ointment	25 g

First, calculate the amount of imiquimod (5%) in the prescription.

$$\frac{5\text{ g}}{100\text{ g}} \times 15\text{ g} = 0.75 \text{ grams of imiquimod}$$

[handwritten: $15g \cdot \frac{5g}{100 g} = 0.75 g$]

The total weight of the prescription is 60 g (15 g + 20 g + 25 g).

$$\frac{0.75\text{ g}}{60\text{ g}} = \frac{X\text{ g}}{100\text{ g}} \quad X = 1.25 \text{ g, which is 1.25\%}$$

[handwritten: $\frac{0.75 g}{(15+20+25) g} \cdot 100\% = 1.25\%$]

Ratio Strength

The concentration of weak solutions can be expressed in terms of ratio strength. Ratio strength describes the drug concentration in terms of a ratio (as the name suggests). It is denoted as one unit of solute contained in the total amount of the solution or mixture (e.g., 1:500).

---

39. Express 0.04% as a ratio strength.

$$\frac{0.04}{100} = \frac{1\text{ part}}{X\text{ parts}} \quad X = 2,500. \text{ Ratio strength is 1:2,500}$$

[handwritten: $\frac{0.04}{100} = \frac{1}{x}$ 1: 2500]

You can go back to 0.04% by taking 1/2500 x 100; try it.

Express 1:4,000 as a percentage strength.

$$\frac{1\text{ part}}{4,000\text{ part}} = \frac{X}{100} \quad X = 0.025, \text{ which is 0.025\%}$$

✱ **40. There are 50 mg of drug in 50 mL of solution. Express the concentration as a ratio strength (% w/v).**

First, convert 50 mg to grams. 50 mg x 1 g/1,000 mg = 0.05 g

Then, find out how many grams per 100 mL.

$$\frac{0.05\text{ g}}{50\text{ mL}} = \frac{X\text{ g}}{100\text{ mL}} \quad X = 0.1 \text{ g}$$

[handwritten: $\frac{50 mg}{50 ml} = \frac{x}{100 ml}$ ⟹ x = 100 mg = 0.1 g]

Now solve for ratio strength.

[handwritten: $\frac{0.1 g}{100 ml} = \frac{1 g}{x}$ 1: 1000]

$$\frac{0.1\ g}{100\ mL} = \frac{1\ part}{X\ parts} \qquad X = 1{,}000,\ or\ 1{:}1{,}000$$

41. How many (milligrams) of iodine should be used in compounding the following prescription?

ITEM	QUANTITY
Iodine	1:400
Hydrophilic ointment ad	10 g
Sig. Apply as directed.	

First, convert the ratio strength to a percentage strength.

1:400 = 0.0025, or 0.25%

Then, multiply by the total amount in the prescription.

10 g x 0.0025 = 0.025 g, or 25 mg

Or, solve another way:

1:400 means 1 g in 400 g of ointment.

$$\frac{1\ g}{400\ g} = \frac{X\ g}{10\ g} \qquad X = 0.025\ g,\ or\ 25\ mg$$

(handwritten) $\frac{1\ g}{400\ g} = \frac{x}{10\ g}$

0.025 g = 25 mg

42. A 10 mL mixture contains 0.25 mL of active drug. Express the concentration as a ratio strength (% v/v).

First, find out how much drug is in 100 mL.

$$\frac{0.25\ mL\ drug}{10\ mL} = \frac{X\ mL\ drug}{100\ mL} \qquad X = 2.5\ mL$$

(handwritten) $\frac{0.25}{10} = \frac{1}{x}$

1:40

Now solve for ratio strength.

$$\frac{2.5\ mL\ drug}{100\ mL} = \frac{1\ part}{X\ parts} \qquad X = 40;\ or\ 1{:}40$$

43. What is the concentration, in ratio strength, of a trituration made by combining 150 mg of albuterol sulfate and 4.05 grams of lactose?

First, add up the total weight of the prescription.

0.150 g + 4.05 g = 4.2 g

Now solve for ratio strength.

$$\frac{0.150\ g}{4.2} = \frac{1}{X} \qquad X = 28,\ or\ 1{:}28$$

(handwritten) 150 mg = 0.15 g

$$\begin{array}{r} 0.15\ g \\ +\ 4.05\ g \\ \hline 4.20\ g \end{array}$$

$\frac{0.15}{4.20} = \frac{1}{x}$

⇒ 1:28

Parts Per Million (PPM)

Parts indicate amount proportions. Parts per million (PPM) and parts per billion (PPB) are used to quantify strengths of very dilute solutions. It is defined as the number of parts of the drug per 1 million (or 1 billion) parts of the whole. The same default units are followed as for percentage systems (% w/w, % w/v and % v/v).

---

44. Express 0.00022% w/v as PPM. Round to the nearest tenth.

$$\frac{0.00022 \text{ g}}{100 \text{ mL}} = \frac{X \text{ g}}{1{,}000{,}000} \qquad X = 2.2 \text{ PPM}$$

$$\frac{0.00022 \text{ g}}{100 \text{ ml}} = \frac{X}{10^6}$$

$$\Rightarrow \quad 2.2 \text{ PPM}$$

---

45. Express 30 PPM of copper in solution as a percentage.

$$\frac{30}{1{,}000{,}000} = \frac{X \text{ g}}{100 \text{ mL}} \qquad X = 0.003\%$$

$$\frac{30}{10^6} = \frac{3 \times 10^{-3}}{100}$$

$$0.003\%$$

---

46. Express 5 PPM of iron in water as a percentage.

$$\frac{5}{1{,}000{,}000} = \frac{X \text{ g}}{100 \text{ mL}} \qquad X = 0.0005\%$$

$$\frac{5}{10^6} = \frac{5 \times 10^{-4}}{100}$$

$$0.0005\%$$

---

47. A patient's blood contains 0.085 PPM of selenium. How many micrograms of selenium does the patient's blood contain if the blood volume is 6 liters?

$$\frac{0.085 \text{ g}}{1{,}000{,}000 \text{ mL}} = \frac{X \text{ g}}{6{,}000 \text{ mL}} \qquad X = 0.00051 \text{ g, or } 510 \text{ mcg}$$

$$\frac{0.085 \text{ g}}{10^6 \text{ ml}} = \frac{X}{6000 \text{ ml}}$$

$$\Rightarrow \quad X = 0.00051 \text{ g} = 510 \text{ μg}$$

---

48. A sample of an intravenous solution is found to contain 0.4 PPM of DEHP. How much of the solution, in milliliters, will contain 50 micrograms of DEHP?

$$\frac{0.4 \text{ g}}{1{,}000{,}000 \text{ mL}} = \frac{0.00005 \text{ g}}{X} \qquad X = 125 \text{ mL}$$

$$\frac{0.4 \text{ g}}{10^6 \text{ ml}} = \frac{50 \times 10^{-6} \text{ g}}{X}$$

$$\Rightarrow \quad 125 \text{ ml}$$

If asked to express something in PPB (parts per billion), you divide by 1,000,000,000 (9 zeros).

Body Mass Index (BMI)

BMI is a measure of body fat based on height and weight that applies to adult men and women. A primary health problem is overweight and obesity which increases the risk of morbidity from hypertension, dyslipidemia, diabetes, coronary heart disease, stroke, gallbladder disease, osteoarthritis and some other conditions. Higher body weights are also associated with increases in all-cause mortality. BMI is a useful measure of body fat, but the BMI can over-estimate body fat in persons who are muscular, and can under-estimate body fat in frail elderly and others who have lost muscle mass. Waist circumference is used concurrently. If most of the fat is around the waist, there is higher disease risk. High risk is defined as a waist size > 35 inches for women or > 40 inches for men. Underweight can be a problem if a person is fighting a disease such as a frail, hospitalized patient with an infection.

BMI is calculated as follows:

$$BMI = \frac{weight\ (kg)}{height\ (m^2)}$$

Alternatively, BMI can be calculated using the following formula:

$$BMI = \frac{weight\ (pounds)}{height\ (in)^2} \times 703$$ — CDC recommendation

BMI Classifications

SCORE	CLASSIFICATION
< 18.5	Underweight
18.5-24.9	Normal weight
25-29.9	Overweight
≥ 30	Obese

49. A male comes to the pharmacy and tells the pharmacist he is 6'7" tall and 250 pounds. His waist circumference is 43 inches. Calculate his BMI. Round to the nearest whole number. Is the patient underweight, normal weight, overweight, or obese?

- Convert weight to kg: 250 pounds x 1 kg/2.2 lbs. = 113.6 kg

- Convert height to cm: 6'7" = 79" x 2.54 cm/inch = 200.66 cm.

- 200.66 cm = 2 m (divide cm by 100 to get the height in meters)

$$BMI\ (kg/m^2) = \frac{113.6}{2^2} = 28.4,\ or\ 28\ which\ is\ overweight.$$

(handwritten) $\frac{250}{79^2} \cdot 703 = 28$ overwt

50. Calculate the BMI for a male who is 6' tall and weighs 198 lbs. Round to the nearest tenth. Is the patient underweight, normal weight, overweight, or obese?

$$BMI\ (pounds/in^2) = \frac{198\ pounds}{(72\ in)^2} \times 704.5 = 26.9,\ or\ 27\ which\ is\ overweight.$$

(handwritten: 703 above 704.5)

(handwritten) $\frac{198}{72^2} \cdot 703 = 26.7$ overwt

Ideal Body Weight (IBW)

IBW is the healthy (ideal) weight for a person. Some medications which are hydrophilic do not distribute much into fat and should be dosed on IBW to prevent giving the patient too much drug. Know these formulas and the creatinine clearance formula below:

- IBW (males) = 50 kg + (2.3 kg)(each inch over 5 feet)

- IBW (females) = 45.5 kg + (2.3 kg)(each inch over 5 feet)

Renal Function and Creatinine Clearance (CrCl) Estimation

A normal range of serum creatinine is approximately 0.6 to 1.2 mg/dL. A serum creatinine above this range usually indicates that the kidneys are not functioning properly. However, the values can appear normal even when renal function is compromised.

Creatinine is a break-down product produced when muscle tissue makes energy. If the kidneys are declining and cannot clear (excrete) the creatinine, the creatinine level will increase in the blood and the creatinine clearance (CrCl) will decrease. This tells us that the concentration of drugs that are renally cleared will also increase and a dose reduction may be required.

Patients should be assessed for dehydration when the serum creatinine value is elevated. Dehydration can cause both the serum creatinine (SCr) and the blood urea nitrogen (BUN) values to increase. Generally, a BUN:SCr ratio > 20 indicates dehydration. Correcting the dehydration will reduce both BUN and SCr, and can prevent or treat acute renal failure. Signs of dehydration should also be assessed and these can include decreased urine output, tachycardia, tachypnea, dry skin/mouth/mucous membranes, skin tenting (skin does not bounce back when pinched into a fold) and possibly fever. Dehydration is usually caused by diarrhea, vomiting, and/or a lack of adequate fluid intake.

---

51. Looking at the laboratory values below, make an assessment of the patient's hydration status.

	NORMAL RANGE	PATIENT'S RANGE
BUN	7-25 mg/dL	54
Creatinine	0.6-1.2 mg/dL	1.8

(handwritten: = 30 ⇒ > 20 ⇒ dehydrated)

    a. The patient appears to be well hydrated given the laboratory results.
    b. The patient appears to be too hydrated given the laboratory results.
    c. The patient is not experiencing dehydration given the laboratory results.
    d. The patient is experiencing dehydration and the patient may need to be started on fluids.
    e. The patient has subjective information indicating dehydration but the patient needs to be assessed objectively as well.

The correct answer is [D]. The patient's BUN:SCr ratio is 54/1.8 = 30. Since 30 > 20, the BUN is disproportionately elevated relative to the creatinine, indicating that the patient is dehydrated.

---

52. Nancy is receiving a furosemide infusion at 5 mg/hr. The nurse notices her urine output has decreased in the last hour. Laboratory values are drawn and the patient has a SCr 1.5 mg/dL and a BUN 26 mg/dL. The nurse wants to know if she should stop the furosemide infusion due to the patient becoming dehydrated. What is the correct assessment of the patient's hydration status?

    a. The patient appears to be too hydrated given the laboratory results.
    b. The patient is not experiencing dehydration given the laboratory results.
    c. The patient is experiencing dehydration and the patient may need to be started on fluids.
    d. The patient has objective information indicating dehydration but the patient needs to be assessed subjectively as well.
    e. None of the above are correct.

(handwritten: $\frac{BUN}{SrCr} = \frac{26}{1.5} = 17.3$ (not > 20))

The correct answer is [B]. The BUN:SCr ratio is 26/1.5 = 17.3, which is < 20. Continue to monitor the patient.

The Cockcroft-Gault Equation

This formula is used commonly by pharmacists to estimate renal function. However, it is (not) commonly used in very young children, ESRD patients or when renal function is fluctuating rapidly. There are different methods used to estimate renal function in these circumstances. The Cockcroft-Gault formula should be known, as it is commonly used in practice.

$$CrCl = \frac{140 - (\text{age of patient})}{72 \times SCr} \times \text{wt in kg} \ (\times 0.85 \text{ if female})$$

A problem may specify which weight to use in the equation. If not, it is advisable to use the following weights:

- If underweight (actual weight is < IBW), use the patient's actual weight

- If normal weight, use the patient's IBW

- If obese or overweight, use the Adjusted Body Weight$_{0.4}$

The adjusted body weight formula should be known:

$$AdjBW_{0.4} = IBW + 0.4(TBW - IBW)$$

ACTUAL
AG (non-obese)
heparin
vanc
LMWHs

obese = > 130% IBW

For dosing a drug, the weight to use may be different. Unless the exam states a specific weight to use, use actual body weight in non-obese patients for aminoglycoside dosing. Heparin, vancomycin, and low molecular weight heparins are dosed on the actual body weight. Theophylline is dosed using the IBW, all the time.

GFR LEVEL (mL/min/1.73m²)	INTERPRETATION
60-89	mild renal insufficiency (Stage 2 CKD)
30-59	moderate renal insufficiency (Stage 3 CKD)
15-29	severe renal insufficiency (Stage 4 CKD)
< 15 or on dialysis	renal failure (Stage 5 CKD)

53. An 87 year old female patient (height 5'4", weight 103 pounds) is placed on levofloxacin, dosing per pharmacy. Her labs include BUN 22 mg/dL and SCr 1 mg/dL. Choose the correct dosing regimen based on the chart below.

CRCL	≥ 50 ML/MIN	20-49 ML/MIN	< 20ML/MIN
Levofloxacin Dose	500 mg Q 24 hours	250 mg Q 24 hours	250 mg Q 48 hours

First, convert weight to kg: 103 pounds x 1 kg/2.2 pounds = 46.8 kg. Use her actual body weight for calculating CrCl since her actual body weight is lower than her IBW.

$$CrCl = 0.85 \left[\frac{(140 - 87) \cdot \frac{103}{2.2}}{72 \cdot 1} \right] = 29.29 \ ml/min$$

$$CrCL = \frac{140-87}{72 \times 1} \times 46.8 \ (x \ 0.85) = 29 \ mL/min. \ \text{The correct dose of levofloxacin is 250 mg Q 24H.}$$

---

54. A 34 year old male (height 6'7", weight 227 pounds) is hospitalized after a motor vehicle accident. He develops a *P. aeruginosa* infection. The physician orders tobramycin 2 mg/kg IV Q8H. Calculate the tobramycin dose. Round to the nearest 10 milligrams.

IBW (males) = 50 kg + (2.3 kg x height in inches over 5 feet):

IBW = 50 kg + (2.3 x 19 in) = 93.7 kg

Handwritten notes:
obese = 93.7 × 1.3 = 121.81 kg
IBW = 50 + 2.3 × 19 = 93.7 kg
actual = 227/2.2 = 103.18 kg

Since the patient is not obese (> 130% of IBW), the tobramycin dose is based on actual weight.

$$227 \ lb \times \frac{1 \ kg}{2.2 \ lbs} = 103.2 \ kg$$

Handwritten notes:
tobra = 2 mg/kg · 103.18 kg = 206.36 mg ≈ 210 mg IV q 8 hrs

Tobramycin 2 mg/kg x 103.2 kg = 206.4 mg, round to 210 mg IV Q8H.

---

55. A 50 year old male (height 6'1", weight 177 pounds) has HIV and is being started on tenofovir, emtricitabine and efavirenz therapy. His laboratory values include K⁺ 4.4 mEq/L, BUN 40 mg/dL, SCr 1.8 mg/dL, and CD4 count of 455 cells/mm³. Using the information below, what is the correct dose of tenofovir for this patient. If the IBW is less than the actual weight, use the actual weight.

CRCL	≥ 50 ML/MIN	30-49 ML/MIN	10-29 ML/MIN	< 10 ML/MIN
Tenofovir Dose	300 mg daily	300 mg Q 48 hours	300 mg Q 72-96 hours	300 mg weekly

First, calculate the patient's IBW.

IBW = 50 kg + (2.3 x 13 in) = 79.9, or 80 kg

The IBW is the same as the actual weight. If the IBW is less than the actual weight, use the actual weight.

Next, calculate the CrCl.

$$CrCL = \frac{140-50}{72 \times 1.8} \times 80 \ kg = 55.5 \ mL/min$$

The dose of tenofovir should be 300 mg daily.

Handwritten notes:
○ actual: 177/2.2 kg = 80.45 kg
○ IBW: 50 + 2.3 · 13 = 79.9 kg
○ CrCl = $\frac{(140-50) \cdot 80.45 \ kg}{72 \cdot 1.8}$ = 55.87 ml/min → dose = 300 mg qd

56. A 64 year old female patient (height 5'5", weight 205 pounds) is hospitalized with a nosocomial pneumonia which is responding to treatment. Her current antibiotic medications include ceftazidime, *Primaxin* and vancomycin. Her morning laboratory values include K⁺ 4.0 mEq/L, BUN 60 mg/dL, SCr 2.7 mg/dL, and glucose 222 mg/dL. Based on the chart below, what is the correct dose of *Primaxin* for this patient? Calculate the dose using the adjusted body weight.

CRCL	≥ 71 ML/MIN	41-70 ML/MIN	21-40 ML/MIN	≤ 20 ML/MIN
Primaxin Dose	500 mg IV Q6H	500 mg IV Q8H	250 mg IV Q6H	250 mg IV Q12H

Since the problem indicates to use the adjusted body weight, use that weight. Calculate her IBW.

IBW = 45.5 kg + (2.3 x 5 in) = 57 kg

Now calculate her adjusted body weight.

$AdjBW_{0.4}$ = 57 + 0.4 (93–57) = 71.4 kg

Then, solve using the Cockcroft-Gault equation.

$$CrCL = \frac{140-64}{72 \times 2.7} \times 71.4 \, (0.85) = 23.7 \, mL/min.$$ Therefore, the correct dose of *Primaxin* is 250 mg IV Q6H.

Handwritten notes:
- actual = 93.18 kg
- IBW = 45.5 + 2.3·5 = 57 kg
- adj = 57 + 0.4 (93.18 - 57) = 71.47 kg

$$CrCl = 0.85 \left[\frac{(140-64) \, 71.47}{72 \cdot 2.7} \right]$$
$$\Rightarrow CrCl = 23.75 \, mL/min$$

---

57. A female patient is to receive 5 mg/kg/d of theophylline. The patient is 5'7" and weighs 243 pounds. Calculate the theophylline dose the patient should receive.

IBW (females) = 45.5 kg + (2.3 x 7 in) = 61.6 kg

Theophylline 5 mg/kg x 61.6 kg = 308 mg

Theophylline and aminophylline are generally dosed on IBW. Check if there were any instructions in the problem regarding rounding, or which weight to use.

Handwritten notes (left margin): theo ALWAYS based on IBW

Handwritten notes:
IBW = 45.5 + 2.3·7 = 61.6 kg
⇒ 5 mg/kg · 61.6 kg = 308 mg/day

Specific Gravity (SG)

Specific gravity is the ratio of the density of a substance to the density of water. SG can be important for calculating IV medications, in compounding, and in urinalysis for use in diagnosis. Water has a specific gravity of 1 where 1 g water = 1 mL water. Substances that have a SG < 1 are lighter than water. Substances that have a SG > 1 are heavier than water. SG does not have units.

$$SG = \frac{weight \, (g)}{volume \, (mL)}$$

---

58. What is the specific gravity of 150 mL of glycerin weighing 165 grams? Round to the nearest tenth.

$$SG = \frac{165 \, g}{150 \, mL} \quad SG = 1.1$$

Handwritten notes:
$$SG = \frac{165 \, g}{150 \, mL} = 1.1$$

Check the answer: 150 mL x 1.1 = 165 g

59. What is the weight of 750 mL of concentrated acetic acid (SG=1.2)?

$$1.2 = \frac{X \text{ g}}{750 \text{ mL}} \qquad X = 900 \text{ g}$$

$1.2 = \frac{x}{750 \text{ ml}} \Rightarrow x = 900 \text{ g}$

Check the answer: 900 g/750 mL = 1.2

---

60. How many mL of polysorbate 80 (SG = 1.08) are needed to prepare a prescription that includes 48 g of the surfactant/emulsifier (polysorbate)? Round to the nearest hundredth.

$$1.08 = \frac{48 \text{ g}}{X \text{ mL}} \qquad X = 44.44 \text{ mL}$$

$1.08 = \frac{48 \text{ g}}{x} \Rightarrow 44.44 \text{ ml}$

Check the answer: 48 g/44.44 mL = 1.08

---

61. What is the specific gravity of 30 mL of a liquid weighing 23,400 milligrams? Round to the nearest hundredth.

$$SG = \frac{23.4 \text{ g}}{30 \text{ mL}} \qquad SG = 0.78$$

$\frac{23.4 \text{ g}}{30 \text{ ml}} = 0.78$

---

62. What is the weight of 0.5 L of polyethylene glycol 400 (SG = 1.13).

$$1.13 = \frac{X \text{ g}}{500 \text{ mL}} \qquad X = 565 \text{ grams}$$

$1.13 = \frac{x}{500 \text{ ml}} \Rightarrow x = 565 \text{ g}$

---

63. Nitroglycerin has a specific gravity of 1.59. How much would 1 quart weigh in grams? Round to the nearest whole number.

- One quart = 946 mL

$$1.59 = \frac{X \text{ g}}{946 \text{ mL}} \qquad X = 1,504 \text{ g}$$

$1 \text{ quart} = 473 \times 2 = 946 \text{ ml}$

$1.59 = \frac{x}{946 \text{ ml}} \Rightarrow x = 1504 \text{ g}$

Check the answer: 1,504 g/946 mL = 1.59

Note that the SG is equivalent to the density in g/mL (with units). If asked for the density in the above problem, the answer would be 1.59 g/mL.

Flow Rates

Intravenous infusions are commonly used to deliver medications in different settings, including hospitals. Flow rates are used to calculate the volume or amount of drug a patient will receive over a given period of time. An order can specify the rate of flow of continuous intravenous fluids in milliliters per minute, drops per minute, milligrams per hour, or as the total time to administer the entire volume of the infusion (e.g., give over 8 hours). Intravenous (IV) tubing is set to deliver a certain number of drops per minute (gtts/min). There are various types of IV tubing and each has a hollow plastic chamber called a drip chamber. One can count the number of drops per minute by looking at the drip chamber. Also, it is important to know how big the drops are to calibrate the tubing in terms of drops/mL. This is called the drop factor.

64. The pharmacist has an order for heparin 25,000 units in 250 mL D5W to infuse at 1,000 units/hour. The pharmacy has the following premixed heparin bags in stock: 25,000 units in 500 mL 1/2 NS, 10,000 units in 250 mL D5W, and 25,000 units in 250 mL D5W. What should the infusion rate be set at in mL/hour?

The pharmacy has the heparin concentration needed in stock. First, calculate units per mL.

$$\frac{25{,}000 \text{ units}}{250 \text{ mL}} = 100 \text{ units/mL}$$

$$\frac{250 \text{ ml}}{25{,}000 \text{ units}} \cdot \frac{1000 \text{ units}}{1 \text{ hr}} = 10 \frac{\text{ml}}{\text{hr}}$$

Since there are 100 units in each mL and 1,000 units/hour must be delivered to the patient, the pump should be programmed for an infusion rate of 10 mL/hr.

$$\frac{1 \text{ mL}}{100 \text{ units}} \times \frac{1{,}000 \text{ units}}{\text{hour}} = 10 \text{ mL/hour}$$

Another way to solve the problem simply is to use the following ratio:

$$\frac{25{,}000 \text{ units}}{250 \text{ mL}} = \frac{1{,}000 \text{ units}}{X \text{ mL}} \quad X = 10 \text{ mL (per hour since we had 1,000 units given in 1 hour)}$$

---

65. If 50 mg of drug are added to a 500 mL bag, what will be the rate of flow, in milliliters per hour, to deliver 5 mg of drug per hour?

$$\frac{50 \text{ mg}}{500 \text{ mL}} = \frac{5 \text{ mg}}{X} \quad X = 50 \text{ mL/hour}$$

$$\frac{500 \text{ ml}}{50 \text{ mg}} \cdot \frac{5 \text{ mg}}{\text{hr}} = 50 \frac{\text{ml}}{\text{hr}}$$

---

66. If 200 mg of drug are added to a 500 mL bag, what will be the rate of flow, in milliliters per hour, to deliver 500 mcg of drug per hour? Round to the nearest hundredth.

$$200 \text{ mg} \times \frac{1{,}000 \text{ mcg}}{1 \text{ mg}} = 200{,}000 \text{ mcg}$$

$$\frac{500 \text{ ml}}{200 \text{ mg}} \cdot \frac{0.5 \text{ mg}}{\text{hr}} = 1.25 \frac{\text{ml}}{\text{hr}}$$

$$\frac{200{,}000 \text{ mcg}}{500 \text{ mL}} = \frac{500 \text{ mcg}}{X} \quad X = 1.25 \text{ mL/hour}$$

---

67. A 68 kg patient is receiving a drug in standard concentration of 400 mg/250 mL of 1/2 NS running at 15 mL/hr. Calculate the dose in mcg/kg/min. Round to the nearest hundredth.

$$\frac{15 \text{ mL}}{\text{hr}} \times \frac{400 \text{ mg drug}}{250 \text{ mL}} = 24 \text{ mg drug/hr}$$

$$\frac{400 \text{ mg}}{250 \text{ ml}} \cdot \frac{15 \text{ ml}}{60 \text{ min}} = 0.4 \frac{\text{mg}}{\text{min}}$$

$$\frac{24 \text{ mg drug}}{\text{hr}} \times \frac{1{,}000 \text{ mcg}}{1 \text{ mg}} = 24{,}000 \text{ mcg/hr}$$

$$\frac{400 \text{ mcg}}{68 \text{ kg min}} = 5.88 \frac{\text{mcg}}{\text{kg min}}$$

$$\frac{24{,}000 \text{ mcg}}{\text{hr}} \times \frac{1 \text{ hr}}{60 \text{ min}} = 400 \text{ mcg/min}$$

$$\frac{400 \text{ mcg/min}}{68 \text{ kg}} = 5.88 \text{ mcg/kg/min}$$

---

68. The pharmacist has an order for heparin 25,000 units in 250 mL D5W to infuse at 1,000 units/hour. How much time, in hours, will be needed to infuse the entire bag?

$$25{,}000 \text{ units} \times \frac{1 \text{ hr}}{1{,}000 \text{ units}} = 25 \text{ hours}$$

(handwritten:) $\dfrac{1000 \text{ units}}{hr} = \dfrac{25\,000 \text{ units}}{x} \Rightarrow 25 \text{ hrs}$

You may need to calculate how many drops will be administered per minute (or per hour). The problem would state the number of drops/mL, which depends on the infusion set.

---

69. A physician orders an IV infusion of D5W 1 Liter to be delivered over 8 hours. The IV infusion set delivers 15 drops/mL. How many drops/min will the patient receive? Round to the nearest whole number.

$$\frac{15 \text{ drops}}{1 \text{ mL}} \times \frac{1{,}000 \text{ mL}}{8 \text{ hr}} \times \frac{1 \text{ hr}}{60 \text{ min}} = 31.25 \text{ drops/min; or } 31 \text{ drops/min}$$

(handwritten:) $15\,000 \text{ drops} = 1000 \text{ ml} = 8 \text{ hrs}$

$\dfrac{15000 \text{ drops}}{8 \cdot 60 \text{ min}} = 31$

---

70. A nurse is hanging a 4% lidocaine solution for a patient. If the dose is 6 mg/min, how many hours will a 250 mL bag last? Round to the nearest tenth.

$$\frac{4 \text{ g}}{100 \text{ mL}} = \frac{X}{250 \text{ mL}} \quad X = 10 \text{ g or } 10{,}000 \text{ mg}$$

(handwritten:) $\dfrac{4g}{100 \text{ ml}} = \dfrac{x}{250 \text{ ml}} \Rightarrow x = 10g$

$$\frac{6 \text{ mg}}{\text{min}} = \frac{10{,}000 \text{ mg}}{X \text{ min}} \quad X = 1{,}666.67 \text{ minutes or } 27.8 \text{ hours}$$

(handwritten:) $6 \text{ mg} = \frac{1}{60} \text{ hr}$

$10\,000 \text{ mg} = ?$

27.8 hrs

Or, solve another way:

$$\frac{1 \text{ hr}}{60 \text{ min}} \times \frac{1 \text{ min}}{6 \text{ mg}} \times \frac{1{,}000 \text{ mg}}{1 \text{ g}} \times \frac{4 \text{ g}}{100 \text{ mL}} \times 250 \text{ mL} = 27.8 \text{ hours}$$

---

71. A patient is to receive *Keppra* at a rate of 5 mg/min. The pharmacy has a 5 mL (100 mg/mL) *Keppra* injection vial to be diluted in 100 mL of NS. What is the rate of infusion, in mL/min, of *Keppra*? Do not include the volume of the 5 mL additive.

First, calculate the amount of *Keppra* in the vial.

$$\frac{100 \text{ mg}}{\text{mL}} = \frac{X \text{ mg}}{5 \text{ mL}} \quad X = 500 \text{ mg}$$

(handwritten:) $5 \text{ ml} \cdot 100 \dfrac{mg}{ml} = 500 \text{ mg vial}$

diluted to $\dfrac{500 \text{ mg}}{100 \text{ ml}} = 5 \dfrac{mg}{ml}$

Then, solve for the answer in mL/min.

$$\frac{100 \text{ mL}}{500 \text{ mg}} \times \frac{5 \text{ mg}}{\text{min}} = 1 \text{ mL/min}$$

(handwritten:) $\dfrac{ml}{5 \text{ mg}} \cdot \dfrac{5 \text{ mg}}{min} = 1 \dfrac{ml}{min}$

72. A physician orders 15 units of insulin to be added to a liter of D5W to be given over 10 hours. What is the infusion rate, in drops/minute, if the IV set delivers 15 drops/mL? Do not round your answer.

$$\frac{15\ drops}{mL} \times \frac{1,000\ mL}{10\ hours} \times \frac{1\ hour}{60\ min} = 25\ drops/min$$

$$\frac{15\ drops}{mL} \cdot \frac{1000\ mL}{10 \cdot 60\ min} = 25$$

73. The pharmacy has insulin vials containing 100 units of insulin/mL. A physician orders 15 units of insulin to be added to a liter of D5W to be given over 10 hours. How many units of insulin will the patient receive each hour if the IV set delivers 15 drops/mL? Do not round the answer.

$$\frac{15\ units}{10\ hours} = \frac{X\ units}{1\ hour} \quad X = 1.5\ units/hour$$

$$\frac{15\ units}{10\ hrs} = 1.5\ \frac{unit}{hr}$$

74. An order is written for 10 mL of a 10% calcium chloride injection and 10 mL of multivitamin injection (MVI) to be added to 500 mL of D5W. The infusion is to be administered over 6 hours. The IV set delivers 15 drops/mL. What should be the rate of flow in drops/minute to deliver this infusion? Round to the nearest whole number.

Total volume of the infusion = 500 mL (D5W) + 10 mL ($CaCl_2$) + 10 mL (MVI) = 520 mL

$$\frac{15\ drops}{mL} \times \frac{520\ mL}{6\ hr} \times \frac{1\ hr}{60\ min} = 22\ drops/min$$

$$\frac{520\ mL}{6 \cdot 60\ min} \cdot \frac{15\ drops}{mL} = 22\ \frac{drops}{min}$$

75. RS is a 45 year old male, 5'5", 168 pounds, hospitalized with a diabetic foot infection. The pharmacist prepared a 500 mL bag of D5W containing 1 gram of vancomycin to be infused over 4 hours using a 20 gtts/mL IV tubing set. How many mg of vancomycin will the patient receive each minute? Round to the nearest tenth.

$$\frac{1,000\ mg\ vanco}{4\ hrs} \times \frac{1\ hr}{60\ min} = 4.16\ mg/min\ or\ 4.2\ mg/min$$

$$\frac{1000\ mg}{4 \cdot 60\ min} = 4.2\ \frac{mg}{min}$$

76. A patient is to receive 600,000 units of penicillin G potassium in 100 mL D5W. A vial of penicillin G potassium 1,000,000 units is available. The manufacture states that when 4.6 mL of diluent is added, a 200,000 units/mL solution will result. How many milliliters of reconstituted solution should be withdrawn and added to the bag of D5W?

$$\frac{200,000\ units}{mL} = \frac{600,000\ units}{X\ mL} \quad X = 3\ mL$$

$$\frac{600,000\ units}{x\ mL} = \frac{200,000\ units}{1\ mL} \Rightarrow x = 3\ mL$$

77. A patient is to receive 1.5 liters of NS running at 45 gtts/min using a 15 gtts/mL IV tubing set. Calculate the total infusion time in hours. Round to the nearest tenth.

$$\frac{45\ gtts}{X\ mL} = \frac{15\ gtts}{1\ mL} \quad X = 3\ mL$$

$$\frac{3\ mL}{min} = \frac{1,500\ mL}{X\ min} \quad X = 500\ min$$

$$\frac{1500\ mL}{x\ min} = \frac{45\ drops}{min} \cdot \frac{1\ mL}{15\ drops}$$

$$x = 500\ min = 8.3\ hrs$$

$$500 \text{ min} \quad \times \quad \frac{1 \text{ hour}}{60 \text{ min}} \quad = 8.3 \text{ hours}$$

---

78. An intravenous infusion contains 2 mL of a 1:1,000 (w/v) solution of epinephrine and 250 mL of D5W. At what flow rate, in mL/min, should the infusion be administered to provide 0.3 mcg/kg/min of epinephrine to an 80 kg patient? Round to the nearest whole number.

- 1:1,000 = 0.1% (w/v)

$$\frac{0.1 \text{ g}}{100 \text{ mL}} = \frac{X \text{ g}}{2 \text{ mL}} \quad X = 0.002 \text{ g, or 2 mg}$$

The patient is 80 kg x 0.3 mcg/kg/min = 24 mcg/min

$$\frac{252 \text{ mL}}{2 \text{ mg}} \times \frac{1 \text{ mg}}{1,000 \text{ mcg}} \times \frac{24 \text{ mcg}}{\text{min}} = 3 \text{ mL/min}$$

Handwritten:
$$\frac{0.3 \text{ µg}}{\text{kg min}} \cdot 80 \text{ kg} = 24 \frac{\text{µg}}{\text{min}}$$
$$\frac{1 \text{ g}}{1000 \text{ ml}} \cdot 2 \text{ ml} = 0.002 \text{ g}$$
$$\frac{252 \text{ ml}}{2000 \text{ µg}} \cdot \frac{24 \text{ µg}}{\text{min}} = 3$$

---

79. A patient is to receive *Flagyl* at a rate of 12.5 mg/min. The pharmacy has a 5 mL (100 mg/mL) *Flagyl* injection vial to be diluted in 100 mL of NS. How much drug in milligrams will the patient receive over 20 minutes?

$$\frac{12.5 \text{ mg}}{\text{min}} \times 20 \text{ minutes} = 250 \text{ mg}$$

Handwritten:
$$\frac{12.5 \text{ mg}}{\text{min}} \cdot 20 \text{ min} = 250 \text{ mg}$$

---

80. A physician has ordered 2 grams of cefotetan to be added to 100 mL NS for a 56 year old female with an anaerobic infection. Using a reconstituted injection containing 154 mg/mL, how many milliliters should be added to prepare the order? Round to the nearest <u>whole</u> number.

$$2,000 \text{ mg} \times \frac{1 \text{ mL}}{154 \text{ mg}} = 13 \text{ mL}$$

Handwritten:
$$\frac{154 \text{ mg}}{\text{ml}} = \frac{2000 \text{ mg}}{x \text{ ml}} \Rightarrow x = 13 \text{ ml}$$

---

81. JY is a 58 year old male who was hospitalized for a total knee replacement. He was given unfractionated heparin and developed heparin-induced thrombocytopenia (HIT). Argatroban was ordered at a dose of 2 mcg/kg/min. The pharmacy mixes a concentration of 100 mg argatroban in 250 mL of D5W. JY weighs 85 kg. How many mL/hour should the nurse infuse to provide the desired dose? Round to the nearest <u>whole</u> number.

First, determine the amount of drug needed based on body weight.

2 mcg/kg/min x 85 kg = 170 mcg/min

Then, calculate mL/hr.

$$\frac{250 \text{ mL}}{100 \text{ mg}} \times \frac{1 \text{ mg}}{1,000 \text{ mcg}} \times \frac{170 \text{ mcg}}{\text{min}} \times \frac{60 \text{ min}}{\text{hr}} = 25.5 \text{ mL/hr, rounded up to 26 mL/hr}$$

Handwritten:
$$\frac{2 \text{ µg}}{\text{kg min}} \cdot 85 \text{ kg} = 170 \frac{\text{µg}}{\text{min}}$$
$$\frac{170 \times 10^{-3} \text{ mg}}{1/60 \text{ hr}} = 10.2 \frac{\text{mg}}{\text{hr}}$$
$$\frac{250 \text{ ml}}{100 \text{ µg}} \cdot 10.2 \frac{\text{µg}}{\text{hr}} = 26 \frac{\text{ml}}{\text{hr}}$$

33

82. The 8 a.m. medications scheduled for your patient include *Tygacil* dosed at 6 mg/kg. The patient weighs 142 pounds. *Tygacil* comes as 500 mg vials to be reconstituted and diluted in 50 mL NS. The dose will be administered over thirty minutes. The IV tubing in the unit delivers 15 drops per milliliter. What is the correct rate of flow in drops per minute? Round to the nearest drop.

$$\frac{142 \text{ pounds}}{2.2 \text{ pounds/kg}} \times \frac{6 \text{ mg}}{\text{kg}} = 387.27 \text{ mg required dose}$$

$$\frac{6 \text{ mg}}{\text{kg}} \cdot \frac{142}{2.2} \text{ kg} = 387.27 \text{ mg}$$

The drug comes as 500 mg in a 50 mL bag: 500 mg/50 mL = 10 mg/mL

$$\frac{500 \text{ mg}}{50 \text{ mL}} = 10 \text{ mg/mL}$$

$$\frac{500 \text{ mg}}{50 \text{ mL}} = \frac{387.27 \text{ mg}}{x \text{ ml}} \Rightarrow x = 38.72 \text{ ml}$$

The patient requires 387.27 mg x 10 mg/mL = 38.727 mL

$$\frac{15 \text{ drops}}{\text{ml}} \cdot \frac{38.72 \text{ ml}}{30 \text{ min}} = 19 \frac{\text{drops}}{\text{min}}$$

$$\frac{38.727 \text{ mL}}{30 \text{ min}} = \frac{1.29 \text{ mL}}{\text{min}} \times \frac{15 \text{ drops}}{\text{mL}} = 19.36 \text{ drops per minute, rounded to 19 drops/minute}$$

---

83. A 165 pound patient is to receive 250 mL of a dopamine drip at a rate of 17 mcg/kg/min. The pharmacy has dopamine premixed in concentration of 3.2 mg/mL in D5W. Calculate the infusion rate in mL/minute. Round to the nearest tenth.

Step 1 – Calculate amount of drug in the 250 mL bag.

$$\frac{3.2 \text{ mg}}{\text{mL}} \times 250 \text{ mL} = 800 \text{ mg}$$

$$\frac{17 \mu g}{kg \text{ min}} \cdot \frac{165}{2.2} \text{ kg} = 1275 \frac{\mu g}{\text{min}}$$

$$\frac{1.275 \text{ mg}}{\text{min}} \cdot \frac{1 \text{ ml}}{3.2 \text{ mg}}$$

Step 2 – Calculate amount of drug the patient needs.

$$\frac{17 \text{ mcg}}{\text{kg/min}} \times \frac{1 \text{ kg}}{2.2 \text{ lbs}} \times 165 \text{ lbs.} = 1,275 \text{ mcg/min or } 1.275 \text{ mg/min}$$

$$= 0.40 \text{ ml/min}$$

Step 3–Solve for milliliters per minute.

$$\frac{250 \text{ mL}}{800 \text{ mg}} \times \frac{1.275 \text{ mg}}{\text{min}} = 0.4 \text{ mL/min}$$

---

84. An order is written for phenytoin to be given by intravenous infusion at a loading dose of 15 mg/kg to be infused at 0.5 mg/kg/min for a 33 pound child. The pharmacy has phenytoin injection solution 50 mg/mL in a 5 mL vial in stock. The pharmacist will put the dose into 50 mL NS. Over how many minutes should the dose be administered? Round to the nearest whole number.

First, calculate the child's body weight in kg.

$$33 \text{ lbs} \times \frac{1 \text{ kg}}{2.2 \text{ lbs}} = 15 \text{ kg}$$

$$LD = \frac{15 \text{ mg}}{kg} \cdot \frac{33}{2.2} \text{ kg} = 225 \text{ mg}$$

$$\text{rate} = \frac{0.5 \text{ mg}}{kg \text{ min}} \cdot \frac{33}{2.2} \text{ kg} = 7.5 \text{ mg/min}$$

Next, find the dose the child will receive.

$$\frac{15 \text{ mg}}{kg} \times 15 \text{ kg} = 225 \text{ mg}$$

$$\frac{225 \text{ mg}}{x \text{ min}} = \frac{7.5 \text{ mg}}{\text{min}}$$

$$\Rightarrow x = 30 \text{ min}$$

Then, calculate the time it will take to infuse this amount of drug at the given rate.

0.5 mg/kg/min x 15 kg = 7.5 mg/min

$$\frac{1 \text{ min}}{7.5 \text{ mg}} \quad x \quad 225 \text{ mg} \quad = \quad 30 \text{ minutes}$$

Dilution and Concentration

Often the strength of a concentration must be increased or decreased. Or, a new quantity is required. This formula can be used to change the strength or quantity. Be careful: the units on each side must match and one or more may need to be changed, such as mg to gram, or vice-versa.

$Q_1 \times C_1 = Q_2 \times C_2$

Q_1 = old quantity

C_1 = old concentration

Q_2 = new quantity

C_2 = new concentration

---

85. How many mL of a 1:2,500 (w/v) solution of aluminum acetate can be made from 100 mL of a 0.2% solution?

1:2,500 is converted to a percentage by making it into a fraction and multiplying by 100.

$$1:2,500 \quad = \quad \frac{1}{2,500} \quad x \quad 100 \quad = \quad 0.04\%$$

Now we can use the formula.

$Q_1 \quad x \quad C_1 \quad = \quad Q_2 \quad x \quad C_2$

100 mL x 0.2% = Q_2 x 0.04%

Q_2 = 500 mL

(handwritten) $100 \text{ ml} \cdot \frac{0.2 \text{ g}}{100 \text{ ml}} = \frac{1 \text{ g}}{2500 \text{ ml}} \cdot x$

$x = 500 \text{ ml}$

---

86. Using 20 g of a 9% boric acid ointment base, the pharmacist will manufacture a 5% ointment. How much diluent is required?

Note the difference from the previous problem where the calculation provided the total volume. Here, you will get the final quantity (weight) but are asked how much diluent should be added to make the final weight.

20 g x 9% = Q_2 x 5%

Q_2 = 36 g total

Then take 36 g – 20 g (already present) = 16 g diluent required

(handwritten)
9%   5p ≅ 20g
  5%
0%   4p ≅ ? 16g
     9p

87. How many grams of petrolatum (diluent) should be added to 250 g of a 20% ichthammol ointment to make a 7% ichthammol ointment? Round to the nearest tenth.

250 g x 20% = Q_2 x 7%

Q_2 = 714.3 g total

714.3 g – 250 g present = 464.3 g petrolatum required

(handwritten: 20% , 7% , 0% ; 7p ≙ 250 g ; 13p ≙ ? 464.3g ; 20 p)

---

88. What is the ratio strength (w/v) of 50 mL containing a 1:20 (w/v) ammonia solution diluted to 1 liter?

1:20 is converted to a percentage by making it into a fraction and multiplying by 100:

1:20 = $\dfrac{1}{20}$ x 100 = 5%

50 mL x 5% = 1,000 mL x C_2

C_2 = 0.25% = 1:400

(handwritten: $50\,ml \cdot \dfrac{1g}{20\,ml} = 2.5g$; $\dfrac{2.5g}{1000\,ml} = \dfrac{1}{x} \Rightarrow 1:400$)

---

89. If 1 gallon of a 20% (w/v) solution is evaporated to a solution with a 50% (w/v) strength, what will be the new volume (in mL)?

3,785 mL x 20% = Q_2 x 50%

Q_2 = 1,514 mL

(handwritten: $3785\,ml \cdot \dfrac{20g}{100\,ml} = 757g$; $\dfrac{50g}{100\,ml} = \dfrac{757g}{x\,ml} \Rightarrow x = 1514\,ml$)

---

90. A pharmacist has an order for parenteral nutrition that includes 550 mL of D70%. The pharmacist checks the supplies and finds the closest strength he has available is D50%. How many mL of D50% will provide an equivalent energy requirement?

(handwritten: $550\,ml \cdot \dfrac{70g}{100\,ml} = x \cdot \dfrac{50g}{100\,ml}$)

550 mL x 70% = X mL x 50%   X = 770 mL

(handwritten: $\Rightarrow x = 770\,ml$)

---

91. A patient has been receiving 200 mL of an enteral mixture that contains 432 mOsm/L. The pharmacist will reduce the contents to 278 mOsm/L. How many mL of bacteriostatic water should be added to the bag? Round to the nearest mL.

200 mL x 432 mOsm/L = X mL x 278 mOsm/L   X = 311 mL

(handwritten: 432 , 278 , 0 ; 278p ≙ 200 ml ; 154p ≙ ? 111 ml ; 432 p)

There are 200 mL in the original bag. The final bag will have 311 mL. The volume that should be added to the original bag is 111 mL.

Alligation

Alligation is used to obtain a new strength (percentage) that is between two strengths the pharmacist has in stock. Occasionally, no math is required to solve this type of problem if the new strength needed is exactly in the middle of the 2 strengths that are given. If the prescription calls for an ingredient that is pure, the concentration is 100%. If you are given a diluent, such as petrolatum, lanolin, alcohol, "ointment base", etc., the concentration of the diluent is 0%.

92. Measure out 100 g of a 50% hydrocortisone powder using the 25% and 75% in stock.

■ Use 50g of the 75%, and 50g of the 25% (total is 100 grams).

[handwritten notes: 25% 50% 25 p ≙ ? 50g; 75% 50% 25 p ≙ ? 50g; 50 p ≙ 100 g]

93. You are asked to prepare 80 g of a 12.5% ichthammol ointment. You have 16% and 12% ichthammol ointments in stock.

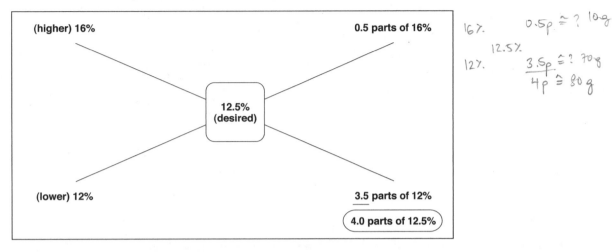

[handwritten notes: 16% 0.5 p ≙ ? 10 g; 12.5% 12% 3.5 p ≙ ? 70 g; 4 p ≙ 80 g]

■ To set up the X method:

  ❏ Put the more concentrated product at the top left (high goes high)

  ❏ Put the less concentrated product at the bottom left (low goes low)

  ❏ Place the desired concentration in the middle of the X

■ Subtract down the "X" lines to obtain the # of parts on the right (16%–12.5% = 3.5 parts; 12%–12.5% = 0.5 parts).

■ Add the # of parts on the right to find the total # of parts (4 parts).

■ Divide by the total weight (80 g) by the number of parts to obtain the weight per part.

$$\frac{80 \text{ g}}{4 \text{ parts}} = \frac{20 \text{ g}}{\text{part}}$$

■ Take the amount per part (20 g) and multiply it by the parts from each of the concentrations (from the high, and from the low).

$$0.5 \text{ parts} \quad \times \quad \frac{20 \text{ g}}{\text{part}} \quad = \quad 10 \text{ g of the 16\% ichthammol ointment}$$

$$3.5 \text{ parts} \quad \times \quad \frac{20 \text{ g}}{\text{part}} \quad = \quad 70 \text{ g of the 12\% ichthammol ointment}$$

Mix together; the end product provides 80 g of a 12.5% ichthammol ointment.

3785 ml

94. You are asked to prepare 1 gallon of tincture containing 5.5% iodine. The pharmacy has 3% iodine tincture and 8.5% iodine tincture in stock. How many mL of each 3% and 8.5% iodine tincture should be used? (Use 1 gallon = 3,785 mL)

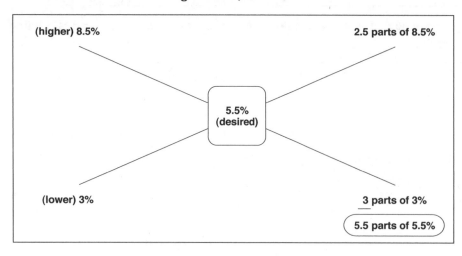

8.5%   2.5p ≟ 1720.5 ml
     5.5%
3%   3p ≟ 2064.5 ml
     5.5p ≟ 3785 ml

- To set up the X method:

  - Put the more concentrated product at the top left (high goes high)

  - Put the less concentrated product at the bottom left (low goes low)

  - Place the desired concentration in the middle of the X

- Subtract down the "X" lines to obtain the # of parts on the right (e.g., 8.5%–5.5% = 3 parts; 3%–5.5% = 2.5 parts for this problem).

- Add the # of parts on the right to find the total # of parts (5.5 parts in this problem).

- Divide the total volume (3,785 mL) by the number of parts to obtain the volume per part.

$$\frac{3,785 \text{ mL}}{5.5 \text{ parts}} = 688.2 \text{ mL per part}$$

$$2.5 \text{ parts} \times \frac{688.2 \text{ mL}}{\text{part}} = 1,720 \text{ mL of the 8.5% iodine tincture}$$

$$3 \text{ parts} \times \frac{688.2 \text{ mL}}{\text{part}} = 2,065 \text{ mL of the 3% iodine tincture}$$

The end product provides 3,785 mL of a 5.5% iodine tincture.

Calorie Sources and Nutrition Calculations

Kilocalories (kcals), "Calories" and "calories"

A calorie is a measurement of the energy, or heat, it takes to raise the temperature of 1 gram of water by 1°C. Calories are associated with nutrition because humans obtain energy from the food they consume, or from enteral nutrition (EN) formulas delivered by "feeding" tubes into the stomach or intestine, or from parenteral nutrition (PN), which is delivered peripherally through a vein, or centrally through an artery. Calories from any of these nutrition sources are provided by these 3 components: carbohydrates, fat and protein.

A calorie is a very small unit, and these are therefore measured in kilocalories, or kcals, where 1,000 calories = 1 kcal. It is common to find the term "calories" used interchangeably for kcals. For example, the "Nutrition Facts" box on the side of a container of Honey Nut Cheerios® states that a serving of ¾ cup of the cereal provides 110 Calories. Precisely, this is 110 kcals. If you were to look at the box, the word "Calories" is written with a capital "C" which is sometimes used to indicate kcals, versus a lower case "c". It is not consistent; for pharmacy calculations, "calories" or "Calories" are meant to refer to kilocalories, or kcals.

Carbohydrates

enteral (EN) = 4 kcal/g
parenteral (PN) = 3.4 kcal/g (dextrose)
4.3 kcal/g (glycerol in insulin impairment)

Glucose is the primary energy source. Unless a patient purchases glucose tablets or gel, carbohydrates are consumed as simple sugars, such as fruit juice, or complex "starchy" sugars, such as legumes and grains. These are hydrolyzed by the gut into the monosaccharides fructose, galactose and glucose, which are absorbed. The liver converts the first two into glucose, and excess glucose is stored as glycogen.

Carbohydrates from food or in EN formulas provide 4 kcal/gram, although the formula calories are measured together (that's the carbs, fat and protein) in total kcal provided by each mL (kcal/mL). In PN, dextrose monohydrate provides the carbohydrate source. This is the isomer of glucose (D-glucose) which can be metabolized for energy. The dextrose in PN provides 3.4 kcal/gram. Occasionally, glycerol is used as an alternative to dextrose in patients with impaired insulin secretion. Glycerol provides 4.3 kcal/gram and comes premixed with amino acids.

Fat

EN = 9 kcal/g
PN = 1.1 kcal/mL (10%)
2 kcal/mL (20%)
3 kcal/mL (30%)

Fats, or lipids, are used by the body for energy or for various critical functions, including being an essential component of cell membranes, a solvent for fat soluble vitamins, in hormone production and activity, in cell signaling, and other functions. In food or from EN formulas, fat is provided as four types: saturated, *trans*, monounsaturated and polyunsaturated. Each of these provides 9 kcal/gram. In PN, lipids are not measured in grams but in kcal/mL due to the caloric contribution provided by the egg phospholipid and glycerol components in the Intravenous Fat Emulsion (IVFE). 10% IVFE provides 1.1 kcal/mL, 20% provides 2 kcal/mL and 30% provides 3 kcal/mL.

Protein

EN/PN = 4 kcal/g

Protein is used either to repair or build muscle cells, or as a source of energy. Protein in enteral intake is present in various forms, and in PN as the constituent amino acids. If adequate energy is provided by carbohydrates and fat, the protein may be "spared" and can be used by muscle, (although the protein calories may not end up in the intended location.) If "protein sparing" is used, the energy required by the patient will come from only the dextrose and lipids, which are the "Non-Protein Calories" (NPC).

Protein calories from food, enteral nutrition formulas or as parenteral amino acid solutions each provide <u>4 kcal/gram. The kcal amounts in the chart below should be known</u>:

USUAL DIET*			EN FORMULAS*		PN FORMULAS	
Carbs	Bread, Rice….	4 kcal/g	Corn syrup solids, cornstarch, sucrose….	The components contribute the same as from the diet, but are measured (together) as kcal/mL	Dextrose Monohydrate	3.4 kcal/gram
					Glycerol/ Glycerin**	4.3 kcal/gram
Fat	Butter, Oil….	9 kcal/g	Borage oil, canola oil, corn oil….		IV Fat Emulsion (IVFE) 10%	1.1 kcal/mL
					IVFE 20%	2 kcal/mL
					IVFE 30%	3 kcal/mL
Protein	Fish, Meat….	4 kcal/g	Casein, soy, whey….		Amino Acid Solutions *(Aminosyn, Freamine….)*	4 kcal/gram

* The diet and enteral formula components are common examples; there are others.

** Glycerol may be used to decrease hyperglycemia; more commonly, the dextrose load is decreased or the insulin dose is increased.

PARENTERAL NUTRITION (PN)

It is preferable to use the <u>least invasive</u> and <u>most physiologic</u> method of feeding. PN is neither and has a higher risk of complications, including infection and thrombosis. It may be indicated when the patient is not able to absorb adequate nutrition via the GI tract for greater than 5 days. Usual conditions that may require PN include bowel obstruction, ileus, severe diarrhea, radiation enteritis and untreatable malabsorption.

There are 2 types of PN admixtures. Mixtures that contain dextrose, amino acids, sterile water for injection, electrolytes, vitamins and minerals are referred to as 2-in-1 formulations, while the intravenous fat emulsion (IVFE) is infused separately. When the IVFE is contained in the same bag, it is referred to as total nutrient admixtures (TNAs), or 3-in-1, or all-in-one formulations.

If the PN is expected to be short-term (<1 week), peripheral access may be possible, but has a high risk of phlebitis and vein damage. Central line placement allows a higher osmolarity and a wider variation in pH. Common types of central lines include peripherally-inserted central catheters ("PICC" lines), Hickman, Broviac, Groshong and others.

The fluid, kcal, protein and lipid requirements, plus the initial electrolyte, vitamin and trace element requirements will be determined. Additional additives may be needed, such as insulin and H2-blockers. PN requires monitoring, including assessing the need, the degree of glucose intolerance and the risk of refeeding syndrome, which is an intracellular loss of electrolytes, particularly phosphate, which causes serious complications. The calculations for PN that follow are basic and should be known by pharmacists who work in the hospital setting. Nutrition pharmacy itself is more complex and is a specialty area.

Determining Fluid Needs

Fluid requirements are often calculated 1st in the PN. Enough (but not too much) fluid needs to be given to maintain adequate hydration. Daily fluid needs can be calculated using this formula:

When weight > 20 kg: 1,500 mL + (20 mL)(Wt in kg – 20)   *per day*

Alternatively, some institutions estimate adult fluid requirements using a general guideline of 30-40 mL/kg/day. The PN and fluid volume should be tailored to the patient. If the patient has problems with fluid accumulation (such as heart failure, renal dysfunction, etc.), the amount of fluid they can handle will be reduced. Fluid volume from medications (including IVPBs) should be included in the overall volume the patient is receiving.

---

95. GG is a 57 year old female admitted to the hospital with bowel obstruction. She is made NPO for the next 5-7 days. The decision was made to start PN therapy. She weighs 65 kg and is 5'6". The SCr is 1.3 mg/dL. Calculate GG's daily fluid requirements.

1,500 mL + (20 mL) (65 − 20) = 2,400 mL/day   *> 20 kg*

1500 + 20 × [65−20] = 2400 ml

---

96. A 76 year old, 154 lbs (IBW) patient is made NPO and needs hydration. She is afebrile and does not have CHF, renal disease, or ascites. What volume of fluid should the patient receive per day?

1,500 mL + (20 mL) (70 − 20) = 2,500 mL/day

$$1500 + 20 \times \left[\frac{154}{2.2} - 20 \right] = 2500 \, ml$$

Calculating Protein Calories

Typical protein requirements for a non-stressed, ambulatory patient are 0.8-1 g/kg/day. Protein requirements increase as the patient is placed under stress, which is defined as illness severity. The more severely ill, the greater the protein requirements will be per day. In patients with a high degree of metabolic stress the protein requirements can be as high as 1.8-2 g/kg/day.

CONDITION	PROTEIN REQUIREMENTS
Ambulatory, non-hospitalized (non-stressed)	0.8-1 g/kg/day
Hospitalized, or malnourished	1.2-2 g/kg/day

↳ *high metabolic stress*   ↳ *1.8 – 2 g/kg/day*

97. MK is a 62 year old female who has been admitted with enteritis and pneumonia. She has a history of Crohn's disease and COPD. The staff gastroenterologist has ordered PN therapy, to be prepared by pharmacy. She is 158 pounds, 5'4". Calculate her protein requirements using her actual weight. She is hospitalized and should receive 1.5 g/kg/day of protein. Round to the nearest whole number.

First, convert pounds to kg. 158 pounds x 1 kg/2.2 lbs = 71.8 kg

$$\frac{1.5 \text{ g}}{\text{kg day}} \cdot \frac{158}{2.2} \text{ kg} = 108 \text{ g/day}$$

Then, calculate the protein requirements. 71.8 kg x 1.5 g/kg/day = 108 g protein/day

---

98. PP is a 46 year old male (207 pounds, 5'11") who has been admitted for bowel resection surgery. Post surgery, he is to be started on PN therapy. The physician wants the patient to receive 1.3 g/kg/day of protein. Calculate his protein requirements using his actual weight. Round to the nearest whole number.

First, convert pounds to kg. 207 pounds x 1 kg/2.2 pounds = 94.1 kg

$$\frac{1.3 \text{ g}}{\text{kg day}} \cdot \frac{207}{2.2} \text{ kg} = 122 \text{ g/day}$$

Then, calculate the protein requirements. 94.1 kg x 1.3 g/kg/day = 122 g protein/day

Calculating Non-Protein Calories

Basal Energy Expenditure (BEE) and Total Energy Expenditure (TEE)

The basal energy expenditure (BEE), otherwise referred to as the basal metabolic rate (BMR), is the energy expenditure in the resting state, exclusive of eating and activity. It is estimated differently in male and female patients using the Harris-Benedict equations (it can also be estimated in adults at 15-25 kcal/kg/day). The Harris-Benedict equations are:

- BEE (males): 66.47 + 13.75 (weight in kg) + 5 (height in cm) - 6.76 (age in years)

- BEE (females): 655.1 + 9.6 (weight in kg) + 1.85 (height in cm) - 4.68 (age in years)

Total energy expenditure (or total daily expenditure or TDE) is a measure of basal energy expenditure plus excess metabolic demands as a result of stress, the thermal effects of feeding, and energy expenditure for activity.

TEE = BEE x activity factor x stress factor

- Once the BEE is calculated, calculate the TEE by taking the BEE calories and multiplying by the appropriate activity factor and stress factor. This will increase the calories required. Energy requirements are increased 12% with each degree of fever over 37° C.

The activity factor is either 1.2 if confined to bed (non-ambulatory), or 1.3 if out of bed (ambulatory). Commonly used stress factors are listed in the table:

STATE OF STRESS	STRESS FACTOR
Minor surgery	1.2
Infection	1.4
Major trauma, sepsis, burns up to 30% BSA	1.5
Burns over 30% BSA	1.5-2

activity factor

confined to bed (non-ambulatory) ⟹ 1.2

out of bed (ambulatory) ⟹ 1.3

99. Using the Harris-Benedict equation, calculate the resting non-protein caloric requirement for a major trauma patient (stress factor 1.5) who is a 66 year old male, 174 pounds and 5'10" in height. Activity factor is 1.2. Round to the nearest whole number.

- Height = 70" x 2.54 cm/inch = 177.8 cm. Weight 174 pounds x 1 kg/2.2 pounds = 79.1 kg.

BEE (males): 66.47 + 13.75(weight in kg) + 5(height in cm)–6.76(age in years)

BEE = 66.47 + (13.75 x 79.1) + (5 x 177.8) - (6.76 x 66)

$$BEE = 66.47 + 13.75\left(\frac{174}{2.2}\right) + 5\left(177.8\right) - 6.76 \times 66$$
$$\Rightarrow BEE = 1596.81 \text{ kcal/day}$$
$$\approx 1597 \text{ kcal/day}$$

BEE = 66.47 + 1,087.6 + 889 - 446.16 = 1,597 kcal/day

The BEE can be estimated using 15-25 kcal/kg (adults). You may want to check your calculations by using the estimates and seeing if the numbers are close. In this case, an estimation using 20 kcal/kg/day would provide 1,582 kcal/day (close to 1,597 kcal/day as above).

---

100. Using the total energy expenditure equation, calculate the total non-protein caloric requirement for a major trauma patient (stress factor is 1.5, activity factor is 1.2) who is a 66 year old male, weighing 174 pounds and measures 5'10" in height. (Use the kcal from the patient in the previous problem.) Round to the nearest whole number.

TEE = BEE x activity factor x stress factor. BEE was calculated above.

TEE = 1,597 x 1.2 x 1.5 = 2,875 kcal/day

TEE = 1.5 x 1.2 x 1597 kcal/day = 2875 kcal

---

101. A 25 year old female major trauma patient survives surgery and is recovering in the surgical intensive care unit. The medical team wants to start PN therapy. She is 122 pounds, 5' 7" with some mild renal impairment. Calculate her BEE using the Harris-Benedict equation and her TEE non-protein caloric requirements (stress factor = 1.7 and activity factor =1.2). Round to the nearest whole number.

- Height = 67" x 2.54 cm/inch = 170 cm. Weight 122 pounds x 1 kg/2.2 pounds = 55.5 kg.

BEE (females): 655.1 + 9.6(weight in kg) + 1.85(height in cm)–4.68(age in years)

BEE = 655.1 + (9.6 x 55.5) + (1.85 x 170) - (4.68 x 25)

$$BEE = 655.1 + 9.6\left(\frac{122}{2.2}\right) + 1.85 \times 170.18 - 4.68 \times 25$$
$$= 1385 \text{ kcal/day}$$

BEE = 655.1 + 532.8 + 314.5 - 117 = 1,385 kcal/day

TEE = BEE x activity factor x stress factor

TEE = 1,385 x 1.2 x 1.7 = 2,825 kcal/day

$$TEE = 1.7 \times 1.2 \times 1385$$
$$= 2825 \text{ kcal/day}$$

Calculating Amino Acids

Amino acids are the source of proteins in PN. Amino acids are used to build muscle mass and may not be counted as an energy source in critically ill patients because they are catabolic. *→ break down*
Amino acids come in stock preparations of 5%, 8.5%, 10%, 15%, and others. Amino acids provide 4 kcal/gram.

102. If the pharmacy stocks *Aminosyn* 8.5%, how many mL will be needed to provide 108 g of protein? Round to the nearest whole number.

$$\frac{8.5 \text{ g}}{100 \text{ mL}} = \frac{108 \text{ g}}{\text{X mL}} \qquad \text{X} = 1,271 \text{ mL}$$

$\frac{8.5 \text{ g}}{100 \text{ ml}} = \frac{108 \text{ g}}{\text{x ml}} \Rightarrow \text{x} = 1271 \text{ ml}$

---

103. How many calories are provided by 108 grams of protein?

$$\frac{4 \text{ kcal}}{\text{g}} \times 108 \text{ g} = 432 \text{ kcal of protein}$$

$\frac{4 \text{ kcal}}{g} = \frac{\text{x kcal}}{108 \text{ g}}$

$\Rightarrow \text{x} = 432 \text{ kcal}$

---

104. The pharmacy stocks *FreAmine* 10%. A patient requires 122 grams of protein per day. How many mL of *FreAmine* will the patient need?

$$\frac{10 \text{ g}}{100 \text{ mL}} = \frac{122 \text{ g}}{\text{X mL}} \qquad \text{X} = 1,220 \text{ mL}$$

$\frac{10 \text{ g}}{100 \text{ ml}} = \frac{122 \text{ g}}{\text{x ml}} \Rightarrow \text{x} = 1220 \text{ ml}$

---

105. JR is requiring 1.4 g/kg/day of protein and the pharmacy stocks *Aminosyn* 8.5%. JR is a 55 year old male (weight 189 pounds) who is confined to bed (activity factor 1.2) due to his current infection (stress factor 1.5). Calculate the amount of *Aminosyn*, in milliliters, JR should receive. Round to the nearest whole number. (The answer will be accurate if rounding is done at the last step; the final number should be 1,415 mL.)

First, convert weight to kg. 189 pounds x 1 kg/2.2 pounds = 85.9 kg

$\frac{1.4 \text{ g}}{\text{kg day}} \cdot \frac{189}{2.2} \text{ kg}$

Next, calculate protein requirements. 1.4 g/kg/day x 85.9 kg = 120.27 g/day

$= 120.2727 \text{ g/day}$

Then, calculate the amount of *Aminosyn* (mL) needed. Note the activity factor and stress factor are not required to calculate the protein requirements.

$$\frac{8.5 \text{ g}}{100 \text{ mL}} = \frac{120.27 \text{ g}}{\text{X mL}} \qquad \text{X} = 1,415 \text{ mL}$$

$\frac{120.2927 \text{ g}}{\text{x ml}} = \frac{8.5 \text{ g}}{100 \text{ ml}}$

$\Rightarrow \text{x} = 1415 \text{ ml}$

---

106. JR is receiving 97 grams of protein in an *Aminosyn* 8.5% solution on day 8 of his hospitalization. How many calories are provided by this amount of protein?

$$\frac{4 \text{ kcal}}{\text{g}} \times 97 \text{ g} = 388 \text{ kcal of protein}$$

$\frac{4 \text{ kcal}}{g} = \frac{\text{x kcal}}{97 \text{ g}} \Rightarrow \text{x} = 388 \text{ kcal}$

---

107. A PN order is written to add 800 mL of 10% amino acid solution. The pharmacy only has 15% amino acid solution in stock. Using the 15% amino acid solution instead, how many mL should be added to the PN bag? Round to the nearest whole number.

First, calculate the the grams that would be provided with the 10% solution.

$$\frac{10 \text{ g}}{100 \text{ mL}} = \frac{\text{X g}}{800 \text{ mL}} \qquad \text{X} = 80 \text{ g}$$

$800 \text{ ml} \cdot \frac{10 \text{ g}}{100 \text{ ml}} = 80 \text{ g}$

$\frac{15 \text{ g}}{100 \text{ ml}} = \frac{80 \text{ g}}{\text{x ml}} \Rightarrow \text{x} = 533 \text{ ml}$

Next, supply the 80 grams of protein with the 15% amino acid solution.

$$\frac{15 \text{ g}}{100 \text{ mL}} = \frac{80 \text{ g}}{\text{X mL}} \quad \text{X = 533 mL}$$

Nitrogen Balance

Determining The Grams Of Nitrogen From Protein

Nitrogen is released during protein catabolism and is mainly excreted as urea in the urine. Nitrogen balance is the difference between the body's nitrogen gains and losses. While grams of protein are calculated in a nutritional plan, grams of nitrogen are used as an expression of the amount of protein received by the patient. There is 1 g of nitrogen (N) for each 6.25 g of protein. To calculate the grams of nitrogen in a certain weight of protein, divide the protein grams by 6.25.

$$\text{Nitrogen intake} = \frac{\text{grams of protein intake}}{6.25}$$

1 g N = 6.25 g protein

---

108. A patient is receiving PN containing 540 mL of 12.5% amino acids per day. How many grams of nitrogen will the patient be receiving? Round to the nearest tenth.

$$\frac{12.5 \text{ g}}{100 \text{ mL}} = \frac{\text{X g}}{540 \text{ mL}} \quad \text{X = 67.5 g of protein}$$

$$\frac{67.5 \text{ g of protein}}{6.25} = 10.8 \text{ g of nitrogen}$$

540 ml · $\frac{12.5 g}{100 ml}$ = 67.5 g

1 g N = 6.25 g protein
10.8 g ? = 67.5 g

Calculating the Non-Protein Calories to Nitrogen (NPC:N) Ratio

The non-protein calorie to nitrogen ratio (NPC:N) is calculated as:

- First, calculate the grams of nitrogen supplied per day (1 g N = 6.25 g of protein).

- Then, divide the total non-protein calories (dextrose + lipids) by the grams of nitrogen.

Desirable NPC:N ratios are:

- 80:1 the most severely stressed patients

- 100:1 severely stressed patients

- 150:1 unstressed patient

---

109. A patient is receiving PN containing 480 mL of dextrose 50% and 50 grams of amino acids plus electrolytes. Calculate the non-protein calories to nitrogen ratio for this patient.

First, calculate the nitrogen intake.

$$\text{Nitrogen} = \frac{50 \text{ g of protein}}{6.25} = 8 \text{ g}$$

480 ml · $\frac{50 g}{100 ml}$ = 240 g

$\frac{3.4 \text{ kcal}}{g} = \frac{x \text{ kcal}}{240 g}$ ⟹ x = 816 kcal

Next, calculate the non-protein calories.

$$\frac{816}{8} = \frac{102}{1}$$

←

1 g N = 6.25 g protein
8 g ? = 50 g

$$\frac{50 \text{ g dextrose}}{100 \text{ mL}} = \frac{X \text{ g}}{480 \text{ mL}} \qquad X = 240 \text{ g dextrose}$$

$$240 \text{ g dextrose} \quad x \quad \frac{3.4 \text{ kcal dextrose}}{1 \text{ g}} = 816 \text{ kcal of dextrose}$$

Then, set up the NPC:N ratio.

NPC:N ratio is 816:8, or 102:1

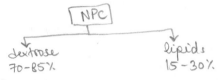

Calculating Dextrose

Dextrose is the source of carbohydrates in PN. The usual distribution of non-protein calories is 70-85% as carbohydrate (dextrose) and 15-30% as fat (lipids). Dextrose comes in concentrations of 5%, 10%, 20%, 30%, 50%, 70% and others. The higher concentrations are used for PN. When calculating the dextrose, do not exceed 4 mg/kg/min (some use 7 g/kg/day). These are conservative estimates of the maximum amount of dextrose that the liver can handle.

---

110. Using 50% dextrose in water, how many mL are required to fulfill a PN order for 405 g of dextrose?

$$\frac{50 \text{ g}}{100 \text{ mL}} = \frac{405 \text{ g}}{X \text{ mL}} = 810 \text{ mL}$$

$$\frac{405 g}{x \, ml} = \frac{50 \, g}{100 ml} \Rightarrow x = 810 \, ml$$

---

111. DF, a 44 year old male, is receiving 1,235 mL of D30W, 1,010 mL of *FreAmine* 8.5%, 200 mL of *Intralipid* 20% and 50 mL of electrolytes/minerals in his PN. How many calories from dextrose is DF receiving from the PN? Round to the nearest whole number.

$$\frac{30 \text{ g}}{100 \text{ mL}} \quad x \quad \frac{1,235 \text{ mL}}{\text{day}} \quad x \quad \frac{3.4 \text{ kcal}}{\text{g}} = 1,260 \text{ kcal/day}$$

$$\frac{30g}{100ml} \cdot 1235 ml = 370.5 g$$

$$\frac{3.4 \, kcal}{g} \cdot 370.5 g = 1260 \, kcal$$

---

112. A pharmacist has mixed 200 mL of D20% with 100 mL of D5%. What is the final concentration in the bag?

The 200 mL bag has 40 g of dextrose (20 g/100 mL x 2).

$$\frac{20g}{100ml} \cdot 200 ml = 40g$$

$$\frac{5g}{100ml} \cdot 100 ml = 5g$$

The 100 mL bag has 5 g of dextrose. There are 45 g dextrose total in the bag.

$$\frac{45 \text{ g}}{300 \text{ mL}} = \frac{X \text{ g}}{100 \text{ mL}} \qquad X = 15 \text{ g; the percentage is 15%}$$

$$\frac{45g}{300 ml} \cdot 100 \% = 15\%$$

---

113. If a 50% dextrose injection provides 170 kcal in each 100 mL, how many milliliters of a 70% dextrose injection would provide the same caloric value? Round to the nearest tenth. Or, to solve more simply: since the calories are from 50 g of dextrose, and the pharmacist is using D70, solve by:

$$\frac{70 \text{ g}}{100 \text{ mL}} = \frac{50 \text{ g}}{X \text{ mL}}$$

$$\frac{70 g}{100 ml} \cdot x \, ml \cdot \frac{3.4 \, kcal}{g} = 170 \, kcal$$

$$2.38 \, kcal \cdot x \, ml = 170 \, kcal$$

$$x = 71.4 \, ml$$

$$\frac{100 \text{ mL}}{70 \text{ g}} \times \frac{1 \text{ g}}{3.4 \text{ kcal}} \times 170 \text{ kcal} = 71.4 \text{ mL}$$

114. AH is receiving 640 mL of D50W in her PN. How many calories does this provide?

$$\frac{50 \text{ g}}{100 \text{ mL}} \times \frac{640 \text{ mL}}{\text{day}} \times \frac{3.4 \text{ kcal}}{\text{g}} = 1,088 \text{ kcal}$$

[handwritten:] $\frac{50g}{100ml} \cdot 640ml = 320 g$

$\frac{3.4 \, kcal}{g} \cdot 320g = 1088 \, kcal$

115. A PN order is written for 500 mL of 50% dextrose. The pharmacy only has D70W in stock. How many mL of D70W would you add to the PN bag? Round to the nearest whole number.

First, calculate the grams of dextrose needed for the PN as written.

$$\frac{50 \text{ g}}{100 \text{ mL}} = \frac{X \text{ g}}{500 \text{ mL}} \quad X = 250 \text{ g}$$

[handwritten:] $\frac{50g}{100ml} \cdot 500ml = 250 g$

Next, supply the 250 grams of dextrose with the 70% dextrose solution.

$$\frac{70 \text{ g}}{100 \text{ mL}} = \frac{250 \text{ g}}{X \text{ mL}} \quad X = 357 \text{ mL of D70W}$$

[handwritten:] $\frac{70g}{100ml} = \frac{250g}{X \, ml} \Rightarrow x = 357 \, ml$

Calculating Lipids

Lipids are the source of fat in PN. The standard distribution of non-protein calories is 70-85% as carbohydrate (dextrose) and 15-30% as fat (lipids). Lipids are available as 10%, 20% or 30% emulsions. Do not exceed 2.5 g/kg/day of lipids. Lipids do not need to be given daily, especially if the triglycerides are high. The recommended hang time limit for IV fat emulsions (IVFE) is 12 hours if infused separately by itself due to the risk of infection. However, an admixture containing IVFE, such as a TNA, may be administered over 24 hours. Patients receiving lipids should have their triglycerides monitored. If lipids are given once weekly, then divide the total calories by 7 to determine the daily amount of fat the patient receives. Lipid emulsions cannot be filtered through 0.22 micron filters; 1.2 micron filters are used in most formulations. PN requires a filter itself due to the risk of a precipitate.

[handwritten margin note:] TNA = total nutrient admixture

116. A patient is receiving 500 mL of 10% lipids. How many calories is the patient receiving from the lipids? Round to the nearest whole number.

[handwritten:] $500ml \cdot \frac{1.1 \, kcal}{ml} = 550 \, kcal$

$$\frac{1.1 \text{ kcal}}{\text{mL}} = \frac{X \text{ kcal}}{500 \text{ mL}} \quad X = 550 \text{ kcal}$$

117. The total energy expenditure (TEE) for a patient is 2,435 kcal/day. The patient is receiving 1,446 kcal from dextrose and 810 kcal from protein. How many kcal should be provided by the lipids?

TEE refers to the non-protein calories. Therefore, 2,435 kcal (total)–1,446 kcal (dextrose) = 989 kcal remaining. 989 kcal should be provided by the lipids.

[handwritten margin note:] TEE = NPC (non protein)

[handwritten:]
```
  2435 kcal   TEE (= dex + lipid)
- 1446 kcal   dex
  989 kcal    lip
```

118. Using a 20% lipid emulsion, how many mL are required to meet 989 calories? Round to the nearest whole number.

$$\frac{2 \text{ kcal}}{\text{mL}} = \frac{989 \text{ kcal}}{X \text{ mL}} \qquad X = 495 \text{ mL}$$

$$\frac{989 \text{ kcal}}{x \text{ ml}} = \frac{2 \text{ kcal}}{1 \text{ ml}} \Rightarrow x = 495 \text{ ml}$$

---

119. A patient is receiving 660 mL of 10% *Intralipid* on Saturdays along with his normal daily PN therapy of 1,420 mL of D20W, 450 mL *Aminosyn* 15%, and 30 mL of electrolytes. What is the daily amount of calories provided by the lipids? Round to the nearest whole number.

$$\frac{1.1 \text{ kcal}}{\text{mL}} = \frac{X \text{ kcal}}{660 \text{ mL}} \qquad X = 726 \text{ kcal/week. Need to divide by 7 to get daily amount} = 104 \text{ kcal/day}$$

$$\frac{1.1 \text{ kcal}}{1 \text{ ml}} = \frac{x \text{ kcal}}{660 \text{ ml}}$$
$$\Rightarrow x = 726 \text{ kcal/wk}$$
$$\Rightarrow 104 \text{ kcal/day}$$

---

120. A patient is receiving 180 mL of 30% lipids. How many calories is the patient receiving from the lipids?

$$\frac{3 \text{ kcal}}{\text{mL}} = \frac{X \text{ kcal}}{180 \text{ mL}} \qquad X = 540 \text{ kcal}$$

$$180 \text{ ml} \cdot \frac{3 \text{ kcal}}{1 \text{ ml}} = 540 \text{ kcal}$$

---

121. A PN order calls for 475 calories to be provided by lipids. The pharmacy has 10% lipid emulsion in stock. How many mL should be administered to the patient? Round to the nearest whole number.

$$\frac{1.1 \text{ kcal}}{\text{mL}} = \frac{475 \text{ kcal}}{X \text{ mL}} \qquad X = 432 \text{ mL}$$

$$\frac{475 \text{ kcal}}{x \text{ ml}} = \frac{1.1 \text{ kcal}}{1 \text{ ml}} \Rightarrow x = 432 \text{ ml}$$

---

122. TE is a 35 year old female who is receiving 325 grams of dextrose, 85 grams of amino acids, and 300 mL of 10% lipids via her PN therapy. What percentage of calories is provided by the protein content? Round to the nearest whole number.

First, calculate the calories from all sources; dextrose, amino acids, and lipids.

DEXTROSE

$$\frac{3.4 \text{ kcal}}{\text{g}} \times 325 \text{ g} = 1{,}105 \text{ kcal of dextrose}$$

$$325 \text{ g} \cdot \frac{3.4 \text{ kcal}}{1 \text{ g}} = 1105 \text{ kcal}$$

PROTEIN

$$\frac{4 \text{ kcal}}{\text{g}} \times 85 \text{ g} = 340 \text{ kcal of protein}$$

$$85 \text{ g} \cdot \frac{4 \text{ kcal}}{1 \text{ g}} = 340 \text{ kcal} \ *$$

LIPIDS

$$\frac{1.1 \text{ kcal}}{\text{mL}} \times 300 \text{ mL} = 330 \text{ kcal of fat}$$

$$300 \text{ ml} \cdot \frac{1.1 \text{ kcal}}{1 \text{ ml}} = 330 \text{ kcal}$$

Then, add up the total calories from all the sources. 1,105 + 340 + 330 = 1,775 kcal

Finally, calculate the percent of protein.

$$\frac{340 \text{ kcal}}{1{,}775 \text{ kcal}} \times 100 = 19\%$$

$$\Rightarrow \frac{340 \text{ kcal}}{1775 \text{ kcal}} \cdot 100\% = 19\%$$

123. WC, a 57 year old male, is receiving 1,145 mL of D30W, 850 mL of *FreAmine* 8.5%, and 350 mL of *Intralipid* 10% in his PN therapy. What percentage of the non-protein calories are represented by dextrose? Round to the nearest <u>whole</u> number.

First, calculate the non-protein calories (dextrose and lipids).

$$\frac{dex}{dex + lip} \cdot 100\%$$

DEXTROSE

$$\frac{3.4 \text{ kcal}}{\text{g}} \times \frac{30 \text{ g}}{100 \text{ mL}} \times 1,145 \text{ mL} = 1,168 \text{ kcal}$$

$$1145 \text{ ml} \cdot \frac{30g}{100 \text{ ml}} = 343.5 \text{ g}$$
$$\downarrow$$
$$\cdot \frac{3.4 \text{ kcal}}{g} = 1167.9 \text{ kcal}$$

LIPIDS

$$\frac{1.1 \text{ kcal}}{\text{mL}} \times 350 \text{ mL} = 385 \text{ kcal}$$

$$350 \text{ ml} \cdot \frac{1.1 \text{ kcal}}{\text{ml}} = 385 \text{ kcal}$$

Then, add up the calories from these non-protein sources. 1,168 + 385 = 1,553 kcal

Finally, calculate the percent from dextrose.

$$\frac{1,168 \text{ kcal}}{1,553 \text{ kcal}} \times 100 = 75\%$$

$$\frac{1167.9 \text{ kcal}}{(385 + 1167.9) \text{ kcal}} \cdot 100\% = 75\%$$

✳ **124.** A 46 year old female with radiation enteritis is receiving 1,800 kcal from her parental nutrition. The solution contains amino acids, dextrose and electrolytes. There are 84.5 grams of protein in the PN and it is running at 85 mL/hour over 24 hours. What is the final concentration of dextrose in the PN solution? Round to the nearest <u>whole</u> number.

First, calculate the amount of dextrose the patient is receiving by subtracting out the protein component.

$$84.5 \text{ g} \times \frac{4 \text{ kcal}}{\text{g}} = 338 \text{ kcal}$$

$$\frac{85 \text{ ml}}{\text{hr}} \cdot 24 \text{ hrs} = 2040 \text{ ml}$$

$$\frac{84.5g}{x \text{ kcal}} = \frac{1g}{4 \text{ kcal}} \Rightarrow x = 338 \text{ kcal}$$

1,800 kcal - 338 kcal of protein = 1,462 kcal from dextrose

$$\begin{array}{r} 1800 \text{ kcal} \\ - \quad 338 \text{ kcal} \\ \hline 1462 \text{ kcal} \text{ dex} \end{array}$$

Next, calculate the grams of dextrose in this PN.

$$1,462 \text{ kcal} \times \frac{1 \text{ g}}{3.4 \text{ kcal}} = 430 \text{ grams of dextrose}$$

$$\frac{1462 \text{ kcal}}{x \text{ g}} = \frac{3.4 \text{ kcal}}{1 \text{ g}}$$
$$\Rightarrow x = 430 \text{ g}$$

Then, calculate the final concentration. This requires calculating the total volume the patient is receiving.

$$\frac{85 \text{ mL}}{\text{hr}} \times 24 \text{ hours} = 2,040 \text{ mL or } 2.04 \text{ L}$$

$$\frac{430 \text{ g}}{2040 \text{ ml}} \cdot 100\% = 21\%$$

$$\frac{430 \text{ g dextrose}}{2,040 \text{ mL}} = \frac{X \text{ g}}{100 \text{ mL}} \quad X = 21\%$$

Determining the Amount of Electrolytes

NaCl => 23.4% (PN) => 4 mEq/L
Na acetate => ↑pH in acidosis => 2 mEq/L

Sodium Considerations

Sodium is the principal <u>extra</u>cellular cation. Sodium may need to be reduced in renal dysfunction or cardiovascular disease, including hypertension. Sodium chloride comes in many concentrations, such as 0.9% (NS), 0.45% (1/2 NS) and others. Sodium chloride 23.4% is used for PN preparation and contains 4 mEq/mL.

Sodium can be added to PN as either sodium chloride or sodium acetate. If a patient is acidotic, sodium acetate should be added. Sodium acetate is converted to sodium bicarbonate and may help correct the acidosis. A patient may require a certain quantity from each formulation. Or, they may get sodium chloride alone. Hypertonic saline (> 0.9%) is dangerous if used incorrectly and is discussed in the Medication Safety chapter.

---

125. The pharmacist is going to add 80 mEq of sodium to the PN; half will be given as sodium acetate (2 mEq/mL) and half as sodium chloride (4 mEq/mL). How many mL of sodium chloride will be needed?

40 mEq will be provided by the NaCl.

$$\frac{4\ mEq}{mL} = \frac{40\ mEq}{X\ mL} \qquad X = 10\ mL$$

$\frac{40\ mEq}{x\ ml} = \frac{4\ mEq}{1\ ml} \Rightarrow x = 10\ ml$

---

126. The pharmacist is making PN that needs to contain 80 mEq of sodium and 45 mEq of acetate. The available pharmacy stock solutions contain 4 mEq/mL sodium as sodium chloride and 2 mEq/mL sodium as sodium acetate. The final volume of the PN will be 2.5 liters to be given at 100 mL/hr. What quantity, in milliliters, of each stock solution should be added to the PN to meet the requirements? Round to the nearest <u>hundredth</u>.

First, calculate the acetate component as this contributes sodium as well.

$$\frac{2\ mEq}{mL} = \frac{45\ mEq}{X\ mL} \qquad X = 22.5\ mL\ of\ sodium\ acetate$$

This amount (22.5 mL of sodium acetate) also supplies 45 mEq of sodium. So, now we only need 35 mEq of sodium (80 mEq–45 mEq = 35 mEq).

$$\frac{2\ mEq}{mL} \times 22.5\ mL\ sodium\ acetate = 45\ mEq\ of\ sodium$$

80 mEq - 45 mEq = 35 mEq of sodium still needed

Supply the remaining needed sodium (35 mEq) with sodium chloride.

$$\frac{4\ mEq}{mL} = \frac{35\ mEq}{X\ mL} \qquad X = 8.75\ mL\ of\ sodium\ chloride$$

$\frac{45\ mEq}{x\ ml} = \frac{2\ mEq}{1\ ml} \Rightarrow x = 22.5\ ml\ acetate\ (45\ mEq\ Na)$

$\begin{array}{r} 80\ mEq\ Na \\ -\ 45\ mEq\ Na \\ \hline 35\ mEq \end{array} \Rightarrow \frac{4\ mEq}{1\ ml} = \frac{35\ mEq}{x\ ml} \Rightarrow x = 8.75\ ml\ Na$

127. A 2 liter PN solution is to contain 60 mEq of sodium and 30 mEq of acetate. The pharmacy has in stock sodium chloride (4 mEq/mL) and sodium acetate (2 mEq/mL). What quantity, in milliliters, of each solution should be added to the PN? Round to the nearest tenth.

First, calculate the amount of sodium acetate needed.

$$\frac{2 \text{ mEq}}{\text{mL}} = \frac{30 \text{ mEq}}{\text{X mL}}$$ X = 15 mL of sodium acetate

acet $\frac{30 \text{ mEq}}{x \text{ ml}} = \frac{2 \text{ mEq}}{1 \text{ ml}}$ =) x = 15 ml

Na $\frac{30 \text{ mEq}}{x \text{ ml}} = \frac{4 \text{ mEq}}{1 \text{ ml}}$ =) x = 7.5 ml

This amount (15 mL of sodium acetate) also supplies 30 mEq of sodium. The additional amount required is 30 mEq of sodium (60 mEq–30 mEq).

Calculate the amount of sodium chloride needed.

$$\frac{4 \text{ mEq}}{\text{mL}} = \frac{30 \text{ mEq}}{\text{X mL}}$$ X= 7.5 mL of NaCl

Potassium, Calcium and Phosphate Considerations

Potassium

Potassium is the principal intracellular cation. Potassium may need to be reduced in renal or cardiovascular disease. Potassium can be provided by potassium chloride (KCl) or potassium phosphate (K Phos) or potassium acetate. The normal range for serum potassium is 3.5-5.0 mEq/L.

Calcium

Calcium is important for many functions including cardiac conduction, muscle contraction, and bone homeostasis. The normal serum calcium level is 8.5-10.5 mg/dL. Almost half of serum calcium is bound to albumin. Low albumin will lead to an incorrect calcium concentration. If albumin is low (< 3.5 g/dL), calcium levels will need to be corrected with this equation prior to the addition of calcium into the PN:

$$Ca_{corrected} = (calcium_{reported(serum)} + [(4.0 - albumin) \times (0.8)]$$

128. Calculate the corrected calcium value for a patient with the following lab values:

LAB	VALUE
Calcium	7.6 mg/dL (normal range 8.5 – 10.5 mg/dL)
Albumin	1.5 g/dL (normal range 3.5 – 5 g/dL)

- $Ca_{corrected} = (calcium_{reported(serum)} + [(4.0 - albumin) \times (0.8)]$

- $Ca_{corrected} = (7.6) + [(4.0 - 1.5) \times (0.8)] = 9.6$ mg/dL

Ca correct = Ca actual + 0.8 (4 - alb)

Ca correct = 7.6 + 0.8 (4 - 1.5)

= 9.6

51

Calcium and Phosphate Solubility

Phosphorus (or phosphate, PO_4) is present in DNA, cell membranes, ATP, acts as an acid-base buffer, and is vital in bone metabolism. Phosphate and calcium need to be added carefully, or they can bind together and precipitate which can cause a pulmonary embolus. This can be fatal. The following considerations can help reduce the risk of a calcium-phosphate precipitate:

- Choose calcium gluconate over calcium chloride ($CaCl_2$) due to being less reactive and lower risk of precipitation with phosphates. Calcium gluconate has a lower dissociation constant compared to calcium chloride, leaving less free calcium available in solution to bind phosphates.

- Add phosphate first (after the dextrose and amino acids), followed by other PN components, agitate the solution, then calcium should be added near the end to take advantage of the maximum volume of the PN formulation.

- The calcium and phosphate added together (units must be the same to do this) should not exceed 45 mEq/L.

- Maintain a proper pH (lower pH; less risk of precipitation) to eliminate binding and refrigerate the bag once prepared (PNs are kept in the refrigerator until they are needed). When temperature increases, more calcium and phosphate dissociate in solution and precipitation risk increases.

An additional safety consideration involves ordering the correct dose of phosphate. Phosphate can be ordered as potassium or sodium salts. The two forms do not provide equivalent amounts of phosphate. The order should be written in mmol (of phosphate), followed by the type of salt form (potassium or sodium).

---

129. The pharmacist has calculated that a patient requires 30 mmol of phosphate and 80 mEq of potassium. The pharmacy has stock solutions of potassium phosphate (3 mmol of phosphate with 4.4 mEq of potassium/mL) and potassium chloride (2 mEq K⁺/mL). How much potassium phosphate and how much potassium chloride will be required to meet the patient's needs?

First, calculate the phosphate required (since potassium comes along with the phosphate in the potassium-phosphate solution).

$$\frac{3 \text{ mmol Phosphate}}{mL} = \frac{30 \text{ mmol Phosphate}}{X \text{ mL}} \qquad X = 10 \text{ mL K-Phos}$$

Each mL of the potassium phosphate (K-Phos) supplies 4.4 mEq of potassium. Calculate the amount of potassium the patient received from the 10 mL of K-Phos.

- 10 mL x 4.4 mEq/mL = 44 mEq potassium

- The remaining potassium will be provided by KCl.

- 80 mEq K required – 44 mEq potassium (from K-Phos) = 36 mEq to be obtained from the KCl.

$$\frac{2 \text{ mEq K}^+}{\text{mL}} = \frac{36 \text{ mEq K}^+}{\text{X mL}} \qquad \text{X = 18 mL KCl}$$

The patient requires 10 mL of potassium phosphate and 18 mL of potassium chloride.

---

130. A patient is to receive 8 mEq of calcium. The pharmacy has calcium gluconate 10% in stock which provides 0.465 mEq/mL. How many mL of calcium gluconate should be added to the PN? Round to the nearest <u>whole</u> number.

$$\frac{1 \text{ mL}}{0.465 \text{ mEq Ca}^{2+}} \times 8 \text{ mEq Ca}^{2+} = 17.2, \text{ or 17 mL calcium gluconate}$$

(handwritten) $\frac{0.465 \text{ mEq}}{\text{ml}} = \frac{8 \text{ mEq}}{x \text{ ml}} \Rightarrow x = 17 \text{ ml}$

---

131. A patient is receiving 30 mmol of phosphate and 8 mEq of calcium. The volume of the PN is 2,000 mL. There are 2 mEq PO_4/mmol. Confirm that the calcium and phosphorus added together does not exceed 45 mEq/L.

First, calculate mEq from the phosphate.

$$\frac{2 \text{ mEq PO}_4}{\text{mmol}} \times 30 \text{ mmol PO}_4 = 60 \text{ mEq phosphate}$$

(handwritten) phos $\frac{2 \text{ mEq}}{1 \text{ mmol}} = \frac{x \text{ mEq}}{30 \text{ mmol}} \Rightarrow x = 60 \text{ mEq}$

$\Rightarrow$ phos + Ca = 8 mEq + 60 mEq = 68 mEq

Then, add the phosphate to the calcium. 60 mEq phosphate + 8 mEq calcium = 68 mEq.

The volume of the PN is 2,000 mL, or 2 L. Find the mEq per liter. 68 mEq/2 L = 34 mEq/L, which is less than 45 mEq/L.

(handwritten) $\frac{68 \text{ mEq}}{2 \text{ l}} = 34 \text{ mEq/L} \checkmark$

QUESTIONS 130-139 RELATE TO PN ORDER BELOW.

132. A pharmacy receives the following PN order. Calculate the amount, in mL, of dextrose 70% that should be added to the PN. Round to the nearest <u>whole</u> number.

ITEM	QUANTITY
Dextrose 70%	250 g
Amino acids	50 g
Sodium chloride	44 mEq
Sodium acetate	20 mEq
Potassium	40 mEq
Magnesium sulfate	12 mEq
Phosphate	18 mmol
Calcium	4.65 mEq
MVI-12	5 mL
Trace elements-5	1 mL
Vitamin K-1	0.5 mg
Famotidine	10 mg
Regular insulin	20 units
Sterile water qs ad	960 mL

(handwritten at left) 3 mmol phos / ml
4.4 mEq K / ml

(handwritten at right)

dex $\frac{70 \text{ g}}{100 \text{ ml}} = \frac{250 \text{ g}}{x \text{ ml}} \Rightarrow x = 357 \text{ ml}$

a.a. $\frac{10 \text{ g}}{100 \text{ ml}} = \frac{50 \text{ g}}{x \text{ ml}} \Rightarrow x = 500 \text{ ml}$

NaCl $\frac{4 \text{ mEq}}{\text{ml}} = \frac{44 \text{ mEq}}{x \text{ ml}} \Rightarrow x = 11 \text{ ml}$

Na acet $\frac{2 \text{ mEq}}{\text{ml}} = \frac{20 \text{ mEq}}{x \text{ ml}} \Rightarrow x = 10 \text{ ml}$

phos $\frac{3 \text{ mmol}}{\text{ml}} = \frac{18 \text{ mmol}}{x \text{ ml}} \Rightarrow x = 6 \text{ ml}$

Mg^{++} $\frac{12 \text{ mEq}}{x \text{ ml}} = \frac{4 \text{ mEq}}{\text{ml}} \Rightarrow x = 3 \text{ ml}$

$$\frac{70\ g}{100\ mL} = \frac{250\ g}{X\ mL} \qquad X = 357\ mL\ of\ dextrose\ 70\%$$

---

133. Using amino acids 10%, calculate the amount of amino acids that should be added to the PN.

$$\frac{10\ g}{100\ mL} = \frac{50\ g}{X\ mL} \qquad X = 500\ mL$$

---

134. Calculate the amount of sodium chloride 23.4% (4 mEq/mL) that should be added to the PN.

$$\frac{4\ mEq}{mL} = \frac{44\ mEq}{X\ mL} \qquad X = 11\ mL$$

**This concentration of NaCl is hypertonic and is a high-alert drug due to heightened risk of patient harm when dosed incorrectly.

---

135. Calculate the amount of sodium acetate 16.4% (2 mEq/mL) that should be added to the PN.

$$\frac{2\ mEq}{mL} = \frac{20\ mEq}{X\ mL} \qquad X = 10\ mL$$

---

136. Using the potassium phosphate (3 mmol of phosphate and 4.4 mEq of potassium/mL) vials in stock, calculate the amount of potassium phosphate that should be added to the PN to meet the needs of the phosphate requirements.

$$\frac{3\ mmol\ Phosphate}{mL} = \frac{18\ mmol\ Phosphate}{X\ mL} \qquad X = 6\ mL\ K\text{-}Phos$$

---

137. The PN contains 6 mL of potassium phosphate (3 mmol of phosphate and 4.4 mEq of potassium/mL). The daily potassium requirement is 40 mEq. How much potassium chloride (2 mEq/mL), in milliliters, should be added to the PN? Round to the nearest tenth.

First, calculate the amount of K^+ already in the PN.

$$\frac{4.4\ mEq\ K^+}{mL} \times 6\ mL = 26.4\ mEq\ K^+$$

Total K^+ needed is 40 mEq. 40 mEq–26.4 mEq = 13.6 mEq still needed.

$$\frac{2\ mEq\ K^+}{mL} = \frac{13.6\ mEq\ K^+}{X\ mL} \qquad X = 6.8\ mL\ KCL$$

Handwritten annotations:

$K^+ \quad 6\ ml \cdot \frac{4.4\ mEq}{ml} = 26.4\ mEq$

$\begin{array}{r} 40\ mEq \\ - 26.4\ mEq \\ \hline 13.6\ mEq \end{array}$

$\frac{2\ mEq}{ml} = \frac{13.6\ mEq}{x\ ml}$

$\Rightarrow x = 6.8\ ml$

---

138. The PN order calls for 4.65 mEq of calcium. The pharmacy has calcium gluconate 10% (0.465 mEq/mL) in stock. How many mL of calcium gluconate 10% should be added to the PN?

$$\frac{0.465\ mEq\ Ca^{2+}}{mL} = \frac{4.65\ mEq\ Ca^{2+}}{X\ mL} \qquad X = 10\ mL\ calcium\ gluconate\ 10\%$$

139. The PN calls for 18 mmol of phosphate and 4.65 mEq of calcium (provided by 10 mL of calcium gluconate 10%, as calculated in the previous problem) in a volume of 960 mL. There are 2 mEq PO_4/mmol. Confirm that the calcium and phosphorus added together do not exceed 45 mEq/L.

First, calculate mEq from the phosphate.

phos $\dfrac{2\,mEq}{1\,mmol} = \dfrac{x\,mEq}{18\,mmol} \Rightarrow x = 36\,mEq$

$$\frac{2\ mEq\ PO_4}{mmol}\ \times\ 18\ mmol\ PO_4\ =\ 36\ mEq\ phosphate$$

$$\begin{array}{r} 36\ mEq \\ +\ 4.65\ mEq \\ \hline 40.65\ mEq \end{array}$$

$$\frac{40.65\ mEq}{\frac{960}{1000}\ l} = 42.34\ \frac{mEq}{l}\ \checkmark$$

Then, add the phosphate to the calcium. 36 mEq phosphate + 4.65 mEq calcium = 40.65 mEq. The volume of the PN is 960 mL, or 0.96 L. 40.65 mEq/0.96 L = 42.3 mEq/L, which is less than 45 mEq/L.

---

140. Calculate the amount of magnesium sulfate (4 mEq/mL) that should be added to the PN.

$$\frac{4\ mEq}{mL}\ =\ \frac{12\ mEq}{X\ mL}\qquad X = 3\ mL\ magnesium\ sulfate$$

---

141. What percentage of the total calories from the above PN are represented by the protein component? Round to the nearest whole number.

First, calculate the total calories.

$250g \cdot \dfrac{3.4\ kcal}{g} = 850\ kcal$

$50g \cdot \dfrac{4\ kcal}{g} = 200\ kcal$

$\dfrac{200\ kcal}{1050\ kcal} \cdot 100\% = 19\%$

DEXTROSE

$$\frac{3.4\ kcal\ dextrose}{g}\ \times\ 250\ g\ dextrose\ =\ 850\ kcal\ of\ dextrose$$

PROTEIN

$$\frac{4\ kcal\ protein}{g}\ \times\ 50\ g\ protein\ =\ 200\ kcal\ of\ protein$$

Total calories = 850 + 200 = 1,050 kcal. Now, calculate the amount of calories from protein.

$$\frac{200\ kcal}{1,050\ kcal}\ \times\ 100\ =\ 19\%$$

Add-in Multivitamins, Trace Elements, and Insulin

B_6 — 25-50 mg po qd to prevent isoniazid neuropathy

Multivitamins: There are 4 fat-soluble vitamins (A, D, E and K) and 9 water-soluble vitamins (thiamine, riboflavin, niacin, pantothenic acid, pyridoxine, ascorbic acid, folic acid, cyanocobalamin, biotin) in the standard MVI-13 mixture. The MVI-12 mixture does not contain vitamin K since certain patients may need less or more of this vitamin. If patients on PN therapy are using warfarin, the INR will need to be monitored.

MVI-13

fat-soluble
A
D
E
K

H2O soluble
thiamine
riboflavin
niacin
pantothenic acid
folic acid
ascorbic acid

biotin
cyanocobalamin
pyridoxine (B6)

* MVI-12
↳ ∅ vit K (pts on warfarin)

Trace Elements

The standard mix includes zinc, copper, chromium and manganese (and may include selenium). Manganese and copper should be withheld in severe liver disease. Chromium, molybdenum and selenium should be withheld in severe renal disease. Iron is not routinely given in a PN.

Insulin

· give ≤ 50% expected to be required + ss
· min dose in PN: 10 units, ↑ by 10-unit incr. ⎫ if need to ↑, only
⎭ + ½ previous day's ss

PNs may contain insulin, usually (50%) or less than what the person is expected to require per day, supplemented by a sliding scale. A minimum dose to add is (10) units, and is usually increased by (10) unit increments. It is important to avoid adding too much insulin. (Half) the previous day's sliding scale or less can be used as a safe amount.

Enteral Nutrition

Enteral nutrition (EN) is the provision of nutrients via the gastrointestinal (GI) tract through a feeding tube. Nasogastric (NG) tubes are often used, primarily for short-term administration. For longer-term, or if the stomach cannot be used, tubes are placed further down the GI tract. EN is the preferred route for patients who cannot meet their nutrition needs through voluntary oral intake. Tube feedings can range from providing adjunctive support to providing complete nutrition support. Several advantages of EN over PN include lower cost, using the gut which prevents atrophy and other problems, and a lower risk of complications (less infections, less hyperglycemia, reduced risk of cholelithiasis and cholestasis). The most common risk associated with enteral feeding is aspiration which can lead to pneumonia. Enteral feedings can cause drug interactions. The general rule for preventing drug/enteral feeding interactions is to hold the feedings one hour before or two hours after the drug is administered. Some drugs may require further separation.

Tube feeds do not, by themselves, provide enough water. Water is given in addition to the tube feeds. If fluid intake is inadequate, it will be uncomfortable for the patient and put them at risk for complications, including hypernatremia.

Drug-Nutrient interactions with enteral feedings (most common problems):

- Warfarin: many enteral products bind warfarin, resulting in low INRs and the need for dose adjustments. Hold tube feeds one hour before and one hour after warfarin administration.

- Tetracycline: will chelate with metals, including calcium, magnesium, and iron, which reduces drug availability, and is separated from tube feeds.

- Ciprofloxacin: the oral suspension is not used with tube feeds because the oil-based suspension adheres to the tube. The immediate-release tablets are used instead; crush and mix with water, flush line with water before and after administration.

- Phenytoin (*Dilantin suspension*): is reduced when the drug binds to the feeding solution, leading to less free drug availability and sub-therapeutic levels. Separate tube feeds by 2 hours.

Tube Names

- A tube in the nose to the stomach is called a nasogastric (NG), or nasoenteral, tube.

- A tube that goes through the skin into the stomach is called a gastrostomy, or percutaneous endoscopic gastrostomy (PEG, or G) tube.

- A tube into the small intestine is called a jejunostomy, or percutaneous endoscopic jejunostomy (PEJ, or J) tube.

142 - 144?

Patient Case (For Questions 140-142)

Wilma is a patient starting enteral nutrition therapy. Wilma has a past medical history significant for diabetes. She will be started on *Glucerna* Ready-to-Drink Vanilla shakes. See the nutrient label provided.

Nutrition Facts	
Serving Size: 8 fl oz (237 mL)	
Amount Per Serving	
Calories	356 kcal
Total Fat 17.8 g	
Protein 19.6 g	
Total Carbohydrate 31.5 g	
Dietary Fiber 3.8 g	
L-Carnitine	51 mg
Taurine	40 mg
m-Inositol	205 mg
Vitamin A	
Vitamin C	
Iron	© RxPrep

142. According to the case above, what percent of calories will Wilma receive from the protein component? Round to the nearest whole number.

First, calculate the amount of calories coming from the protein component.

$$19.6 \text{ g protein} \times \frac{4 \text{ kcal}}{g} = 78.4 \text{ kcal}$$

19.6 g · 4 kcal/g = 78.4 kcal

Next, find the percentage of protein calories.

$$\frac{78.4 \text{ kcal}}{356 \text{ kcal}} \times 100 = 22\%$$

78.4 kcal / 356 kcal · 100% = 22%

143. How many calories will Wilma receive from the fat component of 1 (8 fl oz.) shake? Round to the nearest whole number.

$$17.8 \text{ g} \times \frac{9 \text{ kcal}}{g} = 160.2, \text{ or } 160 \text{ kcal}$$

17.8 g / x kcal = 1 g / 9 kcal => x = 160. kcal

144. What percent of calories are derived from the fat component? Round to the nearest whole number.

$$\frac{160.2 \text{ kcal}}{356 \text{ kcal}} \times 100 = 45\%$$

160 kcal / 356 kcal · 100% = 45%

Patient Case (For Questions 143-145)

Jonathan is a patient receiving *Osmolite* (a high-protein, low-residue formula) enteral nutrition through his PEG tube. See the nutrient label provided.

Nutrition Facts	
Serving Size: 8 fl oz (237 mL)	
Amount Per Serving	
Calories 285 kcal	
Total Fat 9.2 g	
Protein 13.2 g	
Total Carbohydrate 37.4 g	
L-Carnitine	36 mg
Taurine	36 mg
Vitamin A	
Vitamin C	
Iron	© RxPrep

145. According to the case above, how many calories will Jonathan receive from the carbohydrate component in 4 fl oz? Round to the nearest whole number.

First, calculate the total calories from carbohydrates per 1 can (8 fl oz).

37.4 g carbohydrate $\times$ $\dfrac{4 \text{ kcal}}{g}$ = 149.6 kcal from 8 fl oz.

$\dfrac{37.4 \text{ g}}{2}$ = 18.7 g

Then, take half of the amount of calories (4 fl oz).

$\dfrac{149.6}{2}$ = 74.8, or 75 kcal from 4 fl oz.

$\dfrac{4 \text{ kcal}}{g} \cdot 18.7 \text{ g}$ = 75 kcal

---

146. What percent of calories will Jonathan receive from the carbohydrate component? Round to the nearest whole number.

First, calculate the amount of calories coming from the carbohydrate component.

37.$\overset{4}{5}$ g carbohydrate $\times$ $\dfrac{4 \text{ kcal}}{g}$ = 150 kcal

$37.4 \text{ g} \cdot \dfrac{4 \text{ kcal}}{g}$ = 149.6 kcal

Next, find the percentage of carbohydrate calories.

$\dfrac{150 \text{ kcal}}{285 \text{ kcal}}$ $\times$ 100 = 52.6, or 53%

$\dfrac{149.6 \text{ kcal}}{285 \text{ kcal}} \cdot 100\%$ = 52%

---

147. The nurse was administering 1 can (8 fl oz.) of *Osmolite* to Jonathan when she accidentally spilled 2 fl oz. onto the floor. The remaining amount in the can was accurately delivered to Jonathan. How many calories did he actually receive from this can? Do (not) round the answer.

1 can = 8 fl oz

$\dfrac{8 \text{ fl oz}}{285 \text{ kcal}}$ = $\dfrac{6 \text{ fl oz}}{X \text{ kcal}}$ X = 213.75 kcal

$\dfrac{285 \text{ kcal}}{8 \text{ oz}}$ = $\dfrac{x \text{ kcal}}{6 \text{ oz}}$ ⇒ x = 213.75 kcal

Osmolarity

The total number of particles in a given solution is directly proportional to its osmotic pressure. The particles are usually measured in milliosmoles. Osmolarity is the measure of total number of particles (or solutes) per liter (L) of solution, defined as osmoles/Liter (Osmol/L) or, more commonly as milliosmoles/Liter (mOsmol/L). Solutes can be either ionic (such as NaCl, which dissociates into 2 solutes in solution, Na^+ and Cl^-) or non-ionic, which do not dissociate (such as glucose and urea). The term for osmolarity when used to refer to the solute concentration of body fluids is tonicity, and solutions are thus isotonic (osmolarity is the same as blood, which is ~ 300 mOsmol/L), or is lower (hypotonic) or is higher (hypertonic).

If the osmolarity is higher in one cellular compartment, it will cause water to move from the lower to the higher concentration of solutes. If a PN solution is injected with a higher osmolarity than blood, fluid will flow into the vein, resulting in edema, inflammation, phlebitis and possible thrombosis.

Osmolarity ⇒ $\left[\dfrac{m \text{Osmol}}{L} \right]$

mOsmol ⇒ $\left[m \text{Osmo} \right]$

Milliosmole calculation problems differ from osmolarity calculation problems in that osmolarity will always need to be normalized to a volume of 1 liter. Some compounds for which it may be useful to know dissociations are listed to the right:

COMPOUND	# OF DISSOCIATION PARTICLES
Dextrose	1
Mannitol	1
Potassium chloride (KCl)	2
Sodium chloride (NaCl)	2
Sodium acetate ($NaC_2H_3O_2$)	2
Calcium chloride ($CaCl_2$)	3
Sodium citrate ($Na_3C_6H_5O_7$)	4

Osmolarity Calculations

Use this formula to find the mOsmol/L.

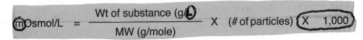

$$mOsmol/L = \frac{\text{Wt of substance (g/L)}}{\text{MW (g/mole)}} \times (\text{\# of particles}) \times 1,000$$

- Add up the number of particles into which the compound dissociates.
- Calculate the number of grams of the compound present in 1 L.
- Use the Molecular Weight (M.W.) to solve the problem.

✳✳ Milliosmole calculations do not normalize to 1 liter. ✳✳

---

148. What is the osmolarity, in mOsmol/L, of normal saline (0.9% NaCl)? M.W. = 58.5. Round to the nearest whole number.

NaCl dissociates into 2 particles; Na^+ and Cl^-.

$$\frac{0.9\,g}{100\,ml} = \frac{9\,g}{1000\,ml}$$

Calculate the number of grams of the compound (NaCl) present in 1 L.

$$\frac{0.9\,g}{100\,mL} = \frac{X\,g}{1,000\,mL} \qquad X = 9\,g$$

$$mOsmol = \frac{9\,g/L}{58.5\,g/mol} \cdot 2 \cdot 1000 = \frac{308\,mOsmol}{L}$$

Use the molecular weight to solve the problem.

$$mOsmol/L = \frac{9\,g/L}{58.5\,g/mole} \times 2 \times 1,000 = 308\,mOsmol/L$$

---

149. What is the osmolarity, in mOsmol/L, of D5W? M.W. = 198. Round to the nearest tenth.

Dextrose does not dissociate and is counted as 1 particle.

$$\frac{5\,g}{100\,ml} = \frac{50\,g}{1000\,ml}$$

$$\frac{5\,g}{100\,mL} = \frac{X\,g}{1,000\,mL} \qquad X = 50\,g$$

$$mOsmol = \frac{50\,g/L}{198\,g/mol} \cdot 1 \cdot 1000$$

Use the molecular weight to solve the problem.

$$= 252.5\,mOsmol/L$$

$$mOsmol/L = \frac{50\,g/L}{198\,g/mole} \times 1 \times 1,000 = 252.5\,mOsmol/L$$

---

150. A solution contains 373 mg Na^+ ions per liter. How many milliosmoles are represented in the solution? M.W. = 23. Round to the nearest tenth.

First, convert the units to match the formula.

$$mOsmol = \frac{0.373\,g/L}{23\,g/mol} \cdot 1 \cdot 1000 = 16.2\,mOsmol$$

$$\frac{373 \text{ mg Na}^+}{\text{L}} \quad \text{x} \quad \frac{1 \text{ g}}{1,000 \text{ mg}} = 0.373 \text{ g/L}$$

$$\text{mOsmol} = \frac{0.373 \text{ g/L}}{23 \text{ g/mole}} \quad \text{x} \quad 1 \quad \text{x} \quad 1,000 = 16.2 \text{ mOsmol}$$

Note that the problem is asking for milliosmoles and not osmolarity. Therefore, the answer is in milliosmoles and not mOsmol/L although the problem is in 1 liter so you would get the same numeric answer.

---

151. Calculate the osmolar concentration, in milliosmoles, represented by 1 liter of a 10% (w/v) solution of anhydrous dextrose (M.W. = 180) in water. Round to the nearest tenth.

$$\frac{10 \text{ g}}{100 \text{ mL}} = \frac{X \text{ g}}{1,000 \text{ mL}} \quad X = 100 \text{ g}$$

$$\text{mOsmol} = \frac{100 \text{ g/L}}{180 \text{ g/mol}} \cdot 1 \cdot 1000 = 555.6 \text{ mOsmol}$$

$$\text{mOsmol} = \frac{100 \text{ g/L}}{180 \text{ g/mole}} \quad \text{x} \quad 1 \quad \text{x} \quad 1,000 = 555.6 \text{ mOsmol}$$

Note that the problem is asking for milliosmoles and not osmolarity. Therefore, the answer is in milliosmoles and not mOsmol/L although the problem is in 1 liter so you would get the same numeric answer.

---

152. How many milliosmoles of $CaCl_2$ (M.W.= 147) are represented in 150 mL of a 10% (w/v) calcium chloride solution? Round to the nearest whole number.

$$150 \text{ ml} \cdot \frac{10 \text{ g}}{100 \text{ ml}} = 15 \text{ g}$$

$$\frac{10 \text{ g}}{100 \text{ mL}} = \frac{X \text{ g}}{150 \text{ mL}} \quad X = 15 \text{ g}$$

$$\text{mOsmol} = \frac{15 \text{ g}}{147 \text{ g/mol}} \cdot 3 \cdot 1000 = 306 \text{ mOsmol}$$

$$\text{mOsmol} = \frac{15 \text{ g}}{147 \text{ g/mole}} \quad \text{x} \quad 3 \quad \text{x} \quad 1,000 = 306 \text{ mOsmol}$$

Note that the problem is asking for milliosmoles and not osmolarity. Therefore, the answer is in milliosmoles and not mOsmol/L. It is not normalized to 1 liter.

---

153. A solution contains 200 mg Ca^+ ions per liter. How many milliosmoles are represented in the solution? M.W = 40

$$\text{mOsmol} = \frac{0.2 \text{ g/L}}{40 \text{ g}} \quad \text{x} \quad 1 \quad \text{x} \quad 1,000 = 5 \text{ mOsmol}$$

$$\text{mOsmol} = \frac{0.2 \text{ g/L}}{40 \text{ g/mol}} \cdot 1 \cdot 1000 = 5 \text{ mOsmol}$$

Please note that the problem is asking for milliosmoles and not osmolarity. Therefore, the answer is in milliosmoles and not mOsmol/L.

✳ **154. Calculate the amount of grams of potassium chloride needed to make 200 mL of a solution contain 250 mOsmol/L. M.W. = 74.5. Round to the nearest hundredth.**

$$250 \text{ mOsmol/L} = \frac{X}{74.5 \text{ g/mole}} \times 2 \times 1{,}000 \quad X = 9.31 \text{ g/L}$$

$$\frac{250 \text{ mOsmol}}{L} = \frac{X \text{ g/L}}{74.5 \text{ g/mol}} \cdot 2 \cdot 1000$$

$$X = 9.3125 \text{ g per liter}$$

$$\frac{9.31 \text{ g}}{1{,}000 \text{ mL}} = \frac{X \text{ g}}{200 \text{ mL}} \quad X = 1.86 \text{ g}$$

$$\frac{9.3125 \text{ g}}{1000 \text{ ml}} = \frac{X \text{ g}}{200 \text{ ml}} \Rightarrow X = 1.86 \text{ g}$$

Isotonicity

Osmolarity is the measure of total number of particles (or solutes) per liter (L) of solution. Tonicity is the term used to describe osmolarity used in the context of body fluids. When solutions are prepared, they need to match the tonicity of the body fluid as closely as possible. Solutions that are not isotonic with the body fluid produce pain upon administration, and cause

NUMBER OF DISSOCIATED IONS	DISSOCIATION FACTOR (OR IONIZATION) i
1	1
2	1.8
3	2.6
4	3.4
5	4.2

fluid transfer. In pharmacy, the terms hypotonic rather than hypo-osmotic, hypertonic rather than hyperosmotic, and isotonic rather than iso-osmotic, are used. Isotonicity is commonly used when preparing eye drops and nasal solutions.

Since isotonicity is related to the number of particles in solution, the dissociation factor (or ionization), symbolized by the letter i, is determined for the compound (drug). Non-ionic compounds do not dissociate and will have a dissociation factor, i, of 1. The chart above shows the dissociation factors (i) based on the percentage that dissociates into ions; for example, a dissociation factor of 1.8 means that 80% of the compound will dissociate in a weak solution.

As mentioned above, body fluids are isotonic, having an osmotic pressure equivalent to 0.9% sodium chloride. When making a medication to place into a body fluid, the drug provides solutes to the solvent and needs to be accounted for in the prescription in order to avoid making the prescription hypertonic. The relationship between the amount of drug that produces a particular osmolarity and the amount of sodium chloride that produces the same osmolarity is called the sodium chloride equivalent, or "E value" for short. This is the formula for calculating the E value of a compound:

$$E = \frac{(58.5)(i)}{(MW \text{ of drug})(1.8)}$$

The "E value" formula takes into account the molecular weight of NaCl (58.5) and the dissociation factor of 1.8 since normal saline is around 80% ionized- adding 0.8 for each additional ion beyond 1 into which the drug dissociates. The reason the compound is compared to NaCl is because NaCl is the major determinate of the isotonicity of body fluid.

Once the "E value" is determined, isotonicity problems can be calculated. The following steps outline the process of doing isotonicity problems:

1. Calculate the total amount of NaCl needed to make the final product/prescription isotonic. This is done by multiplying 0.9% NS by the desired volume of the prescription.

2. Multiply the total drug amount, in grams, by the "E value".

3. Subtract step 2 from step 1 to determine the total amount of NaCl needed to prepare an isotonic prescription.

Isotonicity Calculations

#ions	dis factor
1	1
2	1.8
3	2.6
4	3.4
5	4.2

155. Calculate the E value for mannitol (M.W. = 182). Round to the nearest hundredth.

$$\frac{(58.5)(i)}{(MW\ of\ drug)(1.8)} = \frac{58.5\ (1)}{182\ (1.8)} = 0.18$$

$$E = \frac{58.5 \cdot 1}{182 \cdot 1.8} = 0.18$$

156. Calculate the E value for potassium iodide, which dissociates into 2 particles (M.W. = 166). Round to two decimal places.

$$\frac{(58.5)(i)}{(MW\ of\ drug)(1.8)} = \frac{58.5\ (1.8)}{166\ (1.8)} = 0.35$$

$$E = \frac{58.5 \cdot 1.8}{166 \cdot 1.8} = 0.35$$

157. Physostigmine salicylate (M.W. = 413) is a 2- ion electrolyte, dissociating 80% in a given concentration (therefore, use a dissociation factor of 1.8). Calculate its sodium chloride equivalent. Round to two decimal places.

$$\frac{(58.5)(i)}{(MW\ of\ drug)(1.8)} = \frac{58.5\ (1.8)}{413\ (1.8)} = 0.14$$

$$E = \frac{58.5 \cdot 1.8}{413 \cdot 1.8} = 0.14$$

158. The E-value for ephedrine sulfate is 0.23. How many grams of sodium chloride are needed to make the following prescription? Round to 3 decimal places.

PRESCRIPTION	QUANTITY
Ephedrine sulfate	0.4 g
Sodium chloride	q.s.
Purified water qs	30 mL
Make isotonic soln.	
Sig. For the nose.	

Step 1. Determine how much NaCl would make the product isotonic.

$$\frac{0.9\ g}{100\ mL} = \frac{X}{30\ mL} \qquad X = 0.27\ g$$

$$\frac{0.9\ g}{100\ ml} \cdot 30ml = 0.27\ g\ Na$$

$$0.4\ g \cdot 0.23 = 0.092\ g$$

Step 2. Determine amount of sodium chloride represented from ephedrine sulfate.

■ 0.4 g x 0.23 ("E value") = 0.092 g of sodium chloride

Step 3. Subtract step 2 from step 1.

■ 0.27 g–0.092 g = 0.178 g of NaCl are needed to make an isotonic solution

$$\begin{array}{r} 0.270\ g \\ -\ 0.092\ g \\ \hline 0.178\ g\ Na \end{array}$$

159. The pharmacist receives an order for 10 mL of tobramycin 1% ophthalmic solution. You have tobramycin 40 mg/mL solution. Tobramycin does not dissociate and has a M.W. of 468. Find the E value for tobramycin and determine the amount of NaCl needed to make the solution isotonic. Round to two decimal places.

$$\frac{(58.5)(i)}{(MW \text{ of drug})(1.8)} = \frac{58.5\,(1)}{468\,(1.8)} = 0.07, \text{ which is the "E value" for tobramycin.}$$

Handwritten annotations:

NaCl $\dfrac{0.9\,g}{100\,ml} \cdot 10\,ml = 0.09\,g$

$E = \dfrac{58.5 \cdot 1}{468 \cdot 1.8} = 0.0694$

$\dfrac{1\,g}{100\,ml} \cdot 10\,ml = 0.1\,g$

tobra $0.1\,g \cdot 0.0694 = 6.94 \times 10^{-3}\,g$

$0.09\,g - 6.94 \times 10^{-3}\,g = 0.083\,g$

$\approx 0.08\,g$ (83 mg)

The "E value" for tobramycin is 0.07. The prescription asks for 10 mL of 1% solution.

Step 1. Determine how much NaCl would make the product isotonic (if that is all you were using).

$$\frac{0.9\,g}{100\,mL} = \frac{X}{10\,mL} \qquad X = 0.09\,g, \text{ or } 90\,mg$$

Step 2. Determine amount of sodium chloride represented from tobramycin.

$$\frac{1\,g}{100\,mL} = \frac{X}{10\,mL} \qquad X = 0.1\,g, \text{ or } 100\,mg$$

- 100 mg x 0.07 ("E value") = 7 mg

Step 3. Subtract step 2 from step 1.

You are using tobramycin, so you do not need all the NaCl – subtract out the equivalent amount of tonicity provided by the tobramycin, which is 7 mg.

90 mg-7 mg = 83 mg (83 mg additional sodium chloride is needed to make an isotonic solution)

To calculate how much of the original stock solution is required, use the stock solution that is 40 mg/mL. The prescription is written for 10 mL of a 1% solution. In the previous steps it was found that 100 mg of tobramycin is needed to provide 10 mL of a 1% solution.

$$\frac{40\,mg}{1\,mL} = \frac{100\,mg}{X\,mL} \qquad X = 2.5\,mL \text{ of the original stock solution.}$$

Moles (mols)/Millimoles (mmols)

A mole is the molecular weight of a substance in grams, or g/mole. A millimole is 1/1,000 of the molecular weight in grams, or 1/1,000 of a mole. For monovalent species, the numeric value of the milliequivalent and millimole are identical.

Useful equations

$$mols = \frac{g}{MW} \qquad or \qquad mmols = \frac{mg}{MW}$$

160. How many moles of anhydrous magnesium sulfate (M.W. = 120.4) are present in 250 grams of the substance? Round to the nearest hundredth.

$$mols = \frac{g}{MW}$$

$$\frac{250\ g}{120.4\ g/mol} = 2.08\ mol$$

$$mols = \frac{250\ g}{120.4} = 2.08\ mols$$

161. How many moles are equivalent to 875 milligrams of aluminum acetate (M.W. = 204)? Round to 3 decimal places.

First, convert 875 mg to grams.

$$875\ mg \quad x \quad \frac{1\ g}{1,000\ mg} = 0.875\ g$$

$$\frac{0.875\ g}{204\ g/mol} = 0.004\ mol$$

Next, solve for mols.

$$mols = \frac{g}{MW} = \frac{0.875\ g}{204} = 0.004\ mols$$

162. How many millimoles of sodium phosphate (M.W. = 138) are present in 90 g of the substance? Round to the nearest whole number.

$$\frac{90,000\ mg}{138} = 652\ mmols$$

$$\frac{90\ g}{138\ g/mol} \cdot 1000 = 652\ mmol$$

Or, solve another way:

$$\frac{90\ g}{138} = 0.652\ mols,\ which\ is\ 652\ mmols$$

163. How many moles are equivalent to 45 grams of potassium carbonate (M.W. = 138)? Round to the nearest thousandth.

$$mols = \frac{g}{MW}$$

$$\frac{45\ g}{138\ g/mol} = 0.326\ mol$$

$$mols = \frac{45\ g}{138} = 0.326\ mols$$

164. How many millimoles of calcium chloride (M.W. = 147) are represented in 147 mL of a 10% (w/v) calcium chloride solution?

Step 1: Calculate the amount (g) of $CaCl_2$ in 147 mL of 10% $CaCl_2$ solution.

$$\frac{10\ g}{100\ mL} = \frac{X\ g}{147\ mL} \quad X = 14.7\ g$$

$$147\ ml \cdot \frac{10\ g}{100\ ml} = 14.7\ g$$

Step 2: Calculate the mols of $CaCl_2$ in 147 mL of 10% $CaCl_2$ solution.

$$\frac{14.7\ g}{147\ g/mol} = 0.1\ mol$$

$$= 100\ m\ mol$$

$$\frac{14.7\ g}{147} \qquad X = 0.1\ mol$$

Step 3: Solve the problem by converting moles to millimoles; 0.1 mol x 1,000 = 100 mmols

---

165. How many milligrams of sodium chloride (MW = 58.5) represent 0.25 mmol? Do not round the answer.

$$0.25\ mmols\ =\ \frac{X\ mg}{58.5} \qquad X = 14.625\ mg$$

[handwritten] 0.25 mmol · 58.5 mg/mmol = 14.625 mg

---

166. How many grams of sodium chloride (MW = 58.5) should be used to prepare this solution? Do not round the answer.

PRESCRIPTION	QUANTITY
Methylprednisolone	0.5 g
NaCl solution	60 mL
Each 5 mL should contain 0.6 mmols of NaCl	

[handwritten] 60 mL · $\frac{0.6\ mmol}{5\ mL}$ = 7.2 mmol

$$\frac{0.6\ mmols}{5\ mL}\ =\ \frac{X\ mmols}{60\ mL} \qquad X = 7.2\ mmols$$

[handwritten] 7.2 × 10^{-3} mol · 58.5 g/mol = 0.4212 g

$$7.2\ mmols\ =\ \frac{X\ mg}{58.5} \qquad X = 421.2\ mg\ or\ 0.4212\ g$$

Milliequivalents (mEq)

Drugs can be expressed in solution in different ways:

- **Milliosmoles** refers to the number of particles in solution.

- **Millimoles** refers to the molecular weight (MW).

- **Milliequivalents** represent the amount, in milligrams (mg), of a solute equal to 1/1,000 of its gram equivalent weight, taking into account the valence of the ions. Like osmolarity, the quantity of particles is important – but so is the electrical charge. Milliequivalents refers to the chemical activity of an electrolyte and is related to the total number of ionic charges in solution and considers the valence (charge) of each ion.

COMPOUND	VALENCE
ammonium chloride (NH_4Cl)	1
potassium chloride (KCl^-)	1
potassium gluconate ($KC_6H_{11}O_7$)	1
sodium acetate ($NaC_2H_3O_2$)	1
sodium bicarbonate ($NaHCO_3$)	1
calcium carbonate ($CaCO_3$)	2
calcium chloride ($CaCl_2$)	2
disodium phosphate	2
ferrous sulfate ($FeSO_4$)	2
magnesium sulfate ($MgSO_4$)	2

To count the valence, divide the compound into its positive and negative components, and then count the number of either the positive or the negative charges. For a given compound, the milliequivalents of cations equals that of anions. Some common compounds and their valence are listed in the chart above.

mEq formula

$$mEq = \frac{mg \times valence}{MW} \quad \text{or} \quad mEq = mmols \times valence$$

167. A 20 mL vial is labeled potassium chloride (2 mEq/mL). How many grams of potassium chloride (M.W. = 74.5) are present? Round to the nearest hundredth.

$$20\ mL \times \frac{2\ mEq}{mL} = 40\ mEq\ KCl\ total$$

$$mEq = \frac{mg \times valence}{MW}$$

$$40\ mEq = \frac{mg \times 1}{74.5} = 2{,}980\ mg,\ which\ is\ 2.98\ g$$

Handwritten:
$$20\ ml \cdot \frac{2mEq}{ml} = 40mEq$$
$$\frac{40\ mEq \cdot 74.5}{1} = 2980\ mg = 2.98\ g$$

* Note: if asked to convert KCl liquid to tablets, you can use simple proportion since KCl 10% = 20 mEq/15 mL. For example, if someone is using Klor-Con 20 mEq BID, the total daily dose is 40 mEq, and convert to KCl 10%, solve the following equation to get the 30 mL required dose:

$$\frac{40\ mEq}{X\ mL} = \frac{20\ mEq}{15\ mL}$$

Handwritten: $KCl\ 10\% = \frac{20mEq}{15\ ml}$

168. How many milliequivalents of potassium chloride are present in a 12 mL dose of a 10% (w/v) potassium chloride (M.W. = 74.5) elixir? Round to 1 decimal place.

$$\frac{10\ g}{100\ mL} = \frac{X\ g}{12\ mL} \quad X = 1.2\ g,\ or\ 1{,}200\ mg$$

$$mEq = \frac{1{,}200\ mg \times 1}{74.5} = 16.1\ mEq$$

Handwritten:
$$12\ ml \cdot \frac{10\ g}{100ml} = 1.2\ g = 1200\ mg$$
$$mEq = \frac{1200\ mg \times 1}{74.5} = 16.1\ mEq$$

169. Calculate the milliequivalents of a standard ammonium chloride (M.W. = 53.5) 21.4 mg/mL sterile solution in a 500 mL container.

$$\frac{21.4\ mg}{mL} \times 500\ mL = 10{,}700\ mg$$

$$mEq = \frac{10{,}700\ mg \times 1}{53.5} = 200\ mEq$$

Handwritten:
$$\frac{21.4\ mg}{1\ ml} \cdot 500\ ml = 10700\ mg$$
$$mEq = \frac{10700\ mg \cdot 1}{53.5} = 200\ mEq$$

170. How many milliequivalents of $MgSO_4$ (M.W. = 120.4) are represented in 1 gram of anhydrous magnesium sulfate? Round to the nearest tenth.

$$mEq = \frac{mg \times valence}{MW}$$

$$mEq = \frac{1{,}000\ mg \times 2}{120.4} = 16.6\ mEq$$

Handwritten:
$$mEq = \frac{1000\ mg \times 2}{120.4} = 16.6\ mEq$$

171. How many milliequivalents of sodium are in a 50 mL vial of sodium bicarbonate (M.W. = 84) 8.4%?

$$\frac{8.4\ g}{100\ mL} = \frac{X\ g}{50\ mL} \qquad X = 4.2\ g,\ or\ 4,200\ mg$$

$$mEq = \frac{4,200\ mg \times 1}{84} = 50\ mEq$$

(handwritten)
$$50\ ml \cdot \frac{8.4\ g}{100\ ml} = 4.2\ g$$
$$mEq = \frac{4200\ mg \times 1}{84} = 50\ mEq$$

Temperature Conversions

Converting Fahrenheit to Celsius and Celsius to Fahrenheit

FORMULAS
°C = (°F–32)/1.8

°F = (°C x 1.8) + 32

(handwritten) $F = 1.8\ C + 32$

---

172. Convert 88°F to Celsius. Round to the nearest tenth.

Answer: (88-32)/1.8 = 31.1°C

(handwritten)
$F = 1.8\ C + 32$
$88 = 1.8\ C + 32$
$31.1 = C$

---

173. Convert 26°C to Fahrenheit. Round to the nearest tenth.

Answer: (26 x 1.8) + 32 = 78.8°F

(handwritten)
$F = 1.8\ C + 32$
$F = 1.8 \cdot 26 + 32 = 78.8$

---

174. Convert -15°C to Fahrenheit.

Answer: (-15 x 1.8) + 32 = 5°F

(handwritten)
$F = 1.8\ C + 32$
$F = 1.8\ (-15) + 32 = 5$

(handwritten left margin) Ca gluconate ⇒ PN

Calcium Carbonate and Calcium Citrate Tablet Conversion

Calcium carbonate (*Oscal*, *Tums*, etc) has acid-dependent absorption and should be taken with meals. Calcium carbonate is a dense form of calcium and contains 40% elemental calcium. A tablet that advertises 500 mg of elemental calcium weighs 1,250 mg. If 1,250 mg is multiplied by 0.40 (which is 40%), it will yield 500 mg elemental calcium.

Calcium citrate (*Citracal*, etc) has acid-independent absorption and can be taken with or without food. Calcium citrate is less dense and contains 21% elemental calcium. A tablet that advertises 315 mg calcium weighs 1,500 mg. If 1,500 mg is multiplied by 0.21 (or 21%), it will yield 315 mg elemental calcium. This is why the larger calcium citrate tablets provide less elemental calcium per tablet. They may be preferred if the gut fluid is basic, rather than acidic.

(handwritten notes)

Ca carbonate
- Oscal®, Tums®
- acid-dependent
  ⇒ take w/ food
- 40% elemental Ca++

Ca citrate
- Citracal®
- acid-independent
  ⇒ preferred if gut is basic
- 21% elemental Ca++

175. A patient is taking 3 calcium citrate tablets daily (one tablet, TID). Each weighs 1,500 mg total (non-elemental) weight. She wishes to trade her calcium tablets for the carbonate form. If she is going to use 1,250 mg carbonate tablets (by weight), how many tablets will she need to take to provide the same total daily dose?

1,500 x 0.21 x 3 = 945 mg elemental calcium, daily.

(handwritten: $\frac{21}{100} \cdot 1500$ mg x 3 = 945 mg elemental)

(handwritten: $\frac{40}{100} \cdot 1250$ mg = 500 mg elemental)

Each of the carbonate tablets (1,250 mg x 0.4) = 500 mg per tablet. She would need 2 tablets to provide a similar dose. Calcium absorption increases with lower doses. The tablets should be taken apart with two different meals.

(handwritten: ⇒ 2 carbonate tabs)

Absolute Neutrophil Count (ANC)

(handwritten: normal range = 2,200 - 8000/ μL)

The normal range for the ANC is 2,200-8,000/microliter. The microliter may be written as mm^3, or μL, but it is preferable to avoid this designation for safety reasons. A level < 2,000 is high-risk; for example, clozapine cannot be refilled if the ANC is < 2,000. A level < 500 is very high-risk for developing an infection. A neutropenic patient should be watched for signs of infection, including fever, shaking, general weakness or flu-like symptoms. Precautions to reduce infection risk, such as proper hand-washing and avoiding others with infection, should be followed. Further information is in the Lab Values chapter.

Calculating the ANC

Multiply the WBC by the percentage of neutrophils (the segs plus the bands) and divide by 100.

ANC (cells/mm³) = WBC x (% segs + % bands)/100

(handwritten box: $\text{ANC (cells/mm}^3) = \dfrac{\text{WBC } (\% \text{ segs} + \% \text{ bands})}{100}$)

176. A patient is being followed up at the oncology clinic today after her first round of chemotherapy one week ago. A CBC with differential is ordered and reported back as WBC = 14.8 x 10³ cells/mm³, segs are 10%, bands are 11%. Calculate this patient's ANC.

Segs = 10% Bands = 11%

14,800 x (10% + 11%)/100 = 14,800 x 0.21 = ANC of 3,108

(handwritten: $ANC = \dfrac{14.8 \times 10^3 \,(10\% + 11\%)}{100} = 3,108$)

177. A patient is taking clozapine and is at the clinic for a routine visit. Today's labs include WBC = 4,300 with 48% segs and 2% bands. Calculate this patient's ANC.

Segs = 48% Bands = 2%

4,300 x (48% + 2%)/100 = 4,300 x 0.5 = ANC of 2,150

(handwritten: $ANC = \dfrac{4300 \,(48\% + 2\%)}{100} = 2,150$)

pH, Arterial Blood Gas (ABG), Anion Gap, Buffer Systems and Ionization

pH

The pH refers to the acidity or basicity of the solution. As a solution becomes more acidic (the concentration of protons increases), the pH decreases. Conversely, when the pH increases, protons decrease, and the solution is more basic, or alkaline. Pure water is neutral at a pH of 7, and blood, with a pH of 7.4, is slightly alkaline. Stomach acid has a pH of ~2, is therefore acidic, with many protons in solution.

ABG

The acid-base status of a patient can be determined by an ABG. The primary buffering system of the body is the bicarbonate/carbonic acid system. The kidneys help to maintain a neutral pH by controlling bicarbonate (HCO_3^-) resorption and elimination. Bicarbonate acts as a buffer and a base. The lungs help maintain a neutral pH by controlling carbonic acid (which is directly proportional to the partial pressure of carbon dioxide or pCO_2) retained or released from the body. Carbon dioxide acts as a buffer and an acid. Alterations from the normal values lead to acid-base disorders. Diet and cellular metabolism lead to a large production of H^+ ions that need to be excreted to maintain acid-base balance. See Lab Values, Drug Monitoring & Patient Charts chapter for ABG component reference ranges.

ABG: pH/pCO_2/pO_2/HCO_3^-/O_2 Sat

An acid-base disorder that leads to a pH < 7.35 is called an acidosis. If the disorder leads to a pH > 7.45 it is called an alkalosis. These disorders are further classified as either metabolic or respiratory in origin. The primary disturbance in a metabolic acid-base disorder is the plasma HCO_3^- (bicarbonate) concentration. A metabolic acidosis is characterized primarily by a decrease in plasma HCO_3^- concentration. In a metabolic alkalosis, the plasma HCO_3^- concentration is increased. Metabolic acidosis may be associated with an increase in the anion gap (see below). In respiratory acidosis, the pCO_2 is primarily elevated and in respiratory alkalosis, the pCO_2 is decreased. Each disturbance has a compensatory (secondary) response that attempts to correct the imbalance toward normal and keep the pH neutral.

---

178. A babysitter brings a 7 year old boy to the Emergency Department. He is unarousable. Labs are ordered and an ABG is drawn. The ABG results are as follows: 6.72/40/89/12/94%. What acid base disorder does the child have?

Based on the pH, this is an acidosis. The pCO_2 is normal and the HCO_3^- is decreased. This is a metabolic acidosis.

---

179. An elderly female is admitted to the hospital after a motor vehicle accident. She suffered a head injury and is in the ICU. An ABG is obtained and the results are as follows: 8.25/29/97/26/98%. What acid base disorder does the patient have?

Based on the pH, this is an alkalosis. The pCO_2 is decreased and the HCO_3^- is normal. This is a respiratory alkalosis.

---

pH NOTES

A lower pH means more hydronium ions (H_3O^+, or H^+) in solution and is therefore more acidic. A higher pH is more basic and has less hydronium ions and more hydroxide (OH^-) ions in solution. The pH of 7 is said to be neutral. Blood is just slightly alkaline with a pH that should stay between 7.35-7.45.

Calculating Anion Gap

non-gap acidosis => ↑↑↑ Cl acidosis

When a patient is experiencing metabolic acidosis, it is common to calculate an anion gap. The anion gap is the difference in the measured cations and the measured anions in the blood. An anion gap assists in determining the cause of the acidosis. A mnemonic to remember the causes of a gap acidosis is CUTE DIMPLES [cyanide, uremia, toluene, ethanol (alcoholic ketoacidosis), diabetic ketoacidosis, isoniazid, methanol, propylene glycol, lactic acidosis, ethylene glycol, salicylates]. A gap is considered high if it is > 12 mEq/L (meaning the patient has a gap acidosis). The anion gap can also be low, which is less common. A non-gap acidosis is caused by other factors, mainly hyperchloremic acidosis. Here is the formula to calculate the anion gap:

Anion gap (AG) = $Na^+-Cl^--HCO_3$

---

180. A patient in the ICU has recently developed an acidosis. Using the laboratory parameters below, calculate the patient's anion gap.

Na^+	139
Cl^-	101
K^+	4.6
HCO_3	19
SCr	1.6
BUN	38

anion gap = $Na^+ - Cl^- - HCO_3$
= 139 - 101 - 19
= 19

Cyanide
Uremia
Toluene
Ethanol (alcoholic ketoacidosis)

Diabetic ketoacidosis (DKA)
Isoniazid (INH)
Methanol
Propylene glycol
Lactic acidosis
Ethylene glycol
Salicylates

Anion Gap = 139–101–19

Anion Gap = 19; therefore, the patient has a gap acidosis.

---

181. SJ was recently admitted to the ICU with a pH=7.27. Below is her laboratory data. Calculate SJ's anion gap.

144	95	68	< 414
3.2	21	2.1	

Na	Cl	BUN	glu
K+	HCO₃	SrCr	

anion gap = Na - Cl - HCO3
= 144 - 95 - 21
= 28

Anion Gap = 144–95–21 = 28; therefore, SJ has a gap acidosis.

Buffer Systems/Ionization

Buffer systems help to reduce the impact of too few or too many hydrogen ions in body fluids. These hydrogen ions could cause harm including degrading some drugs, destabilizing proteins, inhibiting cellular functions, and with too much of a change outside of the narrow range, cells die and death can occur. Therefore, buffers minimize fluctuations in pH so that harm is avoided. Buffer systems are common in the body and are composed of either a weak acid and salt of the acid (e.g., acetic acid and sodium acetate), or weak base and salt of the base (e.g., ammonium hydroxide and ammonium chloride). An acid is a compound that dissociates, releasing (donating) protons into solution. Once the proton is released, the compound is now a conjugate base, or its salt form. For example, HCl in solution is an acid and dissociates (giving up the proton) into H^+ and Cl^-. A base picks up, or binds, the proton. For example, NH_3 is a base that can pick up a proton and become NH_4^+.

Acid-base reactions are equilibrium reactions; there is drug moving back and forth between the acid and base state. The pH and the pKa are used to determine if the drug is acting as an acid or a base. When the pH = pKa, the molar concentration of the salt form and the molar concentration of the acid form of the buffer acid-base pair will be equal: 50% of the buffer will be in salt form and 50% in acid form. Notice that the percentage of buffer in the acid form when added to the percentage of buffer in the salt form will equal 100%. When the pH = pKa, this is the point at which half the compound is protonated (ionized), and half is not protonated (un-ionized).

A 'strong' acid or base means that you get 100% dissociation and a 'weak' acid or base means you get very limited dissociation. Any time you are given a pKa, it refers to the acid form losing protons to give to the base, or salt, form.

If you were given the 'pKb' then you would say, 'base' simply because of the definitions of the two terms.

If the pH > pKa, more of the acid is ionized, and more of the conjugate base is un-ionized.

If the pH = pKa, the ionized and un-ionized forms are equal.

If the pH < pKa, more of the acid is un-ionized, and more of the conjugate base is ionized.

The percentage of drug in the ionized versus un-ionized state is important because an ionized drug is soluble but cannot easily cross lipid membranes. An un-ionized drug is not soluble but can cross the membranes and reach the proper receptor site. Most drugs are weak acids. They are soluble, and can pick up a proton to cross the lipid layer.

Most drugs molecules are weak acids (or weak bases). These molecules can exist in either the un-ionized or the ionized state, and the degree of ionization depends on the dissociation constant (Ka) of the drug and the pH of the environment. This leads to the Henderson-Hasselbalch equation, also known as the buffer equation, which is used to solve for the pH.

redo all calculations

WEAK ACID FORMULA

$$pH = pK_a + \log\left[\frac{salt}{acid}\right]$$

[handwritten] $pk_w = pk_a + pk_b = 14$

WEAK BASE FORMULAS

$$pH = pK_w - pK_b + \log\left[\frac{base}{salt}\right], \text{ where } pKw = 14 \quad \text{or} \quad pH = pK_a + \log\left[\frac{base}{salt}\right]$$

---

182. What is the pH of a solution prepared to be 0.5 M sodium citrate and 0.05 M citric acid (pKa for citric acid = 3.13)? Round to the nearest hundredth.

$$pH = pK_a + \log\left[\frac{salt}{acid}\right]$$

$$pH = 3.13 + \log\left[\frac{0.5M}{0.05M}\right]$$

[handwritten]
$$pH = pk_a + \log\left(\frac{salt}{acid}\right)$$
$$= 3.13 + \log\left(\frac{0.5}{0.05}\right)$$
$$= 4.13$$

pH = 3.13 + log[10]

pH = 3.13 + 1

pH = 4.13

---

183. What is the pH of a solution prepared to be 0.4 M ammonia and 0.04 M ammonium chloride (pKb for ammonia = 4.76)? Round to the nearest hundredth.

$$pH = pK_w - pK_b + \log\left[\frac{base}{salt}\right]$$

$$pH = 14 - 4.76 + \log\left[\frac{0.4}{0.04}\right]$$

$$pH = 9.24 + \log(10)$$

$$pH = 9.24 + 1$$

$$pH = 10.24$$

$$pH = 14 - pkb + \log\left(\frac{base}{salt}\right)$$
$$= 14 - 4.76 + \log\left(\frac{0.4}{0.04}\right)$$
$$= 10.24$$

---

184. What is the pH of a buffer solution containing 0.5 M acetic acid and 1 M sodium acetate in 1 liter of solution (pKa for acetic acid = 4.76)? Round to the nearest hundredth.

$$pH = pK_a + \log\left[\frac{salt}{acid}\right]$$

$$pH = 4.76 + \log\left[\frac{1}{0.5}\right]$$

$$pH = 4.76 + \log(2)$$

$$pH = 4.76 + 0.3$$

$$pH = 5.06$$

$$pH = pka + \log\left(\frac{salt}{acid}\right)$$
$$= 4.76 + \log\left(\frac{1}{0.5}\right)$$
$$= 5.06$$

---

185. What is the pH of a solution containing 0.2 mole of a weakly basic drug and 0.02 mole of its salt per liter of solution (pKa of the drug = 9.36)? Round to the nearest hundredth.

$$pH = pK_a + \log\left[\frac{base}{salt}\right]$$

$$pH = 9.36 + \log\left[\frac{0.2}{0.02}\right]$$

$$pH = 9.36 + 1$$

$$pH = 10.36$$

$$pH = 14 - pkb + \log\left(\frac{base}{salt}\right)$$
$$= pka + \log\left(\frac{base}{salt}\right)$$
$$= 9.36 + \log\left(\frac{0.2}{0.02}\right)$$
$$= 10.36$$

---

186. A buffer solution is prepared using 0.3 mole of a weakly basic drug and an unknown quantity of its salt (pKa of the drug = 10.1). The final solution has a pH of 8.99. How much of the salt was used? Round to the nearest hundredth.

$$pH = pK_a + \log\left[\frac{base}{salt}\right]$$

$$8.99 = 10.1 + \log\left[\frac{0.3}{X}\right]$$

$$pH = pka + \log\left(\frac{base}{salt}\right)$$
$$8.99 = 10.1 + \log\left(\frac{0.3}{x}\right)$$
$$-1.11 = \log\left(\frac{0.3}{x}\right)$$
$$10^{-1.11} = \frac{0.3}{x} \implies x = \frac{0.3}{10^{-1.11}} = 3.86$$

$$8.99 - 10.1 = \log\left[\frac{0.3}{X}\right]$$

$$10^{-1.11} = \frac{0.3}{x}$$

X = 3.86 mole of the salt

Percent of Ionization

The Henderson-Hasselbalch equation can be modified to calculate the percent of ionization of a drug.

To calculate the % ionization of a weak acid:

$$\% \text{ ionization} = \frac{100}{1+10^{(pKa-pH)}}$$

To calculate % ionization of a weak base:

$$\% \text{ ionization} = \frac{100}{1+10^{(pH-pKa)}}$$

---

187. What is the % ionization of amitriptyline, a weak base with a pKa = 9.4, at a physiologic pH of 7.4?

Use the weak base formula:

$$\% \text{ ionization} = \frac{100}{1+10^{(pH-pKa)}}$$

$$\% \text{ ionization} = \frac{100}{1+10^{(7.4-9.4)}}$$

$$\% \text{ ionization} = \frac{100}{1+10^{(7.4-9.4)}}$$

$$\% \text{ ionization} = \frac{100}{1.01}$$

$$\% \text{ ionization} = 99\%$$

$$\% \text{ ionization} = \frac{100}{1+10^{(pH-pka)}}$$

$$= \frac{100}{1+10^{(7.4-9.4)}}$$

$$= \frac{100}{1.01} = 99\%$$

---

188. What is the % ionization of naproxen, a weak acid with a pKa of 4.2, in the stomach at a pH of 3?

Use the weak acid formula:

$$\% \text{ ionization} = \frac{100}{1+10^{(pKa-pH)}}$$

$$\% \text{ ionization} = \frac{100}{16.85}$$

$$\% \text{ ionization} = 6\%$$

$$\% \text{ ionization} = \frac{100}{1+10^{(pka-pH)}}$$

$$= \frac{100}{1+10^{(4.2-3)}}$$

$$= 5.9\% \approx 6\%$$

3

COMPOUNDING

We gratefully acknowledge the assistance of Jess Martinez, PharmD, Clinical Associate Professor & Vice Dean, Western University College of Pharmacy, in preparing this chapter.

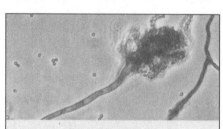

Fungal Meningitis Outbreak Linked to Compounded Medication

In 2012 a compounding pharmacy prepared methylprednisolone injections that were contaminated and caused fungal meningitis (*aspergillis*), with resultant illness and fatalities. In addition to improper aseptic technique there was a lack of proper policies and procedures. The pharmacy prepared multiple batches for mass distribution. Compounding is limited to patient-specific doses (or, in some cases, production of limited quantities of the same product prepared in advance of expected patient prescriptions). The primary purpose of compounding is to provide medications that are not commercially available to meet the unique needs of individual patients.

GUIDELINE

Non-Sterile Preparations: US Pharmacopeia (USP) Chapters <795>, <1151>, <1160>, <1163>, <1176>, <1191>, <1265>, and all applicable compounding laws, guidelines and standards. Sterile Preparations: USP Chapter <797>.

NONSTERILE COMPOUNDING VERSUS FDA-APPROVED DRUGS

Compounding is different from manufacturing since it is patient-specific (ordered by a prescriber for the patient) and regulated by the state boards of pharmacy. For example, a prescriber designates specific percentages of hormone cream for an individual female patient. Or, a hospitalized patient is prescribed a compounded medication for topical administration since she cannot swallow pills.

- Beyond use dates must be applied to each compounded product, using USP <795> guidelines for Nonaqueous Liquids and Solid Formulations and for Water-Containing Formulations. For all other formulations the beyond use date is not later than the intended duration of therapy or 30 days, whichever is earlier.

- The recipe must be kept in a log book (see next section).

- Advertisement of compounded products is not permitted.

- Compounded products do not have NDC numbers.

- In contrast, <u>FDA-approved and regulated drugs must have an approved NDA, must be produced under Good Manufacturing Practices (GMP), have NDC numbers, and carry a set expiration date</u> (provided to the pharmacy).

GENERAL NONSTERILE COMPOUNDING RULES

- Compounding space should be separate and away from the dispensing section.

- A United States Pharmacopeia (USP), including Food Chemicals Codex (FCC) and the National Formulary (NF) are the recommended sources of ingredients for compounding all preparations.

- Required logs that must be in the pharmacy: compounding formulas and procedures, compounded item log, equipment cleaning and calibration and maintenance records (includes ambient, refrigerator and freezer temp logs), record of chemicals, bulk drug substances, drug products, and components used to compound products (which must be obtained from reliable sources).

- For each compounded product, pharmacy records must include: master formula, date the product was compounded, pharmacy personnel who compounded the product, pharmacist with final review, quantity of each product used in compounding the product, manufacturer and lot number of each component, equipment used, pharmacy assigned reference number or lot number, beyond use date, quantity or amount of product compounded.

- Documentation, written or electronic, enables a compounder whenever necessary to systematically trace, evaluate, and replicate the steps included throughout the preparation process of a compounded preparation.

Labels on Pharmacy-Compounded Products

- Expiration Dates (Beyond Use Dates)

  - Solids (non-aqueous) preparations: Label up to 6-months duration if the ingredients are all USP or NF products or use a date that is no later than 25% of the time left on the manufacturer's date, whichever is sooner.

  - Aqueous (water-containing, liquid) preparations: no more than 14 days if the preparation is stored in the refrigerator (2-8°C, 36-46°F).

  - Anything else should expire no more than the intended length of treatment or 30 days, whichever is sooner.

- Auxiliary Labels for Compounded Creams and Lotions

  - Refrigerate, Shake Well (emulsions, suspensions), External Use Only

- The product label must include generic or chemical name of active ingredients, strength or quantity, pharmacy lot number, beyond-use date, and any special storage requirements.

- A statement that the product has been compounded by the pharmacy must be placed on the label of the container.

- For capsules, the label must include mcg or mg/capsule.

- For liquids, the strength should be in concentration (e.g., 125 mg/5 mL), or provided as a percentage.

- The coining of short names for marketing or convenience (e.g., *Johnson's Solution*) is strongly discouraged.

- Purified water (not tap water) is used. Purified water is also used for rinsing equipment.

- If compounding a prescription that calls for alcohol and the type is not specified, use USP 95% ethyl alcohol.

Selected Notes on Sterile Compounding
(see Medication Safety Chapter for further requirements)

- The following products must be compounded in a sterile environment: <u>injections, inhalations, wound and cavity irrigation baths, eye drops and eye ointments. Water used in preparation must be sterile water for injection, or bacteriostatic water for injection.</u>

- Sterile compounding requires personnel trained and evaluated annually for competency in <u>aseptic techniques, environmental control, quality assurance testing and end-product evaluation and sterility testing.</u>

- If the product is an injectable, the certified sterile compounding environment must be either an ISO class 5 (class 100) <u>laminar air flow</u> hood within a <u>ISO class 7</u> (class 10,000) clean room (with <u>positive air pressure</u> differential relative to adjacent areas) or an <u>ISO class 5</u> (class 100) clean room with positive air pressure differential relative to adjacent areas or a barrier isolator that provides a ISO class 5 (class 100) environment for compounding.

- <u>Clean room garb (low-shedding coverall, head cover, face mask and shoe covers) is required and should be put on and taken off outside the designated area. Hand, finger and wrist jewelry is not allowed. Head and facial hair have to be out of the way (tied up) and covered.</u>

- When preparing <u>cytotoxic agents, coated gowns and two pair of ASTM-Tested gloves are worn and a NIOSH-Certified N95 respiratory mask are worn</u>. All cytotoxic agents must be labeled "<u>cytotoxic agents – dispose of properly</u>" and disposal and spill policies and spill kits must be kept in the pharmacy.

- <u>Sterile USP <797> and non-sterile USP <795> compliant areas must be separate.</u>

NONSTERILE COMPOUNDING EQUIPMENT USED IN A COMMUNITY PHARMACY

Balances

Required balances: a torsion balance (a "class A balance") utilizes both internal and external weights and requires the use of external weights for measurements exceeding 1 g), and if compounding routinely, a top-loading electronic balance. Most pharmacists will make their weight measurements on an electronic balance.

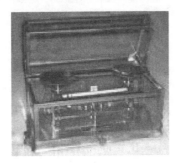

Torsion balance

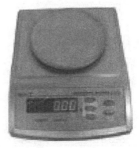

Electronic balance

Measuring Devices

Caution! All equipment, including scales, measuring devices, slabs, spatulas and anything else used must be selected to avoid surfaces that can make contact with reactive, additive, or absorptive materials to avoid altering the safety, strength, quality, or purity of the preparation.

When measuring, select a device equal to or slightly larger than the amount to be measured.

■ If the volume to be measured is viscous use a syringe, rather than a cylinder. Pipettes are long thin tubes made of glass that are used for measuring 1.5 mL or less of liquids.

■ Liquids in a container curve up, therefore measure at the bottom of the meniscus.

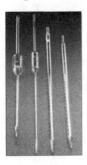

Pipette

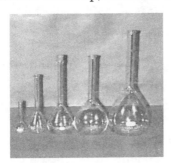

Volumetric Flask

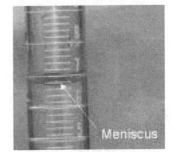

Graduated Cylinder
(measure from the bottom of the meniscus)

Mortar & Pestle

Compounding requires a minimum of two types of mortar and pestles: 1 glass and 1 Wedgewood or porcelain (ceramic). <u>Wedgewood or porcelain is used most commonly and is best for reducing particle size of dry powders and crystals. Porcelain has a smoother surface than Wedgewood and is preferred for blending powders or pulverizing soft materials</u>. If Wedgewood is used for powders or crystals, first coat the inside with lactose to fill in the crevices.

Glass is used for liquids and chemicals that are oily or that will stain the porcelain, including many chemotherapeutics. Glass is preferred for mixing liquids and semi-soft dosage forms.

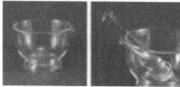
Glass mortar & pestle

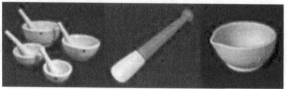
Ceramic mortar and pestle

Surfaces & Spatulas

Glassine weighing paper (as opposed to bond paper) should be used for weighing ointments and some dry chemicals. It is safest not to use ointment paper to prepare creams and lotions (use a slab and spatula instead) because the water content will cause the paper to moisten, and possibly tear.

Generally, large metal (stainless steel) spatula blades are used, but small spatula blades (< 6 inches) can be used for removing product from the large spatula and putting it into the jar.

Plastic spatulas should be used for chemicals (e.g., potassium, iodine) that can react with stainless steel blades. The third type is the rubber spatula. Compounding slabs are also called ointment slabs, they are generally glass, and have nonabsorbent surfaces.

COMPOUNDING TERMINOLOGY AND INGREDIENTS

Levigation

Levigation is the process of reducing the size of a particle of a solid by triturating it (grinding it down to smaller particles) in a mortar or spatulating it on an ointment slab with a small amount of liquid (the wetting agent) in which the solid is not soluble. The goal is to transfer it from a solid to a uniform paste utilizing a levigating agent. This incorporates the solid into a cream or ointment base. It also makes the solid more uniform throughout the base and gets rid of the gritty feeling.

- The levigation agent must be miscible (compatible) with the ointment base. For example, sulfur ointment 10% USP uses 10% mineral oil to prepare a white petrolatum-based ointment. The mineral oil is the levigating agent. The petrolatum is used as the base to deliver the medication (the sulfur, used to treat seborrheic dermatitis (eczema) or scabies) and the petrolatum itself is an effective ointment (barrier) that prevents dehydration and helps protect the skin. "Vaseline" or "petroleum jelly" are common terms for petrolatum.

- Levigating Agents used in preparing ointments are:

  - For aqueous systems (O/W dispersions) – Glycerin, propylene glycol, polyethylene glycol 80.

  - For oleaginous systems (W/O dispersions) – Mineral oil (light and heavy), castor oil, cottonseed oil, *Tween 80*.

- Mineral oil is good to use for levigating a hydrophobic ointment such as white petrolatum.

- If heat is used (to mix things easier), the use should be limited and the ingredient with the higher melting point should be heated. Otherwise, undesired chemical reactions could occur.

- A water bath will help prevent over-heating.

Trituration

Trituration is the process of reducing fracturable powder substances into fine particles by rubbing (or grinding) them with a mortar and pestle, or on an ointment slab.

Extemporaneous

Extemporaneous compounding refers to a compound prepared without a specific formula (not from an official compendium) and made specifically to fill the needs of an individual patient.

Emollients

An emollient is a single agent that is used to soften and smooth the skin. A moisturizer is sometimes referred to as an emollient, but the term emollient is used for single agents, and moisturizers often have coloring, scents, and other ingredients added.

Emulsions & Emulsifiers

Emulsions are a two-phase system of two immiscible liquids, one of which is dispersed through the other as small droplets. Emulsions are immiscible (they do not form a suspension – which means the two liquids stay separate when combined). They can be oil in water, or water in oil. An emulsifier ("emulgent") is used to stabilize the emulsion. Emulsifiers are usually surfactants ("wetting agents") that reduce the surface tension between the two liquids so that the two different substances can move closer to each other.

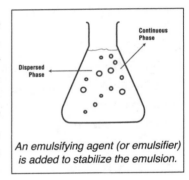

An emulsifying agent (or emulsifier) is added to stabilize the emulsion.

- Emulsifiers include agar, pectin, lipophilic esters of sorbitan (Arlacel and Span) and the hydrophilic esters (Myrj and Tween). Other emulsifier names that may be good to recognize are polyethylene glycol (PEG, which is also commonly used as a laxative), acacia, glyceryl monostearate and sodium laurel sulfate.

- The Continental or dry gum method of preparing an emulsion uses oil, purified water and gum (such as acacia) in the ratio of 4:2:1. The English, or wet gum method uses the same ingredients (oil, water, gum) but the order of mixing is different. In the dry gum method, the gum is mixed rapidly with oil, and then the water is added all at once, while the wet gum method is a slower process in which the gum is dissolved in water first, and then the oil is slowly added.

- The hydrophilic-lipophilic balance (HLB) number is used to choose which surfactant to select when preparing an emulsion to provide good "emulsification." The HLB number is provided for the oil or can be taken from a reference list. Agents with a low HLB number are more oil-soluble. Agents with a high HLB number are more water-soluble. The HLB scale range is 0-20 and a value of 10, the midpoint, is the break-point between water and oil solubility. A value less than 10, therefore, is lipid-soluble, and a value greater than 10 is water-soluble.

Eutectic Mixtures

A eutectic mixture is two or more components that melt at a temperature lower than the melting temperature for the individual components. Eutectic mixtures can be formed between two compounds or between a compound and an excipient, such as salt and water. Traditional ice cream makes take advantage of the mixture of salt and water to make ice cream, which freezes because the melting temperature of the eutectic mixture is lower than either the salt or the water. Eutectic mixtures are in accordance with VantHoff's equation, which is used for calculating the equilibrium constant within certain thermodynamic parameters.

Preservatives

Liquid preparations, unless they are single-use, will commonly contain a preservative to inhibit microbial growth. The preservative must be compatible with the mixture, be relatively stable and have an acceptable color, taste and odor. Antioxidants are used commonly to prevent oxidation, the reaction of a substance with oxygen. Light and temperature catalyze oxidation and many sensitive liquid compounds will require avoidance of light or the use of refrigeration to maintain stability. Unsaturated fatty acids are prone to oxidation and will turn rancid, which produces an odor and discoloration. Common preservatives and antioxidants include benzalkonium chloride (BAK, commonly used in eye drops), benzyl alcohol, chlorhexidine, thimerosal (contains mercury), sodium benzoate, benzethonium chloride, propylparaben and others.

Lotions, Creams, Ointments, Pastes

Lotions, creams, ointments and pastes are all water and oil emulsions (either oil in water, or water in oil), but in different amounts and for different uses. Caution is required when choosing a product for a patient because many come in various formulations. For example, terbinafine (*Lamisil AT*) comes as a cream, gel and solution and mupirocin (*Bactroban*) comes as an ointment and a cream.

Note on medication potency and choice of the delivery vehicle: The Common Skin Conditions chapter reviews how different formulations are used on different types of skin. For example, an antifungal ointment is not applied easily to hairy skin; it will be difficult to spread. Yet, ointments promote medication absorption better than creams and lotions. This is why both site and potency must be considered. A medication delivered in an ointment will have a higher potency than the same medication delivered in a cream or lotion. Example: The topical steroid mometasone (*Elocon*) ointment is high-potency and mometasone (*Elocon*) cream is low-medium potency.

- Lotions have the most water, and are most often oil-in-water (with a small amount of oil). They absorb quickly and are easy to spread on the skin. Since lotions contain a lot of water, they often come in pumps. Some of the lotions contain alcohol, which can be drying. Examples: Most of the OTC moisturizers are lotions, such as *Keri* and *Cetaphil*.

- Creams are emulsions of about half oil and half water. They spread easily and are reasonably hydrating. Creams are packaged in tubes, and sometimes in tubs. Examples: terbinafine *(Lamisil AT)* antifungal cream, docosanol (*Abreva*) antiviral cream.

- Ointments are ~80% oil and 20% water. They do not absorb well and are not easy to use on large areas. They are used for the occlusive benefit – they block (trap in) moisture, and are preferred for dry or dry/cracked skin. They are useful to help injured skin heal from burns or lasers, since moisture is needed for these types of injuries. They are often used for medication delivery and are usually packaged in tubes, and sometimes in tubs. There are five (5) classes or types of ointment bases which are differentiated on the basis of their physical composition. These are oleaginous bases (such as white petrolatum), absorption bases (such as lanolin, *Aquaphor)*, water in oil emulsion bases, oil in water emulsion bases (hydrophilic ointment, *Dermabase)* and water soluble or water miscible bases (PEG ointment).

- Pastes are the thickest ointments and are also used as protective barriers. Example: *Triple Paste* medicated diaper rash ointment.

Gels

Gels are oil in water emulsions, usually with an alcohol base. They are easy to spread and dry into a thin film. Example: Benzoyl peroxide and erythromycin topical acne gel *(Benzamycin)*.

Gels are also used as thickeners. They have a solid and a liquid that are dispersed evenly throughout a material (the suspension is inter-penetrated by the liquid). Example: *BenzaClin* acne gel.

- Common gels used as thickeners are the alginates (including Na$^+$, K$^+$, Ca^{2+} alginate), agar, carrageenan, gelatin, carbomer, tragacanth, bentonite). A commercial product that is used commonly is called *Liqua-Gel*.

Powders

Powders are finely divided drugs, or other chemicals. Powders range in size from very coarse (No. 8) to very fine (No. 80).

Solutions

Solutions are liquid preparations of soluble chemicals dissolved in solvents such as water, alcohol, or propylene glycol. When alcohol is used as a solvent in a systemic formulation, the pharmacist should consider effects on the patient, and if the alcohol could interact with medications.

Suspensions

Suspensions are a two phased-system of a finely divided solid in a liquid medium. The drug must be uniformly dispersed in the medium. The suspension should be deflocculated: this means that the repulsive forces between particles predominate so that the particles in the suspension repel each other and remain as discrete, single particles. Suspensions should settle slowly, be easy to re-disperse by gently shaking and have uniform particles that are of small size. Suspending agents used in suspensions:

- Natural hydrocolloids, including acacia, alginic acid, gelatin, guar gum, alginate, xanthan gum

- Semi-synthetic hydrocolloids, including methylcellulose

- Synthetic hydrocolloids, including carbomers and polyvinyl alcohol

- Clays, including bentonite and veegum

Suppositories

Suppositories are solid dosage forms used to deliver medicine into the rectum, vagina or urethra. They are formed in a mold. They melt, soften or dissolve in the body cavity. Suppositories bypass the oral route and avoid first-pass metabolism.

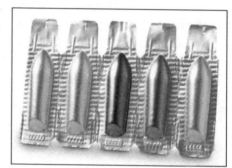

- The base must be compatible with the medication, must not melt too quickly (such as in the hands while inserting), must be stable and must not have a disagreeable look or scent.

- Examples include the following rectal suppositories: acetaminophen suppository, hemorrhoid suppository, mesalamine suppository, and various types of vaginal suppositories. See the Drug Formulations chapter for uses of suppositories.

- Commonly used bases utilized in suppositories include cocoa butter (theobroma oil), glycerin, hydrogenated vegetable oils, and polyethylene glycol (Carbowax).

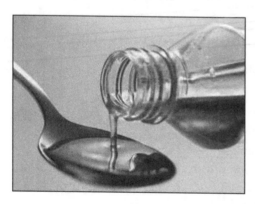

Syrups

Syrups are concentrated, aqueous preparations of sugar or sugar-substitute, medicinal agents, or flavoring in water, such as cough syrups.

Elixirs

Elixirs are clear, sweetened, hydroalcoholic solutions suitable for water-insoluble drugs, such as mouthwashes.

Lozenges/Troches

Lozenges are called troches and deliver drug to the oral mucosa. The lozenge dissolves in the mouth. <u>Example</u>: clotrimazole troche *(Mycelex)* is an antifungal troche that is used to treat oral thrush. Troches are made in molds, with any required flavorings or colorings.

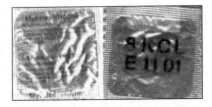

Clotrimazole (Mycelex) Troche

Flavorings/Sweeteners

Products or preparations that have an unpleasant taste are not usually used, or they will result in decreased adherence. Flavor is one of the key attributes in determining the palatability of drugs given in oral liquid and oral semisolid dosage forms. Salty or sweet tastes can be used to mask a bitter flavor. Mint and spices can be used to mask poor flavor. Acids (such as citric acid) are used to enhance fruit flavors. Another option is to put the drug <u>into an emulsion</u> (in the internal phase) where it is less likely to interact with the patient's taste buds. A few concerns with sweeteners used in chewables is described under tablets.

Capsules

Capsules are unit doses made in soluble shells of <u>gelatin</u>, or can be made of hypromellose (a non-animal product) to accommodate cultural and dietary requirements. Unpleasant drug tastes and odors can be masked by the capsule shell. Capsules are made by triturating the powders to a small particle size, mixing by <u>geometric dilution</u>, and calculating the weight needed to fill a capsule. <u>Glycerol</u> and <u>sorbitol</u> are used as "plasticizers" to <u>soften</u> the capsule.

Capsule size: the largest is 000, where the smaller the size, the higher the number. The smallest capsule size is 5.

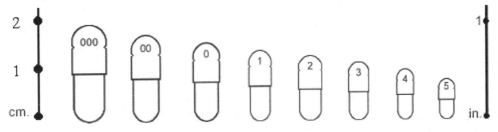

Tablets

In large-scale manufacturing, the formulation that is often the least expensive to make (and the most common dispensed in everyday practice) are compressed tablets. <u>Tablets may contain excipients (also called binders) that hold the tablet together</u>. Capsules may also use similar ingredients as fillers. Sorbitol is used often in chewables because it is sweet. Sorbitol is also used as a plasticizer, and as a thickening agent in liquids. Sorbitol can cause considerable GI distress in some patients with IBS; it has <u>laxative</u> properties. Lactose is a commonly used filler and is a sweetener. <u>Lactose</u> can cause GI issues in patients with lactose-intolerance.

Calculations for compounding require the math skills discussed in the Calculations chapter, which includes compounding problems.

4

PHARMACOKINETICS

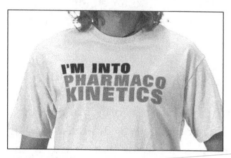

We gratefully acknowledge the assistance of Paul Beringer, PharmD, Associate Professor of Clinical Pharmacy and Clinical Medicine, University of Southern California, in preparing this chapter.

Pharmacokinetics is what the human body does to the drug and pharmacodynamics is what the drug does to the human body. Pharmacokinetics involves the study of the time course of drug absorption, distribution, metabolism and excretion. Pharmacokinetics attempts to use mathematical relationships to describe how drug molecules enter the body, circulate to different tissues and organs, and are then eliminated by metabolic and excretory processes. Pharmacokinetic analysis provides insights into the time course of drug pharmacology by correlating therapeutic and toxic effects with circulating drug levels. Pharmacodynamics refers to the effects of drugs on the patient's body (the mechanism of action, or how they work), the drug's therapeutic benefit and the toxicity profile. Pharmacodynamics is also used to explain the effect of the drug on an organism (such as a bacteriostatic or bactericidal effect).

ABSORPTION, DISTRIBUTION, METABOLISM AND EXCRETION

Absorption

Absorption is the process by which a drug moves from the site of administration to the circulatory system. Sites of drug administration are divided into two main areas, intravascular administration, where the drug is placed directly into the blood either intravenously or intra-arterially, or extravascular administration. Examples of extravascular administration include oral, sublingual, buccal, intramuscular, subcutaneous, dermal, pulmonary, topical ocular, intraocular and rectal. If a drug is administered via intravascular administration, (into the vein, with an IV infusion) there is no drug absorption as the drug is placed directly in the systemic circulation. However, if a drug is administered by extravascular administration, drug absorption occurs as the drug moves from the site of administration to the circulatory system.

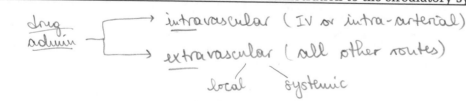

Site of Administration

Extravascular administration can be divided into two groups: drugs intended for local effects and drugs intended for systemic effects. Drugs intended for local effects are often applied topically to the site of action. Examples of drugs intended for local effects include eye drops for glaucoma (e.g., latanoprost), dermal preparations for psoriasis (e.g., coal tar preparations), and nasal sprays for allergies (e.g., fluticasone nasal spray). In general, drug absorption is low with most, but not all, topical products. The extent of topical absorption is affected by other factors, including open wounds on the skin (increases absorption) and the amount that is applied. Therapeutic effects can be observed with local administration, and systemic toxicity can often be avoided due to low systemic exposure. Drugs intended for systemic effects are generally applied in such a way to encourage absorption to the circulatory system. Examples of drugs intended for systemic effects are oral tablets for seasonal allergies (e.g., loratidine), injectables for osteoporosis (e.g., teriparatide), and sublingual tablets for angina chest pain (nitroglycerin SL). With systemic absorption, some percentage of the drug will move from the site of administration into the systemic circulation.

Dosage Form Dissolution and Drug Solubility

When an oral dosage form is ingested, it begins to dissolve in the gastrointestinal (GI) tract and the drug is released from it's dosage form which is typically a compressed tablet or a capsule. This is called dissolution. Dissolution is a function of the inactive matrix that is used to formulate the drug dosage form. Many pharmaceutical companies utilize biocompatible polymers to develop controlled release drug products with a predefined dissolution process. This can provide a more even drug concentration and reduce the dosing frequency. Or, the drug may be given in an immediate release formulation that dissolves fast and is absorbed rapidly. The formulation can be chosen to limit drug degradation in the gut; the drug can be destroyed in the gut (primarily by hydrolysis, or lysis with water) and making less available for absorption. Examples of drugs with "protective" coatings include enteric coated formulations such as bisacodyl and Entocort. Typically, the coating prevents drug dissolution in the acidic gut medium but permits dissolution in the basic medium of the intestine.

EC budesonide (Entocort®)

ASA (Ecotrin®)

micronization ↑ absorption by ↓ particle diameter => ↑ A surface

If the drug has poor absorption, one of the methods used to increase the dissolution rate is to reduce the particle diameter, which increases the surface area. Drugs with very small particle diameters are referred to as micronized, which used to mean the diameter was measured in micrometers, but now may refer to even smaller particle sizes measured in nanometers. Drugs with poor absorption that are "micronized" include progesterone and fenofibrate formulations. Without micronization, these drugs would be poorly absorbed. The rate of dissolution is described by the Noyes-Whitney equation.

micronized glyburide (Glynase®)

fenofibrate (Antara®)

Following dissolution, the drug that is released from the dosage form can be dissolved in GI fluids. The rate and extent to which the drug dissolves in the GI fluid depends on the solubility. Poorly soluble drugs are generally lipophilic, or lipid-loving. Freely soluble drugs are generally hydrophilic, or water-loving. As a drug moves through the GI tract, only dissolved drug is absorbed into the body. Thus poorly soluble drugs generally have poor systemic absorption, and highly soluble drugs often have good systemic absorption.

[handwritten top margin: systemic absorption — passive diffusion ← / → active transport]

Systemic Absorption

Absorption into the systemic circulation occurs via two primary processes, passive diffusion across the gut wall, or active transport via transporter proteins. Passive diffusion occurs when a high concentration of drug in the gut lumen moves to equalize drug concentration (reach an equilibrium) across the gut wall, thus reaching equilibrium. Drug particles move through the gut wall into the portal vein, unassisted by cellular machinery. Active transport occurs when drugs are moved across the gut wall via transporter proteins that are normally used to absorb nutrients from food.

Bioavailability

[handwritten: amount of drug that reaches systemic circulation → available to work @ site of axn]

The extent to which a drug is absorbed into the systemic circulation is called bioavailability. Bioavailability is the percentage of drug absorbed from extravascular administration relative to intravascular administration (e.g., IV bolus). Bioavailability is reported as a percentage from 0 to 100%. If the oral dose of a drug is the same as the IV dose (such as with levofloxacin or linezolid), then the bioavailability is 1, or 100%. With these two drugs, nearly 100% is absorbed and it makes it simple to convert from IV to PO. In many hospitals, these drugs are automatically converted to the same dose orally if the prescriber has written for the IV form and the patient can use the oral dose instead. This is part of the hospital's therapeutic interchange protocol. With most drugs, not all of the dose is absorbed, and the bioavailability is less than 100%; this means that the oral dose will need to be higher than the corresponding IV dose. A drug with good absorption characteristics will generally have a high bioavailability (> 70%), while a drug with poor absorption will have low bioavailability (<10%). Levofloxacin has high bioavailability; the oral and IV drug doses are the same. Bisphosphonates have low bioavailability, and the annual IV dose will be less than the weekly dose of the oral formulation.

[handwritten left margin: AUC → most reliable measure of F]

Bioavailability can be calculated using the area under the plasma concentration time curve, or AUC. The AUC represents the total exposure of drug following administration. The formula is shown here:

Absolute bioavailability, represented by F, is calculated using the following equation:

$$F\,(\%) \;=\; 100 \;\times\; \frac{AUC_{extravascular}}{AUC_{intravenous}} \;\times\; \frac{Dose_{intravenous}}{Dose_{extravascular}}$$

Distribution

Distribution is the process by which drug molecules move from the systemic circulation to the various tissues and organs of the body. Distribution occurs for intravascular and extravascular routes of administration. Distribution to tissues and organs in the body depends on the physical and chemical properties of the drug molecule and its interactions with membranes and tissues throughout the body. In general, drugs distribute evenly throughout the body based on the drug's lipophilicity, molecular weight, solubility, ionization status and the extent of protein binding. Human plasma contains many proteins, and albumin is the primary protein responsible for drug binding. If a drug is highly protein-bound (> 90%) and the albumin is low (< 3.5 g/dL), then a higher percentage of the drug will be in the unbound form, which

[handwritten bottom: distribution depends on: 1) lipophilicity 2) MW 3) solubility 4) ionization 5) protein binding]

"free PHT"
[ionized Ca++] } reflect *true* levels
(regardless of [albumin]) ⟹ no adjustment required

RxPrep Course Book | RxPrep © 2015

is able to interact with receptors and cause therapeutic or toxic effects. For two drugs in particular (phenytoin and valproate), and for calcium, if the albumin is low the true level will be higher than given on the lab report, unless the "free" level of phenytoin or the ionized calcium is reported. If the free phenytoin or ionized calcium is reported, there is no adjustment required. Otherwise, adjustment is required. The formulas to adjust the levels for low albumin are in the Calculation chapter (calcium) and Epilepsy chapter (phenytoin and valproate).

Volume of Distribution

The volume of distribution (V or Vd) is how large an area in the patient's body the drug has distributed into, and is based on the properties of that drug. The volume of distribution relates the amount of drug in the body to the concentration of drug measured in plasma (or serum). A dose of drug is administered (e.g., 10 mg), however, drug is measured as a concentration (amount per volume) from a sample of biological fluid. To convert between amounts and concentrations, a volume is needed. The equation for volume of distribution is:

> **SUBSCRIPTS IN FORMULAS**
>
> Vd can be written as V_d and ke can be written as k_e. In this chapter the subscripts are not used for Vd and Ke for simplicity.

$$Vd = \frac{\text{Amount of drug in body}}{\text{Concentration of drug in plasma}}$$

In the following problem, the Vd formula is used to solve for the amount of drug in the body one hour after the dose has been given: A 500 mg dose of acetaminophen is administered to a patient, and a blood sample is drawn one hour after administration. The concentration of acetaminophen is measured as 8 mcg/mL (which is 8 mg/L). To determine the total amount of drug remaining in the body, we need to multiply the concentration (8 mg/L) by a volume parameter. Acetaminophen has a volume of distribution of 51 L. Therefore, the amount of acetaminophen in the body 1 hour after dose administration is:

$$\text{Amount} = 8 \text{ mg/L} \times 51 \text{ L} = 408 \text{ mg}$$

Volume of distribution and physical volumes

Vd is a theoretical value, which is why it is sometimes called the "apparent" volume of distribution. Vd is not an "exact" physical volume that has been measured, but is a useful parameter because it is used to make inferences regarding the distribution of a drug in the body. The Vd of a drug can be very small, such as with warfarin (Vd = 8 L), or very large, such as with chloroquine (Vd = 15,000 L). Drugs that have a low Vd can be highly protein bound (like warfarin); the protein-binding limits diffusion through the lipid bilayer. More of the drug remains in the intravascular space (within the blood compartment). Chloroquine has an enormous Vd; chloroquine is lipophilic and becomes "sequestered" or "stuck" in the fatty tissue outside of the blood compartment.

high protein binding = ↓ Vd (limits diffusion through lipid bilayer)

Metabolism

Metabolism is the process by which a drug is converted from its original chemical structure into other forms to facilitate elimination from the body. For example, breaking carbon bonds or adding a hydroxyl group to a drug will make the drug more hydrophilic – this means more of the drug will stay in the blood, the blood passes through the kidneys, and the drug can be renally excreted. The original chemical form is called the "parent drug" and the additional forms are called "metabolites". Metabolism can occur throughout the body; however, the gut and liver are primary sites for drug metabolism due to high levels of metabolic enzymes in those tissues.

Metabolism is described in detail in the Drug Interactions chapter.

Excretion

can occur through
1. kidney → urine
2. liver → bile
3. gut → feces
4. lungs → exhaled air
5. skin → sweat

Excretion is the process of irreversible removal of drugs from the body. Excretion can occur via the kidney (urine), liver (bile), gut (feces), lungs (exhaled air) and skin (sweat). The primary routes of excretion for most drugs include the kidney (renal excretion) and the gut/liver (via metabolism). It should be noted that drug that is never absorbed cannot be excreted. Thus only drug that has been absorbed into the systemic circulation can be excreted from the body. Renal excretion is described in detail in the Renal Disease and Dosing Considerations chapter, and in the Calculations chapter.

Clearance and Area Under the Curve (AUC) $\left[\frac{mg \cdot hr}{L} \right]$

Clearance (Cl) describes the rate of drug removal in a certain volume of plasma over a certain amount of time. Since the liver and kidneys clear most of the drug (and these organs do not usually speed up or slow down), drug elimination occurs at a steady rate (the rate of elimination) which is proportional to the amount of the drug that has been taken. For example, example, if a patient takes two 325 mg acetaminophen tablets for a headache, the drug will have worn off in ~6 hours. If the same patient took one 325 mg tablet, it will have worn off in about the same amount of time. The rate of clearance (or elimination) was steady and proportional to the concentration of drug present in the body. The term clearance is used to describe the efficiency of drug removal from the body. Clearance is generally described by the following equation:

$$Cl = \frac{\text{Rate of Elimination (ke)}}{\text{Concentration}} \qquad \frac{L}{h} = \frac{mg/hr}{mg/L} = \frac{mg}{hr} \cdot \frac{L}{mg}$$

The rate of elimination, Ke, has units of mass per time expressed as h^{-1}, and drug concentration has units of concentration (e.g., mg/L); therefore clearance has units of volume per time (expressed as h-1). Because the rate of elimination is difficult to assess clinically, another method is used to calculate the clearance of a drug from the body:

$$F \times Dose = Cl \times AUC$$

Bioavailability, presented by F, is the amount of the drug that reaches the systemic circulation and is available to act at the site of action. The AUC is the most reliable measurement of the drug's bioavailability because it directly represents the amount of the drug that has reached the systemic concentration. The bioavailable dose (F x Dose) is the fraction of an extravascular dose that is absorbed and reaches the systemic circulation. The clearance (Cl/F) for extravascular administration is calculated with this formula:

$$\frac{Cl}{F} = \frac{Dose}{AUC}$$

Following IV administration, F = 1, which can be inserted into the previous equation to determine clearance for a drug given IV:

$$Cl = \frac{Dose}{AUC}$$

ZERO-ORDER, FIRST-ORDER AND MICHAELIS-MENTEN KINETICS

Most drugs follow first-order elimination or "first-order kinetics". The elimination of the drug occurs at a constant rate, which is proportional to the dose or amount of drug remaining in the body. For example, a 325 mg dose of acetaminophen is eliminated at the same rate as a 650 mg dose – but half as much of the lower dose will be eliminated (over a given time) because the elimination is proportional to the dose. With zero-order elimination, a constant amount of drug (mg) is removed per unit of time no matter how much drug is in the body (see table below for example).

Zero-Order vs First-Order Pharmacokinetics

	ZERO-ORDER			FIRST-ORDER		
HOUR	Amount of Drug (mg)	Fraction Removed in Previous Hour	Amount (mg) Removed in Previous Hour	Amount of Drug (mg)	Fraction Removed in Previous Hour	Amount (mg) Removed in Previous Hour
0	2,000			2,000		
1	1,700	0.1500	300	1,600	0.2	400
2	1,400	0.1764	300	1,280	0.2	320
3	1,100	0.2143	300	1,024	0.2	256

Michaelis-Menten

Michaelis-Menten, or saturable kinetics, begins as first-order, but when the metabolism becomes saturated, the concentration increases disproportionately. Drugs with this type of kinetics begin as first-order kinetics, but can change to zero-order once a certain dose is reached and metabolizing enzymes are saturated. Phenytoin, theophylline and voriconazole have this type of saturable kinetics. With saturable kinetics, a small increase in dose may result in a large increase in drug concentration at steady state.

⇒ 0 order

Michaelis-Menten Kinetics – Example

A patient has been using phenytoin 100 mg three times daily. The phenytoin level was taken and found to be 6.8 mcg/mL. The physician increased the dose to 100 mg with breakfast and lunch and 200 mg with dinner. The patient started to slur her words, felt fatigued and returned to the physician's office. The level was retaken and found to be 22.7 mcg/mL. The most likely explanation for the increase in phenytoin level is that although first-order kinetics took place initially, when the dose was increased, the metabolism became saturated, and the steady-state level increased dramatically.

Elimination Rate Constant

The elimination rate constant (ke) is the fraction of the drug that is eliminated (cleared) per unit of time. It is calculated from the Vd and the clearance:

$$ke = \frac{Cl}{Vd} \qquad Cl = Vd \cdot ke$$

For example, if a drug has a Vd of 50 liters and a Cl of 5 liters/hour, the ke is 0.1 hr⁻¹ and 10% of the drug is cleared per hour.

The ke can also be calculated by fitting data points during the elimination phase to a single exponential. The second formula is derived from the definition of C_2:

$$C_2 = C_1 e^{-ket}$$

$$ke = \frac{-\ln(C_1/C_2)}{t} \qquad t = \text{time between } C_1 \& C_2 \; (= t_2 - t_1)$$

where C_1 = the first or higher drug concentration (sometimes the peak concentration), C_2 = the second or lower drug concentration, ke = elimination rate constant, and t = time between C_1 and C_2.

Half-life

The time required for the drug concentration (and drug amount) to decrease by 50% is called the elimination half-life. For example, it takes 5 hours for theophylline concentrations to fall from 16 to 8 mg/L. Thus the half-life of theophylline is 5 hours. It would take 5 more hours for the drug concentration to fall from 8 mg/L to 4 mg/L. It is important to note that the half-life is independent of the drug concentration (for drugs exhibiting first-order kinetics).

The half-life of a drug can be calculated from the ke as shown below

$$t_{1/2} = \frac{0.693}{ke}$$

The half-life of a drug can be used to calculate the time required for drug washout or the time required to achieve steady-state as shown in the following table. Steady state is an important concept in pharmacy, because drug levels are generally (but not always) collected at steady state to obtain clinically useful information. When a fixed dose is administered at regular intervals, the drug accumulates until it reaches steady state where the rate of drug intake equals the rate of drug elimination. The time required to reach steady state depends on the elimination half-life of the drug. If the drug follows first-order kinetics (described previously) in a one-compartment distribution model (the drug is rapidly and evenly distributed throughout the body) and if a loading dose has not been given, it takes ~5 half-lives to reach steady state.

Relationship Between Half-Life, Percent of Drug Remaining and Percent of Steady-State Achieved

# OF HALF-LIVES	% OF DRUG REMAINING	% OF STEADY-STATE ACHIEVED
1	50	50
2	25	75
3	12.5	87.5
4	6.25	93.8
5	3.13	96.9

Half-life example

Tetracycline has a clearance of 7.014 L/hr and a volume of distribution of 105 L. Calculate the half-life of tetracycline and the time required for elimination of greater than 95% of the drug from the body.

Using the equation for the terminal elimination rate constant and the equation for half-life, calculate the following:

$$ke = \frac{Cl}{Vd} = \frac{7.014 \text{ L/hr}}{105 \text{ L}} = 0.0668 \text{ hr}^{-1}$$

$$t_{\frac{1}{2}} = \frac{0.693}{ke}$$

$$t_{\frac{1}{2}} = \frac{0.693}{0.0668 \text{ hr}^{-1}} = 10.4 \text{ hours}$$

Using the values in the table on the preceding page, notice that <u>5 half-lives are required to eliminate more than 95% of the drug</u>. Thus, the time required is 5 x 10.4 hours = 52 hours.

to reach ss of tetracycline

Examples of Various Half-Life Calculations

A patient receives 200 mg of a drug with a half-life of 5 hours. How much of the drug still remains in the patient after 10 hours?

- 10 hours = 2 half-lives:

- 200 mg/2 (or reduced by 50%) = 100 mg (amount of drug left after one half-life)

- 100 mg/2 = 50 mg is left after 10 hours (2 half-lives)

The serum concentration of Drug A over time is plotted below. What is the half-life of Drug A?

Choose two times (in hours) where the drug concentration has decreased by half to find the half-life

- For example, at 2 hours the concentration is 12 mcg/ml and at 4 hours the concentration is 6 mcg/mL.

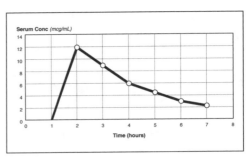

$$ke = \frac{0.693}{5 \text{ hrs}} = 0.1386 \text{ hrs}^{-1}$$

$$C_2 = 200 \text{mg} \cdot e^{-0.1386 \times 10}$$

$$= 50 \text{ mg}$$

91

■ It takes 2 hours for the concentration to decrease by 50%; the half-life is 2 hours.

This problem can also be solved mathematically:

$$C_2 = C_1 e^{-ket}$$

$$6 = 12 e^{-(ke) 2}$$

$$ke = \frac{-\ln \frac{6}{12}}{2} = 0.35 \ hr^{-1}$$

$$t_{1/2} = \frac{0.693}{ke} = \frac{0.693}{0.35} = 2 \ hours$$

Pharmacokinetic Models

The behavior of a drug in the body is complex. In order to attempt to predict both the time and the course of the drug in the body, simplified "compartment" models are used. A one compartment model is used most frequently and is the simplest: the drug enters the body into the one compartment (all the tissues and fluids are part of this one compartment), and then is eliminated. If the drug is given by IV bolus, no absorption is required and the drug rapidly distributes throughout the body. The concentration in the tissues is proportional to the concentration in the body, and the elimination is a first-order process. The figure demonstrates a one compartment model, where b is the IV bolus, Vd is the volume of the compartment and ke is the elimination rate constant:

The concentration of drug in the body at time (t) after the bolus injection is described by the one compartment linear bolus equation:

 after bolus admin

$$C = \frac{D}{Vd} e^{-ket}$$

Where C = concentration at time (t) after the IV bolus administration.

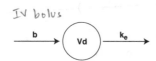 *IV bolus*

Single Dose IV Bolus Example

A patient is to be given a single dose of tobramycin 500 mg by IV bolus injection. His estimated Vd = 20 L and ke = 0.34 h^{-1}. What are the estimated plasma concentrations at 1 hour and 12 hours after the injection?

$$C = \frac{D}{Vd} e^{-ket}$$

$$C = \frac{500}{20} e^{-(0.34)(1)} = 17.8 \ mg/L$$

$$C = \frac{500}{20} e^{-(0.34)ke(12)} = 0.42 \ mg/L$$

NARROW THERAPEUTIC INDEX DRUGS: USE CAUTION
Drugs with a narrow therapeutic index (including aminoglycosides) require careful monitoring of the amount of drug exposure. Why? Because the plasma concentration required for efficacy is close to the concentration that produces toxicity.

Therefore, the estimated plasma concentrations at 1 and 12 hours after the injection are 17.8 and 0.42 mg/L respectively. The level at 12 hours could also be calculated based on the level at 1 hour:

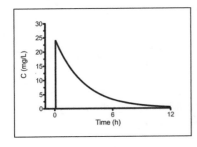

$$C_2 = C_1 e^{-ket}$$

$t_2 - t_1 = 12\ hrs - 1\ hr = 11\ hrs$

$$C_2 = 17.8\ e^{-(0.34)(11)} = 0.42\ mg/L$$

Typically more than one dose of medication is required. The preferred time to take the drug level is at steady state; see the Lab Values chapter. This formula is used to calculate the concentration at steady state when multiple IV doses are given:

Multiple-Dose (Steady State) IV Bolus Equation

$C\ @\ SS$

$$C = \frac{\dfrac{D}{Vd} e^{-ket}}{1 - e^{-ke\tau}}$$

where C = steady state concentration, D = dose, Vd = volume of distribution, ke = elimination rate constant, t = time between injection and when C is targeted, and τ = dosing interval.

Multiple-Dose (Steady State) IV Bolus Example

A 50 kg female patient will be initiated on vancomycin 1,000 mg IV Q12H for empiric treatment of pneumonia due to methicillin-resistant *Staphylococcus aureus*. The population PK parameter estimates for this patient are Vd = 35 L and ke = 0.06 h⁻¹. Calculate the predicted steady state trough concentration.

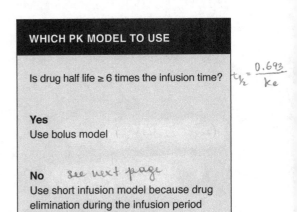

WHICH PK MODEL TO USE

Is drug half life ≥ 6 times the infusion time? $t_{1/2} = \dfrac{0.693}{ke}$

Yes
Use bolus model

No *see next page*
Use short infusion model because drug elimination during the infusion period could be significant

Vancomycin is typically infused over 1 hour (or longer) rather than with a bolus to avoid rapid infusion related "redman" adverse effects (e.g., hypotension, pruritus). Since the 1 hour infusion is short compared to the patient's estimated half-life of 11.6 hours (see side bar), we can utilize the bolus model since no significant drug will be eliminated during the infusion time.

$$C = \frac{\dfrac{D}{Vd} e^{-ke\tau}}{1 - e^{-ke\tau}} \qquad\qquad C = \frac{\dfrac{1,000}{35} e^{-(0.06)12}}{1 - e^{-(0.06)(12)}} = 27\ mg/L$$

Therefore, the steady state vancomycin trough level is estimated to be 27 mg/L. Estimating the trough concentration for vancomycin empirically is important to maximize bacterial killing and minimize the risk for acute kidney injury. The patient in this example is being treated for MRSA pneumonia which requires a target trough concentration of 15 – 20 mg/L, but nephrotoxicity is associated with elevated trough concentrations. The goal is to maintain trough concentrations < 20 mg/L. In the example above the predicted steady state trough is too high. Since the steady state trough concentration is proportional to the dose, a more suitable dose can be calculated by a simple ratio. Vancomycin doses are generally rounded off in 250 mg increments, so the options are to reduce the dose to 750 mg Q12H or 500 mg Q12H. A steady state trough for each regimen can be predicted with a ratio like this:

$$\frac{27\ mg/L}{x} = \frac{1{,}000\ mg}{750\ mg} \quad x = \sim20.3\ mg/L \qquad \frac{27\ mg/L}{x} = \frac{1{,}000\ mg}{500\ mg} \quad x = \sim13.5\ mg/L$$

Remember, these are estimations. Either trough value could come back higher or lower than predicted. In this case, evaluate the patient and decide which to recommend.

The time to reach steady state is based on the half-life (0.693/0.06 = 11.6 hours); therefore, steady state will be achieved in 58 hours (5 half lives x 11.6 hours).

Multiple-Dose (Steady State) Short Infusion Example

A patient is initiated on gentamicin 200 mg IV infusion over 30 minutes Q12H for nosocomial pneumonia. The population PK parameter estimates for this patient are Vd = 17.5 L and ke = 0.3 h^{-1}. What are the estimated steady state plasma concentrations at 1 hour (peak) and 12 hours (trough) after the start of the infusion?

Short Infusion Model

$$C = \frac{\frac{D}{t_{in}}}{Cl}(1-e^{-ke\,t_{in}})}{1-e^{-ke\tau}} e^{-ke\,t^\wedge}$$

$$\frac{\frac{200}{0.5}}{0.3\cdot17.5}\left(1-e^{-0.3\times0.5}\right)}{1-e^{-0.3\times12}}\ e^{-0.3\times1}$$

Where C = steady state concentration, D = dose, t_{in} = infusion time, Cl = clearance (ke x Vd), τ = dosing interval, $t^\wedge$ = time from end of infusion to the time of the drug concentration draw, ke = elimination rate constant.

Therefore, the peak concentration at 1 hour can be calculated as follows:

$$C = \frac{\frac{\frac{D}{t_{in}}}{Cl}(1-e^{-ke\,t_{in}})}{1-e^{-ke\tau}} e^{-ke\,t^\wedge}$$

$$C = \frac{\frac{\frac{200}{0.5}}{17.5(0.3)}\left(1-e^{-0.3(0.5)}\right)}{1-e^{-0.3(12)}} e^{-0.3(1)}$$

$$C = 8.1\ mg/L$$

The trough concentration at 12 hours can be calculated based on the peak concentration as before:

$$C_2 = C_1 e^{-k_e t}$$

$$C_2 = 8.1 e^{-(0.3)(11)} = 0.3 \text{ mg/L}$$

Therefore, the steady state peak and trough gentamicin plasma levels are estimated to be 8.1 mg/L and 0.3 mg/L respectively. Estimating the peak and trough concentrations for the aminoglycoside antibiotics is important to maximize bacterial killing and minimize the risk for acute kidney injury and ototoxicity. The bactericidal activity of the aminoglycoside antibiotics is concentration dependent; therefore, the goal is to maximize the peak concentration. Nephrotoxicity and ototoxicity of the aminoglycosides is associated with elevated trough concentrations; therefore, the goal is to minimize trough concentrations. For traditional multiple daily dosing of gentamicin and tobramycin the peak and trough goals are in the ranges of 5 – 10 mg/L and < 2 mg/L respectively. Therefore, the predicted steady state gentamicin levels for this patient are within goal with the dosing regimen of 200 mg IV Q12H.

The time to reach steady state is based on the half-life.

$T_{1/2} = 0.693/k_e = 0.693/0.3 = 2.3$ hours. After ~12 hours (5 half lives x 2.3 hours) the drug would be expected to reach steady state.

Revised Pharmacokinetic Parameters and Dosing Regimen

The patient continues on gentamicin 200 mg IV bolus Q12H and blood samples obtained 1 hour and 12 hours after the third dose measure 9.5 mg/L and 2.1 mg/L respectively. What are the revised pharmacokinetic parameters and modified dosing regimen to achieve steady state peak (7 - 10 mg/L for pulmonary infection) and trough (< 2 mg/L) concentrations respectively?

While the population models provide a good estimation of the predicted drug concentration, there remains significant interpatient variability. Since the aminoglycosides have the potential to cause acute kidney injury and ototoxicity, we need to be precise in the dosing regimen to minimize the risk of these adverse effects. By obtaining measured drug levels in the patient we can directly assess the levels and use them to determine the revised pharmacokinetic parameters. The revised PK parameters are patient specific and can be used to calculate the optimal dosing regimen for the patient to achieve the targeted drug concentrations.

We can determine the revised elimination rate constant using the measured drug concentrations:

$$C_2 = C_1 e^{-k_e t}$$

$$2.1 = 9.5 e^{-k(11)}$$

$$k_e = 0.14 \text{ h}^{-1}$$

$$0.22 = e^{-k \cdot 11}$$

$$\ln(0.22) = -k \times 11$$

$$k = \frac{\ln(0.22)}{-11}$$

The revised volume of distribution can be calculated from the measured drug level using the steady state IV bolus model, since the revised half-life (5 hours) is long compared with the infusion time (30 minutes).

$$C = \frac{\frac{D}{Vd} e^{-k_e t}}{1-e^{-k_e \tau}}$$

$$9.5 = \frac{\frac{200}{Vd} e^{-0.14(1)}}{1-e^{-0.14(12)}}$$

$$Vd = 22.5 \text{ L}$$

The revised volume of distribution is a bit larger than the population estimate, but the elimination rate constant is much smaller than the population estimate which explains why the measured trough concentration is much higher than expected.

With the revised pharmacokinetic parameters we can now determine a modified dosing regimen to achieve the goal concentrations. We can start by choosing a target peak concentration of 8 mg/L, which is in the middle of the target range of 7-10 mg/L.

$$C = \frac{\frac{D}{Vd} e^{-k_e t}}{1-e^{-k_e \tau}}$$

$$8 = \frac{\frac{D}{22.5} e^{-0.14(1)}}{1-e^{-0.14(12)}}$$

$$D = 168.5, \sim 160 \text{ mg IV Q12H (gentamicin is often rounded in increments of 40 mg)}$$

The trough can be calculated based on the peak concentration and the revised elimination rate constant:

$$C_{trough} = C_{peak} e^{-k_e t}$$

$$C_{trough} = 8 e^{-0.14(11)}$$

$$C_{trough} = 1.7 \text{ mg/L}$$

Therefore, a revised dose of 160 mg IV over 30 minutes Q12H would provide new steady state peak and trough concentrations within the goal range.

The Pharmacokinetic Consult

In practice, pharmacists are consulted to recommend doses that will achieve therapeutic levels. In the examples thus far, ke and Vd have been provided. Population estimates for certain pharmacokinetic parameters are available and widely used as a starting point for empiric calculations. Following are examples of a couple of population PK models for vancomycin and aminoglycosides.

VANCOMYCIN	AMINOGLYCOSIDES
ke = 0.00083(CrCl) + 0.0044	ke = 0.00293 (CrCl) + 0.014
Vd = 0.7 L/kg (use actual body weight*)	Vd = 0.3 L/kg (use actual body weight*)
Usual dose: 15 mg/kg (actual body weight) IV Q12H or Q8H, adjusted for renal insufficiency	Extended-interval aminoglycoside dosing (EIAD) used most commonly for adult dosing in many institutions

* General recommendations – may not apply in all clinical circumstances (e.g., extreme obesity)

Step #1: Do baseline calculations (actual body weight, CrCl, ke, $t_{1/2}$, Vd), estimate dose and interval.

Step #2: Use the dose and interval from Step #1 to solve for estimated steady state peak and trough. Step #2 can be done as many times as needed (with different doses and intervals) until the desired peak and trough are obtained.

Loading Dose Example – Digoxin

A patient is to be initiated on daily oral digoxin for management of atrial fibrillation. The population parameters are F = 0.6, Vd = 500 L, Cl = 120 L/day. What is an appropriate loading dose to rapidly achieve a peak concentration of 1.5 mcg/L?

Administration of a loading dose is needed when the goal is to rapidly achieve therapeutic concentrations. In particular, if the half-life of the drug is long relative to the frequency of administration, it will take several doses before steady state is achieved. In this case, the half life is 0.693/k = 0.693/(Cl/V) = 0.693/(120/500) = 2.9 days. Steady state would be achieved after 5 half-lives = 5 x (2.9) = ~15 days. Therefore, it is beneficial to administer a loading dose to rapidly achieve the targeted levels.

Loading dose   = Desired concentration (Vd)/F

Loading dose   = 1.5 mcg/L (500 L)/0.6

Loading dose   = 1,250 mcg = 1.25 mg

Cl = Vd · ke

$$C = \frac{\frac{D}{Vd}\, e^{-ke\tau}}{1 - e^{-ke\tau}} = \frac{\frac{1250}{59}\, e^{-0.072 \cdot 12}}{1 - e^{-0.072 \cdot 12}} = 15.43 \text{ trough @ 12 hrs}$$

PRACTICE CASE

A 52 y/o male patient with a history a MRSA-positive abscess has been brought to the ER from the local jail. He reports a 3-day history of increasing swelling, pain and erythema of his left lower extremity. Ultrasound of the extremity reveals mild soft tissue swelling and no DVT. He will be admitted for treatment of cellulitis. Orders are entered in the EHR for vancomycin and a pharmacy PK consult. The patient weighs 185 lbs, is 5'10" and his SCr is 1.1 mg/dL.

Questions

$$CrCl = \frac{(140-52)\ SD + 2.3 \times 10}{72 \times 1.1} = 81.11$$

1. Which of the following best represents the patient's vancomycin ke and Vd using population estimates. Use ideal body weight for CrCl and actual body weight for Vd.

   a. $ke = 0.072\ hr^{-1}$, $Vd = 59\ L$ $ke = 0.0717$
   b. $ke = 0.082\ hr^{-1}$, $Vd = 51\ L$ $Vd = 58.86$
   c. $ke = 0.072\ hr^{-1}$, $Vd = 51\ L$
   d. $ke = 0.062\ hr^{-1}$, $Vd = 59\ L$
   e. $ke = 0.082\ hr^{-1}$, $Vd = 129\ L$

2. The patient is started on vancomycin 1250 mg IV Q12H. Vancomycin is infused over 90 minutes and peak levels are drawn 1 hour after the infusion. Which of the following are the estimated steady state peak and trough (using the bolus model)?*

   a. Peak = 15 mg/L and Trough = 8 mg/L
   b. Peak = 13 mg/L and Trough = 9 mg/L
   c. Peak = 34 mg/L and Trough = 12 mg/L
   d. Peak = 42 mg/L and Trough = 21 mg/L
   e. Peak = 34 mg/L and Trough = 15 mg/L

3. What is the goal vancomycin trough for the MRSA abscess? Based on the answer you selected to question #2, is vancomycin 1250 mg IV Q12H an appropriate regimen for this patient?

4. Calculate an expected steady state peak (1 hour after infusion) and trough with this regimen. Use the short infusion model. The hospital infuses vancomycin over 90 minutes and peak levels are drawn 1 hour after the infusion. Use ideal body weight for CrCl and actual body weight for Vd.

   a. Peak = 35 mg/L and Trough = 19 mg/L
   b. Peak = 42 mg/L and Trough = 23 mg/L
   c. Peak = 27 mg/L and Trough = 12 mg/L
   d. Peak = 20 mg/L and Trough = 11 mg/L
   e. Peak = 53 mg/L and Trough = 13 mg/L

5. The patient's nurse calls the pharmacy a few hours after the first dose. The patient only has one IV line and multiple medication compatibility and timing issues. If the dose was changed to vancomycin 2 gm IV Q12H (to avoid compatibility issues with Zosyn), what is the estimated steady state trough? Use the same PK estimates and models from the previous question.

   a. Trough = 5 mg/L
   b. Trough = 7 mg/L
   c. Trough = 9 mg/L
   d. Trough = 10 mg/L
   e. Trough = 12 mg/L

Questions 4-5 apply to the following case.

$$IBW = 50 + 2.3 \times 13 = 80$$

A 46 y/o male patient (205 lbs and 6'1") has been in the ICU for 7 days after a motor vehicle accident. He has been on a ventilator since admission. Today he spiked a temperature to 101.3 F and the CXR shows a new infiltrate. His SCr is 0.8 mg/dL. Orders are written for vancomycin, tobramycin, and prolonged infusion piperacillin-tazobactam. A pharmacy PK consult is ordered to dose the antibiotics and an order for vancomycin 1250 mg IV Q8H is quickly profiled on the EHR.

$$CrCl = \frac{(140-46)\ 80}{72 \cdot 0.8} = 130.56\ ml/min$$

$$Vd = 65.23\ L$$
$$ke = 0.113\ hr^{-1} \Rightarrow$$

$$C = \frac{\frac{D}{Vd}\, e^{-ke\tau}}{1 - e^{-ke\tau}} = \frac{\frac{1250}{65.23} \cdot e^{-0.113 \times 8}}{1 - e^{-0.113 \times 8}} = \frac{\frac{1250}{65.23} \cdot e^{-0.113 \times 8}}{1 - e^{-0.113 \times 8}}$$

$$= 13.04$$

Answers

1-a, 2-e, 3- 10-15 mg/L for treating the abscess. This dose will treat the infection, but may be more than necessary and would require additional calculations to see if a lower dose could provide a trough in the target range without dropping the trough < 10 mg/L, 4-c, 5-d

* Although peak vancomycin levels are not recommended per the ASHP/IDSA guidelines, follow the instructions and calculate them.

DRUG FORMULATIONS & DURABLE MEDICAL EQUIPMENT (DME)

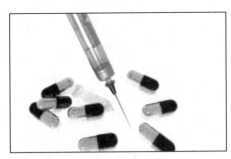

DRUG FORMULATION CONSIDERATIONS

Compressed tablets are the least expensive drug formulation to manufacture and the most common formulation type. Capsules are also relatively inexpensive to make. If a pharmaceutical company develops a drug in any other formulation the cost will be higher – and a patient group that would benefit from the new formulation would be required. Prednisone 10 mg tablets cost < 25¢ per tablet. A similar steroid in an oral disintegrating formulation (ODT), *Orapred ODT*, is branded and is ~$16 per tablet. The higher-priced formulation might be beneficial in a child with facial swelling who might choke on a hard tablet or who cannot yet swallow tablets.

It is helpful to recall a drug's formulation types by asking two questions:

1) Who typically uses this drug?

2) Would there be a reason to have this type of formulation for this patient population?

This can be useful on the exam if unsure if the formulation exists.

Examples

Olanzapine

Olanzapine is an antipsychotic with various formulations available: immediate-release (IR) tablet, oral disintegrating tablet, short-acting injection, and long-acting injection.

Who uses this drug? People with schizophrenia, bipolar disorder or some type of psychosis.

What types of formulations would be beneficial? The majority of patients with schizophrenia discontinue antipsychotics. It is useful to deliver the drug in a long-acting injection to improve adherence. A few of the antipsychotics come as orally disintegrating tablets (ODTs) – these are useful to block the patient from hiding the medication in the mouth ("cheeking") and then spitting it out when no one is watching. The ODT formulations dissolve in the mouth quickly which prevents cheeking. The fast-acting injection works quickly and is useful for acute agitation.

Ondansetron

Ondansetron, a 5-HT$_3$-receptor antagonist used to prevent or treat nausea is available in with various formulations available: IR tablet, short-acting injection, oral solution, ODT and oral film.

Who uses this drug? Patients receiving emetogenic chemotherapy or any other emetogenic drug, post-surgical patients, opioid-naïve patients using opioids acutely or with any condition that causes nausea/vomiting.

What types of formulations would be beneficial? If vomiting is an issue, oral medications would be useless and the injection would be used instead. If there is nausea alone, the ODT or the film or the injection can be given. ODTs are preferred if there is dysphagia, which could be present due to age and/or a medical condition, including cancer. It would be difficult to swallow tablets with painful esophageal ulcers, strictures or tumors. Films can be placed on or under the tongue or along the inside of the cheek and provide similar benefit to ODTs. With some film formulations the loss to first-pass metabolism is reduced. The oral solution would be preferable if the patient has an NG-tube or any dysphagia or pain from solid oral formulations. The solution can be swallowed directly and is sweetened with sorbitol to mask the bitter taste of the medicine. One of the 5-HT$_3$-receptor antagonists comes in a long-acting patch (Sancuso) that reduces nausea for up to seven days; this would be useful for a patient with nausea from chemotherapy that lasts awhile. The patch is put on prior to chemo (not useful for nausea happening when the patch is first applied) since, like most patches, it takes time for drug absorption through the skin. This summary chart contains select medications and the reasoning behind the unique formulation(s).

Select Medications in Unique Formulations

FORMULATION	EXAMPLES	REASONS FOR USE
ODTs – placed on the tongue and disintegrate rapidly in saliva	Niravam – alprazolam Abilify Discmelt – aripiprazole Parcopa – carbidopa/levodopa Zyrtec Allergy Children – cetirizine FazaClo – clozapine Aricept ODT – Donepezil Prevacid SoluTab – lansoprazole Lamictal ODT – lamotrigine Metozolv ODT – metoclopramide Remeron SolTab – mirtazapine Zyprexa Zydis – olanzapine Zofran ODT – ondansetron Orapred ODT – prednisone Risperdal M-TAB – risperidone Maxalt-MLT – rizatriptan Zelapar – selegiline Staxyn – vardenafil Zomig ZMT – zolmitriptan	Dysphagia – trouble swallowing due to a variety of reasons: Stroke is the #1 cause of dysphagia due to paralysis of the throat muscles. Dysphagia can be due to esophagitis, esophageal tumors, ↓ LES pressure/reflux, facial swelling from an allergic reaction, or with other conditions that worsen motor function, including multiple sclerosis and Parkinson disease. Children are often too young to swallow tablets or capsules. Nausea can make it difficult to tolerate anything orally, however, ODTs cause less nausea than oral formulations swallowed whole. If vomiting is present or is likely a non-oral route should be used. Non-adherence – ODTs prevent holding the drug in the corner of the mouth to spit out shortly afterward – the tablet would dissolve quickly and the caregiver could follow with a drink of water.

Common (Select) Medications Given in Unique Formulations Continued

FORMULATION	EXAMPLES	REASONS FOR USE
Films that use gut absorption	*Zuplenz* – ondansetron Many OTC products used for children come as films, and films are used for some adult OTC drugs and for breath fresheners.	Films have similar benefits to ODTs; they dissolve in the mouth easily and do not have issues associated with swallowing.
Lozenges for oral mucosa drug administration	*Mycelex* – clotrimazole troche	Used to treat a condition in the oral mucosa – the drug is held in the mouth while the troche slowly dissolves.
Sublingual (SL) or buccal delivery with tablets, film, or sprays	*Saphris* – asenapine SL tablet *Edluar* – zolpidem SL tablet *Intermezzo* – zolpidem SL tablet *Nitrostat* – nitroglycerin SL tablet *Nitrolingual, NitroMist* – nitroglycerin SL spray *Bunavail* – buprenorphine/naloxone buccal film *Onsolis* – fentanyl buccal film *Subsys* – fentanyl SL spray *Actiq* – fentanyl buccal lozenge *Fentora* – fentanyl buccal tablet *Abstral* – fentanyl SL tablet	SL and buccal absorption has a faster onset than a tablet or capsule that is swallowed; the drug is readily absorbed into the venous circulation right under the absorption site (e.g., under the tongue). Less of the drug is lost to gut degradation and first-pass metabolism.
Nasal sprays (NS)	*Lazanda* – fentanyl NS *Fortical, Miacalcin* – calcitonin NS *Flumist* – influenza live vaccine NS *Nascobal* – cyanocobalamin (vitamin B 12) NS *Sprix* – ketorolac NS *Imitrex* – sumatriptan NS *Zomig* – zolmitriptan NS *Afrin* – oxymetazoline NS *Flonase* – fluticasone NS	Nasal sprays such as *Afrin* and *Flonase* are used primarily to treat localized nasal symptoms. The nasal route has a faster onset than the GI route, and is useful for acute conditions that should be treated quickly, including pain. Nasal sprays bypass gut absorption; proteins that would get destroyed in the gut (calcitonin) can be given nasally. A compound that requires a gut factor for absorption can also be given nasally (vitamin B12).
Creams, ointments, gels, solutions for topical conditions	*Abreva* – docosanol cream *Latisse* – bimatoprost gel *Bactroban* – mupirocin ointment Many others, including topical retinoids and benzoyl peroxide or salicylic acid products for acne, psoriasis treatments, first aid products, steroid creams and ointments & topical antifungals.	Topical treatments used for topical conditions have a decreased incidence of systemic side effects and generally provide faster relief. Common conditions treated topically include cold sores, acne, eczema, inflammation, mild infections, hair loss, rash, fungal infections, viral sores, hypotrichosis.
Topicals for systemic conditions	*Nitro-Bid* – nitroglycerin ointment *AndroGel* and other hormones	

Common (Select) Medications Given in Unique Formulations Continued

FORMULATION	EXAMPLES	REASONS FOR USE
Injections that patients can self-administer (mostly SC)	*Imitrex* – sumatriptan *Arixtra* – fondaparinux *Lovenox* – enoxaparin *Humira* – adalimumab *EpiPen* – epinephrine *Enbrel* – etanercept *Evzio* – naloxone *Simponi* – golimumab *Copaxone* – glatiramer *Peg-Intron, Rebif* – and other interferons *Physicians EZ Use B-12* – cyanocobalamin (vitamin B12) *Aranesp* – darbepoetin alfa *Epogen/Procrit* – epoetin alfa	SC administration is used for acute relief (such as pain, with triptans) or for stat treatment of a severe condition (such as opioid overdose with *Evzio* or bronchoconstriction with the *EpiPen*) or, for drugs that would get destroyed or not absorbed if given by oral administration (enoxaparin). The erythropoiesis stimulating agents (ESAs) are given SC by patients with impaired renal function, and if in ESRD, are given IV at the dialysis center.
Chewable Tablets	Many OTCs (*Pepto-Bismol, Immodium, Claritin*) *Augmentin* – amoxicillin/clavulanate *Suprax* – cefixime *Amoxil* – amoxicillin *Dilantin Infatabs* – phenytoin *Fosrenol* – lanthanum (must chew for drug to bind gut phosphate) *Singulair* – montelukast *Lamictal CD* – lamotrigine *Methylin* – methyphenidate	These are primarily used for children who are unable to swallow tablets. A few are for adults; calcium citrate tablets are large, and chewable calcium products are easier to tolerate. Note that *Pepto-Bismol* and *Immodium* are used for diarrhea; with a gut infection, nausea could be present.
Long-Acting Oral Tablets/Capsules Some capsules can be opened and the beads put in a small amount of soft food-instruct the patient to swallow without chewing. Note the danger if long-acting formulations are crushed: a fatal dose could be released. This includes ER opioids. Be sure to look for the suffix and counsel. There are a few long-acting formulations that can be cut at the score line – but still NOT crushed, such as *Toprol XL* and *Sinemet CR*.	*Concerta* *Detrol LA* Do not crush or chew any drug that has the following suffix that indicates it is a long-acting formulation: XR, ER, LA, SR, CR, CRT, SA, TR, TD, or have 24 in the name, or the ending –cont (for controlled release), or timecaps or sprinkles.	Certain drugs are designed as slow release or are enteric-coated to avoid irritation to the GI lining or are designed to dissolve in the small intestine. Or, the drug may be designed to release drug slowly to avoid nausea or to provide a long-duration of action to avoid repeated day-time dosing. Providing a smooth level of drug release over time reduces high "peaks" which reduces side effects due to too much drug hitting the "wrong" receptor and provides a safe level of drug over the dosing interval. This is required for conditions that require steady drug levels such as with epilepsy, hypertension, and with many others.

Common (Select) Medications Given in Unique Formulations Continued

FORMULATION	EXAMPLES	REASONS FOR USE
Granules, powders or capsules that can be opened and sprinkled into soft food or water Typically these are long-acting beads - if they sit in soft food the liquid will ruin the slow release. The food must not be warm or the beads will dissolve. Instruct patients to consume right after they sprinkle or stir; do not chew if long-acting or an irritant. To swallow <u>without chewing</u> requires that the drug be placed in a <u>small amount of soft food</u>.	*Avinza* – morphine, on applesauce or soft food *Kadian* – morphine, on applesauce or soft food *Monurol* – fosfomycin, in 3-4 ounces cool water *Micro-K* – potassium, on applesauce or pudding *Coreg CR* – carvedilol, on applesauce *Creon, Lip-Prot-Amyl, Pancreaze, Pertzye, Ultresa, Viokace, Zenpep* – pancrelipase, on soft food with low pH (applesauce, pureed pears or banana) *Depakote Sprinkle* – valproic acid, on soft food *Namenda XR* – memantine, on applesauce *Ritalin LA, Metadate CD, Adderall XR* – methylphenidate, on applesauce *Focalin XR* – dexmethylphenidate, on applesauce *Adderall XR* – dextroamphetamine/amphetamine ER, on applesauce *Vyvanse* – lisdexamfetamine, in water, yogurt or orange juice *Singulair* – montelukast granules, in 5 mL baby formula or breast milk or in a spoonful of applesauce, carrots, rice or ice cream *Topamax Sprinkle* – topiramate, on soft food *Dexilant* – dexlansoprazole, in applesauce or acidic juice *Prevacid* – lansoprazole, in applesauce or acidic juice *Nexium* – esomeprazole, in applesauce or acidic juice *Prilosec* – omeprazole, in applesauce or water *Welchol* – colesevelam, in 4-8 oz water, fruit juice or diet soda *Colestid* – colestipol, in at least 3 oz of liquid *Questran, Questran Light, Prevalite* – cholestyramine, in 2-6 oz water or non-carbonated liquid	These are used primarily for geriatric and pediatric patients who have some type of swallowing issue. Sometimes the capsule or tablet is too large to swallow. Instruct patient <u>not to chew</u> any long-acting pellets or beads that are emptied out from a capsule, <u>not to let the mixture sit too long</u> (take within the time directed) and <u>not to add to anything warm or hot</u> (the contents will dissolve too quickly).
Patches	See chart of common patches later in this chapter; a few examples are listed here: *Exelon* – rivastigmine *Duragesic* – fentanyl *Sancuso* – granisetron	Provides drug for a longer period of time (up to 1 week), Less side effects ($\downarrow$ nausea, $\downarrow$ GI irritation) and $\downarrow$ side effects from high peak levels with frequent oral dosing. Useful option if vomiting. Helps with adherence if family member can apply patch.
Intravenous (IV) Infusion	Many, acute care drugs	Fast response, achieves high concentrations and/or avoid poor absorption with critical illness, bypasses the oral route, avoids loss of drug due to N/V.
Long-Acting Intramuscular (IM) Injections	*Haldol* – haloperidol decanoate *Zyprexa Relprevv* – olanzapine *Risperdal Consta* – risperidone *Abilify Maintena* – aripiprazole *Invega Sustenna* – paliperidone *Lupron Depot* – leuprolide	Various drugs come as long-acting injections to improve adherence (such as antipsychotics) or to $\downarrow$ the need for more frequent (painful) injections.

Common (Select) Medications Given in Unique Formulations Continued

FORMULATION	EXAMPLES	REASONS FOR USE
Suppositories/ Enemas	*Rowasa* – mesalamine enema *Canasa* – mesalamine suppository *Babylax* – glycerin suppository *Dulcolax* – bisacodyl suppository *Fleet Enema* – sodium phosphates enema *Preparation H* – phenylephrine/cocoa butter suppository *FeverAll* – acetaminophen suppository	Used either for localized treatment (treating constipation, hemorrhoids) or for systemic treatment (such as mesalamine rectal forms for distal ulcerative colitis. Suppositories can be used when the patient is NPO and systemic treatment is needed (such as acetaminophen for treating pain or fever in an infant).

PATCHES

Medications are increasingly being delivered via transdermal delivery systems. Common concerns with their use includes non-adhesion (patches falling off the skin), patients inappropriately cutting patches, improper disposal, MRI burns, heat exposure leading to toxicity, and lag-time to effect. This list contains the more commonly used patches and how to address common issues concerning patches.

Common Patches, Application Sites

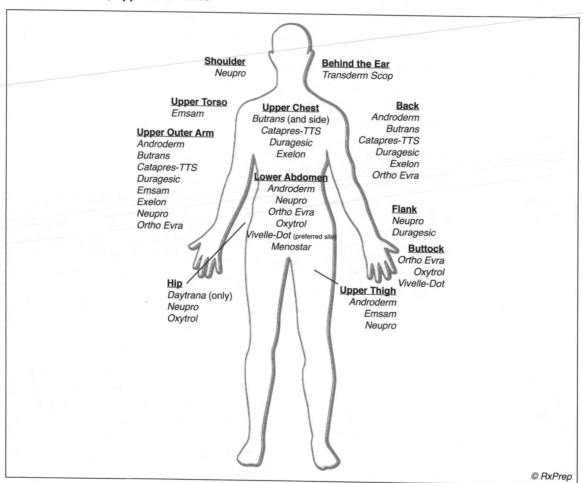

Common Concerns with Patches

QUESTION	RESPONSE
Can I cut the patch into pieces?	■ Usually no, except *Lidoderm*, which is designed to be cut and applied over the painful regions. ■ Some patients are instructed by their healthcare providers to cut matrix patches, such as fentanyl. This is not advisable since prescribed doses can change and medication errors can happen. Fentanyl patches are available in five different doses and as less expensive generics, which should make cutting unnecessary.
Can the patch be exposed to heat from an electric blanket, heating pad, or body temperature > 38 °C (> 100.4 °F)?	In almost all cases no heat exposure; this causes the drug to pour out of the patch, resulting in toxicity. With fentanyl and buprenorphine this can be quickly toxic (fatal).
The patch is bothering my skin. What can I do?	■ Check if the patient is <u>alternating</u> the application site. An alternative site (if permitted) may be beneficial. ■ The skin should not be shaved shortly before applying; shaving is irritating to the skin. ■ In some cases a topical steroid, such as hydrocortisone (OTC) can be applied <u>after</u> the patch is removed; if applied before application it will prevent the patch from sticking well.
Which patches need to be removed prior to an MRI?	Patches containing metal, such as aluminum, need to be removed prior to an MRI or else it will burn the skin. Testosterone *(Androderm)* Clonidine *(Catapres-TTS)* Fentanyl *(Duragesic*, generics) Rotigotine *(Neupro)* Scopolamine *(Transderm-Scop)* *Salonpas Power Plus* (OTC) Nicotine *(NicoDerm CQ)* Check package insert; this can change.

Common Concerns with Patches Continued

QUESTION	RESPONSE
The patch does not stick (it falls or peels off). Can the patch be covered with tape if it will not stick?	With most patches, if it comes off, a new patch is reapplied to the same or a different site. ■ Most patches cannot be covered with tape. A few patches permit tape around the edges. If patches are placed on lubricated skin they will not stick. Place on dry, non-lubricated skin. No moisturizer or bath oils beforehand. Press down for the right amount of time, with palm over the patch. Some require a rather long time, such as the fentanyl patch which takes 30 seconds of pressure to adhere to the skin. ■ Hairy skin will block some of the drug from touching the skin, and can prevent the patch from sticking well. Although patches are not placed on hairy skin, do not shave right before the patch application. This can cause little bumps on delicate skin, and patches cannot be placed on irritated or broken skin. Cut hair close to the skin or shave in advance. Or, use a permitted site that is not hairy. ■ Try not to touch the sticky-side of the patch. ■ Warning: Do not cover patches with the exception of fentanyl (*Duragesic*) or buprenorphine (*Butrans*), which can be covered only with the <u>permitted</u> adhesive film dressings *Bioclusive* or *Tegaderm*. ■ *Catapres-TTS* comes with its own adhesive cover, which goes over the patch to hold it in place. 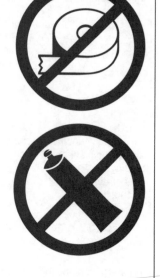
How often do I need to apply my patch?	Clonidine (*Catapres-TTS*): Weekly Estradiol (*Climara, Menostar*): Weekly Estradiol (*Alora, Vivelle-Dot*): Twice weekly Estradiol/levonorgestrel (*ClimaraPro*): Weekly Fentanyl (*Duragesic*): Q72H, if it wears off after 48 hours, change to Q48H Diclofenac (*Flector*): Twice daily Lidocaine (*Lidoderm*): 1-3 patches on for 12 hours, then off 12 hours Methylphenidate (*Daytrana*): Q AM, 2 hours prior to school, alternate hips daily Nicotine (*NicoDerm CQ*): Daily Nitroglycerin (*Minitran, Nitro-Dur*): On 12-14 hours/day, off 10-12 hours/day Ethinyl estradiol/norelgestromin (*Ortho Evra*): Weekly for 3 weeks, off for the 4th week Oxybutynin (*Oxytrol*): Twice weekly Rivastigmine (*Exelon*): Daily Rotigotine (*Neupro*): Daily Scopolamine (*Transderm-Scop*): Q72H, if needed Selegiline (*Emsam*): Daily Testosterone (*Androderm*): Nightly, not on scrotum

Common Concerns with Patches Continued

QUESTION	RESPONSE
Where is the patch applied?	Check individual agent. Common application sites include upper chest or upper/sides of back (below the neck), upper thigh, upper outer arm. Most require alternating sites to reduce skin irritation. ■ *Daytrana* is on hip, alternating right and left hips daily. ■ *Transderm Scop* is behind the ear, alternating ears Q 72H. ■ Estrogen patches are mostly lower abdomen; some can be applied to upper buttock. Never to breasts. ■ Testosterone patch is never to scrotum (testicles and surrounding sac). ■ Topical pain patches, such as *Flector*, *Lidoderm* and *Salonpas* are over the painful area(s). ■ Systemic pain patches, such as *Duragesic*, are applied to the chest, back, flank, or upper arm.
How do I dispose of used patches?	■ In most cases, remove and fold patch to press adhesive surfaces together, then discard but not in the toilet for most patches. The DEA permits flushing of highly potent narcotic patches (*Duragesic, Daytrana, Butrans*), since these are dangerous and a child or animal could ingest a fatal amount. ■ Alternatively, the fentanyl patch can be cut up and mixed with noxious substance, then disposed in the trash. See Drug Disposal chapter for more information. ■ The *Butrans* patch can be placed and sealed into the Patch-Disposal Unit that comes with the drug, then disposed in the trash.

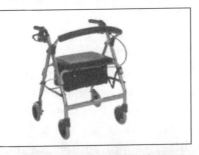

DURABLE MEDICAL EQUIPMENT (DME)

DME is long-lasting (durable) items used for a medical reason in a patient's home. DME requires a prescription and is covered by most insurance. The Center for Medicare and Medicaid Services (CMS) covers DME under the medical insurance component (Part B). The program under which DME is administered at CMS is called DME Prosthetics, Orthotics, and Supplies (DMEPOS).

Diabetic and Pulmonary Supplies Covered under DME

Diabetic supplies covered under Part B as DME includes glucose monitors, test strips, control solution, lancet devices and lancets, and diabetic shoes or inserts. CMS does not cover continuous glucose monitoring (CGM) devices. Part B covers some diabetes services, including self-management training, an annual eye exam, a foot exam every 6 months, glaucoma tests and nutrition therapy. Nebulizers are covered for pulmonary medication delivery.

REFERENCE

HHS CMS DMEPOS Information for Pharmacies. http://www.cms.gov/Outreach-and-Education/Medicare-Learning-Network-MLN/MLNProducts/downloads/DMEPOS_Pharm_FactSheet_ICN905711.pdf (accessed 15 Oct 2014).

NABP's DMEPOS accreditation information. http://www.nabp.net/programs/accreditation/dmepos (accessed 15 Oct 2014).

Pray, S. Durable Medical Equipment: A Challenging Practice. *US Pharm.* 2008; 33(6):10-15.

COMMON COVERED DME ITEMS	
Blood Glucose Monitors and/or Supplies (mail order)	Insulin Infusion Pumps and/or Supplies
Breast Prostheses and/or Accessories	Nebulizer Equipment and/or Supplies
Canes and/or Crutches	Orthotics: Off-The-Shelf
Commodes/Urinals/Bedpans	Ostomy Supplies
Continuous Positive Airway Pressure (CPAP) Devices and/or Supplies	Parenteral Nutrients
	Parenteral Equipment and/or Supplies
Diabetic Shoes/Inserts	Penile Pumps
Diabetic Shoes/Inserts-Custom	Respiratory Assist Devices
Enteral Nutrients	Seat Lift Mechanisms
Enteral Equipment and/or Supplies	Surgical Dressings
External Infusion Pumps and/or Supplies	Urological Supplies
Heat & Cold Applications	Walkers

DMEPOS Accreditation

Expensive equipment is either rented or purchased and there may be a co-pay, depending on the patient's income status. In order for Medicare to cover the DME, the pharmacy must comply with the DMEPOS Quality Standards and obtain accreditation, unless they are granted an exemption. The National Boards of Pharmacy (NABP) is one of the CMS-approved organizations that can provide accreditation for a pharmacy to become a CMS-approved DME provider. This means that the pharmacy can bill for the DME under Part B. NABP collects the documentation from the pharmacy, conducts a site visit, confirms that the pharmacy is licensed and in good standing and reviews the policies and procedures to ensure quality service and accurate billing.

The organization at CMS that reviews the application is the National Supplier Clearinghouse (NSC). NSC issues a billing number which is known as the "Medicare billing number" or the "NSC number". The DMEPOS accreditation is required if the pharmacy or another supplier of DME wishes to bill under Medicare Part B. Drugs that are billed under Part B (e.g. drugs used in a nebulizer) do not require DMEPOS accreditation for Medicare to pay the bill. In some cases, the patient will be asked to pay more than the Medicare-approved item for the DME item. "Accepting Assignment" means that the pharmacy agrees to collect only the Medicare portion and will not for ask for or accept any additional payments from the patient. If the pharmacy agrees to accept assignment, they are called a participating supplier. The other option is to become enrolled but not agree to accept assignment; in this case, the pharmacy could charge above the Medicare reimbursement rate.

Exemption from DMEPOS Accreditation

If the total billing to CMS is < 5% of the total pharmacy sales for previous 3 years and if the pharmacy has been a DMEPOS provider for ≥ 5 years and there have been no adverse actions filed against the pharmacy in the past 5 years, then the pharmacy can submit an attestation to CMS that they meet this criteria. CMS conducts random audits on pharmacies to check that the exemptions are as stated. If there has been a change in the pharmacies taxpayer identification number or any change in their legal business entity information within the past 5 years they will not be able to apply for an exemption. A chain pharmacy with > 25 locations will not be granted an exemption. If the store is part of a franchise, each location is reviewed separately.

CMS Does Not Like Fraud, and Neither do Taxpayers

There has been considerable fraud around two expensive pieces of DME: power wheelchairs and power-operated vehicles. This has led CMS to institute a competitive bidding process for some types of equipment to make sure that CMS is not being over-charged. After all, taxpayers pay for CMS expenses and the competitive bidding process is an effort to keep the taxpayers from being overcharged. Companies that sell glucose meters make money on the strips, not the meters, which are sometimes given at no-cost so that patients need the strips that go with it. Medicare has an anti-switching rule that prohibits suppliers from encouraging patients to switch glucose meters or test strips. If the pharmacy does not have the test strip that the meter requires then the patient can ask about alternative brands but the pharmacy (or any other supplier) cannot initiate the conversation.

Taking Care of the Patients

DME, depending on the type, will require that the staff receive training in order to provide proper care to the patients. The pharmacy should make sure they have all the training materials necessary and the staff can provide competent care. It is not appropriate to sell any equipment without having the staff on board who can help that patient use it safely. Providing ostomy supplies is an area where proper help is essential. Ostomy refers to surgery that diverts part of the bowel through the abdominal wall to the skin to collect urine or stool in a pouch (plastic bag). A stoma (opening) refers to the piece of intestine that is pulled through and sutured to the skin. The characteristics of the stoma and the type of procedure will determine (in part) the type of pouching system the patient requires to collect the urine or stool. Belts are sold that hold the system in place. Stomas commonly become irritated and bleed and a poorly fitting pouching system will worsen bleeding. Skin that is exposed to urine or stool can become irritated or infected and require care.

A new ostomy patient that enters the pharmacy is likely to have emotional issues that will take time to manage. In addition to the discomforting risk of smell, the patient may have comorbidities (including the condition that led to the surgery, such as Crohn's or some type of cancer) and many patients will have difficulty coping with changes in their self-esteem, changes in the ability to comfortably have sexual relations and challenges in finding the additional time required to care for themselves. The last thing an ostomy patient should receive is inexperienced help or be forced to interact with a staff member who lacks compassion. There is a higher level of responsibility required in assisting ostomy patients than simply placing the supplies on a shelf. This extends to other areas of care in which DME is covered since DME patients are coping with some type of chronic illness.

In summary, DME for patients with chronic medical conditions requires a high level of care.

6

BIOSTATISTICS & PHARMACOECONOMICS

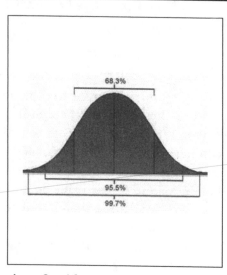

We gratefully acknowledge the assistance of Jeff Lee, PharmD, FCCP, Associate Professor, Lipscomb University College of Pharmacy, and Jan D. Hirsch, BSPharm, PhD, Associate Professor at the University of California San Diego, Skaggs School of Pharmacy and Pharmaceutical Sciences, in preparing this chapter.

BIOSTATISTICS

Background

Health care is evolving at an exponential rate. The development of new technologies and care delivery strategies has contributed to an explosion in the sheer quantity of evidence being created and published in the health care field. As pharmacists, the "drug experts," it is our responsibility to review and evaluate biomedical literature assessing safety, efficacy and value of new drugs and innovative uses of current medications. Biomedical literature presents clinical data, and uses statistical methods and tools to answer research questions and aid in the development of clinical guidelines and consensus statements on the optimal treatment of various medical conditions. While there are a few types of studies that do not require statistical analysis (e.g., case studies, case series), most robust studies include statistical analyses and pharmacists should acquire the basic knowledge of statistical methods to best interpret available data.

Descriptive Statistics

Descriptive statistics are designed to describe the basic features of the data and provide simple summaries in a meaningful way. Measures of central tendency estimate the "center" of a distribution of values. There are three ways of estimating central tendency: the mean, the median and the mode. Although they all estimate the "center" of a group of data, the values obtained can be quite different.

Mean = average   ["μ" in normal distribution]

use for non-skewed data

The mean is the average value of a data set. It is calculated by adding up the values in a list, and dividing by the number of values present. The mean will reflect (or be sensitive to) the outlying (extreme) values – which may not be representative of the norm. For example, in the list 1, 3, 4, 3, 4, 2, 11, the outlier is 11, and the mean would be affected (inflated) by this value. Means can be used when the data are not skewed. The mean is used for continuous data.

$$\text{Mean} = \frac{\text{Sum of all values}}{\text{Number of values}}$$

In this example, the mean would be 4 [(1 + 3 + 4 + 3 + 4 + 2 + 11) divided by 7].

Median = 50th percentile

use for skewed data

The median is the value in the middle of a ranked list – to calculate it, arrange all the observations in numerical order (lowest to highest) and pick the middle value. Half of the values will be above the median, and half will be below. If the list contains an even number of values, then select the 2 values in the middle of the ranked list, add them together and divide by 2 to get the median. Unlike the mean, the median is less influenced by outliers. Another term for the median is the 50th percentile, where 50% of the values are below the median and the other 50% are above the median. For example, if students are ranking a professor from 1-10 (10 being the best) and the class size is small, the median would be more appropriate to represent the data than the mean. If only 1 or 2 students did not like the course, they may rank the professor low (1 or 2). By using the median value to represent the middle, the outlier effect on the data is minimized. Median values should be used when data are skewed. When the mean and the median values are very different, the data set is skewed. The more skewed the data, the larger the difference between the median and the mean. Median values can be used with both continuous and ordinal, or ranked, data.

Mode

The mode is the value that occurs most frequently in a set of data.

Range

The range is the difference between the highest and the lowest values. In the data set 3, 5, 6, 6, 8, 8, 8, 9, 10 the mode would be 8 and the range would be 7 (10 – 3).

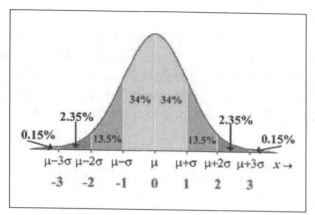

Normal Distribution

A "normal" distribution is also known as a bell-shaped curve or Gaussian curve. Generally, clinical studies rely on "sample" populations that appear to be representative of the population is not available. When researches look at a sample, the entire population is not available and therefore an approximation has to be made. When the sample group is large, the distribution approximates a normal, bell shaped curve (see picture) where μ is the mean, and σ is the standard deviation (SD). In a Gaussian or normal distribution, the mean, mode and median would all have the same (or similar) value and would look like the figure above. Notice the curve is symmetric around the mean and the skew is zero.

Standard Deviation (SD) = $\sqrt{variance}$ ["σ" on normal distribution]

The standard deviation shows how much variation, or dispersion, there is from the mean. The closer the numbers cluster around the mean, the smaller the standard deviation. If the SD is small, one would conclude that the drug being studied had a similar effect on most subjects. SD is expressed in the same units as the data, is used for data that is normally distributed, is always a positive number, and can be used for continuous data only. In a normal distribution, roughly 68% of the values are within 1 standard deviation from the mean and 95% are within 2 standard deviations. Standard deviation is calculated by taking the square root of the variance.

Skewness

Data that do not have a normal distribution are skewed and have an asymmetric curve (see curves A and C below). This means the data has extremes, or outliers. Data that are skewed to the right have a positive skew (curve C below) and data that are skewed to the left have a

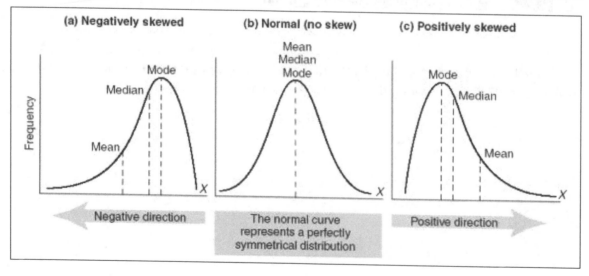

negative skew (curve A below). The direction of the skew refers to the direction of the longer tail, not to the bulk of the data or curve hump. Notice that in curve B, the right and left are perfect mirrors of one another indicating symmetrical data.

Statistical Inference and Error

Null Hypothesis (H_0)   drug A = drug B

The null hypothesis states that there is no difference (or relationship) between groups (i.e., Drug A = Drug B). A study is designed to disprove this assertion by testing for a statistically significant difference between Drug A and Drug B (this is called the alternate hypothesis or H_A). If the study data concluded that there was a statistically significant difference between Drug A and Drug B, then the null hypothesis would fail to be accepted (therefore, it would be rejected).

Alternative Hypothesis (H_A)   drug A ≠ drug B

The alternative hypothesis states that there is a treatment difference (or a relationship among variables) between groups in the trial (i.e., Drug A ≠ Drug B). If you fail to accept (or reject) the null hypothesis (H_0), you are accepting the alternative hypothesis.

P-value

< 0.05 → statistically significant → fail to accept H_0
→ $< 5\%$ (unlikely) result occurred by chance.

The p-value is the likelihood (or probability) that chance would produce a difference as large or larger than the one found in the study, if the null hypothesis is true. In simple terms, it is the probability that the result obtained was due to chance. Generally, a p-value of < 0.05 (and sometimes < 0.01 or other values, depending on the trial design) indicates statistical significance. If the p-value is < 0.05, then there is $\leq 5\%$ probability that the result occurred by chance. In other words, the p-value is the probability of a random difference, given that the null hypothesis is true.

If there is a low probability the result was obtained by chance (e.g., p-value < 0.05) we can state that the conclusion is "statistically significant" (i.e., unlikely to have occurred by chance). When the p-value is smaller than the predetermined significance level (or alpha level), the difference found between groups is statistically significant and the study failed to accept (or reject) the null hypothesis. Again, the study would fail to accept (or reject) the null hypothesis when the p-value is less than the predetermined significance level (say alpha < 0.05), indicating that the observed result is highly unlikely under the null hypothesis.

Confidence Interval (CI) $= 1 - \alpha$ ← type I error

The confidence interval (CI) is a range of values derived from the sample data that has a given probability of encompassing the "true" value. It reflects the margin of error that inherently goes along when a sample statistic is used to estimate the true value of the population. Therefore, CIs help determine the validity of the sample statistic by attempting to capture the true population parameter. The confidence interval states that there is a given probability that the population's true value is contained within this interval. The most common confidence level used in medicine is 95%; however, other levels may be used. As the confidence level increases, the confidence interval becomes wider. A 95% CI can also be stated as a 5% degree of uncertainty. The confidence level is equal to 1 – alpha (type I error), or CI = 1 – type I error.

CIs can be used descriptively or inferentially. An example of descriptive use: a study reports that the mean weight of newborns at one hospital in the past 12 months was 7.7 lbs, with a 95% confidence interval (6.6 – 8.8 lbs) – meaning the researcher is 95% confident that the confidence interval contains the sample statistic. Inferential use looks at the values as a way of comparing groups and determining level of significance. A few rules apply when looking at CIs for inferential use:

- When the 95% CI for the estimated <u>difference</u> between groups (or within the same group over time) does not include <u>zero</u>, the results are <u>significant at the 0.05 level</u>.

- When the 95% CI for an <u>odds ratio, risk ratio or hazard ratio</u> that compares 2 groups does not include <u>1</u>, the results are <u>significant at the 0.05 level</u>.

See examples of inferential use of CIs and p-values using the difference and RR in the tables below. The use of p-values and confidence intervals is complementary. P-values allow a quick decision about whether a result is statistically significant or not. Confidence intervals provide information on statistical significance plus information about the direction and strength of effect.

[handwritten margin note: if p-value not given look @ difference or ratio & determine if results are statistically significant]

LUNG FUNCTION	ROFLUMILAST (N = 745)	PLACEBO (N = 745)	DIFFERENCE (95% CI)	P-VALUE
Change in pre-bronchodilator FEV$_1$ (mL)	46	8	38 (18 – 58)	p = 0.0003
Change in pre-bronchodilator FEV$_1$/FVC (%)	0.314	0.001	0.313 (-0.26 – 0.89)	p = 0.2858

[handwritten: 0 0 ... significant!]
[handwritten: difference includes 0]

EXACERBATIONS	ROFLUMILAST	PLACEBO	RR (95% CI)	P-VALUE
Severe (mean rate, per patient r year)	0.11 (n = 69)	0.12 (n = 81)	RR 0.89 (0.61 – 1.29)	p = 0.5275
Moderate (mean rate, per patient per year)	0.94 (n = 299)	1.11 (n = 343)	RR 0.84 (0.72 – 0.99)	p = 0.0325

[handwritten: ratio includes 1]
[handwritten: 0 1 ... significant!]

Clinical Significance *[handwritten: ≠ statistical significance]*

<u>Note that a measure of statistical significance is not the same as "clinical significance"</u>. Statistical significance reflects the influence of chance on the outcome; clinical significance reflects the clinical value of the outcome. For example, if a blood pressure drug lowers SBP by 3 mmHg, it may be statistically significant (with a p-value < 0.05) versus placebo, but clinically the drug will not be used since other drugs lower BP to a greater degree. It would not be "clinically significant" because it does not measure up to other available drugs and would not have an advantageous clinical benefit.

Correlation

Correlation describes the relationship between two or more variables which is then plotted on a linear scale. The direction and magnitude of the linear correlation can be quantified with a correlation coefficient. The most widely-used type of correlation coefficient is the Pearson Correlation Coefficient, abbreviated r. Values of the correlation coefficient vary from -1 to 1. If the coefficient is 0, then the two variables have no relationship or correlation. If the coefficient is positive, the 2 variables tend to increase or decrease together. If the coefficient is negative, the 2 variables are inversely related, that is, as one variable decreases, the other variable increases. If the coefficient is 1 or -1, the two variables have perfect correlation and the data points form a straight line.

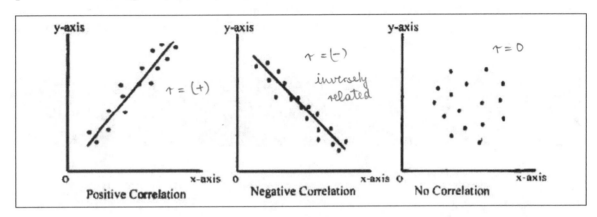

Handwritten annotations: "false (+)" ⟹ drug concluded to be better than placebo when it actually is not

Type I error

Handwritten: H₀ is true yet rejected in error = concluded that drug A ≠ drug B when, in fact, drug A = drug B

The Greek letter, alpha (α) is the probability of a type I error. The alpha value is chosen by the researcher, before the study starts, to be the acceptable threshold of statistical significance (also known as the p-value). Commonly, α is set to = 0.05, which means < 5% of the time the null hypothesis will be rejected in error. A type I error occurs when the null hypothesis is true, yet it is rejected in error. Said another way, it was concluded that there was a difference between two groups when, in fact, there was not. When a researcher chooses the p-value of < 0.05 for statistical significance, the researcher accepts the fact that this error will occur < 5% of the time. A type I error is also known as a false positive (e.g., a drug is concluded to be better than placebo when it is not). Confidence interval is related to the alpha level: CI = 1 – alpha (type I error).

Handwritten annotations: "false (-)" ⟹ drug concluded NOT to have benefit over placebo when it actually does

Type II error

Handwritten: H₀ is false yet accepted in error = concluded that drug A = drug B when, in fact, drug A ≠ drug B

The Greek letter, beta (β) is the probability of a type II error. Beta is generally set at 0.1 or 0.2, indicating a willingness to accept a type II error 10 or 20 times in 100 comparisons. A type II error occurs when the null hypothesis is false, yet it is accepted in error. Said another way, it was concluded that there was no difference between two groups when, in fact, there was. A type II error is also known as a false negative (e.g., a drug is concluded not to have benefit over placebo when it actually has a benefit). Beta is usually expressed in terms of statistical power, which is calculated as 1-beta.

The Importance of Type I and Type II Errors is Dependent on the Situation

For example, consider a screening test for a biological marker known to give a good estimate of whether or not a particular disease will develop within the next 5 years. There is a prophylactic medication that can be given if the patient is at risk, but the medication is very expensive and can have serious side effects. The null hypothesis (H_0) is that the patient does not have the biological marker.

A false positive test (type I error – testing positive for the marker of the disease when indeed the patient does not have the biological marker) may make the patient anxious and seek unnecessary treatments and/or surgery. A false negative (type II error – testing negative for the marker of the disease when indeed the patient has the biological marker) may be more serious since the patient may not seek further treatment that could have prevented or halted the disease.

	UNDERLYING "TRUTH" IS BIOLOGICAL MARKER PRESENT?	
DECISION BASED ON SCREENING TEST	**H_0 TRUE – DO NOT HAVE THE MARKER**	**H_0 FALSE – DO HAVE THE MARKER**
Accept (fail to reject) H_0 No biological marker, therefore, no disease	No error	Type II error *false (−) say pt does not have marker but pt actually has it*
Reject H_0 Have biological marker and will develop disease	Type I error *false (+) say pt has marker but pt actually doesn't*	No error

Statistical Power

Power of a statistical test is the probability that the test will reject the null hypothesis when the null hypothesis is false (avoiding a type II error). As the power increases, the chance of a type II error occurring decreases. Therefore, power is equal to $1 - \beta$. A higher statistical power means that we can be more certain that the null hypothesis was correctly rejected. The power of a study is determined by several factors including the sample size, the number of events (MIs, strokes, deaths, etc.), the effect size and the statistical significance criterion used.

↑ statistical power = ↓ chance of type II error
= ↑ certainty that H₀ was correctly rejected

ways to ↑ statistical power:
1) ↑ events
   - e.g. study looking @ effect of drug on incidence of MI ⇒ enroll pts who've previously had an MI (⇒ more likely to have a 2nd MI than pt w/o hx of MI)
2) ↑ population size (N)

Variables and Data Types

Dependent & Independent Variables

A dependent variable is the outcome of interest, which should change in response to some intervention. An independent variable is the intervention, or what is being manipulated. For example, aspirin is compared against placebo to see if it leads to a reduction in coronary events. The dependent variable (or outcome of interest) is the number of coronary events while the independent variable (the intervention) is aspirin.

Discrete & Continuous Data

NAME	DESCRIPTION

Discrete Data – can have only a limited, or finite, set of values (i.e., not continuous) and can assume only whole numbers. There are 2 types of discrete data:

Nominal	Consists of categories, where the order of the categories is arbitrary (e.g., marital status, gender, ethnicity). The numbers do not have a true numerical, or quantitative, value (e.g., 0 = male, 1 = female).
Ordinal	Consists of ranked categories, where the order of the ranking is important. However, the difference between categories cannot be considered to be equal. These are usually scoring systems that are ranked by severity (e.g., Apgar score, Likert scales, NYHA functional class) but cannot be measured/ quantified. There is no consistent correlation between the rank and the degree of severity. For example, a trauma score of 4 does not necessarily mean you are twice as ill as a trauma score of 2.

Continuous Data – can take an infinite number of possible values (such as height, weight, A1C, blood pressure) within a defined range. Continuous data can include fractional data (e.g., A1C of 7.3%). Types of continuous data include:

Interval	Interval data is used to measure continuous data that have legitimate mathematical values. The difference between 2 consecutive values is consistent along any point of the scale, but the zero point is arbitrary and does not mean "none" of the variable (e.g., Celsius temperature scale).
Ratio	Ratio data has equal intervals between values and a meaningful zero point; meaning there is none of the variable (e.g., height, weight, time, length).

[handwritten margin note: ?? can have (−) value / can't have (−) value]

Determining the appropriate statistical test depends on many factors, including the type of data, the number of groups being compared, whether the samples are independent or paired and the assumptions within a specific test. Below is a chart outlining some of the statistical tests commonly used in clinical trials.

[handwritten note: type of statistical test used depends on: 1) type of data 2) # of groups compared 3) independent or paired samples 4) assumptions within test]

Comparison of Statistical Tests*

NUMBER OF GROUPS COMPARED	INDEPENDENT SAMPLES	PAIRED SAMPLES	CORRELATION
Nominal Data			
2	Chi-squared test or Fisher's Exact test	McNemar test	Phi
3 or more	Chi-squared test	Cochran Q	
Ordinal Data			
2	Wilcoxon rank sum test or Mann-Whitney U test‡	Wilcoxon signed-rank test‡	Spearman's
3 or more	Kruskal-Wallis test‡	Friedman test‡	
Continuous Data			
2	Student's t-test**	Paired Student's t-test** or Wilcoxon signed-rank test‡	Pearson's
3 or more	Analysis of variance (ANOVA)** or Kruskal-Wallis test‡	ANOVA**	

*Other tests may also apply. Specific test utilized also depends on distribution of data.   ** Parametric test   ‡ Nonparametric test

Risk

Relative Risk/Risk Ratio (RR)   "as likely"

The relative risk (or risk ratio) is the probability of an unfavorable event occurring in the treatment group versus the control group. First, the risk of developing the event must be calculated for both the treatment group and the control group. Then the relative risk is calculated by comparing the risk calculated for the treatment group (numerator) to the risk calculated for the control group (denominator). The RR is generally expressed as a decimal but can also appear as a percentage. RR is simply the ratio of risks in the 2 groups.

$$\text{Risk} = \frac{\text{Number of subjects with unfavorable event in that arm}}{\text{Total number of subjects in that arm}}$$

$$\text{RR} = \frac{\text{Risk in treatment group}}{\text{Risk in control group}}$$

"control goes on bottom"

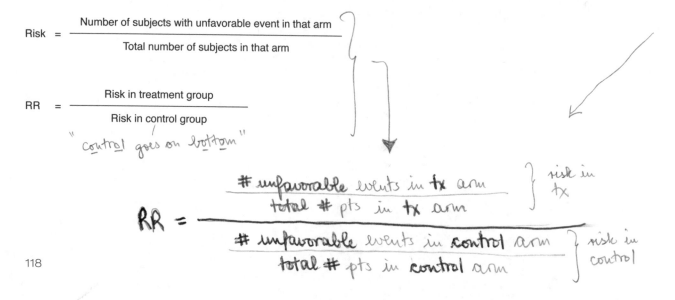

$$RR = \frac{\frac{\#\ \text{unfavorable events in tx arm}}{\text{total}\ \#\ \text{pts in tx arm}}}{\frac{\#\ \text{unfavorable events in control arm}}{\text{total}\ \#\ \text{pts in control arm}}}$$

} risk in tx

} risk in control

INTERPRETING RR

- RR = 1: no difference in risk between the 2 groups

- RR < 1: fewer events are occurring in the treatment group compared to the control group

- RR > 1: more events are occurring in the treatment group compared to the control group

Example #1: A study compared metoprolol vs. placebo in heart failure patients over 12 months. If heart failure progression occurred in 28% of placebo-treated patients and in 16% of metoprolol-treated patients, then the risk ratio is 0.16/0.28 = 0.57, or 57%. Therefore, subjects treated with metoprolol were only 57% as likely as placebo-treated patients to have heart failure progression.

Example #2: Drug A was studied for the prevention of chemotherapy-induced nausea and vomiting (CINV). The trial included 245 patients; 120 patients randomized to Drug A and 125 patients randomized to placebo. There were 20 patients in the placebo group versus 6 patients in the Drug A group who developed CINV. The risk in the Drug A arm is 6 patients divided by 120 patients in this arm, or 5% (6/120 = 0.05 x 100 = 5%). The risk in the placebo arm is 20 patients divided by 125 patients in this arm, or 16% (20/125 = 0.16 x 100 = 16%). The relative risk can be calculated as 0.05/0.16 = 0.3125, or 31%. Therefore, subjects treated with Drug A were only 31% as likely as placebo-treated patients to have CINV. By reporting only the relative risk (as opposed to absolute risk), the value of the treatment may be overstated (as is often done in the lay press).

Here is another formula that can be used for calculating RR:

$$RR = \frac{a/(a+b)}{c/(c+d)}$$

EXPOSURE OR TREATMENT	DISEASE	
	PRESENT	ABSENT
Present (Drug group)	a	b
Absent (Placebo group)	c	d

Example #3: In a group of 100 smokers, 40 people developed lung cancer (CA) while 60 people did not. In a similar group of 100 non-smokers, lung CA developed in 10 people. Calculate the relative risk of developing lung CA from smoking.

$$RR = \frac{40/(40+60)}{10/(10+90)} = 4$$

The RR of 4 means that smokers are 4 times as likely to develop lung CA than non-smokers.

Relative Risk Reduction (RRR)   *" less likely"*

Relative risk reduction measures how much the risk is reduced in the treatment group compared to the control group. It can be calculated by either dividing the absolute risk

** do *not* base decision of whether to include a drug into formulary (assessing clinical benefit in P&T committee) based on RR or RRR ⇒ overstate significance
⇒ INSTEAD, LOOK @ ARR OR NNT !! ⇒ "truer to true picture"

reduction by the control group risk rate or by subtracting the relative risk (expressed as a decimal) from 1.

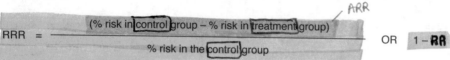

$$RRR = \frac{(\% \text{ risk in control group} - \% \text{ risk in treatment group})}{\% \text{ risk in the control group}}$$

ARR

OR $1 - RR$

Using Example #1 from above: (28% − 16%)/28% = 0.43 or 1 − 0.57 = 0.43, or 43%; meaning there is a 43% relative risk reduction in heart failure progression in patients being treated with metoprolol. Patients taking metoprolol are 43% less likely to experience heart failure progression.

Using Example #2 from above: (16% − 5%)/16% = 0.69 or 1 − 0.31 = 0.69, or 69%; meaning there is a 69% relative risk reduction in CINV in patients being treated with Drug A. Patients taking Drug A are 69% less likely to experience CINV.

Expressing the result as a relative risk reduction is more intuitively understandable, RR and RRR are limited in that these data do not reflect how important, or large, the treatment effect is in the population at-large. They only provide a measure of what the risk of an event is in one group (treatment or exposed) compared to the risk of that event in a comparison (or control) group.

overstate significance of difference

Absolute Risk Reduction (ARR)   " *for every 100 pts treated, ... fewer* "

Absolute risk reduction, or attributable risk, is the difference between the control group's event rate and the treatment group's event rate.

ARR = (% risk in control group) − (% risk in treatment group) = $\dfrac{\# \text{ unfav in control}}{\text{total } \# \text{ in control}} - \dfrac{\# \text{ unfav in tx}}{\text{total } \# \text{ in tx}}$

Using Example #1 from above: 28% − 16% = 12%. The ARR is 12%. This is the difference in risk that can be attributed to the intervention (drug). Therefore, for every 100 patients treated with metoprolol, 12 fewer patients experience heart failure progression.

Using Example #2 from above: 16% − 5% = 11%. The ARR is 11%; therefore, 11% of patients were spared experiencing CINV as a result of receiving drug A rather than placebo. Therefore, for every 100 patients treated with Drug A, 11 fewer patients experience CINV.

Odds

Odds are not the same as risk. Risk is the probability that a person who has not developed the event will develop the event whereas odds represent the probability of the event occurring compared with the probability that it will not occur. Using the example of 100 smokers, if 40 smokers developed lung cancer and 60 smokers did not develop lung cancer, the risk would be 40/100, or 40%, and the odds would be 40:60, 40/60 or 67%.

risk: probability that pt w/o event develops event

$$\frac{\# \text{ event}}{\# (\text{event} + \theta \text{ event})}$$

odds: probability that event occurs vs. probability that event doesn't occur

$$\frac{\# \text{ event}}{\# \theta \text{ event}}$$

OR = (# event in tx/exposure / # ⊖ event in tx / exposure) / (# event in control / # ⊖ event in control)

Odds Ratio (OR)

The odds ratio is the ratio of two odds, or the ratio of the odds of an event occurring in the treatment group to the odds of an event occurring in the control group. It is a measure of association between an exposure and an outcome. Odds ratios are used mostly in case-control studies, but they are the unit of outcome provided by logistic regression analysis which is a valuable statistical tool.

$$\text{Odds Ratio (OR)} = \frac{ad}{bc}$$

	DISEASE	
EXPOSURE OR TREATMENT	PRESENT	ABSENT
Present (Drug group)	a	b
Absent (Placebo group)	c	d

Using Example #3 from above: In a group of 100 smokers, 40 people developed lung CA while 60 people did not. In a similar group of 100 non-smokers, lung CA developed in 10 people. The odds of a smoker developing lung CA would be 40/60 = 0.67, whereas the odds of a non-smoker developing lung CA would be 10/90 = 0.11. The odds ratio is then 0.67/0.11, or 6, meaning that smokers are 6 times as likely to develop lung cancer than non-smokers. An odds ratio of 1 indicates no difference between groups. The smaller the event rate, the closer the odds ratio is to the relative risk.

Hazard Ratio (HR)

Hazard ratios are often used when clinical trials present data related to the time survived to an event (e.g., mortality, cure, specified level of symptom reduction).

A hazard rate is the chance of an unfavorable event occurring by a given point in time. A hazard ratio is the hazard or chance of an event occurring at any given time during the study in the treatment group as compared to a comparator group. Hazard ratios are used in clinical trials with time-to-event (or survival) analysis. Hazard ratios assume that the ratio is constant over time. Hazard ratios are a specific type of RR with the distinction that HR ratios are the relative likelihood of an event in the treated vs comparator group at any given point in time during the trial and the RR is the likelihood of an event in the treated vs comparator group at the end of the trial.

$$\text{HR} = \frac{\text{Hazard rate in the treatment group}}{\text{Hazard rate in the control group}}$$

Interpreting HR

- HR = 1: Event rates are the same in both arms over time
- HR < 1: At any given time, relatively fewer patients in the treatment group have had an event compared to the control group

- HR > 1: At any given time, relatively more patients in the treatment group have had an event compared to the control group

For example, in a clinical trial assessing the cure rate provided by Drug A vs. placebo the hazard ratio (HR) is reported to be 4.0. This means that a treated patient who has not been cured by a certain time point has four times the chance of being cured by the next time point compared to someone in the placebo group.

Number Needed to Treat (NNT)   ROUND UP!

The number needed to treat represents the number of people who would need to be treated with the intervention (drug) for a certain period of time (e.g., one year) in order to achieve the desired outcome (e.g., prevent adverse event) in one patient.

$$NNT = \frac{1}{(\text{risk in control group})^* - (\text{risk in treatment group})^*} \quad or \quad \frac{1}{ARR^*}$$

*expressed as a decimal

NNT => round ↑
NNH =>   ↓

Example #1 from above: 1/0.12 = 8.3, or 9 (must always round up since you cannot divide a person into fractions). Therefore, for every 9 patients who received metoprolol for 1 year, heart failure progression is prevented in one patient.

Example #2 from above: 1/0.11 = 9.09 or 10 (must always round up). Treating 10 patients with Drug A will prevent CINV in 1 patient. The NNT puts the results of a trial in a clinically relevant context. When the treatment or exposure causes harm (e.g., cigarette smoking, *Vioxx*, etc), the term NNT does not work and it is more accurate to report the results as the number needed to harm (NNH) which is calculated the same way as NNT. However, with NNH, we always round down.

Sensitivity and Specificity

Sensitivity and specificity are concepts often applied to diagnostic testing for diseases. Sensitivity is the proportion of time a test is positive in patients who have the disease; also stated as the ability of the test to correctly identify patients who are known to have the disease in question. If a test has high sensitivity, it will pick up nearly everyone with the disease. A test with 100% sensitivity will recognize all patients with the disease by testing positive. Therefore, a negative test would definitely rule out the presence of the disease. Sensitivity is the percentage of "true-positive" results and is equal to 1 – type II error. Specificity is the proportion of time a test is negative in patients who do not have the disease; also stated as the ability of the test to correctly identify patients who are known to not have the disease. If a test has high specificity, it will not mistakenly give a positive result to many people without the disease. A test with 100% specificity will read negative and accurately exclude disease from all healthy patients. Specificity is the percentage of "true-negative" results and is equal to 1 – type I error. In the biological marker example below, the table cells representing true-positives and true-negatives correspond to the sensitivity and specificity of the test, respectively.

Calculating sensitivity and specificity can be described using a simple 2x2 table:

	PATIENTS WITH DISEASE	PATIENTS WITHOUT DISEASE
Test is positive	a (True +)	b (False +)
Test is negative	c (False -)	d (True -)
	a + c	b + d

Using this table, sensitivity may be calculated using the following formula:

$$\text{Sensitivity} = \frac{a}{(a + c)} = \frac{\text{true dz}}{\text{all "dz"}} = 1 - \text{type II error } (\beta) \quad [\text{true (+)}]$$

Specificity, then, can be calculated using the following formula:

$$\text{Specificity} = \frac{d}{(b + d)} = \frac{\text{true health}}{\text{all "health"}} = 1 - \text{type I error } (\alpha) \quad [\text{true(-)}]$$

Overview of Study Designs

There are many types of study designs used in evidence-based medicine. Each trial design has certain strengths and weaknesses. Clinical study designs include observational designs (such as case reports, case series, cross-sectional, case-control, cohort) and experimental designs (such as a randomized, controlled trial). A placebo, or an inert compound indistinguishable from the active drug, may be used in experimental trials to minimize bias.

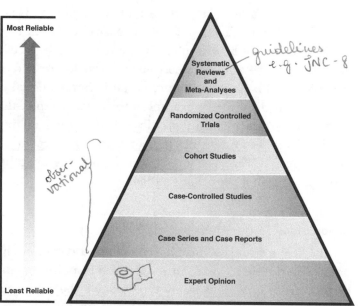

This practice is called "blinding" or "masking" the treatment allocation in a clinical trial. In a single-blind trial, generally the subject (the patient) is unaware of the treatment allocation, whereas the investigator is aware of the treatment the patient is receiving. In a double-blind trial, neither the subjects nor the researchers know who is receiving active drug or placebo. The hierarchy presented in the picture is indicative of the confidence in results that is generally attributed to each type of study.

observational
· case report
· case series
· cross-sectional
· case control
· cohort

experimental
RCT

single blind:
pt does not know
investigator knows

* even observational trials have inclusion/exclusion criteria

123

Observational Studies

An observational study is a type of study in which individuals are observed or certain outcomes are measured under precisely defined conditions in a systematic and objective manner. No attempt is made to affect the outcome (no intervention). Observational studies follow subjects with a certain condition or those who receive a particular treatment over time. They may be compared to another group who are not affected by the condition or are not taking the particular treatment. Large observational studies can clarify the tolerability profile of marketed medicines. An example of an observational study is the Women's Health Initiative trial.

Case Report or Case Series

A simple descriptive account of observations of a single patient (case report) or series of patients (case series) can be useful from a clinical perspective for unusual or rarely observed events. Based on observed clinical aspects of a patient(s) and intervention, the possibility of an association between treatment and effect may be proposed. However, no conclusion can be drawn from these small studies. They may generate hypotheses that can then be studied in larger trials with more robust study designs (e.g., prospective cohort or randomized controlled trial).

Case-Control Study   retrospective → dz vs. θ dz ⌐ exposure / θ exposure

Case-control studies compare patients who have a disease or outcome of interest (the cases) with patients who do not have the disease or outcome (the controls), and look back retrospectively to compare how frequently the exposure to a risk factor is present in each group to determine the relationship between the risk factor and the disease. Case-control studies are observational because no intervention is implemented and no attempt is made to alter the course of the disease. For example, did subjects exposed to statins have a higher incidence of liver damage? Case-control studies are good for studying rare diseases or outcomes, can be conducted in less time since the condition has already occurred, and are useful to establish an association. They are often used to generate hypotheses that can then be studied via a prospective cohort or other studies.

Cohort Study   pro/retrospective → all pts w/ characteristic/exposure   subset w/o exposure

A cohort is a group of people who share a common characteristic or experience within a defined period (e.g., year born, exposure to pollutant/drug/vaccine, or having undergone a certain procedure). This study type follows the cohort over time (longitudinal) and the outcomes are compared to a subset of the group who were not exposed to the intervention such as a drug (e.g., the Framingham studies). They are also good studies for outcomes when a randomized study is unethical. Cohort studies may be prospective in design (carried out into the future) but can be done retrospectively as well (e.g., by reviewing patient medical charts).

Cross-Sectional Study   for epidemiology mostly

Cross-sectional studies are descriptive, observational trials and are used to estimate the relationship between an outcome of interest and population variables as they exist at a cross-section (one point in time). Cross-sectional studies are used to determine prevalence of disease. By identifying associations between exposures and outcomes, they can be used to generate hypotheses about causation that can be tested with other study designs.

Experimental Studies

Randomized Controlled Trial (RCT) *ALWAYS prospective !!*

This experimental trial design involves randomization, which minimizes bias and increases internal validity, thereby increasing the overall strength of the study conclusions. These are generally designed as superiority trials, which aim to determine if one treatment is better than another. RCTs are always prospective and are considered the gold standard trial design in evaluating safety and efficacy of an intervention (e.g., drug). The clinical trial setting can be controlled in many ways.

Within a RCT, there are different study designs and a few are listed below:

PARALLEL STUDY DESIGN

Subjects are randomized to either the treatment group or the placebo group only and stay in that group for the duration of the study. This is the most common design used in Phase III comparative trials for FDA drug approval. A larger sample size is needed compared to the crossover design; however, they can be done in a shorter period of time.

CROSSOVER STUDY DESIGN

Subjects are randomized to a treatment sequence and each subject receives all of the interventions. With this type of design, every patient serves as his or her own control. For example, comparing drugs A and B, half of the subjects are randomly allocated to receive them in the order A then B, and half of the subjects are to receive them in the order B then A. A washout period between treatments is required. This is the time between discontinuing the first treatment and before the initiation of the second treatment and is designed in an attempt to reduce the effects of the 1st drug taken in the 2nd phase of the trial.

FACTORIAL DESIGN

Designed to evaluate multiple interventions in a single experiment. For example, in a simple 2x2 factorial design, patients can be assigned to 1 of 2 drug doses (e.g., 100 mg or 200 mg) and 1 of 2 drugs (Drug A or Drug B).

Intent-To-Treat (ITT) vs. Per Protocol (PP) Analyses

Data from clinical trials can be analyzed in two different ways; intent-to-treat or per protocol. Intention-to-treat analysis includes data for all patients originally allocated to each treatment group (active and control) regardless if the patient did not complete the trial according to the study protocol (e.g., due to non-compliance, protocol deviations or study withdrawal). This method provides a conservative estimate of treatment effect. A per protocol analysis is conducted for the subset of the trial population who completed the study according to the protocol (or at least without any major protocol violations). This method may provide an

ITT
- data for ALL pts allocated to tx regardless of whether/not pt completed trial
- conservative estimate of tx effect

PP
- data ONLY for subset of pts who completed trial according to protocol
- optimistic estimate of tx effect

optimistic estimate of treatment effect since it is limited to the subset of patients who were adherent to the protocol. In practice, both methods are often used to analyze the results of a clinical trial.

[handwritten: "crosses over" drug X control line { w/in margin of error ⇒ non-inferior / outside ⇒ inferior | if drug X doesn't cross over C line, it is superior (won't cross over M line if it doesn't cross over C)]

Non-Inferiority Trial

A non-inferiority trial is another type of RCT where a new treatment is not worse than that of an active control by some pre-specified margin. Non-inferiority trials generally have fewer patients than superiority trials and may be appropriate when a placebo group is unethical.

Clinical trials may not provide "real life" comparisons

Patients in clinical trials may not be reflective of those treated in everyday clinical practice. Patients in clinical trials tend to be younger, more compliant with therapy, more likely to reach target doses of the drug, and do so more quickly than in everyday practice. They are not as likely to have a complex presentation as real-life patients. For example, practitioners may be using a drug that is cleared renally in patients with moderate to severe renal impairment, where this subgroup of patients may have been excluded from clinical trials related to the drug in question. Therefore, we will not know how to use the drug safely in this patient population.

Systematic Reviews and Meta-Analyses

When there are many studies available in the literature, a systematic review and possible meta-analysis is useful to summarize the main findings in order to guide evidence based medical decisions.

A systematic review is a structured literature review that uses a step-by-step protocol with preset criteria for selecting and rigorously evaluating studies. Systematic reviews attempt to identify all studies that meet the pre-defined criteria, evaluate the validity of findings (considering possible bias within the study design), and then synthesize the results into a meaningful, transparent presentation of results. A systematic review study may also conduct a meta-analysis to present a quantitative synthesis of results across studies.

Meta-analysis is a statistical technique that can be used to combine results from multiple studies to develop a single conclusion that has greater statistical power than is possible in the individual smaller studies. The validity and usefulness of a meta-analysis is largely dependent on the quality of the systematic review that identfied which studies to include. A meta-analysis considers the differing sizes and quality of trials for a treatment, giving more weight to the findings from larger, more rigorous studies. The technique also considers how the studies differ and the possible contribution of differing factors to driving treatment outcomes.

Meta-analysis can be used for the following purposes:

- To establish statistical significance with studies that have conflicting results

- To develop a more correct estimate of effect magnitude

- To provide a more complex analysis of harms, safety data, and/or benefits

- To examine subgroups with individual numbers that are not statistically significant

Although there are many potential flaws in this type of pooled data analysis, if the studies included in the meta-analysis are rigorous randomized controlled trials, the results could provide the highest level of evidence for medical decisions.

PHARMACOECONOMICS

Background
Health care costs in the United States rank among the highest of all industrialized countries. In 2012 (the most recent data available), total health care expenditures reached 2.8 trillion dollars, which translates to an average of $8,915 per person, or about 17.2% of the nation's gross domestic product. The increasing costs have highlighted the need to understand how our limited resources can be used most effectively and efficiently in the care of our patients and society as a whole. Therefore, it is necessary to scientifically evaluate the value (e.g., costs vs. outcomes) of interventions such as drug therapy.

Definitions
Pharmacoeconomics is a collection of descriptive and analytic techniques for evaluating pharmaceutical interventions (drugs, devices, procedures, etc.) in the health care system. Pharmacoeconomic research identifies, measures, and compares the costs (direct, indirect and intangible) and consequences (clinical, economic and humanistic) of pharmaceutical products and services. Various research methods can be used to determine the impact of the pharmaceutical product or service. These methods include: cost-effectiveness analysis, cost-minimization analysis, cost-utility analysis, and cost-benefit analysis. Although the term "pharmacoeconomics" is frequently referred to as "outcomes research", they are not the same thing. Pharmacoeconomic methods are specific to assessing the costs and consequences of pharmaceutical products and services, whereas outcomes research represents a broader research discipline that attempts to identify, measure, and evaluate the end result of health care services generally.

Health care providers, payers and other decision makers use these methods to evaluate and compare the total costs and consequences of pharmaceutical products and services. As the results of pharmacoeconomic analyses can vary significantly based on the point of view of the analyst, a critical consideration in evaluating pharmacoeconomic analyses is to clearly identify the study perspective. What may be viewed as good value for society or for the patient may not be deemed as such from an institutional or provider perspective (e.g., the importance of assessing the costs of lost productivity due to illness may be critically important to a patient or employer, but perhaps less so to a health plan).

Pharmacoeconomic analyses can provide useful supplemental evidence to traditional efficacy and safety endpoints. They help translate important clinical benefits into economic and patient-centered terms, and can assist providers and payers in determining where, if at all, a drug fits into the treatment paradigm for a specific condition. Pharmacoeconomic studies serve to guide optimal healthcare resource allocation, in a standardized and evidence-based manner.

The ECHO model (Economic, Clinical and Humanistic Outcomes) provides a broad evaluative framework to assess the outcomes associated with disease and its treatment.

- Economic outcomes: Include direct, indirect and intangible costs of the drug compared to a medical intervention.

- Clinical outcomes: Include medical events that occur as a result of the treatment or intervention.

- Humanistic Outcomes: Include consequences of the disease or treatment as reported by the patient or caregiver (e.g., patient satisfaction, quality of life).

Average and Incremental Cost Effectiveness Ratios

Commonly, the results of a pharmacoeconomic analysis will be expressed in terms of a cost ratio, representing the costs incurred to achieve a particular outcome [e.g., cost per case cured, cost per treatment success, cost per quality-adjusted life year (QALY) gained]. Two fundamental cost ratios are commonly used to communicate results of a pharmacoeconomic analysis.

Average Cost Effectiveness Ratios

Average cost ratios reflect the cost per outcome of one treatment alternative independent of other alternatives. For example, if a treatment costs $50 to generate two successful outcomes, the average cost ratio is $25/treatment success ($50/2 successfully treated).

Incremental Cost Effectiveness Ratios

Incremental cost ratios represent the change in costs and outcomes when two treatment alternatives are compared. An incremental cost ratio is calculated when evaluating costs and outcomes between competing alternatives, and represents the additional costs required to produce an additional unit of effect. Mathematically, it is calculated as (where C is for costs and E is for effects):

$$\text{Incremental Cost Ratio} \ = \ \frac{(C_2 - C_1)}{(E_2 - E_1)}$$

For example, if spending $200 on Drug A results in 5 treatment successes while spending $300 on Drug B results in 7 treatment successes, the incremental cost ratio of Drug B relative to Drug A is $50 for each additional treatment success:

COSTS

Direct Medical Costs
Costs associated with the detection, prevention, or treatment of a disease or illness. Direct cost examples include medications, medication administration, hospitalizations, clinic visits, emergency room visits, and nursing services.

Direct Non-Medical Costs
Costs for non-medical services associated with disease and treatment. Direct non-medical costs include travel costs (gas, bus, hotel stays for family), child care services (for children of patients), or costs for other household services required due to illness.

Indirect Costs
Costs that result from the effects of morbidity or mortality on production capacity, including costs of time lost from work, or working at a lower productivity level due to disease or treatment. Indirect costs can occur at both the patient and caregiver level.

Intangible costs
Costs incurred that represent the nonfinancial outcomes of disease and treatment, including pain and suffering, anxiety, and fatigue.

$$\frac{(\$300 - \$200)}{(7 - 5)} = \frac{\$100}{2} = \$50 \text{ per additional success with Drug B}$$

Pharmacoeconomic Methodologies

Cost-Minimization Analysis

Cost-minimization analysis (CMA) is used when two or more interventions have already demonstrated equivalency in outcomes and the costs of each intervention are being compared. CMA measures and compares the input costs of treatment alternatives that have been deemed as equivalent from an outcomes perspective. This determination of equivalence is a key consideration in adopting this methodology. Ideally, evidence will exist to support the clinical equivalence of the alternatives. In some instances, assumptions will be made in the absence of relevant evidence. For example, two ACE-inhibitors, captopril and lisinopril, are considered therapeutically equivalent in the literature, but the acquisition cost (the price paid for the drug) and administrative costs may be different (captopril is administered TID and lisinopril is administered once daily). A CMA would look at "minimizing costs" when multiple drugs have equal efficacy and tolerability. Another example of CMA is looking at the same drug regimen given in two different settings (e.g., hospital versus home health care). CMA is considered the easiest analysis to perform. However, the use of this method is limited given its ability to compare only alternatives with demonstrated equivalent outcomes.

Cost-Benefit Analysis

Cost-benefit analysis (CBA) is a systematic process for calculating and comparing benefits and costs of an intervention in terms of monetary units. CBA consists of identifying all the benefits from an intervention and converting them into dollars in the year that they will occur. Also, the costs associated with the intervention are identified and are allocated to the year when they occur. All costs are then discounted back to their present day value. Given that all other factors remain constant, the program with the largest present day value of benefits minus costs is the best economic value. In CBA, both benefits and costs are expressed in terms of dollars and are adjusted to their present value. This can be difficult when required to measure the benefits and then assign a dollar amount to that benefit (e.g., when measuring the benefit of patient quality of life, an outcome difficult to measure and assign a dollar value to it). One advantage to using CBA is the ability to determine if the benefits of the intervention exceed the costs of implementation. CBA can also be used to compare multiple programs for similar or unrelated outcomes, as long as the outcome measures can be converted to dollars.

Cost-Effectiveness Analysis *compares within same clinical outcome*

Cost-effectiveness analysis (CEA) is defined as a series of analytical and mathematical procedures that aid in the selection of a course of action from various alternative approaches. Inputs are usually measured in dollars and outputs are usually measured in natural units (e.g., LDL values in mg/dL, % clinical cures, length of stay). The main advantage of this method is that the outcomes are easier to quantify when compared to other analyses, and clinicians and decision makers are familiar with these types of outcomes since they are similar to outcomes seen in clinical trials and practice. Therefore, CEA is the most common methodology seen in the literature today. A disadvantage of CEA is the inability to directly compare different types of outcomes. For example, one cannot compare the cost effectiveness of implementing a diabetes program with implementing an asthma program where the outcome units are different (e.g., blood glucose values versus asthma exacerbations). It is also difficult to combine two or more outcomes into one value of measurement (e.g., comparing one chemotherapeutic agent that prolongs survival but has significant side effects to another chemotherapeutic agent that has less effect on prolonging survival and has fewer side effects).

Cost-Utility Analysis

Cost-utility analysis (CUA) is a specialized form of CEA that includes a quality-of-life component associated with morbidity using common health indices such as quality-adjusted life years (QALYs) and disability-adjusted life years (DALYs). With CEA, you can measure the quantity of life (years gained) but not the "quality" or "utility" of those years. In a CUA, the intervention outcome is measured in terms QALY gained. QALY takes into account both the quality (morbidity) and the quantity (mortality) of life gained. CUA measures outcomes based on years of life that are adjusted by utility weights, which range from 1 for "perfect health" to 0 for "dead". These weights can take into account patient and society preferences for specific health states; however, there is no consensus on the measurement, since both patient and society preferences may vary based on culture. An advantage of CUA is that different types of outcomes and diseases with multiple outcomes of interest can be compared (unlike CEA) using one common unit, like QALY. In addition, CUA combines morbidity and mortality into one unit without having to assign a dollar value to it (unlike CBA).

Four Basic Pharmacoeconomic Methodologies

METHODOLOGY	COST MEASUREMENT UNIT	OUTCOME UNIT
Cost-minimization analysis	Dollars	Demonstrated or assumed to be equivalent in comparative groups
Cost-benefit analysis	Dollars	Dollars
Cost-effectiveness analysis	Dollars	Natural units (e.g., life-years gained, mmHg blood pressure, % at treatment goal)
Cost-utility analysis	Dollars	Quality-adjusted-life-year (QALY) or other utilities

Health-Related Quality of Life

Health-related quality of life (HRQOL) refers to the effects of a disease and its treatment on an individual's functioning and well being as perceived by that individual. It is commonly included under a broad umbrella of assessments known as patient-reported outcomes (PROs). HRQOL is comprised of several important domains, including physical and mental functioning, role functioning, vitality, social functioning, and general health perceptions, among others.

HRQOL assessments can provide important patient-centered information related to the effects of a disease or treatment on patient functioning and well-being. These assessments are typically developed as either general (or generic) health status instruments that can be used across a number of disease areas (e.g., SF-36 Health Survey can be used for asthma and diabetes, among others) or disease-specific measures applicable to a limited disease population (e.g., Asthma Quality of Life Questionnaire). Prior to their use in practice, it is critical that the reliability and validity of HRQOL assessments in specific patient populations has been documented.

PRACTICE CASE

The NEW ENGLAND
JOURNAL of MEDICINE

ESTABLISHED IN 1812   NOVEMBER 15, 2007   VOL. 357 NO. 20

Prasugrel versus Clopidogrel in Patients with Acute Coronary Syndromes

Stephen D. Wiviott, M.D., Eugene Braunwald, M.D., Carolyn H. McCabe, B.S., Gilles Montalescot, M.D., Ph.D.,
Witold Ruzyllo, M.D., Shmuel Gottlieb, M.D., Franz-Joseph Neumann, M.D., Diego Ardissino, M.D.,
Stefano De Servi, M.D., Sabina A. Murphy, M.P.H., Jeffrey Riesmeyer, M.D., Govinda Weerakkody, Ph.D.,
C. Michael Gibson, M.D., and Elliott M. Antman, M.D., for the TRITON–TIMI 38 Investigators*

ABSTRACT

BACKGROUND

Dual-antiplatelet therapy with aspirin and a thienopyridine is a cornerstone of treatment to prevent thrombotic complications of acute coronary syndromes and percutaneous coronary intervention.

METHODS

To compare prasugrel, a new thienopyridine, with clopidogrel, we randomly assigned 13,608 patients with moderate-to-high-risk acute coronary syndromes with scheduled percutaneous coronary intervention to receive prasugrel (a 60-mg loading dose and a 10-mg daily maintenance dose) or clopidogrel (a 300-mg loading dose and a 75-mg daily maintenance dose), for 6 to 15 months. The primary efficacy end point was death from cardiovascular causes, nonfatal myocardial infarction, or nonfatal stroke. The key safety end point was major bleeding.

RESULTS

The primary efficacy end point occurred in 12.1% of patients receiving clopidogrel and 9.9% of patients receiving prasugrel (hazard ratio for prasugrel vs. clopidogrel, 0.81; 95% confidence interval [CI], 0.73 to 0.90; $P<0.001$). We also found significant reductions in the prasugrel group in the rates of myocardial infarction (9.7% for clopidogrel vs. 7.4% for prasugrel; $P<0.001$), urgent target-vessel revascularization (3.7% vs. 2.5%; $P<0.001$), and stent thrombosis (2.4% vs. 1.1%; $P<0.001$). Major bleeding was observed in 2.4% of patients receiving prasugrel and in 1.8% of patients receiving clopidogrel (hazard ratio, 1.32; 95% CI, 1.03 to 1.68; $P=0.03$). Also greater in the prasugrel group was the rate of life-threatening bleeding (1.4% vs. 0.9%; $P=0.01$), including nonfatal bleeding (1.1% vs. 0.9%; hazard ratio, 1.25; $P=0.23$) and fatal bleeding (0.4% vs. 0.1%; $P=0.002$).

CONCLUSIONS

In patients with acute coronary syndromes with scheduled percutaneous coronary intervention, prasugrel therapy was associated with significantly reduced rates of ischemic events, including stent thrombosis, but with an increased risk of major bleeding, including fatal bleeding. Overall mortality did not differ significantly between treatment groups.

QUESTIONS

1. Looking at the results of the trial above, which of the following statements is correct?

   a. Clopidogrel has demonstrated a statistically significant benefit over prasugrel in reducing the primary efficacy endpoint

   b. Prasugrel has demonstrated a statistically significant benefit over clopidogrel in reducing the primary efficacy endpoint

   c. Prasugrel has demonstrated a statistically significant benefit over clopidogrel in preventing major bleeding

   d. Clopidogrel has demonstrated a statistically significant benefit over prasugrel in reducing the primary efficacy endpoint and preventing major bleeding

   e. There is no statistical difference between clopidogrel and prasugrel in the primary efficacy endpoint.

2. In the trial above of the new drug prasugrel vs. the standard (control) drug clopidogrel, what is the absolute risk reduction in the primary efficacy endpoint?

   a. 22%
   b. 2.2%
   c. 9.9%
   d. 200%
   e. 28%

   $$ARR = \left(\begin{array}{c}\text{risk in}\\ \text{control}\end{array}\right) - \left(\begin{array}{c}\text{risk in}\\ \text{tx}\end{array}\right)$$
   $$= 12.1\% - 9.9\%$$
   $$= 2.2\%$$

3. In the trial above, what is the relative risk reduction of experiencing the primary efficacy endpoint?

   a. 81.8%
   b. 50%
   c. 18.2%
   d. 122%
   e. 69%

   $$RRR = \frac{12.1 - 9.9}{12.1} \cdot 100\%$$
   $$= 18.18\%$$

4. In the trial above what is the number of people needed to treat with prasugrel to achieve the primary efficacy measure in one patient?

   round ↑

   a. 40
   b. 45
   c. 4.5
   d. 46
   e. 14

   $$NNT = \frac{1}{ARR} \leftarrow \text{DECIMALS!}$$
   $$= \frac{1}{\left(\begin{array}{c}\text{risk in}\\ \text{control}\end{array}\right) - \left(\begin{array}{c}\text{risk in}\\ \text{tx}\end{array}\right)}$$
   $$= \frac{1}{0.121 - 0.099} = 45.5$$
   $$= 46$$

5. In the trial above the hazard ratio for nonfatal bleeding, 1.25, can be interpreted as

   ✗

   a. At any time a patient in the prasugrel group was 1.25 times as likely to experience nonfatal bleeding as a patient in the clopidogrel group.

   b. At any time a patient in the prasugrel group was 75% more likely to experience nonfatal bleeding as a patient in the clopidogrel group.

   c. At any time a patient in the clopidogrel group was 1.25 times as likely to experience nonfatal bleeding as a patient in the prasugrel group.

   d. At any time a patient in the clopidogrel group was 75% more likely to experience nonfatal bleeding as a patient in the prasugrel group.

   e. At only this point in time a patient in the prasugrel group was 1.25 times more likely to experience nonfatal bleeding as a patient in the clopidogrel group.

Questions 6-14 do not relate to the case.

6. A trial is conducted between 2 different beta blockers, referred to as Drug A and Drug B. The null hypothesis is that both drugs will be equal in their effects on lowering BP. The study concluded that the effects of Drug A were better than Drug B in lowering BP (p-value < 0.01). Which of the following statements is correct?

   a. We can accept the null hypothesis.
   b. We can fail to accept the null hypothesis.
   c. There is a 10% chance that Drug A is superior.
   d. There is a 0.1% chance that Drug B is superior.
   e. This trial did not reach statistical significance.

7. Correlation in a clinical trial describes:

   a. The ability of 1 or more variables to predict another
   b. The relationship between 2 variables
   c. Nominal data
   d. Confounding variables
   e. A cause and effect relationship

8. Which of the following statements concerning a Type I error is correct?

    a. A type I error means that the null hypothesis is accepted in error.
    b. A type I error means that the null hypothesis is rejected in error.
    c. A type I error means failing to reject the null hypothesis in error.
    d. A type I error means that the null hypothesis is accepted.
    e. A type I error is a beta error.

9. Which of the following statements concerning case-control studies is correct? (Select **ALL** that apply)

    a. They are retrospective.
    b. The patient serves as their own control.
    c. The researcher analyzes individual patient cases.
    d. They include cases without the intervention.
    e. They provide conclusive evidence of cause and effect.

10. Which of the following statements regarding the median is correct? (Select **ALL** that apply)

    a. It is the value in the middle of a ranked list.
    b. It is not appropriate to use with skewed data. *use when skewed*
    c. It is not sensitive to outliers.
    d. It is a measure of dispersion.
    e. In a normal distribution, it is the same as the mean.

11. Choose the example that represents a direct medical cost: (Select **ALL** that apply)

    a. Lost productivity *indirect*
    b. Quality of life *intangible*
    c. Clinic visit
    d. Nursing services
    e. Cost of taking the bus to the hospital
    direct non-medical

12. Choose the best description of the purpose of a pharmacoeconomic analysis:

    a. To measure and compare the costs and outcomes of drug therapy and other medical interventions.
    b. To reduce health care expenditures by limiting medication use to only those who need it most.
    c. To get the best treatments available to as many people as possible.
    d. To examine the indirect costs of medical care in each medical specialty within hospitals, clinics, and outpatient surgery centers.
    e. To reduce the pharmacy drug budget within a hospital setting as a way to control health care costs.

13. Which of the following statements regarding average and incremental cost ratios is correct? (Select ALL that apply)

    a. Average cost ratios represent the average cost per outcome between competing alternatives.
    b. Incremental cost ratios represent the cost per additional unit of outcome between competing alternatives.
    c. Average cost ratios represent the average cost per outcome within a single alternative.
    d. Incremental cost ratios represent the cost per additional unit of outcome within a single alternative
    e. In most instances, incremental and average cost ratios are equal.

14. A pharmacist is conducting an analysis to determine the best way to manage patients with diabetes based on A1C values. Three treatment regimens will be evaluated based on cost and effects on A1C reduction. Choose the type of analysis the pharmacist should perform:

    a. A cost-utility analysis
    b. A cost-minimization analysis
    c. A cost-optimization analysis
    d. A cost-benefit analysis
    e. A cost-effectiveness analysis

Answers

1-b, 2-b, 3-c, 4-d, 5-a, 6-b, 7-b, 8-b, 9-a,c,d, 10-a,c,e, 11-c,d, 12-a, 13-b,c, 14-e

PHARMACOGENOMICS

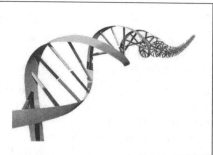

We gratefully acknowledge the assistance of Joseph D. Ma, PharmD, Associate Professor of Clinical Pharmacy at the University of California San Diego, Skaggs School of Pharmacy and Pharmaceutical Sciences, in preparing this chapter.

BACKGROUND

Pharmacogenomics is the science which examines inherited variations in genes that dictate drug response and explores ways that the variations can be used to predict whether a patient will have a good, bad, or no response to a drug. It is estimated that genetic factors contribute between 20-40% of the differences in drug metabolism and response between patients. The goal of pharmacogenomics is to identify these factors and develop optimized treatment strategies to improve efficacy while reducing adverse reactions. Pharmacogenomics is called "personalized medicine" where drugs are tailored for a person's unique genotype.

DEFINITIONS

Deoxyribonucleic acid (DNA): Deoxyribonucleic acid (DNA) is the genetic information, or characteristics of each individual, that has been inherited from both parents. The DNA is composed of long macromolecules that are the main components of the chromosomes. It consists of two long chains of nucleotides twisted into a double helix and joined together by hydrogen bonds.

Chromosome: The DNA is wrapped around proteins and packaged into chromosomes, which appear as threadlike structures. In a human cell there are usually 46 chromosomes, organized into two pairs of 23 – one pair has been inherited from the father and the other pair has been inherited from the mother.

Nucleotides: These consist of a nitrogenous base [adenine (A), thymine (T), guanine (G) and cytosine (C)], a five-carbon sugar, and a phosphate group. Nucleotides are the building blocks of DNA. In DNA, A binds to T and G binds to C, holding the double-helix form together. Similarly, RNA, which is single-stranded, has four bases but uracil (U) replaces the thymine (T).

Gene: The DNA can be divided into specific sequences of nucleotides that code for a single protein. The sequences of the nucleotides are called genes, which are the code, or instructions, for the synthesis of RNA, which is then translated into proteins. The proteins make up the life form; this is why the gene is called the basic unit of heredity.

Allele: The specific form of a gene. The genes have different forms because each person has two alleles (one from the mother and one from the father) for each gene. Alleles are also described as wild-type or variants. A wild-type allele is the usual (or normal) sequence. A mutation and/or polymorphism is referred to as a variant allele.

Genotype: The 2 alleles of a specific gene comprise a genotype. If both alleles are the same, the person is homozygous for that gene or trait. If the alleles are different, the person is heterozygous for that gene or trait.

Phenotype: A phenotype is the set of observable traits of an individual that results from his/her particular genotype. As an example, variations in the cytochrome P450 2D6 gene may result in variant phenotypes of ultra-rapid metabolizers (UMs), extensive metabolizers (EMs), intermediate metabolizers (IMs), and poor metabolizers (PMs) of particular drugs.

Haplotype: A group of genes or DNA variations that exist on the same chromosome and are likely to be inherited together.

Polymorphism: An inherited variation in the DNA sequence. Polymorphisms occur with fairly high frequency, but most do not result in a change in phenotype. Polymorphisms most commonly involve variation at a single base pair within the DNA. This is called a single nucleotide polymorphism (SNP, pronounced "snip"). Polymorphisms can also involve larger stretches of DNA called structural variations (SV). Human leukocyte antigens (HLAs) have structural variations which are clinically significant. HLAs alert the immune system to target a pathogen for destruction, and certain HLA variants put patients at higher risk for hypersensitivity reactions.

SINGLE NUCLEOTIDE POLYMORPHISMS AND STRUCTURAL VARIANTS

SNPs are the most common genetic polymorphisms in DNA. They occur every 100 – 300 base pairs and account for about 90% of all differences in human DNA. SVs are more rare than SNPs; however, they affect a larger region of DNA and have a greater impact on genes than SNPs. Whether the SNP or SV has an effect on function (and subsequent action of a drug) depends on the location and presence within a patient's DNA. Pharmacogenomic testing can identify whether an individual is homozygous or heterozygous for a specific SNP and is used to predict what type of response a patient may have to a drug.

CHANGES IN DRUG RESPONSE OR TOXICITY

Genetic polymorphisms can significantly alter the response or toxicity of a drug. These examples of genetic polymorphisms are well known:

- Variations in CYP2D6 Expression: Based on the presence or absence of CYP2D6 polymorphisms, patients can be CYP2D6 ultra-rapid metabolizers (UMs), extensive metabolizers (EMs), intermediate metabolizers (IMs) or poor metabolizers (PMs). Codeine is metabolized to morphine by CYP2D6; morphine provides the analgesic effect. UMs will have higher morphine levels while PMs will have low, or absent morphine levels and thus minimal analgesic effect from the use of codeine.

- Variations in expression of the solute carrier organic anion transporter family member 1B1 (SLCO1B1) gene: The presence of variant alleles have an increased risk of myalgia when taking statins.

- Variations in the presence or absence of the HLA-B*1502 allele: if present, the risk of a severe skin reaction to carbamazepine or phenytoin is increased from <1% (wild type) to 5-10%.

- Variations in over-expression of the HER2/neu oncogene: If the receptor is over-expressed, the response to trastuzumab *(Herceptin)* and ado-trastuzumab *(Kadcyla)* is positive.

The Drugs With Pharmacogenomic Testing table includes drugs where genetic testing is routinely done and/or required according to the product labeling. Following this list are the drugs known to have genetic factors, but where standardized testing is not yet routine. The FDA has guidelines for drug companies that require diagnostic tests to be approved at the same time as the drug if genetic testing will be required.

Genetic Variation in Warfarin Response

Warfarin consists of two racemic isomers – an S-isomer and an R-isomer. The S-isomer is 3 - 4 times more potent than the R-isomer. The S-isomer is metabolized by CYP2C9, whereby the CYP2C9*1 allele is the wild-type allele and results in normal enzyme activity. The CYP2C9*2 and the 2C9*3 alleles are decreased-function alleles. This results in elevated S-warfarin concentrations leading to increased bleeding. The CYP2C9*2 allele leads to a reduction in metabolism of warfarin whereas the CYP2C9*3 allele causes an even larger reduction in metabolism. Patients who are homozygous for the CYP2C9*3 allele have the greatest risk of bleeding. Lower warfarin doses are needed, at least initially, to reduce bleeding risk.

Vitamin K epoxide reductase (VKOR) is needed for reduction of vitamin K, which, in turn, activates coagulation factors. The liver takes up free warfarin, which inhibits the VCOR complex. By blocking reduction of vitamin K, warfarin interferes with the formation of coagulation factors. The 2nd variation resulting in an increased bleeding risk is a variation in the VKORC1 gene. Several haplotypes are associated with alteration of VKORC1 activity. These are haplotype A and G. Patients with the haplotype A produce less VKORC1 and will require a lower dose of warfarin.

With the patient's genetic information, the warfarin starting dose can be more accurately determined. Genetic testing has been simplified by the availability of several commercial companies that test for these variations; however, testing is not yet routinely performed nor has testing been adequately validated. In warfarin initiation, always proceed cautiously and monitor the INR frequently. The chart below shows the ranges of expected maintenance doses of warfarin based on the presence of the CYP2C9 and VKORC1 alleles.

Expected Warfarin Maintenance Dose Ranges Based on VKORC1 Haplotypes and CYP450 2C9 Genotypes

VKORC1 HAPLOTYPES	CYP2C9 GENOTYPES					
	*1/*1	*1/*2	*1/*3	*2/*2	*2/*3	*3/*3
GG	5-7 mg	5-7 mg	3-4 mg	3-4 mg	3-4 mg	0.5-2 mg
AG	5-7 mg	3-4 mg	3-4 mg	3-4 mg	0.5-2 mg	0.5-2 mg
AA	3-4 mg	3-4 mg	0.5-2 mg	0.5-2 mg	0.5-2 mg	0.5-2 mg

Drugs With Required/Strongly Recommended Genetic Testing

DRUG	INDICATIONS	TESTING AND/OR RECOMMENDATIONS	CLINICAL SIGNIFICANCE
Abacavir (Ziagen) **Abacavir + lamivudine (Epzicom)** **Abacavir + zidovudine + lamivudine (Trizivir)**	HIV	HLA-B*5701 If positive, avoid use of abacavir.	Hypersensitivity to abacavir is a multi-organ clinical syndrome; see HIV chapter Discontinue as soon as a hypersensitivity reaction is suspected.
Clopidogrel (Plavix)	Acute coronary syndromes, PAD, stroke	CYP2C19 genotype Consider alternative treatment in patients identified as poor metabolizers.	Effectiveness of the drug depends on conversion of prodrug to an active metabolite by CYP2C19. Poor metabolizers exhibit higher cardiovascular event rates than patients with normal CYP2C19 function.
Carbamazepine (Tegretol, others)	Seizures, neuralgia	HLA-B*1502 for Asian patients. If positive, do not use unless benefit clearly outweighs risk.	Serious dermatologic reactions with positive HLA-B*1502 alelle, including Toxic Epidermal Necrolysis (TEN) and Stevens-Johnson Syndrome (SJS), have occurred.
Trastuzumab (Herceptin), Ado-trastuzumab emtansine (Kadcyla), Lapatinib (Tykerb), Pertuzumab (Perjeta)	Breast and gastric cancer	HER2/neu oncogene If positive, can use drug	HER2/neu over-expression required for use. The test must be 2+ or 3+ positive on immunohistochemical (IHC) testing, weakly positive (1+) tumors do not respond well to therapy.
Cetuximab (Erbitux), Panitumumab (Vectibix)	Colorectal cancer	K-Ras mutations If positive, do not use drug	These agents are not effective in patients with colorectal cancer who have a K-Ras mutation (~40% of patients). Package inserts state that there is no benefit in patients with K-Ras mutations in codon 12 or 13. Therefore, only patients who are K-Ras mutation-negative (wild type) should receive these medications.
Cetuximab (Erbitux), Erlotinib (Tarceva), Afatinib (Gilotrif)	Non-small cell lung cancer	EGFR If positive, can use drug	These medications have enhanced effectiveness in tumors expressing EGFR or who have EGFR-TK exon 19 deletion or exon 21 substitution mutations.

Drugs With Required/Strongly Recommended Genetic Testing Continued

DRUG	INDICATIONS	TESTING AND/OR RECOMMENDATIONS	CLINICAL SIGNIFICANCE
Imatinib *(Gleevec)*	Gastrointestinal stromal tumors (GIST)	CD117 (KIT, C-Kit) If positive, can use drug	Patients will respond to therapy if GIST is KIT (CD117)+.
Maraviroc *(Selzentry)*	HIV	HIV tropism with Trofile test If CCR5-positive, can use drug	Adult patients infected with only CCR5-tropic HIV-1 should use maraviroc. Do not use in patients with dual/mixed or CXCR-4-tropic HIV-1 disease as efficacy was not demonstrated in a Phase 2 trial of this patient population.
Imatinib *(Gleevec)*, **Dasatinib** *(Sprycel)*, **Nilotinib** *(Tasigna)*, **Bosutinib** *(Bosulif)*, **Ponatinib** *(Iclusig)*	Chronic myelogenous leukemia (CML)	BCR-ABL If positive, can use drug	In CML, the Philadelphia chromosome is a specific abnormality which leads to a fusion protein of abl (Abelson) with bcr (breakpoint cluster region), termed bcr-abl. These drugs target and inhibit this abnormal fusion protein.
Rituximab *(Rituxan)*, **Ofatumumab** *(Arzerra)*	Non-Hodgkin lymphomas, Hodgkin lymphoma, Chronic lymphocytic leukemia, etc.	B-Cell CD20 Expression If positive, can use drug	Directed against CD-20 receptor site on malignant cells but also normal lymphocytes resulting in efficacy and toxicity with antibody dependent cellular cytoxicity (ADCC), complement fixation, natural killer cell activation and apoptosis.
Simeprevir *(Olysio)*	Hepatitis C	NS3 Q80K polymorphism If positive, do not use drug	Screen patients with HCV gentotype 1a infection for the NS3 Q80K polymorphism at baseline. Patients with this polymorphism will not respond and alternative therapy should be given.
Crizotinib *(Xalkori)*, Ceritinib *(Zykadia)*	Locally advanced or metastatic non-small cell lung cancer (NSCLC)	Anaplastic lymphoma kinase (ALK) If positive, can use drug	Tyrosine kinase inhibitors indicated for the treatment of patients with locally advanced or metastatic NSCLC that is ALK positive as detected by an FDA-approved test.
Vemurafenib *(Zelboraf)*, Dabrafenib *(Tafinlar)*, Trametinib *(Mekinist)*	Unresectable or metastatic melanoma	BRAF V600E or BRAF V600K mutation If positive, can use drug	These agents are contraindicated in patients with wild-type BRAF melanoma.
Azathioprine, Mercaptopurine	Solid organ cancers, leukemia, Crohn's disease, ulcerative colitis	Thiopurine methyltransferase (TPMT) If positive (for loss of function TPMT allele), find alternative treatment or start at a very low dose	Patients with a genetic deficiency of TPMT may have ↑ risk of myelosuppressive effects; those patients with low or absent TPMT activity are at risk for severe myelotoxicity; occurs in ~10% of patients.
Lenalidomide *(Revlimid)*	Myelodysplastic syndrome (MDS), others	5q deletion If positive, can use drug	Patients with 5q deletion MDS have increased risk of hematologic toxicity (neutropenia and thrombocytopenia) from their MDS but also a better response to lenalidomide therapy.
Tositumomab	Non-Hodgkin lymphoma after relapse or failure of standard chemotherapies	MS4A1 (CD-20 antigen) If positive, can use drug	Directed against CD-20 receptor site on malignant cells but also normal cells B- and pre-B-lymphocytes resulting in efficacy and toxicity.

Drugs With Required/Strongly Recommended Genetic Testing Continued

DRUG	INDICATIONS	TESTING AND/OR RECOMMENDATIONS	CLINICAL SIGNIFICANCE
Brentuximab vedotin (*Adcetris*)	Hodgkin lymphoma after failure of autologous stem cell transplant. Systemic anaplastic large cell lymphoma after failure of previous chemotherapies.	TNFRSF8 (CD-30 antigen) <u>If positive, can use drug</u>	Directed against CD-30 receptor site on malignant cells but also normal cells resulting in efficacy and toxicity.
Denileukin diftitox (*Ontak*)	Cutaneous T-cell lymphoma	IL2RA (CD-25 antigen) <u>If positive, can use drug</u>	Directed against CD-25 receptor site on positive malignant cells.
Ivacaftor (*Kalydeco*)	Cystic fibrosis transmembrane conductance regulator (CFTR)	CFTR: G551D, G1244E, G1349D, G178R, G551S, S1251N, S1255P, S549N, S549R <u>If positive, can use drug</u>	Patients age six years and older who have the specific mutations in the CFTR gene.

Select Drugs Where Pharmacogenomic Testing Should Be Considered

DRUG	INDICATIONS	TESTING AND/OR RECOMMENDATIONS	CLINICAL SIGNIFICANCE
Allopurinol (*Zyloprim*)	Gout	HLA-B*5801 Consider testing prior to starting therapy in high-risk individuals, such as Korean patients with significant renal impairment or those of Han Chinese or Thai ancestry.	There is increased risk of severe cutaneous reactions in patients testing positive for HLA-B*5801. Discontinue at 1st appearance of skin rash or other signs which may indicate an allergic reaction. In some instances, a skin rash may be followed by more severe hypersensitivity reactions such as exfoliative, urticarial, and purpuric lesions, as well as SJS (and/or generalized vasculitis, irreversible hepatotoxicity, and, on rare occasions, death).
Codeine	Pain, cough	CYP2D6 No recommendation, but use caution – CYP 2D6 ultra-rapid metabolizers are common.	Ultra-rapid metabolizers may have exaggerated response due to extensive conversion to morphine metabolite. Overproduction of morphine can result in ↑ CNS effects, including an ↑ risk of respiratory depression. Use extreme caution in lactating women as most opioids are excreted in breast milk. While use may be acceptable in small amounts, the risk to the infant must be considered. Do not use codeine (in *Tylenol #3*, others), since ultra-rapid metabolizers of the CYP 2D6 enzyme will produce excessive amounts of morphine, which could be fatal to the infant. See contraindications and warnings in Pain chapter.

Drugs Where Pharmacogenomic Testing Should Be Considered Continued

DRUG	INDICATIONS	TESTING AND/OR RECOMMENDATIONS	CLINICAL SIGNIFICANCE
Warfarin (*Coumadin, Jantoven*)	Clot prevention	CYP 2C9 and VKORC1 If not testing, use caution by selecting a low starting dose, increasing slowly, and monitoring INR frequently – especially at initiation. If the test indicates variations, a safer starting dose can be selected.	Increased bleeding risk due to decreased functional (CYP 2C9*2 and CYP 2C9*3) and VKORC1 G > A variant.
Capecitabine (*Xeloda*), Fluorouracil (*Adrucil*)	Breast, colon, pancreatic cancers	Dihydropyrimidine dehydrogenase (DPD) If positive, do not use drug	A deficiency in DPD can increase toxicity associated with these agents. The incidence is low but potentially fatal.
Phenytoin (*Dilantin*), Fosphenytoin (*Cerebyx*)	Seizures	HLA-B*1502 for Asian patients If positive, do not use unless benefit clearly outweighs risk.	Strong association between developing Stevens-Johnson Syndrome (SJS) and Toxic Epidermal Necrolysis (TEN) and the presence of the HLA-B*1502 allele.
Atomoxetine (*Strattera*)	ADHD	CYP2D6 genotype No recommendation, but use caution.	Atomoxetine concentrations have been measured at 5-fold higher concentrations in poor metabolizers versus extensive metabolizers. This can lead to an increase in adverse effects. See ADHD chapter.
Fluorouracil, Methotrexate	Lymphomas, leukemias, psoriasis, RA, others	Methylenetetrahydrofolate reductase (MTHFR) If positive, consider reducing dose	MTHFR polymorphisms influence the metabolism of folates and could modify the pharmacodynamics of antifolates and many other drugs whose metabolism, biochemical effects, or target structures require methylation reactions.
Irinotecan (*Camptosar*)	Colon cancer and other cancers	UGT1A1*28 If positive, consider reducing dose	Patients homozygous for the UGT1A1*28 allele are at risk of neutropenia; initial one-level dose reduction should be considered. Heterozygous carriers of the UGT1A1*28 allele may also be at risk, however, most patients tolerate normal starting doses.
Many pain and psych drugs – see Drug Interactions chapter	Various psychiatric disorders	CYP2D6 genotype If poor metabolizer, consider reducing dose	CYP2D6 poor metabolizers are at risk of variable response to therapies, reduce dosage by 25% for some antipsychotics and reduce doses when co-administered with CYP2D6 inhibitors.
Cisplatin (*Platinol*)	Several cancers	TPMT If positive, can use drug with caution and monitor closely for ototoxicity	TPMT intermediate or poor metabolizers are at risk for severe toxicity. All patients undergoing *Platinol* treatment have a risk of ototoxicity, recommend audiometric testing.
Tamoxifen (*Soltamox*)	Breast cancer	Estrogen receptor 1 If positive, can use drug	Available evidence indicates that patients whose tumors are estrogen receptor positive are more likely to benefit from tamoxifen therapy.

Drugs Where Pharmacogenomic Testing Should Be Considered Continued

DRUG	INDICATIONS	TESTING AND/OR RECOMMENDATIONS	CLINICAL SIGNIFICANCE
Chloroquine *(Aralen)*, Dapsone *(Aczone)*, Methylene blue, Nitrofurantoin, Primaquine, Probenecid, Quinidine, Quinine and Sulfonamides	Infectious diseases	Glucose-6-phosphate dehydrogenase (G6PD) deficiency If positive, can use drug with caution and monitor blood counts	Hemolytic anemia is more common in G6PD deficient patients.
Isoniazid	Tuberculosis	NAT1, NAT2 If positive, can use drug with caution and monitor liver function monthly	Neuropathy and liver toxicity more common in NAT1/NAT2 slow acetylators.

PRACTICE QUESTIONS

1. A 15 year-old female of Asian ancestry presents with a seizure disorder. The physician plans to initiate carbamazepine therapy, but first orders genetic testing in order to determine if she is at an increased risk for the following adverse drug reaction:

   a. Gastrointestinal bleeding
   b. Hemorrhage
   c. Serious skin reactions
   d. Neuropathy
   e. Tendon rupture

2. When initiating carbamazepine in a patient of Asian descent, which is the appropriate allele and/or polymorphism to test for?

   a. VKORC1
   b. HLA-B *1502
   c. CYP450 2C9
   d. HER2/neu
   e. TPMT activity

3. Trastuzumab is indicated in cancers with an overexpression of this gene:

   a. ALK
   b. BCR ABL+
   c. cKIT
   d. HER2/neu
   e. BRCA2

4. A patient was started on warfarin 5 mg once daily. She presents to the clinic 2 weeks later and is found to have an INR of 4.7 with excessive oral bleeding when she brushes her teeth. Which of the following most likely describes the patient's genotype?

   a. CYP 2C9 *1/*1
   b. CYP 2C9 *3/*3
   c. CYP 3A4 *1/*1
   d. CYP 2D6 *1/*1
   e. CYP 2D6 *1/*2

5. Which of the following statements regarding abacavir is correct? (Select **ALL** that apply.)

   a. Testing for HLA-B*5701 is recommended on initiation or re-initiation of therapy.
   b. If the testing is positive for HLA-B*5701, abacavir cannot be used.
   c. Abacavir is a protease inhibitor that should be boosted with ritonavir.
   d. Abacavir can be taken with or without food.
   e. Abacavir is recommended as a preferred first line agent for newly diagnosed HIV+ patients.

Answers

1-c, 2-b, 3-d, 4-b, 5-a,b,d

DRUG ALLERGIES & REPORTING

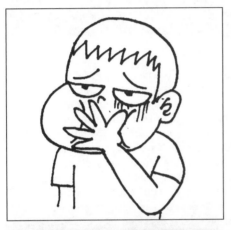

WHAT IS IT? A SIDE EFFECT? AN ADVERSE EFFECT? AN ALLERGY? ANAPHYLAXIS?

Adverse Drug Reactions: Side Effects, Adverse Events and MedWatch Reporting

Side effects or adverse events are not generally avoidable and can occur in anyone with normal doses (although higher doses can increase the side effect severity). Side effects are more common and generally less severe (such as orthostatic hypotension from doxazosin) while adverse events are known complications of a drug but are generally rarer and more severe (such as rash from lamotrigine).

[Note: do not mix these up with medication errors, which are due to someone doing something incorrectly, such as giving the wrong drug to a patient. Medication errors are an important area and are discussed in the Medication Safety chapter.]

True drug allergies, or hypersensitivity reactions, are classified into four types. Type I reactions are immediate (within 15-30 minutes of exposure). The severity can range from minor inconvenience to death. Type II reactions occur minutes to hours after exposure. Examples include hemolytic anemia and thrombocytopenia. Type III reactions are immune-complex reactions. They occur 3-10 hours after exposure. Examples include drug-induced lupus and serum sickness. Type IV reactions are delayed hypersensitivity reactions. They can occur anywhere from 48 hours to several weeks after exposure. The classic example of a type IV reaction is the PPD skin test for tuberculosis, which peaks at 48 hours.

Most drug reactions are characterized as Type A which means that they are dose-dependent and predictable from the drug's pharmacology. For example, if a patient starts doxazosin at 1 mg QHS they will have much less orthostatic hypotension and dizziness than if they began the medication at a 4 mg dose; thus, this drug is slowly titrated upward to reduce the severity of the side effects. Type B reactions [which are idiosyncratic – this means a particular patient has an independent peculiar reaction (or hypersensitivity) to the drug] are not predictable from the known pharmacology of the drug and the reaction is determined by patient-specific susceptibility factors.

Although side effects or adverse effects can occur in anyone, we need to consider that they may be more likely if a drug is given to a patient at high risk for a certain condition. For example, anyone taking an aminoglycoside for longer than a few days would expect to suffer some degree of renal damage. However, if a patient with impaired renal function receives an aminoglycoside they would be more susceptible to further damage sooner.

- Side effects, adverse events and allergies (which are discussed below) should be reported to the FDA's MedWatch program, which is called the FDA's Adverse Event Reporting System (FAERS), that provides a central collection for problems caused by drugs. [Note that vaccines are an exception that are not reported under FAERS; vaccine adverse drug reactions are reported under a different program called VAERS; this is described in the Immunization chapter.]

- The FDA conducts Phase IV (post-marketing safety surveillance programs) for approved drug and therapeutic biologic products and collates the reports to better understand the drug safety profile in a real world setting. When drugs are tested in trials, high-risk patients are typically excluded. Yet, in real life settings high risk patients are often included. If a drug causes a reaction in 1 out of every 3,000 people, you might not even see the reaction appear in a smaller clinical trial. This is why community-based adverse event reporting is critical.

> **EXAMPLE OF "REAL LIFE" ADVERSE EVENT INCIDENCE VERSUS THAT IN A CLINICAL TRIAL SETTING**
>
> When spironolactone was studied in heart failure patients during the RALES trial, patients with renal insufficiency or elevated potassium levels were excluded due to the known risk of additional hyperkalemia from the use of spironolactone. The drug was found to have benefit in advanced heart failure patients and doctors in the community began to use it in their heart failure patients. In this real life setting, patients with renal insufficiency or elevated potassium were occasionally prescribed spironolactone, and arrhythmias and sudden death due to hyperkalemia were reported.

- Reporting is voluntary. Healthcare professionals and patients may also report adverse events to the drug manufacturer, who is required by law to send the report to the FDA's MedWatch program. The MedWatch form that is used for reporting can be found online via the link provided in the references at the beginning of this chapter. We can also report by calling the FDA directly. We can also call in or report online via the link provided in the references at the beginning of this section. MedWatch is not only used to report problems with drugs; it is also used for reporting problems with biologics, medical devices and some nutritional products and cosmetics.

- If the FDA receives enough reports that a drug is linked to a particular problem they may require that the product's drug information, such as the package insert or labeling, be changed. In especially risky cases they will issue safety alerts to prescribers, usually before the labeling is changed.

> **EXAMPLE OF AN ADR THAT WAS ADDED TO THE PACKAGE INSERT MANY YEARS AFTER THE DRUG HAD BEEN RELEASED DUE TO THE ADR REPORTS RECEIVED BY THE FDA**
>
> Oseltamivir *(Tamiflu)* was initially released without any warning of unusual behavior in children. The FDA received enough reports that they issued a warning to prescribers in 2006. After many more reports, in 2008, the FDA required the drug company to update the prescribing information to include a precaution about hallucinations, confusion and other strange behavior in children.

Example of a Posting on the FDA Website of a Drug that is Being Monitored Under Phase IV

DRUG	USAGE	ADVERSE EVENTS	NOTES
Ticagrelor *(Brilinta)*	To reduce the rate of thrombotic cardiovascular events in patients with acute coronary syndrome (ACS) (unstable angina, non-ST elevation myocardial infarction, or ST elevation myocardial infarction).	Adverse event reports of neutropenia, thrombocytopenia, pancytopenia, and clinical gout were identified.	FDA is continuing to evaluate neutropenia, thrombocytopenia, pancytopenia, and clinical gout to determine if regulatory action is required.

Assessing Causality of an Adverse Drug Reaction

When an adverse reaction occurs, it can sometimes be difficult to determine whether a particular drug is the cause. The Naranjo Scale is a validated causality assessment scale that can help pharmacists determine the likelihood that a drug caused an ADR. The pharmacist simply answers the questions on the scale and a probability score is calculated:

QUESTIONNAIRE	YES	NO	DO NOT KNOW
Are there previous conclusive reports on this reaction?	+1	0	
Did the adverse event appear after the suspected drug was given?	+2	-1	
Did the adverse reaction improve when the drug was discontinued or a specific antagonist was given?	+1	0	
Did the adverse reaction appear when the drug was readministered?	+2	-1	
Are there alternative causes that could on their own have caused the reaction?	-1	+2	
Did the reaction reappear when a placebo was given?	-1	+1	
Was the drug detected in any body fluid in toxic concentrations?	+1	0	
Was the reaction more severe when the dose was increased or less severe when the dose was decreased?	+1	0	
Did the patient have a similar reaction to the same or similar drugs in any previous exposure?	+1	0	
Was the adverse event confirmed by any objective evidence?	+1	0	

Scoring > 9 = definite ADR; 5-8 = probable ADR; 1-4 = possible ADR; 0 = doubtful ADR

Characterizing an Adverse Drug Reaction

In order to properly characterize an adverse reaction, sensitivity to a drug or a true drug allergy, pharmacists need to ask the right questions. When patients report an "allergy" to a drug these questions can help place the reaction into the proper context:

- What reaction occurred (was it a mild rash, a severe rash with blisters, trouble breathing?)

- When did it occur? (about how old were you?)

- Can you use similar drugs in the same class (for example, if they report an allergy to penicillin, have they ever used *Keflex*?)

- Ask and include any food allergies and latex allergies in the patient record. Latex allergies should be recorded since some drugs require tubing, have latex vial stoppers, or require gloves for administration.

DRUG SIDE EFFECTS (SENSITIVITIES OR INTOLERANCES)

EXAMPLE OF STOMACH UPSET DUE TO CODEINE BEING REPORTED INCORRECTLY AS A DRUG ALLERGY

Carmen received acetaminophen 300 mg-codeine 30 mg *(Tylenol #3)* for pain relief after a dental extraction several years ago. Carmen got very nauseated from the medicine. When Carmen was admitted to the hospital for a left hip replacement, she reported to the intake coordinator that she was "allergic" to codeine. The intake coordinator did not attempt to clarify the reaction. The hospital's pain management protocol calls for hydromorphone in a patient-controlled analgesic device for post-op pain control. The physician used a less desirable option for pain control due to the reported allergy.

Stomach Upset/Nausea

Stomach upset or nausea is often incorrectly reported as an allergy. The reaction should be listed on the patient profile because the drug bothered the patient and, if possible, the drug should be avoided in the future, but this is not an allergy and should not prevent drugs in the same class from being used. This is more accurately categorized as an intolerance. Modern electronic medical records often allow for documentation of intolerances separate from allergies. An example of an intolerance is the patient who gets stomach upset from codeine (but not hydrocodone or other drugs in the morphine class) or from erythromycin (but not azithromycin or other macrolides).

Mild Rash

Opioids can commonly cause histamine-induced skin rash or itching, particularly in the inpatient setting post-op when opioid-naïve patients are receiving the medication or non-naïve patients are receiving higher-than-normal dosing. Pruritus due to this or other causes, if not severe, can be reduced or avoided if the patient is pre-medicated with an antihistamine before use, such as diphenhydramine.

Photosensitivity

Many drugs can cause photosensitivity, which requires limiting sun exposure and using sunscreens that block both UVA (causes aging, skin cancer) and UVB (causes sunburn). Sunscreens that <u>cover both UVA and UVB are labeled broad-spectrum</u>.

[Note that there is a different type of skin reaction that occurs when sunlight causes the drug to become toxic; this is an allergic reaction and is rare. The reaction looks like a bad sunburn on only sun-exposed skin.]

Another sensitivity that some people have is to the iodine in contrast dyes. This reaction can cause itching, flushing and a drop in blood pressure, but is not technically a true allergy.

NSAIDs can cause issues with either sensitivity or true allergy; these are discussed in the next section.

Severe Skin Rashes

There are several severe skin rashes that can be caused by drugs, including Stevens Johnson syndrome (SJS), toxic epidermal necrolysis (TEN), drug reaction with eosinophilia and systemic symptoms (DRESS) and thrombotic thrombocytopenic purpura (TTP). <u>All of these can be life-threatening and require prompt treatment</u>. SJS and TEN result in severe, explosive mucosal erosions, a high temperature and damage to organs (eyes, liver, kidney, lungs). SJS and TEN are not easily distinguished, SJS can lead to TEN, and the key to treating both is <u>stopping the offending agent as soon as possible</u>. In addition, patients will receive fluid/electrolyte replacement, wound care and pain medications. <u>Corticosteroids</u> may be used in SJS (benefit is controversial) but are <u>contraindicated in TEN</u>. Due to the severity of the mucosal involvement, antibiotics are usually necessary to prevent infection. DRESS can include a variety of skin eruptions as well as systemic symptoms (fever, hepatic dysfunction, renal dysfunction, lymphadenopathy). Treatment is <u>stopping the offending agent</u>, although <u>symptoms may actually worsen</u> for a period of time after the agent has been discontinued. TTP can cause purpura (bruises) and petechiae (dots) on the skin. These are caused by bleeding under the skin. TTP should be treated emergently with

DRUGS MOST COMMONLY ASSOCIATED WITH PHOTOSENSITIVITY

Sulfa antibiotics	Griseofulvin
Tetracyclines	Tacrolimus
NSAIDs	Diuretics, thiazides and loops
Amiodarone	
Chloroquine	Topical fluorouracil
Coal Tar	St John's wort
Oral and topical retinoids	Cyclosporine
Quinine	Tigecycline
Fluoroquinolones	Voriconazole

DRUGS ASSOCIATED WITH SEVERE SKIN RASHES

Not complete; these are well known.

SJS/TEN Sulfamethoxazole	Minocycline, Doxycycline
Allopurinol	Tiagabine
Carbamazepine	Zonisamide
Clindamycin	
Oxcarbazepine	**DRESS** Ethosuximide
Phenobarbital	
Ethosuximide	Carbamazepine
Lamotrigine	Phenytoin/ Fosphenytoin
Phenytoin/ Fosphenytoin	Minocycline, Doxycycline
Clopidogrel	
Ticlopidine	**TTP** Clopidogrel
Quinine	Ticlopidine
Abacavir	
Nevirapine	Sulfamethoxazole
Letrozole	Quinine
Hydroxychloroquine	Acyclovir, valacyclovir, famciclovir
Piroxicam	

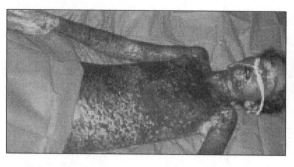

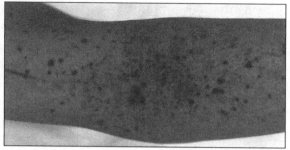

Patient with Stevens-Johnson Syndrome

Patient with Thrombotic Thrombocytopenic Purpura

plasma exchange. The table contains the drugs most commonly associated with severe skin rashes. Note that it is not complete; recently, cases of severe rash were associated with the use of the (generally safe) OTC analgesics acetaminophen and ibuprofen.

TRUE DRUG ALLERGIES AND ANAPHYLAXIS

<u>Penicillins and sulfonamides cause the most drug allergies</u>. For a true drug allergy to occur the person must have taken the drug previously. Initial exposure will cause a Type I hypersensitivity reaction, resulting in IgE production, which primes the body to release excessive histamine at the next drug exposure. This section is describing a drug allergy reaction and treatment, but keep in mind that similar treatment could be necessary for non-drug allergies, and the pharmacist who is dispensing an epinephrine self-injector for other types of allergies will provide the same instructions.

A reaction <u>without breathing difficulty</u> may sometimes be treated by simply <u>stopping the offending drug</u>. <u>Antihistamines</u> can be used to <u>counteract the histamine release</u> that causes itching, swelling and rash. <u>Steroids</u>, and sometimes <u>NSAIDs</u>, can be used to <u>decrease swelling. Severe swelling may necessitate a steroid injection</u>. Epinephrine is used if needed to <u>reverse bronchoconstriction</u> if the patient is wheezing or has other signs of trouble breathing.

Anaphylaxis is a severe, life-threatening allergic reaction that occurs seconds to minutes after taking the drug. Anaphylaxis can occur after an initial exposure and subsequent immune response, but some drugs can cause anaphylaxis with the first exposure.

Signs/Symptoms of Anaphylaxis

A patient experiencing anaphylaxis may have generalized urticaria (hives), swelling of the mouth and throat, difficulty breathing or wheezing sounds, abdominal cramping, hypotension (which can cause dizziness/light-headedness). They can become unconscious or go into shock. Symptoms can develop quickly – within seconds or minutes; treatment needs to be given quickly. Epinephrine instructions for pharmacy use with an immunization protocol are in the Immunizations chapter. Additional information to be provided to patients is included below.

How to Treat Anaphylaxis

If a patient has an anaphylactic reaction, they will need to go to the ED right away (or call 911) and receive an epinephrine injection ± diphenhydramine ± steroids and ± IV fluids. Do not put a pillow under a patient's head because this makes it more difficult to get air into the lungs. Do not attempt to put anything into their mouth.

Swollen airways can be quickly fatal and patients who have had such a reaction should carry injectable single-use epinephrine *(EpiPen, EpiPen Jr, Adrenaclick, Auvi-Q)*, if they may be at future risk. These contain 0.3 mg of epinephrine *(EpiPen Jr is 0.15 mg)*. Their emergency kit should include diphenhydramine tablets (25 mg x 2) and emergency contact information.

EpiPen Injection Instructions (For patients; detailed information on epinephrine use for health care professionals is in the Immunization chapter.)

- If using *Auvi-Q*, pull off the outer case, then follow the voice instructions to administer.

- Grasp the epinephrine shot injector in one fist with the black tip pointing down. Do not touch the black tip. (Color may be different.)

- With the other hand, pull off the cap.

- Hold the tip close to your outer thigh. Swing and jab the tip into your outer thigh (through clothing if necessary). The injector should be at a 90-degree angle to your thigh.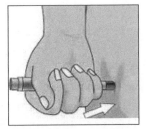

- Keep the injector in your outer thigh while you slowly count to 5.

- Remove the injector and rub the area where the medicine entered your skin.

- Look at the black tip: If the needle is showing, you received the dose. If not, you need to inject again. It is normal for some of the liquid to be left in the injector. Do not try to inject the remaining liquid.

- Patients may have two pens, and may need to use the second (in the opposite thigh) to maintain breathing prior to the arrival of medical help.

- Take the antihistamine tablets (2 x 25 mg) in your allergy kit.

- Anyone with serious allergies to food or drugs should wear a *Medic Alert* bracelet. These are available in the pharmacy, and link the patient and reactions to a 24-hour information line. Patients with serious allergies and medical conditions (including hypoglycemia that may require glucagon) should wear this type of identification.

DRUG CLASSES THAT CAN CAUSE ALLERGIC REACTIONS

While any drug can lead to an allergic reaction, some are more common. These are discussed below. Often the drug that caused the reaction can be replaced with another drug. Rarely this is not possible and desensitization may be recommended. This requires administering the drug in a medical setting in increasing amounts until the patient can tolerate the needed dose. "Patch testing" is occasionally used to try and determine possible rash reactions, including severe skin reactions such as TEN, but the tests do not always work and the research on patch testing is inconsistent.

Beta-Lactam Allergy

Penicillin is a beta-lactam antibiotic and there are many related compounds in this family, including nafcillin, oxacillin, ampicillin, amoxicillin, ticarcillin, piperacillin and others. Anyone who is allergic to one of the penicillins should be presumed to be allergic to all penicillins and should avoid the entire group, unless they have been specifically evaluated for this problem.

Cephalosporins are closely related to penicillin. People with a history of penicillin allergy have a small risk of having an allergic reaction to a cephalosporin or carbapenem. It is prudent on the exam to avoid any beta-lactam with a stated allergy to another, unless there is no alternative agent.

Sulfa Allergies

These are most commonly reported with sulfamethoxazole (in *Bactrim, Septra)*, and the patient should avoid using sulfapyridine, sulfadiazine and sulfisoxazole. "Non-arylamine" sulfonamides (thiazide diuretics, loop diuretics, sulfonylureas, acetazolamide, zonisamide and celecoxib) usually do not cross react with a sulfamethoxazole allergy, but on the exam you will likely have to recognize the reaction. Since the cross-reactivity between sulfamethoxazole and thiazides and loops is very small, the reaction is usually not considered when the need for these drugs is present – but the patient should be aware to watch for a possible reaction. There are other sulfa-type groups that also have low cross-reactivity. Sulfites or sulfate allergies do not cross react with a sulfonamide. The rotigotine patch, orphenadrine injection, the *Rowasa* mesalamine enema and some of the dobutamine formulations and some eye drops contain sulfites.

Opioid Allergy

The following agents cross-react: morphine, oxymorphone, codeine, hydrocodone, hydromorphone, oxycodone, nalbuphine, buprenorphine, butorphanol, levorphanol, naloxone, heroin (diacetyl-morphine). Tapentadol does not have an opioid-allergy contraindication in the US package labeling; tramadol does, however the two agents are structurally similar. Use caution if recommending either in an opioid allergy and if allergy to tramadol an allergy to tapentadol is likely, and vice-versa. If morphine-group allergy, choose (if appropriate): fentanyl, meperidine, methadone, tramadol, tapentadol (meperidine and fentanyl cross-react). Bottom line is safety; if used, monitor the patient.

Breathing Difficulties and NSAIDs

Reactions to NSAIDs, including aspirin, can be either a drug sensitivity (which can cause rhinitis, mild asthmatic type reactions or skin reactions) or a true allergic reaction. If a true allergy is present the patient will experience urticaria and angioedema, and occasionally anaphylaxis. COX-2 selective NSAIDs are used clinically, but on licensing exams it may be prudent to avoid all NSAIDs.

Peanut/Soy Allergy

A food allergy that is important for pharmacists to know is a peanut allergy, since soy is used in some medications. Peanuts and soy are in the same family and can have cross-reactivity. Parents of children with peanut allergies should be trained in CPR. An *EpiPen* may need to be kept within close reach. Most likely, a reaction will be due to consuming peanuts or soy unknowingly in food products. Drugs to avoid with peanut allergy:

- Clevidipine *(Cleviprex)*

- Propofol (*Diprivan*)

- Progesterone in *Prometrium* capsules

Egg Allergy

If a patient has a true allergy to eggs (which means they cannot enjoy birthday cake), they cannot use:

- Clevidipine *(Cleviprex)*

- Propofol (*Diprivan*)

- Influenza vaccine: Per ACIP, people who have experienced only hives from consuming eggs can receive TIV (the shot, given IM), as long as they are treated by a health care provider who is familiar with the potential manifestations of egg allergies and can be observed by a health care professional for at least 30 minutes after receiving each dose. If the person has more severe symptoms (such as wheezing, requiring epinephrine, hypotension, cardiovascular changes) they may not be able to receive the vaccine, but should be evaluated further by an allergist physician. *Flublok* is the first seasonal influenza vaccine made using recombinant techniques and does not use eggs at all in its production.

- Yellow Fever vaccine

- Rabies vaccine (precaution with egg allergy)

9

MEDICATION SAFETY

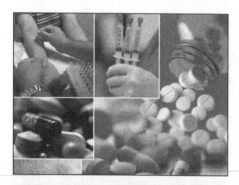

GUIDELINES/REFERENCES

Institute for Safe Medication Practices,
www.ismp.org

Joint Commission,
www.jointcommission.org

MMWR Guideline for Hand Hygiene in
Health-Care Settings October 25, 2002,
51(RR16);1-44.

Addtl guidelines included with the video
files (RxPrep Online).

BACKGROUND

Awareness of the prevalence of medical errors increased after the release of a study from the Institute of Medicine (IOM), *To Err is Human* (1999), which found that up to 98,000 Americans die each year in U.S. hospitals due to preventable medical errors, 7,000 from medication errors alone. These numbers understated the problem because they did not include preventable deaths due to medical treatments outside of hospitals. Since the release of the IOM study, there has been a greater focus on the quality of healthcare provided in the U.S. and the need to reduce medical errors, which are preventable. As pharmacists we are most concerned with errors involving medications.

This chapter begins with an overview of medication errors, followed by specific measures to limit medication errors in the community and institution settings. Included are select "high risk" drugs that require implementation of safety measures to avoid significant patient harm and a discussion of two types of medication devices that have important benefits but known safety risks – patient controlled analgesia (PCA) devices and automated dispensing cabinets (ADCs).

Patient safety includes reducing infection risk. Essential methods to reduce infections, such as proper hand-washing technique, enforcing universal precautions and using safe injection technique are included. The chapter concludes with a discussion of The Joint Commission (TJC), which provides accreditation for healthcare facilities. A primary focus of TJC is patient safety.

Definition of a Medication Error

The formal definition of a medication error developed by the National Coordinating Council on Medication Error Reporting and Prevention (NCC MERP) is "any preventable event that may cause or lead to inappropriate medication use or patient harm while the medication is in the control of the health care professional, patient, or consumer. Such events may be related to professional practice, health care products, procedures, and systems, including prescribing; order communication; product labeling, packaging, and nomenclature; compounding; dispensing; distribution; administration; education; monitoring; and use."

Do not confuse medication errors with adverse drug reactions (ADRs) – these are generally not avoidable although they may be more likely to occur if the drug is given to a patient at high risk for certain complications.

EXAMPLE OF AN ADR (NOT A MEDICATION ERROR)

A 55-year old female had a history of herpes zoster. She has no other known medical conditions. The patient reported considerable "shingles pain" that "run from my back through my left breast." The physician prescribed pregabalin. The patient returned to the physician with complaints of ankle swelling, which required drug discontinuation.

This problem would not be attributable to a medication error made by the physician who prescribed pregabalin or by the pharmacist who dispensed it. Rather, this is a side effect that can occur with the use of this drug.

SYSTEM-BASED CAUSES OF MEDICATION ERRORS

Experts in medication safety concur that the most common cause of medication errors is not individual error but problems with the design of the medical system itself. Currently, instead of blaming the "lousy pharmacist" or the "lousy technician" (or the prescriber), health care professionals should find ways to improve the system in order to reduce the chance that the error will occur again. The idea is to design systems in order to prevent medication errors from reaching the patient.

Root Cause Analysis to Prevent Future Errors

Errors can be prevented from occurring again when the contributing factors are made known and appropriate prevention strategies are employed. A root cause analysis (RCA) is a retrospective investigation of an event that has already occurred which includes reviewing the sequence of events that led to the error. The information obtained in the analysis is used to design changes that will hopefully prevent future errors.

Findings from the RCA (the identification of the factors that contributed to the event and led to a "sentinel event" – the unexpected occurrence involving death or serious physical or psychological injury, or risk thereof) can be applied proactively to analyze and improve processes and systems before they breakdown again.

The RCA can be of enormous value in capturing both the big-picture perspective and the details of the error. This type of analysis facilitates system evaluation and the need for corrective action. Targeting corrective measures at the identified root causes is the best way to prevent similar problems from occurring in the future. However, it is recognized that complete prevention of recurrence by a single intervention is not always possible. Thus, RCA is often considered to be a repetitive process, and is frequently viewed as a continuous quality improvement (CQI) tool.

An analysis can also be done prospectively to identify pathways that could lead to errors and to identify ways to reduce the error risk. Failure Mode and Effects Analysis (FMEA) is a proactive method used to reduce the frequency and consequences of errors. FMEA is used to analyze the design of the system in order to evaluate the potential for failures, and to determine what potential effects could occur when the medication delivery system changes in any substantial way or if a potentially dangerous new drug will be added to the formulary.

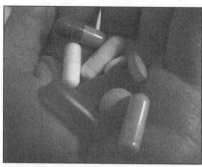

MEDICAL ERROR CLASSIFICATION: ERRORS OF OMISSION AND ERRORS OF COMMISSION

Errors of Omission

An error of omission means leaving something out that is needed for safety, such as missed instructions, or failure to provide a dose at the required time.

Errors of Commission

An error of commission means that something was done incorrectly, such as prescribing bupropion to a patient with a history of epilepsy or dispensing sulfamethoxazole to a patient with a sulfa allergy.

REPORTING MEDICATION ERRORS

Medication errors, preventable adverse drug reactions, close calls, or hazardous conditions should be reported. We report medication errors so that changes can be made to the system to prevent similar errors in the future. Without reporting, such events may go unrecognized and thus will happen elsewhere because others will not learn from the incident.

In a community pharmacy, the staff member who discovers the error should immediately report it (using the established reporting structure) to the corporate office or in the case of an independently owned pharmacy, the owner, who is involved with the quality assurance program. These are mandated by many state boards of pharmacy and have the purpose (in the words of the California state board) "to develop pharmacy systems and workflow processes designed to prevent medication errors." Error investigations need to take place quickly – often as soon as within 48 hours of the incident so that the sequence of events remains clear to those involved. Many states mandate the ethical requirement that errors be reported to the patient and their prescriber as soon as possible.

In a hospital setting, the staff member should report a medication error through the hospital's specific medication event reporting system. Many medication error reporting systems within hospitals are electronic, however some hospitals still maintain a paper reporting system. The hospital's Pharmacy and Therapeutics (P&T) committee should be informed of the error as well as the Medication Safety Committee.

Reporting to Organizations that Specialize in Error Prevention

> **Those who cannot remember the past are condemned to repeat it.**
>
> *Poet and Philosopher George Santayana*
> *1863-1952*

The Patient Safety and Quality Improvement Act of 2005 (Patient Safety Act) authorized the creation of Patient Safety Organizations (PSOs) to improve the quality and safety of health care delivery in the United States. The Patient Safety Act encourages clinicians and health care organizations to voluntarily report and share quality and patient safety information without fear of this information being used in legal proceedings. The Agency for Healthcare Research and Quality (AHRQ) administers the provisions of the Patient Safety Act and the Patient Safety Rule dealing with PSO operations.

Organizations that specialize in error prevention can analyze the system-based causes of the errors and make recommendations to others who can learn from the mistakes. Every pharmacist should make it a practice to read medication error reports in order to use this history to improve their own practice settings. Information sources include the Institute for Safe Medication Practices (ISMP) newsletters which have information about medication-related errors, adverse drug reactions, as well as recommendations that will help reduce the risk of medication errors and other adverse drug events at the practice site.

The ISMP National Medication Errors Reporting Program (MERP) is a confidential national voluntary reporting program that provides expert analysis of the system causes of medication errors and disseminates recommendations for prevention.

On the ISMP website (www.ismp.org), medication errors and close calls can be reported. Click on "Report Errors." Professionals and consumers should be encouraged to report medication errors using this site even if the error was reported internally.

COMMON METHODS USED TO REDUCE MEDICATION ERRORS

Patient Profiles

Pharmacies should maintain current patient profiles that include all prescription drugs, over the counter (OTC) medications, and anything else the patient is taking such as natural products and other supplements. Allergies and the type of allergic reaction (e.g., rash, lip swelling) should be recorded. Intolerances should be noted and the drug avoided, if possible, or the intolerance can be proactively managed (such as using an anti-emetic agent if the intolerance is nausea from an opioid). See the Drug Allergy chapter for pointers on proper documentation. The most common use of the profile is to check for allergies and drug interactions, but it can also be used for monitoring appropriateness of therapy, checking for polypharmacy (polypharmacy means "many drugs" and refers to problems that can occur when a patient is taking more medications than are necessary) and assessing patient adherence with their medication regimen.

Medication Therapy Management

The example above may have been discovered during a more comprehensive medication review (CMR), through the process of medication therapy management (MTM). A personal medication record (PMR) is prepared, and a medication-related action plan (MAP) is developed, preferably by a pharmacist-led team. The next steps involve interventions, referrals, documentation and plans for follow-up. This is a program mandated under the Medicare drug benefit (Medicare Part D) to promote safe and effective medication use. Medicare's drug benefit provides outpatient prescription drug coverage. It is available only through private companies. At a minimum, beneficiaries targeted for MTM include members with multiple chronic conditions who are taking multiple drugs and are likely to incur annual costs for covered drugs that exceed a predetermined level. Computer databases are used to identify patients with certain high-risk conditions (such as heart failure or uncontrolled diabetes) who are generally using many medications (some systems tag patients taking many chronic medications daily) and assign a pharmacist (preferably) to review profiles for proper use. Since this is a Medicare requirement the majority of MTM programs exist within Medicare-funded health care plans. MTM may also apply to populations outside of Medicare.

The pharmacist can form a partnership with the patient and prescriber to remedy any issues or lapses. Often, these reviews identify missed therapy such as lack of an ACE inhibitor or ARB in patients with diabetes, missing beta blocker therapy post-MI, missing bisphosphonate therapy with high-dose chronic steroids, and others, since these are easily searchable in databases. A popular MTM initiative is to improve non-adherence in heart failure patients due to the high-rate of ED visits due to decompensated heart failure. MTM is also used to identify cost-savings, by promoting switches to generics or more affordable brands, or by suggesting patient assistance programs or low income subsidies for eligible members.

Drug Utilization Reviews (DURs) and Retrospective Analysis

DURs are reviews of prescribing used by medical groups, insurance or localities that try to identify some combination of inappropriate medication use, including therapeutic duplications, drug-drug and drug-disease contraindications, incorrect dosage or treatment durations, abuse and clinical misuse, such as prescribing out of formulary for unnecessary indications.

Medication Reconciliation

According to TJC, "Medication reconciliation is the process of comparing a patient's medication orders to all of the medications that the patient has been taking." This reconciliation is done to avoid medication errors such as omissions, duplications, dosing errors, or drug interactions. It should be done at every transition of care in which new medications are ordered or existing orders are rewritten.

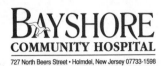

BAYSHORE
COMMUNITY HOSPITAL
727 North Beers Street • Holmdel, New Jersey 07733-1598

MEDICATION RECONCILIATION ORDER FORM

List all patient medications prior to assessment. Include OTCs & alternative meds (herbals). (Alternative meds will not be continued on admission).

Before an outpatient receives any medication as part of their test or procedure, list all of their current home medications looking for allergies, interactions, duplications, or other concerns. A complete reconciliation is required only if the patient is to be admitted to the hospital.

Allergies: _____

DO NOT USE ABBREVIATIONS: .#, #.0, IU, MS, MgSO4, MSO4, QD, QOD, U

Information Source: _____ Patient _____ Family _____ Primary Care Physician
_____ Patient's Pharmacy(s) _____ (See Back)
_____ MAR from _____ _____ Other, specify _____

☐ Check here if patient is not currently on any medication.

Medication Name	Dose	Route	Frequency	Last Dose Date	Time	Physician Decision: Continue? Circle one	
1						Y	N
2						Y	N
3						Y	N
4						Y	N
5						Y	N
6						Y	N
7						Y	N
8						Y	N
9						Y	N
10						Y	N
11						Y	N
12						Y	N
13						Y	N
14						Y	N
15						Y	N

On the lines below, enter orders for new medications that the patient isn't currently taking or changes to their current regimen.

_____
_____
_____
_____

Completed by _____ Nurse Signature _____ Date/Time _____
(print name)

I have reviewed this list of patient medications and to the best of my knowledge, the additional medications I have ordered will not result in any adverse reaction(s).

Completed by _____ MD Signature _____ Date/Time _____
(print name)

Faxed/Given to _____ By _____ Date/Time _____
(sign & print name)

70811 (REV 6/06)   Sheet _____ of _____

Transitions in care include changes in setting, service, practitioner or level of care. This process comprises five steps:

1. Develop a list of current medications;

2. Develop a list of medications to be prescribed;

3. Compare the medications on the two lists;

4. Make clinical decisions based on the comparison; and

5. Communicate the new list to appropriate caregivers and to the patient.

EXAMPLE OF THE BENEFIT OF MEDICATION RECONCILIATION

Ann is an 82 year-old female. Her only medication for the previous ten years has been amlodipine 10 mg daily. Ann recently developed influenza. She began to have trouble breathing and was taken to the hospital. It was discovered that Ann had pneumonia and new-onset atrial fibrillation. She was prescribed diltiazem, dabigatran and digoxin. Ann was discharged to transitional care and received the new medications plus the previous medication amlodipine. The consultant pharmacist conducted a medication review to reconcile the medications and, after discussion with the physician on the patient's rate control, the pharmacist wrote an order to discontinue the diltiazem.

At discharge, give the patient a list of medications and educate about those to be continued at home. Address any discrepancies. Though most often discussed in the hospital context, medication reconciliation can be equally important in ambulatory care, as many patients receive prescriptions from more than one outpatient provider and may go to several pharmacies. Medication reconciliation is a part of the National Patient Safety Goals (NPSGs) issued by TJC.

Medication Guides

Medication Guides (or MedGuides) present important adverse events that can occur with over 300 medications. MedGuides are FDA-approved patient handouts and are considered part of the drug's labeling. If a medication has a MedGuide, it should be dispensed with the original prescription and with each refill. Some medications dispensed while inpatient require MedGuides and these should be available to the patient or family upon request. It is not necessary to dispense them to inpatients routinely as the patient is being monitored. MedGuides are required for many individual agents and some entire classes of medications (including anticonvulsants, antidepressants, long-acting opioids, NSAIDs and the ADHD stimulants and atomoxetine).

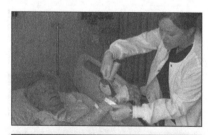

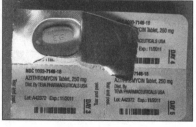

Barcoding

Barcoding may be the most important medication error reduction tool in the arsenal right now. The barcode follows the drug through the medication use process to make sure it is being properly stocked (such as in the right space in the pharmacy or in the right pocket in the dispensing cabinet), through compounding (if required), and to the patient. The barcode is used at the bedside to identify that the correct drug (by scanning the code on the drug's packaging) is going to the right patient (via scanning the patient's wristband) and confirms that the dose is being given at the right time. The nurse may have a badge barcode that can track who administered the dose. Barcodes are now on many pumps and can prevent errors involving medications being given IV that are not meant to be administered in this manner.

Look-Alike, Sound-Alike Medications

Confusing drug names is a common cause of medication errors. Poor handwriting and similar product labeling aggravate the problem of pulling a look-alike or sound-alike agent instead of the intended medication. Drug dictionaries within computer systems are being built with alerts to attempt to double-check that the correct medication is being ordered or withdrawn. For example a warning may appear on the screen of the ADCs which will state: "This is DILAUDID. Did you want hydroMORPHONE? (To avoid confusion with morphine.)

Drugs that are easily mixed up should be labeled with tall man letters (e.g., CeleXA, CeleBREX). Using tall man letters, which mix upper and lower case letters, draws attention to the dissimilarities in the drug names. The letters that are upper cases are the ones that are different between the two look-alike, sound-alike drugs. Tall man lettering makes the drugs with names that look or sound like others less prone to mix-ups. ISMP, FDA, The Joint Commission, and other safety-conscious organizations have promoted the use of tall man letters as one means of reducing confusion between similar drug names. If receiving a verbal order for a drug that is easily confused with another be sure to repeat the drug name back, with spelling if helpful, to the prescriber. It may be possible to remove a drug that is easily confused with another from the institution's formulary.

The FDA's and ISMP's approved tall man lettering information is available at: http://www.ismp.org/tools/tallmanletters.pdf

Do Not Use Error-Prone Abbreviations, Symbols, and Dosage Designations

Abbreviations are unsafe and contribute to many medical errors. TJC standards include recommendations against the use of unsafe abbreviations. The ISMP's list of error-prone abbreviations, symbols, and dosage designations includes those on TJC's do-not-use list (designated by **). Try writing the number 5.0 on a lined paper and you can see how easily the number could be mistaken for 50; this is why trailing zeros (after a whole number) are not permitted. Leading zeros are required because it would be easy to miss a decimal point placed before a number (such as .5) if the leading zero was not present (the correct way to write this is 0.5). The other items on the list are important enough that it is almost misleading to give one example – such as the long history of mix-ups between morphine

Official "Do Not Use" List[1]

Do Not Use	Potential Problem	Use Instead
U, u (unit)	Mistaken for "0" (zero), the number "4" (four) or "cc"	Write "unit"
IU (International Unit)	Mistaken for IV (intravenous) or the number 10 (ten)	Write "International Unit"
Q.D., QD, q.d., qd (daily)	Mistaken for each other	Write "daily"
Q.O.D., QOD, q.o.d, qod (every other day)	Period after the Q mistaken for "I" and the "O" mistaken for "I	Write "every other day"
Trailing zero (X.0 mg)* Lack of leading zero (.X mg)	Decimal point is missed	Write X mg Write 0.X mg
MS	Can mean morphine sulfate or magnesium sulfate	Write "morphine sulfate" Write "magnesium sulfate"
MSO₄ and MgSO₄	Confused for one another	

[1] Applies to all medication-related documentation that is handwritten (including free-text computer entry) or on pre-printed forms.

*Exception: A "trailing zero" may be used only where required to demonstrate the level of precision of the value being reported, such as for laboratory results, imaging studies that report size of lesions, or catheter/tube sizes. It may not be used in medication orders or other medication-related documentation.

and magnesium and resultant fatalities. Review the TJC list carefully. If abbreviations are used within an institution (such as a hospital) they must not be on that institution's unapproved abbreviation list (and not include any on the Joint Commission's do-not use list). The unapproved abbreviations list is supposed to be kept readily accessible in the unit and may be placed at the back of the patient chart. It is best to attempt to avoid abbreviations entirely.

The ISMP's list of error-prone abbreviations is available at: http://www.ismp.org/tools/errorproneabbreviations.pdf

Indications for Use on Prescriptions

An indication for use that is written on the prescription (such as lisinopril 10 mg once daily for hypertension) helps pharmacists ensure appropriate prescribing and drug selection. If the pharmacist does not know the indication for the prescribed medication, the prescriber should be contacted.

Measurements Should be in the Metric System

Measurements should be kept in the metric system only. Prescribers should use the metric system to express all weights, volumes and units.

Provide Instructions on Prescriptions; Avoid Using "As Directed"

Using the term "as directed" is not acceptable on prescriptions because the patient often has no idea what this means and the pharmacist cannot verify a proper dosing regimen. Occasionally, this term is used on the bottle along with a separate dosing calendar, such as with warfarin. It would be preferable to write "use per instructions on the dosing calendar" since the patient may not understand how to take the medication and may not be aware that a separate dosing calendar exists.

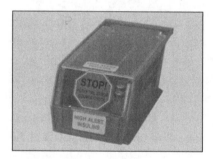

Special Bins and Labeling for High-Alert Drugs

Drugs that bear a heightened risk of causing significant patient harm when used in error should be designated as "High-alert". Any drug that is high risk for significant harm if dispensed incorrectly can be placed in a medication bin that provides a visual alert to the person pulling the medication. The bin can be labeled with warnings and include materials (placed inside the bin) that should be dispensed with the drug (such as oral syringes or MedGuides). In the hospital setting certain drugs are classified as "high-alert" and these can be placed in bins labeled with dispensing requirements.

There are many drugs considered high-alert, including insulin and oral hypoglycemics, opioids, anticoagulants, antiarrhythmics, anesthetics, chemotherapeutics, injectable KCl, phosphate, magnesium and hypertonic saline.

Use the ISMP "high-alert" list to determine which medications require special safeguards to reduce the risk of errors. It is available at: www.ismp.org/tools/highalertmedications. Keep in mind that the ISMP's list represents the most common agents that are high risk, and need special precautions. An institution's list should be based on the experience in that setting.

Select High-Alert Drugs and Safe-Use Precautions

DRUG	PRECAUTIONS
Hypertonic Saline	Allow only commercially available, standard (e.g., isotonic) concentrations of sodium chloride outside the pharmacy
	Limit options – do not stock the 3% sodium chloride injection
	Develop a protocol for administering sodium chloride for use in treating hyponatremia – covering the rate and volume of administration and the frequency of serum sodium monitoring
	Limit addition of sodium to enteral feedings to the pharmacy
	In dialysis units, stock a single hypertonic concentration and store in a locked area with limited access and affix special hazard labeling
Insulin	Eliminate insulin pens from the inpatient setting
	If U-500 is stocked, specify conditions under which it is to be used
	Standardize all insulin infusions to one concentration
	Develop protocols for insulin infusions, transition from infusion to SC and sliding scale orders
	Have standard orders in place for management of hypoglycemia
	Do not use "U" for units; always label with "units" or "units = mL", but never just "mL"
	Do not place in ADCs; all insulin orders should be reviewed by a pharamcist prior to dispensing
Heparin	Standardize heparin solutions – use premixed and reduce the number of concentrations available
	Standardize administration procedures – place dose stickers on heparin bags and double check all rate changes. If a bolus is ordered, give it from a syringe, rather than modifying the rate of the infusion
	Differentiate all look-alike products
	Separate the storage of all drugs ordered in units
	Standardize the dosing using weight-based protocols
	Have infusion pump rate settings and line placement on dual-channel pumps checked by two persons
	Develop and follow standard treatment protocols
	Do not use "U" for units
	Use only 'free flow' protected pumps

High-Alert Drugs and Safe-Use Precautions Continued

DRUG	PRECAUTIONS
Potassium Chloride	Remove all KCl vials from floor stock
	Centralize KCl infusion preparation in the pharmacy
	Use premixed containers
	Use protocols for KCl delivery, including indications for:
	▪ KCl infusion
	▪ Maximum rate of infusion
	▪ Maximum allowable concentration
	▪ Guidelines for when cardiac monitoring is required
	▪ Stipulation that all KCl infusions must be given via a pump
	▪ Prohibition of multiple simultaneous KCl solutions (e.g., no IV KCl while KCl is being infused in another IV)
	Allow for automatic substitution of oral KCl for IV KCl, when appropriate
	Label all fluids containing potassium with a "Potassium Added" sticker
Opioids	Use of tools to screen patients for risk factors for oversedation and respiratory depression
	Monitor vitals, use of telemetry when indicated, and sedation scales per protocol
	Build red flag alerts into e-prescribing systems for dosing limits
	Use of tall man lettering
	Separation of sound-alike and look-alike agents
	Use conversion support systems to calculate correct doses
	Use infusion pump technology when administering IV

EXAMPLE OF AN ERROR DUE TO MISIDENTIFICATION OF A CONCENTRATION BASED ON THE PACKAGING

The intravenous catheters of three neonates in a NICU unit in Los Angeles were flushed with the adult therapeutic dose of heparin (10,000 units/mL) rather than the heparin flush dose of 10 units/mL. This accident did not result in fatalities although two of the babies required the reversal agent protamine. Three babies died from a similar incident the previous year at a different hospital. The overdose was administered because the nurse thought she was using a lower concentration of heparin.

Due to the high risk associated with heparin overdose, high concentration heparin vials should not be present in patient care areas. Instead, therapeutic doses should be sent by the pharmacy department.

Do Not Rely on Medication Packaging for Identification Purposes

Look-alike packaging can contribute to errors. If unavoidable, separate look-alike drugs in the pharmacy and patient care units, or repackage.

Avoid Multiple-Dose Vials, if Possible

These pose risk for cross-contamination (infection) and over-dosing. If used, they should be (ideally) designated for a single patient and labelled appropriately. Discard the remainder when the patient is done with the medication, or is discharged.

Use Safe Practices for Emergency Medications/Crash Carts

Staff must be properly trained to handle emergencies and use crash cart medications. The medications should be unit dose and age-specific, including pediatric-specific doses. A weight-based dosing chart can be placed in the trays used in the pediatric units. If a unit dose medication is not available it is best to have prefilled syringes and drips in the cart as much as possible because it is easy to make a mistake under the stress of a code. The emergency medications should be stored in sealed or locked containers in a locked room and replaced as soon as possible after use (through a cart exchange so that the area is not left without required medications). Monitor the drug expiration dates. Trained pharmacists should be present at codes when possible.

Dedicate Pharmacists to the ICU, Pediatric Units and Emergency Departments

These are units with a high incidence of preventable medication errors, and pharmacist working in these units can assist in identifying and preventing medication errors by developing process improvements designed to reduce drug errors.

Organize Educational Programs

Staff education programs such as "in-services" should be provided whenever new high-alert drugs are being used in the facility, to introduce new procedural changes aimed at preventing medication errors and to introduce any new guidelines. The information provided in these "in-services" should be unbiased and should not be provided in a skewed manner by drug company representatives. Many hospitals now limit the use of pharmaceutical companies to provide drug education due to the inherent bias.

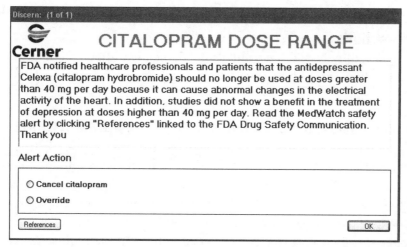

Develop and Use Standard Protocols

Standard protocols for high-risk drugs increase the rate of appropriate prescribing based on published recommended guidelines and reduce the chance of errors due to inappropriate prescribing. The Joint Commission requires that standard order sets be used for all antithrombotics. The standard order sheet should include instructions for initial doses of heparin and other high-risk antithrombotics, monitoring for bleeding, using appropriate antidotes, monitoring for HIT and discontinuing heparin if HIT is suspected. The prescriber should be required to justify any order outside the protocol and a pharmacist should approve the request.

Implement Computerized Prescriber Order Entry (CPOE)

Computerized physician/provider order entry is a computer system that <u>allows direct entry of medical orders</u> by prescribers. Directly entering orders into a computer has the benefit of reducing errors by <u>minimizing the ambiguity</u> resulting from hand-written orders. A much greater benefit is seen with the <u>combination of CPOE and clinical decision support tools</u>. Clinical guidelines and patient labs can be built into the CPOE system and alerts can notify a prescriber if the drug is inappropriate, or if labs indicate the drug could be unsafe (such as a high potassium level and a new order for a potassium-sparing agent). CPOE can include standard order sets. In addition to medication orders, CPOE is used for laboratory orders and procedures. An example of an on-screen alert from a clinical decision support system is shown. The alert in this example pops-up when a prescriber attempts to order citalopram with a dose greater than 40 mg/day.

Educate Patients and their Families

Patients can play a <u>vital role in preventing medication errors</u> when they have been encouraged to ask questions and seek satisfactory answers about their medications before drugs are dispensed at a pharmacy. If a patient questions any part of the medication dispensing process, whether it is about the drug's appearance, or dose, or something else, the pharmacist must be receptive and responsive (<u>not</u> defensive). All patient inquiries should be thoroughly investigated before the medication is dispensed. The written information about the medications should be at a reading level that is comprehensible for the patient.

It may be necessary to provide pictograms or other means of instruction to patients who do not speak English or are unable to read English. Attempts <u>must be made to communicate to the patient in their language</u>, using on-site staff or <u>dial-in</u> services.

Monitor for Drug-Food Interactions

<u>Check for drug-food interactions routinely</u> and have nutrition (also called "dietary") involved with this effort when drugs with a high rate of food interactions (such as warfarin) are ordered.

Follow Requirements for Risk Evaluation and Mitigation Strategies (REMS) Drugs

REMS is an FDA program that requires <u>specified training and various restrictions</u> (patient requirements, user registries, etc.) on certain drugs. Examples include the clozapine patient registry, the APPRISE program for erythropoietin use in oncology, the iPLEDGE program for isotretinoin, and others. In 2011 the FDA began new REMS to reduce the misuse of long-acting opioids due to the inherent danger with these drugs. The list of REMS drugs keeps growing. When working your way through this book note the many drugs that have REMS requirements.

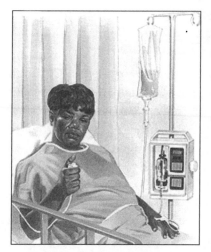

PATIENT CONTROLLED ANALGESIC (PCA) DEVICE OVERVIEW AND SAFETY CONCERNS

Opioids are effective agents used for moderate to severe post-surgical pain and are the mainstay of treatment. These may be administered through PCA devices. PCAs allow the patient <u>to treat pain quickly</u> (there is no need to call the nurse and wait for the dose to arrive) and allow the administration of small doses, which helps reduce side effects (particularly over-sedation). However, as some patients will be opioid-naïve or receiving higher-than-normal doses post-surgically, antiemetics or antihistamines may be required. <u>PCA drug delivery can mimic the pain pattern more closely and provide good pain control</u>. Increasingly, the PCA is administered with anesthetics for a synergistic benefit in pain relief.

PCAs have important safety considerations

- The devices can be complex and require set-up and programming. This is a <u>significant cause of preventable medication errors</u>. PCAs should be used only with well-coordinated health care teams.

- Patients may not be appropriate candidates for PCA treatment. They should be cooperative and should have a cognitive assessment prior to using the PCA to ensure they can follow instructions.

- <u>Friends and family members should not administer PCA doses. This is a Joint Commission requirement.</u>

- PCAs do not frequently cause respiratory depression, but the risk is present. Advanced age, obesity and concurrent use of CNS depressants (in addition to higher opioid doses) increases risk.

With PCAs it is important to follow these safety steps

- <u>Limit the opioids</u> available in floor stock. Use standard orders (set drug dosages, especially for opioid-naïve patients) so that drugs are not over-dosed.

- <u>Educate staff</u> about HYDROmorphone and morphine mix-ups.

- Implement PCA <u>protocols</u> that include independent double-checking of the drug, pump setting, and dosage. The concentration on the <u>Medication Administration Record (MAR)</u> should match the PCA label.

- Use <u>bar-coding</u> technology. Some infusion pumps incorporate bar-coding technology. Scanning the barcode on the PCA bag would help ensure the correct concentration is entered during PCA programming. It will also ensure that the right patient is getting the medication.

- Assess the patient's <u>pain, sedation and respiratory rate</u> on a scheduled basis.

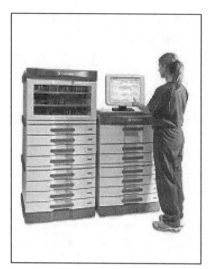

AUTOMATED DISPENSING CABINET OVERVIEW AND SAFETY CONCERNS

Most pharmacy interns will have seen automated dispensing cabinets (ADCs) while on clinical rotations. Common names are *Pyxis, Omnicell, ScriptPro* and *AccuDose.* Over half of the hospitals in the U.S. now use ADCs. In many hospitals the ADCs have replaced patient cassettes that had to be filled at least once daily and exchanged.

ADCs provide practical benefits

The drug inventory and medication can be automated when drugs are placed into the cabinet and removed. Controlled drug security can be improved (versus the previous method of keeping the controlled drugs locked in a metal cabinet or in a drawer in the nurses' station). The drugs are easily available at the unit and do not require individual delivery from the pharmacy. ADCs provide alerts, usage reports and work well with bar-coding.

ADCs have important safety considerations

- Stocking errors, such as a drug being placed in an incorrect drawer or bin, can lead to the wrong drug being dispensed (barcode scanning can be used to make sure that the correct drug is being placed into the ADC or dispensed).

- The wrong drug can be selected from the screen or ADC.

- The wrong dose can be selected from the screen.

- Errors can occur due to overrides that are not subject to a pharmacist's prospective order review.

Methods to improve ADC safety

- The Joint Commission requires that the pharmacist review the order before the medication can be removed from the ADC for a patient, except in special circumstances. The override function should be limited to true emergencies and all overrides should be investigated.

- The most common error associated with ADC use is giving the wrong drug or dose to a patient. The patient medication administration records (MARs) should be accessible to practitioners while they are removing medications from the ADC. Barcode scanning improves ADC safety. The drug can be scanned to make sure it is going into the right place into the cabinet and can ensure that the right drug is being pulled. Prior to administration the patient's wrist band can be scanned to make sure the drug is going to the right patient.

- Look-alike and sound-alike medications should be stored in different locations within the ADC. Using computerized alerts, ideally pop-ups that require a confirmation, when medications with high potential for mix-up in a given setting are selected, can help reduce error risk.

- Certain medications should not be put into the ADCs, including insulin, warfarin and high-dose narcotics (such as hydromorphone 10 mg/mL and morphine 20 mg/mL).

- Do not let nurses put medications back into the medication compartment because it might be placed in the wrong area; it is best to have a separate drawer for all "returned" medications.

- If the machine is in a busy, noisy environment, or in one with poor lighting, errors increase.

The California board specifically states that all drugs that are stocked in the ADC in a nursing facility are restocked by a pharmacist or by an intern or technician working under the supervision of a pharmacist. Removable pockets or drawers transported between the pharmacy and a stocking facility must be <u>transported in a secure tamper-evident</u> container.

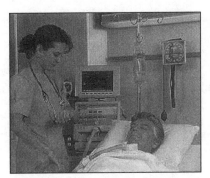

INFECTION CONTROL IN HOSPITALS

Nearly two million infections occur in hospitals annually – about one infection for every twenty patients. It is somewhat incredulous that so many patients enter hospitals for treatment of a condition and contract a different condition at the same facility.

The organisms in healthcare settings are highly pathogenic – this means that resistant bacteria are in the hospitals because that is where the sickest patients are and certain organisms grow in hospital settings, such as *Pseudomonas* in the moist environment of the ventilator.

Hospital infections cause avoidable illness and death and add enormous financial costs. The worst part of this sad state of affairs is that many of these infections are preventable if proper techniques (which are often simple measures) are followed. Many states now require hospitals to report infection rates and Medicare has begun to refuse reimbursement for hospital-acquired infections that are largely avoidable.

Common Types of Hospital (Nosocomial) Acquired Infections

- Urinary tract infections, from indwelling catheters (very common), <u>remove the catheter as soon as possible)</u> – preventing catheter associated infections is a Joint Commission National Patient Safety Goal (NPSG).

- Blood stream infections <u>from IV lines (central lines have the highest risk) and catheters</u>

- Surgical site infections <u>(see the section on antibiotic prophylaxis in the ID chapter)</u>

- Decubitis ulcers

- Hepatitis

- *Clostridium difficile*, other GI infections

- Pneumonia (mostly due to ventilator use), bronchitis

Universal Precautions for the Spread of Infectious Agents in the Healthcare Setting

Universal precautions is an approach to infection control that treats human blood and body fluids as if they are known to be infectious for HIV, HBV and other bloodborne pathogens. Contact with bodily fluids should be avoided through the use of good hand hygiene and, in select cases, the use of gowns, masks, or patient isolation.

There are 3 categories of transmission-based precautions defined by the CDC:

Contact precautions

- Intended to prevent transmission of infectious agents which are spread by direct and indirect contact with the patient and the patient's environment.

- Single patient rooms are preferred. If not available, keep ≥ 3 feet spatial separation between beds to prevent inadvertent sharing of items between patients.

- Healthcare personnel caring for these patients wear a gown and gloves for all interactions that may involve contact with the patient or contaminated areas in the patient's room.

- Contact precautions are recommended for patients colonized with MRSA and VRE.

Droplet precautions

- Intended to prevent transmission of pathogens spread through close respiratory contact with respiratory secretions.

- Single patient rooms are preferred. If not available, keep ≥ 3 feet spatial separation and drawing a curtain between beds is especially important for diseases transmitted via droplets.

- Healthcare personnel wear a mask (a respirator is not necessary) for close contact with the patient. The mask is donned upon room entry.

- Droplet precautions are recommended for patients with active *B. pertussis*, influenza virus, adenovirus, rhinovirus, *N. meningitides*, and group A streptococcus (for the first 24 hours of antimicrobial therapy).

Airborne Precautions

- Intended to prevent transmission of infectious agents that remain infectious over long distances when suspended in the air.

- Patient should be placed in an airborne infection isolation room (AIIR). An AIIR is a single-patient room that is equipped with special air and ventilation handling pressure rooms. The air is exhausted directly to the outside or re-circulated through HEPA filtration before return.

- Healthcare personnel wear a mask or respirator (N95 level or higher), depending on the disease, which is donned prior to room entry.

- Airborne precautions are recommended for patients with rubella virus (measles), varicella virus (chickenpox), or *M. tuberculosis*.

Prevention Of Catheter Associated Bloodstream Infections (CRBSI)

- The most important and most cost-effective strategy to minimize catheter-associated bloodstream infections is through aseptic technique during catheter insertion, including proper handwashing and utilization of standard protocols/catheter insertion checklist.

- It is also important to minimize use of intravascular catheters, if possible, through intravenous to oral route protocols and setting appropriate time limits for catheter use. For example, peripheral catheters should be removed/replaced every 2-3 days to minimize risk for infection.

- Other strategies shown to reduce the risk of CRBSI, include the use of skin antiseptics (2% chlorhexidine), antibiotic impregnated central venous catheters, and antibiotic/ethanol lock therapy, but must be weighed against the potential risk for increased rates of resistance.

Hand Hygiene

Many hospital infections are spread by hospital worker's hands and numerous studies show that proper hand hygiene reduces the spread of nosocomial infection. Patients are often carriers of resistant bacteria, including MRSA and VRE. Alcohol-based hand rubs (gel, rinse or foam) are considered more effective in the healthcare setting than plain soap or antimicrobial soap and water. Review the conditions below in which soap and water are preferable. Do not wear jewelry under gloves – these harbor bacteria and can tear the gloves. Keep fingernails clipped short and clean.

Antimicrobial hand soaps that contain chlorhexidine (*Hibiclens,* others) may be preferable to soap and water to reduce infections in healthcare facilities. Triclosan may also be better but this compound gets into the water supply and has environmental concerns.

When to Wash Hands

- Before entering and after leaving patient rooms.

- Between patient contacts if there is more than one patient per room.

- Before and after removing gloves (new gloves with each patient).

- Before handling invasive devices, including injections.

- After coughing or sneezing.

- Before handling food and oral medications.

Use Soap and Water (not alcohol-based rubs) in these situations

- Before eating.

- After using the restroom.

- Anytime there is visible soil (anything noticeable on the hands).

- After caring for a patient with diarrhea or known *C. difficile* or spore forming organisms – <u>alcohol-based hand rubs have poor activity against spores</u>.

- Before caring for patients with food allergies.

Soap and Water Technique

- Wet both sides of hands, apply soap, rub together for at least 15 (slow) seconds.

- Rinse thoroughly.

- Dry with paper towel and use the towel to turn off the water.

Alcohol-Based Hand Rubs Technique

- Use enough gel (2-5 mL or about the size of a quarter).

- Rub hands together until the rub dries (15-25 seconds).

- Hands should be completely dry before putting on gloves.

Hand-Hygiene for Sterile Compounding

- This is in the Sterile Compounding section later in this chapter.

It is important to properly clean surfaces, including bed rails, eating trays, and other room surfaces. Health care professionals should be careful not to be sources of infection from contaminated clothing (including white coats and ties). Organisms that spread via surface contact include VRE, *C. difficile*, noroviruses and other intestinal tract pathogens.

Safe Injection Practices

Outbreaks involving the transmission of blood borne pathogens or other microbial pathogens to patients (and occasionally to healthcare workers) continue to occur due to unsafe injection technique. The majority of safety breaches involve the reuse of syringes in multiple patients, contamination of IV bags with used syringes, failure to follow basic injection safety when administering IV medications and inappropriate care or maintenance of glucometer equipment that is used on multiple patients.

The following practices ensure safe injection of medications. These recommendations are meant for healthcare facilities; see the Drug Disposal chapter for more information on syringe disposal for patients.

- <u>Never administer an oral solution/suspension IV. Many medication errors (sometimes fatal) have occurred this way. Always label oral syringes "for oral use only."</u>

- <u>Never reinsert used needles into a multiple-dose vial or solution container</u> (whenever possible, <u>use of single-dose vials is preferred over multiple-dose vials</u>, especially when medications will be administered to multiple patients).

- Needles used for withdrawing blood or any other body fluid, or used for administering medications or other fluids should preferably have "engineered sharps protection" which reduces the risk of an exposure incident by a mechanism such as drawing the needle into the syringe barrel after use.

- To avoid contamination to the patient, <u>never touch the tip or plunger of a syringe.</u>

- Disposable needles contaminated with drugs, chemicals or blood products should never be removed from their original syringes unless no other option is available. <u>Throw the entire needle/syringe assembly (needle attached to the syringe) into the red plastic sharps container.</u>

- Never remove a needle by unscrewing it.

- Used disposable needles/sharps should be discarded immediately after use <u>without recapping</u> into a sharps container (a non-reusable plastic container that is puncture resistant, leak proof on the sides and bottom, properly labeled and closable).

- Sharps containers should be easily accessible, replaced routinely, and not allowed to overfill. <u>Never compress or "push down" on the contents of any sharps container.</u>

- If someone is stuck with a needle the proper department at the facility should be contacted immediately.

STERILE MEDICATION PREPARATION AND LAMINAR FLOW HOODS

Medications given intravenously bypass the protective mechanisms of the skin barrier and gastrointestinal tract. About half of medications given in the hospital setting are given IV. If the medication is contaminated the patient will suffer severe adverse effects and possible death. In addition to <u>IV preparations</u>, items that must be prepared in a sterile manner are opthalmics, inhalations, tissue soaks (for organ transplants), other implants, and irrigations.

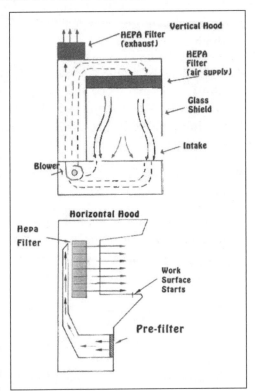

Hoods are ventilation devices used to keep sterile compounded or parenteral drugs free of contaminants, and are used to keep the pharmacy area free of noxious fumes. Vertical flow hoods (also called biological safety cabinets or chemotherapy hoods) blow air <u>from the top down</u> to maintain sterility and to protect the pharmacist or technician preparing the medication from breathing in dangerous fumes. Vertical hoods are used for <u>chemotherapy</u> and other hazardous medications. <u>Laminar flow means that the air is moving in an uninterrupted, constant stream. The air is drawn through a High Efficiency Particulate Air (HEPA) filter that catches particulates.</u> The air may be directed horizontally toward the user, as shown in the picture of the horizontal hood. HEPA filters remove 99.97% of all air particles <u>0.3 mm or larger</u>. This keeps the workspace area free of contaminants, including bacterial and viral organisms. The cabinet is stainless steel with a smooth design to keep out contaminants and is designed to reduce the risk of joints and other spaces where spores might accumulate.

Sterile Compounding Technique and Safety

IV solutions should be isotonic (osmotic pressure matches to human blood by having the same number of particles in solution), measured via milliosmoles (mOsm) or mOsm/Liter. Human blood has 285 mOsm/L. This prevents fluid transfer across the (biological) semipermeable membranes. The pH should be close to neutral (pH of 7); blood is slightly alkaline at a pH of 7.35-7.45. No eating, drinking coughing or talking is permitted. No distractions or interruptions. Non-PVC bags should be used for medications that have leaching or sorption issues (refer to the IV Administration & Storage chapter). The IV set must be sterile and nonpyrogenic.

Proper Procedure for IV Preparation Includes:

■ Hand, finger and wrist jewelry is removed prior to scrubbing. Do not wear make-up if working in the hood. Wash hands using a germicidal agent (such as chlorhexidine gluconate or povidone-iodine) for at least thirty seconds being careful to clean under the fingernails, which should be kept short enough to avoid tearing the gloves. Clean up to the elbows. Dry hands completely.

■ Garb up in the following order: shoe covers, a hair/head cover, facial mask. Wash hands again, dry, put on sterile powder-free gloves. If the gloves rip at any time, replace immediately.

■ Laminar flow hoods are kept running and cleaned as directed. Prior to use (at least at beginning of each work shift and as-scheduled) all surfaces should be thoroughly cleaned with 70% sterile isopropyl alcohol in a side-to-side motion, starting from the back of the hood. In addition, clean whenever there is a spill or if the hood looks like it requires cleaning.

■ Gather all components and check expiration dates, discoloration, particulates (discard) and leaks.

■ Only required items can be placed in the hood, side by side (not behind each other except possibly for items such as consecutive bags that additives are being placed into, for example – if this is done, place the larger items behind the smaller ones and do not put more than a few in this manner) and do not block <u>three inches from the back of the hood</u>.

■ Leave <u>six inches from the front edge of the hood clear (this is where the air starts to mingle)</u>, with no blockage to the HEPA filter. Only essential objects and materials necessary for product preparation should be placed in the airflow hood (no pens or calculators.) Do not tear open components. Open along seal within the hood. Do not touch the syringe tip or plunger, even with gloved hands.

■ Work in the center and place critical items reasonably close to the air source.

- Nothing should pass behind a sterile object and the HEPA filter in a horizontal airflow hood or above a sterile object in a vertical airflow hood. Chemotherapy must be done in a vertical hood.

- For greatest accuracy, use the smallest syringe that can hold the desired amount of solution. The syringe should not be larger than twice the volume to be measured.

- The volume of solution drawn into a syringe is measured at the point of contact between the rubber piston and the side of the syringe barrel.

- Powders are reconstituted by introducing a diluent such as sterile water for injection.

- Prior to withdrawing any liquid from a vial, first inject an equal volume of air to the fluid removed (Exception: do not inject air prior to removing cytotoxic drugs from vials.)

- Swab the rubber top (or ampule neck) with sterile isopropyl alcohol, and wait for it to air-dry; do not blow on or wave over it to dry faster.

- Puncture the rubber top of the vial with the needle bevel up. Then bring the syringe and needle straight up, penetrate the stopper, and depress the plunger of the syringe, emptying the air into the vial. Invert the vial with the attached syringe. Draw up from the vial the amount of liquid required. Withdraw the needle from the vial. In the case of a multi-dose vial, the rubber cap will close, sealing the contents of the vial.

- If the medication is in a glass ampule, open the ampule by forcefully snapping the neck away from you, then tilt the ampule, place the needle bevel of a filter needle or tip of a filter straw in the corner near the opening, and withdraw the medication. Use a needle equipped with a filter for filtering out any tiny glass particles, fibers, or paint chips that may have fallen into the ampule. Before injecting the contents of a syringe into an IV, the needle must be changed to avoid introducing glass or particles into the admixture. A standard needle could be used to withdraw the drug from the ampule; it is then replaced with a filter device before the drug is pushed out of the syringe.

- Instruct the technicians to keep all the additives with the bag and the syringes used (pulled up to the precise volume that was injected into the bag) for the pharmacist to check.

IV Bag Preparation, Label Includes:

- Patient name, location, other identification such as medical record number, DOB

- Active ingredient(s) and quantity of each

- IV solution (diluent)

- Run rate or frequency

- Scheduled hang time, using a 24 hour time scale (described in the Lab Values chapter).

- Any special storage conditions, auxiliary labels, precautions, date prepared

- Expiration date and time and device specific instructions, if needed

- Initials of pharmacist (and tech)

THE JOINT COMMISSION ON ACCREDITATION OF HEALTHCARE ORGANIZATIONS (JOINT COMMISSION, OR TJC)

The Joint Commission is an independent, not-for-profit organization that accredits and certifies more than 17,000 health care organizations and programs in the U.S., including hospitals, healthcare networks, longterm care facilities, homecare organizations, office-based surgery centers and independent laboratories. The Joint Commission focuses on the highest quality and safety of care and sets standards that institutions must meet to be accredited. An accredited organization must undergo an on-site survey at least every three years and surveys can be unannounced.

National patient safety goals (NPSGs) are set annually by the Joint Commission for different types of health care settings in order to improve patient safety. Each goal includes defined measures called "Elements of Performance" that must be met. These will be included in the institution's protocol. There are other NPSGs not discussed here, such as a goal for conducting a preprocedure verification process and another for identifying patients at risk of suicide. Pharmacists focus on medication-related NPSGs. Current hospital NPSGs related to medication safety include the following:

NPSG 03.04.01: Label all medications, medication containers and other solutions on and off the sterile field in perioperative and other procedural settings.

Numerous errors, sometimes fatal, have occurred due to medications and other solutions that were removed from their original containers and placed into unlabeled containers. This is of particular concern in perioperative and other procedural areas. Pharmacists should ensure that all medications and medication containers are labeled. The exception is when an agent is to be immediately administered without a break in the medication use process. Medication and solution labels should contain medication name, strength, quantity, diluent and volume and expiration date/time.

NPSG 03.05.01: Reduce the likelihood of harm associated with anticoagulant therapy.

There are many elements to this goal, including the requirement to use standardized dosing protocols, monitoring INRs, using programmable pumps for heparin, and providing education to patients and families. In the protocol, starting dose ranges are included; if the prescriber requests a dose out of the range the pharmacist will need to confirm agreement. The protocol will note alternative dosing ranges for a drug that increases or decreases the therapeutic effect of the anticoagulant. For example, if a drug that inhibits warfarin metabolism is being used concurrently, a lower starting dose will be required. INR monitoring frequency (plus baseline INR) will be in the protocol, along with the requirement to notify dietary.

NPSG 03.06.01: Maintain and communicate accurate patient medication information.

This includes medication reconciliation, providing written information to the patient and conducting discharge counseling. In conducting the reconciliation the medication name, dose, frequency, route, and purpose (at the minimum) should be confirmed. Refer to Medication Reconciliation earlier in this chapter.

NSPG 02.03.01: Report critical results of tests and diagnostic procedures on a timely basis.

This includes identifying and acting upon critical lab values, blood culture results, and other critical results as defined in the protocol. It should state the acceptable length of time between the availability and the reporting. The process should be evaluated to make sure the time is being met. Pharmacists should play an active role in this communication process.

NPSG 07.01.01: Comply with the Centers for Disease Control (CDC) hand hygiene guidelines.

Proper hand hygiene technique as described previously in this chapter. The goals for improving compliance should be stated, and the frequency of monitoring to ensure the goals are being met must be included.

NPSG 07.03.01; 07.04.01; 07.05.01; 07.06.01: Implement evidence-based practices to reduce health-care associated infections.

These include recommendations to reduce the likely sources of infection, such as from urinary catheters: only use if warranted, proper hand hygiene prior to insertion by qualified personnel only, properly secure the indwelling catheter, use the smallest bore catheter possible, with good drainage (to minimize tissue damage – all insertion and removal should be done according to the institution's protocol), continue to assess the need for continued catheter use in order to remove the catheter as soon as it is no longer needed. To reduce infections with ventilator use: elevate head-of-bed 30-45 degrees, assess readiness to wean off ventilator at least daily, use breaks or reductions in sedation use if possible, consider DVT prophylaxis, use stress-ulcer prophylaxis judiciously and only in patients who meet requirements for use; see the Critical Care chapter.

NPSG 01.01.01: Use at least two patient identifiers when providing care, treatment and services.

There have been countless medication errors (and surgical misadventures) due to patient misidentification. Two identifiers (such as name and medical record number) must be verified prior to administering medications, blood or blood components, taking lab samples or providing any treatment or procedure. The identifiers must be patient-specific – things like doctor's name, zip code or patient location should not be used in a hospital setting. In the community setting (which does not require adherence to NPSG requirements but in which the use of two identifiers is very important to prevent someone receiving someone else's medication) the two identifiers used most commonly are the patient's name and the home address (sometimes DOB is used, but the name and DOB can be the same as another person).

CONCLUSION

We are in an age where medication delivery is becoming more accountable and poor safety routines are no longer acceptable. Proactive assessment of safe medication use involves pharmacists at every step. There is a wide range of resources and information available to help us provide improved medication safety.

10

FDA DRUG DEVELOPMENT

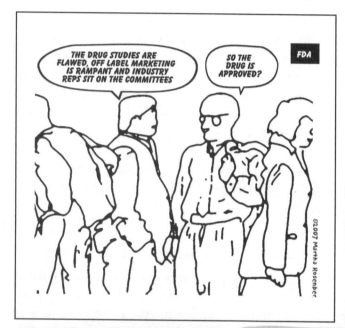

We gratefully acknowledge the assistance of Kelvin Li, R.Ph., Senior Consultant, Global Regulatory Affairs, PAREXEL International, in preparing this chapter.

OVERVIEW

The U.S. drug approval process is overseen by the Food and Drug Administration's (FDA) Center for Drug Evaluation and Research (CDER) for prescription and nonprescription or over-the-counter (OTC) drugs. There are four other FDA centers responsible for medical and radiological devices, food, and cosmetics, biologics, and veterinary drugs. The FDA is an important organization in safeguarding public health. A notable example that emphasizes this point was the refusal of Dr. Frances Oldham Kelsey, a FDA reviewer, to approve thalidomide as an antiemetic for use in pregnancy. In the 1950's and 60's thalidomide was given to pregnant women in other countries, and caused thousands of cases of severe birth defects including missing long bones. This case is considered one of the worst examples of medication-induced tragedy. Fortunately, the American consumer was largely protected by the heroic action of one FDA administrator.

Investigational products seeking medical claims must go through a review and approval process for both nonprescription (OTC) and prescription drugs, before they can be marketed. OTC drugs are defined as "drugs that are safe and effective for use by the general public without seeking treatment by a health professional" with less stringent regulations than

REFERENCE

http://www.fda.gov/drugs/developmentapprovalprocess/default.htm

prescription drugs. Manufacturers and sponsors seeking OTC drug designation can be approved through two routes; the New Drug Approval (NDA) process for new agents or indications or under the OTC monograph process. The OTC drug monograph is a "recipe book" of approved ingredients, doses, indications, formulations, and labeling requirements. If the drug and indication are already found in the approved OTC monograph, it may be marketed without further FDA review.

For prescription drugs, the drug approval process begins with pre-clinical (animal) research, which is followed by an Investigational New Drug (IND) application to conduct human clinical trials. Or, if the company is requesting approval of a generic drug, they file an Abbreviated New Drug Application (ANDA).

Current federal law requires that a drug be the subject of an approved marketing application before it is transported or distributed across state lines. Because an investigator will want to ship the investigational drug to clinical investigators in many states, they must seek an exemption from that legal requirement. The IND is the means through which the sponsor technically obtains this exemption from the FDA in order to conduct clinical trials. There are several phases of clinical trials performed to identify the drug's efficacy and safety. These phases are outlined in the chart on the following page. Note that each phase includes varying safety assessments.

Phase I studies focus on the safety and pharmacology of a compound. Low doses of the compound are given to a small group of healthy volunteers who are closely supervised. In cases of severe or life-threatening illnesses, volunteers with the disease may be used.

Phase II studies examine the effectiveness of a compound. Patients without complications and co-morbidities are often selected for a trial to reduce the number of confounding variables that may influence the trial results. Enrolling healthier individuals allows the potential benefit of the drug to be more clearly demonstrated. It is common in phase II trials to have 3 or 4 arms of the study; each investigating different doses for the best therapeutic benefit and minimal side effect profile.

After phase II, the manufacturer meets with the FDA to pave way for the "pivotal trials." Phase III trial designs and study protocol must obtain FDA approval before enrollment can begin. During phase III, researchers try to confirm efficacy of the new drug for the target indications in a larger population. These studies usually last from 2 to 10 years and typically involve hundreds to thousands of patients across multiple sites.

After Phase III, the manufacturer files a New Drug Application (NDA) for small molecules or a Biologics License Application (BLA) for biologics. Once the NDA is filed, the FDA has one year to review all the data and provide its decision to the manufacturer/researcher. The NDA can either be approved or rejected, or the FDA may request additional requirements before making a decision. Following acceptance, the FDA can also request that the manufacturer conduct additional post-marketing studies (AKA phase IV). Fast-track approval may be given to agents that show promise in treating serious, life-threatening medical conditions for which no other drug either exists or works well. Currently, the FDA is expected to make a decision within 6 months from submission if a drug is fast-tracked. On July 9, 2012, the President signed into law the Food and Drug Administration Safety and Innovation Act (FDA-SIA) of 2012. This new law includes the reauthorization of the Prescription Drug User Fee Act (PDUFA) that provides FDA with the necessary resources to maintain a predictable and efficient review process for human drug and biologic products. For more information see: http://www.fda.gov/ForIndustry/UserFees/PrescriptionDrugUserFee/.

IMPORTANCE OF PHASE IV

For some drugs the total drug approval process is limited to a few hundred patients – while in others, such as cardiovascular drugs, tens of thousands of subjects can be included. If a drug is tested in a relatively small number of patients, the complete safety profile may be missed. Even in larger trials, safety issues may be missed due to the exclusion of certain patient types. The FDA may request a post-marketing, or phase IV, study to examine the risks and benefits of the new drug in a different population or to conduct special monitoring in a high-risk population. The phase IV study can also be used to assess such issues as the longer term effects of drug exposure, to optimize the dose for marketing, to evaluate the effects in pediatric patients, or to examine the effectiveness of the drug for additional indications.

PHASE	PURPOSE	SUBJECTS	SCOPE	LENGTH OF TIME
I	Safety profile and dosing range, PK/PD, open label, often 1 center, may not be done in the US	Healthy volunteers (usually) or patients with illness	20-80 subjects	6-12 months
II	Safety and efficacy (dose response) IIa – proof of concept; pilot study, etc. IIb- well-controlled target population	Used in intended population	100-300 patients	1-2 years
III	Safety and efficacy at the dose and schedule you are seeking approval (package labeling) IIIb – post NDA –submission trial looking at additional indications	Subjects with indications the drug is seeking	Hundreds to thousands of patients	2-3 years 2-10? (previous page)
IV	New indications, QOL, surveillance studies	Subjects with indications the drug is seeking	Hundreds to thousands	1-5 years

For changes to an existing drug, the Supplemental New Drug Application (sNDA) is used. These changes include:

- Labeling changes
- New dose
- New strength
- New manufacturing process

Bioequivalence

Orange Book

The publication, *Approved Drug Products with Therapeutic Equivalence Evaluations* (commonly known as the Orange Book), identifies drug products approved on the basis of safety and effectiveness by the FDA under the Federal Food, Drug, and Cosmetic Act (FDCA). It contains therapeutic equivalence evaluations for approved multisource prescription drug products.

- Can look up by active ingredient, proprietary name, patent, applicant holder or applicant number.

- Published by the FDA Center for Drug Evaluation and Research (CDER).

- Available at www.fda.gov/cder/ob

RATINGS

- **AA** Products in conventional dosage forms not presenting bioequivalence problems.

- **AB** Drugs that have been proven to meet the necessary bioequivalence requirements through in vivo and/or in vitro testing. AB is the most common designation. Drugs coded as AB are therapeutically equivalent and can be interchanged (brand to generic).

- The FDA may not have compared each generic to each brand of the same drug. For example, the Orange Book lists *Cardizem CD*, *Dilacor XR*, and *Tiazac* under the heading for diltiazem. These are not bioequivalent to each other; however, some have generic equivalents.

- For example, *Dilacor XR* is "AB2" and the generic for *Cardizem CD* is "AB3." Products rated AB1 are bioequivalent to each other, products rated AB2 are bioequivalent to each other, and so forth.

- The 2nd letter can also refer to the dosage form:

- **AN** Solutions and powders for aerosolization

- **AO** Injectable oil solutions; these are considered to be pharmaceutically and therapeutically equivalent only when the active ingredient, its concentration, and the type of oil used as a vehicle are all identical.

- **AP** Injectable aqueous solutions and in certain instances, intravenous non-aqueous solutions

- **AT** Topical products, including those for dermatologic, ophthalmic, otic, rectal, and vaginal administration formulated as solutions, creams, ointments, gels, lotions, pastes, sprays, and suppositories

Biologic and Biosimilar Drug Development

Many drugs are biologics, including enzymes, vaccines, insulins, interferons, interleukins, erythropoietins, gonadotropins, granulocyte-colony stimulating factors, growth hormones, monoclonal antibodies and tissue plasminogen activators. Biologics were first developed using recombinant technology, using DNA grown in bacteria, yeast or mammalian cells. The drugs produced are more complex and larger than usual tablets and capsule formulations. For pharmacists, they require considerations for storage (regarding refrigeration), stability concerns (these do not last as long as more stable oral formulations) and instructions for patients on administration and adverse effect management. These drugs have an overall higher risk of safety concerns, including higher incidence of severe reactions. Yet, they are very useful for many conditions. The growth in these agents has fueled the "specialty pharmacy" sector of our profession but many can be dispensed in the community pharmacy. These agents are much more expensive than typical drugs; for example: methotrexate for a year's supply for a patient with rheumatoid arthritis costs ~$750 and adalimumab costs about ~$50,000.

Patents are expiring for some of the common biologics and many "biosimilars" will become available. Biologics are approved under the Public Health Service Act (PHSA) and conventional drugs are approved under the FDCA. The FDCA allows generic drug approvals via the ANDAs. Legislation under the Affordable Care Act established a regulatory pathway for biosimilars to allow approval for drugs that were considered "comparable" and "interchangeable" to the parent compound. Pharmacists look for bioequivalence ratings on drugs using the FDA's Orange Book. Enoxaparin was the first "biosimilar" product but the FDA allowed approval of the "generic" using the ANDA and the "generic" formulations of enoxaparin can be found in the Orange Book. Yet, it could have been classified as a biosimilar. Issues regarding biosimilar approvals and substitutions will continue until the legal issues are resolved. Enoxaparin has been the most costly item in hospital pharmacy budgets and this influenced the FDA's decision to allow approval as a generic drug.

Purple Book

"Purple Book" is published by the FDA. It is meant to be the biological version of the pharmaceutical "Orange Book". The Purple Book lists biological products including any biosimilar and interchangeable biological products by the FDA under the PHS Act. The lists contain the following:

- The BLA number
- Product Name
- Proprietary Name
- Date of Licensure
- Date of First Licensure
- Reference Product Exclusivity Expiration Date
- Interchangeable or Biosimilar
- Withdrawn

Patents and Exclusivity

Typically drugs are given patents from the date of filing (these are for twenty years) and exclusivity, which is exclusive marketing rights granted by the FDA upon approval of a new drug, which typically last for 5 years (on paper) but much longer in practice when the patents are tied up for years in court. Biologics, in contrast, are granted exclusivity for twelve years in order to compensate the manufacturer for the higher cost associated with development. Biosimilars do not need to be biologically identical to the original product and are not expected to be identical since differences in the manufacturing process alter the end product. To gain approval they need to demonstrate that they are not "clinically different" by providing data demonstrating that the biosimilar has no clinically significant differences in "safety, purity and potency." The FDA has considerable flexibility to decide, for each agent, what type of clinical data the manufacturer is required to submit. Since we are now on the "patent cliff" in which many biologics exclusivity is expiring the legality regarding biosimilar approval is expected to remain big drug news. Stay tuned.

NATURAL PRODUCTS & VITAMINS

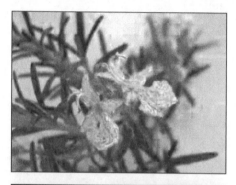

BACKGROUND

Natural product use has a long history of traditional use among native cultures and has become popular today. Many patients supplement their diet or prescription medicines with vitamins or natural products. Natural product is an umbrella term that includes herbals (plant products), vitamins and many substances that are not plant-derived but exist in nature, such as glucosamine from shellfish. The FDA uses the term <u>dietary supplements</u>.

Most natural products act as either mild drugs or are harmless. Pharmacists have accessible sources to check for drug interactions, safety concerns, dosage by indication, and quality. Some natural products pose health risks. A few top safety concerns include manufacturing quality, safety and effectiveness, and the use of a few select agents that can pose specific problems in certain patients:

<u>Manufacturing may not follow good manufacturing practices (GMP);</u> pharmacists need to help consumers choose a reputable product. In recent years quality companies have put in place programs that will put a seal of approval on products made by a company following good manufacturing practices. The website consumerlab.com is useful to help choose a reputable product – this is an independent testing service that analyzes the content of many popular supplements.

<u>A dietary supplement manufacturer does not have to prove a product's safety and effectiveness before it is marketed.</u> For example: late-night TV ads are promoting a thyroid product to help with low energy and fatigue. Perhaps some patients need a thyroid supplement, but this requires lab testing. If people who do not need thyroid hormone take it, they can become hyperthyroid and be subject to cardiovascular and other health risks. The product quality may be poor – this can be a particular issue with thyroid hormone which may contain prions that

can carry mad cow disease. Last but not least, the product used in this example is expensive. Generic levothyroxine, a safer alternative, is pennies per tablet.

By law, the Dietary Supplement Health and Education Act (DSHEA), the manufacturer is responsible for ensuring that their dietary supplement products are safe before they are marketed. In contrast, drugs must be proven safe and effective for the intended use before they can be sold. Under the DSHEA, once the product is marketed, the FDA has the responsibility for showing that a dietary supplement is "unsafe," before it can take action to restrict the product's use or removal from the marketplace. The company selling or distributing the product is required to record, investigate and forward to the FDA reports they receive of serious adverse events.

Dietary supplements can make claims that describe the role of an ingredient that affects normal body structure or function, such as "calcium builds strong bones", "fiber maintains bowel regularity" or "antioxidants maintain cell integrity." They cannot make claims that the product treats or cures a condition.

Three areas of particular safety concern are natural products that increase bleeding risk, interactions between prescription drugs and St. John's wort and natural products that may be hepatotoxic.

- Ginkgo biloba and other agents that can ↑ bleeding risk: Ginkgo biloba increases bleeding risk with no effect on the INR. Refer to the Anticoagulation chapter for additional natural products that increase bleeding risk in patients using warfarin. Warfarin interacts with many natural products. Ginkgo increases bleeding risk with other "bleeding risk" agents, including NSAIDs, antiplatelets and other anticoagulants.

- Ginkgo biloba increases bleeding risk with no effect on the INR. Other natural products that can also pose a risk include bromelains, danshen, dong quai (this product may ↑ INR), vitamin E, evening primrose oil, high doses of fish oils, garlic, ginseng, glucosamine, grapefruit, policosanol, and willow bark.

- Enzyme induction by St. John's wort: this herbal is a "broad-spectrum" inducer and cannot be used with oral contraceptives, transplant drugs, warfarin, among others. St. John's wort induces 3A4 >> 2C9 > 1A2. See the Drug Interactions chapter. SJW causes photosensitivity and is serotonergic; caution with 5HT drugs. Avoid using this agent with anyone with a seizure history.

- Natural products may be hepatotoxic (chaparral, comfrey, kava). If liver enzymes are elevated, check with the patient – sometimes the use of "tea blends" or mixtures can be contributory.

Safety/Financial Comments on Homeopathic Products and Medical Foods

Homeopathic Products: Homeopathy is based on "the law of similars" or the concept that "like is cured by like." This is the belief that giving very small amounts of the illness (so dilute that the original substance cannot be measured) will protect the patient or cure them of an illness. Most evidence does not support validity to homeopathy, however many adherents (including the Queen of England) are advocates. The remedies may be providing a placebo benefit, or, may actually be labeled as homeopathic but contain measurable concentrations of drugs. In 2010, *Hyland's Teething Tablets* were recalled due to cases of belladonna toxicity. The amount of belladonna could be measured and was unsafe. It is tempting to use the term "homeopathic" on a label. It sounds nice, and if a manufacturer labels a product "homeopathic," they are permitted to make health claims, while natural products are not allowed by law to claim benefit for particular conditions. There have been other recent examples of products labeled as homeopathic which actually were not. Check the ingredients.

VITAMINS	NAMES
Vitamin A	Retinol
Vitamin B1	Thiamine
Vitamin B12	Cobalamin
Vitamin B2	Riboflavin
Vitamin B3	Niacin
Vitamin B6	Pyridoxine
Vitamin B9	Folic Acid
Vitamin C	Ascorbic Acid

Medical Foods: These are products that can also make health claims, since they are not FDA-approved drugs. Medical foods are supposed to meet a nutritional need for a group that cannot be met with usual foods, such as specific formulations of enteral nutrition. A recent medical food that many pharmacists will have seen is a formulation of folic acid called *Deplin* that is being marketed for help in treating depression. The ad for this product states that "*Deplin* is a medical food containing L-methylfolate, the active form of the vitamin, folate. It is the only folate that can be taken up by the brain where it helps balance the chemical messengers that affect mood (serotonin, norepinephrine and dopamine)." It is less expensive to use over-the-counter folic acid supplements and there is no evidence that this supplement would provide more benefit, however the manufacturer can make this claim since it is a medical food. In a medical food, all ingredients must be Generally Recognized as Safe (G.R.A.S.) or be approved food additives. Most of the medical foods have Rx-only on the label and have NDC numbers.

COMMONLY USED NATURAL PRODUCTS

CONDITION	TREATMENT
Anxiety	Valerian, lemon balm, glutamine, passion flower and hops (both as teas), chamomile tea, theanine and skullcap. Kava is used as a relaxant but can damage the liver and should not be recommended. Valerian may rarely be hepatotoxic (or some valerian products may have been contaminated with liver toxins); this is unclear at present. Passion flower is rated as "possibly effective" by the Natural Medicines Database. For most of the other agents the evidence is less robust but individual patients may get benefit from the various agents.
Sleep	Melatonin (also used for jet lag – carefully check doses for this use), valerian. Chamomile tea may help people relax. St. John's wort may help if the insomnia is due to depression (worry) but will lower levels of many other drugs. Kava is used but can damage the liver and should not be recommended.
ADHD	Fish oil supplements (which provide omega 3 fatty acids) with or without evening primrose oil (which provides omega-3 fatty acids) may be helpful in some patients.
Aphthous Ulcers (canker sores)	Lysine
Cancer	Beta-carotene, fish oil, black or green tea, garlic, soy, vitamins A and D Colon cancer: calcium Prostate cancer: lycopene (in cooked tomatoes)
Cholesterol	Fish oils (triglycerides), red yeast rice (monitor – may contain small amounts of an HMG CoA reductase inhibitor), plant sterols/stanols, certain probiotics

Commonly Used Natural Products Continued

CONDITION	TREATMENT
Depression	St. John's wort, SAMe (do not use with MAO Is), fish oils, 5-HTP, tryptophan, glutamine, inositol (for OCD and panic disorder). Caution with induction and substrates, with sun exposure and with other 5HT drugs – see above, L-methylfolate.
Colds and Flu	Echinacea (can cause heartburn, allergic reactions), elderberry, garlic, zinc, vitamin C. Caution for loss of smell (possibly permanent) with zinc nasal sprays and swabs.
Dementia/Memory	Ginkgo, huperzine A, vitamin E, phosphatidylserine, acetyl-L-carnitine. Caution with ginkgo for increased bleeding risk. Red palm oil is used for dementia and heart disease; unproven.
Diabetes	Bitter melon, gymnema, chromium, alpha lipoic acid, cinnamon, acetyl-l-carnitine (neuropathy). Green tea may lower DM risk.
Energy/Weight Loss	Bitter orange; caution with bitter orange (similar to ephedra, CVD risk) and guarana (caffeine, caution with excessive intake). Caffeine is in various "natural" weight loss products, including green coffee bean extract. Another popular product is raspberry ketone, which is similar to synephrine.
UTI	Cranberry. Caution on the risk of kidney stones with cranberry supplements.
Gastrointestinal Distress	Peppermint oil, chamomile tea
IBD	Cascara, senna (stimulant laxatives) for constipation. For diarrhea, psyllium (in *Metamucil* and many other formulations) or other "bulk-forming" fiber products can be useful. Peppermint (oil, sometimes teas) can be useful as an antispasmodic. Some use chamomile tea. The probiotic *Lactobacillus* or *Bifidobacterium infantis* may help reduce abdominal pain, bloating, urgency, constipation or diarrhea in some patients. Antibiotics and probiotics are not taken together; separate the dosing by at least two hours. Fish oils (for the EPA and DHA, omega fatty acid components) are being used, although the evidence for benefit is contradictory. Indian frankincense gum resin taken TID may be beneficial for UC, based on preliminary studies. Comfrey is used for GI issues but can damage the liver and should not be recommended.
Probiotics	*Lactobacillus, Bifidobacterium infantis* etc. – check the efficacy of the individual probiotic for the condition – they vary. Separate probiotics from antibiotics or they will get destroyed by the drug. These are used for many conditions, including diarrhea prevention with antibiotics, irritable bowel, cholesterol-lowering, and others. The type of probiotic needs to match the indication, based on efficacy.
Heart Health/Heart Failure	Coenzyme Q10, arginine (do not use with blood pressure meds – additive effect), fish oils, grape seed extract (grape seed extract used as a general health antioxidant and for atherosclerosis), garlic (mild decrease in blood pressure-caution for bleeding, may lower drug levels), hawthorne (caution – has additive effects with other drugs – can cause hypotension, dizziness with beta blockers, digoxin, calcium channel blockers, nitrates and PDE5-Is.)
Inflammation	Fish oils, willow bark (a salicylate)
Liver	Milk thistle
Menopausal Symptoms	Black cohosh (in popular menopause product *Remifemin*, generally safe, but reports of liver toxicity, some get GI upset), dong quai, red clover, evening primrose. Caution with dong quai and increased INR in patients using warfarin.
Migraine/Headache	Feverfew, willow bark, butterbur, guarana (a caffeine product), fish oils, magnesium, coenzyme Q10 and riboflavin. Combinations of these may be helpful.
Motion Sickness/Nausea	Ginger, peppermint
Osteoporosis	Soy, black cohosh, flax seed, evening primrose, calcium, vitamin D
Osteoarthritis	Glucosamine (may raise INR), chondroitin, SAMe (do not use with MAO Is)

Commonly Used Natural Products Continued

CONDITION	TREATMENT
Prostate enlargement	Saw palmetto is used for BPH, but it is rated as "possibly ineffective" by The Natural Medicines Database. If men wish to try saw palmetto, they should be counseled to be seen first to rule out the possibility of prostate cancer and receive treatment, if needed. Pygeum and beta-sitosterol may provide benefit and are considered safe. Other products that may provide mild benefit are African wild potato extract and pumpkin seed. Rye grass pollen is used commonly in Europe. (Lycopene is used for prostate cancer prevention, however there is not good evidence for taking supplements for this purpose.)
Skin	Aloe vera, Tea tree oil is used for a variety of skin conditions. It can be useful for treating acne. It may be helpful for onychomycosis symptoms (depending on the dose and application schedule), but is not useful in eradicating the infection in most patients. Tea tree oil may also be useful for athlete's foot symptoms if the 10% oil is used (not tea tree cream). Higher concentrations (25 or 50%) can cure the infection in up to half of patients, but are not as effective as the recommended antifungal agents. This efficacy data is from the Natural Medicines Database.

VITAMIN SUPPLEMENTATION

People who consume an adequate diet do not require vitamin supplementation. However, many people eat poor diets. It is concerning to health care professionals that calcium and vitamin D intake remains insufficient for the majority of adults and children. Folic acid intake among women of child-bearing age can be insufficient. If thiamine (vitamin B1) is insufficient, this can cause Wernicke's encephalopathy. Symptoms of Wernicke's include ataxia, tremor and vision changes. A lack of vitamin B1 is common in alcoholism, and can be due to malabsorption, including from Crohn's, after obesity surgery, with advanced HIV and from a few other conditions. As the symptoms of Wernicke's fade, Korsakoff syndrome tends to develop (also called Korsakoff psychosis), which is permanent neurologic (mental) damage. Pharmacists are part of the solution to problems associated with vitamin deficiencies. Metformin can contribute to B12 deficiency, and there are other drugs with supplement recommendations (see table at end of chapter).

Calcium & Vitamin D Supplementation

All prescription medicines for low bone density require adequate calcium and vitamin D supplementation taken concurrently (if dietary intake is inadequate). Calcium and vitamin D supplementation is an essential topic for pharmacists since they are often recommended OTC and are required with many prescription drugs; product type and selection is discussed in the Osteoporosis and Hormone Therapy chapter.

Folic Acid

Any woman planning to conceive (and all women of child-bearing age) should be taking a folic acid supplement (400 – 800 mcg/daily, which is 0.4-0.8 mg/daily) to help prevent birth defects of the brain and spinal cord (neural tube defects). Folic acid needs to be taken at least one month before pregnancy and continued for the first 2-3 months of pregnancy. Once pregnant, the woman is likely taking a prescription prenatal vitamin and this is continued throughout since it also contains calcium (not enough, about 200 mg) and some iron. Folic acid is in many healthy foods, including fortified cereals (some of which are not healthy), dried beans, leafy green vegetables and orange juice. Multivitamins usually contain an amount in the recommended range. Prescription prenatal vitamins usually contain 1000 mcg, or 1 mg, of folic acid. The newer birth control pill *Beyaz* contains folate, however it is less expensive to use a different birth control pill with a supplement. *Beyaz* contains the potassium-sparing progestin drospirenone, with ethinyl estradiol and levomefolate.

Vitamin E

It is unusual to have a vitamin E deficiency, since it is present in many foods. Vitamin E in foods is considered healthy, but excess intake in supplements is considered a health risk (particularly CVD risk); patients should not be exceeding 150 IU daily.

Vitamin Requirements For Infants & Children

Most children do not need vitamins, except as listed per the American Academy of Pediatrics:

- Exclusively breastfed infants or babies drinking less than 1 liter of baby formula need 400 IU of vitamin D daily (can use *Poly-Vi-Sol* or generic).

- Older children who do not drink at least 4 cups of Vitamin D fortified milk also need Vitamin D supplements.

Iron Requirements For Infants & Children

0-4 months

- Supplemental iron not required.

4-6 months

- Formulas contain adequate iron; supplementation not required.

- Breast-fed babies need 1 mg/kg/day from 4-6 months old and until consuming iron-rich foods. At about 6 months most breast-fed babies get about half their calories from other foods.

6-12 months

- Need 11 mg/day of iron. Food sources are preferred; supplement as needed.

1-3 years old

- Need 7 mg/day of iron. Food sources are preferred; supplement as needed.

Adolescent girls

- At risk of anemia once they begin menstruating.

Iron-only supplements (generics available) – check bottle on iron drops because the iron mg/dropper ranges from 10-15 mg

- *Fer-In-Sol* Iron Supplement Drops

- *Feosol* Tablets and Caplets

Vitamin Supplements with Iron

- *Poly-Vi-Sol* Vitamin Drops With Iron: use if they need the vitamin D <u>and</u> iron

- Or others, such as: *Flintstones* Children's Chewable Multivitamin plus Iron, *Pokemon* Children's Multiple Vitamin with Iron, and store brands

Supplements that May be Required with Certain Drugs

DRUG	DEPLETED NUTRIENT	CHAPTER
Metformin	Vitamin B12	Diabetes
Valproic Acid/Divalproex	Selenium, zinc, calcium, vitamin D	Epilepsy, Bipolar
Phenytoin	Calcium, vitamin D, folic acid	Epilepsy
Carbamazepine	Calcium, vitamin D	Epilepsy
Oxcarbazepine	Calcium, vitamin D	Epilepsy
Lamotrigine	Selenium, zinc (due to alopecia)	Epilepsy, Bipolar
Phenobarbital/Primidone	Calcium, vitamin D	Epilepsy
Zonisamide	Calcium, vitamin D	Epilepsy
Topiramate	Calcium, vitamin D	Epilepsy, Weight Loss
Acetazolamide	Calcium, vitamin D	Travelers, Glaucoma
Bile Acid Sequestrants (Cholestyramine, Colsevelam, and Colestipol)	Multivitamin with A,D, E and K; separate, folic acid	Dyslipidemia
Orlistat	Multivitamin with A,D, E and K, beta-carotene; separate	Weight Loss
Methotrexate	Folic acid	Autoimmune Conditions, various
Loops	Potassium almost always, magnesium if needed	Hypertension, CHF
Aminoglycosides	Potassium, magnesium, calcium	Infectious Disease
Isoniazid	Vitamin B6	Infectious Disease
Trimethoprim (and *Bactrim*)	Folic acid (if used chronically)	Infectious Disease
Sulfasalazine	Folic acid due to impaired absorption	Autoimmune Conditions, IBD
PPIs	Magnesium, calcium (possibly citrate)	GERD
Oral Contraceptives	Ferrous sulfate, folate	Contraception
Depo-Provera	Calcium, vitamin D	Contraception
Corticosteroids (used in excess)	Calcium, vitamin D	Various
Mineral Oil (possibly other laxatives used in excess)	Vitamins A, D, E, and K; separate	Constipation
Digoxin	Magnesium, potassium	Arrhythmias
Pemetrexed	Folic acid, vitamin B12	Oncology
Heparin (and possibly LMWH)	Calcium supplementation if long-term	Anticoagulation

Conditions that Require Supplements

CONDITION	REQUIRED SUPPLEMENT	CHAPTER
Alcoholism	Vitamin B1, folic acid	Hepatitis
Microcytic Anemia	Ferrous sulfate	Anemia
Macrocytic Anemia	Vitamin B12 and/or folic acid	Anemia
Pregnancy	Folic Acid, calcium, vitamin D, vitamin B6 if nausea	Pregnancy
Osteopenia/Osteoporosis	Calcium, vitamin D	Osteoporosis, Pregnancy
Osteomalacia (Rickets)	Calcium, vitamin D	Vitamin deficiency
Chronic Kidney Disease	Vitamin D	Renal Disease, Bipolar Disorder (for Lithium side effect)
Scurvy	Vitamin C	Vitamin deficiency
Crohn's Disease (and possibly ulcerative colitis)	Patient specific-depends on levels; can require iron, zinc, folic acid, calcium, vitamin D, B vitamins	IBD
Cystic Fibrosis	Pancrealipase ↓ absorption of iron and ↓ concentration of vitamins A,D,E,K and folate	Cystic Fibrosis
Diabetes	Potassium, magnesium	Diabetes
Bariatric Surgery	Various; patient-specific, refer to chapter	Weight Loss
Heart Failure	Potassium, calcium, magnesium due to loop use	Heart Failure

Drugs that Require Supplementation to Work

DRUG	REQUIRED SUPPLEMENT	CHAPTER
Calcium	Vitamin D	Osteoporosis
All osteoporosis drugs	Calcium, vitamin D	Osteoporosis
Epoetin alfa/Darbepoetin alfa	Iron	Anemia

DRUG INTERACTIONS

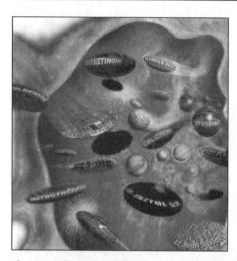

BACKGROUND

The cytochrome P450 enzymes (abbreviated as CYP) contain many forms, but about a dozen of them are involved in the metabolism of most drugs. This discussion begins with the most common isoenzymes that are well known to pharmacists. Enzyme metabolism involves <u>Phase I reactions</u> (oxidation, reduction and hydrolysis), followed by Phase II, which normally terminates the activity of the drug. (Phase I provides a reactive functional group on the compound that permits the drug to be attacked by the Phase II enzymes.) Drugs are considered by the body to be foreign, similar to a toxin, which must be eliminated either through a pump that pushes the drug back into the gut (for elimination in the feces via the P-gp efflux pumps – efflux means "to flow out"), or in the bile (which eliminates through the gallbladder) or through the kidney via renal elimination. For most drugs to be excreted renally, they must be first converted (metabolized) into a more hydrophilic form, which occurs by the process of enzyme metabolism, described here.

CYP enzymes are found in many cells, but are primarily located in the liver and intestines. The majority of medications (75%) are metabolized by CYP 450 enzymes, and of these, greater than 80% are metabolized by CYP 450 <u>3A4</u> alone, or 3A4 <u>and</u> other enzymes.

All enzymes in the body work using an <u>enzyme-substrate system</u>.

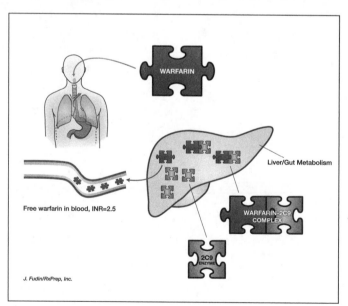

Free warfarin in blood, INR=2.5

Liver/Gut Metabolism

WARFARIN

WARFARIN-2C9 COMPLEX

2C9 ENZYME

J. Fudin/RxPrep, Inc.

The enzyme is a protein that performs some action. The substrate is a chemical that is acted upon. Drug molecules, foods, and toxins are substrates for CYP enzymes. In the following figure, warfarin (the substrate) is joined with the CYP 2C9 enzyme in a manner similar to puzzle pieces. The enzyme converts the warfarin into an inactive metabolite (this is generally the case; however sometimes the conversion produces a toxic metabolite or an active or beneficial metabolite). The metabolite is generally more water-soluble than the parent compound, which facilitates excretion (exit from the body) via filtration through the kidneys. Warfarin causes an increase in the INR (a pharmacologic action), but warfarin metabolites do not. Thus each time warfarin molecules pass through the liver, some are captured by the CYP 2C9 enzyme and converted into inactive metabolites, leaving less warfarin to elicit its beneficial effects of increasing the INR. Most of this reaction occurs during the "first pass" when the drug (substrate) passes through the gut wall and liver prior to reaching the systemic circulation.

Inducers are compounds (many of which are drugs) that either increase the production of the enzyme (by increasing the expression of the gene sequence that codes for the enzyme), or, increase the activity of the enzyme. The net effect of an inducer is to increase the degree of drug metabolism, which results in lower blood levels of the substrate. In the figure to the right, rifampin has caused induction of the enzyme 2C9, which causes more of the enzyme to be present, resulting in more drug metabolism. The warfarin

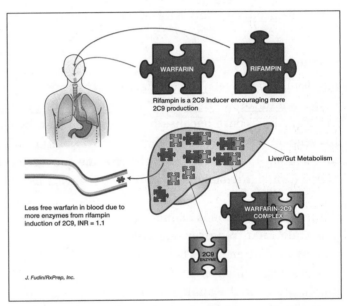

metabolism increases, less warfarin is available systemically, and the INR will decrease. Rifampin is used as an example here because it is one of the strongest inducers and induces many enzymes [1A2, 2C8, 2C9, 2C19, 3A4 and the P-glycoprotein (P-gp) pump]. If rifampin is given to a patient on warfarin the warfarin dose will need to be increased between 100-300% to keep the INR therapeutic.

In the case of prodrugs, the inducer can increase an enzyme that is responsible for converting the substrate into a more active form (instead of a less active or inactive form). Prodrug conversion is technically referred to as bioactivation.

Inhibitors are compounds (many of which are drugs) that inhibit the activity of the enzyme. The enzyme inhibition results in less drug metabolism. The drug serum level (and therapeutic effect) will increase. This can result in drug toxicity. In the next figure, amiodarone, a 2C9 inhibitor is given to a patient using warfarin. Amiodarone inhibits the metabolism of warfarin. The warfarin level in the serum will increase and there will be a corresponding increase in the INR. This interaction would cause a supratherapeutic INR with risk of bleeding. This reaction is well known to pharmacists; when amiodarone is given to a patient who has been using warfarin (which is done commonly) the reaction is anticipated and the INR dose is decreased 30-50%. If they are started concurrently, a lower dose of warfarin will be given.

In the case of a prodrug, an inhibitor of the enzyme involved in bioactivation would block the production of the active form of the drug. Inhibitors <u>decrease</u> the levels of the <u>prodrug's</u> active form.

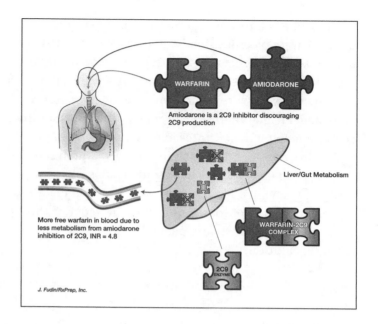

Prodrugs

As discussed above, <u>inducers decrease the concentration of the substrate – except with prodrugs</u>. <u>Inhibitors increase the concentration of the substrate – except with prodrugs</u>. Here, the opposite occurs because prodrugs are taken by the patient in an inactive form and are converted by bioactivation (enzyme conversion) into the active form. With prodrugs, inhibitors decrease the active form (the enzyme conversion is blocked) and inducers increase the active form (more enzymes available to convert more of the drug).

In the figure, codeine is an inactive substrate that requires metabolism by the 2D6 enzymes to various metabolites, which include morphine. Much of the analgesic efficacy of codeine is due to the morphine metabolite. When codeine is dispensed to a patient who has not had a pharmacogenomic analysis the pharmacist will have no way of predicting the dose required of the drug: the 2D6 enzyme is not inducible but is subject to a wide variability in 2D6 expression due primarily to ethnic variations in gene expression. Patients could

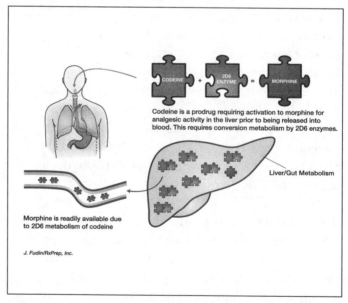

be 2D6 ultrarapid metabolizers (UMs, producing a lot of the enzyme), extensive metabolizers (EMs, producing a lot of the enzyme but less than the UMs), intermediate metabolizers (IMs) or poor metabolizers (PMs). Even within ethnic groups there is wide variability in the gene expression. About 25% of drugs go through the 2D6 system, including many <u>pain and psychiatric</u> drugs. These two conditions, more than most others, typically involve multiple medications given concurrently for the same condition – which makes drug interaction analysis essential. Although diminished analgesic efficacy is a clinical concern, tragedies have occurred repeatedly because of the use of codeine in an UM, and resultant death from morphine overdose. In one case, a breastfeeding mother had taken codeine and (unknown to anyone) she was an UM of 2D6. Morphine passes readily into breast milk and the infant suffered fatal respiratory depression. Recently several children received a morphine overdose after receiving codeine for post-tonsillectomy pain.

In this figure the 2D6 inhibitor paroxetine blocks the conversion of codeine to morphine, resulting in lower analgesia.

<u>Practical Considerations:</u> Discontinuation of an inhibitor or inducer can have dangerous consequences. If a patient is using methadone and the dose has been increased to compensate for induction and the inducer is stopped, the methadone level could become lethal. In the warfarin and rifampin example, if the rifampin is stopped the warfarin levels would become supratherapeutic – and potentially very dangerous.

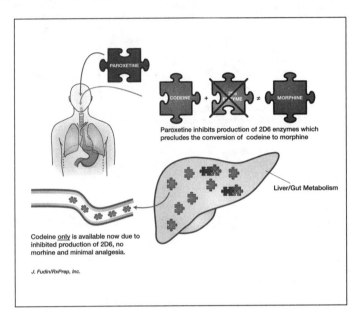

"Lag" time for Inhibition and Induction

<u>Inhibition of an enzyme</u> is fast and at most takes a few days to take effect and will end quickly when the inhibitor is discontinued. <u>Induction</u> most often requires additional enzyme production, which <u>takes time</u>. The full effect may not be present for up to two weeks.

FDA DEFINITIONS		
TERM	**INDUCERS**	**INHIBITORS**
Strong	≥ 80% ↓ in AUC	≥ 5-fold ↑ in AUC
Moderate	50-80% ↓ in AUC	≥ 2 but < 5-fold ↑ in AUC
Weak	20-50% ↓ in AUC	≥ 1.25 but < 2-fold ↑ in AUC

When <u>the inducer is stopped it could take 2-4 weeks for the induction to disappear completely</u>; the enzymes have been produced and will die off based on their half-lives.

P-glycoproteins (P-gp)

P-gp's are efflux transporters found in the gut and other organs. They <u>pump drugs back into the gut</u> (to <u>exit</u> out of the body). If a drug is subject to efflux, and the transporter is inhibited by a different drug, the substrate drug concentration will increase in the plasma. If an inducer is given that causes the production of more pumps, the blood levels of the substrate will decrease. The following figure is a schematic representation of this activity. Many of the

P-gp drug interactions are not yet included in various pharmacy software packages, which warrants caution.

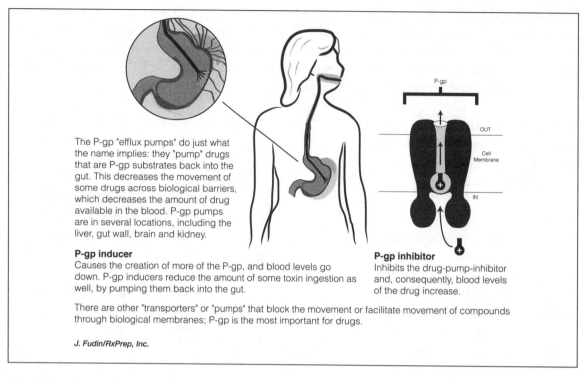

The P-gp "efflux pumps" do just what the name implies: they "pump" drugs that are P-gp substrates back into the gut. This decreases the movement of some drugs across biological barriers, which decreases the amount of drug available in the blood. P-gp pumps are in several locations, including the liver, gut wall, brain and kidney.

P-gp inducer
Causes the creation of more of the P-gp, and blood levels go down. P-gp inducers reduce the amount of some toxin ingestion as well, by pumping them back into the gut.

P-gp inhibitor
Inhibits the drug-pump-inhibitor and, consequently, blood levels of the drug increase.

There are other "transporters" or "pumps" that block the movement or facilitate movement of compounds through biological membranes; P-gp is the most important for drugs.

J. Fudin/RxPrep, Inc.

The following table provides a list of P-glycoprotein efflux pump substrates, inhibitors and inducers. This is not a complete list but includes many clinically important drugs.

P-gp Efflux Pump (Partial List)

STRONG INHIBITORS	STRONG INDUCERS	SUBSTRATES
Itraconazole	Rifampin	Aliskiren
Ketoconazole	Avasimibe	Colchicine
Verapamil	Carbamazepine	Dabigatran
Ritonavir	Phenytoin	Cyclosporine
Lopinavir/Ritonavir	St John's wort	Digoxin
Indinavir/Ritonavir	tipranavir /Ritonavir	Fexofenadine
Conivaptan		Posaconazole
Clarithromycin		Ranolazine
Erythromycin		Rivaroxaban
Amiodarone		Saxagliptin
Quinidine		Tacrolimus

Cytochrome P 450 Substrates, Inducers, and Inhibitors (Partial List)

CLASS	SUBSTRATES	INDUCERS	INHIBITORS
3A4	alfentanil, alfuzosin, alprazolam, amiodarone, amlodipine, amprenavir, apixaban, aprepitant, atazanavir, apomorphine, aripiprazole, atazanavir, atorvastatin, buprenorphine, buspirone, carbamazepine, citalopram, clarithromycin, dapsone, delavirdine, diazepam, diltiazem, dronedarone, dutasteride, efavirenz, eplerenone, erythromycin, escitalopram, esomeprazole, estrogens, felbamate, fentanyl, fosamprenavir, haloperidol, hydrocodone, indinavir, ketoconazole, lansoprazole, levonorgestrel, lidocaine, lopinavir, losartan, lovastatin, mirtazapine, modafinil, nateglinide, nelfinavir, nevirapine, nifedipine, omeprazole, ondansetron, oxycodone, progesterone, propoxyphene, quinidine, rabeprazole, ranolazine, repaglinide, ritonavir, rivaroxaban, saquinavir, sildenafil, simvastatin, sirolimus, tadalafil, tipranavir, tramadol, trazodone, vardenafil, venlafaxine, verapamil, (R)-warfarin, zolpidem	carbamazepine, oxcarbazepine, phenytoin, phenobarbital, primidone, rifabutin, rifampin, rifapentine, smoking, St. John's wort	amiodarone, amprenavir, aprepitant, atazanavir, cimetidine, clarithromycin, cyclosporine, delavirdine, diltiazem, dronedarone, efavirenz, erythromycin, fluconazole, fluvoxamine, fosamprenavir, grapefruit juice, haloperidol, indinavir, isoniazid, itraconazole, ketoconazole, lidocaine, metronidazole, nefazodone, nelfinavir, nevirapine, posaconazole, propofol, quinidine, ranolazine, ritonavir, saquinavir, sertraline, telithromycin, verapamil, voriconazole
1A2	alosetron, amitriptyline, clozapine, cyclobenzaprine, duloxetine, estradiol, methadone, mirtazapine, olanzapine, pimozide, propranolol, rasagiline, ropinirole, theophylline, (R)-warfarin	carbamazepine, estrogen, phenobarbital, phenytoin, primidone, rifampin, ritonavir, smoking, St. John's wort	cimetidine, ciprofloxacin, clarithromycin, erythromycin, fluvoxamine, gemfibrozil, isoniazid, ketoconazole, zileuton
2C8	amiodarone, pioglitazone, repaglinide, rosiglitazone	carbamazepine, phenobarbital, phenytoin, rifampin	atazanavir, gemfibrozil, irbesartan, ritonavir
2C9	carvedilol, celecoxib, diazepam, fluvastatin, phenytoin, ramelteon, (S)-warfarin	aprepitant, carbamazepine, phenobarbital, phenytoin, primidone, rifampin, rifapentine, St. John's wort	amiodarone, cimetidine, trimethoprim/ sulfamethoxazole, fluconazole, fluvoxamine, isoniazid, ketoconazole, metronidazole, voriconazole, warfarin, zafirlukast
2C19	clopidogrel, phenytoin, thioridazine, voriconazole	carbamazepine, phenobarbital, phenytoin, rifampin	cimetidine, esomeprazole, etravirine, efavirenz, fluoxetine, fluvoxamine, ketoconazole, modafinil, omeprazole, topiramate, voriconazole
2D6	amitriptyline, aripiprazole, atomoxetine, carvedilol, clozapine, codeine, desipramine, dextromethorphan, donepezil, doxepin, fentanyl, flecainide, haloperidol, hydrocodone, imipramine, lidocaine, meperidine, methadone, methamphetamine, mirtazapine, nortriptyline, oxycodone, propafenone, propoxyphene, propranolol, thioridazine, tramadol, trazodone, venlafaxine		amiodarone, cimetidine, darifenacin, duloxetine, fluoxetine, paroxetine, propafenone, quinidine, ritonavir, sertraline

QUICK STUDY TOOL FOR CYP INTERACTIONS
SEE MORE COMPLETE LIST OF INDUCERS AND INHIBITORS BELOW

PS PORCS (BIG INDUCERS)

Phenytoin

Smoking

Phenobarbital

Oxcarbazepine

Rifampin (and rifabutin, rifapentine)

Carbamazepine (and is an auto-inducer)

St. John's wort

G ♥ PACMAN (BIG INHIBITORS)

Grapefruit

♥

PIs Protease Inhibitors (don't miss ritonavir) but check all PIs since many are potent inhibitors

Azole antifungals, the agents that are used oral and IV: fluconazole, itraconazole, ketoconazole, posaconazole and voriconazole

C – cyclosporine and cimetidine, the H_2RA that is the most difficult to use due to DIs and androgen-blocking effects (that can cause gynecomastia – swollen, painful breast tissue or impotence)

Macrolides (clarithromycin and erythromycin), not azithromycin, but DO include the related compound telithromycin

Amiodarone (and dronedarone)

Non-DHP CCBs diltiazem and verapamil

SELECT DRUGS WITH SIGNIFICANT INTERACTIONS – WATCH FOR THESE

This is only some, but not all of the common drug interactions – refer to the individual chapters.

Amiodarone

The following medications must have the doses ↓ 30-50% when starting amiodarone: digoxin, warfarin, quinidine and procainamide. Use lower doses of simvastatin, lovastatin and atorvastatin. Digoxin and warfarin are likely drugs to be given with amiodarone (for heart failure, and for arrhythmia). If the drugs are started concurrently the lower dose of the digoxin or warfarin is used. If warfarin or digoxin is on board first, the pharmacist must recognize the interaction and decrease the dose when amiodarone is started.

Digoxin

The digoxin level increases mostly due to a decline in renal function or hypokalemia. The drug interaction with amiodarone is described previously; although a minority of digoxin is hepatically cleared, enzyme interactions are important because digoxin is kept in a narrow therapeutic range. Another consideration with digoxin is additive drugs that lower heart rate (< 60 BPM). These are primarily beta blockers and the non-DHP calcium channel blockers (diltiazem and verapamil). Other drugs that lower heart rate are amiodarone, dexmedetomidine (Precedex), clonidine and opioids. Bradycardia is one of the symptoms of organophosphate poisoning, which occurs most commonly with farm workers due to pesticide exposure.

Grapefruit Juice/Fruit Interactions

Concurrent use with grapefruit and some drugs (including simvastatin, lovastatin and atorvastatin and CCBs) will cause an increase in the drug concentration which may or may not be clinically relevant. With some drugs, it could be quite clinically relevant. For example, with rivaroxaban or ticagrelor there would be increased bleeding risk and with QT prolongers there would be risk of torsades (lurasidone, quinidine, many others). If there is any risk, safety is paramount. Counsel the patient to avoid grapefruit. This is not a "gut interaction" problem; the drug metabolizing enzymes are inactivated.

Lamotrigine & Valproate

This combination has high risk for severe rash and requires a careful titration with patient or parent monitoring. The interaction should not be missed by pharmacists because the rash may occur in children (seizures may require this combination) and the parents need to know that this is an emergency. Any inhibitor of lamotrigine will require a lower dose titration that is included in the packaging. Inducers require a higher dose; this would not cause as much risk with severe rash, but it would impair seizure control.

Monoamine Oxidase Inhibitors (MAO Is)

The non-selective MAO Is have drug interactions that can cause serotonin syndrome, hypertensive crisis, and potentially be fatal. Monoamines that would have reduced metabolism with monoamine oxidase inhibitors include dopamine, epinephrine, norepinephrine, serotonin (and tyramine, which is also a monoamine and thus the problem with foods rich in tyramine). This is mostly a risk with the antidepressants (which raise levels of the monoamines) and other agents that have a similar effect. There is some degree of risk with the Parkinson agents; refer to the chapter for specifics.

- Do not use MAO Is with ephedrine and analogs (pseudoephedrine, etc.), bupropion, buspirone, linezolid, lithium, meperidine, SSRIs, SNRIs, TCAs, tramadol, levodopa, mirtazapine, dextromethorphan, cyclobenzaprine (and other skeletal muscle relaxants), some of the triptans, St. John's wort, procarbazine, lorcaserin, and some others.

- The non-selective MAO Is, the selegiline patch (at the two higher doses) and rasagiline should not be used with tyramine-rich foods, which include aged cheeses, air-dried meats, certain wines and beers and other foods which have been aged, fermented, pickled or smoked.

Hydrocodone and Tramadol

Both of these opioids are metabolized by 2D6; patients without this enzyme (~10% of Caucasians, others) or those on 2D6 inhibitors (fluoxetine, paroxetine, others) would be at increased risk of respiratory depression and, at the least, have increased side effects with hydrocodone. Tramadol requires conversion by 2D6 to the main active (analgesic) metabolite.

Codeine

Codeine is a partial prodrug for morphine and undergoes conversion by the 2D6 enzyme. Patients who have a lot of 2D6 will produce morphine rapidly, which could be fatal to the patient, or to the infant if the mother is using codeine and is breastfeeding. Patients who lack 2D6 or those on 2D6 inhibitors would have a lack of analgesic efficacy from the drug.

Fentanyl, Hydrocodone, Oxycodone, Methadone

These opioids are primarily metabolized by 3A4; patients on 3A4 inhibitors could suffer fatality. This is a black box warning for oxycodone (to avoid use with 3A4 inhibitors) and a product labeling warning for methadone. Using 3A4 inducers could cause a subtherapeutic response.

PDE5-Inhibitors

These are used for erectile dysfunction, pulmonary arterial hypertension, benign prostatic hypertrophy, and a few off label uses. They are contraindicated with nitrates due to severe hypotension. The nitrate most commonly used in the outpatient setting is the sublingual formulations, which are not dosed on a regular basis; it may be necessary to review further back in the dispensing history to find if the patient has the drug. Increasingly, patients use more than one pharmacy and the pharmacy computer will not contain the complete history unless it is collected at intake and entered manually.

These drugs cause orthostasis with headache and dizziness – and are used commonly in older men, who may also be taking alpha blockers for prostate enlargement – and which have similar side effects. The additive effect could be dangerous. When adding one class to another, it is done cautiously with lower dosing. Another complication would occur if too high a dose is given; the product labeling warns against using higher doses with 3A4 inhibitors as these are 3A4 substrates and this interaction would have the effect of providing a higher dose, with more dizziness, orthostasis, flushing and headache. These side effects are related to the action of the drug; blood is moving outward, towards the periphery.

Chelation Risk – Quinolones, Tetracyclines

Antacids, didanosine, sucralfate, bile acid resins, magnesium, aluminum, calcium, iron, zinc, multivitamins or any product containing these multivalent cations can chelate and inhibit absorption; the quinolone separation times vary. The tetracycline class (including doxycycline and minocycline) have the chelation interaction and require separation.

Statins

When the statin dose is increased, the risk is <u>higher for muscle toxicity</u>: muscle aches, soreness, or worse, including a rapid breakdown of muscle tissue (rhabdomyolysis), which can cause renal failure as the muscle "breakdown" products enter the blood and travel to the kidneys, causing damage. The statins that have the most risk for drug interactions are the ones that go through the highest degree of 3A4 metabolism: atorvastatin, simvastatin and lovastatin. Drugs that increase statin levels (including the inhibitor gemfibrozil, macrolides, others) will increase the risk.

Calcineurin Inhibitors (Tacrolimus & Cyclosporine)

The calcineurin inhibitors (CNIs) are important because they are the central immunosuppressants used chronically (with some combination of adjuvants) and they are subject to many drug interactions. Transplant patients are immune-suppressed and this results in illness: fungal infections may be treated with systemic azoles (which are inhibitors), bacterial infections may be treated with macrolides (most are inhibitors) or with rifampin (a strong inducer) or with aminoglycosides or other nephrotoxic drugs – and the calcineurin inhibitors themselves are nephrotoxic. Depression is common post-transplant; many of the SSRIs are inhibitors. Grapefruit juice is an absolute "do not take" with the CNIs. With transplant drugs the serum level needs to remain constant, around-the-clock, to reduce the risk of graft rejection.

ADDITIVE DRUG INTERACTIONS

These involve classes of drugs which may (or may not) pose a problem individually, but can become dangerous when used with other drugs that cause similar side effects. The MAO Is discussed previously could be placed in this section since the toxic effect is generally additive. For example, a patient using fluoxetine 60 mg Q daily, bupropion 150 mg BID and (due to a recent infection) is given linezolid 600 mg IV Q 12. Consider the additive effect with substantial doses.

Bleeding risk

Anticoagulants (warfarin, dabigatran, rivaroxaban, heparin and others) and antiplatelets (aspirin, dipyridamole, clopidogrel, prasugrel, ticagrelor) <u>and</u> other agents that increase bleeding risk have an additive effect: the more agents being used concurrently that increase bleeding risk, the higher the bleeding risk.

In some high-risk cases (such as a patient on warfarin who had a stroke) there may even be use of an anticoagulant with an antiplatelet (such as warfarin plus aspirin). However, the use of this combination may be inadvertent; the cardiologist may have prescribed the warfarin (or other anticoagulant) and the patient is using the aspirin OTC on their own – or is using it based on an old recommendation.

<u>Other agents that increase bleeding risk which should be avoided in patients on the above agents, or at higher bleeding risk for other reasons (such as having had a previous bleed):</u> OTC or prescription NSAIDs, SSRIs (and some SSRIs are inhibitors that will increase warfarin levels) and SNRIs, natural products, including ginkgo biloba (commonly used agent that inhibits platelet activating factor and must be stopped in advance of surgery); ginkgo biloba increases bleeding risk with no effect on the INR. Other natural products that can also pose a risk are in the Anticoagulation chapter.

Hyperkalemia Risk

Potassium is renally cleared; severe renal disease causes hyperkalemia by itself. The largest increases among the drugs listed here would be expected from the aldosterone blockers (spironolactone and eplerenone) since aldosterone regulates potassium excretion; if aldosterone is blocked, hyperkalemia is a significant risk. The American Heart Association has issued recommendations to minimize the risk of hyperkalemia in patients treated with these agents, which includes avoiding use if the potassium is high at baseline (> 5 mEq/L), monitoring renal function and avoiding the use of concurrent NSAIDs. This is discussed further in the Heart Failure chapter.

- Additive potassium accumulation: ACEIs, ARBs, aliskiren, amiloride, triamterene, eplerenone, spironolactone, salt substitutes (KCl), and the drospirenone-containing oral contraceptives.

- Additional drugs that can cause or worsen hyperkalemia include the calcineurin inhibitors (tacrolimus and cyclosporine), canaglifozin, pentamidine and sulfamethoxazole/trimethoprim, due to the trimethoprim component.

CNS Depression

CNS side effects are caused by drugs that enter the CNS (lipophilic) and primarily involve drugs that cause sedation (somnolence), dizziness, confusion (↓ cognitive function) and altered consciousness. CNS side effects can be activating (such as with the use of stimulants), but are primarily sedating. CNS depressants that are legal and dispensed in the pharmacy are one of the top causes of automobile accidents. It is not only alcohol and illicit drug use that causes car crashes. In some cases, the two are mixed, such as the use of opioids and illicit drugs, or opioids taken with alcohol. Any agent will be worse if dosed higher and taken with other CNS depressants. Pain drugs, primarily opioids, cause more accidental death (by overdose) than deaths due to car accidents, whatever the cause. There is regional variance in the risk of death from opioids: this occurs everywhere, but the Southwest and Appalachia region are the hardest-hit. The rate of drug-related deaths more than quadrupled between 1999 and 2010 in several states, including Kentucky, Indiana and Iowa.

- Additive CNS effects: alcohol, most pain medications (all of the opioids, some of the NSAIDs, other pain drugs), skeletal muscle relaxants, anticonvulsants, benzodiazepines, barbiturates, hypnotics, mirtazapine, trazodone, dronabinol, nabilone, propranolol, clonidine, and others, and many illicit substances.

QT Prolongation & Torsade De Pointes (TdP)

QT risk drugs and QT risk conditions are listed in the Arrhythmia chapter. The risk of drug-induced TdP is low relative to other drug-induced effects, but the lethality is high. TdP is always preceded by QT prolongation; yet it is only within the last ten years that the FDA set a requirement that new drugs had to be tested for the effect on the QT interval. In some cases, the drug (alone) has high QT risk (such as with dofetilide and sotalol) but with many others with lower risk the danger develops when the risk is additive, especially in an at-risk patient, such as those with underlying cardiac disease or long QT syndrome. Most commonly, the effect is additive.

Ototoxicity

Many other additive interactions are described in the individual chapters, but ototoxicity is not described elsewhere and is included here. Ototoxicity is disturbing to patients: hearing loss can cause social isolation and impair relationships. Tinnitus can become chronic and cause a large decrease in the quality of life. A loss of equilibrium and dizziness, including increased falls, can decrease confidence and cause injury. The risk increases with concurrent ototoxic drugs, higher drug levels and the duration of exposure. Drugs with known ototoxic risk include:

- Salicylates, vancomycin, aminoglycosides, cisplatin and loop diuretics. If mefloquine (anti-malarial agent) causes tinnitus, it will be present with other symptoms of neurotoxicity.

Additive ototoxic drugs are given inpatient and audiology should be consulted to conduct a baseline hearing exam and throughout treatment on a scheduled basis. With some drugs an audiology consult is ordered after a certain period of time when damage would be expected.

Practice Questions

1. Drug A is a substrate of enzyme X. Drug B is an inducer of enzyme X. A patient has been using Drug A with good results. The patient has now started therapy with Drug B. What will happen to the concentration of Drug A?

    a. Increase
    b. Decrease
    c. Stay the Same
    d. There is not enough information given
    e. None of the above

2. Drug A is a substrate of enzyme X. Drug B is an inhibitor of enzyme X. A patient has been using Drug A with good results. The patient has now started therapy with Drug B. What will happen to the concentration of Drug A?

    a. Increase
    b. Decrease
    c. Stay the Same
    d. This is not enough information given
    e. None of the above

3. Drug A is a substrate of enzyme X. Drug A is also an inducer of enzyme Y. Drug B is a substrate of enzyme Y. Drug B is also an inhibitor of enzyme X. When these drugs are both administered, what will happen to the concentrations of Drug A and Drug B?

    a. Levels of both Drug A and Drug B will increase
    b. Levels of Drug A will increase and levels of Drug B will decrease
    c. Levels of Drug A will decrease and levels of Drug B will increase
    d. Levels of Drug A will increase and levels of Drug B will stay the same
    e. There is not enough information given.

4. A patient with heart failure is using many medications, including digoxin, warfarin and pravastatin. She is started on amiodarone therapy. Which statement is correct?

    a. The INR will increase; the warfarin dose will need to be reduced
    b. The digoxin will increase; the digoxin dose will need to be reduced
    c. The pravastatin level will increase; the pravastatin dose will need to be reduced
    d. A and B
    e. All of the above

5. A patient has been using warfarin for DVT treatment. She was hospitalized for afibrillation and started on amiodarone therapy. While hospitalized, she developed an infection and was prescribed trimethoprim/sulfamethoxazole and ketoconazole. Which of the following agents will increase the INR and could result in bleeding?

    a. Amiodarone
    b. Trimethoprim/sulfamethoxazole
    c. Ketoconazole
    d. A and B
    e. All of the above

6. The pharmacist is dispensing a prescription for ciprofloxacin. The only medication the patient is using is a daily multivitamin, which she takes with breakfast and an iron supplement, which she takes with dinner. She has yogurt or cheese every day with lunch. Which counseling statement is correct?

    a. She will need to separate the ciprofloxacin from the multivitamin
    b. She will need to separate the ciprofloxacin from the iron supplement
    c. She will need to separate the ciprofloxacin from the yogurt and cheese
    d. A and B
    e. All of the above

7. A major drug interaction can occur with the use of grapefruit juice and which of the following medications?

    a. Atorvastatin and Amiodarone
    b. Celecoxib and Felodipine
    c. Lovastatin and Lithium
    d. Levetiracetam and Topiramate
    e. Duloxetine and Mirtazapine

Answers
1-b, 2-a, 3-b, 4-d, 5-e, 6-e, 7-a

LAB VALUES, DRUG MONITORING & PATIENT CHARTS

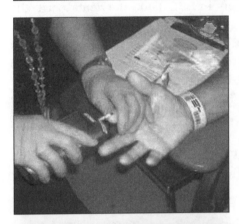

REFERENCES

Lee, M. Basic Skills in Interpreting Laboratory Data. 5th ed. Betheseda, MD: ASHP; 2013.

Schmidt, J and Wieczorkiewicz, J. Interpreting Laboratory Data. Betheseda, MD: ASHP; 2012.

Lab Tests Online. www.labtestsonline.org (accessed 2014 Aug 25).

Berkeley Heart Lab. http://www.bhlinc.com/clinicians/test-descriptions/#a110 (accessed 2014 Sep 2).

BACKGROUND

Laboratory values assist healthcare providers in diagnosing and monitoring diseases and drug therapies. In addition to typical blood or other fluid or tissue samples sent to a hospital or outside laboratory, there are newer ways to obtain drug and tissue samples. Point-of-care testing provides results obtained right at the site of the patient care and includes many tests: A1C, cardiac enzymes, INR, various infection diagnosis kits and others. Home testing kits provide convenience and privacy. There are many, including kits that test for HIV infection, herpes and urine drug analysis kits that identify the presence of illicit substances and opioids.

Therapeutic drug monitoring (TDM) involves testing the drug level and related labs to monitor efficacy and to make sure that the drug is as non-toxic as possible. For example, if a patient is using cyclosporine to prevent graft rejection the health care team will monitor both the cyclosporine trough level and the renal function since cyclosporine causes nephrotoxicity. In California (as of January, 2014) pharmacists, as part of the provider legislation, can order and interpret lab tests for a variety of purposes, including tests to screen for and diagnose disease, to check for medication adherence or to screen for the use of drugs of abuse. Prescribing privilege is advancing in many states.

TEST RESULTS: NORMAL RANGE, REFERENCE RANGE AND CRITICAL VALUES

Test results are usually a numerical value, such as sodium = 139 mEq/L. Other lab results are "positive" or "negative" or indicate a specific item, such as "Gram-positive cocci". Reference ranges can vary slightly from one lab to another due to slight variances in products and techniques. Lab values can indicate normal ranges or may indicate a serious condition that needs to be addressed rapidly. A value that is termed <u>critical</u> can be <u>life-threatening</u> unless a corrective action is taken quickly. The Joint Commission requires that all accredited facilities create and follow a <u>protocol to identify and report critical values to the responsible caregiver</u>, who has an established <u>time frame</u> to manage the result. This applies to critical <u>lab values</u> and diagnostic procedure results.

TEST DEFINITIONS

Complete Blood Cell Count (CBC)

The CBC (see table later in the chapter) is a commonly ordered lab panel that analyzes the white blood cells (WBCs), or neutrophils, the red blood cells (RBCs), and the platelets (PLTs). The CBC includes the hemoglobin (oxygen-carrying protein in RBCs) and the hematocrit (the level of RBCs in the fluid component of the blood, or plasma). A low WBC count is called leukopenia. A high WBC count is leukocytosis. When a CBC with differential is ordered, the types of neutrophils are analyzed. RBCs have an average life span of <u>120 days</u>. A high RBC count is called erythrocytosis. Anemia occurs if there is ↓ production, loss (bleeding), or destruction (hemolysis) of RBCs. PLTs have an average life span of <u>7 – 10 days</u>. A high PLT count is called thrombocytosis and a low PLT count is called <u>thrombocytopenia</u>.

It may be useful to know which values are represented by a stick diagram; this is used in practice when writing up a paper chart note to denote the four primary CBC components:

$$\text{WBC} \diagdown \overset{\textstyle \text{Hgb}}{\underset{\textstyle \text{Hct}}{\times}} \diagup \text{PLT}$$

Basic Metabolic Panel (BMP)/Comprehensive Metabolic Panel (CMP)

The BMP (see table later in the chapter) includes seven or eight tests that analyze the electrolyte and glucose levels, acid/base (with the HCO_3, or bicarbonate) and renal function. Some labs calculate and report the anion gap along with the BMP (see Calculations chapter). The stick diagram below is used to denote seven of the BMP components:

Na^+	Cl^-	BUN	
K^+	HCO_3	SCr	Glucose

A CMP includes the tests in the BMP plus albumin, alanine aminotransferase (ALT), aspartate aminotransferase (AST), total bilirubin and total protein. The additional tests are used primarily to assess liver function. The BMP and CMP are groups of labs that are ordered together for convenience. Clinicians should be aware of cost and not order a panel if single lab tests would be sufficient.

Common Adult Laboratory Reference Ranges

ITEM	COMMON REFERENCE RANGE	CHANGES LEVEL & NOTES
Anticoagulation		
Anti-Xa (Antifactor Xa Activity)	Refer to Therapeutic Drug Monitoring table at end of chapter.	To monitor low molecular weight heparins (LMWHs). Monitoring is recommended in pregnancy and mechanical heart valves and possibly in obesity, low body weight, pediatrics, elderly, or renal insufficiency. ↑ due to heparin, LMWHs and fondaparinux.
PT/INR (Prothrombin Time/International Normalized Ratio)	PT: 10-13 seconds (varies) INR: < 1.2 (for those not on warfarin)	To monitor warfarin. INR increases (without warfarin) due to liver disease. Many drugs ↑ or ↓ INR; see Anticoagulation chapter.
aPTT or PTT (Activated Partial Thromboplastin Time)	22-38 seconds (varies – this is the "control") VTE treatment: 1.5-2.5x control	To monitor unfractionated heparin (UFH) and direct thrombin inhibitors (e.g., argatroban).
ACT (Activated Clotting Time)	70-180 seconds (varies)	To monitor anticoagulation in the cardiac catheterization lab during percutaneous coronary intervention (PCI) and in surgery.
Platelets	150,000-450,000/mm³	To screen for abnormal levels; platelets are required for clot formation. ↓ due to heparin, LMWHs, fondaparinux, glycoprotein IIb/IIIa receptor antagonists, linezolid, valproic acid, chemotherapy that targets the bone marrow, rarely other drugs.
Heparin-induced platelet antibodies: 1st ELISA test, then 2nd SRA serotonin release assay	Negative	To confirm diagnosis of heparin-induced thrombocytopenia (HIT). If the ELISA test is positive, a positive SRA is confirmatory.
Cardiovascular		
CK or CPK (Creatine Kinase or Creatinine Phosphokinase)	55-170 IU/L (male) 30-135 IU/L (female)	To assess muscle inflammation (myositis) or more serious muscle damage or to diagnose cardiac conditions. ↑ due to daptomycin, quinupristin/dalfopristin, statins, fibrates (especially if given with a statin), emtricitabine, tenofovir, tipranavir, raltegravir, dolutegravir, telbivudine.

Common Adult Laboratory Reference Ranges Continued

ITEM	COMMON REFERENCE RANGE	CHANGES LEVEL & NOTES
CK-MB isoenzymes, total	≤ 6.0 ng/mL	These are called "cardiac enzymes" and are used in the diagnosis of MI. The troponins can be elevated with a few other conditions (sepsis, PE, CKD).
TnT (Troponin T)	0-0.1 ng/mL (assay dependent)	
TnI (Troponin I)	0-0.5 ng/mL (assay dependent)	BNP and NT-proBNP are both markers of cardiac stress. They are not HF nor heart disease-specific but the higher the values, the higher the likelihood of HF. Renal failure is the second most common cause of increases in BNP and NT-proBNP.
BNP (B-Type Natriuretic Peptide)	< 100 pg/mL or ng/L	
NT-proBNP (N-terminal-proBNP)	males < 61 pg/mL females 12-151 pg/mL	Myoglobin and CK-MB are not interchangeable; they are 2 separate markers. Myoglobin is a sensitive marker for muscle injury but has relatively low specificity for acute MI and therefore is not routinely used for diagnosis. See ACS chapter.

WBC and Differential

WBC	4,000-11,000/mm³	Used to diagnose and monitor infection/inflammation. Can ↑ as an acute phase reactant – indicating a systemic reaction to inflammation. ↑ due to corticosteroids, colony stimulating factors, epinephrine. ↓ due to clozapine, chemotherapy that targets the bone marrow, carbamazapine, cephalosporins, procainamide, vancomycin.
PMNs or "segs" (Polymorphonuclear neutrophils)	45-73%	Immature neutrophils released from bone marrow to fight infection. Used with WBC in absolute neutrophil count (ANC) calculation.
Bands (Band neutrophils)	3-5%	
Eosinophils	0-5%	↑ in drug allergy, asthma, inflammation, parasite infection.
Basophils	0-1%	↑ in inflammation, hypersensitivity reaction, leukemia.
Lymphocytes	20-40%	↑ in viral infections, lymphoma. ↓ in bone marrow suppression, HIV, or due to corticosteroids.
Monocytes	2-8%	↑ in chronic infections, inflammation & stress.

CBC and Anemia

RBC (Red Blood Cells)	4.5-5.5 x 10⁶cells/μL (male) 4.1-4.9 x 10⁶cells/μL (female)	↑ due to erythropoiesis stimulating agents (ESA), smoking, polycythemia, (a condition that causes high RBCs). ↓ due to chemotherapy that targets the bone marrow, low production, blood loss, deficiency anemias (e.g., B12, folate), hemolytic anemia, sickle cell anemia.

Common Adult Laboratory Reference Ranges Continued

ITEM	COMMON REFERENCE RANGE	CHANGES LEVEL & NOTES
Hgb, Hb (Hemoglobin)	13.5-18 g/dL (male) 12-16 g/dL (female)	Hgb is the iron-containing protein that carries oxygen in the RBCs. The Hct mirrors the Hgb result (providing the same clinical information).
Hct (Hematocrit)	38-50% (male) 36-46% (female)	↑ due to ESAs (see Anemia chapter). ↓ due to bleeding, risk with: anticoagulants, antiplatelets, P2Y$_{12}$ inhibitors, fibrinolytics or due to aplastic anemia from chloramphenicol.
MCV (Mean Corpuscular Volume)	80-100 mm^3	In microcytic anemia (MCV < 80) – due to iron deficiency. In macrocytic anemia (MCV > 100) – due to iron deficiency.
MCH (Mean Corpuscular Hemoglobin)	26-34 pg/cell	Additional tests used in an anemia work-up.
MCHC (Mean Corpuscular Hgb Conc.)	31-37 g/dL	
RDW (RBC Distribution Width)	11.5-14.5%	RDW measures the change in the RBC size.
Iron	65-150 mcg/dL	↑ due to iron supplementation. ↓ due to blood loss or poor nutritional intake.
TIBC (Total iron binding capacity)	250-400 mcg/dL	Monitored as part of the workup and treatment for iron deficiency anemia, anemia of chronic disease or anemia associated with chronic kidney disease (CKD). Often parenteral iron is required in conjunction with an ESA for patients on dialysis (see Anemia chapter).
Transferrin	> 200 mg/dL	
TSAT (Transferrin saturation)	15-50% (male) 12-45% (female)	
Ferritin	11-300 ng/mL	
Erythropoietin	2-25 mIU/mL	
Folic acid (folate)	5-25 mcg/L	B12 and folate are ordered for further workup of a macrocytic anemia. ↓ due to phenytoin/fosphenytoin, methotrexate, phenobarbital, primidone, sulfasalazine, sulfamethoxazole/trimethoprim. Supplement folate in pregnancy, alcoholism; see Natural Products and Vitamins chapter.
Vitamin B12	> 200 pg/mL	↓ due to PPIs, metformin, colchicine, chloramphenicol.
MMA Methylmalonate	Varies	Used for further workup of macrocytic anemia when B12 deficiency is suspected. Schilling test has also been used.
Reticulocyte count	0.5-2.5%	Immature red blood cells; the test can determine if the bone marrow production of RBCs is acceptable.

Common Adult Laboratory Reference Ranges Continued

ITEM	COMMON REFERENCE RANGE	CHANGES LEVEL & NOTES
Coombs Test, Direct Other name for test: Direct Antiglobulin Test (DAT)	Negative Positive Coombs test (risk for hemolytic anemia) If positive, discontinue the offending drug	Used to determine cause of hemolytic anemia (autoimmune vs. drug-induced) and in assessment of transfusion compatibility. Positive in drug-induced hemolysis caused by penicillins and cephalosporins (prolonged use/ high concentrations), isoniazid, methyldopa, nitrofurantoin, quinidine, quinine, rifampin and sulfonamides.
G6PD Glucose-6-phosphate dehydrogenase	5-14 units/g Drugs that can cause hemolysis with G6PD deficiency should not be used in these patients. If hemolysis with these drugs test for G6PD deficiency.	If hemolytic anemia occurs the test can be given to see if due to a G6PD deficiency; the result will be low. The RBC destruction (with the G6PD deficiency) is triggered by stress, foods (fava beans) or these drugs: chloroquine, dapsone, methylene blue, nitrofurantoin, primaquine, probenecid, quinidine, quinine and sulfonamides.
TPMT Thiopurine Methyltransferase	≥ 15 U/mL	Genetic deficiency of thiopurine methyltransferase (TPMT) are at ↑ risk for myelosuppression (bone marrow suppression) and may require lower doses with azathioprine and mercaptopurine.
Vitamin D, serum 25(OH)	> 30 ng/mL	↓ levels increase risk of osteoporosis, osteomalacia (rickets), CVD, diabetes, hypertension, infectious diseases & other conditions. Supplement vitamin D with various conditions; see Osteoporosis/HT and Renal Disease chapters.

BMP and Electrolytes

Calcium (Calcium, ionized)	8.5-10.5 mg/dL 4.5-5.1 mg/dL	Correct calcium if low albumin; see Calculations chapter; correction is not needed with ionized calcium. ↑ due to calcium supplementation, vitamin D, thiazide diuretics. ↓ due to corticosteroids, long-term heparin, loop diuretics, bisphosphonates, calcitonin, foscarnet, topiramate. Supplement in pregnancy and other conditions; see Osteoporosis/HT chapter.
Chloride (Cl⁻)	95-103 mEq/L	Used with other labs to assess acid-base status and fluid balance.
Magnesium (Mg²⁺)	1.3-2.1 mEq/L	↑ due to magnesium-containing antacids and laxatives plus renal impairment. ↓ due to PPIs, diuretics, amphotericin, foscarnet, echinocandins, diarrhea, chronic alcohol intake.
Phosphate (PO4)	2.3-4.7 mg/dL	↑ in renal failure. ↓ due to phosphate binders, foscarnet, oral calcium intake.

Common Adult Laboratory Reference Ranges Continued

ITEM	COMMON REFERENCE RANGE	CHANGES LEVEL & NOTES
Potassium (K⁺)	3.5-5.0 mEq/L	↑ due to ACE Inhibitors, ARBs, aldosterone receptor antagonists (ARAs), aliskiren, NSAIDs, cyclosporine, tacrolimus, everolimus, mycophenolate, potassium supplements, drospirenone-containing oral contraceptives, sulfamethoxazole/trimethoprim, chronic heparin use, canagliflozin, pentamidine ↓ due to corticosteroids, beta-2 agonists, Conivaptan, diuretics, insulin, sodium polystyrene sulfonate, mycophenolate, everolimus, belatacept
Sodium (Na⁺)	135-145 mEq/L	↑ due to lithium, hypertonic saline. ↓ due to carbamazepine, oxcarbazepine, SSRIs, diuretics.
Bicarbonate (HCO3)	24-30 mEq/L	Used to assess acid-base status. ↑ due to loop diuretics, corticosteroids. ↓ due to topiramate, salicylate overdose.
BUN (Blood urea nitrogen)	7-20 mg/dL	Used with SCr (e.g., BUN/SCr ratio) to assess fluid status and renal function.
SCr (Creatinine, serum)	0.6-1. 3 mg/dL	↑ due to many drugs that impair renal function; see Renal Disease and Dosing chapter. False elevations due to sulfamethoxazole/ trimethoprim, H₂RAs. ↓ with low muscle mass, amputation, hemodilution.
Anion Gap (AG)	5-12 mEq/L	A calculated value, but often reported on the BMP. See Calculations chapter.

Liver and Gastroenterology

Albumin	3.5-5.0 g/dL	Reflects liver health, reduced in malnutrition. Highly protein bound drugs are impacted Phenytoin, valproic acid and calcium serum concentration requires correction for low albumin – see Epilepsy/Seizure and Calculations chapters.
Alk Phos (Alkaline phosphatase)	33-131 IU/L	Used with other labs to assess liver, bile duct and bone disease.
AST (Aspartate aminotransferase)	10-40 IU/L	AST and ALT are enzymes released from injured hepatocytes (liver cells). Numerous medications and herbals can ↑ AST and ALT; see Hepatitis and Liver Disease chapter.
ALT (Alanine aminotransferase)	10-40 IU/L	
T Bili (Bilirubin, total)	0.1-1.2 mg/dL	T Bili is used along with other liver tests; used to monitor drug toxicity or to determine other cause of liver damage and to detect bile duct blockage.

Common Adult Laboratory Reference Ranges Continued

ITEM	COMMON REFERENCE RANGE	CHANGES LEVEL & NOTES
Amylase	60-180 units/L	Used to assist in the diagnosis of pancreatitis.
Lipase	5-160 units/L	
Ammonia	19-60 mcg/dL	Though not diagnostic, often measured in suspected hepatic encephalopathy (HE). ↑ due to valproic acid, topiramate. ↓ due to lactulose.

Diabetes

FPG (Fasting Plasma Glucose)	≥ 126 mg/dL is positive for diabetes 100-125 mg/dL is positive for pre-diabetes	Fasting is 8+ hours. See Diabetes chapter for complete information.
EAG (Estimated Average Glucose)	< 154 mg/dL (ADA)	An EAG of 154 corresponds to an A1C of 7%; used to assist patients by making the average glucose over-time correspond to a finger stick value that corresponds to the current glucose level.
A1C (Hemoglobin A1C)	< 7% (ADA), ≤ 6.5% (AACE)	Average blood glucose over the past 3 months; based on attachment of glucose to hemoglobin; ↑ glucose = ↑ BG attached to Hgb = ↑ A1C.
Preprandial blood glucose	70-130 mg/dL (ADA), < 110 mg/dL (AACE)	Blood glucose measurement taken before a meal.
Postprandial blood glucose	< 180 mg/dL (ADA), < 140 mg/dL (AACE)	Blood glucose measurement taken after a meal (1-2 hours after the start of eating).
C-peptide (fasting)	0.78-1.89 ng/mL	Used to distinguish type I from type 2 Diabetes.

Lipids and Cardiovascular Risk Measurements

Cholesterol, total	< 200 mg/dL	Fasting begins 9-12 hours prior to lipid blood draw.
HDL (High Density Lipoprotein)	< 40 mg/dL, low ≥ 60 mg/dL, high	For complete discussion see Dyslipidemia chapter; The guidelines do not support specific CH, HDL or TG goals. The guidelines support a statin intensity level for LDL-C reductions based on those most likely to benefit.
LDL (Low Density Lipoprotein)	LDL: 70-189, depending on risk factors	
Lipoprotein-a, Lp(a)	< 10 mg/dL	↑ Lp(a) and ↑ ApoB are being used more commonly; these are associated with ↑ coagulation and ↑ risk of CVD.
Apoliprotein-B, Apo B	< 130 mg/dL	
TGs (Triglycerides)	< 150 mg/dL	C-reactive protein (CRP) indicates inflammation, which could be due to many inflammatory conditions, including rheumatoid arthritis and heart failure. High-sensitivity CRP (hs-CRP) is more sensitive for CVD.
C-reactive protein	< 2 mg/L; higher is at risk	
Coronary Artery Calcium score	< 300 Agatston units or < 75 percentile for age, sex and ethnicity; higher is at risk	The coronary artery calcium score measures calcium build-up in the coronary arteries.
ABI (Ankle Brachial Index)	1-1.4	The ankle brachial index measures the ratio of the BP in the lower legs to the BP in the arms. It is used to assess severity of peripheral artery disease (PAD). A level < 1 indicates some degree of blockage.

Common Adult Laboratory Reference Ranges Continued

ITEM	COMMON REFERENCE RANGE	CHANGES LEVEL & NOTES

Thyroid Function

ITEM	COMMON REFERENCE RANGE	CHANGES LEVEL & NOTES
TSH (Thyroid stimulating hormone)	0.3-3.0 mIU/L	The TSH test is used with the FT4 to diagnose hypothyroidism and is used alone (sometimes with FT4) to monitor patients being treated. Low iodine intake is a cause of hypothyroidism; this is rare in the U.S. because iodine is added to table salt (NaCl).
Total thyroxine (T4)	4.5-10.9 mcg/dL	T4 and FT4 are two of several tests used for a detailed assessment of thyroid function.
Free thyroxine (FT4)	0.9-2.3 ng/dL	

Uric Acid/Gout Assessment

ITEM	COMMON REFERENCE RANGE	CHANGES LEVEL & NOTES
Uric acid	3.5-7.2 mg/dL (male) 2.0-6.5 mg/dL (female)	Used in diagnosis/treatment of gout. Can ↑ due to diuretics, niacin, high doses aspirin, pyrazinamide, cyclosporine, tacrolimus, ribavirin.

Inflammation/Autoimmune Disease

ITEM	COMMON REFERENCE RANGE	CHANGES LEVEL & NOTES
CRP (C-Reactive Protein)	Normal: < 0.8 mg/dL High risk: > 3 mg/dL	Nonspecific tests used in autoimmune disorders, inflammation and infections. Drug-induced Lupus Erythematosus (DILE) can be caused by many drugs. More likely with hydralazine, methyldopa, minocycline, procainamide, quinidine, methimazole, propylthiouracil, anti-TNF agents, isoniazid and terbinafine. If ANA is positive, histone antibody and anti-dsDNA tests will be help establish diagnosis. Causative drug will require discontinuation.
RF (Rheumatoid Factor, serum)	< 40 IU/mL	
ESR (Erythrocyte sedimentation rate)	≤ 20 mm/hr (male) ≤ 30 mm/hr (female)	
ANA (Antinuclear antibodies)	Negative (titers may be provided)	
Antihistone Antibodies (Detected by ELISA)	Negative	

HIV

ITEM	COMMON REFERENCE RANGE	CHANGES LEVEL & NOTES
HIV Antibody	Negative (non-reactive)	Detects infection with the virus; may not become positive until several weeks after exposure.
HIV DNA PCR	Negative	Useful for early detection.
CD4+ T Lymphocyte Count	800-1,100 cells/mm3	Used to monitor HIV treatment; see HIV chapter.
HIV RNA Concentration (Viral Load)	Undetectable	

Common Adult Laboratory Reference Ranges Continued

ITEM	COMMON REFERENCE RANGE	CHANGES LEVEL & NOTES

Acid-Base

ITEM	COMMON REFERENCE RANGE	CHANGES LEVEL & NOTES
pH	7.35-7.45	Values for arterial blood gas (ABG) sample. See Calculations chapter.
pCO_2	35-45 mmHg	
pO_2	80-100 mmHg	
HCO_3	24-30 mEq/L	
O_2 Sat	~ 95%	

Hormonal

ITEM	COMMON REFERENCE RANGE	CHANGES LEVEL & NOTES
Testosterone total, free	300-950 ng/dL (male)	
PSA (Prostate-specific antigen)	< 4 ng/mL	Can ↑ with testosterone supplementation.
hCG (Human chorionic gonadotropin)	Varies by test	Tested in blood or urine to determine pregnancy.
LH (Luteinizing hormone)	Varies during cycle	Rises mid-cycle causing egg release. Tested in urine with ovulation predictor kits for women attempting pregnancy.

Other

ITEM	COMMON REFERENCE RANGE	CHANGES LEVEL & NOTES
Lactic acid (lactate)	0.5-2.2 mEq/L	Indicates anaerobic metabolism/lactic acidosis. Can ↑ due to NNRTIs (see HIV chapter), metformin (low risk/mostly with renal disease and heart failure), alcohol, cyanide.
Prolactin	1-25 ng/mL	Secretion is regulated by dopamine; Can ↑ with haloperidol, risperidone, paliperidone, methyldopa. Can ↓ with bromocriptine.
Serum osmolality	275-290 mOsm/kg H_2O	Used with Na⁺, BUN/SCr, and clinical volume status to evaluate hypo/hypernatremia.
Cosyntropin Stimulation Test	Baseline and timed increase are measured	Used to test for adrenal suppression; medications that affect baseline cortisol or suppress adrenal response will impact test and may need to be held prior (e.g., corticosteroids).
Mantoux test/PPD (Purified Protein Derivative) test	No induration; induration is measured for diagnosis of TB exposure.	TB test administered by intradermal injection. Response is measured by diameter (mm) of induration at 48 - 72 hours.

THERAPEUTIC DRUG MONITORING (TDM)

Drug levels or other values (such as anti-Xa levels for LMWHs) are used to reach dosing goals and to avoid toxicity. TDM is increasingly common due to the need to target highly resistant organisms and dose medications in overweight and obese patients. Some tests, such as the CBC, are measured directly from whole blood, or, the lab can remove cells from the blood with the use of a centrifuge. The yellowish liquid that remains is the plasma, which contains proteins (including albumin), clotting factors, glucose, electrolytes and other suspended materials in water. Drug levels can be measured in the blood directly or from plasma or, less commonly, from other body fluids, such as saliva or urine.

Drug Levels Must be Taken at the Correct Times

The peak level is the highest concentration in the blood the drug will reach and requires time for the drug to distribute in the body's tissues. The trough level is the lowest concentration the drug will reach in the blood and is drawn right before the next dose.

The steady-state level is often (but not always) the preferred time to take drug levels. Steady-state occurs when the amount of drug going in (for example, when the patient swallows their daily dose) equals the amount of drug going out (from metabolism and clearance). It takes between 4 to 5 half-lives for a drug to reach steady-state.

The following table lists drugs that are commonly monitored. Most are defined as "narrow therapeutic index" (NTI), which means they have a narrow separation between the level at which the drug provides a benefit and the level at which the patient is at risk from too low a level (subtherapeutic) or too high a level (supratherapeutic, and likely toxic). Whether a drug has a NTI can affect generic substitution because a few states do not permit generic substitution of NTI drugs; the FDA, however, does not separate NTI drugs from other drugs in the reference for acceptable generic substitution, the *Orange Book*. The following table does not include the transplant drugs tacrolimus, cyclosporine, sirolimus and everolimus. These are NTI and are monitored but are not listed as single levels since the target level will depend on the transplant type, sampling method, concurrent drugs and time since transplant.

TDM is Common for These Drugs that Require Levels

DRUG	USUAL THERAPEUTIC RANGE
Amikacin (traditional dosing)	Peak: 20 – 30 mcg/mL Trough: < 5 mcg/mL
CarBAMazepine	4 – 12 mcg/mL
Digoxin	0.8 – 2.0 ng/mL (AFib) 0.5 – 0.9 ng/mL (HF)
Gentamicin (traditional dosing)	Peak: 5 – 10 mcg/mL Trough: < 2 mcg/mL
Lithium	0.6 – 1.2 mEq/L (up to 1.5 mEq/L for acute symptoms)
Enoxaparin	VTE treatment with daily therapy: 1 – 2 anti-Xa units/mL VTE treatment with Q12H therapy: 0.6 – 1 anti-Xa units/mL Recurrent VTE prophylaxis in pregnancy: 0.2 – 0.6 anti-Xa units/mL
Phenobarbital/Primidone	20 – 40 mcg/mL (adults)
Phenytoin/Fosphenytoin Free Phenytoin	10 – 20 mcg/mL; if low albumin correct serum level; see Epilepsy/Seizure chapter. 1 – 2.5 mcg/mL

TDM is Common for These Drugs that Require Levels Continued

DRUG	USUAL THERAPEUTIC RANGE
Procainamide	4 – 10 mcg/mL
NAPA	15 – 25 mcg/mL
Combined	10 – 30 mcg/mL
Theophylline	5 – 15 mcg/mL
	5 – 10 mcg/mL (neonates)
Tobramycin (traditional dosing)	Peak: 5 – 10 mcg/mL
	Trough: < 2 mcg/mL
Valproic acid	50 – 100 mcg/mL (up to 150 mcg/mL in some patients); if low albumin correct serum level; see Epilepsy/Seizure chapter.
Vancomycin	Trough: 15 – 20 mcg/mL for most serious infections (pneumonia, endocarditis, osteomyelitis, meningitis, and bacteremia)
	Trough: 10 – 15 mcg/mL for others
Voriconazole	Trough: 1.0 – 5.0 mcg/mL (target trough may vary depending on MIC for pathogen)
Warfarin	Goal INR is 2 – 3 for most indications, use higher range (2.5 – 3.5) with mechanical mitral valves

Patient Charts and the Electronic Health Record (EHR)

Paper charts, which kept all of the patient's medical records in a binder, are being phased out and replaced by electronic health records (EHRs). EHRs, once implemented, save time and provide a more accurate record of the patient's health information. If, for example, a patient has declining renal function, the serum creatinine (SCr) level can be viewed longitudinally by selecting the date range; with a paper chart, time is required to look back through the chart to find the history. With paper charts, papers can be missing – even the entire chart can be lost, and time is required to transport the chart to wherever the patient is going next or to gather history with calls and faxes. Procedures with results recorded on paper can be scanned into the EHR.

The EHR, when linked to Computerized Prescriber Order Entry (CPOE), eliminates the problem of illegible handwriting. Pharmacists do not need to spend as much time clarifying the order or changing to a formulary drug. The CPOE system can be designed to present only formulary drugs as options, without an override from the pharmacist. Clinical decision making tools can be built into the order entry process. Allergies and drug interactions can appear as alerts. Critical results (e.g., aPTT ≥ 150 secs., platelets ≤ 40/mm³) can be linked to alert systems, such as automatic texts. The electronic information is easier to pool together to measure clinical outcomes and quality. EHR implementation at a facility does not occur without complaints; a few primary issues have involved safeguards for patient privacy, the increased time required for training and charting, and the implementation costs for the facility.

CRITICAL RESULTS

Critical results are levels significantly outside the normal range and can indicate a life-threatening situation.

They need to be reported to the caregiver right away and must be responded to quickly.

This is a Joint Commission National Patient Safety Goal.

The Health Insurance Portability and Accountability Act of 1996 (HIPAA) security protections for paper records do not change with electronic records. Access is limited with pins and passwords, information is "encrypted" to prevent documents from being sent electronically out of the institution, and an "audit trail" is used to track access. Even with these safeguards in place security can still be violated: individuals can access medical records for patients they are not involved with, an employee can have the screen visible or forget to log out, and the system can be hacked from the outside. All personnel using the EHR are responsible for the security. As with paper charts, patients have a right to fill out a signed request for their medical records.

Background Papers

The first additions to an EHR (or paper chart) are the admission sheet, a service agreement form ("this is what I am having done at this facility"), a page describing the patient's rights (a Joint Commission requirement), and an advanced directive to document the patient's wishes concerning medical treatment if he or she is unable to make the decisions on their own behalf.

HIPAA & PHI

The HIPAA Privacy Rule covers all individually identifiable health information, which is called "protected health information" (PHI).

The PHI includes the patient's address (anything smaller than the state they live in), the patient's physical and psychological conditions, the care received or planned, and the information that could be used to identify that patient, including name, address, date of birth, medical record number, social security number, phone, fax and email.

It is acceptable to use PHI for treatment decisions, payment (insurance purposes) and for the specific facility operations (such as QA, infection control, etc.) and, if legally warranted (such as with an abuse case) or if required for public health.

Patient's can request their own PHI. If the PHI is used for other purposes (e.g., research), an authorization by the patient is required and identifiers are removed.

Certain religious groups will request a refusal form for blood transfusions and blood products. "Blood products" primarily involve albumin and immune globulins, but some patients will refuse drugs buffered in blood *(Epogen/Procrit, Kogenate* – used for hemophilia), natural clotting factors/tissue adhesives/interferons and a few other uncommon agents. A few vaccines contain porcine-derived gelatin as a stabilizer. The major religious groups consider this use acceptable but a specific patient may not.

Other forms include progress notes, the vital signs record, clinical pathway sheets used for some conditions, medication records used for some medications (such as warfarin to track the INR history), and procedure records, including the diagnostic and operating room (OR) records. The list of "Do Not Use" abbreviations should be easily available. It is important to avoid abbreviations that could be interpreted to mean something else – all hospitals will include their own group of unsafe abbreviations and the Joint Commission's list of unsafe abbreviations, acronyms and symbols; see the Medication Safety chapter for further discussion. Some institutions give prescribers laminated cards of the unapproved abbreviation list to keep in their pocket, hang the list on the wall near the terminal, or make the list visible on the computer screen when making entries. At the end of the hospital stay the planning, and discharge forms, will be added to the EHR.

Requirements for Reimbursement: Documentation and Quality of Care

Pharmacists are involved with various inpatient care activities: reviewing the medication history and use, documenting allergies, assessing vaccination requirements and administering vaccines, providing consults on medication options for the health care team, clarifying drug orders, adjusting the dosages, frequency and routes of administration, managing the investigational drugs, monitoring drug levels and managing toxicities, and managing chronic conditions. All interventions require documentation to get paid since the quality of the care is (increasingly) tied to the reimbursement.

The federal health insurance program is called the Affordable Care Act (ACA) or "Obamacare". The ACA includes a "National Quality Strategy" which assesses the improvement in quality of care by determining if the members are healthier and if the costs are lower. Since the Centers for Medicare and Medicaid Services (CMS) provides the health insurance to many Americans, CMS is directly involved with the quality measurements and cost control. CMS has penalties for poor care and incentives for quality care. Two areas in which the penalties are steep are the rate of hospital-acquired infections and the hospital's readmission rate. These measures are chosen because they are expensive and are often, but not always, avoidable.

The Joint Commission, The Pharmacy Quality Alliance (PQA) and The Agency for Healthcare Research and Quality (AHRQ) are also involved in setting the criteria to measure the quality of care. The PQA quality measurements focus on medications. Specific goals that involve medications include increasing adherence, avoiding unnecessary or unsafe medications (such as high-risk medications in the elderly) and increasing the use of medications indicated for certain conditions.

MEDICARE & MEDICAID

Medicare is the federal health insurance program for ages ≥ 65 and older, < 65 with disability and all ages with end stage renal disease (ESRD).

The prescription drug benefit under Medicare is called Part D.

Part A covers the hospital visit and Part B covers medical costs, such as doctor visits.

Medicaid provides health insurance for all ages with very low income (< 133% of the federal poverty level). Medicaid is a federal and state program.

A senior who qualifies for both Medicare and Medicaid has "dual coverage."

The SOAP Format for Progress Notes

A progress note records a patient encounter. The SOAP note format is organized into four parts: Subjective, Objective, Assessment and Plan (SOAP). Paper charts and EHRs often use this format. Prior to the use of SOAP notes it was difficult to understand patient chart entries because the format was not standardized. The SOAP note was developed to provide a standard structure for recording the patient encounter.

Military Time

In all medical records, including the SOAP note, time is recorded with a 24-hour clock, rather than splitting the day into two 12-hour segments (AM/PM). The 24-hour clock is called "military time." The day begins at midnight, which is called 24:00 (pronounced twenty-four hundred). This is actually the start of the day and is sometimes referred to as 00:00. One minute past midnight is 00:01, thirty minutes is 00:30, one hour is 01:00, and so on. After 12:00 noon the time continues on the same number line for the rest of the day: 1:00 PM is 1300, 2:00 PM is 1400, and so on. The last minute of the day is 23:59, then 24:00 (midnight), and then the next day begins.

MILITARY TIME REFERENCE	
12-Hr clock	**24-Hr clock**
12:00 midnight	24:00
1:00 am	01:00
…(continuing).	(pronounced "Oh-100")
7:00 pm	19:00
8:00 pm	20:00
9:00 pm	21:00
10:00 pm	22:00
11:00 pm	23:00
12:00 midnight	24:00

The 1st section in a SOAP note is the subjective information recorded from the patient. It is the patient's own narrative of their symptoms. Only the relevant information is recorded. The person conducting the interview should use only direct questions and avoid leading questions. For example, the leading question: "You always take your blood pressure pills, right?" is not likely to get a useful response. Phrasing the question in a direct manner that is worded to avoid a yes or no response will elicit a more useful response: "In a typical week, about how mornings do you forget to take the blood pressure pills?"

The subjective section begins with a one-line Chief Complaint (CC), the specific reason the patient is being seen today, such as "I've had a stabbing pain in my right hip for three days" or "I feel like I need to go all the time but nothing much comes out." The subjective section includes the history of the present illness (HPI): the onset and duration of the specific complaint, the quality and severity (for example, with a pain complaint, descriptive words should be used to identify the type of pain, with a numerical pain rating), any modifying factors (what reduces or aggravates the condition), and treatment that has been tried to resolve the condition and the effect of the treatment, if any.

This section includes the past medical history (PMH), social history (alcohol, tobacco and illicit drug use), family history (first-degree relatives only – parents and siblings), allergies and medication use. Medication includes prescriptions, samples, and OTC's, including vitamins and natural products.

The 2nd section in a SOAP note is the objective information obtained by the clinician, either through observation or analysis. This includes the vital signs (respiration rate, heart rate, blood pressure, temperature). Note that on the top of the sample EHR at the end of this chapter the vitals are recorded at the top of the page – but they are part of the objective section. Any other measurements (for example, height and weight, spirometry), physical findings and laboratory results goes into this section.

SIGNS AND SYMPTONS (S/Sx)

A symptom is subjective information, described by the patient, such as "My lower back hurts."

A sign is generally objective (described by the clinician), such as recording the patient's vital signs.

Occasionally objective evidence (such as a skin rash), can be seen by either the patient or family members or the clinician.

The 3rd section is the assessment. This is the provider's thought process of possible causes of the current situation. Many conditions present with similar signs and symptoms; the assessment will often include multiple possible diagnosis. The process of distinguishing the actual condition from others is called the <u>differential diagnosis</u>.

The 4th section is the <u>plan</u>. This is how the problem will be addressed. The plan should be as specific as possible. Labs might be ordered, the patient may be sent out for diagnostic exams, referrals may be requested, or the patient may require education. Education could be required for a variety of reasons, such as suspected non-adherence, to remedy poor device technique or to provide nutritional education or smoking cessation support. If there is a differential diagnosis there will be multiple steps in the plan to "rule out" (eliminate) some of the suspected conditions.

This text contains three EHR SOAP notes; the following page and the patient cases at the end of the Heart Failure and Inflammatory Bowel Disease chapters.

Juanita Burrows (PRN: JB747114): SOAP Note for 09/25/2014
Age on DOS: 40 yrs, DOB: 03/13/1974

San Diego Medical Group
35 La Jolla Drive Suite 100 San Diego, CA 92130
(444) 444-4444

seen by: Alison James
seen on: Thursday 25 September 2014

VS

Height:	Weight:	BMI:	Blood Pressure:	Temp:	Pulse:	Resp Rate:
67.0 in	195.0 lb	30.5	154 / 92 mmHg	97.9 F	80 bpm	12 rpm

CC "I feel limp"

S JB is a 40 y/o female who presents with a 3 month history of increasing fatigue. She first noticed that she felt tired when she was working long hours to get a job done at work, but has been working her usual 8 hours a day for the past 2 months and has not regained her energy. She describes her fatigue as "feeling limp". It is present throughout the day, but worse with significant exertion (e.g., walking > 3-4 blocks or going up stairs). She has tried to go to bed earlier, but even sleeping up to 10 hours/night (increased from 8 hours/night) has not helped. She is concerned that there is something seriously wrong, as she is usually full of energy and her family and friends are starting to ask if she is sick. She has also not been able to exercise, which she usually enjoys. She denies chest pain, SOB, abdominal pain, N/V/D, or changes in her stool. She has no alopecia or skin changes. She has had no fever, chills or night sweats. She has gained about 6-7 lbs in the last few months, which she attributes to inactivity due to fatigue. She denies depressed mood, sadness, or anhedonia. She states that she goes to bed at 10pm and wakes feeling tired at 6am on weekdays and 8am on weekends. Her husband states that she has "always" snored quite loudly. Her menses are regular in timing, heavy flow for 1-2 days, then lighter for another 2-3 days. This pattern is unchanged from prior to the onset of her fatigue. Her last menstrual period was one week ago. When asked about compliance with her medications, she states that she takes everything regularly "except the one for her blood pressure because she doesn't feel like her pressure is high".

She reports a history of GERD, HTN, and depression.
Her medications include: Zantac 150 mg PO QHS, Chlorthalidone 25 mg PO Daily,
Zoloft 100 mg Daily, and Caltrate + D 600 mg BID.

O Well-appearing black female in no acute distress.
SKIN: not pale, no rashes
NECK: no thyromegaly or thyroid nodules
NODES: no cervical, axillary or inguinal lymphadenopathy
CHEST: clear to auscultation and percussion bilaterally
CV: RRR, 2/6 systolic ejection murmur heard best at the LLSB that radiates to the apex, no S3 or S4
ABD: normal active bowel sounds, no hepatosplenomegaly by palpation or percussion, no abdominal tenderness
EXT: no edema, pulses normal

A Recent onset of fatigue with no obvious inciting event. Hypothyroidism is possible especially given her weight gain, though this also may have occurred from her inactivity. It is possible that she is anemic though her menstrual periods have not lengthened or increased and there is no other obvious source of blood loss. A recent menses makes pregnancy unlikely. Given her history of snoring, sleep apnea is possible, but her history of snoring over many years is not entirely consistent with her more recent onset of fatigue. She does not seem to have a recurrence of her depression since she has no new symptoms. She does not have symptoms of infection, nor has her murmur changed, so subacute bacterial endocarditis is possible but unlikely. BP is elevated and she has been noncompliant with prescribed therapy for HTN.

P #1. Check TSH to rule out hypothyroidism
#2. Check CBC to rule out anemia
#3. If the above are unremarkable, consider a sleep study to rule out sleep apnea
#4. Consider blood cultures to rule out subacute bacterial endocarditis
#5. Pharmacy consult for medication adherence
#6. Follow-up visit in 1 week to discuss test results and further work-up

14

RENAL DISEASE & DOSING CONSIDERATIONS

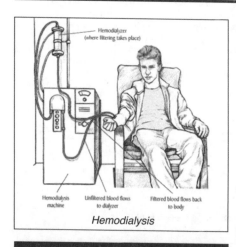

Hemodialyzer
(where filtering takes place)

Hemodialysis machine

Unfiltered blood flows to dialyzer

Filtered blood flows back to body

Hemodialysis

GUIDELINES

Kidney Disease: Improving Global Outcomes (KDIGO) CKD Work Group. KDIGO 2012 Clinical Practice Guideline for the Evaluation and Management of Chronic Kidney Disease. Kidney inter., Suppl. 2013; 3: 1-150, and refer to the KDIGO and KDOQI addtl. guidelines included with the video files (RxPrep Online).

We gratefully acknowledge the assistance of Katie E. Cardone, PharmD, BCACP, FNKF, FASN, Albany Nephrology Pharmacy Group (ANephRx), Albany College of Pharmacy and Health Sciences, in preparing this chapter.

BACKGROUND

The prevalence of chronic kidney disease (CKD) has increased from 12.3% to 14% in the U.S. over the past twenty years. The most common causes of CKD are diabetes and hypertension. Patients with CKD have a higher risk of cardiovascular morbidity and mortality. The pharmacist's role in treating patients with CKD includes modifying medication regimens based on the degree of renal function, initiating treatment to minimize disease progression and treating the complications of CKD (anemia, bone and mineral metabolism disorders, hypertension and acid-base and electrolyte disturbances).

Renal Physiology

Nephron/Glomerulus

The nephron is the functional unit of the kidney and there are roughly one million nephrons in each kidney. Blood is delivered into the glomerulus, a large filtering unit that is located within the Bowman's capsule. Substances with a molecular weight below 40,000 daltons can pass through the glomerular capillaries into the filtrate. Larger substances are not filtered and stay in the blood. If the filter is not damaged, large proteins such as albumin remain in the blood. If the glomerulus is damaged, some of the albumin passes into the urine. The amount of albumin in the urine can be used to gauge the severity of kidney damage in patients with kidney disease or nephropathy. Most drugs are small enough to pass through the filter. Exceptions are large protein compounds and drugs that are bound to albumin.

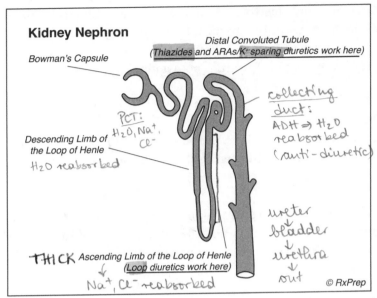

Kidney Nephron

Bowman's Capsule

Distal Convoluted Tubule
(*Thiazides and ARAs/K⁺ sparing diuretics work here*)

collecting duct:
ADH ⇒ H₂O reabsorbed (anti-diuretic)

PCT: H₂O, Na⁺, Cl⁻

Descending Limb of the Loop of Henle

H₂O reabsorbed

ureter
↓
bladder
↓
urethra
↓
out

THICK Ascending Limb of the Loop of Henle
(*Loop diuretics work here*)
↓
Na⁺, Cl⁻ reabsorbed

© RxPrep

A primary function of the nephron is to control the concentration of water and Na⁺. The nephrons reabsorb what is needed (to go back into the circulation) and excrete the remainder as urine. This regulates the blood volume, and in turn, the blood pressure. "Proximal" means close to, and the proximal tubule is the closest part to the Bowman's capsule. Large amounts of water are reabsorbed here, along with Na⁺ and Cl⁻. The pH is regulated by exchange of hydrogen ions and bicarbonate ions. Water, Na⁺ and Cl⁻ absorption continues further along the nephron.

Loop of Henle

The loop of Henle has a descending limb and an ascending limb. As filtrate moves down the loop of Henle (the descending limb), water is reabsorbed, but sodium and chloride ions are not; this concentrates sodium and chloride in the lumen (the inside of the nephron "tube"). As the filtrate moves up the loop of Henle (the ascending limb), sodium and chloride ions are reabsorbed but water is not. If antidiuretic hormone (ADH) is present, water will pass through the walls of the duct and will not be eliminated. The more ADH present, the more water is absorbed back into the blood (anti-diuresis).

digoxin
Na⁺/K⁺
ATPase
pump

Loop diuretics inhibit the Na⁺-K⁺ pump in the ascending limb of the loop of Henle (the part that goes back up). About 25% of the sodium is reabsorbed here and inhibiting these pumps leads to a significant increase in the tubular concentration of sodium and less water reabsorption. By blocking the pump, the electrical gradient is altered and reabsorption of calcium decreases. Loop diuretics used long-term deplete calcium and have a harmful effect on bone.

• loops deplete/waste Ca⁺⁺

• thiazides ↑↑ Ca⁺⁺

Distal Convoluted Tubule

Distal means farthest away and the distal convoluted tubule is the farthest away from the entry point to the nephron. The distal tubule is also involved in regulating K⁺, Na⁺, Ca²⁺ and pH. Thiazide diuretics inhibit the Na-Cl pump in the distal tubule. Only about 5% of the sodium is reabsorbed at this point, which makes thiazides weaker diuretics than loops. Thiazides increase calcium absorption by affecting the calcium pump in the distal convoluted tubule. Consequently, the long-term use of thiazide diuretics have a protective effect on bone.

Collecting Duct

The collecting duct is a network of tubules and ducts that connect the nephrons to the ureter. Urine passes from the ureter into the bladder, and from there out of the body via the urethra. The collecting duct is involved with water and electrolyte balance and is affected by levels of ADH and aldosterone. Aldosterone also works in the distal tubule. The primary function of aldosterone is to increase Na+ and water retention and to lower K+. By blocking aldosterone (with antagonists like spironolactone or eplerenone), serum potassium increases.

↳ aldosterone antag ↓ Na+/H2O , ↑ K+

ESTIMATING KIDNEY FUNCTION

The gold-standard methods to estimate the glomerular filtration rate (GFR) utilize inulin or radioactive substances. These markers are largely limited to the research setting due to the cost, inconvenience and the availability of alternative estimation methods.

Blood urea nitrogen (BUN) measures the amount of nitrogen that comes from urea, a waste product. BUN increases with kidney impairment but is not used independently to measure declines in kidney function because other factors besides renal impairment increase BUN (primarily dehydration).

↑SrCr = ↓ renal fxn

Creatinine, a waste product of muscle metabolism, is commonly used to estimate GFR. Creatinine is easily measured and mostly filtered by the kidneys. Importantly, the concentration correlates inversely with kidney function; as the renal function decreases the creatinine increases. The accuracy of creatinine-based estimation equations is limited when a patient has very low or high muscle mass, is obese, has liver disease, is pregnant or with a few other conditions that cause abnormal muscle turnover. In addition, although creatinine is mostly filtered, it is partially secreted. The contribution of tubular secretion to creatinine elimination is more significant when renal function is impaired.

p. 26
+ very young children
· ESRD
· when renal fxn is fluctuating rapidly

Creatinine Clearance (CrCl) Estimation

normal SrCr = 0.6 - 1.3 mg/dL

A normal range of serum creatinine is approximately 0.6 to 1.3 mg/dL. An important issue clinically is that the renal function can be over-estimated in elderly patients with low muscle mass. This is especially true of frail patients who are bedridden. The Cockcroft-Gault equation is the most commonly used equation for estimating renal function in order to adjust the dose of medications. This equation is reviewed in the Calculations chapter. The Cockcroft-Gault formula may not be preferable in very young children, in end-stage renal disease (ESRD) or when renal function is fluctuating rapidly. Other equations, such as the MDRD and CKD-EPI equations, are more precise for estimating kidney function in CKD and are used to stage the severity of CKD as shown in the following table. CKD is staged based on GFR from stages 1-5 using the KDOQI clinical practice guidelines, with stage 5 being ESRD. The newer guideline (KDIGO 2012) utilize GFR in a similar fashion, but also include the amount of albuminuria and the cause of the kidney disease to stage CKD.

"sarcopenic obesity"
↳ elderly may have fat (wt) but little muscle

Stages of CKD

GFR (ML/MIN/1.73m²)	CKD STAGE (KDOQI 2002)	GFR CATEGORY (KDIGO 2012)
≥ 90 + Kidney Damage	Stage 1	G1
60-89 + Kidney Damage	Stage 2	G2
30-59	Stage 3	G3a (45-59 mL/min/1.73m²)
		G3b (30-44 mL/min/1.73m²)
15-29	Stage 4	G4
< 15 or dialysis dependent	Stage 5	G5

Depending on the extent of renal impairment, drug regimens may need to be modified by reducing the dose and/or extending the dosing interval to avoid accumulation and potential toxicity while maintaining clinically effective serum drug concentrations. Dose reductions lead to reduced peak concentrations but maintain trough concentrations. This strategy is effective for drugs whose pharmacodynamic effect is governed by a minimum concentration over the dosing interval. Beta-lactams are a classic example of drugs that are dosed based on time above the minimum inhibitory concentration (MIC), exhibiting time-dependent killing properties. Extending the interval of a regimen maintains peak concentrations and reduces the trough concentration. This strategy is most useful for drugs that rely on achieving a specific peak concentration, such as quinolones and aminoglycosides, which exhibit concentration-dependent bacterial kill.

COMMON DRUGS & RENAL FUNCTION

COMMON DRUGS THAT REQUIRE DOSAGE REDUCTIONS OR INCREASED DOSING INTERVALS WITH DECREASED RENAL FUNCTION

Acyclovir, valacyclovir

Allopurinol

Amantadine

Amphotericin

Aminoglycosides – increase dosing interval

Azole antifungals

Antiarrhythmics (digoxin, disopyramide, procainamide, sotalol)

Anti-tuberculous medications ethambutol, pyrazinamide

Aztreonam

Beta-lactam antibiotics (most)

Colchicine

Cyclosporine

Dabigatran

Famotidine, ranitidine

Gabapentin, pregabalin

Ganciclovir, valganciclovir

NRTIs, including tenofovir

LMWHs: enoxaparin

Maraviroc

Metoclopramide

Morphine and codeine: use lower starting dose

Penicillins

Quinolone antibiotics (most), including ciprofloxacin and levofloxacin

Statins-most require dose adjustment

Sulfamethoxazole/trimethoprim

Tramadol

Vancomycin

Zoledronic Acid

Proteinuria, Blood Pressure Control, and the Use of ACEIs and ARBs

Uncontrolled blood pressure, diabetes and proteinuria are all risk factors for the progression of CKD. There is strong evidence to support the use of ACE inhibitors or ARBs to prevent the progression of nephropathy in diabetic and non-diabetic patients with proteinuria. It is es-

[handwritten top margin:] ↔ proteinuria ⇒ < 140/90
proteinuria ⇒ < 130/80

sential to control the blood pressure tightly. The goal blood pressure in kidney disease is < 140/90 mmHg if no proteinuria is present, and < 130/80 mmHg if proteinuria is present. Glycemic control, if an issue, will also need to be tightly controlled to preserve kidney function.

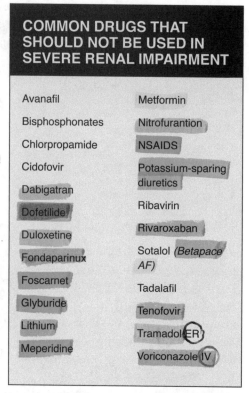

COMMON DRUGS THAT SHOULD NOT BE USED IN SEVERE RENAL IMPAIRMENT

Avanafil	Metformin
Bisphosphonates	Nitrofurantion
Chlorpropamide	NSAIDS
Cidofovir	Potassium-sparing diuretics
Dabigatran	
Dofetilide	Ribavirin
Duloxetine	Rivaroxaban
Fondaparinux	Sotalol (*Betapace AF*)
Foscarnet	Tadalafil
Glyburide	Tenofovir
Lithium	Tramadol ER
Meperidine	Voriconazole IV

ACE inhibitors and ARBs help preserve renal function and reduce proteinuria and provide cardiovascular protection. These drugs inhibit the renin-angiotensin-aldosterone system (RAAS), causing efferent arteriolar dilation. This is described in more detail in the Hypertension chapter. Note that the use of ACEIs and ARBs can cause a 30% rise in serum creatinine during the initiation of treatment. This rise is generally acceptable and is not a reason to stop treatment. If the rise is greater than 30%, the therapy should be discontinued and the patient should be evaluated for hemodynamic factors that may need addressing. Additionally, ACEIs or ARBs may cause hyperkalemia. It is important to counsel patients on adherence to potassium-restricted diets in order to maximize their ACEI/ARB therapy. It is recommended that the serum creatinine and potassium be monitored 1-2 weeks after initiating ACEIs or ARBs in patients with CKD.

[handwritten left margin:] ↑SrCr by 30% when starting ACEI/ARB ⇒ ok! in CKD

Anemia and Bone Metabolism Problems in Advanced Renal Disease

Anemia of Chronic Kidney Disease

Erythropoietin is produced by the kidneys and stimulates production of reticulocytes (immature red blood cells) in the bone marrow. As kidney function declines, the production of erythropoietin declines and anemia results. Further exacerbating the problem is a pro-inflammatory state caused by the chronic kidney disease that can result in anemia of chronic disease. Nutritional deficiencies may be present that could require iron, folate or vitamin B12 supplementation. Anemia identification and treatment is discussed in the Anemia chapter. Key points related to anemia treatment in CKD:

- The treatment of anemia of CKD generally involves a combination of erythropoiesis-stimulating agents (ESAs) and iron supplementation.

- Intravenous iron is preferred over oral iron for patients on hemodialysis, but may also be required for other patients with CKD due to poor iron absorption in the GI tract in advanced CKD.

- ESAs, including epoetin alfa (*Epogen, Procrit*) and darbepoetin alfa (*Aranesp*) are generally necessary to treat anemia of CKD to prevent the need for blood transfusions.

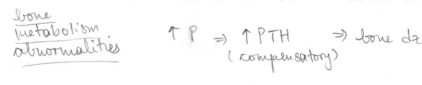

[handwritten bottom:] bone metabolism abnormalities   ↑P ⇒ ↑PTH ⇒ bone dz (compensatory)

PTH ≠ calcitonin; ↓ Ca++ in blood

- For patients using ESAs, the serum hemoglobin concentration should not be corrected to the "normal" concentration for patients without CKD (with CKD they are lower) due to an increased risk of cardiovascular events, stroke and death.

Bone Metabolism Abnormalities

↑ Ca++ in blood
1) parathyroid (PTH)
2) PO4
3) Ca++/vit D

Patients with advanced kidney disease require screening for abnormalities associated with parathyroid hormone (PTH), phosphorus, calcium and vitamin D at regular intervals, according to disease severity. Therapeutic targets for phosphorus, calcium and PTH is dependent on the severity of CKD. These targets are outlined in the following table. The latest KDIGO mineral and bone disease clinical practice guidelines suggest maintaining PTH between 2 and 9 times the normal range for patients on dialysis, but fail to provide specific targets for predialysis CKD patients. Calcium should be maintained in the normal range for all CKD patients. Phosphorus should be maintained in the normal range for non-dialysis CKD patients, and "toward" the normal range in dialysis patients.

should not exceed 45 mEq/L in PN

Target Goals for Bone Mineral and Metabolism Disorders

CKD STAGE	PTH (pg/mL)	Ca²⁺ (mg/dL)	PO4 (mg/dL)	Ca²⁺ x PO4 (mg/dL)
3	35-70	Normal range	2.7-4.6	< 55
4	70-110	Normal range	2.7-4.6	< 55
5	150-300	8.4-9.5	3.5-5.5	< 55

Treatment of Hyperphosphatemia

Bone metabolism abnormalities are initially caused by elevations in phosphorus, which is renally excreted. To compensate for hyperphosphatemia, the parathyroid gland increases the release of PTH. Elevated PTH concentrations over time lead to secondary hyperparathyroidism and high turnover bone disease. Treatment of secondary hyperparathyroidism is initially focused on controlling serum phosphorus by restricting dietary phosphorus by avoiding dairy products, cola, chocolate and nuts. Eventually, phosphate binders may be required. Phosphate binders bind meal-time phosphate in the gut that is coming from the diet. If a dose is missed and the food is absorbed, that dose should be skipped, and the patient should resume normal dosing at the next meal or snack. There are four types of phosphate binders:

AVOID
1) dairy
2) cola
3) chocolate
4) nuts

max 4 weeks

- Aluminum-based agents (ALternaGEL, others): potent phosphate binders, but aluminum can accumulate in CKD and is toxic to the nervous system and bone, and may lead to "dialysis dementia"; should only be used short-term, if at all, and are not used commonly.

- Calcium-based agents (primarily calcium acetate and carbonate): effective first line agents for hyperphosphatemia in CKD. The dose-limiting effect is hypercalcemia, which is especially problematic in patients taking vitamin D (which increases calcium absorption).

- Iron-based agents: the newest agents approved for hyperphosphatemia utilize iron as the cation to bind phosphorus in the gut.

■ **Aluminum-free, calcium-free agents:** effective at controlling phosphorus. Because <u>they do not contain aluminum or calcium</u>, they do not cause problems with excess aluminum load and less of a problem with excess calcium load. They are the most <u>expensive</u>.

PHOSPHATE BINDERS   *ALL DOSED TID W/ MEALS!*

DRUG	DOSE	SAFETY/SIDE EFFECTS/MONITORING

Aluminum-based: one of the most potent phosphate binders but due to risk of accumulation the treatment duration is limited to 4 weeks.

DRUG	DOSE	SAFETY/SIDE EFFECTS/MONITORING
Aluminum hydroxide (*ALternaGEL, Amphojel*, others)	300-600 mg three times daily with meals	**SIDE EFFECTS** Constipation, poor taste, nausea, aluminum intoxication, "dialysis dementia" and osteomalacia **MONITORING** Ca^{2+}, phosphorus, serum aluminum concentrations, PTH

Calcium-based: <u>first line</u> for hyperphosphatemia of CKD.

binds more dietary elemental Ca++

DRUG	DOSE	SAFETY/SIDE EFFECTS/MONITORING
Calcium acetate (*PhosLo, Phoslyra*, others)	667-1,334 mg three times daily with meals	**SIDE EFFECTS** Constipation, nausea, hypercalcemia !! **MONITORING** Ca^{2+}, phosphorus, serum calcium-phosphorus product, PTH
Calcium carbonate (*Tums*, store brands, others)	500 mg three times daily with meals, chewable or not	**NOTES** Calcium acetate binds more dietary phosphorus on an elemental calcium basis compared to calcium carbonate.

Iron-based

DRUG	DOSE	SAFETY/SIDE EFFECTS/MONITORING
Sucroferric oxyhydroxide (*Velphoro*)	500 mg three times daily with meals	**SIDE EFFECTS** Diarrhea, discolored feces **MONITORING** Phosphorus; Iron studies should be monitored with ferric citrate (not sucroferric oxyhydroxide): ferritin and TSAT
Ferric Citrate *monitor ferritin TSAT* *b/c Fe overload possible ⇒ ↓ dose IV*	2,000 mg three times daily with meals, up to 12 g per day	**NOTES** Iron overload possible with ferric citrate, dosage reduction of IV iron may be necessary.

Aluminum-free, calcium-free

DRUG	DOSE	SAFETY/SIDE EFFECTS/MONITORING
Lanthanum carbonate (*Fosrenol*) Bowel obstruction, fecal impaction, ileus	500-1,000 mg three times daily with meals, chewable – <u>must chew thoroughly</u>	**CONTRAINDICATIONS** Bowel obstruction, fecal impaction, ileus **SIDE EFFECTS** Nausea, vomiting, abdominal pain, constipation, diarrhea **MONITORING** Ca^{2+}, phosphorus, PTH **NOTES** Long-term safety has not been established.

Phosphate Binders Continued

DRUG	DOSE	SAFETY/SIDE EFFECTS/MONITORING

Sevelamer: a non-calcium, non-aluminum based phosphate binder that is not systemically absorbed. Also, has the benefit of lowering total cholesterol and LDL by 15-30%. Sevelamer carbonate may have the advantage over sevelamer hydrochloride of maintaining bicarbonate concentrations.

DRUG	DOSE	SAFETY/SIDE EFFECTS/MONITORING
Sevelamer carbonate (*Renvela*) Sevelamer hydrochloride (*Renagel*)	800-1,600 mg three times daily with meals	**CONTRAINDICATIONS** Bowel obstruction **SIDE EFFECTS** Nausea, vomiting, diarrhea (all > 20%), constipation, abdominal pain **MONITORING** Ca²⁺, phosphorus, bicarbonate, Cl, PTH

Handwritten notes:
- CO₃²⁻ maintains [HCO₃⁻] → advantage over HCl
- ∅ systemic absorption
- ↓ TC / LDL 15-30%

Treatment of Vitamin D Deficiency & Secondary Hyperparathyroidism

After controlling hyperphosphatemia, elevations in PTH are treated primarily with vitamin D. Vitamin D deficiency occurs when the kidney is unable to hydroxylate 25-OH vitamin D to its final active form, 1,25-dihydroxy vitamin D. Vitamin D deficiency exacerbates bone disease, impairs immunity and increases cardiovascular disease.

Vitamin D occurs in two primary forms: vitamin D3 or cholecalciferol, which is synthesized in the skin after exposure to ultraviolet light, and vitamin D2 or ergocalciferol, which is produced from plant sterols and is the primary dietary source of vitamin D. Calcitriol (*Rocaltrol*) is the active form of vitamin D3 and is used in patients with CKD to increase calcium absorption from the gut, raise serum calcium concentrations and inhibit PTH secretion. Newer active vitamin D analogs such as paricalcitol and doxercalciferol cause less hypercalcemia than calcitriol. These agents are summarized in the table.

Handwritten notes:
- vit D3 = cholecalciferol
- vit D2 = ergocalciferol

Agents for the Treatment of Secondary Hyperparathyroidism

DRUG	DOSING	SAFETY/SIDE EFFECTS/MONITORING

Vitamin D analogs: increase intestinal absorption of Ca²⁺ and provide a negative feedback to the parathyroid gland.

DRUG	DOSING	SAFETY/SIDE EFFECTS/MONITORING
Calcitriol (*Rocaltrol, Calcijex*) capsule, solution, injection	CKD: 0.25 mcg PO three times weekly to daily Dialysis: 0.5-1 mcg PO daily or 0.5-4 mcg IV three times weekly	**CONTRAINDICATIONS** Hypercalcemia, ↓ vitamin D toxicity **SIDE EFFECTS** Nausea, vomiting, diarrhea (> 10%), hypercalcemia, hyperphosphatemia
Doxercalciferol (*Hectorol*) capsule, injection	CKD: 1 mcg PO three times weekly to daily Dialysis: 2.5-10 mcg PO three times weekly; 1-4 mcg IV three times weekly	**MONITORING** Ca²⁺, Phos, PTH
Paricalcitol (*Zemplar*) capsule, injection	CKD: 1 mcg PO three times weekly to daily Dialysis: 2.8-7 mcg IV three times weekly; 2-4 mcg PO three times weekly	**NOTES** Take with food or shortly after a meal to ↓ GI upset (calcitriol).

Handwritten notes:
- dosed TIW-TID
- after meals
- active D3 w/ food or shortly pc
- cause less hyper Ca²⁺

Agents for the Treatment of Secondary Hyperparathyroidism Continued

DRUG	DOSING	SAFETY/SIDE EFFECTS/MONITORING

Calcimimetic – ↑ sensitivity of calcium-sensing receptor on the parathyroid gland, thereby ↓ PTH, ↓ Ca²⁺, ↓ Phos and preventing progressive bone disease

DRUG	DOSING	SAFETY/SIDE EFFECTS/MONITORING
Cinacalcet (Sensipar) tablets	30-180 mg PO daily with food	**CONTRAINDICATIONS** Hypocalcemia **WARNING** Caution in patients with history of seizure **SIDE EFFECTS** Hypocalcemia, nausea, vomiting, diarrhea, paresthesia, fatigue, depression, anorexia, constipation, bone fracture, weakness, arthralgia, myalgia, limb pain, URTIs **MONITORING** Ca²⁺, Phos, PTH **NOTES** Take tablet whole, do not crush or chew.

Supplementation of vitamin D2 may also be necessary in CKD. The dosing of vitamin D2 depends on the severity of the deficiency and is summarized in the table below. Treatment of vitamin D deficiency can result in hypercalcemia or hyperphosphatemia. These values must be monitored during treatment. Further information on vitamin D is contained in the natural products and vitamins chapter, and the osteoporosis chapter.

Treatment of Vitamin D Deficiency

SERUM 25 (OH) VITAMIN D (NG/ML)	ERGOCALCIFEROL DOSE*	DURATION	COMMENT
< 5	50,000 units PO every week x 12 weeks, then every month	6 months	Measure levels after 6 months
5-15	50,000 units PO every week x 4 weeks, then every month	6 months	Measure levels after 6 months
16-30	50,000 units PO every month	6 months	Measure levels after 6 months

An alternative is to use cholecalciferol (vitamin D3) 2000 units PO daily.

Treatment of Hyperkalemia

A normal potassium level is 3.5-5 mEq/L. Hyperkalemia, depending on the source, can be defined as a potassium level above 5.3 or above 5.5 mEq/L, although clinicians will be concerned with any level above 5 mEq/L.

Potassium is the most abundant intracellular cation and is essential for life. Humans obtain potassium through the diet from many foods, including meats, beans and fruits. Daily intake through the GI tract is about 1 mEq/kg/day. Excess intake is excreted partially via the gut and primarily via the kidneys. Potassium excretion is increased by aldosterone, diuretics (strongly by loops, weakly by thiazides), by a high urine flow (via osmotic diuresis), and by negatively charged ions in the distal tubule (via bicarbonate).

Even if a person intakes a very rich potassium load, the acute rise in potassium would be offset by the release of insulin, which would cause potassium to shift into the cells. This is why excessive intake is not normally a cause of hyperkalemia unless there is significant renal damage. The most common cause of hyperkalemia is decreased renal excretion due to renal failure. This can be in combination with a high potassium intake or can be partially due to the use of drugs that interfere with potassium excretion. Drugs that raise potassium levels include ACE Inhibitors, ARBs, aldosterone receptor antagonists (ARAs), aliskiren, NSAIDs, cyclosporine, tacrolimus, everolimus, mycophenolate, potassium supplements, glycopyrrolate, drospirenone-containing oral contraceptives, sulfamethoxazole/trimethoprim, chronic heparin use, canagliflozin, pentamidine and potassium present in IV fluids, including parenteral nutrition.

Patients with diabetes often have a diet high in sodium and low in potassium and are taking ACE inhibitors or ARBs. The insulin deficiency reduces the ability to shift potassium into the cells. These factors make patients with diabetes higher risk for hyperkalemia. Hospitalized patients, primarily due to the use of drugs, are at higher risk of hyperkalemia than outpatients. Rarely, acute hyperkalemia can be due to tumor lysis, rhabdomyolysis or succinylcholine administration.

A patient with elevated potassium, depending on the level, may be asymptomatic or symptomatic. Muscle weakness and bradycardia may be present. Fatal arrhythmias can develop. The risk for severe, negative outcomes increases as the potassium level increases.

In the Case of Hyperkalemia

If the hyperkalemia is severe the urgent clinical need is to stabilize the myocardial cells and to rapidly shift potassium intracellular: immediately discontinue all potassium sources, 2) give IV calcium (to stabilize the heart; this does not lower potassium), IV bicarbonate and insulin (with dextrose where appropriate). If the potassium is high or the heart rate and rhythm is abnormal, the patient will be hooked up to an ECG.

- Remove sources of potassium intake. This may require dietary changes.
- Enhance potassium uptake by the cells via:
    - Glucose (to stimulate insulin secretion – but not enough by itself).
    - Insulin, given with glucose (to prevent hypoglycemia).
- If metabolic acidosis is present, administer sodium bicarbonate.
- Consider beta-agonists, such as nebulized albuterol. Monitor for tachycardia, chest pain.
- Increase renal excretion with a loop diuretic, such as furosemide. Monitor volume status.

↓K+ by ↑ excretion

- Another option to increase renal excretion is fludrocortisone (*Florinef*), especially in a patient with hypoaldosteronism.

↓K+ by 2 mEq/L
give rectally for acute ER

- Consider the use of the cation exchange resin, sodium polystyrene sulfonate (*Kayexalate*). This works within two hours (but may take much longer) and can decrease potassium by 2 mEq/L with a single enema. SPS is given orally or rectally. Rectal administration is preferred for acute (emergency) treatment. If using oral SPS, do not mix with sorbitol; in 2010 the FDA issued a warning against mixing the drug with sorbitol due to a risk of GI necrosis. Common side effects include ↓ appetite, nausea, vomiting, or constipation (less commonly diarrhea).

- Emergency dialysis can be used if the hyperkalemia could be fatal or for patients with renal failure; setting up dialysis takes time, usually several hours.

INTERVENTION	ROUTE OF ADMINISTRATION	ONSET	MECHANISM OF POTASSIUM LOWERING
Calcium gluconate	IV	1-2 minutes	Reverses electrocardiographic changes; does not lower K+
Furosemide	IV	5 minutes	Urinary elimination
Regular insulin	IV	30 minutes	Intracellular K+ shift
Dextrose	IV	30 minutes	Stimulates insulin release, leading to Intracellular K+ shift
Sodium bicarbonate	IV	30 minutes	Intracellular K+ shift
Albuterol	Nebulized	30 minutes	Intracellular K+ shift
Hemodialysis		Immediate, but may take several hours to set-up procedure	Elimination from blood
Sodium polystyrene sulfonate	Oral or rectal	1 hour; not for acute emergency	Gastrointestinal elimination

TREATMENT OF METABOLIC ACIDOSIS OF CKD   *2° to ↓ renal ability to make HCO₃⁻*

The kidneys' ability to generate bicarbonate decreases as CKD progresses and may result in the development of metabolic acidosis. In the ambulatory care setting, treatment of metabolic acidosis is initiated when the serum bicarbonate concentration is < 22 mEq/L. Agents to replace bicarbonate are summarized below.

DRUG	DOSING	SAFETY/SIDE EFFECTS/MONITORING
Sodium bicarbonate Tablets, granules, powder	1-2 tabs PO 1-3 times a day	**CONTRAINDICATIONS** Alkalosis, hypernatremia, hypocalcemia, pulmonary edema, unknown abdominal pain

WARNINGS Use caution in patients with HTN, cardiovascular disease, fluid retention problems

SIDE EFFECTS Nausea, vomiting, diarrhea, hypernatremia

MONITORING Na+, HCO₃⁻ |

Treatment of Metabolic Acidosis of CKD Continued

DRUG	DOSING	SAFETY/SIDE EFFECTS/MONITORING
Sodium citrate/citric acid (*Bicitra, Cytra-2, Oracit, Shohl's* solution) Solution	10-30 mL PO with water, taken after meals and at bedtime Take after meals and at bedtime to avoid laxative effect Chilled solution improves taste	**CONTRAINDICATIONS** Alkalosis, Na^+ restricted diet, hypernatremia **SIDE EFFECTS** Nausea, vomiting, diarrhea metabolic alkalosis, tetany **MONITORING** Na^+, HCO_3^-, urinary pH **NOTES** Metabolized to bicarbonate by the liver, may not be effective in concomitant liver failure Avoid concurrent use with aluminum containing products (e.g., antacids)

DIALYSIS   *usually, TID @ dialysis center*

If the kidney disease progresses, then renal replacement using dialysis will be required to remove waste products, electrolytes and excess fluid. The two primary types of dialysis are hemodialysis (HD) and peritoneal dialysis (PD).

In HD, the patient is connected to a dialysis machine through a form of vascular access such as catheter or a more permanent form such as an arteriovenous fistula or graft. Blood leaves the patient's body and is pumped through the dialysis circuit in the machine. The blood enters the dialyzer and toxic waste products, electrolytes and water are removed through two processes; diffusion and convection. Solutes diffuse across the semipermeable membrane and the cleansed blood is returned back to the patient. Convection is a process in which the pressure generated in the dialyzer generates filtration of water and solutes. HD is a 3-4 hour process, done several times (usually three times) per week. Increasingly, patients are choosing home HD, which can be done more frequently (typically 5-6 times per week).

In PD, a dialysate solution (usually containing glucose) is pumped into the peritoneal cavity (the abdominal cavity surrounding the internal organs), and the peritoneal membrane acts as the semipermeable membrane (i.e., as the dialyzer). The solution is left in the abdomen to "dwell" for a period of time, then drained. This cycle is repeated throughout the day, everyday. PD is performed by the patient at home. There are two main types of PD: 1. continuous ambulatory peritoneal dialysis (CAPD), which is done without a machine, and which requires the dialysate to be exchanged (by the patient) at scheduled intervals throughout the day, and 2. automated peritoneal dialysis (APD), where the patient uses a machine in the home to exchange the dialysate several times throughout the night.

Factors Affecting Drug Removal during Dialysis

When a patient is on dialysis, the pharmacist needs to consider how much of the patient's medications are removed by dialysis in order to recommend a reasonable dosing regimen and/or schedule replacement dosing post-dialysis. These factors determine the dialyzability of a drug (how much of the drug is removed):

Molecular Size: In HD, the pore size of the dialyzer determines the extent to which compounds can move across the membrane. High efficiency dialyzers are dialyzers with a large surface area, whereas high flux dialyzers are those with larger pore sizes. The use of high flux dialyzers is common and has contributed to the improved clearance of larger drugs such as vancomycin and daptomycin compared with older "conventional" filters with smaller pores. Smaller molecules pass through the dialysis filter more easily.

Protein Binding: Highly protein bound drugs will generally not be removed by dialysis procedures. The unbound fraction in the blood (which can be removed) determines how much is removed by the dialysis procedure. Examples of highly protein bound drugs include ceftriaxone and warfarin.

Volume of Distribution (Vd): Drugs with a large Vd are distributed outside of the plasma and in other tissues. Since the dialysis procedures removes drugs primarily in the blood, if a drug has a large Vd, the dialysis procedure will not be effective at removing the drug. Examples of drugs that have a large Vd are tricyclic antidepressants, digoxin and amiodarone.

Plasma Clearance: The extent to which the drug is eliminated by renal clearance will determine the importance of the dialysis procedure towards drug removal. The dialysis procedure will likely not contribute much to the overall clearance of drugs with high hepatic clearance.

Dialysis Membrane: It is critical to consider the type of membrane when evaluating literature on drug removal. The membranes are characterized as low-flux (or conventional) or high-flux. High-flux membranes have the largest pore size, and larger drugs are cleared with this method, such as vancomycin.

Summary: Drug removal during dialysis depends primarily on the factors in the table below. In general, small, hydrophilic, non-protein bound molecules are readily removed by dialysis. Those with a very high volume of distribution may be removed by the dialysis procedure, only a small fraction of the total drug will reside in the bloodstream, making dialysis removal of the medication insignificant.

FACTOR	EFFECT
Drug Characteristics	
Molecular weight/Size	Smaller molecules tend to be more readily removed by dialysis
Volume of distribution	Drugs with large Vd are less likely to be significantly removed by dialysis
Protein-binding	High protein-binding reduces drug removal by dialysis
Dialysis Factors	
Membrane	High-flux (large pore size) and high-efficiency (large surface area) HD filters remove substances more than conventional/low-flux filters
Blood flow rate	Higher dialysis blood flow rates increase drug removal during dialysis over a given time interval

PRACTICE CASE

DR is a 67 y/o female with a past medical history of diabetes type 2, hypertension, atrial fibrillation, and chronic kidney disease. DR is being seen today by her nephrologist for a regularly scheduled follow-up.

Medications:
Fortamet 1000 mg daily
Glucotrol 10 mg daily
Aleve 1 tablet BID
Pradaxa 150 mg BID
Accupril 20 mg daily
Lorcet 5/325 mg 1 tablet PRN arthritis knee pain NTE 2 daily

Vitals:
Height: 5'6" Weight: 133 lbs
BP: 152/91 mmHg HR: 92 BPM RR: 17 BPM Temp: 37.8°C Pain: 3/10

Labs:
Na (mEq/L) = 140 (135 - 145)
K (mEq/L) = 5.0 (3.5 - 5)
Cl (mEq/L) = 100 (95 - 103)
HCO_3 (mEq/L) = 26 (24 - 30)
BUN (mg/dL) = 26 (7 - 20)
SCr (mg/dL) = 2.4 (0.6 - 1.3)
Glucose (mg/dL) = 230 (100 - 125)
Ca (mg/dL) = 10.1 (8.5 - 10.5)
Mg (mEq/L) = 2.4 (1.3 - 2.1)
PO_4 (mg/dL) = 7.2 (2.3 - 4.7)
WBC (cells/mm^3) = 8.2 (4 - 11 x 10^3)
Hgb (g/dL) = 12.1 (13.5 - 18 male, 12 - 16 female)
Hct (%) = 32.8 (38 - 50 male, 36 - 46 female)
Plt (cells/mm^3) = 199 (150 - 450 x 10^3)
A1C (%) = 12.3

New prescriptions for Fosrenol and Sensipar. Follow-up appointment in 2 weeks.

Questions:

1. DR's nephrologist wrote a prescription for Fosrenol 500 mg TID. Which of the following is true of Fosrenol? (Select **ALL** that apply.)

   a. It ↓ serum phosphorus
   b. Hypercalcemia limits the use of Fosrenol
   c. It ↑ hemoglobin
   d. The tablets must be chewed thoroughly
   e. The dose should be 500 mg three times weekly

2. Sensipar 30 mg daily was also prescribed for DR. Which of the following is true of Sensipar? (Select **ALL** that apply.)

   a. It ↓ PTH
   b. It ↑ serum calcium
   c. It ↓ serum phosphorus
   d. It ↓ serum potassium
   e. In the presence of dysphagia, crush and mix with a small amount of soft food

3. Which of DR's home medications is contra-indicated or is unsafe and discontinuation should be recommended by the pharmacist? (Select **ALL** that apply.)

   a. *Fortamet*

   b. *Glucotrol*

   c. *Aleve*

   d. *Lorcet*

   e. *Accupril*

4. What is the correct dose of *Pradaxa* for DR given her current renal function?

   a. 150 mg BID

   b. 75 mg BID

   c. 150 mg daily

   d. 75 mg daily

   e. *Pradaxa* is contraindicated

5. How would you characterize DR's renal function according to KDOQI Guidelines with the information given in the case?

   a. Stage 1

   b. Stage 2

   c. Stage 3

   d. Stage 4

   e. Stage 5

Answers:

1-a,d, 2-a,c, 3-a,c, 4-b, 5-d

HEPATITIS & LIVER DISEASE

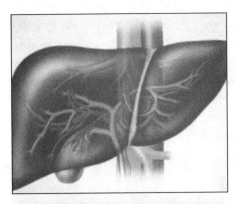

We gratefully acknowledge the assistance of Paulina Deming, PharmD, University of New Mexico College of Pharmacy, in preparing this chapter.

BACKGROUND

The term hepatitis means inflammation of the liver. There are many possible causes of hepatitis, including viral hepatitis and liver inflammation due to drugs, including alcohol.

Symptoms of Liver Disease

GUIDELINES

American Association for the Study of Liver Diseases (AASLD) Guidelines at www.hcvguidelines.org/

Symptoms can include nausea, loss of appetite, vomiting, diarrhea, malaise, pain in the upper right quadrant of the abdomen, yellowed skin and yellowed whites of the eyes (jaundice), darkened urine and/or lightened color (white or clay-colored) stool caused by low bile in the stool due to decreased production or a blocked bile duct.

Objective Criteria

Alanine aminotransferase (ALT) and asparatate aminotransferase (AST) are liver enzymes. The ALT normal range is 10 - 40 units per liter (units/L), and the AST normal range is 10 - 40 units/L. There is some slight variance in these ranges on different lab reports. In general, the higher the values, the more active the liver disease. Clinical signs of liver disease, in addition to ↑ ALT and ↑ AST, include ↓ albumin (protein produced by the liver; normal range 3.5-5.5 g/dL), ↑ alkaline phosphatase (Alk Phos), ↑ total bilirubin (Tbili), ↑ lactate dehydrogenase (LDH), and ↑ in prothrombin time (PT). Albumin and PT/INR are markers of synthetic (production ability) liver function. Liver disease can be classified as hepatocellular (↑ ALT and ↑ AST), cholestatic (↑ Alk Phos and ↑ Tbili), or mixed (↑ ALT, AST, Alk Phos and Tbili).

DRUGS THAT CAN CAUSE LIVER DAMAGE

Below are some drugs for which patients should be monitored for symptoms of liver disease. Patients may require blood tests to check their liver function.

Acarbose	Nefazodone
Acetaminophen (acute, high doses)	Niacins
Amiodarone	NNRTIs (highest risk with nevirapine)
Atomoxetine	NRTIs (highest risk with didanosine, stavudine, zidovudine)
Azathioprine	
Bicalutamide	
Bosentan	Oxymorphone
Carbamazepine	Phenobarbital/ Primidone
Dronedarone	
Estrogen	Phenytoin
Etanercept and other TNF-blockers	Pioglitazone, Rosiglitazone
Febuxostat	PIs (highest risk with tipranavir)
Felbamate	
Fenofibrates	Propylthiouracil
Flutamide	Pyrazinamide
Gemfibrozil	Quinidine
Griseofulvin	Ribavirin
Imatinib & other "ibs"	Rifampin
Interferons	Tamoxifen
Isoniazid	Tasimelteon
Isotretinoin	Telithromycin
Ketoconazole (highest risk), other azoles	Terbinafine
	Testosterone
Ketorolac	Tigecycline
Leflunomide and Teriflunomide	Tizanidine
	Tolcapone
Lomitapide	Tolvaptan
Macrolides	Valproic acid
Maraviroc	Zileuton
Metaxalone	
Methimazole	**Natural Products** Comfrey, Flavocoxid (Limbrel), a medical food
Methotrexate	
Methyldopa	
Mipomersen	Kava
Mycophenolate	

Severity of Liver Disease

It is important to assess the severity of the liver disease as it serves as a predictor of patient survival, surgical outcomes, and the risk of complications such as variceal bleeding. The Child-Pugh classification system is widely used which has a scoring system that ranges from 0 - 15. Class A (mild disease) is defined as a score < 7; Class B (moderate disease) is a score of 7 - 9, and Class C (severe disease) is a score of 10 - 15. The model for end-stage liver disease (MELD) is another scoring system with a scoring system that ranges from 0 - 40, with higher numbers indicating a greater risk of death within three months. Noninvasive tests are increasingly used to predict fibrosis and cirrhosis. Unlike drug dosing in renal failure, little data is available to guide drug dosing of hepatically cleared agents with liver failure. In general, caution is advised when using hepatically cleared agents in severe liver disease (Class C) and, in select cases, dose adjustment may be necessary.

Natural Product

Milk thistle, an extract derived from a member of the daisy family, is often used by patients with liver disease. Although there are limited data to demonstrate efficacy of milk thistle for alcoholic liver disease, hepatitis B or C, milk thistle does not appear to be harmful. A possible side effect is mild diarrhea and there are concerns for possible drug interactions with milk thistle and antiviral hepatitis C medications.

OTC Analgesics in Patients with Cirrhosis

Acetaminophen is a known hepatotoxic agent and can cause severe injury. Acetaminophen may be used by patients with cirrhosis, however for limited periods of time and at lower dosages. Patients with alcoholic cirrhosis who are actively drinking and/or malnourished may be more susceptible to further liver damage.

NSAIDs should be avoided with cirrhosis because these agents can lead to decompensation, including bleeding.

Drug-Induced Liver Damage

If a drug is damaging the liver, the primary treatment (in most cases) is to stop the drug. Many drugs that are hepatotoxic are discontinued when the liver enzymes are > 3 times the upper limit of normal (> 150 ALT or AST), however clinical judgment is warranted. Rechallenging with the potential agent can be considered if clinically necessary.

ALCOHOLIC LIVER DISEASE

Alcoholic liver disease is caused by excessive drinking, and can include fatty liver, alcoholic hepatitis, and chronic hepatitis with hepatic fibrosis or cirrhosis. Chronic alcohol ingestion over a long period of time causes "steatosis" or fatty liver, due to fat deposition in the hepatocytes. This can be reversible and self-limited (if drinking is stopped) or can lead to to fibrosis and cirrhosis. Some patients develop alcoholic hepatitis, an acute process with poor short-term survival. Of all chronic heavy drinkers, only 15–20% develop hepatitis or cirrhosis, which can occur simultaneously or in succession.

Alcohol-induced liver disease is the most common type of drug-induced liver disease. Risk increases with amount consumed, and duration. Women have higher risk than men. Treatment programs use mainly benzodiazepines for alcohol withdrawal in inpatients whereas anticonvulsants are used for outpatients. Naltrexone *(ReVia)*, acamprosate *(Campral)* and disulfiram *(Antabuse)* are used to prevent relapses. There are a few off-label treatments.

Chronic consumption of alcohol results in the secretion of pro-inflammatory cytokines (TNF-alpha, IL-6 and IL-8), oxidative stress, lipid peroxidation, and acetaldehyde toxicity. These factors cause inflammation, apoptosis (cell death) and eventually fibrosis of liver cells. This can cause portal hypertension, ascites, variceal bleeding and hepatic encephalopathy (discussed in the next section). Drinking habits of patients need to be assessed routinely. If the alcohol consumption is ceased the liver can possibly regenerate to some extent.

Treatment

The most important part of treatment is alcohol cessation. Maintenance of abstinence is essential to improving outcomes and should include the use of drug treatment to control cravings. An alcohol rehabilitation program and a support group whose members share common experiences and problems are extremely helpful in breaking the addiction to alcohol. Proper nutrition is essential to help the liver recover. Vitamins and trace minerals, including vitamin A, vitamin D, thiamine (vitamin B1), folate, pyridoxine (vitamin B6) and zinc can help reverse malnutrition. Thiamine is used to prevent and treat Wernicke-Korsakoff syndrome. Wernicke's encephalopathy and Korsakoff syndrome are different conditions that are both due to brain damage caused by a lack of vitamin B1. Last, avoidance of hepatotoxic agents and/or adjusting/limiting the dose of hepatotoxic agents should be utilized.

COMPLICATIONS OF LIVER DISEASE

Portal Hypertension and Variceal Bleeding

Portal hypertension, or increased blood pressure in the portal vein, can cause further complications including the development and bleeding of esophageal varices. These are enlarged veins in the lower part of the esophagus. They are most commonly caused by cirrhosis. The scarring blocks the blood flow through the liver, which causes blood to flow up through the veins in the esophagus. The veins balloon out and will bleed if they break open. Non-selective beta-blockers (such as nadolol and propranolol) or Endoscopic Variceal Ligation (EVL) are used for primary prevention. Beta-blockers reduce portal pressure by reducing portal venous inflow by two mechanisms: 1) they decrease cardiac output (via beta-1 blockade), and 2) they decrease splanchnic blood flow by vasoconstriction (via beta-2 blockade and unopposed alpha activity). The beta-blocker should be titrated to the maximal tolerated dose (target HR 55-60 BPM) and continued indefinitely.

DRUG	DOSING	SAFETY/SIDE EFFECTS/MONITORING
Nadolol (Corgard)	20-40 mg PO daily	Refer to Hypertension chapter for a complete review of beta blockers. **BOXED WARNING** Do not withdraw beta blockers abruptly (particularly in patients with CAD), gradually taper over 1-2 weeks to avoid acute tachycardia, HTN, and/or ischemia. **CONTRAINDICATIONS** Sinus bradycardia, 2nd or 3rd degree heart block, sick sinus syndrome (unless patient has a functioning artificial pacemaker) or cardiogenic shock. Do not initiate in patients with active asthma exacerbation.
Propranolol (Inderal LA, Inderal XL, InnoPran XL)	20 mg PO BID	These are non-selective agents; use extreme caution with asthma or severe COPD or peripheral vascular disease and Raynaud's disease. May mask signs of hyperthyroidism; may aggravate psychiatric conditions, and use caution in patients with diabetes particularly with recurrent hypoglycemia. Monitor HR and BP.

Managing Acute Variceal Bleeding

Patients with acute variceal bleeding should be stabilized by providing supportive therapy such as blood volume resuscitation/blood products, mechanical ventilation, correction of coagulopathy, and attempts to stop the bleeding and preventing rebleeding. Band ligation or sclerotherapy are recommended first-line treatments for bleeding varices. In addition, vasoactive therapy is used to stop or minimize the bleeding by decreasing portal blood flow and pressure by splanchnic vasoconstriction. Octreotide is selective for the splanchnic vessels whereas vasopressin is non-selective. Surgical interventions may be considered if the patient is not responding to treatment or to prevent future rebleeding episodes. Common surgical procedures include balloon tamponade (may help control current bleeding) or transjugular intrahepatic portosystemic shunt (TIPS). In general, the addition of antimicrobial therapy (ceftriaxone) for 5 days to prevent subsequent infection and albumin (1.5 mg/kg IV on day 1 and 1 mg/kg IV on day three) are recommended as they are both associated with mortality benefits. <u>Non-selective beta-blockers should be added after resolution of variceal bleeding</u> for secondary prevention of variceal bleeding recurrence.

DRUG	DOSING	SAFETY/SIDE EFFECTS/MONITORING
Octreotide *(SandoSTATIN)* Analogue of somatostatin – has greater potency and longer duration of action	25-50 mcg IV bolus, followed by 25-50 mcg/hr continuous IV infusion x 2-5 days	**SIDE EFFECTS** Bradycardia, chest pain, fatigue, headache, pruritus, hyperglycemia, hypoglycemia (highest risk in type 1 diabetes), N/V/D, hypothyroidism, abdominal pain, malaise, fever, dizziness, flatulence, cholelithiasis, biliary sludge, constipation, injection site pain, arthropathy, myalgias, URTIs **MONITORING** Blood glucose, HR, ECG
Vasopressin *(Pitressin)* <u>Antidiuretic hormone analog</u> Not 1st line (usually used with nitroglycerin IV to prevent myocardial ischemia)	0.2-0.4 units/min (max 0.8 units/min) IV continuous infusion for max of 24 hours	**SIDE EFFECTS** Arrhythmias, chest pain, MI, ↓ cardiac output, ↑ BP, nausea, vomiting **MONITORING** BP, HR, ECG, fluid balance

Hepatic Encephalopathy

Hepatic encephalopathy (HE) is a syndrome of neuropsychiatric abnormalities caused by acute or chronic hepatic insufficiency. Symptoms include <u>musty odor of the breath</u> and/or urine, <u>changes in thinking, confusion, forgetfulness</u>, mood changes, poor concentration, drowsiness, disorientation, worsening handwriting and hand tremor (asterixis), sluggish movements, and many others, including risk of coma. The <u>symptoms of HE result from an accumulation of gut-derived nitrogenous substances in the blood</u> (such as <u>ammonia</u>, glutamate, others) due to decreased hepatic functioning and shunting through the porto-systemic collaterals, which bypass the liver. Treatment includes identifying and treating precipitating factors and <u>reducing blood ammonia levels through diet (limiting the amount of animal protein) and drug therapy</u>.

Patients should get a daily protein intake of 1-1.5 g/kg. Vegetable and dairy sources of protein are preferred to animal sources due to the lower calorie to nitrogen ratio. Branched-chain amino acids (BCAAs) (e.g., leucine, isoleucine, valine) are favored over aromatic amino acids (AAAs); they interfere with AAAs ability to cross the blood-brain barrier and increase hepatocyte growth factor synthesis.

Drug therapy consists of nonabsorbable disaccharides (such as lactulose) and antibiotics (rifaximin, neomycin, others) for acute and chronic therapy. <u>Lactulose is first line therapy for both acute and chronic (prevention) therapy, followed by rifaximin</u>. Lactulose works by converting ammonia produced by intestinal bacteria to ammonium, which is polar and therefore cannot readily diffuse into the blood. Lactulose also enhances diffusion of ammonia into the colon for excretion. Antibiotics work by inhibiting the activity of urease-producing bacteria, which decreases the ammonia production. Zinc (220 mg PO BID) may be used; it can serve as a cofactor for enzymes of the urea cycle and further decrease ammonia concentrations and correct a zinc deficiency.

DRUG	DOSING	SAFETY/SIDE EFFECTS/MONITORING
Lactulose (Constulose, Enulose, Generlac, Kristalose)	Treatment: 30-45 mL (or 20-30 g powder) PO every hour until evacuation; then 30-45 mL (20-30 g powder) PO 3-4 times/day titrated to produce 2-3 soft bowel movements daily Enema: given Q4-6H PRN Prevention: 30-45 mL (or 20-30 g powder) PO 3-4 times/day titrated to produce 2-3 soft bowel movements daily	**SIDE EFFECTS** <u>Flatulence, diarrhea, dyspepsia, abdominal discomfort,</u> dehydration, hypernatremia, hypokalemia **MONITORING** Mental status, bowel movements, ammonia, fluid status, electrolytes
Rifaximin (Xifaxan)	Treatment (off-label): 400 mg PO Q8H x 5-10 days Prevention: 550 mg PO BID	**SIDE EFFECTS** Peripheral edema, dizziness, fatigue, nausea, ascites, flatulence, headache **MONITORING** Mental status, ammonia
Neomycin (Neo-Fradin)	500-2,000 mg PO Q6-8H x 5-6 days	**BOXED WARNINGS (3)** Neurotoxicity, (hearing loss, vertigo, ataxia); nephrotoxicity (particularly in renal impairment or with concurrent use of other nephrotoxic drugs); may cause neuromuscular blockade and respiratory paralysis especially when given soon after anesthesia or with muscle relaxants **SIDE EFFECTS** <u>GI upset</u>, ototoxicity, nephrotoxicity, irritation/soreness of mouth/rectal area **MONITORING** Mental status, renal function, hearing, ammonia
MetroNIDAZOLE (Flagyl, Flagyl ER, Metro) off-label	250 mg PO Q6-12H Do not use long term due to peripheral neuropathies	For a complete review see Infectious Disease I chapter.

Ascites

Ascites is fluid accumulation within the peritoneal space that can lead to the development of spontaneous bacterial peritonitis (SBP) and hepatorenal syndrome (HRS). Ascites is a common occurrence when the portal hypertension leads to an increase in systemic and splanchnic vasodilation, which results in increased arterial pressure, sodium and water retention, and renal vasoconstriction.

There are many treatment approaches to managing ascites, which are chosen based on the severity. Patients with ascites due to portal hypertension should restrict dietary sodium intake to < 2 grams/day, avoid sodium-retaining medications (including NSAIDs), and use diuretics to increase fluid loss. Restriction of fluid is recommended only in patients with symptomatic severe hyponatremia (serum Na^+ < 120 mEq/L).

Diuretic therapy for ascites can be initiated with either spironolactone monotherapy or with a combination of furosemide and spironolactone. Spironolactone is initiated at a single daily dose of 50-100 mg and increased to a maximum of 400 mg per day. When used in combination, the drugs should be titrated to a maximal weight loss of 0.5 kg/day with a ratio of 40 mg furosemide to 100 mg spironolactone to maintain potassium balance, if possible. Furosemide by itself is ineffective. All patients with cirrhosis and ascites should be considered for liver transplantation. In severe cases abdominal paracentesis may be needed to directly remove ascitic fluid. Large volume paracentesis (removal of > 5 L) has been associated with significant fluid shifts and the addition of albumin is recommended to prevent progression to hepatorenal syndrome.

Spontaneous Bacterial Peritonitis (SBP)

SBP is an acute infection of the ascitic fluid. Diagnosis is guided by cell and microbiologic analysis. In general, targeting *Streptococci* and enteric Gram-negative pathogens with ceftriaxone (or equivalent) for 5-7 days is recommended. Primary prophylaxis with norfloxacin or sulfamethoxazole/trimethoprim to prevent SBP is indicated in select cases. The same agents are used to prevent SBP recurrence. Norfloxacin is not readily available and ciprofloxacin is used as an alternative.

Hepatorenal Syndrome (HRS)

HRS is the development of renal failure in patients with advanced cirrhosis. HRS is the result of renal vasoconstriction mediated by activation of the renin-angiotensin-aldosterone system (RAAS) and the sympathetic nervous system (SNS) through a feedback mechanism known as hepatorenal reflux. Appropriately treating the various stages and complications of cirrhosis helps prevent progression to HRS; however HRS can be directly treated with renal vasodilators such as fenoldopam or dopamine.

VIRAL HEPATITIS

Viruses that damage the liver include hepatitis A through E (most cases of viral hepatitis are caused by hepatitis A, B and C), along with herpes, CMV, Epstein-Barr virus, and adenoviruses.

Hepatitis A virus (HAV) is a vaccine preventable disease that causes an acute, self-limiting illness in most patients. Transmission is primarily via the fecal-oral route through improper hand washing after exposure with an infected person or via contaminated food/water. The hepatitis A vaccine *(Havrix, Vaqta)* is given to children beginning at one year of age (2 shots are required), and to older persons if risk factors are present: household members and close personal contacts of adopted children from high or intermediate HAV endemicity, men who have sex with men, users of illegal injection and noninjection drugs, if someone lives in or travels to areas with high prevalence, if liver disease is present, if receiving blood products, or if working with HAV infected animals. <u>Treatment of hepatitis A is supportive and no antiviral agents are needed.</u> Immunoglobulin (IgG) can be given for post-exposure prophylaxis in select cases.

<u>Hepatitis B virus (HBV) is a vaccine preventable disease that causes acute illness and may lead to chronic infection,</u> cirrhosis of the liver, liver cancer, liver failure, and death. Transmission requires contact with infectious blood, semen, or other body fluids by having sex with an infected person, sharing contaminated needles to inject drugs, or from an infected mother to her newborn (perinatal transmission). For persons recommended to receive HBV vaccination and the vaccination schedules see the Immunizations chapter. <u>Many antiretrovirals (NRTIs) and interferons are used for chronic therapy of HBV. Treatment duration is not well defined. Hepatitis B reactivation is a concern in patients with prior HBV exposure undergoing certain immunosuppressive therapies and requires screening, monitoring, and managing patients to minimize the risk of HBV reactivation.</u>

<u>Hepatitis C virus (HCV) is a non-vaccine preventable disease that can cause acute disease, but more commonly is associated with chronic disease,</u> with consequences similar to hepatitis B. Transmission is through blood and is most commonly transmitted in the United States via intravenous drug use. <u>There are 6 different</u> hepatitis C genotypes (1-6) and various subtypes (for example 1a or 1b). Treatment options and duration of therapy depend on the genotype and include peginterferons, ribavirin, sofosbuvir, simeprevir, and the combination of ledipasvir/sofosbuvir.

INTERFERON ALFA

Interferon alfas are indicated for <u>treatment of HBV and HCV</u>. The interferons cause substantial toxicities and laboratory abnormalities limiting their use. The pegylated forms (*Pegasys* or *Peg-Intron*) have polyethylene glycol added to the interferon via pegylation, which prolongs the half-life, reducing the dosing frequency to once weekly. Interferons are naturally-produced cytokines that have antiviral, antiproliferative, and immunomodulatory effects. Interferon-βs are used for Multiple Sclerosis; see Autoimmune chapter.

DRUG	DOSING	SAFETY/SIDE EFFECTS/MONITORING
Interferon-α-2b (*Intron A*) – for HBV, HCV, many cancers Pegylated interferon–α-2b (*Peg-Intron*) – for HCV Pegylated interferon–α-2a (*Pegasys*) – for HBV and HCV Interferon Alfacon-1 (*Infergen*) – for HCV Combo product: Interferon-α-2b and ribavirin (*Rebetron*) Interferon-βs are used for Multiple Sclerosis; see Autoimmune chapter	Dosing varies based on indication. HCV dosing example: *Intron A:* 3 million units SC 3 times weekly *Peg-Intron:* 1.5 mcg/kg SC weekly *Pegasys:* 180 mcg SC weekly + ribavirin (different doses depending on interferon type used) Treatment duration depends on the genotype (which determines disease severity) Dose reduction required in the setting of thrombocytopenia and neutropenia (withhold treatment when ANC < 500/mm^3 or platelets < 25,000/mm^3) and for renal dysfunction (CrCl < 50 for *Peg-Intron* and CrCl < 30 for *Pegasys*)	**BOXED WARNINGS (4)** <u>May cause or exacerbate autoimmune disorders; may cause or aggravate infectious disorders; may cause or aggravate ischemic and hemorrhagic cerebrovascular events; combination treatment with ribavirin may cause birth defects and/or fetal mortality and/or hemolytic anemia.</u> **CONTRAINDICATIONS** Autoimmune hepatitis, decompensated liver disease in cirrhotic patients, infants and neonates **WARNINGS** Neuropsychiatric events, cardiovascular events, endocrine disorders (aggravates hypo/hyperthyroidism, hypo/hyperglycemia), ophthalmologic disorders (retinopathy, decrease in vision), pancreatitis, myelosuppression and serious skin reactions **SIDE EFFECTS** Interferons can cause <u>many</u> adverse effects. <u>Flu-like syndrome 1-2 hrs after administration (fever, chills, headache, malaise, arthralgia, myalgia, diaphoresis – can last 24 hrs) – can pre-treat with acetaminophen, antihistamine; CNS effects (fatigue, anxiety, depression, weakness), GI upset (nausea, vomiting, anorexia, weight loss), ↑ LFTs (5-10x ULN during treatment), myelosuppression, mild alopecia</u> **MONITORING** CBC with differential and platelets, LFTs, uric acid, SCr, electrolytes, TGs, thyroid function tests, serum HBV DNA or HCV-RNA levels **NOTES** MedGuide required with each new prescription and refill.

NUCLEOSIDE REVERSE TRANSCRIPTASE INHIBITORS

These agents inhibit HBV replication by inhibiting HBV polymerase resulting in DNA chain termination. Prior to starting HBV therapy, all patients should be tested for HIV. Antivirals used for HBV can have activity against HIV and if a patient is co-infected with both HIV and HBV, it is important that the chosen therapy is appropriate for both viruses to minimize risk of HIV antiviral resistance developing.

DRUG	DOSING	SAFETY/SIDE EFFECTS/MONITORING
Entire Class	↓ in CrCl < 50 mL/min	**BOXED WARNINGS (2) (ADDITIONAL BOXED WARNINGS FOR INDIVIDUAL AGENTS BELOW)** Lactic acidosis and severe hepatomegaly with steatosis, which may be fatal Exacerbations of HBV may occur upon discontinuation, monitor closely See HIV chapter for further information.
LamiVUDine (Epivir HBV)	100 mg PO daily 150 mg BID or 300 mg daily if co-infected with HIV CrCl < 50 mL/min: ↓ dose	**BOXED WARNING** Do not use Epivir HBV for treatment of HIV (contains lower doses of lamivudine) **SIDE EFFECTS** Headache, N/V/D, fatigue, insomnia, myalgias, ↑ LFTs, rash
Adefovir (Hepsera)	10 mg PO daily CrCl < 50 mL/min: ↓ frequency	**BOXED WARNING** May cause HIV resistance in patients with unrecognized or untreated HIV infection Use caution in patients with renal impairment or those at risk of renal toxicity (including concurrent nephrotoxic agents or NSAIDs) **SIDE EFFECTS** Headache, weakness, abdominal pain, hematuria, rash, nephrotoxicity
Tenofovir (Viread) 1st line agent	300 mg PO daily CrCl < 50 mL/min: ↓ dose	**SIDE EFFECTS** Fanconi syndrome, renal insufficiency, osteomalacia and ↓ bone density, GI upset, ↑ LFTs
Entecavir (Baraclude) 1st line agent	Nucleoside-treatment naïve: 0.5 mg PO daily Lamivudine-resistant: 1 mg PO daily Take on empty stomach CrCl < 50 mL/min: ↓ dose or frequency	**BOXED WARNING** May cause HIV resistance in patients with unrecognized or untreated HIV infection **SIDE EFFECTS** Peripheral edema, pyrexia, ascites, ↑ LFTs, hematuria, nephrotoxicity, ↑ SCr **NOTES** Food reduces AUC by 18-20%; take on an empty stomach (2 hours before or after a meal)
Telbivudine (Tyzeka)	600 mg PO daily CrCl < 50 mL/min: ↓ frequency	**SIDE EFFECTS** ↑ CPK, fatigue, headache, ↑ LFTs **MONITORING** CPK

Nucleoside Reverse Transcriptase Inhibitor Drug Interactions

■ Ribavirin can ↑ hepatotoxic effects of all NRTIs

■ Lamivudine: SMX/TMP can ↑ lamivudine levels due to reduced excretion

■ Tenofovir: Avoid concomitant treatment with didanosine due to increased risk of virologic failure and potential for increased side effects.

Nucleoside Reverse Transcriptase Inhibitor Counseling

■ *Epivir HBV* tablets and oral solution are not interchangeable with *Epivir* tablets and solution (which have higher doses).

■ Entecavir: Food ↓ the absorption of this drug; take on an empty stomach (take 2 hours before or after a meal).

■ Some people (rarely) have developed a serious condition called lactic acidosis (a buildup of an acid in the blood). Lactic acidosis is a medical emergency and must be treated in the hospital. Be seen right away if you feel very weak or tired, have unusual muscle pain, have trouble breathing, have stomach pain with nausea and vomiting, and/or feel dizzy or light-headed.

■ Lamivudine: Some people (rarely) have developed pancreatitis, which is a medical emergency and must be treated in the hospital. Be seen right away if you have upper abdominal pain that radiates to your back, or abdominal pain that feels worse after eating with or without nausea or vomiting.

RIBAVIRIN

Ribavirin is an oral antiviral agent that inhibits replication of RNA and DNA viruses. It is indicated for HCV in combination with interferon alfa, simeprevir, and/or sofosbuvir. Aerosolized ribavirin has been used for respiratory syncytial virus.

DRUG	DOSING	SAFETY/SIDE EFFECTS/MONITORING
Ribavirin *(Copegus, Rebetol, Ribasphere, Ribasphere RibaPak, Virazole)* 200 mg capsules and tablets	MedGuide required with each new prescription and refill. Dose (400-600 mg PO BID) varies based on indication, patient weight and genotype. Take with food (better tolerated). Dose reductions are needed for Hgb < 10 g/dL (avoid for hemoglobin < 8.5 g/dL).	**BOXED WARNINGS (4)** Significant teratogenic effects (avoid in pregnancy or women wishing to become pregnant) Monotherapy not effective for HCV and should not be used alone Hemolytic anemia (primary toxicity of oral therapy mostly occurring within 4 weeks of therapy) Caution with inhalation formulation in patients on a ventilator (precipitation of drug may interfere with ventilation) **CONTRAINDICATIONS** Pregnancy, women of childbearing age who will not use contraception reliably, male partners of pregnant women, hemoglobinopathies, CrCl < 50 mL/min, autoimmune hepatitis, concomitant use with didanosine **SIDE EFFECTS** Hemolytic anemia – primary toxicity, can worsen cardiac disease and lead to MIs; do not use with unstable cardiac disease. Fatigue, headache, insomnia, N/V/D, anorexia, myalgias, hyperuricemia **MONITORING** CBC with differential and PLTs, electrolytes, uric acid, bilirubin, LFTs, serum HCV-RNA levels, TSH, monthly pregnancy tests. **NOTES** Highly teratogenic; Pregnancy Category X Can stay in body for as long as 6 months. Avoid pregnancy in female patients and female partners of male patients during therapy and for 6 months after completing therapy. At least two reliable forms of effective contraception must be utilized during treatment and during the 6-month post-treatment follow-up period. Capsule should be not be crushed, chewed, open, or broken.

Ribavirin Drug Interactions

- Do not use with didanosine due to cases of fatal hepatic failure, peripheral neuropathy and pancreatitis.

- Ribavirin can ↑ hepatotoxic effects of NRTIs.

- Zidovudine can enhance the adverse effect of anemia from ribavirin.

Ribavirin Patient Counseling

- Ribavirin can cause birth defects or death of an unborn child. If you are pregnant or your sexual partner is pregnant, do not use. If you could become pregnant, you must not become pregnant during therapy and for 6 months after you have stopped therapy. During this time, you must use 2 forms of birth control, and you must have pregnancy tests that show that you are not pregnant.

- Female sexual partners of male patients being treated must not become pregnant during treatment and for 6 months after treatment has stopped. Therefore, you must use 2 forms of birth control during this time.

- If you or a female sexual partner becomes pregnant, you should tell your health care provider. There is a Ribavirin Pregnancy Registry that collects information about pregnancy outcomes in female patients and female partners of male patients exposed to ribavirin. You or your healthcare provider should contact the Registry at 1-800-593-2214. All information is confidential.

- If using the oral solution, wash the measuring cup or spoon to avoid swallowing of the medicine by someone other than the person to whom it was prescribed.

- This medicine can cause a dangerous drop in your red blood cell count, called anemia. Your healthcare provider should check your red blood cell count before you start therapy and often during the first 4 weeks of therapy. Your red blood cell count may be checked more often if you have any heart or breathing problems.

- Do not take ribavirin alone to treat hepatitis C infection. Ribavirin is used in combination for treating hepatitis C infection.

PROTEASE INHIBITORS

These direct-acting antiviral agents (DAA) are <u>indicated for the treatment of chronic HCV genotype 1 infection</u> in combination with peginterferon alfa and ribavirin in adult patients. These agents bind reversibly to protein 3 (NS3) serine protease and inhibit replication of HCV. Telaprevir is no longer available in the U.S. and boceprevir use has been supplanted by simeprevir. Simeprevir is also used in combination with sofosbuvir for treatment of HCV.

DRUG	DOSING	SAFETY/SIDE EFFECTS/MONITORING
Boceprevir (Victrelis)	800 mg 3 times/ day (every 8 hours) with food (a meal or light snack) starting on week 5 of peginterferon α plus ribavirin for 24-44 weeks With compensated cirrhosis – treat for 44 weeks Without cirrhosis – treat for 24 to 44 weeks	**CONTRAINDICATIONS** All contraindications to peginterferon α and ribavirin also apply since must be administered with these agents. Due to co-administration with ribavirin, <u>pregnancy (use of 2 non-hormonal contraceptives and negative pregnancy test before use and monthly is required) and men whose female partner is pregnant</u>. Concurrent administration of drugs dependent on 3A4 for clearance where ↑ concentrations result in serious or life-threatening events and concurrent use of 3A4 inducers. **SIDE EFFECTS** <u>Fatigue, anemia (requiring ESA use), neutropenia, dysgeusia</u>, N/V/D, headache, chills, insomnia, dizziness, alopecia, arthralgia, weakness, dyspnea **MONITORING** CBC with differential (to monitor anemia and neutropenia), HCV-RNA levels, electrolytes, LFTs, all laboratories as required for concomitant use with peginterferon and ribavirin apply **NOTES** <u>Never reduce the dose or interrupt therapy as treatment failure may result. Never use as monotherapy; must always be combined with peginterferon and ribavirin</u>. If HCV-RNA >100 units/mL at week 12 or detectable at week 24 (treatment futility), discontinue treatment (boceprevir, peginterferon α, and ribavirin).

Protease Inhibitors Continued

DRUG	DOSING	SAFETY/SIDE EFFECTS/MONITORING
Simeprevir *(Olysio)* If given with *Sovaldi* eliminates the need for ribavirin/ interferon (new indication)	150 mg PO daily with food	**CONTRAINDICATIONS** All contraindications to peginterferon α and ribavirin also apply when adminstered with these agents. <u>Due to co-administration with ribavirin, pregnancy (use of 2 non-hormonal contraceptives and negative pregnancy test before use and monthly is required) and men whose female partner is pregnant.</u> **SIDE EFFECTS** Rash (photosensitivity), pruritus, myalgia, dyspnea, ↑ serum bilirubin and nausea **MONITORING** CBC with differential (to monitor anemia and neutropenia), HCV-RNA levels, electrolytes, LFTs, all laboratories as required for concomitant use with peginterferon and ribavirin apply **NOTES** Screening patients with HCV genotype 1a infection for the presence of virus with the NS3 Q80K polymorphism at baseline is strongly recommended. Patients with this polymorphism will have a reduced response and alternative therapy should be given. If HCV-RNA level ≥ 25 units/mL at treatment weeks 4 or 12 (treatment futility), discontinue treatment (simeprevir, peginterferon alfa and ribavirin). <u>Never use as monotherapy; must always be combined with peginterferon and ribavirin or in combination with sofosbuvir (no treatment futility rules apply).</u>

Protease Inhibitor Drug Interactions

- Boceprevir is a strong CYP3A4 inhibitor and 3A4 substrate as well as P-glycoprotein inhibitor. Strong 3A4 inhibitors and inducers are contraindicated with the use of boceprevir. There are many drug interactions.

- Simeprevir mildly inhibits 1A2 activity and intestinal 3A4 activity, but does not affect hepatic 3A4 activity.

- Simeprevir is a 3A4 substrate; do not administer with moderate or strong 3A4 inhibitors or inducers.

SOFOSBUVIR AND SOFOSBUVIR/LEDIPASVIR

Sofosbuvir is an inhibitor of the HCV NS5B RNA-dependent RNA polymerase, which is essential for viral replication. Sofosbuvir is a nucleotide prodrug and is <u>indicated for hepatitis C only</u> with activity against HCV genotypes 1-4. The combination of sofosbuvir and ledipasvir, an NS5A inhibitor in a single table is approved for HCV genotype 1 infections.

DRUG	DOSING	SAFETY/SIDE EFFECTS/MONITORING
Sofosbuvir (Sovaldi)	400 mg PO daily with or without food HCV Genotype 1 & 4: give with peginterferon alfa + ribavirin x 12 weeks Or in patients who are interferon ineligible, give with simeprevir +/-ribavirin x 12 weeks HCV Genotype 2: give with ribavirin x 12 weeks HCV Genotype 3: give with ribavirin x 24 weeks	**CONTRAINDICATIONS** All contraindications to peginterferon α and ribavirin also apply when administered with these agents. Due to co-administration with ribavirin, pregnancy (use of 2 non-hormonal contraceptives and negative pregnancy test before use and monthly is required) and men whose female partner is pregnant. **SIDE EFFECTS** Fatigue, headache, nausea, insomnia, anemia, chills, irritability, pruritus, skin rash, weakness, myalgia **MONITORING** CBC with differential, HCV-RNA levels, LFTs **NOTES** For HCV genotype 1, the combination pill of sofosbuvir and ledipasvir is available (see ledipasvir/sofosbuvir)
Ledipasvir/Sofosbuvir (combination of ledipasvir and sofosbuvir in single tablet) (Harvoni)	90 mg ledipasvir combined with 400 mg sofosbuvir in single tablet taken PO daily x 12 weeks Patients who are previously treatment experienced (including prior pegylated interferon or prior HCV protease inhibitor) and cirrhotic require 24 weeks of treatment	**SIDE EFFECTS** Fatigue, headache **MONITORING** CBC with differential, HCV-RNA levels, liver function tests **NOTES** Requires acidic environment for absorption. Acid suppressive therapy should be avoided or minimized during therapy. Treatment naïve patients with no evidence of cirrhosis and a viral load of < 6 million IU/mL can be considered for an abbreviated course of therapy of 8 weeks.

Sofosbuvir Drug Interactions

- Sofosbuvir is a substrate of drug transporter P-gp; avoid with potent intestinal P-gp inducers (e.g., St. John's wort, rifampin). Avoid co-administration with carbamazepine, oxcarbazepine, phenobarbital, phenytoin, rifapentine, rifabutin and tipranavir/ritonavir.

PRACTICE CASE

PM is a 44 y/o male patient being seen in the gastroenterology clinic for follow-up. He was recently diagnosed with HCV and started treatment 2 weeks ago. The Patient Assistance Program at the clinic pharmacy is getting the medication for him free of charge. He is experiencing many side effects, but managing them well so far because he was counseled to expect them. His past medical history is significant for depression and GERD. PM stopped using alcohol and IV drugs 5 years ago. He has repeatedly tested negative for HIV over many years.

Allergies: NKDA

Medications:
Celexa 40 mg daily
Pepcid 20 mg daily
Tums 1-2 tabs PRN heartburn
Sovaldi 400 mg daily
Ribasphere 600 mg BID
Peg-Intron Redipen 150 mcg SC once weekly

Vitals:
Height: 5'9" Weight: 196 pounds
BP: 131/82 mmHg HR: 75 BPM RR: 13 BPM Temp: 98.2°F Pain: 3/10

Labs:

Na (mEq/L) = 140 (135 - 145)	WBC (cells/mm^3) = 6.1 (4 - 11 x 10^3)
K (mEq/L) = 4.1 (3.5 - 5)	Hgb (g/dL) = 14.1 (13.5 - 18 male, 12 - 16 female)
Cl (mEq/L) = 101 (95 - 103)	
HCO$_3$ (mEq/L) = 29 (24 - 30)	Hct (%) = 42.3 (38 - 50 male, 36 - 46 female)
BUN (mg/dL) = 17 (7 - 20)	
SCr (mg/dL) = 1.1 (0.6 - 1.3)	Plt (cells/mm^3) = 187 (150 - 450 x 10^3)
Glucose (mg/dL) = 132 (100 - 125)	AST (IU/L) = 87 (1 - 40)
Ca (mg/dL) = 10.1 (8.5 - 10.5)	ALT (IU/L) = 75 (1 - 40)
Mg (mEq/L) = 1.5 (1.3 - 2.1)	Albumin (g/dL) = 3.7 (3.5 - 5)
PO$_4$ (mg/dL) = 4.2 (2.3 - 4.7)	T Bili (mg/dL) = 1.5 (0.1 - 1.2)
	TSH (mIU/L) = 1.9 (0.3 - 3)

Refer to the clinical pharmacist for review of medication side effects and additional counseling.

Questions

1. PM is receiving treatment with *Sovaldi, Ribasphere* and *Peg-Intron* and experiencing many side effects. Which side effect would not be expected on this regimen?

   a. Depression
   b. Fatigue
   c. Flu-like syndrome
   d. Headache
   e. Dysgeusia

2. PM is taking *Ribasphere*. He is in a sexual relationship with a female partner. Which of the following statements is correct?

   a. No precautions are required since she is not using the medication.
   b. Female sexual partners of male patients being treated must not become pregnant during treatment and for 6 months after treatment has stopped. Therefore, 2 forms of birth control are required during this time.
   c. Female sexual partners of male patients being treated must not become pregnant during treatment and for 60 days after treatment has stopped. Therefore, 2 forms of birth control are required during this time.
   d. If she becomes pregnant, she should notify the Centers for Disease Control.
   e. If she becomes pregnant, the baby will be fine, however, the mom will develop anemia.

3. Which of the following is the most serious and primary toxicity of ribavirin?

   a. Hemolytic anemia
   b. Hemorrhagic cystitis
   c. Pancreatitis
   d. Agranulocytosis
   e. Gastrointestinal hemorrhage

Questions 4-7 do not apply to the above case.

4. A patient is scheduled to start immunosuppressive therapy for chronic inflammatory bowel disease. Testing for which of the following is indicated? (Select **ALL** that apply.)

   a. Latent Hepatitis A virus infection
   b. Latent Hepatitis B virus infection
   c. Latent Hepatitis C virus infection
   d. HIV
   e. Herpes Simplex Virus

5. A patient with liver failure presents with acute hepatic encephalopathy. Which of the following is considered first-line treatment for acute hepatic encephalopathy?

   a. Decreasing protein intake to < 1 gram/kg/day
   b. Lactulose
   c. Furosemide
   d. Neomycin
   e. Rifaximin

6. Which of the following is correct regarding sofosbuvir/ledipasvir treatment? (Select **ALL** that apply.)

   a. Test for Q80k polymorphism prior to starting treatment
   b. Avoid acid suppressive therapy while on treatment
   c. Duration of treatment depends on the 4 week viral load
   d. The brand name is *Harvoni*
   e. It is indicated for hepatic encephalopathy

7. Which of the following medications can lead to renal insufficiency and osteomalacia?

   a. Telaprevir
   b. Tenofovir
   c. Boceprevir
   d. Lamivudine
   e. Entecavir

Answers

1-e, 2-b, 3-a, 4-b, 5-b, 6-b,d, 7-b

DRUG USE IN PREGNANCY

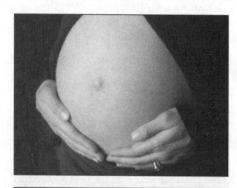

FDA PREGNANCY CATEGORIES

Note: The letter categories listed below (A, B, C, D and X) will be replaced in 2015 with three detailed subsections that describe risks within the real-world context of caring for pregnant women who may need medication. The subsections in the labeling are titled "Pregnancy," "Lactation" and "Females and Males of Reproductive Potential." When this has been incorporated, and if it seems reasonable for "testing" purposes, RxPrep will include an update on the "Errata and Updates" page that is kept under the "Student Resources" tab on the RxPrep website.

Pregnancy Category A

Controlled studies in animals and women have shown no risk in the 1st trimester, and possible fetal harm is remote.

Pregnancy Category B

Either animal studies have not demonstrated a fetal risk but there are no controlled studies in pregnant women, or animal studies have shown an adverse effect that was not confirmed in controlled studies in women in the 1st trimester.

Pregnancy Category C

No controlled studies in humans have been performed and animal studies have shown adverse events, or studies in humans and animals are not available; give only if potential benefit outweighs the risk.

Pregnancy Category D

Positive evidence of fetal risk is available, but the benefits may outweigh the risk if life-threatening or serious disease.

Pregnancy Category X

Studies in animals or humans show fetal abnormalities; use in pregnancy is contraindicated.

As a General Rule: Try to avoid all drugs if possible during 1st trimester (organogenesis) and use lifestyle recommendations first, if reasonable.

Encourage Enrollment in the Pregnancy Registries

Pregnancy exposure registries exist for select disease states (cancer, autoimmune conditions, HIV, epilepsy) and for many individual drugs. They are designed to collect health information from women who take various drugs when they are pregnant and breastfeeding. Information is also collected on the newborn baby. This information is compared with women who have not taken medicine during pregnancy and the health of their babies.

The FDA pregnancy categories listed above do not always correctly define risk: consider that many drugs have had pregnancy categories changed recently in light of data that the drugs were not as safe as previously thought, including older drugs such as NSAIDs and SSRIs. Clinicians need real-life data on the effect of these drugs; only with this information can clinicians help parents make informed decisions. This is why the new rating system described earlier has been developed and is currently being implemented. Search for "pregnancy registries" at www.fda.gov.

Common Teratogens

If a case indicates hCG+, the patient is pregnant and teratogenic drugs should be discontinued, if possible. Well-known teratogens include alcohol, ACE inhibitors, angiotensin receptor blockers, benzodiazepines, carbamazepine, ergot-derivatives, isotretinoin, leflunomide, lithium, methimazole, nafarelin, NSAIDs, paroxetine, phenytoin, phenobarbital, propylthiouracil, quinolones, ribavirin, tazarotene, tetracyclines, topiramate, valproic acid, misoprostol, methotrexate, statins, dutasteride, finasteride, warfarin, lenalidomide and thalidomide.

Many psychiatric drugs have risk in pregnancy. The drug's potential harm must be weighed against the risk of the condition not being treated adequately. In bipolar disorder, lithium and valproate are considered among the highest risk. The treatment of depression during pregnancy, and postpartum depression, has changed recently. Although SSRIs have historically been the preferred agents, in December of 2011 the FDA issued a warning regarding SSRI use during pregnancy and the potential risk of persistent pulmonary hypertension of the newborn (PPHN). Paroxetine is considered to have the highest risk in the class. Tricyclics, also pregnancy category C, are the second group most commonly used. Pregnancy-related depression and treatment is discussed further in the Depression chapter.

Folic Acid in Women of Child-Bearing Age

Whenever a young woman enters the pharmacy, the pharmacist can ask if she is consuming adequate folic acid (400-800 mcg daily, which is 0.4-0.8 mg/day), calcium (1,000 mg daily) and vitamin D (600 IU daily).

It is a safe and reasonable recommendation to women planning to conceive (and all women of child-bearing age, since many pregnancies are not planned) to take a folic acid supplement (at least one month prior to pregnancy) to help prevent birth defects of the brain and spinal cord (neural tube defects). Folic acid should be continued for the first 2-3 months of pregnancy. Folic acid is in many healthy foods, including fortified cereals (some of which are not healthy), dried beans, leafy green vegetables and orange juice. An OTC prenatal vitamin that contains 600-800 mcg would supply the recommended amount. Prescription prenatal vitamins (*Prima-Care ONE*, *Zenate*, others) usually contain 800 mcg. Folic acid at 1 mg and higher is usually by prescription, although there are a few OTC products with this dose available.

Common OTC-Treatable Conditions in Pregnancy

Nausea/Vomiting

First, recommend eating smaller, more frequent meals, avoiding spicy or odorous foods, taking more frequent naps, and reducing stress, including working long hours. If this does not work recommend pyridoxine, which is vitamin B6. This is the 1st line recommendation by ACOG, with or without doxylamine. A natural product which may be helpful is ginger, in tea form, or cooked, but do not recommend supplements. Dried, salted plums are used by certain ethnic groups. *Hyperemesis gravidarum* is severe N/V in pregnancy and causes weight loss, dehydration and electrolyte imbalance. It will be treated under the care of an obstetrician and may require hospitalization.

GERD/Heartburn/Gas Pains

First recommend eating smaller, more frequent meals, avoiding foods that worsen GERD, and if symptoms occur while sleeping, recommend elevating the head of the bed and not eating three hours prior to sleep. If this does not work, calcium antacids are first-line, such as calcium carbonate in *Tums* or store brands. This is a good antacid choice since calcium intake is often deficient in pregnancy. Use caution with excessive use of antacids containing aluminum or magnesium if renal disease is present. Do not recommend sodium bicarbonate or magnesium trisilicate (which comes in combination with aluminum hydroxide in *Gaviscon*).

If gas is a concern, simethicone is considered safe *(Gas-X, Mylicon)* – and the *Mylicon* infant drops are considered safe for infants. H_2 antagonists *(Pepcid, Tagamet, Axid, Zantac)* are all pregnancy category B; many doctors recommend OTC or Rx doses. PPIs are B's or C's.

Constipation

First recommend increasing fluid intake, increasing fiber in the diet, increasing physical activity, such as walking. If this does not work fiber is 1st-line and psyllium is pregnancy category B *(Metamucil*, store brands).

Cough/Cold/Allergies

The first-generation antihistamines are the usual first-line recommendation. Chlorphenira-mine (drug of choice) and diphenhydramine are pregnancy category B. The non-sedating 2nd generation agents loratadine and cetirizine are often recommended by obstetricians during the second and third trimesters. If nasal steroids are needed for chronic allergy symptoms, budesonide *(Rhinocort)* and beclomethasone *(Beconase AQ)* are considered safest; both are prescription only. Decongestants (pseudoephedrine, phenylephrine, oxymetazoline), the cough-suppressant dextromethorphan and the mucolytic guaifenesin are pregnancy category C, but may be recommended by the physician. The oral decongestants should not be recommended during the first trimester.

Pain

Acetaminophen is pregnancy category C and is the analgesic and antipyretic drug of choice during pregnancy and is considered safe to use if breast feeding. Ibuprofen is pregnancy category C/D > 30 weeks gestation, and naproxen is pregnancy category C; pharmacists should not recommend OTC NSAIDs in pregnancy. Acetaminophen is considered safe for treating mild pain in women who are breast feeding. Consider carefully safety with opioid metabolism in pregnant or lactating women (reviewed in the Drug Interactions and Pain chapters); for example, if codeine is given to a breast feeding mother who is a rapid metabolizer of CYP450 2D6, the infant could suffer fatality. Any opioid used should be at the lowest possible dose. in a short-acting formulation taken after feedings, to reduce the risk to the infant.

SELECT CONDITIONS AND FIRST-LINE TREATMENT

Vaccine Use During Pregnancy

- Influenza vaccine (shot, inactivated): each fall, whether pregnant or not – this is recommended in all stages of pregnancy.

- No live vaccines [MMR, varicella (chickenpox), live influenza nasal, etc.] one month before and during pregnancy.

- Pregnant women should receive Tdap between weeks 27-36, each pregnancy. If the woman has not been vaccinated or if the history is unclear, a 3-dose series is needed (one with Tdap, the other two with Td only). If the woman delivers and has not received vaccination, she should receive it post-delivery. Vaccination protects the baby (and the mother) from pertussis (whooping cough).

- Other vaccines may be needed in unusual circumstances, such as a need for a tetanus update, or foreign travel; refer to CDC guidelines.

Antibiotic Use During Pregnancy

Generally considered safe to use:

Penicillins (including amoxicillin and ampicillin, both B's) and cephalosporins, erythromycin and azithromycin (B's, but not clarithromycin, which is C)

Do not use during pregnancy:

Quinolones (due to cartilage damage) and tetracyclines (due to teeth discoloration)

Vaginal Fungal Infections

Use topical antifungals (creams, suppositories), at least 7 days.

Urinary Tract Infections

Beta lactams that cover the organism can be used, such as cephalexin (500 mg QID) or ampicillin. Nitrofurantoin 100 mg BID is used, but not in the last several weeks of pregnancy. Another option is fosfomycin (*Monurol*) 3 grams (1 packet, mixed with water) x 1. Must treat bacteriuria in pregnant women (for 7 days) even if asymptomatic with negative urinalysis. If not, the infection can lead to premature birth, pyelonephritis, and neonatal meningitis. In pregnant women, avoid quinolones (cartilage toxicity and arthropathies) and tetracyclines (teratogenic). SMX/TMP can cause hyperbilirubinemia and kernicterus in 3rd trimester, and is Pregnancy Category D.

Chlamydia

Azithromycin 1 g x 1, or amoxicillin 500 mg PO TID x 7 days.

Gonorrhea

Cephalosporin, or if contraindicated, azithromycin 2 g PO x 1

Bacterial Vaginosis

Clindamycin 300 mg PO BID or metronidazole (500 mg PO BID or 250 mg PO TID), all x 7 days. Topical (vaginal) therapy for bacterial vaginosis is not recommended during pregnancy.

Vaginal Trichomoniasis

2 g PO metronidazole x 1 (or 250 mg PO TID or 500 mg PO BID x 7d) at any stage of pregnancy. Treatment may be deferred after 37 weeks.

Asthma in Pregnancy

- Inhaled corticosteroids are first-line controller therapy for persistent asthma during pregnancy.

- Budesonide is the preferred inhaled corticosteroid for use during pregnancy (and is the preferred steroid for infants in the *Respules*, which are put in a nebulizer).

- Inhaled albuterol is the recommended rescue inhaler in pregnancy.

Venous Thromboembolism/Mechanical Valves

Heparin (UFH) or LMWH, convert to shorter half-life UFH during last month of pregnancy or if delivery appears imminent. Use pneumatic compression devices prior to delivery in women with thrombosis if they are getting a C-section. No warfarin during pregnancy (category X), the newer anticoagulants are pregnancy category B or C and are not currently in the recommendations.

Hypothyroidism

Must test for and treat, with levothyroxine, which is pregnancy category A.

Hyperthyroidism

Mild cases will not require treatment. If drugs are needed, such as with Graves', both hyperthyroid drugs are pregnancy category D: propylthiouracil is used if trying to conceive and in 1st trimester, then it is generally reasonable to switch to methimazole. Both are high risk for liver injury and there is risk with either to the neonate: both of these drugs readily cross the placenta and cause congenital defects, however, uncontrolled maternal hyperthyroidism causes adverse neonatal outcomes, including premature delivery and low birth weight. This is why it is preferable to normalize the mother's thyroid function prior to pregnancy. Contraception should be used until the disease is controlled.

Anemia

Anemia due to iron deficiency can occur during pregnancy and will be treated with supplemental iron, in addition to prenatal vitamins (which contain some iron).

Do not use tobacco during pregnancy/encourage cessation: Smoking in pregnancy can cause adverse outcomes for the child, including spontaneous abortion, low birth weight and sudden infant death. If women smoke 5 or less cigarettes (occasional, "nervous" type smokers) they should be encouraged to quit with behavioral support. If they smoke more than 5 cigarettes daily, ACOG recommends bupropion (pregnancy category C), and other sources recommend nicotine replacement in pregnancy, however the efficacy is not as high in non-pregnant patients. Nicotine gum and lozenges are pregnancy category C.

Do not use alcohol during pregnancy/encourage cessation: No amount of alcohol is safe during pregnancy.

PEDIATRIC CONDITIONS

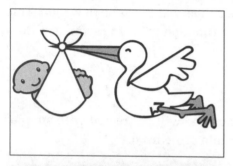

REFERENCES

Chery JD. Clinical practice: Croup. *N Engl J Med.* 2008; 358(4):384-391.

Vande Walle J, Rittig S, Bauer S, et al. Practical consensus guidelines for the management of enuresis. *Eur J Pediatr.* 2012; 171(6):971-983.

Addtl guidelines included with the video files (RxPrep Online).

AGE CLASSIFICATIONS

Neonate	0 – 28 days
Infant	1 month – 12 months
Child	1 – 12 years
Adolescent	13 – 18 years

We gratefully acknowledge the assistance of Allison Provine, PharmD, BCPS, Lipscomb University College of Pharmacy, in preparing this chapter.

BACKGROUND

Pediatric patients have unique and important differences in pharmacokinetic and pharmacodynamic properties that change as they mature. Several conditions common in younger patients are covered in this chapter. Additional pediatric topics are covered elsewhere in this text: Iron and vitamin D recommendations for infants and children are in Natural Products and Vitamins, various ID conditions are in Infectious Diseases, vaccines are in Immunizations, childhood asthma treatment is in Asthma, cough & cold is covered in Allergic Rhinitis, Cough & Cold and head lice and diaper rash are covered in Common Skin Conditions.

An infant can become seriously ill – very quickly. The box indicates conditions in which a child should be referred for urgent care.

Various studies have demonstrated that when parents measure liquid doses the dose is often incorrect. Household spoons should not be used for measuring medication. All liquid medications should be dispensed with an oral dosing syringe or dosing cup. The parent (or caregiver) should be able to read the markings on the device when it contains medication. Instruct the parents how to draw up the correct dose.

When dispensing liquid medications that carry high risk, follow safe practice recommendations:

- Stock one strength if a dangerous drug comes in a variety of strengths. Place the container into a high-risk bin with instructions attached to the container.

- The prescription should be written in terms of total mg and in mg/kg dose.

- The pharmacist should check that the dose is accurate with the child's weight. Ask the parent for the child's weight if it is not available.

- The container label should include the weight (mg) and the volume (mL). Dispense with a measuring device.

With some high-risk drugs it is preferable to administer at a medical facility where help is available if needed.

REFER FOR URGENT CARE WITH ANY OF THE FOLLOWING SIGNS OR SYMPTOMS
Age < 3 months old with a temperature of 100.4°F (rectal)
Age 3 – 6 months with a temperature of 101°F (rectal)
Age > 6 months with a temperature of 103°F (rectal)
Any cough/cold that worsens or does not improve in several days
Unusual, severe, or persistent pain that does not go away after several hours
Blood in the urine or stool
Inability to sleep or drink
Rash that looks severe, or any rash with fever
Abrasions that are dirty or deep (requiring sutures)
Limping or unable to move an extremity or seizure

BACTERIAL MENINGITIS

This infectious disease topic is included in the Infectious Disease chapter, and is additionally covered here for 3 primary reasons that are specific to neonates: the fatality rate if untreated is close to 100%, organisms that cause the condition differ and this changes the drug treatment, and the need for emphasis regarding safety issues with ceftriaxone use in neonates.

The classic signs of meningitis are uncommon in neonates. Bulging fontanelles and nuchal rigidity will be present in < 25% of cases; otherwise, the symptoms are non-specific and a definite diagnosis in a suspected case can be made with a lumbar puncture.

The organisms more likely to cause bacterial meningitis in a neonate differ from other ages due to the vertical transmission of pathogens from the mother to the baby. The predominant pathogens are Group B streptococcus (GBS – predominantly type III), *Escherichia coli* and *Listeria monocytogenes*. A few other common organisms that should be treated empirically and the recommended treatment is specified in the table. Ceftriaxone, which is used in adults, is generally avoided in neonates: ceftriaxone displaces bilirubin from albumin, which can cause bilirubin-induced brain damage (kernicterus). There is risk of an embolus from a ceftriaxone-calcium precipitate; a critically ill neonate will be receiving various IV fluids.

Bacterial Meningitis Empiric Treatment

AGE	COMMON BACTERIAL PATHOGENS	EMPIRIC TREATMENT
< 1 month	*Streptococcus agalactiae (Group B strep), Escherichia coli, Listeria monocytogenes, Klebsiella*	Ampicillin + Cefotaxime or Ampicillin + Aminoglycoside
1 – 23 months	*Streptococcus pneumoniae, Neisseria meningitides, S. agalactiae, Haemophilus influenza, E. coli*	Vancomycin + 3rd generation cephalosporin (Ceftriaxone or Cefotaxime)
2+ years	*N. meningitides, S. pneumoniae*	Vancomycin + 3rd generation cephalosporin (Ceftriaxone or Cefotaxime)

Respiratory Syncytial Virus (RSV)

RSV infection occurs commonly and nearly all children have been infected by the age of two years. In older, healthier children the symptoms mimic the common cold, but in premature babies and neonates RSV can be deadly. Symptoms include low-grade fever, cough, dyspnea and cyanosis (bluish skin due to lack of oxygen). Similar to other viral infections the treatment is primarily supportive [supplemental oxygen, IV fluids].

RSV Prophylaxis

Palivizumab (*Synagis*) is a humanized monoclonal antibody indicated for the prevention of serious lower respiratory tract disease caused by RSV in children at high risk of the disease. The American Academy of Pediatrics (AAP) recommends considering palivizumab prophylaxis during RSV season (late fall, early winter, early spring) for infants born before 29 weeks gestation who are younger than 12 months at the start of the RSV season, and for infants with chronic illness [primarily congenital heart disease or chronic lung disease (CLD)]. Palivizumab is dosed monthly at 15 mg/kg per dose. Infants should not receive more than 5 monthly doses during the RSV season. In addition to premature infants, palivizumab is used for certain infants and children < 24 months with select medical conditions that affect respiration.

Palivizumab is given by intramuscular (IM) injection. In neonates and infants, the IM injection site is the anterolateral thigh muscle. The deltoid can be used in children > 1 year if the muscle mass is adequate, but this is unlikely until the child is older.

Croup (Laryngotracheobronchitis)

Croup is a viral or bacterial infection which causes inflammation of the upper airway, larynx, trachea and bronchi. The inflammation results in the hallmark signs of inspiratory stridor (high pitched breathing sound), barking cough, and hoarseness. Croup is most common in children < 6 years old and is often worse at night. The illness is classified and treated by the severity of the symptoms.

Mild Illness: Supportive Care Only

For mild cases a child may present with only a croupy cough, which can be managed at home and should resolve within a few days. Cool mist or steam (avoid spilling hot water on infants) and adequate hydration will help alleviate symptoms.

Drug Treatment for Mild (if Warranted), Moderate or Severe Illness

Corticosteroids and nebulized epinephrine are used in mild, moderate, and severe cases of croup. Some severe symptoms can require breathing support, including intubation.

In a typical croup case presenting to an acute care setting with moderate-to-severe symptoms, a patient having difficulty breathing will be given nebulized racemic epinephrine and a steroid (oral if tolerated, or by injection). Antibiotics are used only if there is lack of improvement due to a secondary bacterial infection. Nebulized racemic epinephrine is a 1:1 mixture of dextro (D) isomers and levo (L) isomers (the L-isomer is the active component). If racemic epinephrine is not available L-epinephrine is used; this is ½ of the drug (one of the isomers) and the dose is, consequently, ½ of the racemic formulation.

Epinephrine is an adrenergic agonist that will relax the bronchial smooth muscle and cause bronchodilation. When given with a nebulizer (or as an injection – these are used occasionally in an outpatient self-administered device) the onset of action is fast but lasts at most up to 2 hours; a child receiving epinephrine will need to be monitored for a return of bronchospasm, and for tachycardia. The child should not be discharged until the breathing is easy with no stridor at rest and after receiving steroids to reduce the inflammation (usually dexamethasone).

DRUG	DOSING	SAFETY/SIDE EFFECTS/MONITORING
Dexamethasone Oral solution, injection (other forms not used in infants)	0.6 mg/kg x1 PO/IM/IV, max 16 mg/dose	See Asthma chapter for steroid safety issues. This is acute use only.
Either given via nebulizer: Racemic epinephrine 2.25% solution L-epinephrine solution 10 mg racemic epinephrine = 5 mg L-epinephrine	Racemic epinephrine 0.05 – 0.1 mL/kg (max 0.5 mL) diluted in 2 mL NS, can repeat Q 20 min PRN L-epinephrine 0.5 mL/kg of 1:1000 solution (maximum dose: 5 mL) diluted in NS, can repeat Q 20 min PRN	**WARNINGS** Caution with cardiovascular disease,, cerebrovascular disease, Parkinson disease, thyroid disease, diabetes (can ↑ blood glucose), extravasation (IV) **SIDE EFFECTS** ↑ BP, HR, anxiety **NOTES** Monitor for recurrent bronchospasm.

NOCTURNAL ENURESIS (BED WETTING)

Bed-wetting is a normal part of a child's development and is not generally treated before age 5. Boys (more often than girls) can still be developing nighttime bladder control until 7 years old. The two "treatments" are alarm therapy and desmopressin. Prior to either of these, behavioral approaches are used first. Embarrassment should be minimized. Bladder training exercises (such as attempting to hold the urine during the day for a set time period) are not recommended.

Behavioral approaches that can be effective include positive reinforcement, establishing a normal daytime voiding pattern and a normal bowel pattern, and establishing a normal hydration pattern. Fluid intake should be limited prior to bedtime. Behavioral approaches are effective in many children and should be tried for up to 3 months. If behavioral methods do not result in dryness, either alarm therapy or alarm therapy with drug treatment (desmopressin) can be tried.

Alarm therapy can be useful and should be considered for a minimum of 3 consecutive months. If unsuccessful initially, alarm therapy might work when the child is older and more motivated. Alarm therapy is effective in about 2/3 of children initially; many will relapse and require the intervention repeated. There are numerous alarms available that attach to the underwear or pajamas and sound an alarm when wet. The child may sleep through the alarm but will generally stop voiding. When the alarm sounds a parent should wake the child and escort him or her to the bathroom.

Drug Treatment

Desmopressin (oral tablets) is the only preferred medication for enuresis. Desmopressin is a synthetic analogue of antidiuretic hormone (ADH); simulating ADH will ↓ nocturnal urine production. Desmopressin can be used in combination with alarm therapy.

DRUG	DOSING	SAFETY/SIDE EFFECTS/MONITORING
Desmopressin *(DDAVP)* – used in tablets for enuresis, and in tablets, nasal spray or injection for diabetes insipidus and hemophilia A (to control bleeding)	Start 0.2 mg PO QHS, can titrate to 0.6 mg max	**CONTRAINDICATIONS** Hyponatremia or history of hyponatremia CrCl < 50 mL/min **SIDE EFFECTS** Headache, fatigue, possible ↓ sodium due to water retention **NOTES** Limit fluid intake 1 hour before dose and until the next morning.

OVER THE COUNTER (OTC) PRODUCTS FOR CHILDREN < 12 MONTHS OLD

If the condition does not require urgent care, there are several OTC products approved that are deemed generally safe for use in the pediatric population.

Intestinal Gas

Intestinal gas is a common condition with infants and causes distress post-feedings. Simethicone drops can offer mild, if any, benefit. The drug is not absorbed and is safe to use. Typically, as the child's digestive tract grows, the crying and fussiness will resolve. Parents can be comforted that symptoms will generally dissipate when the child is around 6 – 8 months old.

Nasal Congestion

Nasal congestion is very common in babies and is generally not serious. Children < 2 years old breathe mostly through their nose; they have not yet learned to breathe through their mouths. Smoke, including that from e-cigarettes, will cause irritation; do not permit anyone to smoke near children. Using a car seat indoors to sit the child upright will help. A cool mist humidifier near the bedside may reduce congestion – especially in the winter months when the home is heated. Some parents will help reduce congestion by steaming the bathroom up with the shower while a parent sits with the baby outside of the shower (in the steamy bathroom). Be careful not to let hot steam get near the child's skin.

Over-the-counter cough and cold medicines are not used in children < 2 years old (per the FDA) and < 6 years old (per the AAP). Compared to placebo (sweet syrup with no medicine in it) these are no more effective in babies but do have more toxicities. Gentle suctioning with saline drops or spray to loosen the mucus can provide relief. Suction bulbs are sold in pharmacies.

Mild Pain and Fever

Never recommend aspirin or any salicylate-containing product (bismuth subsalicylate, others) for ages < 16 years who are recovering from chickenpox or flu symptoms due to the association with Reye's syndrome. It is best not to recommend these at all because it may not be clear if the child is recovering from a virus. The infant drops and children's suspensions both contain the same dosage for acetaminophen to help reduce toxicity in older children; previously, the infant drops were more concentrated. Acetaminophen is the most common cause of liver failure when used in doses above the safe amount. Accidental acetaminophen overdose can be due to the parent's inadvertent use of acetaminophen in multiple products. Take the time to counsel parents about this danger and the various names under which acetaminophen is packaged. This is discussed further in the Allergic Rhinitis, Cough & Colds chapter. Ibuprofen comes in different dosage strengths for infants and children. With either acetaminophen or ibuprofen infant drops the medicine can be squirted into the child's mouth. It is acceptable to mix with a small amount of formula but if the child might not drink the entire dose it will be difficult to know how much of the dose was taken. The branded acetaminophen or ibuprofen are more expensive than the store's own formulations, which contain the same active ingredients and are less costly.

Constipation

Community pharmacists commonly recommend pediatric-size glycerin suppositories for "stat" removal of feces in a quite uncomfortable baby. Previously, there had not been a recommendation available for treating constipation in the youngest patients. In 2011, a guideline on the use of laxatives in children by the Canadian Paediatric Society was developed. This guideline recommends oral polyethylene glycol (Miralax) as an option for intermittent constipation prevention. This is an unlabeled use and assumes the child will be able to swallow the medication. Miralax (or the less-expensive store brand) is started at 0.5 to 1 g/kg/day and titrated up, if needed. Dietary measures (prunes or pears, as the fruit or juice) is helpful and a regular toileting schedule (in children who have not established a regular routine) can be recommended in older children who are using the bathroom. Any child with continuing issues with constipation should be seen by the pediatrician.

Select OTC Products for Infants

DRUG	DOSING	SAFETY/SIDE EFFECTS/MONITORING
Intestinal Gas		
Simethicone *(Mylicon Infants' Gas Relief Drops, Baby Gas-X Infant Drops)*	20 mg, 1-4 times/day PRN	Take after meals for mild gas pains. Shake drops before using. Can mix with water, formula, or other liquids.
Nasal dryness/congestion		
NaCl 0.9% intranasal saline solution *(Little Remedies Saline Nasal Drops, Ocean for Kids)*	2-6 drops per nostril PRN	See Allergic Rhinitis chapter; saline can be used with a suction bulb.
Fever		
Acetaminophen *(Children's Tylenol, PediaCare Infants' Fever Reducer/Pain Reliever)*	10-15 mg/kg/dose every 4-6 hours (max 75 mg/kg/day) All acetaminophen liquid (infants and children) is the same dosage: 160 mg/5 mL	For simplicity, age and weight-based dosing for infants is on the side of the dropper container. Caution for overdose from a variety of products, or incorrect dosing.
Ibuprofen *(Motrin Infant Drops, Infants' Advil Drops, Motrin or Advil children's suspension)*	5-10 mg/kg/dose every 6-8 hours Infant drop strength: 50 mg/1.25 mL	Indicated for infants > 6 months old. Caution for nausea.
Constipation		
Glycerin suppositories *(Babylax, Pedia-Lax)*	1 pediatric suppository. Insert high into the rectum and on the side of the stool. Retain for ~15 minutes.	Instruct parent to check with the pediatrician if using more than infrequently.
Polethylene glycol *(MiraLax)*	Age ≥ 6 months: 0.5-1 g/kg. Dissolve in at least 4 oz water or other beverage. The capful, which is ~1 heaping tablespoon, contains ~17 grams.	Instruct parent to check with the pediatrician if using more than infrequently.

Systemic Drugs Not Generally Used in Pediatrics

- Fluoroquinolones are not routinely used in pediatric patients due to the possibility of adverse musculoskeletal adverse effects. In special cases, such as anthrax treatment, cystic fibrosis or in the treatment of multidrug-resistant organisms, they are used on a case-by-case basis.

- Tetracyclines are not used in children < 8 years of age due to permanent discoloration of teeth and retardation of skeletal development and bone growth.

- Promethazine is contraindicated in children < 2 years of age due to the potential for severe and potentially fatal respiratory depression.

- Codeine is metabolized to morphine by the CYP450 2D6 enzyme; certain children over-express this enzyme – and consequently, would produce a higher than expected amount of morphine. This can result in toxicity and a possible lethal overdose. Codeine has a boxed warning to avoid use with two childhood surgeries that are done routinely (tonsillectomy, adenoidectomy); codeine is dangerous if used for any condition if the child over-expresses this enzyme. It is preferable to avoid this analgesic in children.

- Several OTC products are not safe in young children; even OTC diphenhydramine can quickly become toxic if used in ages < 6 years. Consult drug information sources prior to recommending OTC or Rx drugs for use in children.

Primary Toxicities From Accidental Overdose in Children

Iron and acetaminophen are two common culprits of accidental overdose in children. Toddlers put anything in their mouths, especially if it looks like it could be candy. One dose of several drug classes, including sulfonylureas, can be fatal to an infant. Taking care of our smallest patients, therefore, requires counseling to the older patients about safe storage of medication. If the child has ingested anything that could be toxic (even if the ingestion is suspected only) the poison control center should be contacted immediately for advice. Review the Antidote chapter for further information on pediatric poisoning.

Vaccine-Preventable Childhood Diseases

Vaccine-preventable illness is, unfortunately, being seen more commonly than in previous years due to a lack of immunizations in certain communities. Additionally, recent immigrants who have not received vaccination in their home countries can bring in disease. The vaccine information on these conditions is in the Immunization chapter. The symptoms of the more common vaccine-preventable illnesses are listed below so that the pharmacist can recognize the illness if it presents in a child. Each of the conditions below can lead to severe, permanent damage except for chickenpox, which generally dissipates without long-term consequences for most of the person's life. Eventually, when the child who has had chickenpox when younger becomes an older person (> 50 years old) they will be at risk for shingles, which can be quite painful. Shingles only occurs in patients who have had chickenpox.

ILLNESS	EMBLEMATIC SYMPTOMS	SYMPTOM DESCRIPTION
Measles	Koplik spots are small white spots on the inside of the cheeks (inside the mouth) and appear 2-5 days prior to the rash seen below. 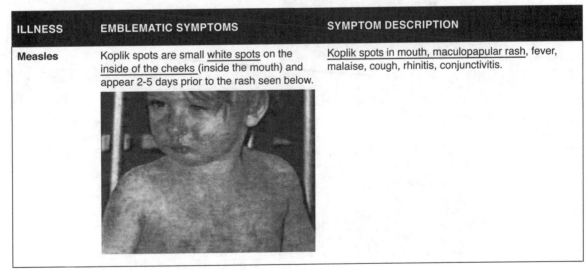	Koplik spots in mouth, maculopapular rash, fever, malaise, cough, rhinitis, conjunctivitis.

Vaccine-Preventable Childhood Diseases Coninued

ILLNESS	EMBLEMATIC SYMPTOMS	SYMPTOM DESCRIPTION
Mumps	Swollen and tender salivary glands under the ears (parotitis)	Swollen salivary glands, fever, headache, myalgia, fatigue, loss of appetite; up to 50% of patients have mild or no symptoms.
Rubella		Fever, rash, swollen glands, cold-like symptoms, aching joints; up to 50% of patients have mild or no symptoms.
Polio	Child with poliomyelitis	Fever, sore throat, fatigue, nausea, headache, abdominal pain; the majority have no symptoms and never know they were infected – others get severe nerve damage (paralytic polio) and later in life, post-polio syndrome, which causes progressive weakness and cognitive issues.
Pertussis	"WHOOP" Listen to a child making whooping sounds on youtube; several parents have posted videos. The condition is most dangerous in infants.	Sudden cough outbursts, fever, rhinitis, blueish skin (cyanosis), vomiting, fatigue.
Chicken Pox (Varicella)	Chicken pox rash (spots)	<u>Itchy</u> rash, fever, malaise. The rash appears as crops of sores (head, then trunk, then arms & legs), that turn into blisters, burst, then form crusts.

Questions

1. An 8 year old male weighs 55 pounds. Select an appropriate acetaminophen dose to recommend for this child:

   a. 1000 mg PO Q6 hours PRN pain

   b. 650 mg PO Q6 hours PRN pain

   c. 325 mg PO Q6 hours PRN pain

   d. 120 mg PO Q6 hours PRN pain

   e. 80 mg PO Q6 hours PRN pain

2. HY is a 2 year old female who presents to the emergency department with a frequent barking cough, prominent inspiratory stridor, marked sternal retractions, and agitation. She is afebrile with some rhinorrhea. Which of the following drug treatments is most likely warranted for her severe condition, based on the presentation?

   a. Dexamethasone and nebulized racemic epinephrine

   b. Dexamethasone only

   c. Nebulized budesonide and dextromethorphan

   d. Dexamethasone, pseudoephedrine, and nebulized racemic epinephrine

   e. Nebulized racemic epinephrine

3. MS is a 6 year old female (37.4 pounds) who presents to your pharmacy with a prescription for cefpodoxime written by her pediatrician for presumed bacterial pneumonia. She has a history of rash with penicillin. The pediatrician chose to use a cephalosporin. The dose of cefpodoxime recommended in the drug information reference is 10 mg/kg/day divided every 12 hours. The pharmacist should counsel the parent/caregiver to give the following milligrams for each dose:

   a. 15 mg

   b. 25 mg

   c. 55 mg

   d. 85 mg

   e. 115 mg

4. A 4 day-old male presents to the hospital with increased lethargy, poor feeding, and hypothermia. Blood and urine cultures are obtained along with a lumbar puncture to evaluate his cerebrospinal fluid. The most appropriate empiric regimen for suspected meningitis would be:

   a. Vancomycin and ampicillin

   b. Ampicillin and ceftriaxone

   c. Vancomycin and ceftriaxone

   d. Ampicillin and gentamicin

   e. Ceftriaxone and gentamicin

5. Which of the following statements concerning respiratory syncytial virus (RSV) are correct? (Select **ALL** that apply.)

   a. A patient presenting with RSV should be given nebulized corticosteroids early in the course to improve respiratory function.

   b. All patients requiring hospital admission due to RSV should be given nebulized ribavirin.

   c. An 11 month old infant with chronic lung disease on home oxygen should receive prophylaxis against RSV with pavilizumab (*Synagis*).

   d. Pavilizumab (*Synagis*) should be given once a week for the duration of RSV season for patients who meet criteria for prophylaxis.

   e. The treatment for RSV infection is primarily supportive and does not routinely require drug treatment.

6. Which of the following statements concerning croup are correct? (Select **ALL** that apply.)

   a. Clinical manifestations are caused by inflammation of the upper airway leading to narrowing of the trachea.

   b. Croup is most common in children 6-10 years of age.

   c. Croup is most commonly caused by a fungal infection.

   d. Mild cases are treated with supportive care, including possible use of nebulized albuterol or an albuterol MDI.

   e. Antibiotics should generally be given in children presenting with croup in order to prevent severe consequences.

7. A 14 year old male who weighs 132 lbs is diagnosed with a deep vein thrombosis and started on a heparin continuous infusion at 20 units/kg/hour. The heparin concentration in the IV bag is 25,000 units in 250 mL. How many milliliters of heparin should this patient receive each hour?

    a. 12 mL
    b. 22 mL
    c. 32.5 mL
    d. 55 mL
    e. 111.5 mL

8. A father brings his 2 month old daughter to the pharmacy. The girl weighs 14 pounds. The father states she has a rectal temperature of 100.6°F (38.1°C) and wants advice on an over-the-counter medication to treat her fever. The most appropriate recommendation is:

    a. Recommend ibuprofen 5-10 mg/kg/dose every 6-8 hours as needed until her fever subsides.
    b. Recommend putting his daughter in a cold bath to lower her temperature.
    c. Recommend acetaminophen 10-15 mg/kg/dose every 4-6 hours as needed until her fever subsides.
    d. Recommend he seek immediate medical care for his daughter.
    e. Recommend he continue monitoring her and seek medical care only if her temperature rises to 103°F (39.4°C).

9. Which of the following would be an appropriate over-the-counter recommendation for an infant?

    a. Simethicone drops for gas
    b. Dextromethorphan for a dry cough
    c. Bisacodyl suppository for constipation
    d. Fexofenadine (*Allegra Allergy Chidren's*) for runny nose/sneezing
    e. Loperamide for diarrhea

Answers

1-c, 2-a, 3-d, 4-d, 5-c, e, 6-a, d, 7-a, 8-d, 9-a

DRUG REFERENCES

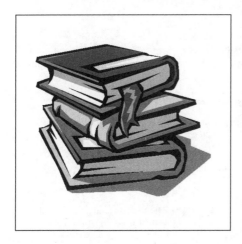

BACKGROUND

Providing drug information to patients as well as other healthcare professionals is one of the critical functions of pharmacists, regardless of the practice setting. In order to perform this function effectively and efficiently, it is important to be able to choose the most appropriate and specific resources based on the type of information needed. The following section is intended to highlight some of the key resources based on the type of information needed. It is not intended to be a comprehensive review of drug information resources available, but should provide a basic understanding for licensure.

It is important to continually evaluate new drug information resources and technology, and incorporate them into your practice to insure the resources being reviewed are current, and are reflecting the most current information available.

It is also important to recognize that patients also have access to many of the same drug information resources. As healthcare providers, pharmacists need to be aware of what patients are reading and be able to provide context as-needed to clarify the information as it applies to their case. Pharmacists must also be able to recognize when the medical information requested is outside the scope of normal pharmacy practice/expertise. These questions should be referred to the appropriate healthcare provider for follow up.

SOURCES, BY CATEGORY

General Drug Information

American Hospital Formulary Service (AHFS) Drug Information

Lexicomp's Drug Information Handbook, and online resource

Drug Topics: Red Book

- The Red Book is a useful resource to determine product presentations (i.e., dosage form, strength, and package size) and availability

Food and Drug Administration (FDA): Orange Book:

- Indicates if a generic is therapeutically equivalent to the brand at www.accessdata.fda.gov/scripts/cder/ob/ See FDA Drug Approval & Therapeutic Equivalence chapter for more information.

FDA: National Drug Code (NDC) Directory

- The National Drug Code (NDC) is the universal product identifier for human drugs at http://www.accessdata.fda.gov/scripts/cder/ndc/default.cfm

FDA: Purple Book: lists biological products, including any biosimilar and interchangeable biological products at www.fda.gov

Facts and Comparisons

FDA: Drugs Home page at www.fda.gov/Drugs

FDA: Drugs@FDA at www.accessdata.fda.gov/scripts/cder/drugsatfda

Micromedex

National Library of Medicine (NLM): Dailymed

- Database of Product Package Inserts at dailymed.nlm.nih.gov/dailymed

NLM: Drug Information Portal at druginfo.nlm.nih.gov/drugportal

Physician's Desk Reference (PDR)

- Collection of product package inserts

Pharmacist's Letter

Drugs of Choice from the Medical Letter

Sanford Guide to Antimicrobial Therapy

Toxicology

Micromedex: POISINDEX

Lexicomp's: Poisoning and Toxicology: Lexi-Tox

NLM: TOXNET at toxnet.nlm.nih.gov/

Adverse Drug Reactions

Individual product package inserts, PDR, *DailyMed, Lexicomp*, or in any of the general drug resources

ASHP: Drug-Induced Diseases: Prevention, Detection, and Management

Drug Shortages

ASHP: Drug Shortages at www.ashp.org/drugshortages

FDA: Drug Shortages at www.fda.gov/drugs/drugsafety/drugshortages/

Centers for Disease Control and Prevention (CDC): Vaccines and Immunizations –
Current Vaccine Shortages & Delays at www.cdc.gov/vaccines/vac-gen/shortages/

FDA Drug and Biologic Recalls

Drug Recalls at www.fda.gov/Drugs/DrugSafety/DrugRecalls/default.htm

Biologic Recalls at www.fda.gov/BiologicsBloodVaccines/SafetyAvailability/Recalls/

Professional Medical Information

CDC: Diseases & Conditions at www.cdc.gov/diseasesconditions

Harrison's Principles of Internal Medicine

National Cancer Institute (NCI) at www.cancer.gov

The Merck Manual at www.merckmanuals.com/professional/

Washington Manual of Medical Therapeutics

Pink Book – epidemiology & prevention of vaccine-preventable dz

SOURCES, BY CATEGORY *Continued*

Consumer Medical and Drug Information
CDC: Diseases & Conditions at
www.cdc.gov/diseasesconditions

FDA: Consumer pages at
www.fda.gov/ForConsumers

NIH: MedlinePlus at
www.nlm.nih.gov/medlineplus

Medication Safety (see Medication Safety chapter)
FDA: Drug Safety Communications at
www.fda.gov/Drugs/DrugSafety

FDA: Medication Guides at
www.fda.gov/Drugs/DrugSafety/ucm085729.htm

FDA: MedWatch at
www.fda.gov/Safety/MedWatch

Institute for Safe Medication Practices (ISMP) at
www.ismp.org

Reporting Adverse Drug Reactions
Drugs/Devices: FDA: MedWatch Adverse Event Reporting System (FAERS) at www.fda.gov/medwatch or 1-800-FDA-1088 (1-800-332-1088)

Vaccines: CDC/FDA: Vaccine Adverse Event Reporting System (VAERS) at vaers.hhs.gov/index

Reporting Medical Errors
In Hospital

- To the P&T Committee, at staff meetings (as defined by facility), to the Medication Safety Committee

In any setting

- ISMP's Medication Errors Reporting Program (MERP)
- FDA's MedWatch
- MedMARx program

Drug Interactions
Drug Interaction Facts

Hansten and Horn's Drug Interactions Analysis and Management

Micromedex

Lexicomp's Online Database

IV Stability/Compatibility
AHFS Drug Information

King Guide

Micromedex

Product Package Inserts

Trissel's Handbook on Injectable Drugs

Compounding and Manufacturing
Allen's Compounded Formulations

Extemporaneous Formulations for Pediatric, Geriatric, and Special Needs Patients

International Journal of Pharmaceutical Compounding, bimonthly publication

Pediatric Drug Formulations

Remington: The Science and Practice of Pharmacy

- Includes a chapter on extemporaneous prescription compounding

Trissel's Stability of Compounded Formulations

US Pharmacopoeia National Formulary (USP-NF)

- Includes chapters on Pharmacy Compounding; Non-Sterile Compounding is USP Chapter 795 and Sterile Compounding is USP Chapter 797
- USP sets standards for quality, purity, identity, and strength of medicines, food ingredients and dietary supplements

Drug Identification
Facts and Comparisons

Therapeutic Research Center's Ident-A-Drug at ident-adrug.therapeuticresearch.com

Micromedex: IDENTIDEX

PDR

NLM: PillBox at pillbox.nlm.nih.gov

SOURCES, BY CATEGORY *Continued*

Foreign Drug Identification
Diccionario de Especialidades Farmacéuticas, printed in Spanish

International Drug Directory (Index Nominum)

Martindale

Micromedex

USP Dictionary of USAN and International Drug Names

Natural Products/Alternative Medicine
Micromedex

Natural Medicines Comprehensive Database

Natural Standard

PDR for Herbal Medicines

US Pharmacopoeia

Travel Medicine *Yellow Book*
CDC: Travelers' Health at www.cdc.gov/travel

International Society of Travel Medicine (ISTM) at www.istm.org

Association For Medical Assistance To Travelers (IA-MAT) at www.iamat.org

Pregnancy and Lactation
Breastfeeding: A Guide for the Medical Profession

Briggs' Drugs in Pregnancy and Lactation

CDC: Medications and Pregnancy at www.cdc.gov/pregnancy/meds/

Hale's Medications and Mothers' Milk at www.medsmilk.com/

Micromedex

NLM: LactMed at toxnet.nlm.nih.gov/newtoxnet/lactmed.htm

Women's Health
CDC: Women's Health at www.cdc.gov/women

Department of Health and Human Services (DHHS) Women's Health at http://www.hrsa.gov/womenshealth/index.html

FDA: For Women at www.fda.gov/ForConsumers/ByAudience/ForWomen

NLM: Women's Health at www.nlm.nih.gov/medlineplus/womenshealth.html

World Health Organization (WHO): Women's Health at www.who.int/topics/womens_health/en

Geriatrics
FDA: Medicines and You: A Guide for Older Adults at www.fda.gov/Drugs/ResourcesForYou/ucm163959.htm

Lexicomp: Geriatric Dosage Handbook

NIH: Senior Health at nihseniorhealth.gov

The American Geriatrics Society (AGS) Guidelines & Recommendations at www.americangeriatrics.org/health_care_professionals/clinical_practice/clinical_guidelines_recommendations/

Pediatrics
AHFS Drug Information

CDC: Vaccines & Immunizations at www.cdc.gov/vaccines

Harriet Lane Handbook

Micromedex

Nelson: Textbook of Pediatrics

Neofax

Lexicomp's Pediatric & Neonatal Dosage Handbook

ASHP: Pediatric Injectable Drugs

Psychiatry
Clinical Handbook of Psychotropic Drugs

Diagnostic and Statistical Manual of Mental Disorders: Fifth edition (DSM-5)

SOURCES, BY CATEGORY *Continued*

Pharmacology/Pharmacy Text Books
Koda-Kimble's Applied Therapeutics: The Clinical Use of Drugs

Goodman and Gilman's: The Pharmacological Basis of Therapeutics

Handbook of Nonprescription Drugs (OTC)

DiPiro's Pharmacotherapy: A Pathophysiologic Approach

Pharmaceutics
Handbook of Pharmaceutical Excipients

Merck Index

Remington: The Science and Practice of Pharmacy

Guidelines
National Guideline Clearinghouse at www.guideline.gov

Select Key Guidelines

- ACC/AHA Guideline on the Treatment of Blood Cholesterol to Reduce Atherosclerotic Cardiovascular Risk in Adults (2013)

- 2014 Evidence-based guideline for the management of high blood pressure in adults. Report from the panel members appointed to the Eighth Joint National Committee (JNC 8)

- American Diabetes Assoc (ADA) Clinical Practice Recommendations and American Association of Clinical Endocrinologists/American College of Endocrinology Consensus Statement (AACE), both for diabetes

- CHEST guidelines for antithrombotic therapy

Refer to the professional organization websites (e.g., AACE, ACG, ACOG, others)

Clinical Trials
NIH: ClinicalTrials.gov at www.clinicaltrials.gov

Professional Organizations
American Academy of Pediatrics (AAP) at www.aap.org

American Cancer Society (ACS) at www.cancer.org

American Diabetes Association (ADA) at www.diabetes.org

American Heart Association (AHA) at www.heart.org

American Society of Clinical Oncology (ASCO) at www.asco.org

Infectious Diseases Society of America (IDSA) at www.idsociety.org/

For Additional Professional Organizations
NLM: Professional Organizations at: www.nlm.nih.gov/medlineplus/organizations/all_organizations.html

Pharmacy Organizations
Academy of Managed Care Pharmacy (AMCP) at www.amcp.org

American College of Clinical Pharmacy (ACCP) at www.accp.com

American Pharmacists Association (APhA) at www.pharmacist.com

American Society of Health-System Pharmacists (ASHP) at www.ashp.org

Literature Search
Excerpta Medica (EMBASE)

International Pharmaceutical Abstracts (IPA)

NLM: PubMed at www.ncbi.nlm.nih.gov/pubmed

Miscellaneous Resources
NLM: Gallery of Mobile Apps and Sites www.nlm.nih.gov/mobile

Legislative and Business Developments
The Pink Sheet: biopharma regulatory, legislative, legal & business developments

Pharmacist's Letter

FDA: Center for Drug Evaluation and Research (CDER) at www.fda.gov

19

DISPOSAL OF PRESCRIPTION DRUGS

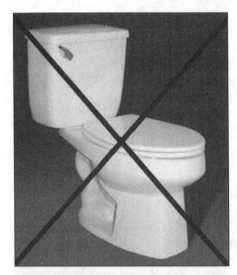

GUIDELINES

US EPA Disposal of Medical Sharps, available at: http://www.epa.gov/waste/nonhaz/industrial/medical/disposal.htm

Medical Waste Disposal information from NABP, available at: http://www.nabp.net/news/tagged/medication-collection-program-disposal

PROPER DISPOSAL OF PRESCRIPTION DRUGS

Common prescription agents, including beta-blockers and ACE Inhibitors, can be measured in fish in the Pacific basin. This region is not alone; drug concentrations in the ocean are an environmental disaster. It is important to realize that proper disposal is critical, but only part of the solution. The majority of drugs and drug metabolites end up in the oceans from the patient's urine and stool – the best way to reduce this exposure is to improve the health of the population to reduce the amount of drugs people are using. The federal prescription drug disposal guidelines recommend (in the absence of a "take-back" program – described below) mixing unwanted drugs (including controlled drugs) with unpalatable substances and placing them in a non-descript container before discarding in the trash unless the prescribing information specifically states the drug is to be flushed down the toilet or sink (see list of "okay to flush" drugs at the end of this section). The list of drugs that are acceptable to flush include only certain controlled drugs.

Some environmental experts disagree with the FDAs recommendations for flushing certain high-risk drugs and instead advise consumers to dispose of unwanted medications in their original prescription containers with any identifying information removed, and to not flush any medications, even if the patient information instructs otherwise. Note that the FDA is particularly concerned with the risk of the wrong person getting or taking the controlled drug – and subsequent harm.

Instruct patients: Do not flush prescription drugs down the toilet or drain unless the label or accompanying patient information specifically instructs you to do so.

To dispose of prescription drugs not labeled to be flushed, patients should be advised to take advantage of community drug take-back programs or other programs, such as household hazardous waste collection events, that collect drugs at a central location for proper disposal. In 2010, the FDA started the first national "Take Back" day for unwanted drugs. Pharmacies have been involved, in all 50 states, in notifying patients where to take unused medications for destruction. These are annual events and have been very successful. The first four years of the program collected over 2,400 tons of unused drugs; that's 4,800,000 pounds! They continue to grow.

The DEA's Take-Back events are a significant piece of the government's prescription drug abuse prevention strategy. Purging America's home medicine cabinets of unwanted or expired medications is one of four action items outlined in the strategy for reducing prescription drug abuse and diversion. The other action items include education of health care providers, patients, parents and youth; establishing prescription drug monitoring programs in all the states; and increased enforcement to address "doctor shopping" and pill mills.

Pharmacy Involvement in Taking Back Unwanted Drugs (this is ongoing, and not "Take Back Days" as described above)

In many states, pharmacies, and other designated sites, have the ability to help patients dispose of unwanted prescription and over-the-counter drugs – but not controlled substances, which must be returned only to law enforcement – without flushing them down the toilet or tossing them in the garbage. These are voluntary programs for community pharmacies.

The pharmacies can either:

- Use postage pre-paid envelopes so that consumers can return unwanted drugs to licensed waste disposal facilities, away from pharmacies where health care is provided, or

- Establish a collection bin for ongoing collection at pharmacies.

Drugs should not be reviewed by staff at a collection site (whether a pharmacy or community event) before being deposited into a secured collection bin. The patient or patient's agent should deposit the drugs themselves, thereby preventing staff from knowing what is being returned.

Drugs that are collected should be separated from their containers by patients or their agents before being placed in the collection bin, which reduces the disposal costs because the containers will not be part of the pharmaceutical waste.

Locking the "Take Back" Container

- There should be two separate locks on the secured collection bin: one key should be in the possession of the pharmacy, the other key in the possession of the licensed integrated waste hauler who will pick up what is now classified as "hazardous household waste."

- This dual lock ensures that the pharmacy cannot open the collection bin without the presence of the integrated waste hauler, and vice versa.

Some pharmacies do not participate in Take Back Programs, but offer services for disposal by mail, including the common "TakeAway" mailers that are processed by companies, such as Sharps, Inc.

The "TakeAway" mailers are popular in many pharmacies and include return shipping and handling. They are for Rx (not controlled) and OTC drugs. At the receiving end the products are processed by law enforcement. Pharmacies can also have bins for medication drop off in the store. These services can also be used by pharmacies for their own medical waste, such as syringes during flu season.

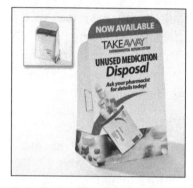

Patient either gives TakeAway envelope to US postal service or UPS driver, or store – this picture is a display box that contains the mailing envelopes

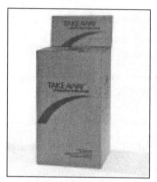

Or, the patient drops off in the box of a pharmacy that has the container – neither option is for controlled drugs

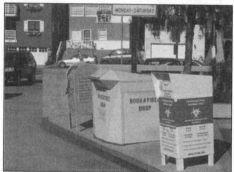

Some communities have locked boxes for controlled drugs – if putting medicine into this container, the drug name must be visible (but not patient info)

If the patient uses the mailer (rather than the drop-off box in a pharmacy) they put the medications into the brown mailing envelope, then put in the US mail or bring to a UPS store or driver. The return shipping is paid. Up to 4 ounces of liquids or gels can be put in a *Ziploc* bag into the envelope.

In the absence of a Take Back Program or access to mailers, instruct patients to follow local guidelines for Home Hazardous Waste (HHW) Collection.

Find the phone number of the local HHW collection site in the government section of the local white pages of the telephone directory. It is important for patients to know their local regulations. It may be that the locality requires drugs to be dropped off at certain sites, or be placed in the trash. If drugs are placed in the trash the following procedures should be followed:

- Keep medicine in its original child-resistant container. Scratch or mark out the patient information on the label.

- Place some water into solid medications, such as pills or capsules. Then add something nontoxic and unpalatable such as sawdust, kitty litter, charcoal, *Comet* or powdered spices (such as cayenne pepper).

- Close and seal the container lids tightly with packing or duct tape. If discarding blister packs of unused medicines, wrap in multiple layers of duct tape.

- Place medicine containers in durable <u>packaging that does not show what's inside</u> (such as a cardboard box).

- Place in the trash close to garbage pickup time.

SYRINGE DISPOSAL

Safe injection technique in a health care setting, including sharp disposal, is discussed in the Medication Safety chapter. This section is for patient (home) syringe disposal.

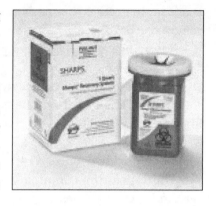

Improper management of discarded needles expose waste workers to potential needle stick injuries and infection risk when containers break open inside garbage trucks or needles are mistakenly sent to recycling facilities. Janitors, housekeepers and family members risk injury if loose sharps poke through plastic garbage bags. Used needles can transmit diseases, including HIV and hepatitis.

Options for Safe Syringe Disposal

Drop Box or Supervised Collection Sites

Sharps users can take their own sharps containers filled with used needles to appropriate collections sites: doctors' offices, hospitals, pharmacies, health departments, or fire stations. Services are free or have a nominal fee. Check the options in your area as they vary.

Mail-Back Programs

Sharps users place their used sharps in special containers and return the container by mail to a collection site for proper disposal. Fees depend on the size of the container. These are available in many pharmacies. Sharps, Inc. is a commonly used source for sharps mail-in containers, among others.

Syringe Exchange Programs (SEP)

Sharps users can exchange used needles for new needles. This is a proven method to decrease the transmission of blood-borne pathogens (HIV, hepatitis) by injection drug users. It is run by the North American Syringe Exchange Network at www.nasen.org. Currently, federal funds are not available for syringe exchange programs; this is why, in some states, a small number of syringes can be purchased without a prescription.

At-Home Needle Destruction Devices

There are products patients use to destroy used needles at home. These devices sever, burn, or melt the needle. In general these are not recommended for places where others can be infected with a condition, because people can be pricked removing the needle. On the other hand, if the patient is in their own home and infection risk is low, this process reduces the cost of disposal because the plastic syringe can be disposed of in the trash if the needle has been removed. For example, this can be a cost-effective method for a patient injecting insulin several times daily.

Used Needle-Syringe Safety Tips

Disposable needles contaminated with drugs, chemicals or blood products should never be removed from their original syringes unless no other option is available. Throw the entire needle/syringe assembly (needle attached to the syringe) into the red plastic sharps container.

Never remove a needle by unscrewing it with your hands in a health care facility. At home, if infection risk is low, it may be possible to remove the needle by one of the devices described above.

Used disposable needles/sharps should be discarded immediately after use without recapping into a sharps container (a non-reusable plastic container that is puncture resistant, leak proof on the sides and bottom, properly labeled and closable).

Sharps containers should be easily accessible, replaced routinely, and not allowed to overfill. Never compress or "push down" on the contents of any sharps container.

If someone is stuck with a needle that someone else has used, they should be seen by a health care provider immediately to assess infection risk and consider prophylactic therapy.

This is the list from the FDA of unused or expired medicines that should be flushed down the sink or toilet in order to help prevent danger to people and pets in the home. Please note that there are other options for disposal, but the FDA feels that the risk permits the flushing of these medications only. These are all controlled substances and must be disposed of according to DEA law.

ACTIVE INGREDIENT	DRUG
Acetaminophen; Oxycodone Hydrochloride	*Percocet*, tablets *
Aspirin; Oxycodone Hydrochloride	*Percodan*, tablets *
Buprenorphine	*Butrans*, transdermal patch (extended release)
Buprenorphine Hydrochloride	Buprenorphine Hydrochloride, tablets (sublingual) *
Buprenorphine Hydrochloride; Naloxone Hydrochloride	Buprenorphine Hydrochloride; Naloxone Hydrochloride, tablets sublingual
	Zubsolv, tablets (sublingual)
Diazepam	*Diastat/Diastat AcuDial*, rectal gel
Fentanyl	*Abstral*, tablets (sublingual)
	Duragesic, patch (extended-release) *
Fentanyl Citrate	*Actiq*, oral transmucosal lozenge *
	Fentora, tablets (buccal)
	Onsolis, soluble film (buccal)
Hydromorphone Hydrochloride	Dilaudid, tablets *
	Dilaudid, oral liquid *
	Exalgo, tablets (extended release)
Meperidine Hydrochloride	*Demerol*, tablets *
	Demerol, oral solution *
Methadone Hydrochloride	*Dolophine* Hydrochloride, tablets *
	Methadone Hydrochloride, oral solution *
	Methadose, tablets *
Methylphenidate	*Daytrana*, transdermal patch system
Morphine Sulfate	*Avinza*, capsules (extended release)
	Kadian, capsules (extended release)
	Morphine Sulfate, tablets (immediate release) *
	Morphine Sulfate, oral solution *
	MS Contin, tablets (extended release) *
Morphine Sulfate; Naltrexone Hydrochloride	*Embeda*, capsules (extended release)
Oxycodone Hydrochloride	*Oxecta*, tablets (immediate release)
	Oxycodone Hydrochloride, capsules
	Oxycodone Hydrochloride, oral solution
	Oxycontin, tablets (extended release)
Oxymorphone Hydrochloride	*Opana*, tablets (immediate release)
	Opana ER, tablets (extended release)
Sodium Oxybate	*Xyrem*, oral solution
Tapentadol	*Nucynta ER*, tablets (extended release)

* These medicines have generic versions available or are only available in generic formulations.

List revised: November 2013

20

TOXICOLOGY & ANTIDOTES

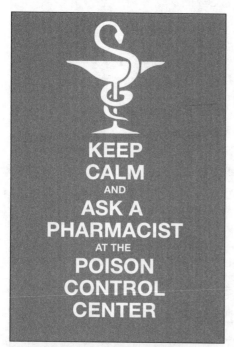

KEEP CALM AND ASK A PHARMACIST AT THE POISON CONTROL CENTER

REFERENCES

National Library of Medicine's TOXNET. http://toxnet.nlm.nih.gov/(accessed 2014 Oct 1).

Lexi-Comp's Toxicology Online. http://online.lexi.com/lco/action/home/tox (accessed 2014 Oct 1).

Mowry, JB, Spyker, DA, et al. 2012 Annual Report of the American Association of Poison Control Centers' National Poison Data System (NPDS). *Clinical Toxicology.* 2013; 51:949–1229.

We gratefully acknowledge the assistance of Susan E. Gorman, PharmD, MS, DABAT, FAACT, President, American Board of Applied Toxicology, and Cynthia L. Morris-Kukoski, PharmD, DABAT, FAACT, Past-President, American Board of Applied Toxicology, in preparing this chapter.

BACKGROUND

Toxic means poisonous, and toxicology is the study of poisonous chemicals, which includes drugs at unsafe doses. Antidotes are substances that stop the harmful effects of the poison (or overdosed drug).

Children are the most common victims of accidental poisoning in the United States. The top categories of substances in accidental pediatric exposures are cosmetics/personal care products, analgesics and cleaning substances. Accidental poisoning is common among the elderly due to mental or physical impairment, the use of multiple drugs, and reduced elimination. Poisoning can be intentional, such as with attempted suicide or as an act of revenge, or in situations such as rape (drug-facilitated sexual assault).

Prevention of Accidental Poisoning

To reduce accidental poisoning in children, child-resistant (C-R) containers are helpful, but are not foolproof. These are required for prescription drugs unless waived by the patient or with specific substances that are excluded from this requirement, such as nitroglycerin sublingual tablets. <u>Non-prescription drugs that require C-R containers</u> include anything containing iron, diphenhydramine, acetaminophen, salicylates, NSAIDs, "imidazoline" vasoconstrictors such as naphazoline and oxymetazoline and drugs that have been switched from Rx to OTC. Non-drug compounds that are dangerous if swallowed require C-R packaging, such as turpentine. Common C-R packaging includes <u>screw caps</u> that require more than a simple turn to open (such as having the user press down with the palm when turning to open), <u>unit-dose packaging</u> and the card adherence and safety packaging that require the user to press on

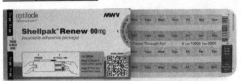

one side while pulling the medication card out of the other side. The picture demonstrates the *Optilock* packaging, which, additionally, can help with adherence when the day of the week is indicated.

Early Suspicion, Actions and Decontamination

For any questionable exposure the national poison control line (phone # 800-222-1222) can be contacted. With topical exposure, <u>remove any contaminated clothing and run water over the skin for 10 minutes</u>, then soap and rinse. For ocular exposure, remove contact lenses and rinse eye (or eyes) with water from a tap or hose with a gentle stream for at least 15 minutes. With oral ingestion, remove anything in the mouth and <u>collect any suspect containers to bring to the emergency department</u>. If unconscious, place the patient on the left side to more easily clear vomit if emesis (vomiting) occurs. <u>Ipecac syrup</u> was used previously to induce emesis for certain exposures, but <u>is no longer commercially available, and is no longer recommended</u>. Instruct others not to give ipecac syrup (it remains in many home medicine cabinets) or use any other mechanism to induce vomiting.

If the patient is unconscious, having difficulty breathing, appears agitated or is seizing emergency help should be contacted (call 911). If the patient is not breathing and/or has no pulse CPR should be initiated. Upon arrival to the acute care facility cardiovascular support and breathing support, including assisted ventilation, may be required. Cardiac monitoring with an ECG will be needed with drugs that affect heart rate or rhythm or with any cardiac abnormality present. With some substances, specific antidotes or dialysis may be used.

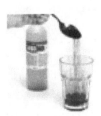

Decontamination with Activated Charcoal

For some orally ingested compounds taken in potentially toxic amounts, <u>activated charcoal can be administered</u> and is most effective within one hour of the ingestion. Activated charcoal can be aqueous, or combined with sorbitol as a cathartic and sweetener. <u>Sorbitol should be avoided</u> because it can induce vomiting and cause electrolyte disturbances. It may be necessary to protect the airway in patients who are unconscious or likely to become unconscious with intubation to prevent vomiting and aspiration. Activated charcoal is contraindicated when the airway is unprotected, or if the ingested compound may increase the risk of aspiration (i.e., hydrocarbons). Drugs should be separated from the activated charcoal by at least two hours. The dose of activated charcoal is 1 g/kg. Alcohols, heavy metals (iron, lead, lithium, mercury) and corrosives (alkalis, acids) do not bind to charcoal.

Caution: Symptoms of Overdose May Not Be Present

Several of the most dangerous compounds do not cause immediate symptoms when toxic. To identify whether a patient is at risk, the clinician should determine the time(s) of ingestion, the quantity, and the formulation ingested. For example, in an acetaminophen overdose the patient can remain asymptomatic for up to two days – until end organ toxicity (liver failure) is apparent. Due to the asymptomatic presentation the serum acetaminophen level is used as the basis for diagnosis and treatment. In certain overdoses, drug levels can be useful to guide treatment and monitoring of the patient; however, in most drug overdose situations, clinical evaluation of the patient's signs and symptoms will guide treatment.

Antidotes for Common Drug and Non-Drug Poisonings

DRUG	ANTIDOTE	COMMENTS
Acetaminophen	**N-acetylcysteine** (oral or *Acetadote*, IV)	N-acetylcysteine restores hepatic glutathione (acts as a glutathione substrate). It should be initiated immediately if overdose is suspected regardless of symptoms.
		Oral: 140 mg/kg x 1, followed by 70 mg/kg every 4 hours x 17 additional doses. Repeat the dose if emesis occurs within 1 hour of administration.
		Intravenous: 150 mg/kg IV over 60 minutes, followed by 50 mg/kg IV over 4 hours, followed by 100 mg/kg IV over 16 hours.
Organophosphates (OPs), include industrial insecticides (malathion, others) and nerve (warfare) gases (sarin, others)	**Atropine** and **pralidoxime**, or in combination (*DuoDote*)	OPs block acetylcholinesterase, which increases acetylcholine (Ach) levels. Atropine is an anticholinergic and blocks the effects of Ach to reduce the cholinergic SLUDGE symptoms: salivation, lacrimation, urination, diarrhea, gastrointestinal distress and emesis.
		Pralidoxime treats the muscle weakness and relieves paralysis of respiratory muscles secondary to the toxicity.
Botulism	Botulism antitoxin, heptavalent	Heptavalent botulism antitoxin is only available through the CDC. BabyBIG (botulism immune globulin) is used for infant botulism (different than foodborne botulism) and is available through the California Department of Public Health.
Black Widow spider bites	Antivenin *for Latrodectus mactans*, supportive care	Predominantly found in southern and western states. Children and frail elderly at highest risk for severe injury. The spiders are non-aggressive if left alone. Supportive care is the mainstay of therapy (opioids for pain management and benzodiazepines for muscle spasms).
Carbon monoxide (CO)	Oxygen, possibly hyperbaric	Accidental exposure from gas heaters, wood or charcoal stoves, CO-emitting kerosene heaters (colorless, odorless) or automobile exhaust.
Ethanol (alcoholic drinks)	Supportive care, correct hypoglycemia	If any question if chronic alcohol user, administer thiamine (vitamin B1) to prevent Wernicke syndrome (neurological damage).

Antidotes for Common Drug and Non-Drug Poisonings Continued

DRUG	ANTIDOTE	COMMENTS
Ethylene glycol, diethylene glycol, methanol	**Fomepizole (Antizol)**, preferred or Ethanol (2nd line)	Fomepizole and ethanol inhibit alcohol dehydrogenase (ADH). Caution: children are very prone to hypoglycemia. Methanol or ethylene glycol toxicity should be suspected with anion-gap metabolic acidosis along with an osmolar gap.
Anticholinergic overdose (atropine, diphenhydramine, dimenhydrinate, *Atropa belladonna* (deadly nightshade), jimson weed, scopolamine	Supportive care, rarely physostigmine	Physostigmine inhibits acetylcholinesterase, which increases the affects of acetylcholine, reducing the anticholinergic toxicity but is not routinely recommended. It may be used in severe cases of delirium if no contraindications are present (cardiac conduction defects, seizures). Benzodiazepines/anticonvulsants if seizures present. Anticholinergic overdose symptoms can be remembered with the mnemonic, "red as a beet, dry as a bone, blind as a bat, mad as a hatter, and hot as a hare" for the symptoms of flushing, dry skin and mucous membranes, mydriasis with double or blurry vision, altered mental status and fever. Severe symptoms include tachycardia, hypertension, psychosis, seizures, respiratory and cardiovascular collapse.
Benzodiazepines	**Flumazenil**	Flumazenil is used off-label for non-benzodiazepine hypnotic overdose (e.g., zolpidem) but is not routinely recommended. Flumazenil can precipitate seizures when used in benzodiazepine-dependent patients.
Beta blockers	Supportive care, possibly glucagon and/or high dose insulin with glucose	Treat bradycardia, hypotension and seizures. Glucagon may be used if unresponsive to standard supportive care. High dose insulin with glucose may be used in patients refractory to glucagon therapy.
Calcium channel blockers	Supportive care (see beta blockers above), Calcium (chloride or gluconate), possibly glucagon and/or high dose insulin with glucose	Administer calcium IV only, avoid fast infusion, monitor ECG, do not infuse calcium in same line as phosphate-containing solutions. Glucagon may be used if unresponsive to standard care. High dose insulin with glucose may be used in patients refractory to glucagon therapy.
Cyanide	2 IV antidotes: Hydroxocobalamin (Cyanokit) Sodium thiosulfate + Sodium nitrite (Nithiodote)	Cyanide overdose is due to high dose, or long treatment duration or renal impairment treatment with nitroprusside, or from ingestion of amygdalin, a synthetic form of laetrile (used as a cancer remedy – is ineffective), or most commonly, due to smoke inhalation. Do not use *Cyanokit* if solution is not dark red.
Digoxin, oleander, foxglove	**Digoxin Immune Fab (DigiFab)**	*DigiFab* 40 mg vial binds ~0.5 mg digoxin. Interferes with digoxin levels drawn after its use. When neither amount ingested nor digoxin level is known, adult dose is 20 vials.
Heavy metals, including arsenic, copper, gold, lead, mercury	**Dimercaprol** or Penicillamine or Calcium disodium edetate (EDTA) **Succimer** (Dimercaptosuccinic acid, DMSA)	Succimer is a water-soluble, oral chelating agent that is used in asymptomatic children with serum lead levels > 45 mcg/dL. EDTA is a parenteral chelating agent. It does not cross the blood-brain barrier and can exacerbate encephalopathy; dimercaprol, which does cross the blood-brain barrier, is given first. Do not use disodium EDTA; use CaNa$_2$ EDTA. Lead poisoning is initially asymptomatic; toxicity results in cognitive deficits, highest risk in children with exposure to lead-containing paint chips.

Antidotes for Common Drug and Non-Drug Poisonings Continued

DRUG	ANTIDOTE	COMMENTS
Heparin, Low Molecular Weight Heparin (LMWH)	**Protamine**	<u>1 mg will reverse ~100 units of heparin, and is used as a reversal agent for LMWHs.</u> See Anticoagulation chapter.
Insulin or other hypoglycemics, severe low blood glucose	**Dextrose** Glucagon if unconscious and outpatient	Dextrose injection or infusion (drip): do not exceed 12.5 or 25% peripherally due to risk of thrombosis, may require co-administration of potassium (IV dextrose will result in hypokalemia). Sulfonylureas: octreotide (*SandoSTATIN*) may be given with dextrose.
Isoniazid	**Pyridoxine (Vitamin B6)**	Oral pyridoxine 10 – 50 mg is used daily with isoniazid to prevent neuropathies, and in higher intravenous doses to treat toxicity.
Iron Aluminum (unlabeled)	**Deferoxamine *(Desferal)*** Deferiprone *(Ferriprox)* and Deferasirox *(Exjade)* – for iron overload from blood transfusions	Overdose can be due to accidental ingestion or secondary to multiple transfusions. Childhood iron overdose: iron tablets look like candy and toddlers put almost anything into their mouths; most lethal ingestion is due to exposure to prenatal multivitamins and OTC iron tablets. Deferoxamine is used for iron and aluminum toxicity (off label use).
Methotrexate	Leucovorin (Folinic acid), Levoleucovorin *(Fusilev)* Glucarpidase *(Voraxaze)*	Leucovorin/levoleucovorin: For rescue after high-dose methotrexate treatment (in cancer treatment) and to diminish the toxicity and counteract the effects of impaired methotrexate elimination or with a change to accidental overdose. Note: Glucarpidase availability may be limited.
Methemoglobinemia	Methylene blue	Drugs that cause methemoglobinemia (an altered form of hemoglobin) include anesthetics, dapsone, phenytoin, chloroquine and silver sulfadiazene; this condition is rare, and is more likely to occur if multiple drugs listed are used together or can be due to a congenital condition. Chemicals that can cause methemoglobinemia include amyl nitrate and nitrites. Antidote is contraindicated in patients with G6PD deficiency.
Amatoxin-containing mushrooms	Supportive care, Silibinin (*Legalon SIL*) ± Atropine	There are various types of mushrooms; some are poisonous, many are not. Treatment is guided by symptoms, such as hallucinations. Atropine if severe muscarinic symptoms (bradycardia). Silibinin is the flavonoid in milk thistle, sometimes used for hepato-protection.
Napthalene, from mothballs	Supportive care, Methylene blue	Methylene blue is indicated for drug-induced methemoglobinemia and as an indicator dye; this is off-label use.
Neostigmine, pyridostigmine	Pralidoxime	Pralidoxime counteracts the muscle weakness and/or respiratory depression secondary to overdose of anticholinesterase medications used to treat myasthenia gravis.
Nicotine, including e-cigarettes in teenagers	<u>Supportive care</u>, **Atropine**	Atropine is a nicotinic receptor antagonist and should be given to treat symptomatic bradycardia. Benzodiazepines should be given to treat seizures.
Opioids, legal and illicit (e.g., heroin)	**Naloxone *(Narcan, Evzio)***	*Evzio* is an auto injector for emergency treatment outside of the hospital. See Pain chapter.

Antidotes for Common Drug and Non-Drug Poisonings Continued

DRUG	ANTIDOTE	COMMENTS
Petroleum distillates (gasoline, kerosene, mineral oil, paint thinners)	Oxygen, supportive care	Do not use gastric emptying. Keep patient NPO.
Plants: Castor beans, jequirity beans, oleander and foxglove, hemlock	Supportive care, *DigiFab* if oleander or foxglove	Castor beans contain ricin. Jequirity beans contain abrin; structurally has the same two-subunit configuration as ricin. Oleander and foxglove contain digitalis glycosides.
Salicylates	**Sodium bicarbonate**	Salicylates are acidic; sodium bicarbonate is an alkalinizing agent.
Scorpion stings	Antivenin immune FAB *Centruroides (Anascorp)*, supportive care.	Scorpions producing clinical symptoms are found mainly in the southwest.
Snake bites: Eastern coral snake, Texas coral snake, Copperhead snake, Rattlesnake	Antivenin *Micrurus fulvius* for coral snake bites; *CroFab* for Copperhead and Rattlesnake bites	
Stimulant overdose from amphetamines, including ADHD and weight loss drugs, cocaine, ephedrine, caffeine, theophylline, MDMA (ecstasy), alcohol withdrawal	Supportive care, possibly Benzodiazepines	Symptoms of overdose include tachycardia, hypertension, mydriasis, agitation, possible seizures, hyperthermia and psychosis. Benzodiazepines (e.g., lorazepam) may be administered for agitation and/or seizures.
Tricyclic Antidepressants	Supportive care	IV hypertonic sodium bicarbonate can be administered to decrease a widened QRS complex. Benzodiazepines may be used for symptom relief, seizures. Vasopressors may be used for hypotension.
Valproate-induced hyperammonemia	L-Carnitine (Levocarnitine)	Treat if symptomatic (changes in mental status, elevated ammonia level).
Warfarin, rat poison (rodenticides)	**Phytonadione (vitamin K) (Mephyton)**	See Anticoagulation chapter (note this is given as vitamin K1, the precursor of other vitamin K forms).

21

IV DRUG STORAGE, COMPATIBILITY & ADMINISTRATION

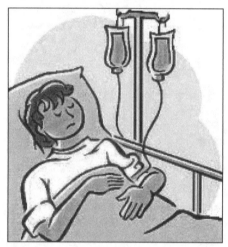

BACKGROUND

The pharmacist is the primary consult for questions concerning the compatibility and stability of parenteral medications. There are many drugs and the information changes; reputable resources are required. *Trissel's* or *King's* are the primary compatibility and stability resources, with the drug's package insert. Drug reference sources (such as *Micromedex* and *Lexi-Comp*) list container compatibility (mixed in the same IV container or in a syringe) and Y-site compatibility separately. A reputable group of pharmacists prepares lists of compatibility issues on a periodic basis that are published in *Pharmacy Practice News* and in *Hospital Pharmacy*; however, these lists are used for handy reference purposes. The pharmacist on site must verify the information as it may have changed.

Chemical incompatibility causes drug degradation or toxicity due to a hydrolysis, oxidation or decomposition reaction. Physical incompatibility is commonly due to compounds binding together and forming a precipitate which may be visible or not, and can be quickly fatal if the precipitate travels to the lungs.

Physical Incompatibilities can occur with either of the following:

- The containers (drugs that cannot be placed into PVC containers)

- The solutions (diluents – primarily dextrose or saline) and

- The other drugs, such as phenytoin binding to dextrose or calcium binding to phosphate; drug-drug incompatibility can occur when drugs are mixed in the same syringe or container, or during Y site administration (described further).

FILTERS

In-line filters are used with drugs that have a risk of particles, precipitates, crystals, some type of contaminant or entrapped air in the final solution. The size of the filter required is determined by the size of the particles to be removed. The majority of drugs in which filters are necessary use a 0.22 micron filters (1 micron = 1/1,000 mm); another common filter size is 1.2 microns which is used for lipids. A few drugs require larger filters and some drugs come packaged with the filter that should be used. If compounding IV medications in a sterile hood and glass ampules are used, filter needles are used to prevent particulates from getting into the IV bag and a filter may be required in the line.

COMMON DRUGS THAT REQUIRE FILTERS DURING ADMINISTRATION	
Abatacept (Orencia)	Infliximab (Remicade)
Abciximab (ReoPro)	Golimumab (Simponi)
Albumin	Lipids
Amiodarone (continuous infusion)	Lorazepam (Ativan)
Amphotericin B Liposomal (AmBisome)	Mannitol (Osmitrol)
	Phenytoin (Dilantin)
Diazepam (Valium)	Parenteral Nutrition
Digoxin Immune Fab (DigiFab)	

Drugs and Intravenous Polyvinyl Chloride (PVC) Containers

The majority of PVC containers use diethylhexyl phthalate (DEHP) as a "plasticizer" to make the plastic flexible. The DEHP compound is considered environmentally unsafe, is a potential human carcinogen and may affect human fertility. The two primary concerns with the use of PVC containers are leaching (DEHP leaches from the PVC container into the solution) and sorption (the drug moves into the PVC container). Drugs that have incompatibility with PVC containers can be placed in polyolefin containers, or with some of drugs, in glass containers (glass is heavy and can break).

Drugs that leach into PVC include tacrolimus, temsirolimus, teniposide, cabazitaxel, docetaxel, etoposide, ixabepilone and paclitaxel. The rhyme "tic tac toe, craving delicious, excellent, irresistible pho" (pho is Vietnamese soup) may be helpful.

Drugs with sorption issues include amiodarone (for infusions greater than 2 hours), carmustine, lorazepam, sufentanil, thiopental, regular human insulin and nitroglycerin. The mnemonic ACLS TIN may be helpful.

Drugs and Incompatible IV Solutions (Saline or Dextrose)

When drugs are put into solution for IV administration in the pharmacy they are commonly placed into 50 mL IV "piggy-backs" that contain 5% dextrose or 0.9% saline. With many drugs either solution is acceptable but with others only dextrose or only saline is compatible (see table).

Incompatibility During Y-Site Administration

A drug can mix with an incompatible solution or incompatible drug during "Y site" administration (see figure). This type of administration is common in acute care settings where the amount of drugs required exceed the number of available ports (the opening into the patient) for the catheter (the soft plastic tube that enters the port). Notice that the two catheter lines in the figure merge together; this is where incompatibility can occur.

When a pharmacist is referencing a resource to check if drugs can be co-administered, "compatibility" is listed separately from "Y-site compatibility", which involves a shorter duration of time. There are many incompatibilities of both types and the nursing staff (who hang the infusion bags) commonly consult with the pharmacy to check for compatibility issues.

COMMON DRUGS THAT GO INTO EITHER DEXTROSE OR SALINE	
Dextrose Only (No Saline)	**Saline Only (No Dextrose)**
Amphotericin B (Amphotec)	Ampicillin
Carfilzomib (Kyprolis)	Abatacept (Orencia)
Lorazepam (Ativan)	Ampicillin/Sulbactam (Unasyn)
Mycophenolate (CellCept IV)	Azacitidine (Vidaza) NS or LR
Pentamidine	Belimumab (Benlysta)
Quinupristin/Dalfopristin (Synercid)	Bevacizumab (Avastin)
Sulfamethoxazole/Trimethoprim (Bactrim)	Caspofungin (Cancidas) NS or LR
	Daptomycin (Cubicin) NS or LR
	Phenytoin
	Ertapenem (Invanz)
	Infliximab (Remicade)
	Iron Sucrose (Venofer)
	Sodium Ferric Gluconate Complex (Ferrlecit)
	Natalizumab (Tysabri)
	Trastuzumab (Herceptin)

Additive Compatibility

DRUG*	MFR*	CON/L*	MFR	CONC/L	TEST SOLN	REMARKS	REF	C/I
Ciprofloxacin	MI	2 g		400 mg	NS	C for 24 hrs at 25°C	888	C

Y-Site Injection Compatibility (1:1 Mixture)

DRUG*	MFR*	CON/L*	MFR	CONC/L	REMARKS	REF	C/I
Cefepime	BMS	20 mg/mL	AST	3.2 mg/mL	Haze and precipitate form in 1 hr	1689	I
	BMS	120 mg/mL		0.4 mg/mL	Physically compatible with < 10% cefepime loss	2513	C
Heparin	ES	100 units/mL	AB	3.2 mg/mL	Visually compatible for 4 hr at 27°C	2062	C

*Info on the test drug (e.g., ciprofloxacin, cefepime, heparin)

Y-site incompatibilities are important in pharmacy because this type of administration is common and many drugs that would not be mixed in the same container can mix in the line.

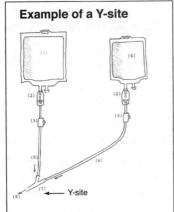

Example of a Y-site

Y-site

There are many incompatibilities; this is a discussion of a select few: aminoglycoside antibiotics are often given with other agents for synergy; this includes some of the beta-lactams which are not compatible with aminoglycosides in the same infusion container or with Y-site administration. Amphotericin is incompatible with the majority of IV drugs with any type of IV administration. The common hospital IV drug piperacillin/tazobactam (discussed further below) forms a precipitate when it makes contact with acyclovir, amphotericin B and many other IV drugs.

Heparin is incompatible when administered with many drugs – including those which would be given concurrently in a patient requiring heparin (nitroglycerin, alteplase and hydromorphone). Caspofungin, another common hospital drug for treating *Candida* infections, has many Y-site incompatibilities. All of the IV quinolones are incompatible with Y-site infusion with <u>many</u> drugs. The list is extensive and explains why *Trissel*'s is long (with small type).

IV AGENTS THAT ARE NOT REFRIGERATED

Acetaminophen (*Ofirmev*)

Acyclovir – refrigeration causes crystallization

Clindamycin – refrigeration causes crystallization

Deferoxamine (*Desferal*)

Furosemide – refrigeration causes crystallization

Hydralazine

Metronidazole

Pentamidine

Moxifloxacin (*Avelox*)

Phenytoin

Phenylephrine

Sulfamethoxazole/Trimethoprim (*Bactrim*)

Store at Room Temperature ("excursions" to cold storage permitted, but not required)

Dexmedetomidine (*Precedex*)

Enoxaparin (*Lovenox*)

Propofol (*Diprivan*)

Stability is Affected by Time, Temperature, Light, Agitation

A drug that is "stable" at room temperature will be stable only for a certain time, at a certain temperature and with a certain degree of light exposure.

<u>The longer the time a drug is in solution increases the likelihood that a chemical reaction will occur</u>. Compatibility concern due to longer infusion times has become an important issue in recent years with <u>piperacillin/tazobactam (Zosyn) continuous infusions</u>. *Zosyn* is also commonly used with shorter, intermittent infusions (which cause less interaction issues). The longer infusion period is used to obtain a higher MIC in order to counter drug resistance with some of the common nosocomial pathogens, including *Pseudomonas*, *Enterobacter* and *Acinetobacter*. The higher MIC is beneficial, but the other side to consider is that the longer infusion times result in more significant compatibility issues with some of the many other drugs that the hospitalized pa-

tient is receiving. Interactions with piperacillin/tazobactam, azithromycin, ciprofloxacin, tobramycin, vancomycin, other antibiotics, insulin, chemotherapeutics and vasopressors are more common with this type of administration.

Higher temperatures promote chemical reactions, which is why the majority of IV drugs are kept cold (refrigerated) in order to extend the time that the drug is stable. There are exceptions; for example, furosemide crystallizes if kept cold and is stored at room temperature. IV drugs that are not refrigerated are listed in the table.

Light exposure causes photo-degradation that can destroy the drug and in some cases will increase the toxicity. Light sensitive drugs either come in light-resistant packaging or can be protected (by the pharmacy staff, after preparation) with an amber light-sensitive cover that is placed over the IV container. Additionally, in some cases, light-protective tubing (generally amber colored) is required. The table includes "photosensitive" drugs that require light-protection after the drug is prepared in solution.

Agitation destroys some drugs, particularly proteins. Drugs that are easily destroyed include alteplase, immune globulins, insulins, rasburicase and some vaccines, including zoster. Quinupristin/dalfopristin (Synercid), etanercept (Enbrel) vials (and a few other drugs) are swirl only (when reconstituting), which makes foam; do not shake. Wait for the foam to dissolve.

COMMON DRUGS THAT REQUIRE LIGHT PROTECTION DURING ADMINISTRATION

Abatacept (Orencia)	Doxycycline	Levothyroxine	Promethazine
Argatroban	Epinephrine – Oxidation turns drug pink, then a brown color. Do not use if discolored or contains a precipitate.	Linezolid (Zyvox)	Sulfamethoxazole/ Trimethoprim (Bactrim)
Belimumab (Benlysta)		Metronidazole (Flagyl)	Thiamine
Bumetanide, Furosemide		Morphine	Thiotepa (Tepadina)
Buprenorphine (Buprenex)	Epoprostenol (Flolan)	Micafungin (Mycamine)	Verapamil
Butorphanol	Esomeprazole (Nexium I.V.)	Natalizumab (Tysabri)	
Chlorpromazine – A slightly yellowed solution does not indicate potency loss, but a markedly discolored solution should be discarded.	Isoproterenol (Isuprel) – Exposure to air, light, or increased temperature may cause a pink to brownish pink color to develop.	Nicardipine (Cardene IV)	**Oncology**
		Nitroprusside (Nitropress)	Anthracyclines
			Dacarbazine
		Norepinephrine (Levophed)	Irinotecan
Dopamine – Do not use if darker than slightly yellow.	Ketamine (Ketalar)	Pentamidine	
		Octreotide (Sandostatin)	
	Ketorolac	Phytonadione (vitamin K)	

IV Drug Discoloration. What Does it Mean?

In some cases, not much. In most cases, discoloration indicates oxidation or another type of decomposition. Here are some examples:

- Nitroprusside – Light causes decomposition, which is visible as an orange, dark brown or blue liquid. A blue color indicates almost complete decomposition. If discolored, do not use.

- Chlorpromazine, dopamine – a slightly yellowed color is acceptable, but <u>anything darker</u> than light yellow is not.

- Dacarbazine – Turns pink if drug has decomposed; do not use.

- Norepinephrine – <u>Oxidation</u> turns the liquid <u>brown</u>. If discolored, do not use.

- Epinephrine – <u>Oxidation</u> turns the liquid pink, then <u>brown</u>. If discolored, do not use.

- Isoproterenol – If the liquid turns pink or darker, do not use.

- Morphine – If the solution is dark, do not use.

- Tigecycline – reconstituted solution is yellow/orange, do not use if green/black.

<u>And the opposite</u>: Do not use the antidote *Cyanokit* if the solution is not dark red.

What About "Particulate" Matter in the Solution?

Do not inject particles; do not use. Drugs in solution decompose faster than other formulations. The clinician (or the patient if using a self-injectable) should be instructed to check for color changes and for particulate matter and discard if present.

22

CRITICAL CARE & FLUIDS/ ELECTROLYTES

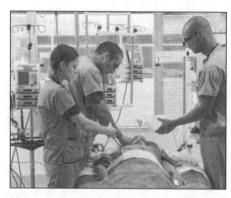

We gratefully acknowledge the assistance of Stacy A. Voils, PharmD, MSc, BCPS, Clinical Assistant Professor at the University of Florida College of Pharmacy, in preparing this chapter.

BACKGROUND

Medicine can be divided into chronic care (ideally at home), acute care (in the hospital on a general floor) and critical care. Critical care usually takes place in an intensive care unit (ICU) where patients have life-threatening injuries or illnesses like car accidents, serious infections, and breathing problems that require mechanical ventilation. Special equipment needed to take care of the patient is in the patient's room. Large hospitals have specialized ICUs for certain types of patients: surgical, cardiovascular, trauma, pediatric, neonatal, etc. Patients in the ICU receive most of their medications by the intravenous (IV) route. This avoids gut/absorption issues and allows for easy titration and access when the patient is sedated. Although patients in the ICU are very sick, many recover and eventually go home. The ICU mortality rate in the U.S. is ~15%. This chapter addresses conditions that are common in the ICU.

IV FLUIDS

Hospitalized patients frequently receive IV fluids to replace losses and treat various conditions requiring intravascular volume replacement. For instance, IV fluids are considered first line therapy for patients with hypovolemic or distributive (e.g. septic) shock. There are 2 types of IV fluids: crystalloids and colloids.

Crystalloids And Colloids

Crystalloids contain various concentrations of sodium and/or dextrose that <u>pass freely</u> between <u>semipermeable membranes</u>. Most of the administered volume <u>does not remain</u> in the intravascular space (inside the blood vessels). It goes into the <u>extravascular</u> space or <u>interstitial</u> space. Crystalloids are <u>less costly</u> and generally have <u>fewer adverse reactions</u> than colloids. Some data suggest balanced (chloride-restrictive) solutions may be preferred in certain disease states like sepsis. The chloride load provided to ICU patients can be high enough to contribute to cell injury, including renal damage. Colloids are large molecules (typically protein or starch) dispersed in solutions that primarily remain in the intravascular space. Colloids provide greater intravascular volume expansion than equal volumes of crystalloids, but are more expensive and provide questionable clinical benefit over crystalloids.

FLUID	COMMENTS

Crystalloids

FLUID	COMMENTS
Dextrose 5% (D5W)*	Slightly hypotonic, equivalent to "free water"-crosses membranes easily, useful in dehydration
NaCl 0.9% (normal saline, NS)*	Isotonic, useful for fluid resuscitation, risk of hypernatremia and hyperchloremic metabolic acidosis
Lactated Ringer's (LR) Chloride-restrictive	Isotonic, contains NaCl, Na-lactate, KCl, CaCl. Lactate converted to bicarb to help correct acidosis, risk for hyperkalemia, equally effective to NS
Multiple electrolyte injection (*Plasma-Lyte A*, others) Chloride-restrictive	Isotonic, *Plasma-Lyte A* contains electrolytes and acetate (converted to bicarb to help correct acidosis), risk for hyperkalemia

Colloids

FLUID	COMMENTS
Albumin 5%, 25% (Albuked, Flexbumin, Albutein, AlbuRx, others)	Natural colloid, more expensive than hydroxyethyl starch or crystalloids with no evidence of superiority
	Remains in the extravascular space; useful with significant edema (5% albumin and 25% albumin are isotonic; 25% albumin pulls water into the intravascular space; do not use to replace albumin with low albumin states
	Prepare 5% albumin by diluting 25% albumin with normal saline, not sterile water (sterile water used as a diluent may cause hemolysis/renal damage due to hypotonicity), filter required
Dextran (Dextran 40, Dextran 70)	High risk for ADRs (urticaria, acute renal failure, increased bleeding time), can cause anaphylaxis, impairs hemostasis (sometimes used as an anticoagulant), used infrequently
Hydroxyethyl starch (Hespan, Hextend)	Semi-synthetic colloid, can cause anaphylaxis, impairs coagulation/platelets, not recommended in sepsis

*There are various crystalloid combinations including: D5NS, D51/2NS, 1/2NS

CONDITIONS AND CONCERNS IN THE ICU

Shock Syndromes

GUIDELINE

Dellinger RP, Levy MM, Rhodes A, et al. Surviving Sepsis Campaign: international guidelines for management of severe sepsis and septic shock: 2012. *Crit Care Med.* 2013; 41(2):580-637.

Shock is a medical emergency characterized by hypoperfusion and usually hypotension (SBP < 90 mmHg). Shock can be the final result of many medical conditions including MI, anaphylaxis, sepsis, pulmonary embolism, and others. There are four main types: 1) Hypovolemic (e.g., hemorrhagic), 2) Cardiogenic, 3) Distributive (e.g., septic), and 4) Obstructive (e.g., massive pulmonary embolism). Fluid resuscitation with crystalloids or colloids is generally recommended as first-line therapy in patients with hypovolemic shock. Blood products may also be appropriate in these patients. If the patient does not respond to this fluid challenge, then vasopressor therapy should be initiated. Vasopressors will not be effective without adequate fluids (at least 30 mL/kg). Patients with cardiogenic shock require the use of vasopressors and/or inotropes. Sepsis is the presence of an infection with Systemic Inflammatory Response Syndrome (SIRS). Septic shock is the development of IV fluid-resistant hypotension in a patient with sepsis, and typically requires vasopressor administration. The mortality rate of septic shock is 30-50%; prompt interventions are necessary. These patients also require immediate infection source control (such as surgery) and antibiotic administration within an hour of presentation, and may be given corticosteroids.

Vasopressors work via vasoconstriction (think "pressing down on the vasculature") and therefore they increase systemic vascular resistance (SVR). This raises the blood pressure. Phenylephrine is a pure alpha agonist that increases SVR without increasing heart rate. Epinephrine and norepinephrine are mixed alpha and beta agonists. Norepinephrine is considered the vasopressor of choice in septic shock, while epinephrine is a mainstay in advanced cardiac life support and anaphylactic shock states. Dopamine is a natural precursor of norepinephrine that stimulates different receptors depending on the dose (see table). High doses of dopamine are required to stimulate alpha receptors and exert vasopressor effects. At medium doses, dopamine stimulates beta-1 receptors and acts as a positive inotrope along with other actions. At low doses, dopamine stimulates D_1 receptors in the kidney causing vasodilation.

Inotropes work by increasing contractility of the heart. Dobutamine is a beta-agonist and increases heart rate and force of contraction, which increases cardiac output. Milrinone is a selective phosphodiesterase-3 inhibitor in cardiac and vascular tissue. It produces inotropic effects with vasodilation and less chronotropic effect (less of an effect on heart rate) compared to dobutamine. The vasodilatory properties of milrinone make it more suitable for treatment of acute decompensated heart failure and cardiogenic shock than other shock syndromes. Drugs used for shock are also used for advanced cardiac life support, hypotension during surgery/anesthesia, and acute decompensated heart failure.

Vasopressors & Inotropes Used in Shock Syndromes

DRUG	DOSING/MOA	SAFETY/SIDE EFFECTS/MONITORING

Vasopressors: Obtain central line for administration as quickly as possible.

DRUG	DOSING/MOA	SAFETY/SIDE EFFECTS/MONITORING
DOPamine	**Low dose: D1 agonist** 1-3 mcg/kg/min **Med dose: Beta-1 agonist** 5-10 mcg/kg/min **High dose: Alpha-1 agonist** 10-20 mcg/kg/min	**BOXED WARNING** Dopamine, norepinephrine, and epinephrine (IV): vesicants, if extravasation occurs, treat with phentolamine **SIDE EFFECTS** Arrhythmias, tachycardia (especially with dopamine and epinephrine), bradycardia (with phenylephrine), tachyphylaxis, peripheral/gut ischemia, necrosis (gangrene), hyperglycemia (epinephrine)
EPINEPHrine (*Adrenalin*)	**Alpha-1, beta-1, beta-2 agonist** 0.1-0.5 mcg/kg/min	**MONITORING** Requires continuous BP monitoring, HR, MAP, urine output, infusion site for extravasation
Norepinephrine (*Levophed*)	**Alpha-1 agonist > beta-1 agonist** 0.1-3 mcg/kg/min	**NOTES** Epinephrine used for IV route is 0.1 mg/mL or 1:10,000 ratio strength. Epinephrine used for the IM route is 1:1,000 ratio strength. Phenylephrine: Do not refrigerate. Norepinephrine: Protect from light.
Phenylephrine (*Vazculep*)	**Alpha-1 agonist** 0.5 mcg/kg/min	Solutions should not be used if they are discolored or contain a precipitate. Dopamine renal dosing is not considered beneficial for kidney protection.
Vasopressin (*Vasostrict*)	**Vasoconstrictor, no inotropic or chronotropic effects** 0.01-0.03 units/min for septic shock; cardiac arrest: 40 units x 1 Vesicant; use central line, treat extravasation with phentolamine	**SIDE EFFECTS** Arrhythmias, necrosis/gangrene. Doses > 0.04 units/min cause more cardiovascular side effects (asystole, MI); hyponatremia **MONITORING** BP, HR, CO, ECG, fluid balance, sodium concentration **NOTES** Taper dose to avoid rebound hypertension.

Inotropes

DRUG	DOSING/MOA	SAFETY/SIDE EFFECTS/MONITORING
DOBUTamine	**Beta-1 agonist, beta-2 agonist (weak)** 2-20 mcg/kg/min	**SIDE EFFECTS** Dobutamine: hypotension, premature ventricular beats, tachycardia, angina Milrinone: ventricular arrhythmias, supraventricular arrhythmias, hypotension
Milrinone	**Phosphodiesterase-3 (PDE3) inhibitor** 0.125-0.75 mcg/kg/min; may consider a 50 mcg/kg loading dose (loading dose often omitted due to propensity to cause hypotension)	**MONITORING** Requires continuous BP monitoring, HR, ECG, CVP, MAP, urine output, LFTs and renal function (with milrinone) **NOTES** Milrinone: dose must be reduced for renal dysfunction. Because of risk of hypotension, dobutamine may be used for inotropic effect only after adequate perfusion is achieved. Dobutamine and milrinone often referred to as "inodilators". Dobutamine may turn slightly pink due to oxidation, but potency is not lost.

Treatment of Extravasation

Vasopressors are vesicants that cause severe tissue damage/necrosis with extravasation. This is a medical emergency. For all, treat with phentolamine, an alpha-adrenergic blocker that antagonizes the effects of the vasopressor. Due to this risk dopamine vials are diluted and given in a central line. If extravasation occurs with norepinephrine, epinephrine or phenylephrine, stop the infusion but do not disconnect the needle/canula and do not flush the line. Gently aspirate out the drug.

GUIDELINE

Barr J, Fraser GL, Puntillo K, et al. Clinical practice guidelines for the management of pain, agitation, and delirium in adult patients in the intensive care unit. *Crit Care Med.* 2013; 41(1):263-306.

Pain, Agitation and Delirium in the ICU

Pain, agitation and delirium (PAD) are so inseparable in the ICU that they have a single abbreviation to represent them.

Pain

IV opioids (such as morphine and fentanyl) are first-line for analgesia (to reduce pain) in the ICU, but the principles of pain management are the same for all patients (see Pain chapter for a full discussion of the opioids). The pharmacokinetic properties of the drug and the renal/hepatic function of the patient will dictate the choice of agent, because all IV opioids exhibit similar analgesic efficacy. Adjuvants (acetaminophen, NSAIDs, others) may be appropriate depending on the type of pain. Assessment of pain (with a validated scale) will be performed as frequently as every 2-4 hours in the ICU, and all ICU patients should be evaluated for pain at rest.

Agitation

Sedation (to reduce distress, fear and anxiety) is necessary in most ICU patients to maintain synchronized breathing if on a ventilator (prevent "bucking" the ventilator), and to limit suffering in the harsh ICU environment. Agitation is managed with benzodiazepines (lorazepam, midazolam) and/or hypnotics (propofol, dexmedetomidine). Nonbenzodiazepines (propofol and dexmedetomidine) are associated with improved ICU outcomes, shorted duration of mechanical ventilation, and ↓ length of stay (LOS), though they are more expensive than benzodiazepines. Dexmedetomidine *(Precedex)* is the only sedative approved for use in non-intubated patients. Benzodiazepines will always have an important role in sedation of the ICU patient with seizures or alcohol/benzodiazepine withdrawal. Benzodiazepines are discussed in more detail in Anxiety chapter.

Sedatives are used with validated sedation scales that allow for titration to light or deep sedation. Light sedation (unless contraindicated) is associated with improved outcomes. Some commonly used sedation scales include the Richmond Agitation Sedation Scale (RASS – see figure), the Ramsay Agitation Scale (RAS), and the Riker Sedation-Agitation Scale (SAS). Patients are generally monitored every 2-3 hours while receiving a sedation protocol to make sure they are receiving the minimal amount of drug(s) to keep them calm and pain-free. Many ICUs have sedation protocols that are based on validated assessment tools. Daily interruptions of continuous infusions of sedative drugs ("sedation vacations") are used to assess the readiness to wean off the sedative and to stop the drip as soon as medically feasible.

Richmond Agitation and Sedation Scale (RASS)

SCORE	TERM	DESCRIPTION
+4	Combative	Overtly combative, violent, immediate anger to staff
+3	Very agitated	Pulls or removes tube(s) or catheter(s); aggressive
+2	Agitated	Frequent non-purposeful movement, fights ventilator
+1	Restless	Anxious but movements not aggressive, vigorous
0	Alert and calm	
-1	Drowsy	Not fully alert, but has sustained awakening (eye opening/eye contact) to voice (≥ 10 seconds)
-2	Light sedation	Briefly awakens with eye contact to voice (< 10 seconds)
-3	Moderate sedation	Movement or eye opening to voice (but no eye contact)
-4	Deep sedation	No response to voice, but movement or eye opening to physical stimulation
-5	Unarousable	No response to voice or physical stimulation

Delirium

Delirium affects up to 80% of ventilated ICU patients and is associated with ↑ mortality and ↑ LOS. Delirium assessment is required. Early mobilization and control of the patient's environment (light, noise, stimuli) is recommended to ↓ incidence of delirium, but no medications are recommended for prevention. There is little evidence to support the use of haloperidol for treatment of ICU delirium, although this practice is commonplace. Atypical antipsychotics (primarily quetiapine, which is mildly sedating and has little risk for movement disorders) can be useful. Providing sedation with dexmedetomidine as opposed to benzodiazepines may ↓ incidence of delirium and shorten the duration in patients who already have it. Antipsychotics are discussed in more detail in the Schizophrenia/Psychosis chapter.

Agents for Pain, Agitation, and Delirium (PAD) in the ICU

DRUG	DOSING	SAFETY/SIDE EFFECTS/MONITORING

Sedation/Agitation

DRUG	DOSING	SAFETY/SIDE EFFECTS/MONITORING
LORazepam (Ativan, LORazepam Intensol)	LD: 0.02-0.04 mg/kg IV push (max 2 mg) MD: 0.02-0.06 mg/kg IV Q2-6H PRN or an infusion 0.01-0.1 mg/kg/hr (max 10 mg/hr)	See Anxiety chapter. In critical care patients monitor BP, HR and sedation scale. Benzodiazepine use to control delirium should be limited.

DRUG	DOSING	SAFETY/SIDE EFFECTS/MONITORING
Midazolam Benzodiazepine used specifically in acute care settings, injection only	LD: 0.01-0.05 mg/kg IV push MD: 0.02-0.1 mg/kg/hr IV Shorter acting than lorazepam if patient has preserved organ function (no hepatic or renal impairment or CHF) Highly lipophilic and can accumulate in obese patients Active metabolite that accumulates in renal dysfunction (caution with continuous infusion) Major 3A4 substrate; caution/lower dose if used with 3A4 inhibitors	**BOXED WARNINGS (3)** May cause severe respiratory depression, respiratory arrest, or apnea. Start at lower end of dosing range in debilitated patients and geriatric population. Do not administer by rapid IV injection in neonates. **CONTRAINDICATIONS** Intrathecal or epidural administration due to benzoyl alcohol in the formulation, acute narrow angle glaucoma, concurrent use of potent CYP450 3A4 inhibitors **SIDE EFFECTS** Respiratory depression, apnea, oversedation, hypotension **MONITORING** BP, HR, sedation scale
Propofol *(Diprivan)* FDA permits importation of propofol formulation *Fresenius Propoven* due to drug shortage	Initial Infusion: 5 mcg/kg/min IV, ↑ by 5-10 mcg/kg/min until desired level of sedation achieved MD: 5-50 mcg/kg/min IV In oil-in-water emulsion (provides 1.1 kcal/mL)	**CONTRAINDICATIONS** Hypersensitivity to egg, egg product, soy and soy product **SIDE EFFECTS** Hypotension, apnea, hypertriglyceridemia, green urine/hair/nail beds, propofol-related infusion syndrome (PRIS – rare but can be fatal) myoclonus, pancreatitis, pain on injection (particularly peripheral vein) **MONITORING** BP, respiration, triglycerides (if administered longer than 2 days), signs and symptoms of pancreatitis, sedation scale **NOTES** Shake well before use. Use strict aseptic technique due to potential for bacterial growth. Discard vial and tubing within 12 hours of use. If transferred to a syringe prior to administration, must discard syringe within 6 hours. Do not use if there is separation of phases in the emulsion. Do not use filter of < 5 micron for administration. Does not require refrigeration.
Dexmedetomidine *(Precedex)* Alpha-2 adrenergic agonist Used for sedation in intubated and non-intubated patients; patients are arousable and alert when stimulated (less respiratory depression than other sedatives)	LD: 0.5-1 mcg/kg IV over 10 minutes (may be omitted) MD: 0.2-1.5 mcg/kg/hr IV for 24 hours Duration of infusion should not exceed 24 hours	**WARNINGS** Use with caution in patients with hepatic impairment, diabetes, heart block, bradycardia, severe ventricular dysfunction, hypovolemia or chronic hypertension **SIDE EFFECTS** Transient hypertension during loading dose (may need to ↓ infusion rate), hypotension, bradycardia, dry mouth, nausea **MONITORING** BP, HR, sedation scale **NOTES** Does not require refrigeration.

Agents for Pain, Agitation, and Delirium (PAD) in the ICU Continued

DRUG	DOSING	SAFETY/SIDE EFFECTS/MONITORING
Etomidate (*Amidate*) Nonbarbiturate hypnotic Ultra short-acting; used as an induction agent for anesthesia Minimal cardiovascular effects	Initial: 0.2-0.6 mg/kg IV over 30-60 seconds, then 5-20 mcg/kg/min	**WARNING** Inhibits 11-B-hydroxylase which can lead to ↓ cortisol production for up to 24 hours **MONITORING** Monitor for adrenal insufficiency (hypotension, hyperkalemia), respiratory status, BP, HR, infusion site, sedation scale
Ketamine (*Ketalar*) NMDA receptor antagonist	1-4.5 mg/kg IV over 0.5 mg/kg/min (may follow with continuous infusion) Pretreatment with benzodiazepine can ↓ incidence of emergence reactions (see warnings) by 50%.	**WARNINGS** Emergence reactions (vivid dreams, hallucinations, delirium), cerebrospinal fluid (CSF) pressure elevation, respiratory depression/apnea, may cause dependence/tolerance **MONITORING** BP, HR, respiratory status, emergence reactions, sedation scale **NOTES** Used as an induction agent for anesthesia. Protect from light.

Pain/Analgesia

DRUG	DOSING	SAFETY/SIDE EFFECTS/MONITORING
Morphine	LD: 2-4 mg IV push MD: 2-30 mg/hr	See Pain chapter. In critical care patients monitor BP, HR, respiration, pain and sedation.
FentaNYL	LD: 25-35 mcg slow IV push (for ~70 kg patient) MD: 0.7-10 mcg/kg/hr	See above. Less hypotension than morphine due to no histamine release. Fast onset of action and short duration of action (half-life increases with duration of infusion). 100 times more potent than morphine. Preferred if unstable hemodynamics. Can accumulate in hepatic impairment; 3A4 substrate and potential for numerous drug interactions.
HYDROmorphone (*Dilaudid*)	LD: 0.2-0.6 mg IV push MD: 0.5-3 mg/hr	See Pain chapter. In critical care patients monitor BP, HR, respiration, pain and sedation. Potent; dose carefully.
Remifentanil (*Ultiva*)	LD: 1.5 mcg/kg over 1 min MD: 0.5-15 mcg/kg/hr	See Pain chapter. In critical care patients monitor BP, HR, respiration, pain and sedation.

Delirium

DRUG	DOSING	SAFETY/SIDE EFFECTS/MONITORING
Haloperidol (*Haldol*)	0.5-10 mg IV push at 5 mg/minute; may repeat Q15-30 minutes until calm, then administer 25% of last dose Q6H	See Schizophrenia/Psychosis chapter. Not recommended for treatment of delirium in recent guidelines.
QUEtiapine (*SEROquel*)	50 mg PO Q12H; may increase by 50-100 mg/day every 24 hours up to 200 mg Q12H	See Schizophrenia/Psychosis chapter. May decrease duration of delirium.

RISK FACTORS FOR THE DEVELOPMENT OF STRESS ULCERS
Mechanical ventilation
Coagulopathy
Sepsis
Traumatic brain injury
Burn patients
Acute renal failure
High dose corticosteroids

Stress Ulcer Prophylaxis

Stress ulcers can result from the metabolic stress experienced by a patient in an ICU. Patients with critical illness have reduced blood flow to the gut as blood flow is diverted to the major organs of the body. This results in a breakdown of gastric mucosal defense mechanisms including prostaglandin synthesis, bicarbonate production and cell turnover.

Histamine-2 receptor antagonists (H_2RAs) and proton pump inhibitors (PPIs) are the recommended agents for prevention of stress-related mucosal damage. H_2RAs can cause thrombocytopenia and mental status changes in the elderly or those with renal/hepatic impairment. Tachyphylaxis (tolerance) has also been reported. PPIs have been associated with an increased risk of GI infections *(C. difficile)*, fractures and nosocomial pneumonia. These agents are discussed in the GERD and PUD chapters. Patients without risk factors for stress ulcers should not receive stress ulcer prophylaxis (see risk factors in the box).

ADDITIONAL DRUGS USED IN THE ICU/OR

COMMONLY USED ANESTHETICS
Topical, local – lidocaine *(Xylocaine)*, benzocaine
Inhaled – desflurane *(Suprane)*, sevoflurane *(Ultane)*, isoflurane *(Forane)*, nitrous oxide, others
Injectable – bupivacaine *(Marcaine, Sensorcaine)*, lidocaine *(Xylocaine)*, ropivacaine *(Naropin)*, others

Anesthetics

Anesthetics are used for a variety of effects including numbing of an area (local anesthesia), to block pain (regional anesthesia), or to cause a reversible loss of consciousness and sleepiness during surgery (general anesthesia). Anesthetics can be given via several routes of administration: topical, inhaled, intravenous, epidural or spinal. Increasingly, anesthetics are being used concomitantly with opioids to reduce the opioid requirement for pain control. They work by blocking the initiation and conduction of nerve impulses by decreasing the neuronal permeability to sodium ions. Patients receiving anesthetics must be continuously monitored (vital signs and respiration).

The main side effects of anesthetics include hypotension, bradycardia, nausea and vomiting and a mild drop in body temperature that can cause shivering. Overdose can cause respiratory depression. Allergic reactions are possible. Inhaled anesthetics can rarely cause malignant hyperthermia (MH). See side bar for some commonly used anesthetics. Epidurals containing bupivacaine can quickly be fatal if given via the intravenous route. Do not give bupivacaine epidurals via IV infusion. ISMP has issued warnings about topical lidocaine absorption (up to 35%) when applied to mucous membranes during bronchoscopy – avoid using dual routes of administration (IV and topical).

Neuromuscular Blocking Agents (NMBAs)

These agents cause skeletal muscle paralysis. Patients can require the use of a paralytic agent to facilitate mechanical intubation, i.e., rapid sequence intubation (RSI), manage increased intracranial pressure, treat muscle spasms (tetany) and prevent shivering in patients undergoing therapeutic hypothermia after cardiac arrest. The use of NMBAs is typically recommended when other methods have proven ineffective; they are not to be routinely used in critically ill patients. These agents do not provide sedation or analgesia. Therefore, patients should receive adequate sedation and analgesia prior to starting a NMBA. Patients must be mechanically ventilated as these agents paralyze the diaphragm. These are considered high risk medications by ISMP. All NMBAs should be labeled with bright red auxiliary labels stating "WARNING, PARALYZING AGENT".

There are 2 types of NMBAs – depolarizing and non-depolarizing. Succinylcholine is the only available depolarizing agent and is typically reserved for intubation. It is not used for continuous neuromuscular blockade. Succinylcholine has been rarely associated with causing malignant hyperthermia (particularly with the use of inhaled anesthetics). Resembling acetylcholine, succinylcholine binds to and activates the acetylcholine receptors and desensitizes them. The non-depolarizing NMBAs work by binding to the acetylcholine receptor and blocking the actions of endogenous acetylcholine.

DRUG	SAFETY/SIDE EFFECTS/MONITORING

Non-depolarizing NMBAs

For all non-depolarizing NMBAs	**SIDE EFFECTS** Flushing, bradycardia, hypotension, tachyphylaxis, acute quadriplegic myopathy syndrome (AQMS) with long-term use **MONITORING** Peripheral nerve stimulator to assess depth of paralysis during continuous infusions [also called train-of-four (TOF)], vital signs (BP, HR, RR)
Atracurium	Short t½; intermediate acting; metabolized by Hofmann elimination (independent of renal and hepatic function)
Cisatracurium (Nimbex)	Short t½; intermediate acting; metabolized by Hofmann elimination (independent of renal and hepatic function)
Pancuronium	Long-acting agent, can accumulate in renal or hepatic dysfunction, ↑ HR
Rocuronium (Zemuron)	Intermediate-acting agent
Vecuronium	Intermediate-acting agent; can accumulate in renal or hepatic dysfunction

Depolarizing NMBA

Succinylcholine (Anectine, Quelicin, Quelicin-1000)	Short-acting, fast onset (30-60 seconds)

Hemostatic Agents

The term "hemostasis" means causing bleeding to stop. A variety of hemostatic methods can be used, ranging from simple manual pressure with one finger to electrical tissue cauterization, or the systemic administration of blood products (transfusions) or "hemostatic" agents. The systemic hemostatic drugs work by inhibiting fibrinolysis or enhancing coagulation.

Several factor products are available to treat hemorrhage in patients with hemophilia. One of the hemostatic drugs, prothrombin complex concentrate (PCC – *KCentra)*, is an approved agent for warfarin overdose.

Systemic Hemostatic Agents

DRUG	SAFETY/SIDE EFFECTS/MONITORING
Aminocaproic acid *(Amicar)* Tablet, solution, injection	**CONTRAINDICATIONS** Disseminated intravascular coagulation (without heparin); evidence of an active intravascular clotting process **SIDE EFFECTS** Injection-site reactions, thrombosis **NOTES** FDA-approved for excessive bleeding associated with cardiac surgery, liver cirrhosis, and urinary fibrinolysis. Do not use if active clotting process, do not give with factor IX complex concentrates due to ↑ risk for thrombosis.
Tranexamic acid *(Cyklokapron, injectable)* *(Lysteda, oral)*	**CONTRAINDICATIONS** IV: acquired defective color vision, active intravascular clotting, subarachnoid hemorrhage Oral: previous or current thromboembolic disease, current use of combination hormonal contraception **SIDE EFFECTS** Injection: vascular occlusion, thrombosis Oral: retinal clotting *Lysteda* (oral) is approved for menstrual heavy bleeding (menorrhagia). The injection is approved for bleeding with hemophilia and is often used off-label to control surgical bleeding.
Recombinant Factor VIIa *(NovoSeven RT)* Injection	**BOXED WARNING** Risk of thrombotic events, particularly when used off-label **NOTES** FDA-approved for hemophilia and factor VII deficiency; has been used successfully for patients with hemorrhage from trauma and warfarin-related bleeding events.
Factor eight inhibitor bypassing activity *(FEIBA NF)* Injection Contains Factors II, IX, X (non-activated) and VIII (activated); contains no heparin	**CONTRAINDICATIONS** Disseminated intravascular coagulation (DIC); acute thrombus or embolism including myocardial infarction, patients with normal coagulation mechanisms, bleeding episodes from factor deficiencies in the absence of inhibitors to Factor VIII or IX **WARNING** Thrombotic and thromboembolic events (esp. with high doses and in patients with thrombotic risk factors)
Factor IX complex *(Bebulin, Bebulin VH, Profilnine SD)*, Injection	**WARNINGS** Thromboembolic events, DIC, anaphylaxis/hypersensitivity, transmission of infectious agents **NOTES** Contains Factors II, IX, and X (low or non-therapeutic level of Factor VIII and a small amount of heparin)
Prothrombin complex concentrate or PCC *(KCentra)* Injection	See Anticoagulation chapter. Contains Factors II, VII, IX, X, Protein C & S and a small amount of heparin.

Topical Agents: There are many and most are used surgically. These include thrombin in bandages, liquids and spray forms, fibrin sealants, acrylates and a few others (names often include "throm": _Recothrom, Evithrom)_. A few topical hemostats are OTC.

Intravenous Immunoglobulin (IVIG)

Intravenous immune globulin (IVIG or IGIV) contains pooled immunoglobulin (IgG), administered intravenously. The IgG is extracted from the plasma of a thousand or more blood donors (this is the FDA's minimum; typically the IVIG is derived from between 3,000-10,000 donors). IVIG is given as a plasma protein replacement therapy (IgG) for immune deficient patients who have decreased or abolished antibody production capabilities. Initially, IVIG was used only for immunodeficiency conditions. Currently, IVIG has several FDA-approved indications and is used for a variety of off-label indications, with varying results.

DRUG	DOSING	SAFETY/SIDE EFFECTS/MONITORING
Intravenous immunoglobulin (Carimune NF, Bivigam, Flebogamma, **Flebogamma DIF**, **Gammagard**, Gammagard S/D, Gammaked, Gammaplex, **Gamunex-C**, **Octagam**, Privigen)	400 mg/kg – 2,000 mg/ kg per IV infusion; dose and interval depend on indication. Use IBW to calculate dose Use slower infusion rate in renal and cardiovascular disease	**BOXED WARNINGS (2)** Acute renal dysfunction can rarely occur and has been associated with fatalities; usually within 7 days of use (more likely with products stabilized with sucrose). Use with caution in the elderly, patients with renal disease, diabetes mellitus, volume depletion, sepsis, paraproteinemia, and nephrotoxic medications due to risk of renal dysfunction. Thrombosis may occur with IVIG products even in the absence of risk factors. For patients at risk, administer at the minimum dose. Monitor all patients. **CONTRAINDICATIONS** IgA deficiency (can use product with lowest amount of IgA) **WARNINGS** Use with caution in patients with cardiovascular disease (use isotonic products and low infusion rate) **SIDE EFFECTS** Headache, nausea, diarrhea, injection site reaction, infusion reaction (facial flushing, chest tightness, fever, chills, hypotension – slow/stop infusion), renal failure or blood dyscrasias (both rare) **MONITORING** Renal function, urine output, volume status, Hgb **NOTES** Patients should be asked about past IVIG infusions, including product used and any reactions that occurred. The pharmacy must keep track of IVIG lot numbers used for each patient.

ELECTROLYTE DISORDERS

Critically ill patients are especially prone to electrolyte abnormalities which can also be present in other patients, including outpatients. Some of the drugs deplete electrolytes and cause acute deficiency. Some electrolyte abnormalities can be fatal when severe (seizures, cardiac arrhythmias, coma). Protocols to replace electrolytes should be followed in order to avoid toxicity. Electrolytes and their reference ranges are discussed in the Lab Values, Drug Monitoring, and Patient Charts chapter.

Sodium

Hyponatremia

Hyponatremia (Na^+ < 135 mEq/L) may develop from many causes and is usually not symptomatic until < 120 mEq/L unless the sodium falls rapidly. Hyponatremia is classified according to osmolality:

- <u>Hypertonic</u> – is a state in which serum osmolality is increased and is caused by hyperglycemia or use of hypertonic solutions that do not contain sodium.

- <u>Isotonic</u> – has normal osmolality and can be associated with hyperlipidemia.

- <u>Hypotonic – may occur with changes in volume status</u>:

  - Hypovolemic hyponatremia (diuretic use, salt-wasting syndromes, adrenal insufficiency, blood loss, vomiting/diarrhea). The treatment is typically to correct the underlying cause and to administer saline solutions.

  - Hypervolemic hyponatremia is caused by fluid overload, usually with cirrhosis, heart failure, or renal failure. Diuresis with fluid restriction is the preferred treatment.

  - Isovolemic (euvolemic) hyponatremia is usually caused by the syndrome of inappropriate antidiuretic hormone (SIADH). It is treated with fluid restriction or diuresis.

The <u>arginine vasopressin (AVP) receptor antagonists (conivaptan or tolvaptan)</u> may be used to treat <u>SIADH and hypervolemic hyponatremia</u>. They increase excretion of free water while maintaining sodium. The role for these agents is still being determined, as they are <u>more expensive than 3% saline</u> and use beyond 30 days with the oral product *(Samsca)* is not recommended.

DRUG	DOSE	SAFETY/SIDE EFFECTS/MONITORING
Conivaptan *(Vaprisol)* Injection Dual AVP antagonist (V1A and V2)	LD: 20 mg IV over 30 minutes MD: 20 mg IV continuous infusion over 24 hours. May increase to 40 mg IV daily if Na⁺ does not ↑ at desired rate. Do not exceed 4 days. Do not use if CrCl < 30 mL/min Reduce dose in moderate hepatic impairment	**CONTRAINDICATIONS** Allergy to corn/corn products, hypovolemic hyponatremia, concurrent use with strong 3A4 inhibitors, anuria **WARNING** Overly rapid correction of hyponatremia (> 12 mEq/L/24 hours) associated with osmotic demyelination syndrome (life-threatening) **SIDE EFFECTS** Orthostatic hypotension, fever, hypokalemia, infusion site reactions (> 60%) **MONITORING** Rate of Na⁺ increase, BP, volume status, urine output
Tolvaptan *(Samsca)* Tablet Selective AVP antagonist (V2)	15 mg PO daily; max 60 mg PO daily; for up to 30 days due to hepatotoxicity Not recommended if CrCl < 10 mL/min Avoid fluid restriction in first 24 hours of therapy	**BOXED WARNINGS (2)** Should be initiated and re-initiated in a hospital under close monitoring of serum Na⁺ Overly rapid correction of hyponatremia (> 12 mEq/L/24 hours) associated with osmotic demyelination syndrome (life-threatening) **CONTRAINDICATIONS** Patients who are unable to sense or respond appropriately to thirst, urgent need to raise Na⁺, hypovolemic hyponatremia, concurrent use with strong 3A4 inhibitors, anuria **WARNINGS** Hepatotoxicity (avoid use > 30 days and in liver disease/cirrhosis) **SIDE EFFECTS** Thirst, nausea, dry mouth, polyuria, weakness, hyperglycemia, hypernatremia **MONITORING** Rate of Na⁺ increase, BP, volume status, urine output; signs of drug-induced hepatotoxicity

Hypernatremia

Hypernatremia (Na⁺ > 145 mEq/L) is associated with a water deficit and hypertonicity.

- Hypovolemic is caused by dehydration, vomiting, diarrhea and is treated with fluids.

- Hypervolemic is caused by hypertonic and is treated with diuresis.

- Isovolemic (euvolemic) is frequently caused by diabetes insipidus (DI), which can ↓ antidiuretic hormone (ADH). It is treated with desmopressin.

Caution should be taken in treating patients with sodium disorders to prevent correcting too quickly. Corrections of sodium > 12 mEq/L over 24 hours can cause osmotic demyelination syndrome or central pontine myelinolysis, which can cause paralysis, seizures and death.

Potassium

Treatment of hyperkalemia is discussed in the Renal Disease and Dosing Considerations chapter. Hypokalemia (K^+ < 3.5 mEq/L) is a common occurrence in hospitalized patients. Management includes treating the underlying cause [e.g., metabolic alkalosis, overdiuresis, some medications (amphotericin, insulin)] and administering oral or IV potassium. The oral route is preferred when available. In most cases 100 mEq of potassium (oral or IV) raises potassium by 1 mEq/mL. In general, a drop of 1 mEq/L in serum K^+ below 3.5 mEq/L represents a total body deficit of 100 – 400 mEq. Hospitals use K^+ sliding scales that allow a healthcare provider (usually a nurse) to administer a certain dose of potassium based on various ranges of low serum K^+ (e.g., for K^+ 3.5 – 3.7 mEq/L, give 20 mEq KCl PO x 2 doses; for K^+ 3.3 – 3.4 mEq/L, give 20 mEq KCl PO x 3 doses). When hypokalemia is resistant to treatment, serum magnesium should be checked and replaced as needed. Magnesium is necessary for potassium uptake. IV potassium should be administered no faster than 10-20 mEq/hr with intermittent doses. Concentrations above 80 mEq/L should be administered through a central line. Potassium salt formulations are in the Heart Failure chapter.

Magnesium

Hypomagnesemia (Mg^{2+} < 1.3 mEq/L) is more common than hypermagnesemia. Common causes of hypomagnesemia include chronic alcohol use, diuretics, vomiting, and diarrhea. Hypermagnesemia is most commonly due to renal insufficiency. When serum Mg^{2+} is < 1 mEq/L with life-threatening symptoms (seizures or arrhythmias), IV replacement is recommended. When serum Mg^{2+} is < 1 mEq/L without life-threatening symptoms, therapy can be administered IV or IM. When serum Mg^{2+} is > 1 mEq/L and < 1.5 mEq/L, there are many options including oral replacement. Magnesium replacement regimens should continue for 5 days to fully replace body stores.

Phosphorous

Treatment of hyperphosphatemia is discussed in the Renal Disease and Dosing Considerations chapter. Hypophosphatemia is considered severe and usually symptomatic when serum PO_4 is < 1 mg/dL. Hypophosphatemia can be associated with phosphate-binding drugs (calcium, sevelamer, anatacids), chronic alcohol intake, and hyperparathyroidism. When serum PO_4 is < 1 mg/dL, IV phosphorus is used for replacement. Many regimens can be used, but 0.08 – 0.16 mmol/kg in 500 mL of NS over 6 hours is common. Patients must be carefully monitored and additional doses may be necessary. Patients with hypophosphatemia often have hypokalemia and hypomagnesemia that will require correction. Less severe hypophosphatemia can be treated orally and full replacement often takes one week or longer.

PRACTICE CASE

JL is a 65 y/o female in the ER with pneumonia. Over the past hour, she has had increasing difficulty breathing and oxygen saturation is not markedly improving with nasal administration of O_2. ER staff believes she will require admission to the ICU for intubation and mechanical ventilation. Past medical history includes COPD, chronic kidney disease, and diabetes.

Home Medications:
Lantus 30 units SC at HS
Novolog 5 units TID with meals
Lisinopril 10 mg daily
Symbicort 2 inhalations BID
Albuterol nebulizer PRN
Oxygen at 1 liter (delivered via home health company)

Labs:
Na (mEq/L) = 138 (135-145)
K (mEq/L) = 5.1 (3.5-5)
Cl (mEq/L) = 100 (95-103)
HCO_3 (mEq/L) = 33 (24-30)
BUN (mg/dL) = 24 (7-20)
SCr (mg/dL) = 1.7 (0.6-1.3)
Glucose (mg/dL) = 202 (100-125)
WBC (mm^3) = 14.6 (4,000-11,000)
Hgb (g/dL) = 11.2 (13.5-18 male, 12-16 female)
Hct (%) = 33.5 (38-50 male, 36-46 female)
Plt (mm^3) = 227,000 (150,000-450,000)
PMN (%) = 85 (45-73)
Bands (%) = 1 (3-5)
MCV (mm^3) = 78 (80-96)
RDW (%) = 15 (11.5-14.5)

Vitals and Tests:
BP: 138/87 HR: 98 RR: 25 Temp: 101.2°F O_2 Saturation on 1 liter = 92%
CXR: RML infiltrate

QUESTIONS

1. Based on this patient's past medical history, which of the following medications may accumulate and cause over sedation?

   a. Dexmedetomidine

   b. Lorazepam

   c. Midazolam

   d. Propofol

   e. Remifentanil

2. Propofol and fentanyl continuous IV infusions were started for this patient. What general principle is correct regarding management of these medications for this patient?

   a. Heavier sedation is preferred to minimize risk to staff

   b. Pain and sedation should be monitored with validated scales at least weekly

   c. Daily sedation vacations are recommended to minimize the dose of these medications

   d. Propofol may be sufficient as a single agent since it also has analgesic properties

   e. Benzodiazepines are preferred over propofol or dexmedetomidine because they cause less delirium

3. The patient's respiratory status worsened and she is now requiring cisatracurium to maintain adequate oxygenation. Which of the following is correct regarding the propofol and fentanyl?

   a. Propofol may be discontinued since the patient should not be agitated while receiving a neuromuscular blocking drug

   b. Fentanyl may be discontinued since pain should be well controlled while receiving a neuromuscular blocking drug

   c. Haloperidol should be added to propofol and fentanyl since cisatracurium may cause delirium

   d. Propofol and fentanyl should be continued and sedation and analgesia assessed prior and during cisatracurium therapy

   e. Propofol and fentanyl should be continued, but succinylcholine is a better choice of neuromuscular blocking drug for this patient

Questions 4-15 do not apply to the case.

4. Which of the following statements about colloids is/are true? (Select **ALL** that apply.)

   a. 0.9% sodium chloride is a colloid

   b. Approximately 25% of the volume of a colloid remains intravascularly after administration

   c. Colloids are significantly more expensive than crystalloids

   d. Patients receiving colloids have a higher risk of developing pulmonary edema compared to patients receiving crystalloids.

   e. 25% albumin is a colloid

5. Which of the following vasopressors is considered first-line in treating patients with sepsis?

   a. Norepinephrine

   b. Vasopressin

   c. Epinephrine

   d. Phenylephrine

   e. Ephedrine

6. Which of the following is an antidote for morphine overdose?

   a. Naloxone

   b. Sodium thiosulfate

   c. Flumazenil

   d. Protamine

   e. Deferoxamine

7. Which of the following statements is true regarding neuromuscular blocking agents?

   a. Cisatracurium is a non-depolarizing agent

   b. Patients receiving these drugs do not require sedation/analgesia

   c. These drugs should be used routinely in critically ill patients

   d. NMBAs are not associated with significant adverse effects

   e. NMBAs are monitored using the Ramsay agitation scale

8. Which of the following statements is true regarding dexmedetomidine?

    a. It causes respiratory depression
    b. It induces deep levels of sedation
    c. It may cause urine to turn green
    d. It is associated with more delirium compared to benzodiazepines
    e. It may cause bradycardia

9. What effect can be expected from dopamine at medium doses (5 – 10 mcg/kg/min)?

    a. Alpha-1 antagonist, vasoconstriction
    b. Alpha-1 agonist, vasoconstriction
    c. Beta-1 agonist, positive inotropic effect
    d. Beta-2 agonist, positive inotropic effect
    e. D1 agonist, vasodilation

10. Which of the following electrolyte disorders is conivaptan recommended to be used to treat?

    a. Hypovolemic hypotonic hyponatremia
    b. Euvolemic hyponatremia
    c. Hypervolemic hypernatremia
    d. Diabetes insipidus
    e. Euvolemic hypernatremia

11. How much of a change in sodium should be avoided in patients with sodium imbalances?

    a. > 4 mEq/L
    b. > 6 mEq/L
    c. > 10 mEq/L
    d. > 12 mEq/L
    e. > 20 mEq/L

12. Which of the following medications contains clotting Factors II, VII, XI, X, and Protein C & S?

    a. Amicar
    b. NovoSeven
    c. Cyklokapron
    d. Profilnine
    e. KCentra

13. Which of the following medications used for rapid sequence intubation may cause adrenal insufficiency?

    a. Midazolam
    b. Ketamine
    c. Succinylcholine
    d. Etomidate
    e. Cisatracurium

14. Which of the following medications used for ICU sedation has a high concentration of propylene glycol, which may lead to metabolic acidosis?

    a. Propofol
    b. Dexmedetomidine
    c. Lorazepam
    d. Haloperidol
    e. Midazolam

15. Which of the following is important to monitor before and during haloperidol administration for ICU delirium?

    a. Blood glucose
    b. Potassium
    c. Cortisol
    d. QT interval
    e. Lactate

Answers

1-a 2-c, 3-d, 4-c,e, 5-a, 6-a, 7-a, 8-e, 9-c, 10-b, 11-d, 12-e, 13-d, 14-c, 15-d

23

IMMUNIZATIONS

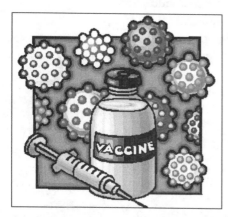

We gratefully acknowledge the assistance of Jeff Goad, PharmD, MPH, FAPhA, FCPhA, FCSHP, Chapman University School of Pharmacy, in preparing this chapter.

BACKGROUND

Immunizations in the United States over the past century are one of public health's greatest achievements. Since vaccines are medications, pharmacists should review immunization histories with patients. Vaccines prevent patients from acquiring serious or potentially fatal diseases. Many formerly prevalent childhood diseases (diphtheria, measles, meningitis, polio, tetanus) are rare because many children are vaccinated to prevent the illness, and others are protected by herd immunity (people around them are protected – thus they are less likely to catch the illness). If immunization rates drop below 85% to 95%, vaccine-preventable diseases may once again become common threats, as recent scattered pertussis outbreaks in the United States demonstrate.

GUIDELINES/REFERENCES

Immunization recommendations are written by the CDC Advisory Committee on Immunization Practices (ACIP) and the Committee on Infectious Diseases of the American Academy of Pediatrics (AAP). The pediatric and adult schedules are updated annually and published in January. Since the ACIP meets several times throughout the year to review new information, updates are published in Morbidity and Mortality Weekly Report (MMWR). Updated immunization schedules are available at www.cdc.gov.

The CDC's Pink Book, Epidemiology and Prevention of Vaccine Preventable Disease. is published every 2 years and is available at www.cdc.gov.

Helpful resources for immunizing pharmacists are available on the following three websites:

- www.pharmacist.com/imz (American Pharmacists Association)

- www.cdc.gov/vaccines (Centers for Disease Control and Prevention/Vaccines and Immunizations)

- www.immunize.org (Immunization Action Coalition)

Read through the background information before reviewing the individual vaccines. Immunization is currently taught in most pharmacy schools and has become standard pharmacy practice in many settings, especially in the community pharmacy. Principles of immunization should be well understood.

The <u>CDC Advisory Committee on Immunization Practices (ACIP)</u> develops written recommendations for the routine administration of vaccines to children and adults in the civilian population. The Immunization Action Coalition's website has useful information for clinicians, such as vaccine records and clinic tools.

Safety Concerns

Some parents withhold vaccines due to misconceptions about the risk of autism, a developmental disorder. There is <u>no evidence that vaccines cause autism</u>. Thimerosal, a mercury-containing preservative used in vaccines, was thought to be a possible cause since mercury has been linked to some brain disorders. Evidence does not suggest that thimerosal poses a risk for or is linked to autism. Thimerosal has been removed from most childhood vaccines. Others thought the risk was due to providing multiple vaccines concurrently at an early age. Although the autism rates have not decreased among communities with a high rate of vaccine refusal, there are parents who remain concerned. This will likely continue to be an issue until the causes of autism are better understood. Promoting vaccination requires open communication and education.

Usually, vaccine adverse effects are minor and include mild fever, soreness or swelling at the injection site. Some vaccines may cause headache, loss of appetite and dizziness – but these quickly dissipate. Very rarely, anaphylaxis can occur. Anyone giving vaccines must screen for previous reactions and be prepared to treat a severe reaction. Some vaccines have specific contraindications to use, such as a true egg allergy with the some of the influenza vaccines (this has been "softened" in recent years; see allergy discussion in this chapter), and with yellow fever and rabies vaccine.

<u>Federal law requires that patients receive the most up-to-date version of the Vaccine Information Statement (VIS) BEFORE EACH vaccine is administered</u>. The VIS standardized forms describe the risk and benefit of the vaccines, purpose of the vaccine, who should receive it and who should not, and what the patient can expect for both mild and serious adverse effects. VISs are created by the CDC and updated versions are available on the CDC and IAC websites.

Gelatin in Vaccines

Gelatin is used in some vaccines as a stabilizer, which is porcine-derived. For observant Muslims, Jews and Seventh Day Adventists who follow dietary rules that prohibit pork products, most religious leaders permit the use of gelatin-containing vaccines because the gelatin is injected, not ingested, and the end-product has been rendered pure.

Pharmacist's Role in Immunization

Pharmacists in the community setting have increased immunization rates, particularly by providing influenza, meningococcal, pneumococcal, pertussis (in Tdap) and herpes zoster (shingles) vaccinations. The pharmacist's role is expanding to include more vaccines and management of immunization clinics in health care settings. Pharmacists have become increasingly involved in pre-travel health services, providing travel advice, medications and immunizations per protocol for international travel. During comprehensive medication therapy management (MTM) sessions and in many inpatient and community pharmacy settings, pharmacists routinely screen and order vaccines (e.g., pneumococcal, Tdap, and influenza), per protocols.

Principles of Immunity

Immunity is the ability of the human body to tolerate the presence of material indigenous to the body ("self"), and to eliminate foreign ("nonself") material. This discriminatory ability provides protection from infectious disease, since most microbes are identified as foreign by the immune system. Immunity to a microbe is usually indicated by the presence of antibody to that organism. There are two basic mechanisms for acquiring immunity, active and passive.

Active and Passive Immunity

Active immunity is protection that is produced by the person's own immune system. This type of immunity is usually permanent. One way to acquire active immunity is to survive an infection. Another way to produce active immunity is by vaccination. Passive immunity is protection by antibody containing products produced by an animal or human and transferred to a human, usually by injection. This protection wanes with time, usually within a few weeks or months. The most common form of passive immunity is the antibodies an infant receives from the mother. Many types of blood products contain antibody, including intravenous immune globulin and plasma products.

Live Attenuated and Inactivated Vaccines

Live attenuated (weakened) vaccines are produced by modifying a disease-producing ("wild") virus or bacterium in a laboratory; they retain the ability to replicate (grow) and produce immunity, but usually do not cause illness. Administering live vaccines to immunocompromised patients may be contraindicated since uncontrolled replication of the pathogen could take place (see other chapters for immunization recommendations in specific populations, such as with HIV/AIDS). Live attenuated vaccines produce a strong immune response since the body's response to the vaccine is similar to actual disease.

Inactivated vaccines can be composed of either whole viruses or bacteria, or fractions of either. Antibody titers against inactivated antigens diminish with time. As a result, some inactivated vaccines may require periodic supplemental doses to increase, or "boost" antibody titers.

SEPARATION TIME BETWEEN LIVE VACCINES AND ANTIBODY-CONTAINING PRODUCTS

PRODUCT GIVEN FIRST	ACTION
Vaccine	Wait 2 weeks before giving antibody
Antibody	Wait 3 months or longer before giving vaccine

*Except zoster vaccine

General rule

The more similar a vaccine is to the disease-causing form of the organism, the better the immune response to the vaccine.

Timing and Spacing of Vaccines

Vaccines and antibody products may require a separation period. The presence of circulating antibody to a vaccine antigen may reduce or completely eliminate the immune response to the vaccine. The amount of interference produced by circulating antibody generally depends on the type of vaccine administered and the amount of antibody.

Inactivated antigens are generally not affected by circulating antibody, so they can be administered before, after, or at the same time as the antibody. Live vaccines, however, must replicate in order to cause an immune response and antibody against injected live vaccine antigen may interfere with replication. If the live vaccine is given first, it is necessary to wait at least 2 weeks (i.e., an incubation period) before giving the antibody.

The necessary interval between an antibody-containing blood product and MMR or varicella-containing vaccine (except zoster vaccine – this is not affected by circulating antibody) is a minimum of 3 months and may be up to 11 months. The specific blood product and dose administered determines the time interval. Consult "The Pink Book" to determine the specific recommended interval. During pregnancy maternal antibodies are passed from the mother to the baby and may reduce the subsequent live vaccine response in the baby. This is why live vaccines are withheld until the child is 12 months. Inactivated vaccines may be started at the age of 2 months, with the exception of Hepatitis B vaccine which can be started at birth.

Simultaneous administration of antibody (in the form of immune globulin) and vaccine is recommended for postexposure prophylaxis of certain diseases, such as hepatitis A and B, rabies and tetanus.

Simultaneous Administration

Administering the most common live or inactivated vaccines simultaneously (on the same day or at the same visit) does not decrease antibody responses and does not increase the rate of adverse reactions. Simultaneous administration of all vaccines for which a child is eligible is very important in childhood vaccination programs. It increases the probability that a child will be fully immunized at the appropriate age.

According to the ACIP, there are no contraindications to simultaneous administration of any of the vaccines currently available in the United States and every effort should be made to provide all necessary vaccinations at one visit to improve compliance.

Non-Simultaneous Administration of Different Vaccines

In some situations, vaccines that could be given at the same visit are not. If live injected vaccines (MMR, MMRV, varicella, zoster, and yellow fever) and live intranasal influenza vaccine (LAIV) are not administered at the same visit, they should be separated by at least 4 weeks.

Intervals of Doses between Vaccines given in Series

Increasing the interval between doses of a multidose vaccine does not diminish the effectiveness of the vaccine after completion of all doses. It may, however, delay more complete protection. Decreasing the interval between doses of a multidose vaccine may interfere with antibody response and protection.

INTERVAL FOR ADMINISTRATION OF LIVE VACCINES AND TB TEST

The tuberculin skin test (TST) is used to determine if a person is infected with Mycobacterium tuberculosis. The test is performed by injecting 0.1 ml of tuberculin purified protein derivative (PPD) into the inner surface of the forearm. Live vaccines can be administered on the same day and is the preferred method to avoid a false negative response to the skin test. Although a theoretical risk, interferon-gamma release assay (IGRA) tests (which may be used to detect TB infection) and live vaccines should be done on the same day or the IGRA drawn before administration of a live vaccine. If a live vaccine has been given recently (but not on the same day) as the PPD, wait 4 weeks before placing the PPD in order to avoid a false negative TB test result. False negative TB test results delay treatment of tuberculosis infection and are a significant risk to the patient and to public health. Alternatively, administer the PPD test first, then wait 48-72 hours and determine the PPD results before administering the live vaccine.

Vaccine Adverse Reactions

Vaccine adverse reactions fall into three general categories: local, systemic, and allergic. Local reactions are generally the least severe and most frequent. Allergic reactions can be the most severe, but are the least frequent.

The most common type of adverse reactions are local reactions, such as pain, swelling and redness at the site of injection. Local reactions may occur with up to 80% of vaccine doses, depending on the vaccine type. Local reactions are most common with inactivated vaccines, particularly those, such as DTaP, that contain an adjuvant. These reactions generally occur within a few hours of the injection and are usually mild and self-limited. Rarely, local reactions may be very exaggerated or severe.

Systemic adverse reactions are more generalized events and include fever, malaise, myalgias (muscle pain), headache, loss of appetite, and mild manifestations similar to the actual disease being prevented (such as a few chicken pox vesicles after receiving the varicella vaccine). These symptoms are common and may be nonspecific. Systemic adverse reactions following live vaccines are usually mild, and often occur 7–21 days after the vaccine was given (i.e., after an incubation period of the vaccine virus). Intranasal LAIV is cold adapted, meaning it can replicate in the cooler temperatures of upper airways (nose and throat) but not in the higher temperatures of the lower airways and the lungs. Mild cold-like symptoms such as a runny nose may occur.

A third type of vaccine adverse reaction is an allergic reaction. The allergic reaction may be caused by the vaccine antigen itself or some other component of the vaccine, such as cell culture material, stabilizer, preservative, or antibiotic used to inhibit bacterial growth. Minor allergic reactions are self-limited and can be treated with diphenhydramine. Minor allergic reactions are <u>not</u> a contraindication to subsequent vaccination. Severe allergic reactions, like anaphylaxis, may be life-threatening if not managed correctly. <u>Fortunately, they are rare, occurring at a rate of less than one in half a million doses. The risk of an allergic reaction can be minimized by good screening prior to vaccination</u>. A severe, anaphylactic allergic reaction following a dose of vaccine is a <u>contraindication to a subsequent dose of that vaccine</u>. Anaphylactic allergies are those that are mediated by IgE, occur within minutes or hours of receiving the vaccine, and require immediate medical attention. <u>Examples of symptoms and signs typical of anaphylactic reactions are generalized urticaria (hives), swelling of the mouth and throat, difficulty breathing, wheezing, abdominal cramping, hypotension, or shock</u>. In the event of an anaphylactic reaction, the appropriate emergency protocols should be followed and epinephrine should be immediately accessible. Immunizations should never be administered if epinephrine is not available.

Providers should report clinically significant adverse events to the FDA's <u>Vaccine Adverse Event Reporting System (VAERS)</u> even if they are unsure whether a vaccine caused the event.

<u>All providers who administer vaccines must have emergency protocols and supplies to treat anaphylaxis</u>. If symptoms are generalized, a second person should activate the emergency medical system (EMS), by calling 911 and notifying the on-call physician. The primary health care provider should remain with the patient, assessing the airway, breathing, circulation, and level of consciousness.

- Administer aqueous epinephrine 1:1000 dilution intramuscularly, 0.01 mg per kg of body weight per dose, up to a 0.5 mg maximum per dose.

- Most pharmacies use *EpiPens* or another epinephrine injection device are stocked, at least three adult (0.3 mg) should be available. Patients taking beta blockers may need higher or more frequent doses of epinephrine. Most adults will require 1 to 3 doses spaced every 5-10 minutes until paramedics arrive.

- In addition, for systemic anaphylaxis such as generalized urticaria, diphenhydramine may be administered either orally or by injection. Due to the risk of choking, no drug should be administered orally if the patient is exhibiting signs of mouth, throat or lip swelling or difficulty breathing.

- Monitor the patient closely until EMS arrives. Perform cardiopulmonary resuscitation (CPR), if necessary, and maintain the airway. Keep patient in a supine position (flat on back) unless he or she is having breathing difficulty. If breathing is difficult, the patient's head may be elevated, provided blood pressure is adequate to prevent loss of consciousness. If blood pressure is low, elevate legs. Monitor blood pressure and pulse every 5 minutes.

- If EMS has not arrived and symptoms are still present, repeat dose of epinephrine.

- Record all vital signs, medications administered to the patient, including the time, dosage, response, the name of the medical personnel who administered the medication and other relevant clinical information.

- Notify the patient's primary care physician.

- Report reaction to VAERS.

- Immunizing pharmacists should always maintain a current basic life support (BLS or CPR) certification.

Contraindications and Precautions

Contraindications and precautions to vaccination generally dictate circumstances when vaccines will not be given. Most precautions are temporary, and the vaccine can be given at a later time.

A contraindication is a condition that greatly increases a potential vaccine recipient's chance of a serious adverse reaction. It is a condition related to the recipient, not with the vaccine per se. For instance, administering influenza vaccine (except *Flubok)* to a person with a true anaphylactic allergy to egg could cause serious illness or death. In general, vaccines should not be administered when a contraindicated condition is present.

Two conditions are absolute contraindications to vaccination with live vaccines: pregnancy and immunosuppression. Two conditions are temporary precautions to vaccination: moderate or severe acute illness (all vaccines), and recent receipt of an antibody-containing blood product. The latter precaution applies only to live vaccines.

Immunosuppression

Live vaccines can cause severe or fatal reactions in immunocompromised people due to uncontrolled replication of the vaccine virus or reduced vaccine efficacy. Live vaccines should not be administered to severely immunosuppressed persons for this reason. Certain drugs may cause immunosuppression. For instance, persons receiving most cancer treatments

---

STEROID-INDUCED IMMUNOSUPPRESSION

CORTICOSTEROIDS

- 20 mg or more per day of prednisone*

- 2 mg/kg or more per day of prednisone*

- NOT intra-articular injections, metered-dose inhalers, topical, alternate day or short course for less than 14 days

For 14 days or longer

INVALID CONTRAINDICATIONS TO VACCINATION

VACCINATIONS MAY BE GIVEN, IF REQUIRED & INDICATED

- Mild acute illness (slight fever, mild diarrhea)

- Antimicrobial therapy (exceptions are certain antiviral medications and oral typhoid vaccine)

- Local skin reactions (mild/moderate)

- Bird feather allergies

- Recent infectious disease exposure

- Penicillin allergy

- Disease exposure or convalescence

- Breastfeeding

- Pregnant or immunosuppressive person in the household

- Preterm birth

- Allergy to products not present in vaccine or allergy that is not anaphylactic

- Family history of adverse events

- Tuberculin skin test (see above for timing and spacing with live vaccines only)

- Multiple vaccines

should not be given live vaccines. Live vaccines can be given after chemotherapy has been discontinued for at least 3 months. Anyone receiving large doses of corticosteroids should not receive live vaccines (see the sidebar). Live vaccines, MMR and Varicella, are only contraindicated for HIV patients with CD4 T lymphocyte counts < 200 cells/mm³. In general, the same vaccination recommendations apply as with other types of immunosuppression. While live-virus vaccines are usually contraindicated, patients may need other inactivated vaccines such as penumococcal and influenza vaccines. Both pneumoccocal conjugate vaccine (PCV13) and the 23-valent pneumococcal vaccine (PPSV) should be given to adult patients with altered immune competence (immunocompromised and asplenic).

VACCINATION OF PREGNANT WOMEN

- Live vaccines should not be administered to women 1 month before or during pregnancy

- In general, inactivated vaccines may be administered to pregnant women for whom they are indicated

- HPV vaccine should be deferred during pregnancy

- Pregnant women should receive the influenza vaccine (in season) and Tdap

Vaccinations During Pregnancy

The most frequent vaccine administered to pregnant women is the influenza (inactivated) vaccine. It is indicated in all trimesters of pregnancy. Pregnant women should receive Tdap with each pregnancy. The optimum time for Tdap vaccination is between weeks 27 and 36 of the pregnancy. If the woman has not been vaccinated or her vaccination history is unclear, a 3-dose series is needed; one Tdap then two Td doses at 1-2 months and 6 months. If the woman delivers and has not received vaccination, she should receive it post-delivery. Vaccination protects the baby and the mother from pertussis (whooping cough).

VACCINATIONS FOR HEALTHCARE PROFESSIONALS

Hepatitis B

If there is no documented evidence of a complete hepatitis B vaccine series or no serologic evidence of immunity then the healthcare professional should:

- Get the 3-dose series (dose #1 now, #2 in 1 month, #3 approximately 5 months after #2).

- Get anti-HBs antibody tested 1–2 months after dose #3.

Flu (Influenza)

- Get 1 dose of influenza vaccine annually.

MMR (Measles, Mumps, & Rubella)

- If born in 1957 or later and have not had the MMR vaccine or if lacking an up-to-date blood test showing immunity to measles, mumps, and rubella, get 2 doses of MMR, 4 weeks apart.

Varicella (Chickenpox)

- If no varicella vaccine received, or without positive serology to varicella, get 2 doses of varicella vaccine, 4 weeks apart.

Tdap (Tetanus, Diphtheria, Pertussis)

- Get a one-time dose of Tdap as soon as possible if no Tdap previously (regardless of when previous dose of Td was received). Get Td boosters every 10 years thereafter. Pregnant health care workers need to get a dose of Tdap during each pregnancy.

Screening Prior to Vaccine Administration

Use a screening form to rule out specific contraindications and precautions to the vaccine in adults. Note that a "yes" response to some of these questions will indicate a type of vaccine to use, rather than a contraindication to all (e.g., if a person has diabetes and selects "yes" to question #4, they should receive the inactivated influenza vaccine rather than the live influenza vaccine).

1. Are you sick today?

2. Do you have allergies to medications, food, a vaccine component, or latex?

3. Have you ever had a serious reaction after receiving a vaccination?

4. Do you have a long-term health problem with heart disease, lung disease, asthma, kidney disease, metabolic disease (e.g., diabetes), anemia, or other blood disorder?

5. Do you have cancer, leukemia, AIDS, or any other immune system problem?

6. Do you take cortisone, prednisone, other steroids, or anticancer drugs, or have you had radiation treatments?

7. Have you had a seizure or a brain or other nervous system problem?

8. Do you have cochlear implants or a cerebrovascular leak?

9. During the past year, have you received a transfusion of blood or blood products, or been given immune (gamma) globulin or an antiviral drug?

10. For women: Are you pregnant or is there a chance you could become pregnant during the next month?

11. Have you received any vaccinations in the past 4 weeks?

Immunization Registries

Immunization registries are computerized information systems that collect vaccination histories and help ensure correct and timely immunizations, especially for children. They are useful for healthcare providers who use the registries to obtain the patient's history, produce vaccine records, manage vaccine inventories, among other benefits. It helps the community at-large to identify groups who are not receiving vaccines in order to target outreach efforts. Some systems are able to notify parents if vaccines are needed. Where allowed, pharmacists should strive to report all vaccines administered to their state or local registry.

VACCINE	ADMINISTER TO	STORAGE/ADMINISTRATION

Diphtheria Toxoid-, Tetanus Toxoid- and acellular Pertussis-Containing Vaccines

DTaP: *DAPTACEL, Infanrix, Tripedia* DTaP-IPV: *KINRIX* DTaP-HepB-IPV: *Pediarix* DTaP-IPV/Hib: *Pentacel*	<u>DTaP series given to children younger than 7 years of age.</u>	Store in the refrigerator. Do not freeze. Shake the prefilled syringe or vial before use. Give IM.

Haemophilus influenzae type b-Containing Vaccines

Hib: *ActHIB, Hiberix, PedvaxHIB* Hib-HepB: *Comvax (may be withdrawn by the manufacturer)* DTaP-IPV/Hib: *Pentacel* MenCY-Hib: *Menhibrix* (Meningococcal serogroups C and Y-Hib)	Hib: Given to children. Sometimes in adults after splenectomy. *Menhibrix* is only for high risk infants ages 6 weeks-18 months.	Store in the refrigerator. Do not freeze. Shake the prefilled syringe or vial before use. Give IM.

Hepatitis-Containing Vaccines

HepA: *Havrix, Vaqta* **HepB: *Engerix-B, Recombivax HB*** **HepA-HepB: *Twinrix*** DTaP-HepB-IPV: *Pediarix* Hib-HepB: *Comvax* (may be withdrawn by the manufacturer)	Hep A is given to children at 1 year of age as a routine vaccination (2 doses). Hep A in adults for men who have sex with men, IV drug abusers, chronic disease, travelers to countries with high Hep A incidence. **Hep B** Health care workers (required by OSHA), men who have sex with men, anyone who has sex with multiple partners, IV drug users, ESRD, chronic liver disease. Hep B is a 3-dose series given at 0, 1 and 6 months for all children and adolescents and certain adults. Infants – dose 1: given at birth; dose 2: 1-2 months of age; dose 3: no earlier than 24 weeks (only if administering HBV vaccine by itself. Does not apply to pediatric combination products such as *Comvax*) If combined Hep A/Hep B vaccine (*Twinrix*) is used, administer 3 doses at 0, 1, and 6 months for those 18 years and older; a 4-dose *Twinrix* schedule is approved for accelerated dosing, administered on days 0, 7, and 21 to 30, followed by a booster dose at month 12.	Store in refrigerator. Do not freeze. Shake the vial or prefilled syringe before use. Give IM. HepA: Older than 18 years inject 1 mL intramuscularly. The two available brands can be used interchangeably. HepB: 20 years and older inject 1 mL intramuscularly. The two available brands have varying dosing indications. Check prior to administration.

Vaccines Continued

VACCINE	ADMINISTER TO	STORAGE/ADMINISTRATION

Human Papillomavirus Vaccines: Prevents 70% of cervical cancers, as well as vulvar, vaginal, oropharyngeal and anal cancers.

HPV2: *Cervarix* Bivalent vaccine. Only provides immunity against the HPV strains that cause cancer. Female only. **HPV4: *Gardasil*** Quadrivalent vaccine. Provides immunity against HPV strains responsible for causing certain cancers and genital warts. Either vaccine recommended for females. Only *Gardasil* is indicated for males. Primary prevention of cervical CA is via vaccination. PAP smears are still necessary in sexually active women. Cervical CA has high mortality.	HPV vaccine is indicated for females age 9-26 years. ACIP recommends the 3 dose series between the age of 11-12 years, with catch-up vaccination at age 13-26 years. Vaccination can begin at age 9 years and ideally prior to sexual activity. Males 9-26 years to reduce the likelihood of genital warts or anal cancers. (HPV4) Requires 3 doses. The 2nd dose is 1-2 months after the 1st and the 3rd 6 months after the 1st.	Store in the refrigerator. Do not freeze. Protect from light. Shake the prefilled syringe or vial before use. Give IM.

Vaccines Continued

VACCINE	ADMINISTER TO	STORAGE/ADMINISTRATION

Influenza Vaccines: Most illness occurs in young children, most severe illness occurs in people > 65 years or those with comorbid conditions.

<u>Quadrivalent nasal spray</u>: live, for healthy people ages 2-49 years (LAIV) *FluMist*

<u>Quadrivalent flu shots</u>: *Fluarix, Flulaval, Fluzone*

<u>Trivalent, standard dose</u>: various ages (youngest 6 months), grown in eggs (IIV3) *Afluria, Fluarix, Flulaval, Fluvirin, Fluzone*

<u>Trivalent, intradermal</u>: approved for 18-64 years (IIV3) *Fluzone Intradermal*

<u>Trivalent, grown in cell culture</u>: approved for ≥ 18 years (ccIIV3) *Flucelvax*

<u>Trivalent, high-dose</u>: approved for ≥ 65 years (IIV3) *Fluzone High-Dose*

<u>Trivalent, recombinant, egg-free</u>: approved for 18-49 years (RIV3) *Flublok*

Fluzone Intradermal uses smaller needle (30 gauge, 1.5 mm vs 22 to 25 gauge, 15.8- 38.1 mm), but more redness, swelling, itching. Preg B (other influenza shots are Preg C)

The CDC recommends that everyone 6 months of age and older get a seasonal flu vaccine. Children ages 6 months – 8 years who are receiving the vaccine for the 1st time require two doses – the 1st dose primes the immune system and should be given as soon as vaccine is available. The 2nd dose is 28 days after the first dose. If a child did not get the 2009 H1N1 vaccine in 2009-2010 or a seasonal flu vaccine in 2010 or later they will not be fully protected against the 2009 H1N1 unless they receive two doses of the 2014-2015 flu vaccine.

The Live Attenuated Influenza Vaccine, Quadrivalent (<u>LAIV4, nasal spray</u>) is <u>preferred</u> over the inactivated influenza vaccine (IIV, flu shots) when immediately available for <u>children 2-8 years of age</u>. Other than LAIV4 in children, the CDC does not have a preference for use of any particular flu vaccine when indicated. LAIV4 has specific indications: healthy (no underlying medical conditions that predisposes them to influenza complications), ages 2-49 years.

All patients should be monitored for at least 15 minutes after vaccination.

Trivalent flu vaccines protects against three influenza viruses: two influenza A's (an H1N1 and an H3N2) and one influenza B. The quadrivalent flu vaccines protect against two influenza A's and two influenza B's.

Store all influenza vaccines in the refrigerator. Do not freeze.

Give vaccine as soon as it is available, even if it arrives in late summer and preferably before October. Offer throughout the influenza season; Outbreaks usually peak in February or later.

Revaccinate each year.

PRECAUTIONS:
1.Defer if patient has a moderate-severe acute illness.

2. Refer to physician if patient had Guillain-Barré within 6 weeks of a prior dose of flu vaccine.

Those who can eat lightly cooked eggs without reactions or if they experience only hives after eating eggs can receive inactivated vaccine and be observed for 30 minutes. See "Allergy to Vaccine Components" for details. *FluBlok* is completely egg-free (recombinant vaccine).

Afluria: Note the product is labeled for children > 5 years old, but ACIP recommends giving it after age 9 years or older due to reports of febrile illness in young children. If vaccine shortage occurs, discuss risks/benefits of using *Afluria* in younger children with parents.

Flumist Quadrivalent is given as 0.2 mL, divided between the two nostrils; see diagram later in chapter.

Vaccines Continued

VACCINE	ADMINISTER TO	STORAGE/ADMINISTRATION

Measles, Mumps and Rubella-Containing Vaccines

MMR: *M-M-R II* MMRV: *ProQuad*	Given to children and non-immune adults. Adults born before 1957 generally are considered immune to measles and mumps. Health care providers born before 1957 must prove immunity or receive 2 doses MMR vaccine at least 4 weeks apart. Live vaccine, not used in pregnancy.	MMR: Refrigerator or freezer MMRV: Freezer only due to varicella component. Always store diluents in refrigerator. Protect from light. Give SC.

Meningococcal Vaccines

MCV4: *Menactra, Menveo* MPSV4: *Menomune* Adults usually 1 dose but 2 doses for HIV+, asplenia, complement component deficiencies	Vaccinate: ■ 1 dose for 11-12 year old adolescents with one booster dose at age 16-18 years. ■ 2-55 years old if at high risk, such as: College freshman in dormitories, asplenia, military service, immunodeficiencies (specifically complement deficiency), travelers to high-risk countries like the meningitis belt in Sub-Saharan Africa, lab workers with *N. meningitidis* exposure. People with continued risk of meningococcal disease should be revaccinated every five years. *Menomune:* use in ≥ 56 years old *Menactra:* 9 months-55 years *Menveo:* 2 months-55 years	Refrigerate. Protect from light. MCV give IM, MPSV give SC. Required by Saudi Arabia for annual travel during the period of the Hajj and Umrah pilgrimages, with proof of vaccination.

Vaccines Continued

VACCINE	ADMINISTER TO	STORAGE/ADMINISTRATION

Pneumococcal Vaccines

13-valent pneumococcal conjugate vaccine (PCV13): *Prevnar 13*

Minimum age at immunization: 6 weeks

23-serotype polysaccharide vaccine (PPSV23): *Pneumovax 23*

Minimum age at immunization: 2 years; PPSV23 does not invoke immunity in patients < 2 years old.

PREVNAR 13/PNEUMOVAX 23
RECOMMENDATIONS

Children
Routine vaccination, all, beginning at 2 months:

- *Prevnar 13* at 2, 4, 6 and 12-15 months. (4 doses)

Immunocompromised children 24 months-5 years (any immunocompromised condition, sickle cell disease, HIV, CSF leak, cochlear implant):

- *Prevnar 13* x 1 or 2 doses if the series PCV13 was not completed when younger and *Pneumovax 23*.

Immunocompromised children 6-18 years (any immunocompromised conditions, sickle cell disease, HIV, CSF leak, cochlear implant):

- *Prevnar 13* x 1, if the series was not completed when younger even if they received *Pneumovax 23* or the older conjugate vaccine (*Prevnar 7*).

Adults
Immunocompromised adults 19-64 years:

- (Assuming PCV13 naive) give *Prevnar 13* first, followed by *Pneumovax 23* at least 8 weeks later. If *Pneumovax 23* was given 1st, wait at least 1 year before giving *Prevnar 13*.

- Repeat *Pneumovax 23* 5 years after the initial *Pneumovax 23*.

Immunocompetent adults ≥ 19 years with CSF leak or cochlear implant:

- (Assuming PCV13 naive) give *Prevnar 13* first, followed by *Pneumovax 23* at least 8 weeks later was given 1st, wait at least 1 year before giving *Prevnar 13* (assure there is at least 5 years between doses of PPSV23).

Immunocompetent adults 19-64 years with chronic illness, habits or living conditions that put them at risk for pneumococcal disease (smoking, asthma, long-term care resident, alcoholism, liver disease, pulmonary disease, diabetes, heart disease):

- *Pneumovax 23* x 1

Adults ≥ 65 years, all:

- *Prevnar 13* (if not given previously) followed by *Pneumovax 23* 6 to 12 months later by a dose of *Pneumovax 23*. If *Pneumovax 23* was given first, wait at least 1 year before giving *Prevnar 13*.

Store in refrigerator. Do not freeze.

PCV13
Shake the vial or prefilled syringe prior to use. Do not mix with other vaccines in the same syringe. Give IM.

PPSV23
Shake the vial or prefilled syringe prior to use. Do not mix with other vaccines in the same syringe. Give IM or SC.

Vaccines Continued

VACCINE	ADMINISTER TO	STORAGE/ADMINISTRATION

Poliovirus-Containing Vaccines

IPV: *IPOL* DTaP-HepB-IPV: *Pediarix* DTaP-IPV: *KINRIX* DTaP-IPV/Hib: *Pentacel*	Vaccine series to ALL children.	**Inactivated Poliomyelitis Vaccines (IPV)** Store in the refrigerator. Do not freeze. Shake the prefilled syringe or vial before use. Give IM or SC.

Rotavirus Vaccines

RV1: *Rotarix* RV5: *RotaTeq*	Vaccine series to ALL children. Do not initiate the series after age 15 weeks	Store in refrigerator. Do not freeze. Protect from light. Oral suspensions.

Tetanus Toxoid- and Diphtheria Toxoid-Containing Vaccines

Td: *DECAVAC* DT: *Diphtheria and Tetanus Toxoid*	May be used in wound prophylaxis and for routine boosting. If the patient has received 3 or more doses of tetanus, and the wound is NOT clean or minor, revaccination with Td if more than 5 years since the last dose. They may also require tetanus immunoglobulin (TIG). If less than 3 doses or unclear history with serious wound, they may require both.	Store in refrigerator. Do not freeze. DT is for primary series in infants and children < 7 years old who have a contraindication to the acellular pertussis antigen. Give IM.

Vaccines Continued

VACCINE	ADMINISTER TO	STORAGE/ADMINISTRATION
Tdap: *Adacel, Boostrix* See above for DTaP series, indicated for children 6 weeks to 6 years of age. Single Tdap dose for ages 7-10 years who were not fully vaccinated with DTaP series (missed dose in series). Tdap is the one time booster for ages 11-64 years with no previous record of Tdap, then one dose of Td every 10 years.	Administer a one-time dose of Tdap to adults who have not received Tdap previously, and as soon as feasible to all 1) pregnant or postpartum women, 2) close contacts of infants younger than age 12 months (e.g., grandparents and child-care providers), and 3) health-care personnel with direct patient contact. Pregnant women (weeks 27-36) should receive Tdap with each pregnancy. If the woman has not been vaccinated or the history is unclear, a 3-dose series is needed (one with Tdap, the other 2 with Td only at 0, 1 month, and 6-12 months). If the woman delivers and has not received vaccination, she should receive it post-delivery. Vaccination protects the baby and mother from pertussis (whooping cough).	All tetanus, diphtheria, and pertussis containing vaccines: Store in the refrigerator. Do not freeze. Shake the prefilled syringe or vial before use. Give IM. The pediatric formulations (with the upper-case D, as in DTaP) have 3-5 times as much of the diphtheria component than the adult formulation. The adult formulations have a lower case d (Tdap, or Td).

Varicella-Containing Vaccines

VAR: *Varivax* **(chickenpox)** **ZOS:** *Zostavax* **(herpes zoster/shingles)** MMRV: *ProQuad*	Children get varicella vaccine at 12 months & again at 4-6 yrs. All adults without evidence of immunity to varicella should receive 2 doses of varicella vaccine at least 4 weeks apart. Varicella vaccines are live vaccines; do not use in pregnancy or if immunocompromised. Herpes zoster vaccination (potency 14 times greater than varicella in order to elicit needed immune response) In May, 2011 the FDA licensed zoster vaccine for adults 50 years of age and older. ACIP continues to recommend herpes zoster vaccine for patients 60 years and older. *Zostavax* is indicated for prevention of shingles and not for treatment of active case. Also reduces complications such as severity of postherpatic neuralgia following infections. Vaccinate even if history of zoster infection since you can get it again.	Varicella-containing vaccines have 2 components: vaccine & diluent. Store vaccine in freezer & protect from light (keep in original container). Store diluent in refrigerator or room temp. LIVE vaccines: do not give if immunocompromised, pregnant or if pregnancy is expected within 4 weeks. Do not give if hypersensitivity to gelatin or neomycin. Give SC. Reconstituted; reconstitute immediately upon removal from freezer and inject; short stability. SC injection in adults for vaccines is in the fatty tissue at triceps; see diagram at end of chapter.

Other Vaccines

DRUG	ADMINISTER TO	STORAGE/ADMINISTRATION
Japanese Encephalitis *Ixiaro*	Not recommended for all travelers to Asia. May be given if spending 1 month+ in endemic areas during transmission season, especially if travel will include rural areas.	2 doses 28 days apart, complete at least 1 week prior to potential exposure. Give IM.
Rabies *Imovax, RabAvert*	May be given preventively if high risk exposure (animal handlers, traveling to high risk area, etc.) or given with rabies exposure.	Reconstitute with provided diluent, 3 doses for prevention. If exposed to rabies with no rabies vaccination history: 4 doses vaccine + rabies immune globulin with 1st dose If exposed to rabies and had vaccination: 2 doses vaccine only. Give IM.
Tuberculosis bacille Calmette-Guerin (BCG)	Not used often in U.S. Often given to infants and small children in countries with higher TB incidence. Protection provided by the vaccine for pulmonary TB is poor. Can cause false positive reaction to TB skin test.	
Typhoid *Vivotif Berna* (oral capsules, refrigerate) *Typhim Vi, Typherix* (Injections)	Typhoid fever caused by *Salmonella Typhi* exposure from food or drink beverages handled by infected person who is shedding or from contaminated sewage. Travelers from U.S. to Asia, Africa, and Latin America at risk. To reduce risk:"Boil it, cook it, peel it, or forget it."	4 capsules: 1 on alternate days (day 1, 3, 5 & 7); take on an empty stomach with cold or lukewarm water, complete at least 1 week prior to exposure.
Yellow Fever After vaccination provide International Certificate of Vaccination (yellow card) valid 10 days after vaccine for 10 years, may be required to enter endemic areas.	In tropical and subtropical areas South America and Africa. Transmitted by mosquito. Use insect repellent, wear protective clothing, and consider vaccination.	Give SC. Reconstituted. Contraindicated with a severe (life-threatening) allergy to eggs or gelatin. Avoid donating blood for 2 weeks after receiving vaccine.

Vaccines: Miscellaneous Tips

- If the wrong vaccine is chosen the patient is not covered for the intended disease.

- Review the brand name/components for vaccines that can be confused, including combos.

- If the vaccine is stored incorrectly, it may lose its potency and leave patients unprotected. Use vaccines quickly if removed from cold storage. Reconstituted vaccines have short stability.

- The CDC does not require gloves when giving vaccines, unless likely to come into exposure with blood/bodily fluids. However, this is possible and most wear gloves. If using gloves they must be changed between each patient.

- The CDC does not recommend using acetaminophen routinely before or at vaccination as it may decrease the immune response. It can be used to treat pain and fever <u>after</u> vaccination.

- Never mix vaccines in the same syringe yourself – they have to come mixed.

- Do not aspirate – this is when you see a flash of blood come up into the syringe upon retraction of the plunger.

- All vaccines can be given simultaneously. If a vaccine is missed, then any 2 live vaccines not given at the same time must be given at least 4 weeks apart.

- You can vaccinate through a tattoo.

STORAGE

Store refrigerated vaccines immediately upon arrival. Vaccines are stored in refrigerator and freezer units designed for storing biologics, including vaccines, or the frozen and refrigerated vaccines are stored in separate, free-standing freezer and refrigerator units. At a minimum, a household-style unit can be used if there is a separate exterior door for the freezer and separate thermostats for the freezer and refrigerator. Dormitory-style refrigerators should not be used. Keep a calibrated thermometer or a digital data logger connected to a glycol encased probe in the refrigerator and freezer. Post "Do Not Unplug" signs next electrical outlets and "Do Not Stop Power" signs near circuit breakers to maintain a consistent power source. Store vaccines on the shelves away from the walls. Vaccines should never be stored in the door of the freezer or refrigerator. The temperature there is unstable. Read and document refrigerator and freezer temperatures at least twice each workday: in the morning and before the end of the workday. Keep temperature logs for at least 3 years. Rotate stock so vaccine and diluent with the earliest expiration date is used first. Place vaccine with the longest expiration date behind the vaccine that will expire the soonest.

Store refrigerated vaccines between 35°F and 46°F (2°C and 8°C). Store frozen vaccines between -58°F and +5°F (-50°C and -15°C).

Administration

See the chart at the end of this chapter for injection technique. In adults intramuscular (IM) injections are given in the deltoid muscle at the central and thickest portion above the level of the armpit and below the acromion. Adults require a 1" syringe (or a 1½" needle for women greater than 200 lbs or men greater than 260 pounds). Use a 22-25 gauge needle inserted at a 90 degree angle. The higher the gauge, the thinner the needle.

Subcutaneous (SC) vaccinations are given in the fatty tissue over the triceps with a 5/8", 23-25 gauge syringe at a 45 degree angle.

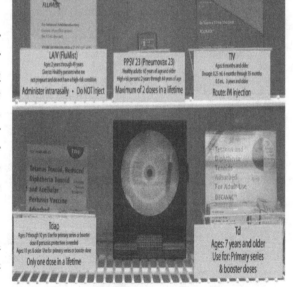

Staff can easily confuse the vaccines within the storage unit. Use labels & separate containers.

Influenza (the Flu)

Influenza is the most common vaccine preventable illness in the U.S.

Make sure patients know:

- The influenza vaccine cannot cause the flu. They may get a sore arm, or mild systemic reactions that go away.

- The only patients who can use the nasal mist vaccine are healthy (no chronic disease) non-pregnant females and males from age 2 to 49 years. This is a live vaccine; the others are inactivated injections.

- Everyone 6 months and older should be vaccinated annually – patients at highest risk will get vaccinated first if there is a vaccine shortage; check the CDC vaccination website if a shortage is present.

- Pregnant women are at risk for severe disease and should be vaccinated.

- Individuals can and should be vaccinated for influenza even if it is late in the season.

Influenza A and B are the two types of influenza viruses that cause epidemic human disease. Influenza A viruses are further categorized into subtypes on the basis of two surface antigens: hemagglutinin and neuraminidase. Immunity to the surface antigens, particularly the hemagglutinin, reduces the likelihood of infection and severity of disease if infection occurs. Frequent development of antigenic variants through antigenic drift is the virologic basis for seasonal epidemics and the reason for the usual incorporation of one or more new strains in each year's influenza vaccine, which is made as a trivalent vaccine. More dramatic antigenic changes, or shifts, occur approximately every 30 years and can result in the emergence of a novel influenza virus with the potential to cause a pandemic.

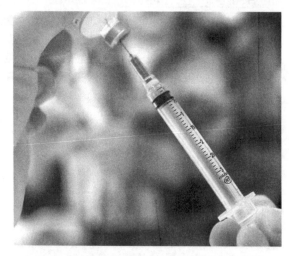

Influenza (inactivated) injection – annually, each fall

The virus spreads from person to person, primarily through respiratory droplet transmission. This can happen when an infected person coughs or sneezes in close proximity to an uninfected person. If someone sneezes in their hands and touches something it is possible to spread illness.

Uncomplicated influenza illness is characterized by the abrupt onset of these symptoms: fever, myalgia, headache, malaise, non-productive cough, sore throat, and rhinitis.

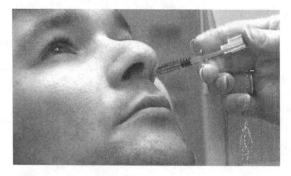

Influenza – live nasal vaccine, annually, each fall, if healthy, ages 2-49 years

Among children, otitis media, nausea, and vomiting also are commonly reported with influenza illness.

Uncomplicated influenza illness typically resolves after 3-7 days for the majority of persons, although cough and malaise can persist for more than 2 weeks. However, for certain people, influenza can exacerbate underlying medical conditions (e.g., pulmonary or cardiac disease), leading to secondary bacterial pneumonia or primary influenza viral pneumonia, or occur as part of a co-infection with other viral or bacterial pathogens.

Antiviral treatment of patients with influenza
- See Infectious Disease chapter.

How to Administer IM and SC Vaccine Injections to Adults

Intramuscular (IM) Injections

Administer these vaccines via IM route:
Tetanus, diphtheria (Td), or with pertussis (Tdap); hepatitis A; hepatitis B; human papillomavirus (HPV); trivalent inactivated influenza (TIV); and quadrivalent meningococcal conjugate (MCV4). Administer polio (IPV) and pneumococcal polysaccharide vaccine (PPSV23) either IM or SC.

Injection site:
Give in the central and thickest portion of the deltoid—above the level of the armpit and below the acromion (see the diagram).

Needle size:
22–25 gauge, 1–1½" needle (*see note at right*)

Needle insertion:

- Use a needle long enough to reach deep into the muscle.
- Insert the needle at a 90° angle to the skin with a quick thrust.
- Separate two injections given in the same deltoid muscle by a minimum of 1".

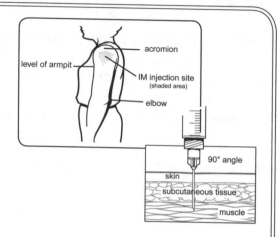

Note: A ⬜ " needle is sufficient in adults weighing <130 lbs (<60 kg); a 1" needle is sufficient in adults weighing 130–152 lbs (60–70 kg); a 1–1½" needle is recommended in women weighing 152–200 lbs (70–90 kg) and men weighing 152–260 lbs (70–118 kg); a 1½" needle is recommended in women weighing >200 lbs (>90 kg) or men weighing >260 lbs (>118 kg). A ⬜ " (16mm) needle may be used only if the skin is stretched tight, the subcutaneous tissue is not bunched, and injection is made at a 90-degree angle.

Subcutaneous (SC) Injections

Administer these vaccines via SC route:
MMR, varicella, meningococcal polysaccharide (MPSV4), and zoster (shingles). Administer polio (IPV) and pneumococcal polysaccharide vaccine (PPSV23) either SC or IM.

Injection site:
Give in fatty tissue over the triceps (see the diagram).

Needle size:
23–25 gauge, 5/8" needle

Needle insertion:

- Pinch up on the tissue to prevent injection into the muscle. Insert the needle at a 45° angle to the skin.
- Separate two injections given in the same area of fatty tissue by a minimum of 1".

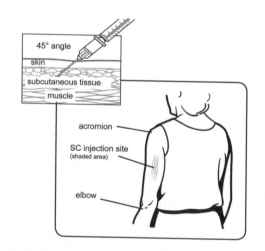

Adapted by the Immunization Action Coalition, courtesy of the Minnesota Department of Health

Technical content reviewed by the Centers for Disease Control and Prevention, November 2010.

www.immunize.org/catg.d/p2020A.pdf Item #P2020A (11/10)

Immunization Action Coalition • 1573 Selby Ave. • St. Paul, MN 55104 • (651) 647-9009 • www.immunize.org • www.vaccineinformation.org

TRAVELERS

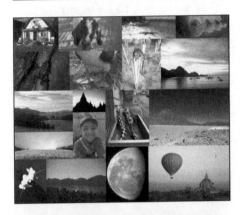

We gratefully acknowledge the assistance of Catrina Derderian, BS, PharmD, Clinical Pharmacist, Cambridge Health Alliance, Boston MA, in preparing this chapter.

BACKGROUND

International travel involves millions of travelers to all places in the world. Travelers often do not recognize the associated health risks and may not seek consultation with an appropriate health professional prior to travel. Pharmacists offer formal advice to the traveling public, provide recommended vaccinations and medications and, in some settings, charge for consultative services, which include awareness of country-specific risks and ways to prevent and address them.

GUIDELINES

Centers for Disease Control (CDC) Center on Travelers Health. Available at http://wwwnc.cdc.gov/travel (accessed 2014 Sept 23).

International Society of Travel Medicine (ISTM), Pharmacist Professional Group of the ISTM, Available at www.istm.org (accessed 2014 Sept 23).

Patients should be advised to <u>pack medications and medical supplies in carry-on luggage</u>, in the original prescription bottles. They should bring copies of all prescriptions and a <u>list of all medications and conditions</u>. It is prudent for travelers to check with their health insurance company to find out if their policy will cover medical care in another country or on board a ship. Travel health information, including insurance recommendations, is available on the CDC's travel information website where the "<u>Yellow Book</u>" (the CDC's <u>standard resource on travel information</u>) is located. Travel advisories and visa requirements can be checked on the U.S. State Department website. Additional information on vaccinations is in the Immunizations chapter.

MAJOR CONCERNS FOR TRAVELING INDIVIDUALS

When preparing a patient for travel, a few topics are routinely considered. Common concerns include 1) diseases spread through <u>food and water</u>, 2) diseases spread through <u>blood</u>

and bodily fluids, and 3) diseases transmitted by insects. Traveler's risk for contracting disease should be assessed based upon travel duration, country and region specific risks, and patient specific health concerns.

THE RETURNED TRAVELER

The 2014 Ebola outbreak in West Africa has heightened awareness regarding contagion risks from returned travelers. Ebola is transmitted by direct contact with blood or bodily fluids of a person who is symptomatic. The Ebola symptoms (fever, headache, diarrhea, and hemorrhaging) can appear from 2 to 21 days after exposure – which means that a person can be infected but have an asymptomatic presentation when entering the U.S. There is a fear (at the time this text has gone to press) that the virus could mutate into a form that can be transmitted more easily, such as with aerosolized transmission. If the disease can be transmitted by coughing or sneezing it will be more easily spread. Whether this turns out to be accurate or not, pharmacists can obtain current information from the CDC website and will be involved with measures to assist staff and patients to reduce transmission risk.

If a patient is ill upon returning from travel they may require immediate isolation, such as with Ebola, or require less intensive measures. The risk of disease spread from initially asymptomatic patients must be considered. Important information for a patient to relay to the healthcare provider includes the travel itinerary (where they went), the trip duration, where they stayed, what they did and what precautions they took to reduce infection risk, including vaccination history prior to leaving the U.S.

Diseases Transmitted through Contaminated Food and Water

Travelers' Diarrhea Prevention

Contracting travelers' diarrhea (TD) is the most common concern of patients who travel abroad. TD is caused by unclean food and water. Most cases (> 80%) are bacterial and *E. coli* is the primary bacterial pathogen. Travelers to developing countries are at highest risk due to limited access to sanitary water and inadequate practices for handling foods. Areas of highest risk include most of Asia, the Middle East, Africa, Mexico, and Central and South America.

Patients can follow safe food and water habits to reduce risk. Patients are often told to "cook it, peel it, or forget it" when discussing food consumption when traveling. The following food and water precautions can be recommended to traveling patients:

- Eat only food that is cooked and served hot. Avoid food that has been sitting on a buffet.

- Avoid raw or undercooked meats/fish.

- Eat raw fruits and vegetables only if washed in clean water or peeled (e.g., oranges).

- Drink from factory-sealed containers; avoid ice. Water should be boiled or purified.

- Keep hands clean; wash hands often with soap and water, especially after using the bathroom and before eating. If soap and water are not available, use an alcohol-based hand sanitizer. Keep hands out of the mouth.

If traveler's diarrhea develops, <u>hydration is essential</u>. In serious cases with prolonged diarrhea or vomiting, oral rehydration solution can be used for fluid replacement. The packets are available in pharmacies throughout the world and can be prepared by mixing 1 packet with 1 liter of boiled purified water. <u>Over-the-counter loperamide *(Imodium)* can be used to decrease the frequency and urgency of bowel movements</u>, and can make it easier for a person with diarrhea to ride on a bus or airplane while waiting for an antibiotic to take effect. It should <u>not be used in children < 2 years old without a physician's authorization</u> due to the risk of toxic megacolon. Another option to help symptoms of TD is bismuth subsalicylate, which is the active ingredient in *Pepto Bismol*. This should not be used with <u>anticoagulants or with a salicylate allergy</u>, renal insufficiency, or in children who are < 12 years old or who may have a viral infection (due to the risk of Reye's syndrome). Bismuth subsalicylate turns the tongue (and possibly stool) <u>black</u>, which resolves with drug discontinuation. If used excessively or with other salicylates, toxicity could present as tinnitus.

TD caused by a bacterial infection can be treated with antibiotics; options are discussed in the Infectious Diseases chapter.

Typhoid Fever

Typhoid fever is potentially severe and can be life-threatening. Typhoid is caused by the bacterium *Salmonella* Typhi. Areas of risk include east and southeast Asia, Africa, the Caribbean, and Central and South America.

Humans are the only source of the bacteria, which is spread primarily through <u>consumption of water or food that has been contaminated by the feces</u> of someone with <u>an acute infection</u> or from a <u>chronic, asymptomatic carrier</u>. Transmission through <u>sexual contact</u>, especially among men who have sex with men, can occur but is not the common cause of transmission.

The incubation period of typhoid (and paratyphoid infection, a similar disease) is 6 – 30 days. Symptoms of illness include gradually increasing fatigue, malaise, fever, earache and anorexia, with possible hepatosplenomegaly. A transient, macular rash may be present on the trunk. Intestinal hemorrhage or perforation can occur 2 – 3 weeks later and can be fatal.

Typhoid vaccines are recommended but are only 50 – 80% effective; therefore, even vaccinated travelers should follow <u>safe food and water precautions and wash hands frequently</u>. These precautions are the only prevention method for paratyphoid fever, for which there is no vaccine. There are two typhoid vaccines: *Vivotif Berna*, taken as oral capsules, or *Typhim Vi*, an intramuscular injection.

<u>Vivotif Berna</u> is an <u>oral, live, attenuated</u> vaccine and consists of <u>4 capsules, 1 taken every other day</u>. The capsules are <u>refrigerated</u> (not frozen). Each capsule is <u>taken with cool liquid</u> (not warm), 1 hour before a meal. The oral vaccine should not be considered if a patient is on

antibiotics or has an extremely sensitive stomach. The regimen should be completed 1 week prior to travel and is not used in children < 6 years.

Typhim VI, the injectable vaccine, is one 0.5-mL dose given intramuscularly ≥ 2 weeks before expected exposure. The injectable vaccination is not recommended for children < 2 years.

Hepatitis A

Hepatitis A is one of the most common vaccine-preventable infections acquired during international travel. Persons from developed countries who travel to developing countries are at highest risk. The virus is transmitted when a person ingests fecal matter, even in microscopic amounts, from objects, food, or drinks contaminated by the feces of an infected person. The patient can be asymptomatic or present with fever, malaise, jaundice, nausea and abdominal discomfort.

Vaccination is recommended for susceptible travelers to countries with high or intermediate risk of hepatitis A. There are two monovalent (hepatitis A only) vaccines *(Havrix, Vaqta)* and a combination hepatitis A/B vaccine *(Twinrix)*. Immunoglobulin is given with the Hepatitis A vaccine in some high-risk groups.

Diseases Transmitted Through Blood and Bodily Fluids

Hepatitis B

Hepatitis B is a DNA virus that is transmitted through contact with contaminated blood or other body fluids. The risk for travelers who do not participate in high risk behaviors is low. Hepatitis B has an incubation period of about 90 days. Infection may present as malaise, jaundice, nausea and abdominal discomfort. Chronic infection with Hepatitis B can result in chronic liver disease and liver cancer.

Vaccination for Hepatitis B is extremely important to consider for travelers who plan to have sexual encounters with new partners, patients who may be traveling to receive medical care, or patients who may be volunteering to provide medical work. Piercings and tattoos can transmit the virus and should be avoided.

The vaccine is a 3-dose series on a 0-, 1-, and 6-month schedule. Due to the extended amount of time needed to receive the full vaccination series, many travelers are unable to receive all three doses before departure. Therefore, as many doses as possible should be administered before departure and the series should be completed when the traveler returns to the United States. In instances of high risk, an accelerated series may be administered. There are two vaccines available *(Engerix-B, Recombivax HB)* and the Hepatitis A/B *Twinrix* combination.

Diseases Transmitted By Insect Bites

Insects that transmit disease are vectors. The vector carries the disease to the individual, causing infection. A reservoir is any place (such as an animal, insect, soil or plant) in which the disease lives and can multiply. The primary insect that causes infection to travelers are various types of <u>mosquitos</u>, which carry parasites for <u>Japanese encephalitis, yellow fever, dengue and malaria</u>. The tsetse fly spreads African sleeping sickness. Insect bites should be avoided as much as possible.

Mosquito-Borne Illness Prevention: Recommendations to Reduce Insect Bites

- Stay and sleep in screened or air-conditioned rooms.

- Cover exposed skin by wearing long-sleeved shirts, long pants and hats.

- Use a bed net, which can be pre-treated with mosquito repellant.

- Use proper application of mosquito repellents containing 20% to 50% <u>DEET</u> as the active ingredient on exposed skin and clothing. DEET also protects against ticks. Other insect repellants that can be used topically for mosquitos (but not for ticks) are picaridin, oil of lemon, eucalyptus or IR3535. <u>Permethrin</u> can be used to treat clothing, gear and bed nets but <u>should not be applied directly to the skin</u>.

Dengue: No Vaccine, Transmitted By Mosquito

Dengue (den' gee) is transmitted between people by the mosquitoes *Aedes aegypti* and *Aedes albopictus*. In many parts of the tropics and subtropics, dengue is endemic; it occurs every year, usually during a season when mosquito populations are high and rainfall is optimal for breeding. Sequential infections put people at greater risk for <u>dengue hemorrhagic fever</u> and dengue shock syndrome, both of which can be fatal. <u>Protection from mosquito bites with non-drug measures is essential</u>.

Malaria: Prophylactic Medication Available, Transmitted By Mosquito

<u>Malaria</u> is transmitted by the bite of an infected <u>*Anopheles* mosquito</u>. It is endemic to tropical and subtropical areas of Asia, North and South America, the Middle East, North Africa, and the South Pacific. Travelers to sub-Saharan Africa have the greatest risk. The CDC website includes maps of malaria presence by country, the species of malaria and medication recommendations. *Plasmodium vivax* is the most common of four human malaria species (*P. falciparum, P. malariae, P. ovale,* and *P. vivax*). <u>*P. vivax*</u> causes up to 65% of malaria cases in India and is becoming increasingly resistant to malaria drugs. By contrast, <u>*P. falciparum*</u> is the most deadly species and the subject of most malaria-related research.

Several medications are available for malaria prophylaxis and some of these are used for treatment. When deciding on which drug to use for prevention, clinicians should consider the <u>resistance, date of departure</u> (some must be started longer in advance of travel), <u>cost, allergies, pregnancy, if an infant or child, and concurrent conditions</u>.

<u>Mefloquine</u> is dosed once weekly. It is started 1 – 2 weeks prior to travel and is taken for 4 weeks post-travel. There is a high degree of <u>resistance in many areas</u>, which must be checked prior to dispensing. This drug can cause a range of side effects, including psychiatric symptoms (<u>anxiety, paranoia, depression, hallucinations, and psychosis</u>) and neurologic symp-

toms (seizures, dizziness or vertigo, tinnitus, and loss of balance). Mefloquine cannot be used with cardiac conditions, however it is an option during pregnancy and for children.

Atovaquone/Proguanil *(Malarone)* is quick-acting and dosed once daily. It is started 1 - 2 days before travel and is taken for 7 days post-travel. It is well tolerated but cannot be used during pregnancy.

Chloroquine *(Aralen)* is dosed once weekly. It is started 1 – 2 weeks before travel and is taken for 4 weeks post-travel. Chloroquine can cause visual problems (retinopathy), can exacerbate psoriasis, cause GI upset and is best avoided in pregnancy and with severe renal impairment. It should not be used in areas with high chloroquine or mefloquine resistance.

Primaquine is effective for *P. vivax*. It is dosed once daily. It is started 1 – 2 days before travel and taken for 7 days post-travel. It cannot be used in pregnancy or in a G6PD deficient patient; use in G6PD+ patients can cause bleeding. The CDC requires screening for G6PD deficiency prior to initiating treatment with primaquine.

Doxycycline is sometimes used and some patients may be using it for other conditions already, primarily for acne. This is usually a good option for patients who may need malaria prophylaxis for an extended amount of time. These drugs are included in the Infectious Diseases chapter.

Japanese Encephalitis: Vaccine Available, Transmitted By Mosquito

The Japanese Encephalitis (JE) vaccination is occasionally recommended. JE can cause asymptomatic infection, or can develop into encephalitis, with rigors and risk of seizures, coma and death. Travelers are most likely to become infected when visiting rural agricultural areas. The best prevention is to reduce exposure to mosquitos. The vaccine is recommended for travelers > 17 years who plan to spend at least 1 month in endemic areas during the JE virus transmission season or for those with extended exposure to the outdoors (e.g., campers). The vaccine *(IXIARO)* is a two-dose series. The last dose should be given at least 1 week before travel.

Yellow Fever: Vaccine Available, Transmitted By Mosquito

Yellow fever is caused by a virus found in tropical and subtropical areas in South America and Africa. Reducing mosquito exposure is essential. Most infections are asymptomatic. If symptoms develop, the initial illness presents as an influenza-like syndrome. Most patients will improve, but ~15% progress to a more toxic form of the disease with risk of shock and organ failure. There is no specific treatment for acute infection except symptomatic relief with fluids, analgesics and antipyretics. Aspirin and other NSAIDs cannot be used due to the increased risk for bleeding. Infected patients should be protected from further mosquito exposure (staying indoors or under a mosquito net) during the first few days of illness, or they will contribute to the transmission cycle.

Clinicians should only vaccinate travelers who are at a high risk of exposure (including some travelers to South America and Africa) or to those travelers who require proof of vaccination to enter a country. This is due to the high risk of serious adverse effects after yellow fever vaccination, including low grade fever, headache, and in rare cases, yellow fever vaccine-associated neurologic disease. After vaccination, the patient is provided an "International Certificate of Vaccination or Prophylaxis", which is called the "yellow fever card." The card is valid only if the vaccination is completed 10 days before arrival.

The vaccine is contraindicated in infants < 6 months who are at higher risk for significant complications, and in patients with hypersensitivity to eggs, egg products, chicken proteins, or gelatin. Additional contraindications include a thymus disorder or myasthenia gravis. This is a live vaccine and cannot be used with immunosuppression, including HIV patients with a CD4+ count < 200/mm^3, anyone using strong immune-suppressants (TNF-inhibitors, high-dose systemic steroids, certain chemotherapy agents, and IL-1 and IL-6 antagonists). Clinicians should review the contraindications and precautions to the yellow fever vaccine before administration.

ACIP recommends that a woman wait 4 weeks after receiving the vaccine before conceiving. Yellow fever vaccine safety has not been tested during pregnancy. The CDC recommends advising pregnant women who would require vaccination to avoid travel to at-risk regions.

African Sleeping Sickness: No Vaccine, Transmitted By Tsetse Fly

The tsetse fly lives in sub-Saharan Africa and spreads African sleeping sickness (African trypanosomiasis). Tsetse fly protection is different from mosquito protection. The insect can bite through thin fabric. Clothing should be medium-weight and be neutral in color as the fly is attracted to bright colors, dark colors, metallic fabric and the color blue. Insect repellants described above should be used, but there is limited evidence they work against this insect.

ADDITIONAL CONCERNS FOR TRAVELING INDIVIDUALS

Meningitis

Meningitis is spread by respiratory secretions and is widespread in many parts of the world. The vaccine is recommended by the CDC for people who travel to or reside in countries where *N. meningitidis* is hyperendemic or epidemic, particularly if contact with the local population will be prolonged. Hyperendemic regions include the meningitis belt of Africa during the dry season (December – June). Additionally, the meningococcal vaccine is required by the government of Saudi Arabia for annual travel during the period of the Hajj and Umrah pilgrimages.

Bacterial meningitis has high fatality and is a medical emergency. Patients with symptoms of fever, severe, unrelenting headache, nausea, stiff neck and mental status changes require urgent treatment to avoid the risk of permanent brain damage and death. There are three vaccines: ages 9 – 23 months *(Menactra-*2 doses), ages 2 – 55 years *(Menveo)*, and ages 56+ *(Menomune)*. 7 – 10 days are required after vaccination for protective antibody levels.

Polio

Most people in the U.S. have received polio vaccination as children. The virus has not been eradicated and there have been recent outbreaks. Three countries remain endemic (Afghanistan, Nigeria and Pakistan) and there is wild poliovirus circulation (WPC) in other places; the CDC recommends that adult travelers to regions with WPC receive a single lifetime booster dose.

Venous Thromboembolism Prevention

Travelers are at increased risk for deep vein thrombosis (DVT) and pulmonary embolism (PE) due to limited movement with intercontinental air travel. Wearing compression stockings during long trips reduces risk; these are sold in pharmacies. Travelers should be instructed to get up and walk (choosing an aisle seat is helpful) and to perform lower leg exercises when sitting.

Patients should know symptoms of DVT and PE and be instructed to seek immediate medical care if suspected. DVT risk factors, symptoms and treatment are discussed in the Anticoagulation chapter.

Motion Sickness, Altitude Sickness, Jet Lag

Motion Sickness is common among travelers and is discussed in the Motion Sickness chapter. Acute mountain sickness (AMS) occurs when people climb rapidly to a high altitude. It occurs commonly above 8,000 feet and is more likely in persons who live close to sea level or who have had the condition previously. Primary symptoms are dizziness, headache, tachycardia and shortness of breath. The primary prophylactic medication is acetazolamide (Diamox) 125 mg twice daily, started the day before (preferred) or on the day of ascent. Higher doses are used for treatment. This can improve breathing, but is not without side effects (polyuria, taste alteration, risk of dehydration, photosensitivity, urticaria and a possibility of severe skin rashes). Acetazolamide is contraindicated with a sulfa allergy. Sun protection and hydration is recommended. In acute cases, oxygen, inhaled beta-agonists and dexamethasone is given to reduce cerebral edema.

For treatment of jet lag see the Natural Products & Vitamins chapter.

cold: cough, mild weakness, stuffy nose, sore throat, ⊖ fever

flu: sudden onset high fever (~ 3-4 days), dry cough, prominent h/a, myalgia, weakness, fatigue (can last for wks), occasional stuffy nose & sore throat

* flu shot ⇒ inactivated ⇒ cannot cause flu
- may cause mild illness × [1-2 days] afterwards
  ↳ DO NOT TX IN ADVANCE/AT TIME OF SHOT! ⇒ ↓ vaccine effectiveness

INFECTIOUS DISEASES I: ANTIBACTERIALS, ANTIFUNGALS & ANTIVIRALS

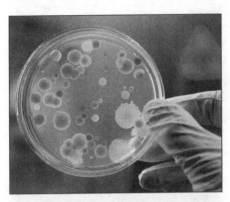

We gratefully acknowledge the assistance of Craig Martin, PharmD, BCPS, Clinical Associate Professor at the University of Kentucky and Brett Heintz, PharmD, BCPS-ID, AAHIVE, Infectious Diseases/Internal Medicine Pharmacist at Iowa City VA Medical Center and Associate Clinical Professor at the University of Iowa College of Pharmacy, in preparing this chapter.

BACKGROUND

An infectious disease is caused by one or more pathogenic viruses, bacteria, fungi, protozoa, parasites, and/or aberrant proteins known as prions. Transmission of disease can occur through various mechanisms including physical contact with an infected individual, food, body fluids, contaminated objects, airborne inhalation, or spread via a vector (carrier). Transmissible diseases, which occur through contact with an ill person or their secretions (or objects touched by them), are especially infective and are sometimes referred to as contagious diseases.

REFERENCES

Barlett JG, Auwaerter PG, Pham PA. Johns Hopkins *Antibiotic Guide: Diagnosis & Treatment of Infectious Diseases* 3rd Ed. Massachusetts: Jones and Bartlett Learning; 2012.

Bacterial Organism Identification

Bacterial organisms stain differently on a Gram stain depending if they are Gram-positive or Gram-negative organisms. Gram-positive organisms have a thick cell wall and stain purple, or bluish in color from the crystal violet stain, whereas Gram-negative organisms have a thin cell wall and take up the safranin counterstain, resulting in a pink or reddish color. The Gram stain, while not providing a definitive organism identification, can provide an important clue. Often patients will have been placed on broad spectrum antibiotic therapy to cover multiple possible organisms, and the Gram stain results can be used to streamline therapy. Streamlining, or de-escalating, therapy is a core component of antimicrobial stewardship, which is discussed later in this chapter.

Bacterial Organism Classification

The results of a Gram stain will help determine the appropriate antibiotic regimen for the infection. Clinically important Gram-positive bacteria consist mainly of the following species: *Staphylococcus, Streptococcus, Enterococcus, Clostridium*, and *Listeria*. Following is a select list of bacterial organisms.

Bacterial Organisms

CLASSIFICATION	ORGANISMS	
Gram-positive Cocci	*Enterococcus*	*Staphylococcus saprophyticus*
	Peptostreptococcus spp.	*Streptococcus agalactiae* (Grp. B)
	Staphylococcus aureus	*Streptococcus bovis* (Grp. D)
	Staphylococcus epidermidis	*Streptococcus pneumoniae*
	Viridans Streptococcus	*Streptococcus pyogenes* (Grp. A)
Gram-positive Rods	*Propionibacterium acnes*	*Corynebacterium jeikeium*
	Bacillus anthracis	*Listeria monocytogenes*
	Clostridium difficile	*Nocardia asteroides* (branched)
	Clostridium perfringens	*Actinomyces israelii* (branched)
	Corynebacterium diphtheriae	*Mycobacterium* species (acid-fast)
Gram-negative Cocci	*Neisseria gonorrhoeae*	*Neisseria meningitidis*
Spirochetes	*Borrelia burgdorferi*	*Treponema pallidum*
Atypicals	*Chlamydia/Chlamydophilia*	*Mycoplasma pneumoniae*
Gram-negative Coccobacillus	*Acinetobacter baumannii*	*Pasteurella multocida*
	Bordetella pertussis	*Moraxella catarrhalis*
Gram-negative Rods	*Bacteroides fragilis*	*Helicobacter pylori* (curved rod)
	Burkholderia cepacia	*Klebsiella pneumoniae*
	Campylobacter jejuni (curved rod)	*Legionella pneumophilia*
	Citrobacter freundii	*Morganella morganii*
	Eikenella corrodens	*Prevotella melaninogenica*
	Enterobacter cloacae	*Proteus mirabilis*
	Pseudomonas aeruginosa	*Proteus* spp.
	Providencia spp.	*Salmonella* spp.
	Enterobacter aerogenes	*Yersinia pestis*
	Escherichia coli	*Serratia* spp.
	Gardnerella vaginalis	*Shigella* spp.
	Haemophilus influenzae	*Stenotrophomonas maltophilia*
	Vibrio cholerae	

COMMON BACTERIAL PATHOGENS FOR SELECTED SITES OF INFECTION

CNS/Meningitis
Streptococcus pneumoniae
Neisseria meningitidis
Haemophilus influenzae
Streptococci/*E. coli* (young)
Listeria (young/old)

Upper Respiratory
Moraxella catarrhalis
Haemophilus influenzae
Streptococci

Bone & Joint
Staphylococcus aureus
Staphylococcus epidermidis
Streptococci
Neisseria gonorrhea
± GNR

Mouth/ENT
Peptostreptococcus
Actinomyces
Anaerobic GNRs
± *Haemophilus influenzae* and aerobic GNR

Skin/Soft Tissue
Staphylococcus aureus
Streptococcus pyogenes
Staphylococcus epidermidis
Pasteurella
± aerobic/anaerobic GNR (diabetics)

Intra-abdominal Tract
E. coli, Proteus, Klebsiella
Enterococci/Streptococci
Bacteroides species

Lower Respiratory (Community)
Streptococcus pneumoniae
Haemophilus influenzae
Atypicals: *Legionella, Mycoplasma*
Enteric GNRs (Alcoholics, IC, HCA)

Lower Respiratory (Hospital)
Enteric GNRs (*E. coli, Klebsiella, Proteus*)
Streptococcus pneumoniae
Pseudomonas aeruginosa
Enterobacter species
S. aureus, including MRSA

Urinary Tract
E. coli, Proteus, Klebsiella
Staphylococcus saprophyticus
Enterococci/Streptococci

CNS = *central nervous system*, ENT = *ear, nose and throat*, GNR = *Gram-negative rods*, HCA = *healthcare associated*, IC = *immunocompromised*

ANTIBACTERIAL AGENTS

All antibacterial agents carry a warning of the risk of superinfection with prolonged use including *C. difficile*-associated diarrhea (CDAD) and pseudomembranous colitis. This is due to killing of normal, healthy flora in the gastrointestinal tract and the resulting overgrowth of *Clostridium difficile*, which is resistant to most antibiotics. It is important to optimize therapy with the right drug and dose for an appropriate duration to reduce this and other complications.

Aminoglycosides (AMGs)

[handwritten margin notes: • Gram (-) • [ ] • cidal + Enterococcus]

AMGs interfere with bacterial protein synthesis by binding to the 30S and 50S ribosomal subunits resulting in a defective bacterial cell membrane. AMGs exhibit concentration-dependent killing and have a post-antibiotic effect (PAE). The PAE is defined as the continued suppression of bacterial growth when antibiotic levels are below the MIC of the organism. Due to concentration-dependent killing activity and a long post-antibiotic effect, AMGs are generally dosed once daily (extended interval dosing) for Gram-negative organisms. Extended interval dosing has also been shown to ↓ nephrotoxicity relative to traditional dosing.

- Coverage: Mainly active against Gram-negative bacteria (e.g., *Pseudomonas*); gentamicin and streptomycin are used for synergy in treating Gram-positive cocci (e.g., *Staphylococcus* and *Enterococcus*, in the setting of endocarditis) in combination with a beta-lactam or vancomycin.

[handwritten note: gent or strep + β-lactam or vanco → synergy for Gram (+)]

DRUG	DOSING	SAFETY/SIDE EFFECTS/MONITORING
Gentamicin IV, IM, ophthalmic, topical **Tobramycin** IV, IM, ophthalmic, inhaled Tobramycin inhalation for CF – *TOBI, TOBI Podhaler, Bethkis* **Amikacin** IV, IM **Streptomycin** IM	Use total body weight, unless the patient is obese (> 130% of IBW) If obese, use adjusted body weight **Traditional Dosing** Gent/tobra: 1-2.5 mg/kg/dose (lower doses for Gram-positive infections; higher doses for Gram-negative infections) Amikacin: 5-7.5 mg/kg/dose CrCl > 60 mL/min: Q8H CrCl 40-60 mL/min: Q12H CrCl 20-40 mL/min: Q24H CrCl < 20 mL/min: give loading dose, then monitor levels **Extended Interval Dosing** Gent/tobra: 4-7 mg/kg/dose Amikacin: 15-20 mg/kg/dose Frequency determined by nomogram (example on next page)	**BOXED WARNINGS (4)** AMGs may cause neurotoxicity (hearing loss, vertigo, ataxia), nephrotoxicity (particularly in renal impairment or with concurrent use of other nephrotoxic drugs), fetal harm if given in pregnancy **WARNINGS** Use with caution in patients with impaired renal function, in the elderly, and those on other nephrotoxic drugs (amphotericin B, cisplatin, colistimethate, cyclosporine, loop diuretics, NSAIDs, radiocontrast dye, tacrolimus and vancomycin). May ↑ the respiratory depressant effect of neuromuscular blocking agents. **SIDE EFFECTS** Nephrotoxicity (acute tubular necrosis), hearing loss (early toxicity associated with high-pitched sounds), vestibular toxicity (resulting in balance deficits). **MONITORING** Renal function, urine output, hearing tests, and peak and trough levels if using traditional dosing or a random level with extended interval dosing Traditional dosing: Take trough level right before 3rd dose, take a peak level ½ hour after the end of drug infusion of the 3rd dose Extended interval dosing: take random level per timing on the nomogram (example of nomogram on next page) **NOTES** Pregnancy Category D Extended interval dosing is less nephrotoxic and more cost-effective. Amikacin has the broadest spectrum of activity. Streptomycin: protect from light.

Traditional Dosing Target Drug Concentrations

DRUG	PEAK	TROUGH
Gentamicin		
Gram-negative infection:	5-10 mcg/mL	< 2 mcg/mL
Gram-positive infection:	3-4 mcg/mL	< 1 mcg/mL
Tobramycin	5-10 mcg/mL	< 2 mcg/mL
Amikacin	20-30 mcg/mL	< 5 mcg/mL

Organism specific peak goals are typically 8-10 times the MIC of the bacteria causing the infection. (J. Infect. Dis. 155:93–99.)

Example of Extended Interval Dosing Nomogram

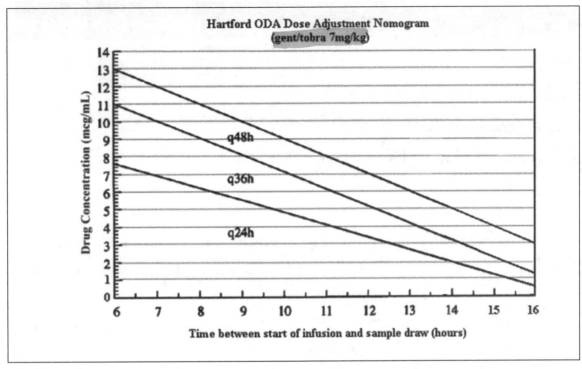

Hartford ODA Dose Adjustment Nomogram
(gent/tobra 7mg/kg)

handwritten left margin:
- Gram (+)
- time
- **cidal**
  (except
  Enterococcus
  ⇒ AG)

PENICILLINS (PCNs)

Penicillins are beta-lactams that <u>inhibit bacterial cell wall synthesis</u> by binding to one or more penicillin-binding proteins (PBPs), which in turn prevents the final transpeptidation step of peptidoglycan synthesis in bacterial cell walls. Penicillins exhibit <u>time-dependent killing</u> and are <u>bactericidal, except against</u> *Enterococci* species where aminoglycosides (gentamicin and streptomycin) are needed for bactericidal activity.

- Coverage: Mainly active against Gram-positive cocci and some Gram-negative bacilli; no atypical coverage. Ampicillin, amoxicillin and piperacillin have activity against *Enterococci*. Nafcillin and oxacillin have enhanced activity against methicillin susceptible *Staphylococcus aureus* (MSSA). The addition of a beta-lactamase inhibitor adds anaerobic *(Bacteroides)*, *Haemophilus*, *Neisseria* and other coverage. Piperacillin and ticarcillin have extended Gram-negative coverage including *Pseudomonas aeruginosa*.

handwritten notes:
★ Ampicillin, amoxicillin, piperacillin } cover Enterococci

nafcillin, oxacillin } enhanced coverage for MSSA

★ adding β-lactamase inhib. ⇒ + anaerobes (Bacteroides) + Haemophilus + Neisseria ? + Staph

piperacillin, ticarcillin } cover ext. Gram (−) ⇒ Pseudo

Select Penicillins

(handwritten: ↓ dose or ↑ interval in renal impairment EXCEPT)

(handwritten left margin: stable @ room temp x 14 d)

(handwritten left margin: stable @ room temp x 8 hrs (NOT for continuous infusion))

(handwritten left margin: anaerobic coverage (BLI))

DRUG	DOSING	SAFETY/SIDE EFFECTS/MONITORING
Aminopenicillins		**BOXED WARNING** Penicillin G benzathine: Not for intravenous (IV) use, can cause cardiorespiratory arrest and death.
Amoxicillin (Amoxil, Moxatag) *(handwritten: after, take 1 hr meals)* Tablet, capsule, chewable, suspension *(handwritten: fridge to ↑ taste)* Amoxicillin – DOC in acute otitis media, *H. pylori* regimen, prophylaxis for endocarditis **+ clavulanate (Augmentin, Augmentin ES-600, Augmentin XR, Amoclan)** Tablet, chewable, suspension *(handwritten: fridge)* Chewable tablets contain phenylalanine	Amoxicillin: 250-500 mg PO Q8H or 500-875 mg PO Q12H or 775 mg XR (Moxatag) PO daily *H. pylori* treatment (as part of a multidrug combination): 1,000 mg PO BID IE prevention: 2 grams PO 30-60 min before dental procedure Amox/Clav: 500 mg TID, 875 mg BID, or 2,000 XR PO BID with food	**CONTRAINDICATIONS** *Augmentin XR*: history of cholestatic jaundice or hepatic dysfunction; severe renal impairment (CrCl < 30 mL/minute) **WARNINGS** Anaphylaxis/hypersensitivity reactions, do not use in PCN-allergic patients **SIDE EFFECTS** GI upset, diarrhea, taste disturbance (oral), acute interstitial nephritis, rash/allergic reactions/anaphylaxis, bone marrow suppression with prolonged use, ↑ LFTs, seizures with accumulation
Ampicillin IV/IM, capsule, suspension **+ sulbactam (Unasyn)** IV *Unasyn* 3 g = 2 g ampicillin/1 g sulbactam *Unasyn* 1.5 g = 1 g ampicillin/0.5 g sulbactam	Ampicillin: 250-500 mg PO Q6H on empty stomach 1 hr before or 2 hrs after meals or 1-2 grams IV Q4-6H Amp/Sulbactam: 1.5-3 grams IV Q6H *(handwritten: mix w/ NS ONLY)*	**MONITORING** Renal function, symptoms of anaphylaxis with 1st dose, CBC, LFTs **NOTES** Pregnancy Category B Test Interactions: can cause false (+) urinary glucose test.
Natural Penicillins		Can cause positive direct Coombs test
Penicillin (Pen VK) *(handwritten: susp → fridge)*	125-500 mg PO Q6-8H on empty stomach	*Augmentin* oral suspension must be refrigerated, *Amoxil* oral suspension is refrigerated to improve taste, but is stable for 14 days at room temperature.
Penicillin G Benzathine (Bicillin L-A) Pen G Benzathine and Pen G Procaine *(Bicillin C-R)* Penicillin G Aqueous *(Pfizerpen-G)*	1.2-2.4 MU IM x 1 (frequency varies) *(handwritten: not IV (BBW))* *(handwritten: cardioresp. arrest death)* 2-4 MU IV Q4-6H	Take *Moxatag* within 1 hour of finishing a meal. Take extended release amox/clav tablets with food. Take ampicillin PO on an empty stomach 1 hour before or 2 hours after meals. Ampicillin IV is compatible with NS only; stable for 8 hours at room temperature (not suitable for continuous infusion).
Ureidopenicillins		*Unasyn* is compatible with NS only.
Piperacillin **+ tazobactam (Zosyn)** *Zosyn* 3.375 g = 3 g piperacillin/0.375 g tazobactam	Piperacillin: 3-4 grams IV Q4-6H Pip/Tazo: 3.375 grams IV Q6H or 4.5 grams IV Q6-8H	Take *Pen VK* on an empty stomach. *Pen VK* suspension should be refrigerated after reconstitution. Piperacillin and ticarcillin have activity against *Pseudomonas*.
Carboxypenicillins		Nafcillin is a vesicant – if extravasation occurs, use cold packs and hyaluronidase injections. Administration through a central line is preferred.
Ticarcillin **+ clavulanic acid (Timentin)** *Timentin* 3.1 g = 3 g ticarcillin/0.1 g clavulanic acid	Ticarcillin/Clav: 3.1 grams IV Q4-6H	Reduce dose and/or extend interval in renal impairment except for nafcillin, oxacillin and dicloxacillin. Cefazolin, cefuroxime, cefotaxime, ceftriaxone and cefepime IV: protect from light.

(handwritten right margin: monitor renal + hepatic fxn)

(handwritten bottom:)
- amoxicillin/clav (Augmentin®)
- ampicillin/sulb (Unasyn®)
- cover Pseudo { pip/tazo (Zosyn®) ticar/clav (Timentin®)

Select Penicillins Continued

DRUG	DOSING	SAFETY/SIDE EFFECTS/MONITORING
Antistaphylococcal Penicillins		⊖ renal adj
Nafcillin vesicant	1-2 grams IV/IM Q4-6H	↑ warfarin metabolism
Oxacillin	250-2,000 mg IV Q4-6H	↓ INR
Dicloxacillin	125-500 mg PO Q6H	

Penicillin Drug Interactions

- Probenecid can ↑ levels of PCNs by interfering with renal excretion. This combination may be used to ↑ penicillin levels for severe infections.

- Penicillins can ↑ the serum concentration of methotrexate.

- Tetracyclines and other bacteriostatic agents may ↓ effectiveness of penicillins by slowing bacterial growth (penicillins work best against actively growing bacteria).

- Dicloxacillin and nafcillin can ↓ INR through ↑ metabolism of warfarin; other PCNs may ↑ anticoagulant effect of warfarin.

- Penicillins can ↓ serum concentrations of the active metabolites of mycophenolate due to impaired enterohepatic recirculation.

CEPHALOSPORINS

• time
• cidal

Cephalosporins are beta-lactams that inhibit bacterial cell wall synthesis by binding to one or more penicillin-binding proteins (PBPs), which in turn prevents the final transpeptidation step of peptidoglycan synthesis in bacterial cell walls. Cephalosporins exhibit time-dependent killing with bactericidal activity.

- Coverage: The spectrum of activity is dependent upon the generation of the cephalosporin. For example, early generation cephalosporins often excel against Gram-positive pathogens (*Staphylococcus* spp.), while later generation agents provide enhanced Gram-negative coverage.

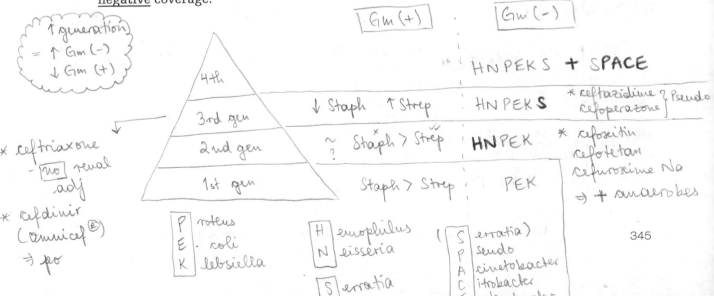

345

↓ dose or ↑ interval in renal impairment [EXCEPT] ceftriaxone !

DRUG	DOSING	SAFETY/SIDE EFFECTS/MONITORING
1st Generation – ↑ *Staphylococci* activity, but ↓ *Streptococci* and Gram-negative activity compared to 2nd/3rd generation; covers *Proteus mirabilis*, *E. coli* and *Klebsiella* species (PEK).		**CONTRAINDICATIONS** Ceftriaxone: Hyperbilirubinemic neonates (causes biliary sludging), concurrent use with calcium-containing IV products in neonates ≤ 28 days years old
Cefadroxil	500-1,000 mg PO Q12H	
CeFAZolin *(Kefzol)* Ancef®	1-1.5 g IV/IM Q8H	**WARNINGS** Anaphylaxis/hypersensitivity reactions
Cephalexin *(Keflex)*	250-1,000 mg PO Q6H	Some agents may ↑ INR if patient is taking warfarin
2nd Generation – ↑ Gram-negative activity compared to 1st generation with similar Gram-positive activity including PEK, *Haemophilus* and *Neisseria* species (HNPEK). Cefotetan and cefoxitin have anaerobic activity (*Bacteroides fragilis*), but ↓ Gram-positive activity.		Cross sensitivity (< 10%) with PCN allergy – do not use in patients who have a type 1 mediated PCN allergy (swelling, angioedema, anaphylaxis)
Cefaclor *(Ceclor®)*	250-500 mg PO Q8H	Cefotetan contains a N-methylthiotetrazole (NMTT or 1-MTT) side chain, which can ↑ risk of hypoprothrombinemia (bleeding) and a disulfiram-like reaction with alcohol ingestion.
CefoTEtan *(Cefotan®)*	1-2 grams IV/IM Q12H	
CefOXitin *(Mefoxin®)*	1-2 grams IV/IM Q6-8H	
Cefprozil *(Cefzil®)*	250-500 mg PO Q12-24H	**SIDE EFFECTS** GI upset, diarrhea, rash/allergic reactions/anaphylaxis, acute interstitial nephritis, bone marrow suppression with prolonged use, ↑ LFTs, seizures with accumulation, drug fever
Cefuroxime *(Ceftin, Zinacef)* axetil Na⊕	250-1,500 mg PO/IV/IM Q8-12H, take suspension with food	
3rd Generation – ↑ Gram-negative activity compared to 2nd generation, including HNPEK ± *Serratia* (HNPEKS) and some additional enteric Gram-negative rods; ↓ *Staphylococcal* activity compared to 1st generation but ↑ *Streptococcal* activity. Note that ceftazidime has ↓ Gram-positive activity, but ↑ Gram-negative activity including *Pseudomonas*.		**MONITORING** Renal function, signs of anaphylaxis with 1st dose, CBC, LFTs
		NOTES Pregnancy Category B
Cefdinir *(Omnicef®)*	300 mg PO Q12H or 600 mg PO daily	Test Interactions – positive direct Coombs test, false positive urinary glucose test.
Cefditoren *(Spectracef)*	200-400 mg PO Q12H with food	↓ dose and/or extend interval in renal impairment except for ceftriaxone.
Cefixime *(Suprax)* also chewable	400 mg PO divided Q12-24H	Cefditoren tablets should be taken with food. Take cefuroxime suspension with food. Take ceftibuten suspension on an empty stomach.
Cefotaxime *(Claforan)*	1-2 grams IV/IM Q4-12H	
Cefpodoxime	100-400 mg PO Q12H	
CefTAZidime *(Fortaz, Tazicef)*	1,000–2,000 IV/IM mg Q8-12H	Cefixime is available as 100 and 200 mg chewable tablets; these contain phenylalanine.
Ceftibuten *(Cedax)*	400 mg PO daily on empty stomach *suspension*	
CefTRIAXone *(Rocephin)*	1-2 grams IV/IM Q12-24H	
4th Generation – Best Gram-negative activity, including HNPEKS, *Citrobacter*, *Acinetobacter*, *Pseudomonas*, *Enterobacter* and *Serratia* species (CAPES) and Gram-positive activity similar to 3rd generation.		
Cefepime *(Maxipime)*	1-2 grams IV/IM Q8-12H	
5th Generation – Best Gram-positive activity; covers MRSA, some Gram-negative similar to ceftriaxone (no *Pseudomonas* coverage).		
Ceftaroline fosamil *(Teflaro)*	600 mg IV Q12H	

(margin notes:)

⊕ intra-abdom. (anaerobes)

Pseudo + cefo-perazone (Cefobid®)
⊖ renal adj.

Same as PCN ⊕ taste disturbance

↳ Micromedex: 2 hrs before / 1 hr after meal

→ only IV cephalo that can be dosed qd

some ↑INR by inhibiting vit K-dependent CF production

Cephalosporin Drug Interactions

- Probenecid can ↑ levels of cephalosporins by interfering with renal excretion. This combination may be used to ↑ cephalosporin levels.

- Cephalosporins may enhance the anticoagulant effect of warfarin by inhibiting the production of vitamin K-dependent clotting factors.

time
cidal

CARBAPENEMS   DOC for ESBL producers!

Carbapenems are beta-lactams that inhibit bacterial cell wall synthesis by binding to one or more penicillin-binding proteins (PBPs), which in turn prevents the final transpeptidation step of peptidoglycan synthesis in bacterial cell walls. Carbapenems exhibit time-dependent killing with bactericidal activity.

- Coverage: Very broad spectrum with activity against most Gram-positive, Gram-negative, and anaerobic pathogens. They do not cover atypical pathogens, MRSA, VRE, *C. difficile* and *Stenotrophomonas*. Ertapenem does not have activity against *Pseudomonas* or *Acinetobacter*.

↓ dose or ↑ interval in renal impairment!

Seizures

++++

+++

+++

DRUG	DOSING	SAFETY/SIDE EFFECTS/MONITORING
Imipenem/ Cilastatin (*Primaxin*)	250-1,000 mg IV Q6-8H	**CONTRAINDICATIONS** Anaphylactic reactions to beta-lactam antibiotics
Meropenem (**Merrem**)	500-1,000 mg IV Q8H Dilute with SWFI – stable for 3 hours at room temp.	**WARNINGS** Carbapenems have been associated with CNS adverse effects, including confusional states and seizures Doripenem: do not use for the treatment of pneumonia including healthcare-associated pneumonia (HAP) and ventilator-associated pneumonia (VAP) Do not use in patients with PCN allergy, cross-reactivity has been reported to be as high as 50%, but newer studies show rates < 10%.
Ertapenem (**INVanz**)	1,000 mg IV/IM daily Stable in NS Ertapenem is not active against *Pseudomonas* or *Acinetobacter*	**SIDE EFFECTS** Diarrhea, rash, and seizures with higher doses and in patients with impaired renal function (mainly imipenem), bone marrow suppression with prolonged use, ↑ LFTs **MONITORING** Renal function, symptoms of anaphylaxis with 1st dose, CBC, LFTs
Doripenem (*Doribax*)	500 mg IV Q8H	**NOTES** Pregnancy Category B/C (imipenem) Imipenem is combined with cilastatin to prevent drug degradation by renal tubular dehydropeptidase. ↓ dose and/or extend interval in renal impairment.

NOT for pneumonia
(HAP / VAP)

Carbapenem Drug Interactions

- Probenecid can ↑ levels of carbapenems by interfering with renal excretion. This combination may be used to ↑ carbapenem levels.

- Carbapenems can ↓ serum concentrations of valproic acid leading to a loss of seizure control.

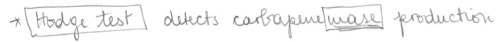

* Hodge test detects carbapenemase production

- Use with caution in patients at risk for seizures or with other agents known to lower seizure threshold (e.g., ganciclovir, fluoroquinolones, bupropion, tramadol). See Epilepsy chapter for a complete list.

FLUOROQUINOLONES (FQs)

[handwritten left margin: · [ ] · cidal]

Fluoroquinolones inhibit bacterial DNA topoisomerase IV and inhibit DNA gyrase (topoisomerase II). This prevents supercoiling of DNA and promotes breakage of double-stranded DNA. Fluoroquinolones exhibit concentration-dependent killing with bactericidal activity.

- Coverage: Extensive activity against Gram-negative, Gram-positive, and average-to-excellent atypical coverage (levofloxacin, moxifloxacin and gemifloxacin). Ciprofloxacin and levofloxacin have enhanced Gram-negative activity, including *Pseudomonas*, while moxifloxacin has enhanced Gram-positive and anaerobic activity and is often used for mixed infections alone (intra-abdominal infections). Gemifloxacin, levofloxacin and moxifloxacin are often referred to as respiratory fluoroquinolones due to enhanced coverage of *Streptococcus pneumoniae* and atypical coverage. It is important to note that any use of fluoroquinolones for the treatment of *Pseudomonas* infections generally requires the use of another agent (typically a beta-lactam) in combination.

[handwritten notes:]

* cipro / levo } enhanced Gm (-) =) Pseudo

* use w/ β-lactam for dual Pseudo coverage

* moxi ⇒ enhanced Gm (+) + anaerobes (intraabd.)   monotx

* gemi / levo / moxi } resp. FQ ↑↑↑ atypical + Strep. pneumo

↑ interval (and may ↓ dose) in renal impairment [EXCEPT] moxi

DRUG	DOSING	SAFETY/SIDE EFFECTS/MONITORING
Ofloxacin Tablet, ophthalmic, otic	200-400 mg PO Q12H CrCl < 30 mL/min: 400 mg Q24H	**BOXED WARNINGS (2)** Tendon inflammation and/or rupture (most often in Achilles tendon) – ↑ risk with concurrent corticosteroid use, organ transplant patients, > 60 years of age May exacerbate muscle weakness related to myasthenia gravis
Norfloxacin *(Noroxin)* Tablet	400 mg PO BID or 800 mg PO daily CrCl ≤ 30 mL/min: 400 mg daily	**CONTRAINDICATIONS** Concurrent administration of tizanidine (with ciprofloxacin) **WARNINGS** Fluoroquinolones can prolong the QT interval; avoid use in patients at risk for QT prolongation. Use caution with agents that prolong QT interval including Class Ia and Class III antiarrhythmics.
Ciprofloxacin *(Cipro, Cipro XR, Ciloxin* eye drops, *Cetraxal* ear drops)* + dexamethasone *(Ciprodex* ear drops)* Tablet, suspension, injection, ointment, ophthalmic, otic	250-750 mg PO or 200-400 IV Q8-12H CrCl 30-50 mL/min: Q12H CrCl < 30 mL/min: Q18-24H *IR – can crush + H₂O ⇒ feeding tube ⊖ other feedings 1hr/2hrs*	Peripheral neuropathy (with oral and IV formulations) – may last months to years after the drug has been discontinued. In some cases, it may become permanent. If symptoms occur, stop the drug. CNS effects: Tremor, restlessness, confusion, and very rarely hallucinations, ↑ intracranial pressure (including pseudotumor cerebri) or seizures may occur; use with caution in patients with known or suspected CNS disorder Hypoglycemia/Hyperglycemia Hepatotoxicity
Levofloxacin *(Levaquin, Quixin* eye drops)* Tablet, solution, injection, ophthalmic *light protect*	250-750 mg IV/PO daily CrCl < 50 mL/min: ↓ dose and/or extend dosing interval, dose adjustment varies depending on dosage strength and renal function	Photosensitivity/phototoxicity Risk of arthropathy, use in children should be avoided due to concerns of musculoskeletal toxicity but may use if benefit outweighs the risk (such as anthrax) per the American Academy of Pediatrics
Gatifloxacin *(Zymaxid* eye drops)*	Oral formulation not available	**SIDE EFFECTS** GI upset/diarrhea, headache, dizziness, insomnia, crystalluria and interstitial nephritis (rare)
Moxifloxacin *(Avelox, Avelox ABC Pack, Moxeza* eye drops, *Vigamox* eye drops)* Tablet, injection, ophthalmic	400 mg IV/PO Q24H	**NOTES** Pregnancy Category C *Cipro Oral Susp* should not be given through a NG or other feeding tube (the oil-based suspension adheres to the tubing). Shake vigorously for 15 seconds each time before use. Do not chew the microcapsules. Do not refrigerate the oral suspension.
Gemifloxacin *(Factive)* Tablet	320 mg PO daily CrCl ≤ 40 mL/min: 160 mg daily	*Cipro IR* – can crush immediate release tablets, mix with water and give via feeding tube. Hold tube feedings at least 1 hour before and 2 hours after dose. Ciprofloxacin and levofloxacin IV: protect from light. Take levofloxacin oral solution on an empty stomach (1 hour before or 2 hours after a meal); maintain adequate hydration to prevent crystalluria; store at room temperature. Extend interval (and may reduce dose) in renal impairment except for moxifloxacin. These agents can be used in PCN-allergic patients.

≠ tizanidine

• po only
• ⊖ NG tube (sticks)
• shake ×15 sec
• ⊖ chew microcaps
• ⊖ fridge

most QT prolong in class

Quinolone Drug Interactions

- Antacids, didanosine, sucralfate, bile acid resins, magnesium, aluminum, calcium, iron, zinc, multivitamins or any product containing these multivalent cations can chelate and inhibit absorption. Separate as follows:

  cipro 2/6
  - Give ciprofloxacin 2 hours before or 6 hours after these agents

  levo 2/2
  - Give levofloxacin 2 hours before or 2 hours after these agents

  moxi 4/8
  - Give moxifloxacin 4 hours before or 8 hours after these agents

- Although it is usually recommended that concomitant intake of calcium-rich foods (dairy products) be avoided because of the potential for chelation, the actual influence of dairy products on fluoroquinolone absorption varies. In general, recommend to avoid administration with dairy products.

- Lanthanum *(Fosrenol)* can ↓ the serum concentration of quinolones; take oral quinolones at least 2 hours before or after lanthanum.

- Can ↑ the effects of warfarin, sulfonylureas/insulin and QT-prolonging drugs (moxifloxacin prolongs the QT interval the most).

- Probenecid and NSAIDs can ↑ FQ levels.

- Ciprofloxacin is a P-glycoprotein substrate, strong 1A2 inhibitor and weak 3A4 inhibitor; ciprofloxacin can ↑ the levels of caffeine and theophylline by reducing metabolism.

- Levofloxacin is primarily renally cleared.

static **MACROLIDES**

Macrolides bind to the 50S ribosomal subunit, resulting in inhibition of RNA-dependent protein synthesis with bacteriostatic activity related to total exposure of the drug (AUC/MIC).

- Coverage: Activity against Gram-positive pathogens, namely *Streptococci* species, and some Gram-negative pathogens, namely *Haemophilus, Neisseria* and *Moraxella* species, and good atypical coverage (*Legionella, Chlamydia, Mycoplasma* and some *Mycobacterium* species); suitable for treatment of community-acquired upper and lower respiratory tract infections and certain sexually transmitted infections.

DRUG	DOSING	SAFETY/SIDE EFFECTS/MONITORING
Azithromycin (Zithromax, Z-Pak, Zmax, Zithromax Tri-Pak, AzaSite ophthalmic)** Tablet, suspension, injection, ophthalmic Better Gram-negative coverage compared to erythromycin	500 mg PO on day 1, then 250 mg on days 2-5 (Z-Pak) or 500 mg PO daily x 3 days or 1-2 grams x 1 250-500 mg IV daily No adjustment in renal impairment	**CONTRAINDICATIONS** History of cholestatic jaundice/hepatic dysfunction with prior use Clarithromycin and erythromycin: concomitant use with pimozide, ergotamine or dihydroergotamine, lovastatin or simvastatin Clarithromycin: concurrent use with colchicine in patients with renal or hepatic impairment, history of QT prolongation or ventricular cardiac arrhythmia **WARNINGS** Macrolides have been associated with QT prolongation and ventricular arrhythmias, including torsade de pointes; use with caution in patients at risk of prolonged cardiac repolarization; avoid use in patients with uncorrected hypokalemia or hypomagnesemia, clinically significant bradycardia, and patients receiving Class Ia or Class III antiarrhythmic agents Hepatotoxicity
Clarithromycin (Biaxin, Biaxin XL, Biaxin XL Pac) Tablet, suspension Better Gram-positive coverage	250-500 mg PO Q12H or 1 gram PO daily CrCl < 30 mL/minute: ↓ dose by 50%	**SIDE EFFECTS** GI upset (diarrhea, abdominal pain and cramping especially with erythromycin), taste perversion, ↑ LFTs, ototoxicity (reversible and rare) **NOTES** Pregnancy Category B/C (clarithromycin) *AzaSite* – viscous solution for ophthalmic use. Store at room temp once dispensed (cold makes solution more viscous).
Erythromycin (E.E.S., Ery-Tab, EryPed, Erythrocin, PCE) Capsule, tablet, suspension, injection, ophthalmic, topical	E.E.S.: 400-800 mg PO Q6-12H Erythromycin base/stearate: 250-500 mg PO Q6-12H Erythromycin lactobionate: 15-20 mg/kg/day IV Q6H (max 4 grams/day) No adjustment in renal impairment IV is stable in NS	These agents can be used in PCN-allergic patients. Azithromycin ER suspension (*Zmax*) is not bioequivalent with *Zithromax* and should not be interchanged. *Zmax* must be consumed within 12 hours of reconstitution on an empty stomach. Do not refrigerate azithromycin oral suspension (*Zmax*). Take *Biaxin XL* with food. Do not refrigerate *Biaxin* oral suspension (can gel). Must refrigerate erythromycin ethylsuccinate (E.E.S.) oral granule suspension and use within 10 days. Erythromycin powder suspension stable at room temperature x 35 days.

Handwritten margin notes:

↓↓ interaxns than other 2

ER susp

Zmax® ≠ Zithromax® (not bioeq)
- empty stomach
- w/in 12 hrs of recon.
- ⊘ fridge

≠ pimozide (dihydro-) ergotamine lovastatin simvastatin

→ ⊘ fridge → gel

≠ ① colchicine + renal/hepatic imp.
② hx of QT prolongation
③ hx of ventr. ♡ arrhythmia

Biaxin® XL – w/ food

→ fridge *

SE:
GI upset (diarrhea, abdomin. pain, cramping)

major 3A4 inhib

* use w/in 10 days (powder stable @ room temp x 35 days)

351

Macrolide Drug Interactions

- Erythromycin and clarithromycin are substrates of 3A4 (major) and 3A4 inhibitors (moderate/strong); use caution or avoid with many medications metabolized by 3A4 including apixaban, colchicine, conivaptan, cyclosporine, dabigatran, digoxin, quinidine, rivaroxaban, theophylline, warfarin and others. See Drug Interactions chapter for more information.

- Azithromycin is a substrate of 3A4 (minor) and inhibitor of 1A2 (weak) and P-gp; it does not have as many clinically significant drug interactions.

- All macrolides: do no use concurrently with agents that can prolong the QT interval.

TETRACYCLINES

static

Tetracyclines inhibit bacterial protein synthesis by reversibly binding to the 30S ribosomal subunit with bacteriostatic activity related to the total exposure of the drug (AUC/MIC). Doxycycline is used more often in practice due to improved tolerability and broader coverage, including for respiratory tract infections, tick-borne/rickettsial diseases, spirochetes and *Chlamydia* infections. Doxycycline is also an option for the treatment of MRSA in mild skin infections and VRE in urinary tract infections. Minocycline has enhanced Gram-positive coverage and is often preferred for skin infections, including acne. Tetracycline is rarely used in practice, but can be used as part of *H. pylori* regimens.

- Coverage: Activity against many Gram-positive bacteria, including *Staphylococci, Streptococci, Enterococci, Nocardia, Bacillus* and *Propiobacterium* specius, Gram-negative bacteria, including respiratory tract flora *(Haemophilus, Moraxella,* atypicals) and other unique pathogens *(spirochetes, Rickettsiae, Bacillus anthracis, Treponema pallidum,* etc.).

DRUG	DOSING	SAFETY/SIDE EFFECTS/MONITORING
Doxycycline *(Adoxa, Atridox, Doryx, Monodox, Oracea, Vibramycin,* others) Capsule, tablet, suspension, syrup, injection	100-200 mg PO/IV in 1-2 divided doses Take *Oracea* on an empty stomach (1 hr before or 2 hrs after meals). Take other forms with food to ↓ GI irritation No adjustment in renal impairment	**WARNINGS** Children < 8 years of age, pregnancy and breastfeeding (Preg Category D – suppresses bone growth and skeletal development, permanently discolors teeth) Drug Rash with Eosinophilia and Systemic Symptoms syndrome (DRESS), exfoliative dermatitis ↑ BUN Photosensitivity Drug-induced lupus erythematosus (DILE) with minocycline
Minocycline *(Minocin, Solodyn)* Capsule, tablet, injection	200 mg PO/IV x 1, then 100 mg PO/IV Q12H No adjustment in renal impairment	**SIDE EFFECTS** Nausea, vomiting, diarrhea, rash **MONITORING** LFTs, BUN, SCr, CBC
Tetracycline Capsule	250-500 mg PO Q6H on an empty stomach CrCl ≤ 80 mL/min: extend dosing interval	**NOTES** Pregnancy Category D Take with 8 oz water to minimize GI irritation. Doxycycline IV to PO ratio is 1:1. Doxycycline oral suspension should not be refrigerated. Doxycycline IV: requires light protection during administration.

Tetracycline Drug Interactions

- Tetracycline absorption is impaired by antacids containing magnesium, aluminum, or calcium or medications that contain divalent cations such as iron-containing preparations, sucralfate, bile acid resins, or bismuth subsalicylate – separate doses (take 1-2 hours before or 4 hours after). Doxycycline and minocycline are less likely to be of clinical concern. These can be taken with food to reduce GI upset, but do not administer with dairy products (calcium). Do not eat or drink dairy products within 1 hour before or 2 hours after tetracycline products.

- Lanthanum *(Fosrenol)* can ↓ the concentration of tetracycline derivatives; take at least 2 hours before or after lanthanum.

- Tetracycline is a substrate of 3A4 (major) and 3A4 (moderate) inhibitor. Caution with the use of 3A4 inhibitors which ↑ levels and 3A4 inducers which ↓ levels.

- Doxycycline is a weak 3A4 inhibitor.

- Can enhance the anticoagulant effects in patients taking warfarin.

- Tetracycline derivatives can enhance the effects of neuromuscular blocking agents.

- Avoid concomitant use with retinoic acid derivatives due to the risk of pseudotumor cerebri.

- Tetracyclines can ↓ the effectiveness of penicillins by slowing bacterial growth (penicillins work best against actively growing bacteria).

cidal

SULFONAMIDES

Sulfamethoxazole (SMX) interferes with bacterial folic acid synthesis via inhibition of dihydrofolic acid formation from para-aminobenzoic acid and trimethoprim (TMP) inhibits dihydrofolic acid reduction to tetrahydrofolate resulting in inhibition of enzymes of the folic acid pathway. Individually they are bacteriostatic, however collectively they are bactericidal.

- Coverage: SMX/TMP has activity against Gram-positive bacteria, including *Staphylococci/MRSA*, and many Gram-negative bacteria, including *Haemophilus, Enterobacter, Acinetobacter, Shigella, Salmonella, Stenotrophomonas*; active against some opportunistic pathogens (*Nocardia, Pneumocystis, Toxoplasmosis*); but no *Pseudomonas, Enterococci,* atypical or anaerobic coverage.

DRUG	DOSING	SAFETY/SIDE EFFECTS/MONITORING
Sulfamethoxazole/ Trimethoprim *(Bactrim, Bactrim DS, Septra DS, Sulfatrim,* others) **Single Strength (SS)** 400 mg SMX/80 mg TMP **Double Strength (DS)** 800 mg SMX/160 mg TMP Sulfamethoxazole: Trimethoprim dose is always a 5:1 ratio	Dose is based on the TMP component **Severe Infections** 10-20 mg/kg/day TMP (2 DS tabs BID-TID) **Adult Female Uncomplicated UTI** 1 DS tab BID x 3 days **PCP Prophylaxis** 1 DS or SS tab daily **PCP Treatment** 15-20 mg/kg TMP IV/PO divided Q6H CrCl 15-30 mL/min: ↓ dose by 50% CrCl < 15 mL/min: not recommended	**CONTRAINDICATIONS** Sulfa allergy, pregnancy (at term), breastfeeding, anemia due to folate deficiency, marked renal or hepatic disease, infants < 2 months of age **WARNINGS** Blood dyscrasias including agranulocytosis and aplastic anemia SJS/TEN, thrombotic thrombocytopenic purpura, and other dermatologic reactions G6PD deficiency - use caution **SIDE EFFECTS** Nausea, vomiting, anorexia, diarrhea, skin reactions (rash, urticaria), crystalluria (take with 8 oz of water), interstitial nephritis, photosensitivity, bone marrow suppression with prolonged use, false elevations in SCr due to inhibition of tubular secretion of creatinine (pseudoazotemia), hyperkalemia, hypoglycemia, CNS (confusion, drug fever, seizures), ↑ LFTs, QT prolongation, ↓ folic acid, positive Coombs test **MONITORING** SCr, BUN, LFTs, electrolytes, CBC **NOTES** To avoid confusion, mg/kg doses should always reference the trimethoprim component. Pregnancy Category D: risk for kernicterus and spinal cord defects. *Bactrim IV* – store at room temp, short stability (~6 hrs; however, the more concentrated the solution, the shorter the stability), dilute with D5W. Requires light protection during administration. Infuse over 60-90 minutes. *Bactrim* suspension should be stored at room temp and protected from light. IV to PO ratio is 1:1.

(handwritten left margin: works best on empty stomach (light snack if stomach upset))

(handwritten right margin: ↑ K+ ↓ BG)

(handwritten table:)

indication	dose	interval
PCP proph	1 DS or SS	qd
UTI	1 DS	BID
severe infxn	2 DS	BID-TID

Sulfonamide Drug Interactions

- Sulfonamides are inhibitors of 2C8/9 (moderate/strong), caution with concurrent use of warfarin. See Drug Interactions chapter for more 2C8/9 substrates.

(handwritten bottom of page:)

PABA
SMX ↳→ dihydrofolic acid
     ↳→ tetrahydrofolic acid
TMP   ↳ DNA/RNA

- Can ↑ levels/effects of sulfonylureas, metformin, fosphenytoin/phenytoin, dofetilide, aza-thioprine, methotrexate, mercaptopurine and warfarin.

- Levels of SMX/TMP can be ↓ by 2C8/9 inducers and the therapeutic effects may be diminished by the use of leucovorin/levoleucovorin.

- ACE inhibitors, ARBs, aliskiren, potassium-sparing diuretics, drospirenone-containing oral contraceptives, cyclosporine, tacrolimus and canagliflozin will ↑ risk for hyperkalemia when used concurrently; monitor.

- Additive QT prolongation with other agents that prolong the QT interval (refer to the Antiarrhythmics chapter for complete list).

ADDITIONAL AGENTS TO TREAT GRAM-POSITIVE INFECTIONS

Vancomycin   *↑ interval in renal imp.*

• time
• cidal

Inhibits bacterial cell wall synthesis by blocking peptidoglycan polymerization by binding to the D-alanyl-D-alanine portion of cell wall precursor. Vancomycin exhibits time-dependent killing and is bactericidal.

- Coverage: Active against most Gram-positive bacteria, including *Staphylococci* (MRSA), *Streptococci* and *Enterococci* (not VRE) and *Clostridium difficile*.

DRUG	DOSING	SAFETY/SIDE EFFECTS/MONITORING
Vancomycin (Vancocin)	MRSA infections: 15-20 mg/kg IV Q8-12H Extend interval in renal impairment: CrCl 20-49 mL/min: Q24H CrCL < 20 mL/min: give loading dose, then monitor levels *C. difficile*-associated diarrhea 125-500 mg PO QID x 10-14 days (higher if recurrent or severe, complicated disease) Infuse peripheral IV at a concentration not to exceed 5 mg/mL	**WARNINGS** Caution with the use of other nephrotoxic or ototoxic drugs (AMGs, cisplatin, others) **SIDE EFFECTS** *angio-edema, dyspnea* GI upset (oral route), infusion reaction/red man syndrome (maculopapular rash from too rapid of an infusion rate, hypotension, flushing, chills – give 30 min infusion for each 500 mg of drug), nephrotoxicity, bone marrow suppression (neutropenia/thrombocytopenia), drug fever, ototoxicity **MONITORING** Renal function, WBC, trough concentration at steady state (generally before the 4th dose) *AG → trough before 3rd dose* Target troughs of 15-20 mcg/mL – pneumonia, endocarditis, osteomyelitis, meningitis, bacteremia Target troughs of 10-15 mcg/mL for other infections **NOTES** Pregnancy Category B (oral)/C (IV) Consider alternative agent when MIC of organism ≥ 2 mcg/mL *↳ if vanc used ⇒ clinical failure*

troughs
○ *15-20 µg/ml { pneumo, endoCD, osteo meningitis bacteremia }*
○ *10-15 µg/ml → other infxns*

Vancomycin Drug Interactions

- Vancomycin can ↑ toxicity of other nephrotoxic drugs (e.g., AMGs, amphotericin B, cisplatin, colistimethate, cyclosporine, loop diuretics, NSAIDs, radiocontrast dye, tacrolimus, vancomycin). Vancomycin can ↑ toxicity of other ototoxic drugs (e.g., AMGs, cisplatin, loop diuretics, others).

✱ despite [time]-dependent killing, parameter best correlated w/ vanc efficacy is AUC/MIC   355

·[ ]
·cidal

Daptomycin *(Cubicin)*

Cyclic lipopeptide class – binds to cell membrane components causing rapid depolarization, inhibiting all intracellular replication processes including protein synthesis. Daptomycin exhibits concentration-dependent killing and bactericidal activity.

- Coverage: Active against most Gram-positive bacteria, including *Staphylococci* (MRSA) and *Enterococci* including VRE *faecium* and *faecalis.* Approved for complicated skin and soft-tissue infections and *Staphylococus aureus* bloodstream infections, including right-sided endocarditis.

DRUG	DOSING	SAFETY/SIDE EFFECTS/MONITORING
DAPTOmycin *(Cubicin)*	4-6 mg/kg IV daily CrCl < 30 mL/min: extend dosing interval to Q48H	**WARNINGS** May cause eosinophilic pneumonia – generally develops 2-4 weeks after therapy initiation Myopathy – discontinue in patients with signs and symptoms of myopathy in conjunction with an increase in CPK > 1,000 units/L (5 times ULN) or in asymptomatic patients with a CPK ≥ 2,000 units/L (10 times ULN) **SIDE EFFECTS** Diarrhea, constipation, vomiting, nausea, anemia, headache, dizziness, ↑ CPK and myopathy, dyspnea, hypokalemia, hyperkalemia, hyperphosphatemia, ↑ LFTs **MONITORING** CPK level weekly (more frequently if on a statin); muscle pain/weakness **NOTES** Pregnancy Category B Do not use to treat pneumonia as drug is inactivated by surfactant. Compatible with NS and LR only. Can cause false elevations in PT/INR (but no ↑ in bleeding risk).

handwritten notes:

myopathy ⇒ d/c if

- Sx + CPK > 1,000

OR

- ⊖ Sx + CPK ≥ 2,000

↑↓K⁺
↑PO₄

Daptomycin Drug Interactions

- Daptomycin can have additive risk of muscle toxicity when used in conjunction with statins.

• [ ]
• cidal

Telavancin *(Vibativ)*

Lipoglycopeptide and derivative of vancomycin – inhibits bacterial cell wall synthesis by blocking polymerization and cross-linking of peptidoglycan by binding to the D-Ala-D-Ala portion of the cell wall. Unlike vancomycin, telavancin has an additional mechanism involving disruption of membrane potential and changes in cell permeability due to the presence of a lipophilic side chain moiety. Telavancin exhibits concentration-dependent killing and is bactericidal.

- Coverage: Active against most Gram-positive bacteria, including *Staphylococci* and *Enterococci* (but not VRE). Approved for complicated skin and soft-tissue infections caused by Gram-positive organisms and for hospital acquired pneumonia (HAP) due to Gram-positive pathogens, including MRSA, when alternative treatments are not appropriate.

DRUG	DOSING	SAFETY/SIDE EFFECTS/MONITORING
Telavancin (*Vibativ*)	10 mg/kg IV daily CrCl ≤ 50 mL/min: reduce dose or extend interval	**BOXED WARNINGS (3)** Fetal risk – obtain pregnancy test prior to starting therapy Nephrotoxicity – new onset or worsening renal impairment has occurred Patients with pre-existing moderate-to-severe renal impairment (CrCl ≤ 50 mL/minute) treated for hospital-acquired/ventilator-associated bacterial pneumonia (HABP/VABP) had ↑ mortality versus vancomycin **WARNINGS** Can prolong the QT interval Rapid IV administration may result in red man syndrome (flushing, rash, urticaria, and/or pruritus) – infuse over 60 minutes to prevent infusion reaction. **SIDE EFFECTS** Metallic taste, nausea, vomiting, ↑ SCr, QT prolongation, red man syndrome **MONITORING** Renal function, pregnancy status **NOTES** Pregnancy Category C Can interfere with coagulation tests MedGuide Required

Jv ??

Telavancin Drug Interactions

- Avoid in patients with congenital long QT syndrome, known QT prolongation, or uncompensated heart failure. Caution with the use of other medications known to prolong the QT interval.

[ ]
cidal

Oritavancin (Orbactiv)

Oritavancin is a lipoglycopeptide that inhibits cell wall biosynthesis by inhibiting the polymerization step by binding to stem peptides of peptidoglycan precursors, by inhibiting cross-linking by binding to bridging segments, and by disrupting bacterial membrane integrity, leading to cell death. Oritavancin exhibits the concentration-dependent bactericidal activity.

- Coverage: Active against Gram-positive organisms including *Staphylococci* (both MSSA and MRSA), *Streptococci*, and *Enterococcus faecalis* (vancomycin susceptible strains only).

DRUG	DOSING	SAFETY/SIDE EFFECTS/MONITORING
Oritavancin *(Orbactiv)*	1,200 mg IV x1 Infuse over 3 hours CrCl < 30 mL/min: has not been studied, use with caution	**CONTRAINDICATIONS** Use of intravenous unfractionated heparin for 48 hours after oritavancin administration due to artificial interference with aPTT laboratory results. **WARNINGS** May ↑ risk of bleeding in patients receiving warfarin. Enhanced monitoring is recommended. Additionally, oritavancin may artificially prolong PT/INR for up to 24 hours after a dose. If infusion-related reactions occurs, slow or interrupt infusion. **SIDE EFFECTS** Nausea, vomiting, diarrhea, infusion-related reactions **NOTES** Pregnancy Category C Compatible with D5W only

Oritavancin Drug Interactions

- Weak inhibitor of CYP2C9 and CYP2C19 and weak inducer of CYP3A4 and CYP2D6. Use caution when coadministered with drugs metabolized by these enzymes.

[ ] dependent
AG
FQ
dapto
telavancin
oritavancin
dalbavancin
telithro
polymixins
↓
dosed less frequently
(in higher doses)

time dependent ⇒ dosed more frequently
PCN
cephalos } β-lactams
CBPs
vanco

cidal
AG   polymixins
PCN   chloramph
cephalos   telithro
CBP   Flagyl®
FQ   Tindamax®
sulfonamides   rifamixin
vanco   Dificid®
dapto   fosfomycin
telavancin   nitrofuran
oritavancin   ampho B
dalbavancin   flucytosine
Synercid®   echinocand

static
macrolides
tetras
Zyvox®
Sivextro®
Tyacil®
clinda

azoles (cidal?)

Dalbavancin *(Dalvance)*

· [ ]
- *cidal* Dalbavancin is a lipoglycopeptide which binds to the D-alanyl-D-alanine terminus of cell wall peptidoglycan, preventing cross-linking and interfering with cell wall synthesis. It exhibits concentration-dependent bactericidal activity.

- Coverage: Active against Gram-positive organisms such as *Staphylococci* (including MSSA and MRSA) and *Streptococci*

DRUG	DOSING	SAFETY/SIDE EFFECTS/MONITORING
Dalbavancin *(Dalvance)*	1,000 mg IV x 1, then 500 mg IV x 1 one week later CrCl < 30 mL/min: 750 mg IV x 1, followed by 375 mg IV x 1 one week later Infuse over 30 minutes	**WARNINGS** Infusion reactions: rapid IV administration may result in red man syndrome (flushing, rash, urticaria, and/or pruritus) – infuse over 30 minutes. ↑ ALT levels > 3 times the upper limit of normal. **SIDE EFFECTS** Nausea, headache, diarrhea, rash **MONITORING** Liver function, renal function **NOTES** Pregnancy Category C Compatible with D5W only

Dalbavancin Drug Interactions

- None reported.

Linezolid *(Zyvox)*

static

Oxazolidinone class – binds to the bacterial 23S ribosomal RNA of the 50S subunit inhibiting bacterial translation and protein synthesis and is mainly bacteriostatic.

- Coverage: Active against most Gram-positive bacteria, including *Staphylococci* (MRSA) and *Enterococci* (VRE *faecium* and *faecalis*). Approved for pneumonia and uncomplicated/complicated skin and soft-tissue infections including diabetic foot infections and infections caused by *Staphylococcus aureus* and *Streptococcus* species and for VRE infections.

DRUG	DOSING	SAFETY/SIDE EFFECTS/MONITORING
Linezolid *(Zyvox)*	600 mg PO/IV Q12H No adjustment in renal impairment	**CONTRAINDICATIONS** Concurrent use or within 2 weeks of MAO inhibitors **WARNINGS** Duration-related myelosuppression, peripheral and optic neurpathy when treated > 28 days, serotonin syndrome, hypoglycemia – caution on diabetes patients on insulin or hypoglycemia agents **SIDE EFFECTS** Anemia (↓ Hgb), thrombocytopenia, headache, diarrhea, nausea, insomnia, taste alteration, ↑ pancreatic enzymes, ↑ LFTs, neuropathy **MONITORING** Weekly CBC, visual function **NOTES** Pregnancy Category C IV to PO ratio is 1:1. Store oral suspension at room temp and use within 21 days of reconstitution. Prior to administration mix gently by inverting bottle; do not shake. IV: requires light protection during administration.

oral susp
- *store @ room temp*
- *use w/in 21 days of recon*
- *gently invert bottle to mix before use (⊘ shake)*

↓ BG

Linezolid Drug Interactions

- Linezolid is a weak monoamine oxidase inhibitor. Caution in patients taking concurrent serotonergic or adrenergic drugs. Avoid tyramine containing foods and serotonergic drugs. See Drug Interactions chapter.

- Linezolid can exacerbate hypoglycemic episodes, caution in patients receiving insulin or oral hypoglycemic agents.

Tedizolid *(Sivextro)*

static

Oxazolidinone class – binds to the bacterial 23S ribosomal RNA of the 50S subunit inhibiting bacterial translation and protein synthesis and is bacteriostatic.

- Coverage: Gram-positive organisms such as *Staphylocci* (including MSSA and MRSA), *Streptococci*, and *Enterococcus faecalis*.

DRUG	DOSING	SAFETY/SIDE EFFECTS/MONITORING
Tedizolid *(Sivextro)*	200 mg IV/PO daily for 6 days Infuse over 1 hour, stable in NS No adjustment in renal impairment	**WARNINGS** Consider alternative therapy in patients with neutropenia. **SIDE EFFECTS** Headache, diarrhea, nausea, myelosuppression, dizziness **NOTES** Pregnancy Category C Tedizolid is a weak MAOI, similar to linezolid. Clinical relevance of this interaction with tedizolid has yet to be determined.

Tedizolid Drug Interactions

- Potential interaction with serotonergic drugs.

Quinupristin/Dalfopristin *(Synercid)*

cidal

Streptogramin class – binds to different sites on the 50S bacterial ribosomal subunit inhibiting protein synthesis and is bactericidal.

- Coverage: Active against most Gram-positive bacteria, including *Staphylococci, Enterococcus faecium* (not *E. faecalis*). Also approved for complicated skin and soft-tissue infections caused by *Staphylococcus aureus* and *Streptococcus pyogenes*.

DRUG	DOSING	SAFETY/SIDE EFFECTS/MONITORING
Quinupristin/Dalfopristin *(Synercid)*	7.5 mg/kg IV Q8-12H No adjustment in renal impairment	**SIDE EFFECTS** Arthralgias/myalgias (up to 47%), infusion reactions, including edema and pain at infusion site (up to 44%), phlebitis (40%), hyperbilirubinemia (up to 35%), GI upset, CPK elevations, ↑ LFTs **NOTES** Pregnancy Category B Must be in a volume of 250 mL or greater (D5W only) to be given peripherally. IV formulation should be refrigerated after reconstitution.

Quinupristin/Dalfopristin Drug Interactions

- Quinupristin/Dalfopristin is a weak 3A4 inhibitor; can ↑ levels of CCBs, cyclosporine, dofetilide and others.

ADDITIONAL AGENTS TO TREAT GRAM-NEGATIVE INFECTIONS

Aztreonam

A monobactam that inhibits bacterial cell wall synthesis by binding to one or more of the penicillin-binding proteins (PBPs), which in turn inhibits the final transpeptidation step of peptidoglycan synthesis in bacterial cell walls, thus inhibiting cell wall synthesis; bactericidal. The monobactam structure makes cross-allergenicity with beta-lactams unlikely.

- Coverage: Active against many Gram-negative organisms including *Pseudomonas*; no Gram-positive activity.

DRUG	DOSING	SAFETY/SIDE EFFECTS/MONITORING
Aztreonam *(Azactam IV, Cayston* – inhaled for CF)	500-2,000 mg IV Q6-12H CrCl 10-30 mL/min: ↓ dose by 50% CrCl <10 mL/min: ↓ dose by 25%	**SIDE EFFECTS** Similar to penicillins, including rash, diarrhea, nausea, vomiting, ↑ LFTs **NOTES** Pregnancy Category B Can be used in PCN-allergic patients

Polymyxins

The polymyxin class consists of two main agents, colistin and polymyxin B. Colistimethate is the inactive prodrug that is hydrolyzed to colistin, which acts as a cationic detergent and damages the bacterial cytoplasmic membrane causing leaking of intracellular substances and cell death. These agents exhibit concentration-dependent killing and are bactericidal.

- Coverage: Cover Gram-negatives such as *Enterobacter* spp., *E. coli*, *Klebsiella pneumonia*, and *Pseudomonas aeruginosa* – used primarily in setting of multidrug resistant Gram-negative pathogens. These agents do not cover *Proteus* spp.

- Should be used in combination with another agent due to emergence of resistance.

DRUG	DOSING	SAFETY/SIDE EFFECTS/MONITORING
Colistimethate sodium *(Coly-Mycin M)* PRODRUG hydrolyzed to colistin	2.5-5 mg/kg/day IV/IM in 2-4 divided doses CrCl < 80 mL/min: reduce frequency and extend interval	**WARNING** Dose-dependent nephrotoxicity (monitor renal function and electrolytes), neurotoxicity **SIDE EFFECTS** Nephrotoxicity (proteinuria, ↑ SCr), neurologic disturbances (dizziness, tingling, numbness, paresthesia, vertigo) **NOTES** Pregnancy Category C Solutions for inhalation must be mixed immediately prior to administration.

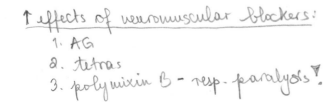

↑ effects of neuromuscular blockers:
1. AG
2. tetras
3. polymixin B - resp. paralysis!

Polymyxins Continued

DRUG	DOSING	SAFETY/SIDE EFFECTS/MONITORING
Polymyxin B Sulfate IM/IV, intrathecal	15,000-25,000 units/kg/day IV divided every 12 hours CrCl < 80 mL/min: reduce frequency and extend interval	**BOXED WARNINGS (6)** Nephrotoxicity (dose-dependent) – monitor renal function/electrolytes closely Neurotoxicity Safety in pregnancy is not established Intramuscular/intrathecal administration only to hospitalized patients. The concurrent or sequential use of other neurotoxic or nephrotoxic drugs such as bacitracin, streptomycin, neomycin, kanamycin, gentamicin, tobramycin, amikacin, cephaloridine, paromomycin, viomycin, and colistin should be avoided. The neurotoxicity of polymyxin B sulfate can result in respiratory paralysis from neuromuscular blockade. **SIDE EFFECTS** Nephrotoxicity, neurologic disturbances (dizziness, tingling, numbness, paresthesia, vertigo) fever, urticaria **NOTES** 1 mg = 10,000 units polymyxin B Compatible with D5W

Polymyxin Drug Interactions

Other nephrotoxic agents can enhance the nephrotoxic effect.

ADDITIONAL BROAD SPECTRUM AGENTS

Chloramphenicol

Reversibly binds to the 50S ribosomal subunit of susceptible organisms inhibiting protein synthesis; bactericidal.

- Coverage: Activity against Gram-positives, Gram-negatives, anaerobes, and atypicals.

DRUG	DOSING	SAFETY/SIDE EFFECTS/MONITORING
Chloramphenicol Rarely used due to side effects	50-100 mg/kg/day IV in divided doses Q6H (max 4 g/day) No adjustment in renal impairment but use with caution	**BOXED WARNING** Serious and fatal blood dyscrasias (aplastic anemia, thrombocytopenia) **WARNINGS** Gray syndrome – characterized by circulatory collapse, cyanosis, acidosis, abdominal distention, myocardial depression, coma, and death; associated with high serum levels **SIDE EFFECTS** Myelosuppression (pancytopenia), aplastic anemia, dermatologic (angioedema, rash, urticaria), diarrhea, ↓ vitamin B12 **MONITORING** CBC at baseline and every 2 days during therapy, liver and renal function, serum drug concentrations

*[ ]
: cidal

Telithromycin *(Ketek)*

Ketolide class – inhibits bacterial protein synthesis by binding to 2 sites on the 50S ribosomal subunit (structurally related to macrolides). Telithromycin exhibits concentration-dependent killing and is bactericidal.

- Coverage: Activity against Gram-positives, primarily *Streptococci* species, including macrolide resistant strains, Gram-negatives, some anaerobes, and *Mycobacteria* atypicals; FDA approved for community acquired pneumonia only.

DRUG	DOSING	SAFETY/SIDE EFFECTS/MONITORING
Telithromycin *(Ketek)*	800 mg PO daily CrCl < 30 mL/min: 600 mg PO daily CrCl < 30 mL/min + hepatic impairment: 400 mg PO daily	**BOXED WARNING** Do not use in myasthenia gravis due to respiratory failure **CONTRAINDICATIONS** Allergy to macrolides, history of hepatitis or jaundice from macrolides, myasthenia gravis, concurrent use with colchicine (if patient has renal or liver impairment), lovastatin, simvastatin or pimozide **WARNINGS** Acute hepatic failure (can be fatal), QT prolongation, visual disturbances (blurry vision, diplopia), syncope **SIDE EFFECTS** Diarrhea, nausea, vomiting, dizziness, headache, ↑ LFTs, rash **MONITORING** LFTs and visual acuity **NOTES** Pregnancy Category C

FQ also worsen MG (muscle weakness)

Telithromycin Drug Interactions

- Telithromycin is a substrate of 1A2 (minor), 3A4 (major) and an inhibitor of 2D6 (weak) and 3A4 (strong). Avoid with moderate/strong 3A4 inhibitors and 3A4 substrates with a narrow therapeutic window or significant toxicity (e.g., simvastatin, lovastatin). Avoid with class Ia and class III antiarrhythmics and other major QT prolonging drugs. See Drug Interactions chapter for more information.

static ## Tigecycline *(Tygacil)*

Glycylcycline class – binds to the 30S ribosomal subunit inhibiting protein synthesis; structurally related to the tetracyclines; bacteriostatic.

- Coverage: Activity against Gram-positives such as *Staphylococci* (including MSSA and MRSA), *Enterococci* (including VRE *faecium* and *faecalis*), Gram-negatives, anaerobes, and atypicals. Among the Gram-negatives, tigecycline does not have activity against the "3 P's": *Pseudomonas, Proteus, Providencia* species. Tigecycline is approved for adults with complicated skin and soft-tissue infections/intraabdominal infections and for community acquired pneumonia; however, a recent FDA warning suggests to use it only when other alternatives are not possible. ↑ death

DRUG	DOSING	SAFETY/SIDE EFFECTS/MONITORING
Tigecycline *(Tygacil)* Derivative of minocycline	100 mg IV x 1 dose, then 50 mg IV Q12H Severe hepatic impairment: 100 mg IV x 1, then 25 mg IV Q12H No adjustment in renal impairment	**BOXED WARNING** ↑ risk of death, should only be used in situations when alternative treatments are not suitable **WARNINGS** Hepatotoxicity, pancreatitis, photosensitivity, teeth discoloration in patients < 8 years old (avoid use) **SIDE EFFECTS** Nausea, vomiting, diarrhea, headache, dizziness, insomnia, ↑ LFTs, pruritus, rash **NOTES** Pregnancy Category D Lower cure rates in ventilator-associated pneumonia. Avoid use in bloodstream infections as it does not achieve adequate concentrations in the blood due to its lipophilicity (drug remains concentrated in tissues). Reconstituted solution should be yellow-orange; discard if not this color.

Handwritten notes:
the 4 Ts
1) related to tetras
2) concentrates in tissues
3) Three Gm (-) Ps NOT covered
   1. Pseudomonas
   2. Proteus
   3. Providencia
4) tummy ↑ SE (N/V/D)

Tigecycline Drug Interactions

- Tigecycline can ↑ INR in patients taking warfarin.

OTHER ANTIBACTERIAL AGENTS

Clindamycin *(Cleocin)*

Handwritten: static

Lincosamide class – reversibly binds to the 50S ribosomal subunit and inhibits bacterial protein synthesis; bacteriostatic.

- Coverage: Activity against most aerobic Gram-positives (not *Enterococcus*) and anaerobic Gram-negative and Gram-positives.

DRUG	DOSING	SAFETY/SIDE EFFECTS/MONITORING
Clindamycin *(Cleocin)* Topical: *Cleocin, Cleocin-T, Clindacin ETZ, Clindacin Pac, Clindacin-P, Clindagel, ClindaMax, Clindesse, Evoclin*	150-450 mg PO Q6H 600-900 mg IV Q8H No adjustment in renal impairment	**BOXED WARNING** Can cause severe and possibly fatal colitis **WARNING** Severe or fatal reactions like SJS/TEN **SIDE EFFECTS** GI upset (nausea, vomiting, diarrhea); rash, urticaria, ↑ LFTs (rare) **NOTES** Pregnancy Category B

Handwritten: susp ⊘ fridge

cidal

Metronidazole *(Flagyl)* and Tinidazole *(Tindamax)*

These agents cause a loss of helical DNA structure and strand breakage resulting in inhibition of protein synthesis; bactericidal.

- Coverage: Metronidazole has activity against anaerobes and protozoal infections; effective for bacterial vaginosis, trichomoniasis, giardiasis, amebiasis and *Clostridium difficile* infection. Tinidazole has activity against protozoa (giardiasis, amebiasis), trichomoniasis and bacterial vaginosis organisms – structurally related to metronidazole.

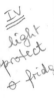

IV light protect & fridge

DRUG	DOSING	SAFETY/SIDE EFFECTS/MONITORING
Metronidazole *(Flagyl, Flagyl ER, Metro)* Topical: *MetroCream, MetroGel, MetroGel Vaginal, MetroLotion, Noritate, Vandazole* *IR- w/ food* *XR- empty stomach* *≠ disulfiram w/in past 2 wks*	500-750 mg IV/PO Q8-12H or 250-500 mg IV/PO Q6-8H **Mild-to-Moderate *C.diff* infections** 500 mg IV/PO TID for 10-14 days No adjustment in renal impairment Take immediate release tablets with food to ↓ GI upset. Take extended release tablets on empty stomach	**BOXED WARNING** Possibly carcinogenic based on animal data **CONTRAINDICATIONS** Pregnancy (1st trimester), breastfeeding (tinidazole), use of disulfiram within the past 2 weeks (metronidazole), use of alcohol or propylene glycol-containing products during therapy or within 3 days of therapy discontinuation **WARNINGS** CNS effects – seizures, peripheral/optic neuropathies, aseptic meningitis (metronidazole), encephalopathy (metronidazole)
Tinidazole *(Tindamax)* *≠ breastfeeding*	2 grams PO daily Take with food to minimize GI effects No adjustment in renal impairment	**SIDE EFFECTS** Nausea, vomiting, diarrhea, metallic taste, furry tongue, darkened urine, rash, headache, dizziness **NOTES** Metronidazole IV: PO ratio is 1:1 and requires light protection during administration. Do not refrigerate (metronidazole) IV (crystals may form which may dissolve upon warming to room temperature). Pregnancy Category B metronidazole/C (tinidazole)

Metronidazole/Tinidazole Drug Interactions

- Metronidazole is an inhibitor of 3A4 (weak) and 2C9 (weak) whereas tinidazole is a substrate of 3A4 (minor).

- Metronidazole and tinidazole should not be used with alcohol (during and for 3 days after discontinuation of therapy) due to a potential disulfiram-like reaction.

- Metronidazole, and potentially tinidazole, can ↑INR in patients taking warfain.

7:15 - 4:15

cidal ## Rifaximin *(Xifaxan)*

Rifaximin inhibits bacterial RNA synthesis by binding to bacterial DNA-dependent RNA polymerase. It is structurally related to rifampin and is bactericidal.

minimal systemic absorption (not strong hepatic enzyme inducer)

- Coverage: Rifaximin is indicated for treatment of travelers' diarrhea caused by non-invasive *E. coli* and prevention of hepatic encephalopathy. Although not an FDA-approved indication, it may sometimes be used as a salvage therapy option in patients with recurrent or refractory *Clostridium difficile* infection.

DRUG	DOSING	SAFETY/SIDE EFFECTS/MONITORING
Rifaximin *(Xifaxan)*	**Travelers' Diarrhea** 200 mg PO TID x 3 days	**SIDE EFFECTS** Peripheral edema, dizziness, headache, flatulence, nausea, abdominal pain, rash/pruritus
	Reduction of Hepatic Encephalopathy Recurrence 550 mg PO BID	**NOTES** Pregnancy Category C
	No adjustment in renal impairment	Not effective for systemic infections – < 1% oral absorption

cidal ## Fidaxomicin *(Dificid)*

Inhibits RNA polymerase resulting in inhibition of protein synthesis and cell death; bactericidal.

- Coverage: Used for *Clostridium difficile* associated diarrhea. Although it has shown benefit in preventing recurrence of disease, it is currently used most often in select cases due to high cost (e.g., resistance and/or failure to vancomycin or metronidazole).

DRUG	DOSING	SAFETY/SIDE EFFECTS/MONITORING
Fidaxomicin *(Dificid)*	200 mg PO BID x 10 days No adjustment in renal impairment	**SIDE EFFECTS** Nausea, vomiting, abdominal pain, GI bleeding, anemia
		NOTES Pregnancy Category B
		Not effective for systemic infections – absorption is minimal

cidal ## Fosfomycin *(Monurol)*

Inhibits bacterial cell wall synthesis by inactivating the enzyme, pyruval transferase, which is critical in the synthesis of cell walls; bactericidal.

- Coverage: Single dose used to treat uncomplicated UTI (cystitis only) due to *E. coli* and *E. faecalis* (active against VRE).

DRUG	DOSING	SAFETY/SIDE EFFECTS/MONITORING
Fosfomycin *(Monurol)* 1 packet of granules = 3 grams	**Female, Uncomplicated UTI** 3 grams PO x 1, mixed in 3-4 oz of cold water	**SIDE EFFECTS** Headache, diarrhea, nausea
		NOTES Pregnancy Category B

Nitrofurantoin *(Macrodantin, Macrobid, Furadantin)*

cidal

Bacterial cell wall inhibitor; bactericidal.

- Coverage: Used for uncomplicated UTI (cystitis only) due to *E. coli, S. aureus, Enterococcus, Klebsiella* and *Enterobacter.*

serum [ ]s not adequate to tx systemic/ uncompx UTIs

DRUG	DOSING	SAFETY/SIDE EFFECTS/MONITORING
Nitrofurantoin *(Macrodantin, Macrobid, Furadantin)*	*Macrodantin* 50-100 mg PO QID with food x 3-7 days; 50-100 mg PO QHS with food for prophylaxis *MacroBID* 100 mg PO BID x 7 days ≠ CrCl < 60 mL/min: contraindicated	**CONTRAINDICATIONS** Patients with renal impairment (CrCl < 60 mL/min) due to concerns of inadequate urinary concentrations and risk for accumulation of neurotoxins, pregnancy (at term) **WARNINGS** Optic neuritis, hepatotoxicity, peripheral neuropathy, pulmonary toxicity, hemolytic anemia (use caution in patients with G6PD deficiency) and positive Coombs test **SIDE EFFECTS** GI upset, headache, rash, brown urine discoloration (harmless) **NOTES** Pregnancy Category B (contraindicated at term)

SELECT ORAL ANTIBIOTIC (SOLUTIONS, SUSPENSIONS) REFRIGERATION REQUIREMENTS AND ANTIBACTERIALS THAT DO NOT NEED TO BE ADJUSTED IN RENAL IMPAIRMENT

Oral antibiotics (solutions, suspensions) that need to be refrigerated after reconstitution

Amoxicillin/Clavulanate (Augmentin)

Cefaclor

Cefadroxil

Cefpodoxime

Cefprozil

Cefuroxime *(Ceftin)*

Ceftibuten *(Cedax)*

Cephalexin *(Keflex)*

Erythromycin/Benzoyl peroxide (Benzamycin)

Erythromycin ethylsuccinate/ Sulfisoxazole *(E.S.P.)*

Penicillin VK

Refrigeration recommended

Amoxicillin *(Amoxil)* – improves taste

Keflex ® – use w/in 14 days • shake well • take w/ food if stomach upset

Do not refrigerate

Azithromycin *(Zmax)*

Cefdinir

Clarithromycin *(Biaxin)* – bitter taste and thickening/gels

Clindamycin *(Cleocin)* – thickening and may crystallize

Ciprofloxacin *(Cipro)*

Doxycycline *(Vibramycin)*

Fluconazole *(Diflucan)*

Levofloxacin *(Levaquin)*

Linezolid *(Zyvox)*

Sulfamethoxazole/Trimethoprim *(Septra, Sulfatrim)*

Voriconazole *(VFEND)*

Chewable Tablets

Amoxicillin

Amoxicillin/Clavulanate

Cefixime

Common antibacterials that do not require renal dose adjustment

Azithromycin

Ceftriaxone

Chloramphenicol

Clindamycin

Dicloxacillin

Doxycycline

Erythromycin

Fidaxomicin

Linezolid

Metronidazole

Minocycline

Moxifloxacin

Nafcillin

Oxacillin

Quinupristin/Dalfopristin

Rifaximin

Rifampin

Tedizolid

Tigecycline

Tinidazole

SYSTEMIC FUNGAL INFECTIONS

Background

- Certain types of fungi (including yeasts such as *Candida)* may colonize body surfaces and are considered to be normal flora in the intestine. They do not normally cause serious fungal infections unless the immune system is weakened, or compromised, by drugs or diseases.

- Invasive fungal infections are associated with high morbidity and mortality. Candidemia, the 4th most common cause of nosocomial bloodstream infections in the U.S., has a mortality rate up to 30%.

- Some fungi reproduce by spreading microscopic spores. These spores are often present in the air, where they can be inhaled or come into contact with the skin, therefore, causing lung and skin infections and in some cases central nervous system infections.

- Fungi are classified as either yeasts (e.g. *Candida, Cryptococcus),* molds *(Aspgergillus, Mucor),* or dimorphic *(Histoplasma, Blastomyces).*

- *Blastomyces, Coccidioides* and *Histoplasma* are considered dimorphic fungi as they can exist in both mold (lower temperatures) and yeast forms (higher temperatures).

- Some common fungal organisms include *Aspergillus* spp., *Blastomyces* spp., *Candida* spp., *Crytococcus* spp., *Coccidioides* spp., *and Histoplasma* spp.

Drug Treatment

cidal (handwritten, left margin)

Amphotericin B Deoxycholate and Lipid Formulations

Amphotericin B binds to ergosterol, altering cell membrane permeability in susceptible fungi and causing cell death; fungicidal. Lipid formulations are a complex of the active medication and a lipid component, which are used clinically because they lessen the toxicity of the drug. Amphotericin B deoxycholate (the conventional form) is very toxic.

premedicate! (handwritten, left margin)

AMPHOTERICIN B FORMULATIONS	DOSING	SAFETY/SIDE EFFECTS/MONITORING
Conventional Formulations		**BOXED WARNINGS (2)** Medication errors from confusion between lipid-based forms of amphotericin *(Abelcet, Amphotec, AmBisome)* and conventional amphotericin B for injection have resulted in death. Conventional amphotericin B for injection doses should not exceed 1.5 mg/kg/day, verify product name and dosage if dose exceeds 1.5 mg/kg/day. Overdose may result in cardiopulmonary arrest.
Amphotericin B deoxycholate Injection Broad spectrum: covers yeasts, molds, dimorphic fungi	0.1-1.5 mg/kg/day *light protect* (handwritten)	
		SIDE EFFECTS Fever, chills, headache, malaise, rigors, hypokalemia, hypomagnesemia, nephrotoxicity, anemia, hypotension/hypertension, thrombophlebitis, nausea, vomiting *AmBisome* has had rare reports of severe back/chest pain with 1st dose
Lipid Formulations *"fierce on the fungus, kinder to the kidneys"* (handwritten)		
Amphotericin B Lipid Complex *(Abelcet)* Injection	5 mg/kg/day No renal adjustment needed	**MONITORING** Renal function, LFTs, electrolytes (especially K+ and Mg2+), CBC **NOTES** Pregnancy Category B Compatible with D5W only; all products should be refrigerated.
Liposomal Amphotericin B *(AmBisome)* Injection *Severe back/chest pain w/ 1st dose* (handwritten)	3-6 mg/kg/day No renal adjustment needed	Lipid formulations has ↓ infusion reactions and ↓ nephrotoxicity compared to conventional formulation. While lipid formulations are more expensive than conventional amphotericin B, most institutions use lipid formulations due to ↓ toxicity and ↓ premedication use. Amphotericin B conventional requires light protection during administration and pre-medication is needed to reduce infusion-related reactions (fever, chills, hypotension, nausea). Give 30-60 minutes prior to infusion:
Amphotericin B cholesteryl sulfate complex *(Amphotec)* Injection	3-4 mg/kg/day No renal adjustment needed	■ Acetaminophen or NSAID ■ Diphenhydramine and/or hydrocortisone ■ Meperidine to ↓ duration of severe rigors ■ Fluid boluses to ↓ risk of nephrotoxicity

↓ K+ (handwritten, right margin)
↓ Mg++ (handwritten, right margin)

Amphotericin B Drug Interactions

■ Additive ↑ risk of nephrotoxicity when used with other nephrotoxic agents such as AMGs, cisplatin, colistimethate, cyclosporine, flucytosine, loop diuretics, NSAIDs, radiocontrast dye, tacrolimus, vancomycin and others. May ↑ risk of digoxin toxicity due to hypokalemia.

■ Use caution with any agent that ↓ potassium or magnesium since amphotericin decreases both. Scheduled replacement of potassium or magnesium should be considered.

K+, Mg++ (handwritten)

cidal ## Flucytosine

Flucytosine penetrates fungal cells and is converted to fluorouracil which competes with uracil, interfering with fungal RNA and protein synthesis; fungicidal.

DRUG	DOSING	SAFETY/SIDE EFFECTS/MONITORING
Flucytosine, 5-FC (Ancobon) Spectrum: covers yeasts, including *Candida* and *Cryptococcus*	50-150 mg/kg/dose PO Q6H CrCl < 40 mL/min: reduce dose and extend interval	**BOXED WARNING** Use with extreme caution in patients with renal dysfunction. Closely monitor hematologic, renal, and hepatic status. **SIDE EFFECTS** Dose-related bone marrow suppression, many CNS effects, hypoglycemia, hypokalemia, aplastic anemia, hepatitis, ↑ bilirubin, ↑ SCr, ↑ BUN and others **NOTES** Avoid use as monotherapy due to rapid resistance. Ampho B can ↑ effect of flucytosine; may be used for synergy with ampho B for certain fungal infections (*Cryptococcus* spp.).

↓ BG
↓ K+

Localized Therapy for Oral Candidiasis

DRUG	DOSING	SAFETY/SIDE EFFECTS/MONITORING
Clotrimazole 10 mg troche/lozenge	**Oral Candidiasis** Prophylaxis: 10 mg 3x/day Treatment: 10 mg 5x/day x 14 days Allow troche to dissolve slowly over 15-30 minutes	**SIDE EFFECTS** ↑ LFTs, nausea, dysgeusia **MONITORING** LFTs **NOTES** Pregnancy Category C Inhibitory concentrations remain in the saliva for up to 3 hours after dissolution of the troche/lozenge.
Nystatin Swish and Swallow (Bio-Statin) Suspension, tablet	**Oral Candidiasis** Suspension (swish and swallow): 400,000-600,000 units 4 times/day; swish in the mouth and retain for as long as possible (several minutes) before swallowing **Intestinal infections** Oral tablets: 500,000-1,000,000 units Q8H	**SIDE EFFECTS** Diarrhea, nausea, stomach pain, vomiting **NOTES** Pregnancy Category C Shake suspension well before using.

↳ topical azole x 7 days ⇒ DOC in pregnancy vaginal fungal infxns

[handwritten top margin: for all azoles — ↑LFTs / QT prolong / ↓K+ / drug interaxns]

[handwritten left margin: static / cidal]

Azole Antifungals

Azole antifungals decrease ergosterol synthesis and inhibit cell membrane formation and are typically fungistatic, but may be fungicidal for select fungal pathogens. Fluconazole is the drug of choice for oropharyngeal candidiasis (thrush) in HIV patients or in moderate-severe disease in non-HIV infected patients. Voriconazole is the drug of choice for Aspergillus infections.

DRUG	DOSING	SAFETY/SIDE EFFECTS/MONITORING
Itraconazole (*Sporanox, Sporanox PulsePak, Onmel*) Tablet, capsule, solution Spectrum: covers yeasts, dimorphics, *Aspergillus*	200-400 mg PO daily-BID Capsules and oral solution are not interchangeable Take capsule/tablet with food. Take solution on empty stomach. Limited data on use in renal impairment, use with caution	**BOXED WARNINGS** **Itraconazole (2)** Use is contraindicated for treatment of onychomycosis in patients with ventricular dysfunction or a history of HF. Coadministration with itraconazole can cause ↑ plasma concentrations of certain drugs and can lead to QT prolongation and ventricular tachyarrhythmias, including torsade de pointes. Coadministration with methadone, disopyramide, dofetilide, dronedarone, quinidine, ergot alkaloids, irinotecan, lurasidone, oral midazolam, pimozide, triazolam, felodipine, nisoldipine, ranolazine, eplerenone, cisapride, lovastatin, simvastatin and, in subjects with renal or hepatic impairment, colchicine, is contraindicated.
Ketoconazole (*Nizoral, Nizoral AD, Ketodan, Extina, Xolegel* – all brands are topicals) Used off-label to treat advanced prostate cancer due to anti-androgenic activity	200-400 mg PO daily No adjustment in renal impairment	**Ketoconazole (3)** Ketoconazole has been associated with hepatotoxicity which have led to liver transplantation and/or death. Concomitant use with cisapride, dofetilide, pimozide, and quinidine is contraindicated due risk of life-threatening ventricular arrhythmias such as torsade de pointes. Use oral tablets only when other effective antifungal therapy is unavailable or not tolerated and the benefits outweigh risks.
		SIDE EFFECTS Headache, nausea, abdominal pain, vomiting, rash/pruritus, ↑ LFTs, hypertriglyceridemia, QT prolongation, hypokalemia, hypertension, edema, dizziness, hair loss (or possible hair growth) and altered hair texture with ketoconazole shampoo
Fluconazole (*Diflucan*) Tablet, suspension, injection Spectrum: covers yeasts, including *Candida albicans* and *Cryptococcus* and dimorphic fungi	150-800 mg PO/IV daily CrCl ≤ 50 mL/min: ↓ dose by 50%	**NOTES** *Sporanox PulsePak* should be taken in "pulses" of 200 mg PO BID for 1 week, then 3 weeks off (then repeat) for treatment of onychomycosis. All azoles are cleared hepatically except fluconazole. Only fluconazole and voriconazole penetrate the CNS adequately to treat fungal meningitis and are often associated with CNS toxicities (headache, dizziness, hallucinations or ocular toxicity as with voriconazole). Fluconazole IV should not be refrigerated. Fluconazole IV to PO ratio is 1:1. Pregnancy Category C – itraconazole, ketoconazole, fluconazole 150 mg single dose, posaconazole/D – fluconazole (not 150 mg) and voriconazole

[handwritten left margin near Itraconazole: pH-dependent absorption (avoid w/ antacids)]

[handwritten below Itraconazole cell: caps/tabs – w/ food / solution – empty stomach]

[handwritten right margin near Itraconazole: (-) ionotropic effect]

[handwritten under Ketoconazole dosing: ↑INR]

[handwritten below Ketoconazole: shampoo can cause altered hair texture / Nizoral AD – 1%]

[handwritten right margin near Side Effects: ↑LFTs / HTN / ↑TGs / ↓K+]

[handwritten left margin near Fluconazole: ✱ only azole not hepatically cleared]

[handwritten under Fluconazole dosing: ↑INR]

[handwritten below Fluconazole: DOC – oropharyngeal candid. / ✱ HIV pts / ✱ moderate-severe dz in non-HIV / ⊝ fridge IV]

[handwritten bottom: ✱ ONLY fluconazole / voriconazole } penetrate CNS ⇒ tx fungal meningitis]

Polymyxins Continued

DRUG	DOSING	SAFETY/SIDE EFFECTS/MONITORING
Voriconazole (VFEND) Tablet, suspension, injection Spectrum similar to itraconazole with enhanced mold coverage, drug of choice for *Aspergillosis.* No activity against *Mucormycosis* and *Zygomycosis*	Loading dose: 6 mg/kg IV Q12H x 2 doses Maintenance dose: 4 mg/kg IV Q12H or 200 mg PO Q12H – use actual body weight for dosing **Therapeutic Range** 1-5 mcg/mL Take 1 hour before or 1 hour after meals (empty stomach) In patients with CrCl < 50 mL/min, the IV vehicle, SBECD (sulfobutyl ether beta-cyclodextrin), may accumulate. Use oral dosing after the initial IV loading doses Suspension – shake for 10 seconds before each use. Do not refrigerate.	**CONTRAINDICATIONS** Coadministration with barbiturates (long-acting), carbamazepine, efavirenz (≥ 400 mg/day), ergot alkaloids, pimozide, quinidine, rifabutin, rifampin, ritonavir (≥ 800 mg/day), sirolimus and St. John's wort **WARNINGS** QT prolongation – correct K^+, Ca^{2+}, and Mg^{2+} prior to initiating therapy **SIDE EFFECTS** Visual changes (~20% – blurred vision, photophobia, altered color perception, altered visual acuity) ↑ SCr, CNS toxicity (hallucinations, headache, dizziness), rash, photosensitivity, ↑ LFTs, hypokalemia **MONITORING** LFTs, renal function, electrolytes, visual function, CBC, trough concentrations **NOTES** Caution driving at night due to vision changes. Avoid direct sunlight. Hold tube feedings for 1 hour before and 1 hour after an oral dose. More active against *Aspergillus* species, *C. glabrata,* and *C. krusei,* compared to itraconazole/fluconazole.
Posaconazole (Noxafil) Tablet, suspension, injection Spectrum similar to voriconazole with *Mucormycosis* and *Zygomycosis* activity	PO: 100-400 mg QD-TID IV: 300 mg BID x 1 day, then 300 mg daily In patients with CrCl < 50 mL/min, the IV vehicle, SBECD (sulfobutyl ether beta-cyclodextrin), may accumulate. Oral formulations are preferred. Must be taken with a full meal (during or within 20 minutes following a meal)	**CONTRAINDICATIONS** Coadministration with sirolimus, ergot alkaloids, pimozide, quinidine, atorvastatin, lovastatin or simvastatin **WARNINGS** QT prolongation – correct K^+, Ca^{2+}, and Mg^{2+} prior to initiating therapy **SIDE EFFECTS** Diarrhea, nausea, vomiting, fever, headache, ↑ LFTs, rash, hypokalemia, hypomagnesemia, hyperglycemia **MONITORING** LFTs, renal function, electrolytes, CBC

Handwritten margin notes (left): tablets contain lactose; DoC - Aspergillus infxns; ↑INR

Handwritten margin notes (right): ↓ Mg++; ↓ K+; ↑ BG

Azole Antifungals Drug Interactions

- <u>All azoles are 3A4 inhibitors</u> (moderate-strong). Itraconazole is an inhibitor of 3A4 (strong) and P-gp. Ketoconazole inhibits 1A2 (weak), 2C9 (moderate), 2C19 (moderate), 2D6 (moderate), 3A4 (strong) and P-gp. Fluconazole is an inhibitor of 2C9 (moderate), 2C19 (strong), and 3A4 (moderate). Voriconazole is an inhibitor of 2C9 (moderate), 2C19 (moderate) and 3A4 (strong). Posaconazole is an inhibitor of 3A4 (strong).

Handwritten margin notes (right): Plavix Ⓔ; Plavix Ⓔ

- <u>Itraconazole and ketoconazole have pH-dependent absorption;</u> ↑ pH causes ↓ absorption; avoid using with antacids, H_2RAs, PPIs.

- **Voriconazole** is metabolized by several CYP 450 enzymes (2C19, 2C9 and 3A4); the concentration of voriconazole can ↑ dangerously when given with drugs that inhibit voriconazole's metabolism or with small dose increases – it is first-order, followed by zero-order (non-linear) kinetics.

- Avoid concurrent use of voriconazole and the following drugs: barbiturates (long-acting), carbamazepine, efavirenz (≥ 400 mg/day), ergot alkaloids, pimozide, quinidine, rifabutin, rifampin, ritonavir (≥ 800 mg/day), sirolimus and St. John's wort.

- All azoles can ↑ INR in patients on warfarin – greatest risk with fluconazole, ketoconazole and voriconazole.

cidal

Echinocandins IV, ⊖ renal adj

Echinocandins inhibit synthesis of β(1,3)-D-glucan, an essential component of the fungal cell wall, and are considered to be fungicidal. They are effective against most *Candida* spp., including non-albicans strains resistant to azole antifungals. They have activity against *Aspergillus* spp., but should be used as part of a combination regimen.

infuse over 1 hr

DRUG	DOSING	SAFETY/SIDE EFFECTS/MONITORING
Caspofungin (Cancidas) IV	70 mg IV on day 1, then 50 mg IV daily Moderate hepatic impairment: 70 mg IV on day 1, then 35 mg IV daily ↑ dose to 70 mg IV daily when used in combination with rifampin or other strong enzyme inducers Stable in NS and LR, do not mix with dextrose-containing solutions	**WARNINGS** Histamine-mediated symptoms (rash, pruritus, facial swelling, flushing, hypotension) have occurred; anaphylaxis **SIDE EFFECTS** ↑ LFTs, hypotension, fever, diarrhea, hypokalemia, hypomagnesemia, hypoglycemia, anemia, ↑ SCr, rash, nausea, vomiting
Micafungin (Mycamine) IV *light protect*	**Candidemia** 100 mg IV daily **Esophageal Candidiasis** 150 mg IV daily	**MONITORING** LFTs **NOTES** All 3 agents are given once daily and do not require dose adjustment in renal impairment. Very few drug interactions. Micafungin requires light protection during administration.
Anidulafungin (Eraxis) IV	**Candidemia** 200 mg IV on day 1, then 100 mg IV daily **Esophageal Candidiasis** 100 mg IV on day 1, then 50 mg daily	Caution use of caspofungin with cyclosporine due to ↑ hepatotoxicity. Pregnancy Category C/B (anidulafungin)

↓ K+
↓ Mg++
↓ BG

Other Antifungal Agents

DRUG	DOSING	SAFETY/SIDE EFFECTS/MONITORING
Griseofulvin *(Grifulvin V, Gris-PEG)* Tablet, suspension Griseofulvin binds to the keratin precursor cells, which prevents fungal invasion; indicated for dermatomycosis and Tinea infections of skin, hair and nails	*Grifulvin V:* 500-1,000 mg/day in 1-2 divided doses *Gris-PEG:* 375-750 mg/day in 1-2 divided doses Take with a fatty meal to ↑ absorption or with food/milk to avoid GI upset	**CONTRAINDICATIONS** Severe liver disease, porphyria, pregnancy **SIDE EFFECTS** Headache, rash, urticaria, dizziness, photosensitivity, ↑ LFTs, leukopenia, severe skin reactions **MONITORING** LFTs, renal function, CBC **NOTES** Pregnancy Category X Cross reaction possible with PCN allergy.
Terbinafine *(LamISIL, Terbinex)* Tablet, oral granule, topical Inhibits squalene epoxidase, a key enzyme in sterol biosynthesis in fungi, resulting in a deficiency of ergosterol within the cell wall leading to cell death Topical forms (Rx, OTC)	250 mg in 1-2 divided doses without regards to meals Confirm fungal infection prior to use for onychomycosis or dermatomycosis	**WARNINGS** Taste disturbance (including loss of taste) may occur with severe cases resulting in weight loss. Depression has been reported. Loss of smell has been reported. Can exacerbate systemic lupus erythematosus **SIDE EFFECTS** Headache, skin rashes, diarrhea, dyspepsia, taste disturbance, ↑ LFTs **MONITORING** CBC, LFTs

[handwritten note in margin: Exacerbate SLE]

Drug Interactions

- Griseofulvin: Induces 1A2, 2C9, 3A4 (all weak/moderate). Griseofulvin may ↑ the metabolism of contraceptives which may lead to contraceptive failure. Use an alternative, non-hormonal form of contraception.

- Terbinafine is a strong 2D6 inhibitor and a weak/moderate 3A4 inducer.

VIRAL INFECTION OVERVIEW

Virus Replication Cycle

Viruses are obligate intracellular parasites, depending on the host cell metabolic processes for survival. Antivirals treat viral infections by targeting viral specific steps in the replication process. As viruses depend on hosts for metabolism/replication, antivirals may injure or destroy the host cells.

Antiviral Treatment of Patients with Influenza

- The Centers for Disease Control and Prevention (CDC) frequently updates treatment recommendations based on the type of circulating virus during influenza season.

- Neuraminidase inhibitors should be started within 48 hours of illness onset.

Neuraminidase Inhibitors

Inhibit the <u>neuraminidase</u> enzyme which affects the release of viral particles, thereby reducing the amount of virus in the body. They are active against both influenza A and B.

DRUG	DOSING	SAFETY/SIDE EFFECTS/MONITORING
Oseltamivir (*Tamiflu*) 30, 45, 75 mg capsules 6 mg/mL (60 mL) suspension	**Treatment > 12 years** <u>75 mg BID x 5 days</u> **Prophylaxis > 12 years** <u>75 mg daily x 10 days</u> Pediatric patients (2 weeks-12 years) are dosed on body weight CrCl ≤ 60 mL/min: ↓ dose and/or extend interval	**WARNINGS** CNS – rare side effects of neuropsychiatric events (sudden confusion, delirium, hallucinations, unusual behavior, or self-injury) **SIDE EFFECTS** <u>Vomiting</u>, nausea, abdominal pain, diarrhea **NOTES** Pregnancy Category C <u>Start within 48 hours of symptoms</u> or contact with an infected individual.
Zanamivir *(Relenza Diskhaler)*	**Treatment ≥ 7 years** 10 mg (two 5-mg inhalations) BID x 5 days **Prophylaxis ≥ 5 years** 10 mg (two 5-mg inhalations) once daily x 10 days (household setting) or 28 days (community outbreak)	**WARNINGS** CNS – rare side effects of neuropsychiatric events (sudden confusion, delirium, hallucinations, unusual behavior, or self-injury) <u>Bronchospasm risk:</u> Do not use in asthma/COPD or with any breathing problems. Stop the drug if wheezing or breathing problems develop. **SIDE EFFECTS** Headache, throat pain, cough **NOTES** Pregnancy Category C Start within 48 hours of symptoms or contact with an infected individual.

OTHER ANTIVIRALS	DOSING	SAFETY/SIDE EFFECTS/MONITORING
Rimantadine *(Flumadine)* – for Influenza A only Amantadine can be used but has higher incidence adverse effects and greater dose reductions in renal impairment	Treatment/ Prevention: 100 mg BID CrCl < 30 mL/min: 100 mg daily	**WARNINGS** Seizures – use with caution in patients with a history of seizure disorder Psychosis – avoid use **SIDE EFFECTS** Nausea, vomiting, loss of appetite, dry mouth, insomnia, impaired concentration. Amantadine has greater incidence of these side effects. **NOTES** See Parkinson Disease chapter for further information on amantadine.

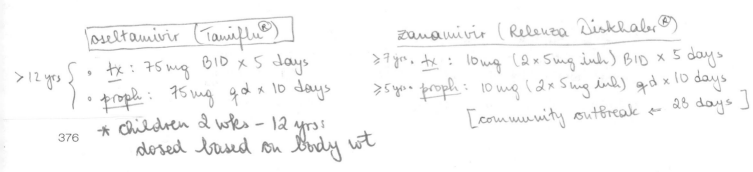

oseltamivir (Tamiflu®)

> 12 yrs { • tx : 75 mg BID x 5 days
    { • proph : 75 mg qd x 10 days

* children 2 wks - 12 yrs:
    dosed based on body wt

Zanamivir (Relenza Diskhaler ®)

≥ 7 yrs • tx : 10 mg (2 x 5 mg inh) BID x 5 days
≥ 5 yrs • proph : 10 mg (2 x 5 mg inh) qd x 10 days
    [community outbreak ⟵ 28 days]

See p.415 *(handwritten)*

Antivirals Used for Treatment of Herpes Simplex Virus (HSV), Varicella Zoster Virus (VZV) & Cytomegalovirus (CMV)

↓ dose or ↑ interval in renal impairment ! *(handwritten)*

ANTIVIRAL	COMMON TREATMENT DOSING RANGE (ADULTS)*	SAFETY/SIDE EFFECTS/MONITORING
Acyclovir (Zovirax) Capsule, tablet, suspension, injection, topical HSV, VZV *Zovirax* cream, *Denavir, Sitavig* – for cold sores (herpes simplex labialis)	200-800 mg PO Q4-8H* 5-10 mg/kg IV Q8H* <u>Dose based on IBW in obese patients</u> Infuse over 1 hour to prevent renal damage *+ maintain hydration (handwritten)*	**WARNINGS** Thrombocytopenic purpura/hemolytic uremic syndrome (TTP/HUS) has been reported in immunocompromised patients Caution in patients with renal impairment, the elderly, and/or those receiving nephrotoxic agents; infuse acyclovir over at least 1 hour and maintain adequate hydration to reduce risk of renal tubular damage **SIDE EFFECTS** Malaise, headache, nausea, vomiting, diarrhea, rash, pruritus, ↑LFTs, neutropenia, ↑ SCr/BUN (crystal nephropathy), ↑ seizures especially with IV formulation, transient burning or stinging with topical formulation
ValACYclovir (Valtrex) Tablet prodrug of acyclovir HSV, VZV *PRODRUG (handwritten)*	500-4,000 mg/day in a single or divided dose *Susp → fridge (handwritten)*	**MONITORING** BUN, SCr, LFTs, CBC **NOTES** Pregnancy Category B Reduce dose and/or extend interval in renal impairment. Store acyclovir IV at room temperature (do not refrigerate). Store valacyclovir oral suspension in a refrigerator.
Famciclovir (Famvir) Tablet prodrug of penciclovir HSV, VZV *PRODRUG (handwritten)* *if resistant to acyclovir, resistant to famciclovir (handwritten)*	250-500 mg Q8-12H*	
Ganciclovir (Cytovene IV, Zirgan ophthalmic gel) Injection, ophthalmic gel CMV	5 mg/kg IV daily or BID Prepare in sterile water (<u>not</u> bacteriostatic) and in laminar flow hood (toxic agent)	**BOXED WARNINGS (2)** Myelosuppression; carcinogenic and teratogenic effects and inhibition of spermatogenesis in animals **SIDE EFFECTS** Fever, nausea, vomiting, diarrhea, anorexia, thrombocytopenia, neutropenia, leukopenia, anemia, ↑ SCr, seizures (rare), retinal detachment (valganciclovir)
ValGANciclovir (Valcyte) Tablet, suspension prodrug of ganciclovir CMV *PRODRUG (handwritten)*	900 mg daily-BID* with food *SE: retinal detachment (handwritten)*	**MONITORING** CBC with differential, PLT, SCr, retinal exam (valganciclovir) **NOTES** Pregnancy Category C Extend interval and reduce dose when CrCl < 60 mL/min. Ganciclovir and valganciclovir are the <u>drugs of choice for CMV</u>.

Handwritten left margin notes: Store IV @ room temp — results in ↑↑ [ ] than — results in ↑↑ [ ] than

Antivirals Continued

ANTIVIRAL	COMMON TREATMENT DOSING RANGE (ADULTS)*	SAFETY/SIDE EFFECTS/MONITORING
Cidofovir *(Vistide)* Injection CMV treatment in HIV patients only	5 mg/kg/wk IV x 2 weeks, then 5 mg/kg once every 2 weeks	**BOXED WARNINGS (3)** Dose-dependent nephropathy, neutropenia, carcinogenic/teratogenic **CONTRAINDICATIONS** SCr > 1.5 mg/dL, CrCl < 55 mL/min, urine protein ≥ 100 mg/dL (> 2+ proteinuria), sulfa allergy, use with or within 7 days of other nephrotoxic drugs, direct intraocular injection **SIDE EFFECTS** Similar to ganciclovir with ↑ risk of nephrotoxicity and lower risk for bone marrow suppression **NOTES** Pregnancy Category C
Foscarnet *(Foscavir)* Injection Resistant HSV, CMV	90 mg/kg IV Q12H or 60 mg/kg Q8H x 2-3 weeks, then 90-120 mg/kg/day*	**BOXED WARNINGS (2)** Renal impairment occurs to some degree in majority of patients, seizures due to electrolyte imbalances **SIDE EFFECTS** Electrolyte abnormalities (↓ K+, ↓ Ca2+, ↓ Mg2+, ↓ Phos), ↑ SCr, ↑ BUN **NOTES** Vesicant (use central line), handle as a chemotherapeutic agent.

Handwritten annotations:
reserved for refractory or resistant virus

≠ ① SrCr > 1.5
② CrCl < 55
③ urine protein ≥ 100 (> 2+)
④ sulfa allergy
⑤ nephrotoxic drugs w/in 7d
⑥ direct intraocular inj

↓ K+
↓ Ca++
↓ Mg++
↓ phos

GI: gastrointestinal, INH: inhaled, IO: intraocular, PO: oral, Inj: intravenous, TTP/HUS: Thrombotic Thrombocytopenic Purpura and Hemolytic Uremic Syndrome

* *Depends on indication, phase of treatment (induction, recurrence, or suppressive therapy)*

Patient Counseling

Counseling That Applies to All Antibiotics

- Antibiotics only treat bacterial infections. They do not treat viral infections such as the common cold and most cases of acute bronchitis and sinusitis.

- Skipping doses or not completing the full course of therapy may ↓ effectiveness of treatment, cause the infection to return, and increase the likelihood that this medicine will not work for you in the future.

- If your symptoms worsen, contact your healthcare provider.

- Many antibiotics can cause rash. If you experience a rash, contact your healthcare provider.

- Many antibiotics cause GI upset. Taking medication with food will usually help, however some antibiotics need to be taken on an empty stomach.

- Measure liquid doses carefully using a measuring device/syringe which came with the medicine. Ask your pharmacist if you do not have one. Do not to use a household spoon because it may not give you the correct dose.

- For all antibiotics, contact your healthcare provider if you have watery diarrhea several times a day, with or without mild abdominal cramping. This can occur during treatment, or weeks after the antibiotic treatment has finished. You should not self-treat with anti-diarrheal medicine.

• amox — w/ food (q8 or 12 hrs)
• Moxatag® — w/in 1 hr of finishing meal
• Augmentin® — w/ food ⟹ ↑ absorption, ↓ tumm
• Augmentin XR — w/ food

RxPrep Course Book | RxPrep © 2015

Amoxicillin products

- Amoxicillin may be taken with food, usually every 8 or 12 hours. *Moxatag* is taken within 1 hour of finishing a meal. *Augmentin* is taken with food to ↑ absorption and ↓ stomach upset. Amoxicillin/clavulanate extended release tablets should be administered with food.

- The suspensions should be refrigerated (especially important for *Augmentin*).

[fridge Amoxil® susp to ↑ taste]

Azithromycin *(Zithromax)*

- Common dosing is two 250 mg tablets on day 1, followed by one 250 mg tablet daily on days 2-5 or 500 mg daily for 3 days.

- The tablets and immediate release oral suspension can be taken with or without food, extended release suspension should be taken on an empty stomach (1 hour before or 2 hours after a meal). The suspension should be stored at room temperature and should not be refrigerated. — *Zmax*® ⊖ fridge

Cefdinir/Cefuroxime *(Ceftin)*/Cephalexin *(Keflex)*

3rd   2nd   1st

- Cefdinir: The suspension should <u>not</u> be refrigerated. Can be taken with or without food.

- Cefuroxime: Take this medication by mouth with a meal or snack every 12 hours. The suspension should be refrigerated.

- Cephalexin: Take this medication by mouth with or without a meal or snack every 6 hours. The suspension should be refrigerated.

Clarithromycin *(Biaxin)*

- Common side effects include abnormal (metallic) taste, diarrhea and GI upset.

- The tablets and oral suspension are taken with or without food and can be taken with milk twice daily.

- *Biaxin XL* tablets should be taken with food.

- The liquid suspension should not be refrigerated. ⟹ gel

Ciprofloxacin *(Cipro)*

- Rarely, seizures can occur, especially in those with seizure disorders (quinolones should be avoided with a seizure history).

- This medicine can make your skin more sensitive to the sun, and you can burn more easily. Use sunscreen, wear protective clothing, and avoid the sun.

- This medicine can rarely cause a serious problem called tendon rupture or swelling of the tendon (tendinitis). If you notice, pain, swelling and inflammation of the tendons on the back of the ankle (Achilles), shoulder, hand or other sites, stop the medicine and be seen right away. This occurs more frequently in people over age 60, and in patients who have had transplants and use steroid medicine, such as prednisone.

- This medicine can rarely cause weakness or tingling/painful sensations in the arms and legs. If this occurs, contact your healthcare provider immediately.

- This medicine should be taken 2 hours before or 6 hours after taking antacids, vitamins, magnesium, calcium, iron or zinc supplements, dairy products, bismuth subsalicylate or the medicines sucralfate or didanosine *(Videx)*.

- This is not a first choice medicine in patients under 18 years of age due to a risk of bone and joint problems. However, it is used occasionally on a short-term basis for certain conditions.

- Do not use this medicine if you take a different medicine called tizanidine *(Zanaflex)*. Please tell your pharmacist about all medicines you are using, since this medicine can interact with many others. <u>The liquid suspension should not be refrigerated.</u> Maintain adequate hydration to prevent crytalluria.

Clindamycin (Cleocin)

- Take by mouth with or without food, 3-4 times a day.
- Take with a full glass of water.
- The liquid suspension should not be refrigerated.

Doxycycline (Doryx, others)

- This medicine can make your skin more sensitive to the sun, and you can burn more easily. Use sunscreen, wear protective clothing, and avoid the sun.
- Drink plenty of fluids while using this medicine. ↓ GI irritation
- This medicine should be taken twice daily 1-2 hours before, or 4-6 hours after taking antacids, vitamins, magnesium, calcium, iron or zinc supplements, dairy products, bismuth subsalicylate.
- The liquid suspension should be stored at room temperature and not refrigerated.
- Do not use this medicine if you are pregnant, if you could become pregnant, or if you are breastfeeding.

Erythromycin

- The liquid suspension combination with sulfisoxazole should be refrigerated. E.S.P.

Levofloxacin (Levaquin)

- This medication is taken once daily, with or without food. The suspension is taken 1 hour before or 2 hours after eating. Maintain adequate hydration to prevent crystal formation in the urine.
- If you use blood sugar-lowering medicines, your blood sugar may get unusually low. Be sure to check your blood sugar level frequently and treat a low blood sugar if it occurs.
- This medicine should be taken 2 hours before, or 2 hours after taking antacids, vitamins, magnesium, calcium, iron or zinc supplements, dairy products, bismuth subsalicylate or the medicines sucralfate (Carafate) or didanosine (Videx).
- The liquid formulation should be stored at room temperature.

Metronidazole (Flagyl)

IR - w/ food
XR - empty stomach

- Common side effects include nausea and unusual (metallic) taste.
- Do not use any alcohol products while using this medicine, and for at least 3 days afterward.
- Immediate-release tablets and capsules may be taken with food to minimize stomach upset. Take extended release tablets on an empty stomach (1 hour before or 2 hours after meals); do not split, crush, or chew.

Minocycline (Minocin, Solodyn)

- Take this medication with or without food, 1-2 times daily.
- Do not use this medication if you are pregnant, if you could become pregnant, or if you are breastfeeding.

Mupirocin (Bactroban)

- The most common side effects are burning and itching.
- The nasal ointment is used to prevent the spread of a bacteria known as MRSA and should be administered into each nostril twice daily for 5 days, or as directed by your healthcare provider.

Nitrofurantoin *(Macrodantin, Macrobid)*

- Take this medication with food to improve absorption and ↓ side effects. Swallow the medication whole.
- Do not use magnesium trisilicate-containing antacids while taking this medication. These antacids can bind with nitrofurantoin, preventing its full absorption into your system.
- Side effects including nausea and headache may occur.
- This medication may cause your urine to turn dark yellow or brown in color. This is usually a harmless, temporary effect and will disappear when the medication is stopped. However, dark brown urine can also be a sign of liver damage. Seek immediate medical attention if you notice dark urine along with any of the following symptoms: persistent nausea or vomiting, pale stools, unusual fatigue or if your skin and whites of your eyes become yellow.
- This medication may rarely cause very serious (possibly fatal) lung problems. Lung problems may occur within the first month of treatment or after long-term use of nitrofurantoin (generally for 6 months or longer). Seek immediate medical attention if you develop symptoms of lung problems including: persistent cough, chest pain, shortness of breath/trouble breathing, joint/muscle pain or bluish/purplish skin.

[handwritten margin note: hepatotox]
[handwritten margin note: pulm. tox]

Penicillin VK

- Take this medication by mouth one hour before or two hours after a meal, usually every 6 hours.
- The suspension should be refrigerated.

Sulfamethoxazole and Trimethoprim *(Bactrim, Septra)*

[handwritten note: (light snack if stomach upset) works best on empty stomach]

- Do not use this medication if you have an allergy to sulfa medicines.
- Take with a full glass of water to prevent crystal formation in the urine. Take with or without food. If stomach upset occurs, take with food or milk.
- Do not use this medication if you are pregnant, if you could become pregnant, or if you are breastfeeding.
- This medicine can make your skin more sensitive to the sun, and you can burn more easily. Use sunscreen, wear protective clothing, and avoid the sun.
- Shake the suspension prior to use. The suspension should be kept at room temperature.

Fluconazole *(Diflucan)*, ketoconazole *(Nizoral)* and itraconazole *(Sporanox)*

- Common side effects include headache, nausea and abdominal pain.
- Generally taken once daily with or without food (or given as a single 150 mg tablet for a vaginal fungal infection). *[handwritten note: → Diflucan]*
- Contact your healthcare provider right away if you are passing brown or dark-colored urine, pale stools, unusual fatigue or if your skin and whites of your eyes become yellow. These may be symptoms of liver damage.
- The liquid suspension should not be refrigerated.
- Ketoconazole tablets and itraconazole capsules should be taken with food (itraconazole solution should be taken on an empty stomach). Do not use with antacids (need two hour separation) and stop the use of PPIs or H$_2$RAs while using this medicine. These other medicines will reduce the amount of the antifungal medicine that gets absorbed.

Nystatin

- If you are using the suspension form of this medication, shake well before using. Be sure to swish the medication around in your mouth for several minutes before swallowing.

Terbinafine *(Lamisil)*

- Terbinafine is used to treat certain types of fungal infections (e.g., fingernail or toenail). It works by stopping the growth of fungus.

- Take this medication by mouth with or without food, usually once a day. Dosage and length of treatment depend on the location of the fungus and the response to treatment.

- It may take several months after you finish treatment to see the full benefit of this drug. It takes time for your new healthy nails to grow out and replace the infected ones.

- Skipping doses or not completing the full course of therapy may ↓ effectiveness of treatment, cause the infection to return, and increase the likelihood that this medicine will not work for you in the future.

- The most common side effect is headache. Temporary change or loss of taste and appetite may also occur.

- This drug has rarely caused very serious (and fatal) liver disease. Liver function tests may be monitored during the course of therapy. Tell your healthcare provider immediately if you develop symptoms of liver disease including persistent nausea, loss of appetite, severe stomach/abdominal pain, dark urine, yellowing of eyes/skin, or pale stools.

Voriconazole *(VFEND)*

- Avoid driving at night because this medicine may cause vision problems like blurry vision. If you have any change in your eyesight, avoid all driving or using dangerous machinery. Vision changes are temporary and reversible.

- Avoid sunlight. Your skin may burn more easily. Your eyes may hurt in bright sunlight.

- Discuss with the pharmacist if you have trouble digesting dairy products, lactose, or regular table sugar. The tablets contain lactose (milk sugar). The liquid contains sucrose (table sugar). *[handwritten: lactose intolerance (tablets)]*

- Take this medication by mouth on an empty stomach, at least 1 hour before or 1 hour after meals, usually every 12 hours or as directed.

- The liquid suspension should not be refrigerated.

- There are many interactions with this drug and other medicines. Please discuss with your pharmacist to make sure this will not pose a problem.

- Do not use this medication if you are pregnant, if you could become pregnant, or if you are breast-feeding.

- Contact your healthcare provider right away if you are passing brown or dark-colored urine, feeling more tired than usual or if your skin and whites of your eyes become yellow. These may be symptoms of liver damage.

Acyclovir *(Zovirax)* – Antiviral

- This medicine works best when taken at the first sign of an outbreak within the first day.

- The most common side effects are malaise, headache, nausea and diarrhea.

- Take this medication by mouth with or without food, usually 2 to 5 times daily, as directed. The intervals should be evenly spaced.

- Drink plenty of fluids while taking this medication.

- The topical cream may cause temporary burning or stinging.

Oseltamivir *(Tamiflu)*

- Treatment should begin within 2 days of onset of influenza symptoms.

- Adult treatment dose is 75 mg twice daily for 5 days. Prophylaxis is 75 mg once daily for 10 days. Children (2 weeks-12 years) are dosed based on body weight.

- The most common side effects are nausea and vomiting. Take with or without food. There is less chance of stomach upset if you take it with a light snack, milk, or a meal.

- Please let your healthcare provider know if you have received the nasally administered influenza virus vaccine during the past two weeks (risk that drug may inhibit replication of the live virus vaccine).

- Patients with the flu, particularly children and adolescents, may be at an ↑ risk of self-injury and confusion shortly after taking this medicine and should be closely monitored for signs of unusual behavior. Contact your healthcare provider immediately if you or your loved ones show any signs of unusual behavior.

Valacyclovir *(Valtrex)*

- *Valtrex* is used daily to manage herpes simplex along with the following safer sex practices can lower the chances of passing genital herpes to your partner.

  - Do not have sexual contact with your partner when you have any symptom or outbreak of genital herpes.

  - Use a condom made of latex or polyurethane whenever you have sexual contact.

- This medication does not cure herpes infections (cold sores, chickenpox, shingles, or genital herpes).

- This medication can be taken with or without food. If GI upset occurs, take with meals.

- Start treatment during prodrome or within 24 hours of the onset of symptoms. This medication is not helpful if you start treatment too late.

- The most common side effects are tiredness and headache. These side effects are usually mild and do not cause patients to stop taking the medication.

- Store suspension in a refrigerator. Discard after 21 days.

26

INFECTIOUS DISEASES II: TERMINOLOGY & INFECTIONS

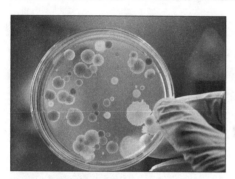

We gratefully acknowledge the assistance of Brett Heintz, PharmD, BCPS-ID, AAHIVE, Infectious Diseases/ Internal Medicine Pharmacist at Iowa City VA Medical Center and Associate Clinical Professor at University of Iowa College of Pharmacy and Craig Martin, PharmD, BCPS, Clinical Associate Professor at the University of Kentucky, in preparing this chapter.

KEY DEFINITIONS

- **Minimum inhibitory concentration (MIC):** lowest drug concentration that prevents visible microbial growth after a 24 hour incubation.

- **Breakpoint:** the level of MIC at which a bacterium is deemed either susceptible or resistant to an antibiotic. Breakpoints vary for different antimicrobial classes. Breakpoints are established by the FDA and Clinical and Laboratory Standards Institute (CLSI) and can change based on clinical data in order to optimize antimicrobial therapy and patient outcomes.

- **Minimum bactericidal concentration (MBC):** lowest drug concentration that reduces bacterial density by 99.9% in 24 hours (kills bacteria).

- **Synergy:** effect of two or more agents combined to produce a greater effect than the sum of their individual effects.

ANTIMICROBIAL STEWARDSHIP PROGRAMS (ASP)

- Antimicrobial stewardship has been defined as the optimal selection, dosage, route of administration, and duration of antimicrobial treatment that results in the best clinical outcome. Promoting the appropriate use of antimicrobials will improve clinical outcomes by reducing the emergence of resistance, limiting drug-related adverse events, and minimizing risk of unintentional consequences associated with antimicrobial use.

[handwritten margin notes: E-test; MBC test; cidal; synergy test]

- Antimicrobial stewardship programs are a team effort among infectious diseases physicians, infectious diseases pharmacists, staff from microbiology, infection control, pharmacy, information technology, and others.

- Most programs contain an auditing component to review prescribing habits of providers and an educational component to change suboptimal prescribing habits and improve patient care. These programs often oversee guideline development with the goal of optimal antibiotic use.

- Other common aspects of an ASP include 1) a restriction and/or pre-authorization policy, 2) automatic intravenous-to-oral medication interchange, and 3) de-escalation or streamlining of therapy based on patient response and culture/susceptibility results.

ANTIBIOGRAM

An antibiogram is a chart that contains the susceptibility patterns of local bacterial isolates to antimicrobial agents at a single institution (hospital) over a specific period of time (generally 1 year). Antibiograms aid in the selection of empiric antibiotic therapy and in monitoring resistance trends over time within an institution. They can also be used to compare susceptibility rates across institutions and track resistance trends in the community. An example of an antibiogram for Gram-negative organisms is provided below.

Antibiogram Example (abridged)

GRAM-NEGATIVE ORGANISM (#) – ALL SOURCES (EXCLUDING URINE)																
CATEGORY	BETA-LACTAMS							CARBAPENEM	B-LACTAM/B-LACTAMASE INHIBITOR COMBINATION		FLUOROQUINOLONES		AMINOGLYCOSIDES			OTHER
MICROBIOLOGIC PATHOGEN (# OF ISOLATES)	AZTREONAM	CEFAZOLIN	CEFEPIME	CEFOTAXIME	CEFTAZIDIME	CEFTRIAXONE	PIPERACILLIN	MEROPENEM	AMPICILLIN/ SULBACTAM	PIPERACILLIN/ TAZOBACTAM	CIPROFLOXACIN	LEVOFLOXACIN	AMIKACIN	GENTAMICIN	TOBRAMYCIN	SULFAMETHOXAZOLE/ TRIMETHOPRIM
Acinetobacter baumannii (65)			71	8	68	38	0	94			69	86	85	71	82	85
Enterobacter cloacae (142)	72		92	70	70	68	64	100		74	95	95	98	96	91	85
Escherichia coli (431)	87	76	88	86	85	85	46	100	46	91	74	75	99	91	88	68
Klebsiella oxytoca (49)	96	67	96	96	96	96	80	100	61	98	92	92	100	100	100	85
Klebsiella pneumoniae (158)	87	87	87	87	87	87	77	100	75	90	91	97	98	98	87	86
Proteus mirabilis (84)	99	75	100	100	100	99		100		86	81	85	100	92	87	87
Pseudomonas aeruginosa (474)	64		74		80		87	88		88	79	79	99	92	96	
Serratia marcescens (104)	99		100	93	98	96	83	99		93	91	98	99	91	72	
Stenotrophomonas maltophilia (75)					29			0f				61				98

Data source: The Surveillance Network – hospital name has been intentionally deleted

Drug Therapy Considerations

FACTORS TO CONSIDER WHEN SELECTING A DRUG REGIMEN	MONITORING FOR THERAPEUTIC EFFECTIVENESS	LACK OF THERAPEUTIC EFFECTIVENESS REASONS
Etiology/epidemiology (community vs. hospital-acquired infection, exposures to pathogens) Site/severity of infection Known patient colonization with resistant bacteria Patient characteristics (age, body weight, renal/liver function, allergies, pregnancy status, immune function) Spectrum of activity and pharmacodynamics/pharmacokinetics of the drug regimen	Fever trend WBC count Radiographic findings Pain/inflammation – elevated markers of inflammation include procalcitonin levels (more specific to inflammation from bacterial infection), C-reactive protein, Erythrocyte Sedimentation Rate (ESR) Reduction in signs and symptoms of infection Microbiologic cure	Antibiotic factors: inadequate coverage and/or dose, lack of penetration, drug-drug interaction, non-adherence Host factors: length of therapy not adequate, misdiagnosis Microbiologic factors: resistance, superinfection (C. difficile), antibiotic unresponsive infection (viral)

Culture and Susceptibility Report

Once cultures and susceptibilities are reported, the empiric antimicrobial regimen will need to be evaluated and streamlined, as appropriate. For example, a hospitalized patient is experiencing urinary urgency and burning upon urination. The patient has no known drug allergies and was started on *Unasyn* as empiric treatment. Based on the urine culture and sensitivities provided below, what would be the best antibiotic regimen for this patient?

Sample Culture and Susceptibility Report

DRUG	ORGANISM 1 – PSEUDOMONAS	MIC (MG/L) FOR ORGANISM 1	ORGANISM 2 – MORGANELLA	MIC (MG/L) FOR ORGANISM 2
Ampicillin	-	-	R	> 16
Ampicillin/Sulbactam	-	-	R	> 16
Cefazolin	-	-	R	> 16
Cefoxitin	-	-	R	> 16
Ceftazidime	S	2	I	16
Ceftriaxone	-	-	S	8
Cefuroxime	-	-	S	8
Ciprofloxacin	S	≤ 0.5	R	> 2
Ertapenem	-	-	S	2
Gentamicin	I	8	S	2
Imipenem	S	< 1	I	8
Levofloxacin	R	> 4	R	> 4
Meropenem	S	< 1	I	8
Nitrofurantoin	-	-	R	> 64
Piperacillin/Tazobactam	S	8	R	> 16
Tobramycin	S	< 1	S	2
Sulfamethoxazole/Trimethoprim	-	-	R	> 2/38

S = susceptible; I = intermediately susceptible; R = resistant

To treat the urinary tract infection effectively, choose the narrowest spectrum antimicrobial to limit the spread of resistance (e.g., low dose tobramycin based on culture and susceptibility results and urinary source). Given the patient is in the hospital and can receive IV therapy, tobramycin is appropriate. If the patient was treated as an outpatient where oral therapy is used, ciprofloxacin targeting the *Pseudomonas* and cefuroxime targeting the *Morganella* would be the best choice.

Considerations When Evaluating a Patient for Antibiotic Therapy

- Determine the presence of infection based on clinical signs and symptoms. A urine culture report does not determine the presence or absence of an infection. Oftentimes patients are only colonized and not infected, therefore will not need antimicrobial therapy.

- Be aware of drug allergies, history of antibiotic use and patient characteristics.

- Ensure the antibiotic being considered will have adequate penetration to the site of infection. Lipophilic antimicrobials have enhanced tissue penetration. Hepatically cleared antimicrobials may not achieve adequate drug concentrations in the urine.

- Absence of susceptibility results reported as "-" does not mean resistance; it means the drug was not tested against the bacteria.

- If available, use MICs to guide definitive therapy. It is best to use the lowest MIC relative to the breakpoint for susceptibility. Generally, choose the most active antimicrobial agent to treat the infection. However, if the patient is responding to a less active agent based on MIC findings, it may be appropriate to continue that agent.

- For empiric therapy, a broad spectrum regimen is often necessary to ensure adequate therapy for likely pathogens.

- When susceptibilities are available, narrow spectrum therapy should be chosen to limit the collateral damage associated with broad therapies.

ANTIMICROBIAL PRINCIPLES

The appropriate selection of an antimicrobial regimen requires an understanding of pharmacokinetic principles (absorption, distribution, metabolism and excretion) as well as pharmacodynamic principles (concentration-dependent or time-dependent killing). Refer to Pharmacokinetics chapter for a review on pharmacokinetic principles.

Antimicrobial Pharmacokinetics: Hydrophilic or Lipophilic Agents

Hydrophilicity or lipophilicity of the antimicrobial agent can be used to predict a number of pharmacokinetic features (see figure below). Lipophilic agents generally have enhanced penetration of bone, lung, and brain tissues.

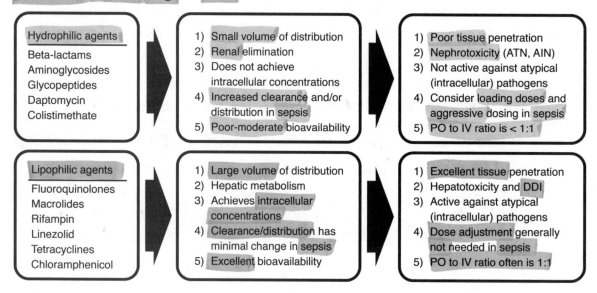

Hydrophilic agents		
Beta-lactams Aminoglycosides Glycopeptides Daptomycin Colistimethate	1) Small volume of distribution 2) Renal elimination 3) Does not achieve intracellular concentrations 4) Increased clearance and/or distribution in sepsis 5) Poor-moderate bioavailability	1) Poor tissue penetration 2) Nephrotoxicity (ATN, AIN) 3) Not active against atypical (intracellular) pathogens 4) Consider loading doses and aggressive dosing in sepsis 5) PO to IV ratio is < 1:1
Lipophilic agents		
Fluoroquinolones Macrolides Rifampin Linezolid Tetracyclines Chloramphenicol	1) Large volume of distribution 2) Hepatic metabolism 3) Achieves intracellular concentrations 4) Clearance/distribution has minimal change in sepsis 5) Excellent bioavailability	1) Excellent tissue penetration 2) Hepatotoxicity and DDI 3) Active against atypical (intracellular) pathogens 4) Dose adjustment generally not needed in sepsis 5) PO to IV ratio often is 1:1

ATN = acute tubular necrosis, AIN = acute interstitial nephritis, PO = oral, IV = intravenous, DDI = drug-drug interaction

Antimicrobial Pharmacodynamics: Dose Optimization

Antimicrobial pharmacodynamics of selected antimicrobial agents is displayed in the following figure. Agents that exhibit time-dependent killing (such as beta-lactams) are generally dosed more frequently to maximize the time above the MIC, while concentration-dependent agents (such as aminoglycosides) are generally dosed less frequently and in higher doses to maximize the concentration above the MIC. Beta-lactam antibiotics may be maximized by more frequent dosing, extending the infusion time (such as over 4 hours) or given as a continuous infusion which can lead to greater time above the MIC. Numerous studies have documented that extended/continuous infusion of beta-lactams can reduce length of stay, mortality, and costs particularly when treating Gram-negative pathogens like *Pseudomonas*.

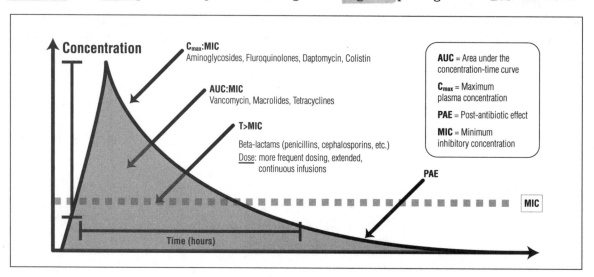

Antibacterial Mechanism of Action: Bacteriostatic or Bactericidal Activity

Knowledge of the mechanism of action generally predicts the bacteriostatic (bacterial inhibition by antimicrobial agent) or bactericidal (bacterial killing by antimicrobial agent) activity of antimicrobial agents (see figure below). In general bactericidal agents are preferred for immunocompromised patients and/or for deep-seated infections (e.g. endocarditis). However, for most mild infections, bactericidal activity does not imply improved patient outcomes in an immunocompetent host. Further, while bactericidal activity can be predicted by the mechanism of action, it is also dependent on a number of microbiologic, pharmacologic and host factors (culture and susceptibility results, achievable concentrations of the antimicrobial agent at the site of infection, duration of exposure, and size of bacteria inoculum).

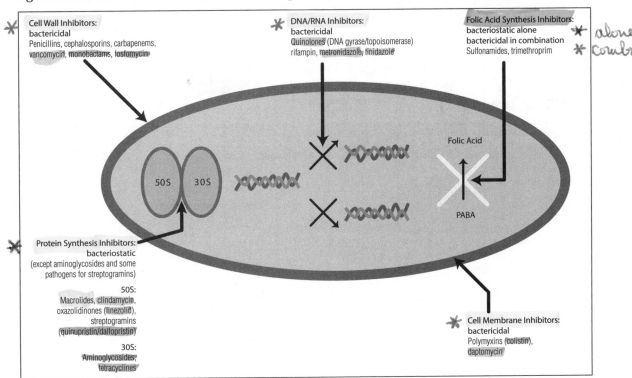

Cell Wall Inhibitors:
bactericidal
Penicillins, cephalosporins, carbapenems, vancomycin, monobactams, fosfomycin

DNA/RNA Inhibitors:
bactericidal
Quinolones (DNA gyrase/topoisomerase) rifampin, metronidazole, tinidazole

Folic Acid Synthesis Inhibitors:
bacteriostatic alone
bactericidal in combination
Sulfonamides, trimethroprim

alone
combo

Protein Synthesis Inhibitors:
bacteriostatic
(except aminoglycosides and some pathogens for streptogramins)

50S:
Macrolides, clindamycin, oxazolidinones (linezolid), streptogramins (quinupristin/dalfopristin)

30S:
Aminoglycosides, tetracyclines

Folic Acid

PABA

50S   30S

Cell Membrane Inhibitors:
bactericidal
Polymyxins (colistin), daptomycin

ANTIMICROBIAL AGENTS FOR SELECT INFECTIOUS DISEASE SYNDROMES

Background

Knowledge of the likely pathogens at the suspected site of infection will guide initial empiric therapy. When the specific pathogens and susceptibilities are identified, therapy can be streamlined. Always consider local resistance patterns and antibiotic use guidelines.

Perioperative Antimicrobial Prophylaxis

- A very brief course of an antimicrobial agent initiated within 60 minutes before the incision (or 120 minutes before the incision if using fluoroquinolones or vancomycin) to obtain therapeutic levels in both serum and tissue.

■ In order to maintain therapeutic levels throughout the surgery, longer surgeries (> 3-4 hours) may require additional intraoperative doses. In cases of major blood loss during procedure, an additional dose may also be necessary. Controversy exists regarding the duration of prophylaxis necessary after the surgery is complete. In most circumstances, no additional doses are required. Quality measures dictate that prophylactic agents are discontinued within 24 hours. In general, first or second generation cephalosporins (e.g., cefazolin) are the drugs of choice for most procedures. Vancomycin is used as an alternative in beta-lactam allergic patients or when MRSA is a concern.

Ancef®

■ While cefazolin and some other agents may be administered rapidly just prior to incision, vancomycin and fluoroquinolones require longer administration times to avoid serious adverse effects. Care must be taken to account for these considerations early enough prior to the procedure.

■ Surgeries that involve the bowel or have risk of an anaerobic infection will commonly require antibiotics with broader coverage such as cefotetan, ertapenem or ceftriaxone with metronidazole.

1st & 2nd gen cephalos typically DOC for most procedures

SURGICAL PROCEDURE	RECOMMENDED ANTIBIOTICS	IF BETA-LACTAM ALLERGY
CABG, other cardiac or vascular surgeries	Cefazolin or cefuroxime	Vancomycin* or clindamycin
Hip fracture repair/total joint replacement	Cefazolin	Vancomycin* or clindamycin
Colon (colorectal)	Cefotetan, cefoxitin, ampicillin/ sulbactam, ertapenem or Metronidazole + (cefazolin or ceftriaxone)	Clindamycin + (aminoglycoside or fluoroquinolone or aztreonam) or Metronidazole + (aminoglycoside or fluoroquinolone)
Hysterectomy	Cefotetan, cefazolin, cefoxitin or ampicillin/sulbactam	Clindamycin or vancomycin* + (aminoglycoside or fluoroquinolone or aztreonam) or Metronidazole + (aminoglycoside or fluoroquinolone)

* For procedures and/or patients where MRSA is a likely pathogen consider using vancomycin.
Bratzler DW, Dellinger EP, Olsen KM et al. Clinical practice guidelines for antimicrobial prophylaxis for surgery.
Am J Health-Syst Pharm. 2013; 70:195-283.

Meningitis

Meningitis is inflammation of the meninges (membranes) that cover the brain and spinal cord. The meninges swell, causing the classic triad of symptoms: severe headache, nuchal rigidity (stiff neck) and altered mental status. Not all patients will demonstrate all three classic symptoms. Other symptoms could include chills, vomiting and photophobia. Most cases are due to viral infections, but can be due to bacteria or fungi as well. Meningitis symptoms must be recognized quickly to avoid severe complications, including death.

- A lumbar puncture (LP) is required for most patients with suspected bacterial meningitis, and ideally, should be performed prior to the initiation of antimicrobial therapy. The LP will help provide data for an accurate diagnosis, differentiation of viral and bacterial meningitis, and determination of the causative pathogen and susceptibilities. In some patient populations, a computed tomography (CT) scan is necessary prior to LP to avoid potentially fatal complications. These patients include those with a clinical exam consistent with a mass-occupying cranial lesion. In such patients, risk of cerebral herniation after lumbar puncture precludes the procedure until such a lesion can be ruled out by imaging. While an LP is important from a diagnostic perspective, do not delay starting antibiotics until the LP can be performed or while awaiting the results from the LP.

- Antibiotic dosages must be maximized to optimize penetration of the CNS.

- The most likely organisms causing bacterial meningitis are *Streptococcus pneumoniae*, *Neisseria meningitidis*, *Haemophilus influenzae* and *Listeria monocytogenes*.

- Likely pathogens and empiric antimicrobial selection depends on patient's age (see table).

ANTIBIOTIC	SUSCEPTIBLE (S)	INTERMEDIATE (I)	RESISTANT (R)
Penicillin	≤ 0.06 mcg/mL	–	≥ 0.12 mcg/mL
Ceftriaxone	≥ 0.5 mcg/mL	1 mcg/mL	≥ 2 mcg/mL

Definitive therapy for the most common bacterial pathogen, *Streptococcus pneumoniae*, is dictated by the susceptibility results as follows:

- Penicillin-S: use penicillin or ampicillin

- Penicillin-I and ceftriaxone/cefotaxime-S: use ceftriaxone or cefotaxime

- Ceftriaxone/cefotaxime-I or -R and penicillin-R: use vancomycin + ceftriaxone or cefotaxime ± rifampin

Generally, the duration of treatment is 7-14 days, but can vary based on the pathogen severity of infection and clinical response.

Acute Bacterial Meningitis

EMPIRIC THERAPY	NOTES
Treatment in Patients 2-50 Years Old (primarily *S. pneumoniae* and *N. meningitidis*)	
Cefotaxime 2 grams IV Q4-6H or Ceftriaxone 2 grams IV Q12H or Meropenem 2 grams IV Q8H (alternative to 3rd gen. ceph) PLUS Vancomycin 30-45 mg/kg/day in divided doses ± Dexamethasone 0.15 mg/kg IV Q6H x 2-4 days	Give dexamethasone 15-20 min prior to or concomitantly with 1st dose of antibiotic Need high doses of vancomycin to penetrate CSF Add ampicillin 2 grams IV Q4H if age < 1 month or > 50 years, has impaired cellular immunity, and suspect *Listeria*

Acute Bacterial Meningitis Continued

EMPIRIC THERAPY	NOTES

Treatment in Immunocompromised Patients or Age > 50 years old *(S. pneumoniae, N. meningitidis, L. monocytogenes)*

Vancomycin + ampicillin + ceftriaxone or Vancomycin + ampicillin + cefotaxime	

For Severe PCN Allergy

Chloramphenicol 4,000-6,000 mg/day in 4 doses PLUS Vancomycin 30-45 mg/kg/day in divided doses ± SMX/TMP 10-20 mg/kg IV Q6-12H	Chloramphenicol and vancomycin will provide adequate coverage for *Neisseria* and *Streptococcus pneumoniae*. SMX/TMP can be added for suspected *Listeria*.

Tunkel AR, Hartman BJ, Kaplan SL et al. Practice Guideline for Management of Bacterial Meningitis. Clin Infect Dis 2004; 39:1367-1289.

UPPER RESPIRATORY TRACT INFECTIONS

Acute Otitis Media (AOM)

AOM is the most common childhood infection in the United States requiring antibiotic treatment. Signs and symptoms of the infection include bulging tympanic membrane, otorrhea (middle ear effusion/fluid), otalgia (ear pain), a rapid onset of symptoms, fever, crying and tugging or rubbing the ears. Many of the infections are viral, therefore antibiotics will be ineffective.

- Treat the pain with acetaminophen or ibuprofen. Can use topical benzocaine, procaine or lidocaine *(Americaine Otic)* in children > 5 years of age.

- Observation without antibiotics may be an option for non-severe AOM depending on age, diagnostic certainty, and illness severity. The observation period is 48-72 hours and is used to assess clinical improvement without antibiotics. The decision for observation should be a joint decision of the pediatrician and parents.

AGE	OTORRHEA WITH AOM	UNILATERAL OR BILATERAL AOM WITH SEVERE SYMPTOMS*	BILATERAL AOM WITHOUT OTORRHEA	UNILATERAL AOM WITHOUT OTORRHEA
6 months-2 years	Antibiotic therapy	Antibiotic therapy	Antibiotic therapy	Antibiotic therapy or additional observation
≥ 2 years	Antibiotic therapy	Antibiotic therapy	Antibiotic therapy or additional observation	Antibiotic therapy or additional observation

*Severe symptoms include otalgia > 48 hrs, temperature ≥ 39°C (102.2°F) in past 48 hrs

INITIAL TREATMENT		ANTIBIOTIC TREATMENT AFTER 48-72 HOURS OF FAILURE OF INITIAL THERAPY
Recommended First-line Treatment	Alternative Treatment (if Penicillin Allergy)	Recommended First-line Treatment
Amoxicillin 80-90 mg/kg/day in 2 divided doses or	Cefdinir 14 mg/kg/day in 1 or 2 doses	Amox/Clav* (90 mg/kg/day of amoxicillin with 6.4 mg/kg/day of clavulanate) in 2 divided doses or
Amox/Clav [90 mg/kg/day of amoxicillin with 6.4 mg/kg/day of clavulanate (amoxicillin to clavulanate ratio is 14:1)] in 2 divided doses	Cefuroxime 30 mg/kg/day in 2 divided doses	Ceftriaxone 50 mg/kg IM/IV daily for 3 days
	Cefpodoxime 10 mg/kg/day in 2 divided doses	
	Ceftriaxone 50 mg/kg IM/IV daily for 1 or 3 days	

*May be considered in patients who have received amoxicillin in the past 30 days

Lieberthal AS, Carroll AE, Chonmaitree T et al. The Diagnosis and Management Acute Otitis Media; Pediatrics. 2013; 131:e964-e999.

- First line treatment is high-dose amoxicillin (80-90 mg/kg/day divided Q12H) or amoxicillin/clavulanate (90 mg/kg/day of amoxicillin divided Q12H). The higher dose will cover most *S. pneumoniae*.

- Recommended agents in setting of amoxicillin failure include amoxicillin/clavulanate 90 mg/kg/day of amoxicillin component x 5-10 days (see recommendations for duration below) or ceftriaxone 50 mg/kg IM/IV x 3 days.

- Recommended duration of treatment for amoxicillin, amox/clavulanate and oral cephalosporins: < 2 years of age = 10 days; 2-5 years of age = 7 days; and ≥ 6 years of age = 5-7 days.

- When giving high dose amoxicillin/clavulanate, the clinician should prescribe the formulation with a relatively lower amount of clavulanate such as *Augmentin ES-600* (amoxicillin 600 mg and clavulanate 42.9 mg per 5 mL) to avoid increased risk of GI side effects associated with higher levels of clavulanate. The 600 mg/5 mL concentration has a lower ratio of amoxicillin/clavulanate than the other strengths.

- Ceftriaxone (50 mg/kg) can be given IM/IV daily for 1 or 3 days (1 or 3 days for initial treatment or 3 days for treatment failure) for those who cannot tolerate oral medication due to GI side effects.

Prevention

- *Prevnar 13*, the pneumococcal conjugate vaccine (PCV) which contains 13 serotypes, is now given to all children 2-23 months. Children receive four doses of PCV13 intramuscularly at age 2, 4, 6, and 12 to 15 months old. *Pneumovax* is the adult polyvalent vaccine which contains 23 serotypes.

- ACIP recommends the *Pneumovax* vaccine for children aged ≥ 24 months who are at increased risk for pneumococcal disease (sickle cell disease, HIV, and other immunocompromising or chronic medical conditions).

- Annual influenza vaccine should be given at ≥ 6 months of age and older.

- Clinicians should not prescribe prophylactic antibiotics to reduce frequency of AOM.

Overview of Upper Respiratory Tract Infection Management

The majority of upper respiratory tract infections are caused by viruses, antibacterials will have no benefit. In select cases of more severe/chronic symptoms and/or microbiologic/diagnostic evidence of a bacterial etiology, antibacterials may be indicated in the setting of pharyngitis and sinusitis (see table below).

	COMMON COLD	INFLUENZA	PHARYNGITIS	SINUSITIS
Typical Etiology	Resp viruses: Rhinovirus Coronavirus RSV	Influenza virus	Resp viruses *S. pyogenes*	Resp viruses; *S. pneumoniae; H. influenzae; Moraxella catarrhalis; Staphylococci* species anaerobes, and Gram-negative rods may also be implicated in chronic sinusitis
Indications for Anti-infective Treatment	None	< 48h since symptom onset Risk factors for severe disease Outbreak scenario	Positive rapid antigen diagnostic test or positive *S. pyogenes* culture	> 7-10 days of symptoms Tooth/face pain Nasal drainage/discharge Congestion or severe/worsening symptoms
Anti-infective Choice	None	Oseltamivir Zanamavir	Penicillin Amoxicillin 1st/2nd generation cephalosporin Clarithromycin or azithromycin or clindamycin in patients allergic to penicillin	**First Line** Amox/clav, doxycycline **Second Line if Failure to Above** Oral 2nd or 3rd generation cephalosporins + clindamycin Respiratory fluoroquinolone
Duration	Per symptoms	5 days	10 days unless using azithromycin (5 days)	Variable depending on severity and chronicity Acute sinusitis: Adults: 5-7 days Children: 10-14 days Chronic sinusitis: ≥ 21 days ± surgical intervention

Shulman ST, Bisno AL, Clegg HW et al. Clinical Practice Guideline for the Diagnosis and Management of Group A Streptococcal Pharyngitis: 2012 Update by the Infectious Diseases Society of America. Clin Infect Dis. 2012; 55:1279-82.

Chow AW, Benninger MS, Brook I et al. IDSA Clinical Practice Guideline for Acute Bacterial Rhinosinusitis in Children and Adults. Clin Infect Dis. 2012; 54:1041-45.

CDC Get Smart Campaign

LOWER RESPIRATORY TRACT INFECTIONS

Bronchitis

Bronchitis, inflammation of the mucous membranes of the bronchi, can be divided into 2 categories: acute and chronic.

Acute Bronchitis

- Acute bronchitis is primarily caused by respiratory viruses and is almost always self-limiting. Bacterial etiology should be considered for more severe cases of acute bronchitis and likely pathogens include *Mycoplasma pneumoniae, Streptococcus pneumoniae, Haemophilus influenzae, Bordetella pertussis*, and others.

- In mild-moderate disease, treatment is supportive with the use of fluids to prevent dehydration, antipyretics for fever, cough suppressants, vaporizers to thin secretions, etc. In more severe disease and/or known bacterial etiology, antibiotics are indicated (see box).

- Signs and symptoms of acute bronchitis include cough (generally lasts > 2 weeks), sore throat, coryza, malaise, headache, low-grade fever, and/or purulent sputum production.

[handwritten: stuffy nose, irritation/swelling of mucous membrane in nose]

Chronic Bronchitis – Acute Exacerbation of Chronic Bronchitis (AECB)

- Antibiotics are indicated in more severe cases of chronic bronchitis, especially among patients with at least two of the following symptoms: increased dyspnea, increased sputum production, and increased sputum purulence. These episodes are distinct from acute bronchitis and are termed acute exacerbation of chronic bronchitis (AECB).

[handwritten: abx when 2+ of: 1) ↑ dyspnea 2) ↑ sputum prod 3) ↑ sputum purulence]

BRONCHITIS NOTES & TREATMENT

Acute Bronchitis – expect cough to last 2 weeks
Mild-to-moderate disease:

- Usually viral – antibiotics not indicated. Recommend antitussive ± inhaled bronchodilators

Persistent Cough (> 14 days)/Pertussis (whooping cough)
Severe disease:

- Azithromycin 500 mg x 1, then 250 mg daily x 2-5 days or
- Erythromycin estolate 500 mg QID x 14 days or
- SMX/TMP DS 1 tab BID x 14 days or
- Clarithromycin 500 mg BID or 1 gm ER daily x 7 days

Acute Bacterial Exacerbation of Chronic Bronchitis (ABECB)
Mild-to-moderate disease:

- No antibiotic treatment or if used, choose: amoxicillin, doxycycline, SMX/TMP, or a cephalosporin

Severe disease with two or more of the following: increased dyspnea, increased sputum production, and increased sputum purulence:

- Inhaled anticholinergic bronchodilator plus oral corticosteroid, taper over 2 weeks.
- Role of antibiotic therapy debated even for severe disease. If used, choose: doxycycline or macrolide or SMX/TMP or 3rd generation cephalosporin or amoxicillin/clavulanic acid or antipneumococcal FQ (moxi, gemi or levo). In general, amox/clav or FQ should be reserved for patients at risk for drug-resistant *S. pneumoniae* (age > 65 years, multiple comorbidities, etc.). Treat 5-7 days or longer if needed.

Martinez FJ, Anzueto A. Appropriate outpatient treatment of acute bacterial exacerbations of chronic bronchitis. Am J Med. 2005; 118:39S-44S.

5-10 days (handwritten, left margin)

COMMUNITY-ACQUIRED PNEUMONIA (CAP)

Community-acquired (occurring outside of health care facilities) pneumonia is one of the most common types of pneumonia. Causes could be bacterial, viral or fungal (rare). Most bacterial cases are caused by *Streptococcus pneumoniae, Haemophilus influenzae* and *Moraxella catarrhalis*. Patients often present with fever, productive cough with purulent sputum and pleuritic chest pain. Rales (crackling noises) can be heard over the infected lobe on auscultation. A chest x-ray is the gold standard for the diagnosis of CAP.

RECOMMENDED EMPIRICAL ANTIBIOTIC COVERAGE FOR CAP

Outpatient Treatment

Previously healthy and no use of antimicrobials within the past 3 months:

- Macrolide* (azithromycin, clarithromycin, erythromycin) or

- Doxycycline

At risk for drug-resistant *S. pneumoniae* (comorbidities such as HF, DM, cancer, renal/liver dysfunction, alcoholism, malignancies, asplenia, immunosuppression – and use of antibiotics within past 3 months):

- A respiratory fluoroquinolone (moxifloxacin, gemifloxacin, or levofloxacin [750mg]) or

- Beta-lactam PLUS a macrolide (high-dose amoxicillin or amoxicillin/clavulanate is preferred, alternatives include ceftriaxone, cefpodoxime, cefuroxime; doxycycline is an alternative to the macrolide)

Inpatient (non-ICU)

- Beta-lactam PLUS a macrolide (preferred beta-lactam agents include ceftriaxone, cefotaxime, ampicillin; doxycycline as an alternative to the macrolide) or

- Respiratory fluoroquinolone (moxifloxacin, gemifloxacin, or levofloxacin) – IV or PO (consider reserving fluoroquinolones for beta-lactam allergies)

Inpatient (ICU) – IV therapy preferred

- Beta-lactam (ceftriaxone, cefotaxime, ampicillin/sulbactam) PLUS azithromycin or a fluoroquinolone. For penicillin-allergic patients, a respiratory FQ and aztreonam are recommended.

If *Pseudomonas* is a consideration, use an antipneumococcal, antipseudomonal beta-lactam (piperacillin/tazobactam, cefepime, imipenem, meropenem or doripenem) plus either ciprofloxacin or levofloxacin

or

the above beta-lactam plus an aminoglycoside and (azithromycin or respiratory FQ)

If CA-MRSA is a consideration, add vancomycin or linezolid

Handwritten notes:

outpt
→ healthy
~~⊕ abx past 3 mo~~
⇒ macrolide
OR doxy

→ risk for MDR Strep. pneumo
⇒ resp. FQ
OR β-lactam + macrolide
↓
amoxi
Augmentin®   OR
ceftriaxone   doxy
cefpodoxime
cefuroxime

inpt (non-ICU)
⇒ β-lactam + macrolide
↓   ↓
ceftriaxone   OR
cefotaxime   doxy
amp

OR resp. FQ (IV/po)
↳ reserve for β-lactam allergy

inpt (ICU)
⇒ β-lactam + [azithro or FQ]
↓
ceftriaxone
cefotaxime
Unasyn®

*if Pseudo
⇒ antipseudo β-lactam + [cipro/levo]
↓   OR
pip/tazo   [AG + azithro
cefepime   OR
CBP (⊖ erta)   resp. FQ]

* + vanc OR Zyvox® for MRSA

Oral Antibiotics for Community Acquired Pneumonia (CAP)

DRUG	USUAL ADULT DOSE
Cephalosporins	
Cefpodoxime	200 mg Q12H
Cefuroxime (*Ceftin*)	500 mg Q12H
Cefdinir	300 mg Q12H
Macrolides	
Azithromycin (*Zithromax*)	500 mg x 1, then 250 mg daily (days 2-5)
Clarithromycin (*Biaxin*)	250 mg Q12H
Clarithromycin (*Biaxin XL*)	1,000 mg daily
Erythromycin base	250 mg Q6H or 500 mg Q12H
Fluoroquinolones	
Gemifloxacin (*Factive*)	320 mg daily
Levofloxacin (*Levaquin*)	500-750 mg daily
Moxifloxacin (*Avelox*)	400 mg daily
Tetracyclines	
Doxycycline (*Vibramycin*)	100 mg Q12H
Penicillins	
Amoxicillin (*Amoxil*)	875 mg Q12H or 500-1,000 mg Q8H
Amoxicillin/clavulanate (*Augmentin*)	875/125 mg Q12H or 500/125mg Q8H
Amoxicillin/clavulanate (*Augmentin XR*)	2 grams Q12H

(handwritten annotations: q12 next to Cephalosporins, Tetracyclines, and Penicillins)

MOST COMMON ETIOLOGIES OF CAP

Outpatient
Streptococcus pneumoniae

Mycoplasma pneumoniae

Haemophilus influenzae

Chlamydophila pneumoniae

Respiratory viruses

Inpatient (non-ICU)
Streptococcus pneumoniae

Mycoplasma pneumoniae

Chlamydophila pneumoniae

Haemophilus influenzae

Legionella sp.

Aspiration

Respiratory viruses

Inpatient (ICU)
Streptococcus pneumoniae

Staphylococcus aureus

Legionella sp.

Gram-negative bacilli

Haemophilus influenzae

Duration

The duration of treatment can be as short as 5 days, or longer, depending on the patient's condition. Most are treated successfully in 5-10 days.

Mandell LA, Wunderink RG, Anzuetto A et al. Guidelines adapted from the Infectious Diseases Society of America/ American Thoracic Society Consensus Guidelines on the Management of CAP in Adults. Clin Infect Dis. 2007; 44 suppl 2:S27-72.

[handwritten left margin: 7-8 days (14 if Pseudo/ Acineto bacter- emia)]

Hospital Acquired Pneumonia (HAP)/Ventilator Associated Pneumonia (VAP)

HAP is pneumonia that occurs during the hospital stay. Because hospitalized patients tend to have different oropharyngeal flora than their community-dwelling counterparts, the causative agents are different. Ventilated patients are at especially high-risk. HAP is the leading infectious cause of death in ICUs.

- In addition to proper hand-washing, HAP can be reduced by elevating the head of bed by 30 degrees or more, weaning off ventilator as quickly as possible, removing nasogastric (NG) tubes when possible, and discontinuing use of stress ulcer prophylaxis if not needed.

- HAP that occurs < 5 days (early onset) after admission is often caused by pathogens similar to that of CAP except for the fact that the incidence of enteric Gram-negative bacteria is more prevalent and atypical pathogens (e.g., *Legionella, Mycoplasma*) are less prevalent. Nosocomial pathogens (MRSA, *Pseudomonas aeruginosa*) are more prevalent with hospitalization ≥ 5 days (late onset).

Overview of Hospital-Acquired Pneumonia (HAP) Etiology and Management

ONSET	COMMON PATHOGENS	RECOMMENDED REGIMEN		
Early hospital-acquired pneumonia (< 5 days) and no risk factors for multidrug-resistant pathogens	*Streptococcus pneumoniae* MSSA *Haemophilus influenzae* E. coli, Proteus, Klebsiella, Enterobacter, Proteus, Serratia	Ceftriaxone or Ampicillin/sulbactam (*Unasyn*) or Ertapenem or Levofloxacin, moxifloxacin (preferred) or ciprofloxacin *[handwritten: use in severe β-lactam allergy]*		
Late hospital-acquired pneumonia (≥ 5 days or risk for multidrug resistant pathogens)	Above pathogens PLUS MRSA *Pseudomonas aeruginosa* *Acinetobacter sp.* *Enterobacter sp.* + other nosocomial pathogens	Antipseudomonal Beta-lactam (choose 1) +	2nd Antipseudomonal Agent (choose 1) +	Anti-MRSA if patient has risk factors for MRSA (choose 1)
		Cefepime Ceftazidime Imipenem Meropenem Piperacillin/ tazobactam	Gentamicin Tobramycin Amikacin Levofloxacin Ciprofloxacin *[handwritten: anti Pseudo FQs]*	Vancomycin Linezolid

American Thoracic Society, Infectious Disease Society. Guidelines for the management of adults with hospital-acquired, ventilator-associated, and healthcare-associated pneumonia. Am J Respir Crit Care Med. 2005; 15;171:388-416.

Severe Beta-lactam Allergy

- Early onset: levofloxacin or moxifloxacin

- Late onset: Substitute aztreonam 2 grams IV Q8H for the antipsdeudomonal choices listed above

Duration of Treatment

Treat for 7-8 days, except when caused by *Pseudomonas* and *Acinetobacter* or when concomitant bloodstream infection is present (14 days recommended).

Tuberculosis (TB)

handwritten margin note: 6 wo (MDR-TB ⇒ 24 wo)

Tuberculosis is caused by the bacterium *Mycobacterium tuberculosis* (aerobic, non-spore forming bacillus). It is transmitted by aerosolized droplets (via sneezing, coughing, talking, etc.) and is highly contagious. TB primarily attacks the lungs, and occasionally other organs. There are strains resistant to multiple drugs (MDR-TB and XDR-TB), and these have been increasing in incidence. Tuberculosis can be fatal if not treated properly.

The disease has two phases: latent and active. Latent disease is characterized by a complete lack of symptoms. Active disease is most often manifested in coughing, fever and purulent sputum.

Latent Tuberculosis

- Latent disease is diagnosed by tuberculin skin test (TST), also called a purified protein derivative (PPD) test. The solution is injected intradermally and the area is inspected for induration 48-72 hours after injection.

  - A TST test ≥ 5 mm is considered positive for patients with close contacts of recent TB cases or patients with significant immunosuppression (e.g., HIV).

  - A TST ≥ 10 mm is considered positive for recent immigrants, IV drug users, residents/ employees of "high-risk" congregate settings (e.g., healthcare workers or inmates) and patients with moderate immunosuppression.

  - A TST ≥ 15 mm is considered positive for patients with no risk factors.

  - A newer diagnostic test for latent tuberculosis has become available in recent years. The interferon-gamma release assay (IGRA) has the benefit of not requiring a follow-up visit for reading, and can be used in patients who have received BCG vaccine (in areas of the world with high TB rates).

  - Latent Disease Treatment:

    - Isoniazid (INH) 300 mg daily (or twice weekly) for 9 months (typical regimen, preferred for HIV+ or children),

    - Rifampin 400 mg daily for 4 months,

    - INH and Rifapentine *(Priftin)* once weekly for 12 weeks (not if HIV+ or in children < 2 years old) – The older recommendation of rifampin + pyrazinamide is no longer used due to hepatotoxicity.

Active Tuberculosis

- Active tuberculosis is not diagnosed with a TST but rather through a sputum sample.

- *M. tuberculosis* (MTB) are acid fast bacilli and can be detected by staining methods in the laboratory. However the acid fast result is not specific to MTB. Final diagnosis must be made through PCR testing or culture results. Final results can take several weeks.

❑ <u>Active disease</u> is generally treated with a <u>4-drug regimen of</u> rifampin, isoniazid, pyrazinamide and ethambutol (RIPE) and divided into two treatment phases (initial and continuation phases). When MDR-TB is of concern, the addition of moxifloxacin is often added (RIPE becomes PRIME regimen).

TB Disease Treatment Regimens

PREFERRED REGIMEN

Initial Phase – Take all 4 drugs for ~8 weeks (when cultures and susceptibilities are available)

RIPE × 8 wks (56 days)	Rifampin (RIF) + Isoniazid (INH) + Pyrazinamide + Ethambutol* (RIPE) for 56 daily doses (8 weeks)

Continuation Phase – Take once susceptibilities are known

If susceptible to INH and RIF	Continue INH and RIF daily or twice weekly (18 weeks)
	Total duration of therapy = 26 weeks (6 months)
If resistant to INH	RIF + Pyrazinamide + Ethambutol ± Moxifloxacin
	Total duration of therapy = 26 weeks (6 months)
If resistant to RIF	Isoniazid + Ethambutol + FQ + (Pyrazinamide x 2 months)
	Total duration of therapy = 12-18 months
If MDR-TB (resistant to 2 or more drugs including INH and RIF)	FQ + Pyrazinamide + Ethambutol + AMG (streptomycin/amikacin/kanamycin) ± alternative agent**
	Total duration of therapy = 18-24 months

* *Ethambutol can be discontinued if drug susceptibility studies demonstrate susceptibility to first-line drugs. FQ = fluoroquinolone (levofloxacin or moxifloxacin)*

** *Alternative agents include cycloserine, capreomycin, ethionamide and others*

- <u>Use Direct Observed Therapy (DOT), if possible</u>. DOT regimens are preferred for regimens dosed 2 or 3 times per week instead of daily.

- <u>Many variations in dosing intervals exist; however</u> daily dosing is strongly encouraged unless DOT is possible. Less frequent dosing can be used in this setting.

- Patients with active TB should be <u>isolated in a single negative pressure room</u>. Healthcare workers should wear N95 respirator masks when entering the room of a patient suspected to have active tuberculosis.

- <u>Isoniazid carries a risk of</u> neuropathy <u>which can be reduced by taking</u> pyridoxine (vitamin B6) 25-50 mg PO daily.

- Rifabutin can be used instead of rifampin in cases of unacceptable drug-drug interactions with rifampin. *Concurrent use w/ PIs*

DRUG	MOA	DOSING	SAFETY/SIDE EFFECTS/MONITORING
Rifampin *(Rifadin)* + isoniazid *(Rifamate)* + isoniazid + pyrazinamide *(Rifater)*	Inhibits RNA synthesis by blocking RNA transcription in susceptible isolates	10 mg/kg (max 600 mg) daily or 2-3x/week Take on an empty stomach 1 hour before or 2 hours after a meal	**CONTRAINDICATIONS** Concurrent use with PIs (switch to rifabutin) **SIDE EFFECTS** ↑ LFTs, GI upset, rash/pruritus, orange-red discoloration of body secretions, flu-like syndrome, positive Coombs test **MONITORING** LFTs, CBC, mental status, sputum culture, chest X-ray **NOTES** Orange-red discoloration of body secretions – can stain contact lens and clothing. Rifabutin dosed 5 mg/kg/day (300 mg) can replace rifampin to avoid significant drug-drug interactions (e.g., HIV patient on protease inhibitors).
Isoniazid (INH) + rifampin *(Rifamate)* + pyrazinamide/ rifampin *(Rifater)*	Inhibits cell wall synthesis of susceptible isolates	5 mg/kg (max 300 mg) daily or 15 mg/kg (max 900 mg) 2-3x/week Take on an empty stomach 1 hour before or 2 hours after a meal	**BOXED WARNING** Severe (and fatal) hepatitis may occur; usually within first 3 months of treatment **CONTRAINDICATIONS** Active liver disease, previous severe adverse reaction to INH **SIDE EFFECTS** Headache, GI upset, ↑ LFTs, peripheral neuropathy, drug-induced lupus erythematosus (DILE), hyperglycemia, agranulocytosis, hemolytic and aplastic anemia, thrombocytopenia, positive Coombs test **MONITORING** LFTs, sputum culture, chest X-ray **NOTES** Add pyridoxine 25-50 mg/day to reduce risk of peripheral neuropathy. Store oral solution at room temp.
Pyrazinamide + rifampin + isonazid *(Rifater)*	Converts to pyrazinoic acid in susceptible strains of *Mycobacterium* which ↓ pH	20-25 mg/kg/day 40-55 kg: 1 g/d 56-75 kg: 1.5 g/d 76-90 kg: 2 g/d (max dose); 3-4 grams given 2-3x/week Extend interval for CrCl < 30 mL/min	**CONTRAINDICATIONS** Acute gout, severe hepatic damage **SIDE EFFECTS** GI upset, malaise, hepatotoxicity, arthralgias, myalgias, rash, hyperuricemia, gout **MONITORING** LFTs, uric acid, sputum culture, chest X-ray, SCr
Ethambutol *(Myambutol)*	Suppresses mycobacteria replication by interfering with RNA synthesis	15-20 mg/kg (max 1.6 grams) daily or 25-30 mg/kg (max 2.4 grams) 3x/week or 50 mg/kg (max 4 grams) 2x/week Take without regards to meals Extend interval for CrCl < 50 mL/min	**SIDE EFFECTS** Optic neuritis, ↓ visual acuity, scotoma and/or color blindness (usually reversible); rash, headache, confusion, hallucinations, N/V, abdominal pain **MONITORING** Routine vision tests (monthly), SCr

Handwritten margin notes:

LUPUS

↑ dietary intake:
① folic acid
② niacin
③ Mg++

↑ BG

↑ UA

Tuberculosis Agents Continued

DRUG	MOA	DOSING	SAFETY/SIDE EFFECTS/MONITORING
Streptomycin	Binds to 30S ribosomal subunit and inhibits bacterial protein synthesis	15 mg/kg (max 1 gram) daily or 25-30 mg/kg (max 1.5 grams) 2-3x/week Extend interval for CrCl < 50 mL/min	**BOXED WARNING** Neurotoxicity, nephrotoxicity, and neuromuscular blockade/respiratory paralysis **SIDE EFFECTS** Nephrotoxicity, ototoxicity (especially with IV) **MONITORING** Vestibular/audio tests, renal function and streptomycin levels
Bedaquiline (*Sirturo*) Indicated for MDR-TB	Inhibits the proton transfer chain of mycobacterial ATP synthase required for energy generation in *M. tuberculosis*	Weeks 1-2: 400 mg once daily Weeks 3-24: 200 mg 3 times weekly (total weekly dose: 600 mg). Space doses at least 48 hours apart Take with food	**BOXED WARNINGS (2)** May prolong QT interval Increased risk of death versus placebo; only use if no other effective treatment regimen is available. **SIDE EFFECTS** Nausea, arthralgia, headache, hemoptysis, chest pain, ↑ LFTs

Tuberculosis Agents Drug Interactions

- **Rifampin** – Potent inducer of 1A2, 2C8, 2C9, 2C19, 3A4 and P-glycoprotein. Avoid concomitant use with protease inhibitors, apixaban, dabigatran, dronedarone, lurasidone, mycophenolate, nilotinib, ranolazine, ticagrelor, voriconazole and alcohol. Can ↓ levels of warfarin (very large decrease in INR), antiretroviral agents, corticosteroids, quinidine, benzodiazepines, methadone, sulfonylureas, calcium channel blockers, digoxin, cyclosporine, amiodarone, and 100+ others. Rifampin will decrease the effectiveness of oral contraceptives. Rifabutin can replace rifampin to avoid significant drug-drug interactions such as HIV patients requiring protease inhibitors.

- **INH** – Inhibitor of 1A2 (weak), 2C19 (moderate), 2C9 (weak), 2D6 (moderate), and 3A4 (weak). Can ↑ levels of benzodiazepines, carbamazepine, citalopram, fosphenytoin/phenytoin, metoprolol, theophylline, and other 2C19 and 2D6 substrates; can ↓ effects of clopidogrel, codeine, tamoxifen and other drugs requiring conversion to active metabolite via pathways inhibiting by INH. Manufacturer recommends avoiding tyramine and histamine containing foods (low clinical significance). ↑ dietary intake of folic acid, niacin, and magnesium while taking INH.

- **Pyrazinamide** – Can ↑ cyclosporine levels; can cause fatal hepatotoxicity with rifampin; monitor liver function tests and uric acid.

- **Streptomycin** – Can ↑ effects of neuromuscular blocking agents; ↑ nephrotoxicity with other nephrotoxic drugs.

Infective Endocarditis (IE)

4-6 wks

IE is an infection of the inner tissue of the heart, which can include the heart valves, and is generally fatal if untreated. The majority of patients present with fever and heart murmur. The three most common organisms that cause IE are *Staphylococcus*, *Streptococcus*, and *Enterococcus* species. IE is diagnosed by the Modified Duke Criteria which includes an echocardiogram, allowing for visualization of the vegetation. Empiric treatment generally should include vancomycin and ceftriaxone. Definitive treatment is dependent on the pathogen, presence or absence of a prosthetic valve, and susceptibility results. In general, 4-6 weeks of treatment is required. Penicillin, ampicillin, or ceftriaxone are preferred options for Streptococcal IE. Nafcillin or cefazolin are preferred options for MSSA IE. Vancomycin is generally reserved for MRSA IE or for other Gram-positive IE if the patient has a severe beta-lactam allergy. Rifampin may be used in cases of prosthetic valve endocarditis due to its activity against biofilm-dwelling organisms. Gentamicin is often added to primary antimicrobial therapy for synergy for a varied duration depending on the pathogen (such as 4-6 weeks for *Enterococcus*) and/or presence of a prosthetic valve (2 weeks). When gentamicin is used for synergy, target peak levels of 3-4 mcg/mL and trough levels < 1 mcg/mL. Do not use extended interval dosing for AMG when treating endocarditis.

Baddour LM, Wilson WR, Bayer AS et al. Infective Endocarditis. Circulation. 2005; 111:e394-e433.

Dental Procedures and IE Prophylaxis

The mouth contains bacteria that are released during dental work and travel into the bloodstream where they can settle on the heart lining, a heart valve or a blood vessel. IE after dental procedures is rare, but certain cardiac conditions increase the risk. Antibiotics should be used before dental procedures in patients with the highest risk of contracting IE (see the following indications).

- An artificial (prosthetic) heart valve or heart valve repaired with artificial material.

- A history of endocarditis.

- A heart transplant with abnormal heart valve function.

- Certain congenital heart defects including:

  - Cyanotic congenital heart disease (birth defects with oxygen levels lower than normal), that has not been fully repaired, including children who have had surgical shunts and conduits.

  - A congenital heart defect that has been completely repaired with artificial material or a device for the first six months after the repair procedure.

  - Repaired congenital heart disease with residual defects, such as persisting leaks or abnormal flow at or adjacent to a prosthetic patch or prosthetic device.

AGENT	ADULTS	CHILDREN

Prophylactic Regimens: Take a single dose 30-60 minutes before dental procedure

Oral

Amoxicillin	2 grams	50 mg/kg

Unable to take oral medication

Ampicillin or	2 grams IM/IV	50 mg/kg IM/IV
Cefazolin or ceftriaxone	1 grams IM/IV	50 mg/kg IM/IV

Allergic to penicillins and can take oral medication

Cephalexin or cefadroxil* or	2 grams	50 mg/kg
Clindamycin or	600 mg	20 mg/kg
Azithromycin or clarithromycin	500 mg	15 mg/kg

Allergic to penicillins and unable to take oral medication

Cefazolin or Ceftriaxone or	1 grams IM/IV	50 mg/kg IM/IV
Clindamycin	600 mg IM/IV	20 mg/kg IM/IV

* *Cephalosporins should not be used in an individual with a history of anaphylaxis, angioedema, or urticaria with penicillins or ampicillin.*

Wilson W, Taubert KA, Gewitz M et al. Prevention of Infective Endocarditis Guidelines. Circulation. 2007; 116:1736-54.

Intra-Abdominal Infections

Intra-abdominal infections are a common cause of hospital admissions and the second most common cause of infectious mortality in ICUs. They are characterized as primary (spontaneous bacterial), secondary, and tertiary peritonitis, and biliary tract infections (cholecystitis and cholangitis).

- Primary peritonitis (aka spontaneous bacterial peritonitis, SBP) is an infection of the peritoneal space and often occurs in patients with liver disease. The most likely pathogens are *Streptococci* and enteric Gram-negative organisms (PEK) and, rarely, anaerobes. The drug of choice is ceftriaxone for 5-7 days. Alternatives include ampicillin, gentamicin or a fluoroquinolone, among other options. SMX/TMP, ofloxacin and/or ciprofloxacin can be used for primary or secondary prophylaxis of SBP.

- Secondary peritonitis is caused by a traumatic event (e.g. ulceration, ischemia, obstruction, or surgery). Abscesses are common and should be drained and damaged tissue may require surgery. The most likely pathogens are *Streptococci*, enteric Gram-negatives and anaerobes *(Bacteroides fragilis)*. In more severe cases (critically ill patients in the ICU), coverage of *Pseudomonas* and CAPES organisms may be necessary.

- Cholecystitis is an infection of the gallbladder and is generally surgically managed through cholecysectomy. Likely pathogens and antimicrobial selection (if needed) are similar to primary peritonitis. Cholangitis is an infection of the biliary ductal system and is generally managed with bile decompression and antimicrobial therapy. Likely pathogens and antimicrobial selection is similar to secondary peritonitis.

Management of Secondary Peritonitis and Cholangitis* *[handwritten: ICU, APACHE >15, ↑↑ age, malignancy, comorbid + organ dysfxn, ⊖ source control]*

[handwritten left margin: 4-7 days]

[handwritten right margin: 7-14 days]

MILD-TO-MODERATE INFECTIONS	HIGH-SEVERITY INFECTIONS/ICU#
Cover PEK + anaerobes + Streptococci ± Enterococci	Cover PEK + CAPES + anaerobes + Streptococci ± Enterococci

*[handwritten left margin: ** intraabd. abscess → tx ≥ 14 days **]*

Single Agent Regimens

Ticarcillin/clavulanate or	Imipenem or
Ertapenem or	Meropenem or
Cefoxitin or	Doripenem or
Tigecycline or	Piperacillin/tazobactam
Moxifloxacin	

[handwritten right: COVER FOR PSEUDO IN ICU]

Combination Regimens

(Cefazolin or cefuroxime or ceftriaxone) + metronidazole	(Ceftazidime or cefepime) + metronidazole
(Ciprofloxacin or levofloxacin) + metronidazole	(Ciprofloxacin or levofloxacin) + metronidazole
	(Aztreonam or AMG) + metronidazole

AMG = aminoglycosides; CAPES (nosocomial GNRs) = Citrobacter, Acinetobacter, Pseudomonas, Enterobacter, Serratia; ICU = intensive care unit; PEK (enteric GNRs) = Proteus, E. coli, Klebsiella

*Duration of treatment is generally 4-7 days, especially for mild to moderate cases with adequate source control. Longer courses (7-14 days) may be needed in more severe cases. In the setting of intra-abdominal abscess ≥ 14 days may be required.

#High severity: ICU, APACHE II > 15, advanced age, comorbidity and organ dysfunction, malignancy, lack of source control

Solomkin JS, Mazuski JE, Bradley JS et al. Diagnosis and management of complicated intra-abdominal infection in adults and children: guidelines by the Surgical Infection Society and the Infectious Diseases Society of America. Clin Infect Dis. 2010; 50:133-64.

Skin and Soft-Tissue Infections (SSTIs)

Skin and soft-tissue infections may involve any or all layers of the skin (epidermis, dermis, and subcutaneous fat), fascia, and muscle. Most primary infections, including cellulitis and impetigo, are superficial and mild. Secondary infections involve areas of previously damaged skin. Multiple organisms are usually involved.

Cellulitis affects all layers of the skin and is a serious type of SSTI. *S. pyogenes* and *S. aureus* are the most frequent pathogens, with community-acquired MRSA on the rise. Lesions are usually painful, erythematous, and feel hot and tender. The infected area has poorly defined margins and may extend. Non-pharmacologic treatment consists of elevation and immobilization of the area to decrease swelling and cool sterile saline dressings to decrease the pain. Mild to moderate infections without systemic symptoms may be treated with oral therapy. If possible, skin abscesses should be incised and drained (I & D) and may be all that is required for mild cases of purulent cellulitis. In cases of non-purulent cellulitis, no locus of fluid exists, making drainage impossible.

INFECTION	ADULT TREATMENT OPTIONS	COMMENTS

Empiric oral therapy options for _purulent cellulitis_. **If non-purulent, treat with a beta-lactam (e.g., penicillin, dicloxacillin or cephalexin or clindamycin in setting of beta-lactam allergies)**

| Outpatient SSTI | Clindamycin 300-450 mg TID or SMX/TMP 1-2 DS tabs BID or Doxycycline 100 mg BID or Minocycline 200 mg x 1, then 100 mg BID or Linezolid 600 mg BID Duration of therapy = 5 to 10 days | Target Gram-positive organisms (_Staphylococci, Streptococci_) Primary treatment for cutaneous abscess is incision and drainage (I & D) Use IV antibiotics for severe infections, rapid progression, systemic illness, etc. For recurrent SSTIs in patients with nasal MRSA colonization, consider decolonization with intranasal mupirocin (_Bactroban_ Nasal) BID for 5 days, daily chlorhexidine washes, and daily decontamination of personal items. |

[handwritten annotations: "5-10 days", "purulent"]

Empiric therapy options for _complicated_ **SSTIs (pending culture results)**

| Inpatient SSTI | Vancomycin 15 mg/kg IV Q12H (goal trough 10-15 mg/L) or Linezolid 600 mg IV/PO BID or Daptomycin 4 mg/kg/dose once daily or Telavancin 10 mg/kg/dose once daily or Ceftaroline 600 mg IV Q12H Tedizolid 200 mg IV/PO once daily Dalbavancin 1,000 mg IV x1, then 500 mg IV one week later Duration of therapy = 7 to 14 days | MRSA risk high compared to outpatient Broader spectrum therapy, including antipseudomonal coverage, may be required for severe/complicated cases of non-purulent cellulitis, in particular among immunocompromised patients and/or for management of diabetic foot ulcers/infections (see table below). Bite infections generally requires broader therapy to include coverage of aerobic Gram-negative and Gram-positive pathogens, along with anaerobes (e.g. ampicillin-sulbactam). Necrotizing infections generally require the addition of clindamycin for toxin suppression. |

[handwritten annotations: "7-14 days", "complex SSTIs", "MRSA!!"]

Stevens DL, Bisno AL, Chambers, HF et al. Practice Guidelines for the Diagnosis and Management of Skin and Soft Tissue Infections: 2014 Update by the Infectious Diseases Society of America. Clin Infect Dis. 2014; 59(2):147-159.

Liu C, Bayer A, Cosgrove SE et al. Clinical Practice Guidelines for MRSA Infections. Clin Infect Dis. 2011; 52:1-38.

Diabetic Foot Infections

Diabetics are at high-risk for foot infections because of compromised blood flow to the lower extremities and neuropathic damage. Infections are the most common cause of amputation in diabetics. It is imperative that patients to follow proper foot care and evaluation, as discussed in the Diabetes chapter.

ETIOLOGY	GRAM-POSITIVE	GRAM-NEGATIVE
Aerobic	_S. epidermidis_ _S. aureus_ (including MRSA) Group A _Streptococcus_ Viridans _Streptococci_	_E. coli_ _Klebsiella pneumoniae_ _Proteus mirabilis_ _Enterobacter cloacae_ _Pseudomonas aeruginosa_
Anaerobic	_Peptostreptococcus_ _Clostridium perfringens_	_Bacteroides fragilis_ and others

[handwritten annotation: "↳ gas gangrene"]

7-14 days *2-4 wks* *→ 4-6 wks*

Treatment of Moderate-Severe (Life or Limb-threatening) Diabetic Foot Infections

TYPE OF REGIMEN	TREATMENT REGIMEN	COMMENTS
Combination	3rd or 4th generation cephalosporin + (metronidazole or clindamycin) ± vancomycin or Clindamycin + fluoroquinolone (ciprofloxacin or levofloxacin) or Vancomycin + ceftazidime + metronidazole or (Daptomycin or linezolid) + (aztreonam or aminoglycoside) + (metronidazole or clindamycin)	Duration: 7-14 days More severe, deep tissue infection = treat for 2-4 weeks Severe, limb-threatening or bone/joint infection = treat 4-6 weeks Chronic osteomyelitis may require longer courses of therapy, including chronic suppressive therapy
Monotherapy	Ampicillin/sulbactam (Unasyn) or Piperacillin/tazobactam (Zosyn) or Ticarcillin/clavulanate (Timentin) or Imipenem/cilastatin or Meropenem or Doripenem or Ertapenem or Tigecycline or Moxifloxacin	

Lipsky BA, Berendt AR, Deery HG et al. Diagnosis and treatment of diabetic foot infections. Clin Infect Dis. 2012; 54(12):132–173.

Urinary Tract Infection (UTI)

Most UTIs occur in the bladder (cystitis) and urethra, which is called the lower urinary tract. More severe infections can occur in the kidneys (pyelonephritis), or the upper urinary tract. UTIs are more common in females than males due to the shorter urethra and the shorter route for organisms to travel up into the urethra. Sexual intercourse can facilitate this movement and women who develop UTIs commonly after intercourse may require prophylactic antibiotics after sexual intercourse. UTIs are uncommon in younger males but increase in incidence with age. An infection in males is considered to be complicated because it is likely due to some type of abnormality or obstruction, such as an enlarged prostate. In females, the majority of infections are not associated with an abnormality or obstruction and are most often uncomplicated. Complicated infections result from a neurogenic bladder (e.g., spinal cord injury, stroke, multiple sclerosis) or obstruction (e.g., a stone, indwelling catheter). Both genders are at risk for catheter-associated infections, see the Medication Safety chapter for a discussion of ways to reduce this common type of (often preventable) infection.

- Typical signs and symptoms of lower urinary tract infections (cystitis) are dysuria, urgency, frequency, burning, nocturia, suprapubic heaviness, and/or hematuria (fever is uncommon). A urinalysis is considered positive when there is evidence of pyuria (positive leukocyte esterase or ≥ 10 WBC/mL) and bacteriuria (≥ 10^5 bacteria/mL in uncomplicated patients and ≥ 10^3 bacteria/mL in complicated patients, including in men).

(+) urinalysis

pyuria = (+) leukocyte esterase OR ≥ 10 WBC/ml

+ bacteriuria = ≥ 10^5 bact/ml (uncomplex)
≥ 10^3 bact/ml (complex)

- Typical signs and symptoms of upper urinary tract infections (pyelonephritis) are flank pain, abdominal pain, fever, nausea, vomiting, costovertebral angle pain, and malaise.

- Must treat bacteriuria in pregnant women (for 7 days) even if asymptomatic with negative urinalysis. If not, the infection can lead to premature birth, pyelonephritis, and neonatal meningitis. In pregnant women, avoid quinolones (cartilage toxicity and arthropathies) and tetracyclines (teratogenic). SMX/TMP can cause hyperbilirubinemia and kernicterus in 3rd trimester (Pregnancy Category D near term); otherwise, category C. Generally, beta-lactams are used (amox/clav or oral cephalosporins) and, if penicillin-allergic, nitrofurantoin or fosfomycin can be used. See Drug Use in Pregnancy chapter for more information.

[handwritten margin note: 7 days]

UTI Treatment

DIAGNOSIS	PATHOGENS	DRUGS OF CHOICE/GUIDELINES	COMMENTS
Acute uncomplicated cystitis in females of child bearing age (~15-45 years of age)	E. coli (vast majority), Proteus, Klebsiella (PEK) S. saprophyticus, Enterococcus	Nitrofurantoin 100 mg BID x 5 days or SMX/TMP 1 DS tab BID x 3 days (avoid if resistance > 20% to E. coli or sulfa allergy) or Fosfomycin x 1 (3 grams in 4 oz water – lower efficacy) or If ≥ 20% local E. coli resistant to SMX/TMP or sulfa allergy: Ciprofloxacin 250 mg BID x 3 days or Ciprofloxacin ER 500 mg daily x 3 days or Levofloxacin 250 mg daily x 3 days	May add phenazopyridine 200 mg PO TID x 2 days to the regimen to relieve symptoms (dysuria) Usually empirically treated as an outpatient Prophylaxis: ≥ 3 episodes in 1 yr; use 1 SMX/TMP SS daily, nitrofurantoin 50 mg PO daily, or 1 SMX/TMP DS post coitus If no response on 3-day course, perform urinary culture and treat for 2 weeks Do not recommend moxifloxacin (does not reach high levels in the urine) or gemifloxacin (poor to limited activity against normal UTI pathogens) Beta-lactam agents (amoxicillin/clavulanate and oral cephalosporins) x 3-7 days are appropriate choices when other recommended agents cannot be used. Treat pregnant women for 7 days
Acute uncomplicated pyelonephritis	E. coli, Enterococci, P. mirabilis, K. pneumoniae, P. aeruginosa	Moderately ill outpatient (PO): For FQ resistance < 10%: Ciprofloxacin 500 mg PO BID or ciprofloxacin ER 1,000 mg daily x 7 days or levofloxacin 750 mg daily x 5 days For FQ resistance > 10%: ceftriaxone 1 gram x 1 or 24 hours of AMG initially followed by SMX/TMP (if susceptible) or beta-lactam (amox/clav, cefdinir, cefaclor, or cefpodoxime) – treat for 14 days Severe – hospitalized tx (IV): FQ, AMP + Gent, Pip/Tazo, or ceftriaxone, then stepdown to similar oral options above based on susceptibility results; treat for 14 days of total antibiotic duration (IV and PO)	If risk for or documented Pseudomonas infection, consider piperacillin/tazobactam or meropenem ± aminoglycoside

[handwritten margin notes: "x 3 days"; "Bactrim ®"; table with "indication / dose / interval" — "PCP proph: 1DS or SS, qd"; "UTI: 1DS, BID"; "severe infxn: 2DS, BID – TID"; "14 days"; "14 days (IV + po)"]

UTI Treatment Continued

DIAGNOSIS	PATHOGENS	DRUGS OF CHOICE/GUIDELINES	COMMENTS
Complicated UTI	E.coli, Klebsiella, Enterobacter, Serratia, Pseudomonas, Enterococcus, Staphylococcus	Similar to options noted above for pyelonephritis or If ESBL producers are present, use carbapenems	Need urinalysis, urine and blood cultures May be due to obstruction, catheterization – remove or change catheter if possible Treat for 7 days if there is prompt symptom relief Treat for 10-14 days with delayed response regardless of catheterization or not

handwritten left margin: 7 days (10-14 days if delayed response)

Gupta K, Hootan TM, Naber KG et al. International Clinical Practice Guidelines for the Treatment of Acute Uncomplicated Cystitis and Pyelonephritis in Women: A 2010 Update by the Infectious Diseases Society of America and the European Society for Microbiology and Infectious Diseases. Clin Infect Dis. 2011; 52:e103-e120

Hooton TM, Bradley SF, Cardenas DD et al. Diagnosis, Prevention, and Treatment of Catheter-Associated Urinary Tract Infection in Adults: 2009 International Clinical Practice Guidelines from the Infectious Diseases Society of America. Clin Infect Dis. 2010; 50:625-663

Bader MS, Hawboldt J, Brooks A. Management of complicated urinary tract infections in the era of antimicrobial resistance. Postgrad Med. 2010; 122:7-15.

Urinary Analgesic

Phenazopyridine may be given to reduce the symptoms of pain or burning with urination. It is occasionally given to reduce pain from vaginal procedures.

DRUG	DOSING	SAFETY/SIDE EFFECTS/MONITORING
Phenazopyridine (Azo, Uristat, Pyridium)	100-200 mg TID (OTC and Rx) x 2 days (max)	**CONTRAINDICATIONS** Do not use in patients with CrCl < 50 mL/min or liver disease **SIDE EFFECTS** Headache, dizziness, stomach cramps, body secretion discoloration **NOTES** Pregnancy Category B Take with or following food and 8 oz of water to minimize stomach upset May cause red-orange coloring of the urine and other body fluids. Contact lenses and clothes can be stained Can cause hemolytic anemia in patients with G6PD deficiency

Clostridium Difficile Infection (CDI)

The GI tract contains > 1,000 species of organisms. The use of antibiotics will eliminate much of the "healthy" bacteria, allowing an overgrowth of *Clostridium difficile* bacteria. This organism releases toxins that attack the intestinal lining, causing colitis. Symptoms of CDI include abdominal cramps, bloody, soft, or watery stool, and fever. Pseudomembraneous colitis occurs when the overgrowth has inflamed the colon. This infection is one of the causes of toxic megacolon, which can be quickly fatal. Rates of CDI have increased in recent years. In addition to the antibiotic, other risk factors include previous CDI, advanced age, immunocompromised state and obesity.

handwritten: risk factors:
1) abx use
2) hx of CDI
3) ↑↑ age
4) immuno suppression
5) obesity

Treatment Principles of CDI Include

- Discontinue the offending agent immediately, if possible.

- Avoid antimotility agents due to the risk of toxic megacolon.

- Wash hands with soap and water to prevent transmission. Hand sanitizers containing alcohol do not kill *C. difficile* spores.

- Isolate patients to prevent transmission (single patient rooms, gloves, gowns).

- Metronidazole should not be used beyond the 1st recurrence or for long-term therapy due to the potential for cumulative neurotoxicity.

- Probiotics *(Lactobacillus)* are not beneficial for treatment, but may have some benefit for prophylaxis.

Treatment of *C. difficile**

10-14 days

SEVERITY OF INFECTION	TREATMENT OF 1ST INFECTION	TREATMENT OF 2ND INFECTION (1ST RECURRENCE)	TREATMENT OF 3RD INFECTION (2ND RECURRENCE)
Mild-moderate disease	Metronidazole 500 mg PO TID x 10-14 days	Same as 1st infection if same severity	Vancomycin taper/pulse therapy 125 mg PO QID x 10-14 days, BID x 1 week, daily x 1 week, then 125 mg every 2-3 days/ week for 2-8 weeks
Severe disease (WBC ≥ 15,000 or SCr > 1.5x baseline level)	Vancomycin 125 mg PO QID x 10-14 days	Same as 1st infection if same severity	Vancomycin taper/pulse therapy
Severe, complicated disease (Hypotension, shock, ileus, or toxic megacolon)	Vancomycin 500 mg PO QID + metronidazole 500 mg IV Q8H If complete ileus, add vancomycin per rectum (500 mg in 100 mL NS PR Q6H)	Same as 1st infection if same severity	Vancomycin taper/pulse therapy

Handwritten margin notes:
① 125 mg QID x 10-14 d
② BID x 1 wk
③ qd x 1 wk
④ 2-3 d/wk x 2-8 wks

* *In clinical trials, fidaxomicin was non-inferior to vancomycin oral therapy, but with lower recurrence rates. Consider fidaxomicin instead of vancomycin for patients at high risk of recurrence (patients receiving chemotherapy or immuno-suppressed patients) – place in therapy not fully established. Cohen SH, Gerding DN, Johnson S et al. Clinical practice guidelines for Clostridium difficile infection in adults: 2010 update by the SHEA and the IDSA. Infect Control Hosp Epidemiol. 2010; 31:431-55.*

Traveler's Diarrhea (TD)

TD is the most common travel-related illness. Bacteria causes 80% of TD cases, including en-terotoxigenic *Escherichia coli*, followed by *Campylobacter jejuni*, *Shigella spp.*, and *Salmonella spp.* Viral diarrhea can be caused by a number of pathogens, most commonly norovirus and ro-tavirus. Less commonly, protozoa including *Giardia, Entamoeba histolytica, Cryptosporidium* and *Cyclospora*, may result in TD. Bacterial and viral diarrhea presents with sudden onset of symptoms, including cramps and urgent loose stools to severe abdominal pain, fever, vomit-ing, and bloody diarrhea. Protozoal diarrhea, such as that caused by *Giardia* or *E. histolytica*, generally has a more gradual onset of low-grade symptoms, with 2–5 loose stools per day.

The primary source of infection is ingestion of fecally contaminated food and water. Most cas-es are benign and resolve in 1-2 days without treatment. Preventive measures should be taken:

- Avoid eating foods or drinking beverages from street vendors or other places of unhygienic conditions

- Avoid eating raw or undercooked meat/ seafood

- Avoid eating raw fruits (e.g., oranges, bananas, avocados) and vegetables unless the traveler peels them

- Avoid tap water, ice, unpasteurized milk and dairy products

A simple rule is "boil it, cook it, peel it, or forget it." Well-cooked and packaged foods are generally safe. Safe beverages include bottled, carbonated drinks, hot tea or coffee, beer, wine, boiled water or treated water (with iodine or chlorine).

Prophylactic antibiotics are not recommended due to concerns of toxicity, resistance, lack of activity against viral pathogens and the fact that most cases of TD are self-limiting without antimicrobial therapy. Bismuth subsalicylate (BSS) taken as either 2 tablets QID (or liquid) reduces the incidence of TD (not to be used longer than 3 weeks). BSS commonly causes blackening of the tongue and stool and may cause nausea, constipation, and rarely tinnitus. BSS should be avoided in those with an aspirin allergy, renal insufficiency, and by those taking anticoagulants, probenecid, or methotrexate. The role of probiotics for the prevention of TD is unclear at this time. The most important treatment is oral rehydration therapy, especially in young children, elderly or those with chronic medical conditions. A 1-3 day course of fluoroquinolones or macrolides are generally effective in treating TD (see table above). Adjunctive therapy, including antimotility agents (loperamide) provide symptomatic relief, but generally should be avoided for bloody diarrhea or for patients with a fever. Diphenoxylate is no longer recommended due to concerns of toxicity (risks > benefits).

TRAVELER'S DIARRHEA TREATMENT

Drug Therapy – FQs are the drugs of choice
Ciprofloxacin 500 mg PO BID x 3 days or

Norfloxacin 400 mg BID x 3-5 days

Ofloxacin 200 mg BID x 3 days or

Levofloxacin 500 mg daily x 1-3 days or

Rifaximin 200 mg TID x 3 days or

Azithromycin 1,000 mg x 1 or 500 mg daily x 1-3 days – drug of choice for pregnancy and children

Bismuth subsalicylate 524 mg (2 tablets) every 30 min to 1 hour up to 8 doses/day x 2 days

PLUS

Loperamide 4 mg x 1, then 2 mg after each loose stool – max 8 mg/d (loperamide is not recommended if patient has signs of dysentery, high fever or blood in stool)

* Metronidazole, tinidazole, and nitazoxanide should be reserved for TD caused by Protozoa (e.g., Giardia or Cryptosporidia)

Sexually Transmitted Infections (STIs)

INFECTION	DOC	DOSING/DURATION	ALTERNATIVES/NOTES
Syphilis – caused by *Treponema pallidum*, a spirochete Primary, secondary, or early latent (< 1 year duration)	Penicillin G benzathine *(Bicillin L-A – do not substitute with Bicillin C-R)*	2.4 million units IM x 1	Doxycycline 100 mg PO BID or Tetracycline 500 mg PO QID x 14 days Pregnant patients allergic to PCN should be desensitized and treated with PCN
Syphilis – Late latent (> 1 year duration), tertiary, or latent syphilis of unknown duration	Penicillin G benzathine *(Bicillin L-A – do not substitute with Bicillin C-R)*	2.4 million units IM weekly x 3 weeks (7.2 MU total)	Doxycycline 100 mg PO BID or Tetracycline 500 mg PO QID x 28 days Pregnant patients allergic to PCN should be desensitized and treated with PCN

Sexually Transmitted Infections (STIs) Continued

INFECTION	DOC	DOSING/DURATION	ALTERNATIVES/NOTES
Neurosyphilis (including ocular syphilis)	Penicillin G aqueous crystalline	3-4 million units IV Q4H or continuous infusion (18-24 million units/day) x 10-14 days	Penicillin G procaine 2.4 million units IM daily + probenecid 500 mg PO QID x 10-14 days
Congenital syphilis	Penicillin G aqueous crystalline	Newborns: 50,000 units/ kg IV Q12H x 7 days, then Q8H for 10 days total Infants ≥ 1 month old: 50,000 units/kg IV Q4-6H x 10 days	Penicillin G procaine 50,000 units/kg IM daily x 10 days
Gonorrhea – caused by *Neisseria gonorrhea*, a Gram-negative diplococcus Urethral, cervical, rectal, pharyngeal	Ceftriaxone PLUS Azithromycin (preferred) or Doxycycline – for co-infection with Chlamydia*	250 mg IM x 1 1 gram PO x 1 100 mg PO BID x 7 days	*Ceftriaxone is most effective for pharyngeal infections If ceftriaxone is not available, can use Cefixime *(Suprax)* 400 mg PO x 1 + azithromycin (or doxycycline); test for cure in 1 week If severe cephalosporin allergy, azithromycin 2 g PO x 1 – effective for both gonorrhea and chlamydia but poorly tolerated (GI effects), more expensive and rapid emergence of resistance. Test for cure in 1 week
Chlamydial Infections – caused by *Chlamydia trachomatis*, intracellular obligate parasite	Azithromycin or Doxycycline PLUS Ceftriaxone for co-infection with Gonorrhea*	1 gram PO x 1 or 100 mg PO BID x 7 days	Erythromycin base 500 mg PO QID x 7 days or Levofloxacin 500 mg PO daily x 7 days
Bacterial Vaginosis – caused by many different organisms	Metronidazole or Metronidazole 0.75% gel or Clindamycin 2% cream	500 mg PO BID x 7 days 5 g intravaginally daily x 5 days 5 g intravaginally at bedtime x 7 days	Clindamycin 300 mg PO BID x 7 days or Clindamycin ovules 100 mg intravaginally at bedtime x 3 days or Tinidazole 2 g PO daily x 2 days or Tinidazole 1 g PO daily x 5 days
Trichomoniasis – caused by *Trichomonas vaginalis*, a flagellated protozoan	Metronidazole or Tinidazole	2 g PO x 1 2 g PO x 1	Metronidazole 500 mg PO BID x 7 days
Herpes Simplex Virus (HSV)			See Viral Section

Coinfection with C. trachomatis frequently occurs among patients who have gonococcal infection (and vice versa); therefore, presumptive treatment for both pathogens is appropriate.

Workowski KA, Berman S. Sexually Transmitted Diseases Treatment Guidelines, 2010. MMWR Recommendations and Reports. 2010; 59:1-110 and 2012 update.

All sexual partners must also be treated concurrently to prevent re-infection

Rickettsial Diseases

Rickettsial organisms are carried by many ticks, fleas, and lice and cause diseases in humans such as those found below. Rocky Mountain spotted fever is the most common and most fatal rickettsial illness in the U.S. Initial signs and symptoms include fever, headache, muscle pain followed by the development of a rash.

DISEASE	TREATMENT
Rocky Mountain Spotted Fever	Doxycycline 100 mg PO/IV BID x 5-7 days
Lyme Disease	Doxycycline 100 mg PO BID x 10-21 days or amoxicillin 500 mg PO TID or cefuroxime axetil 500 mg BID x 14-21 days
Typhus	Doxycycline 100 mg PO/IV BID x 7 days
Ehrlichiosis	Doxycycline 100 mg PO/IV BID x 7-14 days
Tularemia	Gentamicin or tobramycin 5 mg/kg/d divided Q8H IV x 7-14 days

Wormser GP, Dattwyler RJ, Shapiro ED et al. The clinical assessment, treatment, and prevention of lyme disease, human granulocytic anaplasmosis, and babesiosis: clinical practice guidelines by the IDSA. Clin Infect Dis. 2006; 43:1089-134.

SYSTEMIC FUNGAL INFECTIONS

Treatment Recommendations for Selected Fungal Pathogens

PATHOGEN	1ST-LINE
Candida	Oropharyngeal and vaginal: fluconazole or topicals (clotrimazole or nystatin)
	Esophageal and invasive: fluconazole or echinocandin or amphotericin B
Aspergillus	Voriconazole
Cryptococcus neoformans	Induction in serious infections (primarily causes meningitis): amphotericin B + flucytosine (5-FC)
	Consolidation: fluconazole (prolonged)
Coccidioides immitis	Amphotericin B or fluconazole
Histoplasma capsulatum	Amphotericin B or itraconazole
Zygomycetes class (*Rhizopus*, *Mucor*, etc.)	Amphotericin B ± posaconazole
Dermatophytes	Nail bed infections: itraconazole, terbinafine, or fluconazole (confirm fungal infection prior to treatment)

DRUGS USED TO TREAT DIFFICULT PATHOGENS

Agents used for skin and skin structure infections caused by Community-Associated methicillin-resistant *Staphylococcus aureus* (CA-MRSA)

SMX/TMP *(Bactrim DS)*

Doxycycline

Minocycline

Clindamycin ☺ *perform susceptibility test (resistance!)*

Linezolid

Daptomycin

Tigecycline

Ceftaroline

Vancomycin

Telavancin

Dalbavancin

Tedizolid

Agents used to treat nosocomial-associated methicillin-resistant *Staphylococcus aureus*

Vancomycin (If VISA, then use agents listed below or consider agents below if MIC ≥ 2)

Linezolid

Quinupristin/Dalfopristin

Daptomycin (not for pneumonia)

Ceftaroline

Telavancin

Tigecycline

Dalbavancin

Tedizolid

Rifampin (combination therapy for prosthetic infections)

SMX/TMP

Agents used to treat VRE. *faecalis*

Pen G or ampicillin

Linezolid

Daptomycin

Tigecycline

Cystitis only per susceptibilities: nitrofurantoin, fosfomycin, doxy-cycline

Agents used to treat VRE. *faecium*

Daptomycin

Linezolid

Quinupristin/Dalfopristin

Tigecycline

Cystitis only per susceptibilities: nitrofurantoin, fosfomycin, doxy-cycline

Agents used to treat *Pseudomonas aeruginosa* (double cover except in urine)

Imipenem

Meropenem

Doripenem

Cefepime

Ceftazidime

Ciprofloxacin

Levofloxacin

Aztreonam

Ticarcillin/Clavulanic acid

Piperacillin

Piperacillin/Tazobactam

Colistimethate

Amikacin

Tobramycin

Gentamicin

Agents used to treat extended spectrum beta-lactamase producing enteric gram-negative rods (ESBL GNR) – *E. coli*, *Klebsiella pneumoniae*, *P. mirabilis*

Carbapenems

Cefepime (high dose)

Piperacillin/Tazobactam

Fluoroquinolones

Aminoglycosides (per susceptibilities)

Agents used to treat *Acinetobacter baumannii*

Imipenem

Meropenem

Doripenem

Ampicillin/Sulbactam

Colistimethate

Minocycline

Tigecycline

Fluoroquinolones

SMX/TMP

Agents used to treat *Bacteroides fragilis*

Metronidazole

Carbapenems

Beta-lactam/Beta-lactamase inhibitor combos

Tigecycline

Cefoxitin

Cefotetan

Others but reduced activity: clindamycin, moxifloxacin

Agents used to treat *Clostridium difficile*

Metronidazole

Vancomycin (oral)

Fidaxomicin

☺ *Before using clindamycin, an induction test (D test) should be performed on isolates sensitive to clindamycin but resistant to erythromycin – look for a flattened zone between the disks → this signifies that inducible clindamycin resistance is present. Also, never use FQs regardless of susceptibility profile.*

suscept. test w/ clinda

↳ D-test determines presence of constitutive (already present) resistance in MRSA

See p. 377.

VIRAL INFECTIONS

Herpes Simplex Virus (HSV)

- HSV-1 is most commonly associated with oropharyngeal disease, and HSV-2 is associated more closely with genital disease. However, each virus is capable of causing infections clinically indistinguishable in both anatomic areas.

- Genital herpes is a chronic, life-long viral infection. 1 in 6 people in the U.S. have HSV-2.

- The first episode of genital herpes usually begins within 2-14 days post exposure, but up to 50% of patients are asymptomatic. First episode symptoms can include flu-like symptoms, fever, headache, malaise, myalgia, and development of pustular or ulcerative lesions on external genitalia.

- Lesions usually begin as papules or vesicles that rapidly spread and clusters of lesions form, crust, and re-epithelialize. Lesions are described as painful. Itching, dysuria, and vaginal or urethral discharge are common symptoms.

- Recurrent infections are not associated with systemic manifestations. Symptoms are localized to the genital area, milder, and of shorter duration. Patients typically experience a prodrome prior to symptoms. Treatment must be initiated during prodrome or within 1 day of lesion onset for the patient to experience the full benefit.

- Suppressive therapy reduces the frequency of genital herpes recurrences by 70-80% among patients who have frequent recurrences (e.g., > 6 recurrences/yr) and many report no symptomatic outbreaks. Viral transmission is also reduced.

- Acyclovir (Zovirax) is usually the least expensive regimen. Valacyclovir (Valtrex) is a pro-drug of acyclovir that results in higher concentrations than with oral acyclovir and less frequent dosing that may enhance adherence. In general, 5 mg/kg IV acyclovir = 1,000 mg PO valacyclovir. If the virus is found to be resistant to acyclovir, it will be resistant to valacyclovir. Famciclovir (Famvir) is a pro-drug of penciclovir. Strains resistant to acyclovir are generally resistant to famciclovir.

Following is a table summarizing the treatment of herpes simplex virus infections.

Herpes Simplex Virus Treatment In Non-HIV Patients

HSV INFECTION	ACYCLOVIR	VALACYCLOVIR	FAMCICLOVIR
Primary – initial episode			
Genital HSV	200 mg PO 5x daily x 10 days or 400 mg PO TID x 7-10 days	1 g PO BID x 10 days	250 mg PO TID x 7-10 days
Oral HSV	200 mg PO 5x daily or 400 mg TID x 7-10 days		

Herpes Simplex Virus Treatment In Non-HIV Patients Continued

HSV INFECTION	ACYCLOVIR	VALACYCLOVIR	FAMCICLOVIR
Recurrent episodes			
Genital HSV	400 mg PO TID x 5 days or 800 mg PO BID x 5 days or 800 mg PO TID x 2 days	500 mg PO BID x 3 days or 1 g PO daily x 5 days	125 mg PO BID x 5 days or 1g PO BID x 1 day
Oral HSV	200 mg PO 5x/d x 5 days or 400 mg PO TID x 5 days or 800mg PO BID x 5 days	1-2 g PO BID x 1 day	1.5 g PO x 1 dose
Chronic suppression (daily therapy)			
Genital HSV	400 mg PO BID	500 mg PO daily or 1 g PO daily	250 mg PO BID
Oral HSV	400 mg PO BID		

Workowski KA, Berman S. Sexually Transmitted Diseases Treatment Guidelines, 2010. MMWR Recommendations and Reports. 2010; 59:1-110. Barlett JG, Auwaerter PG, Pham PA, eds. Johns Hopkins Antibiotic Guide: Diagnosis & Treatment of Infectious Diseases. 3rd ed. Massachusetts; 2012.

Varicella Zoster Virus and Herpes Zoster

Most adults in the U.S. have had chickenpox infection, which is caused by varicella zoster virus. The virus can lie dormant for decades without causing any symptoms. An outbreak may occur as the patient ages, and is often due to acute stress. The recurrence of viral symptoms is called herpes zoster or shingles. The shingles rash is distinctive and very painful. Pharmacists should be able to recognize a shingles rash and inform patients to see a physician; refer to the following image.

Therapy should be initiated at the earliest sign or symptom of shingles and is most effective when started within 72 hours of the onset of zoster rash.

Shingles vaccine (*Zostavax*) is not used for treatment, but can be given to patients who have experienced an outbreak (recurrence is common). The vaccine is FDA-approved for use in patients 50+ years; the ACIP recommendation is for 60+ years.

Antiviral therapy is in table below; pain can be treated with topical agents (*Lidoderm* patch, lidocaine viscous gel) or with pain agents with neuropathic efficacy (anticonvulsants, antidepressants), and sometimes with NSAIDs or opioids. Most recover without long-term sequelae; 5-10% have chronic pain, which can be debilitating.

[handwritten note: FDA → gabapentin (Gralise®, Horizant®) - postherpetic neuralgia]

*[handwritten note: * varicella transmitted via droplet particles]*

Herpes Zoster Treatment

DRUG	DOSING	DESCRIPTION
Acyclovir *(Zovirax)* or Famciclovir *(Famvir)* or Valacyclovir *(Valtrex)*	Acyclovir 800 mg PO 5 times daily for 7-10 days; Famciclovir 500 mg PO TID for 7 days; Valacyclovir 1,000 mg PO TID for 7 days	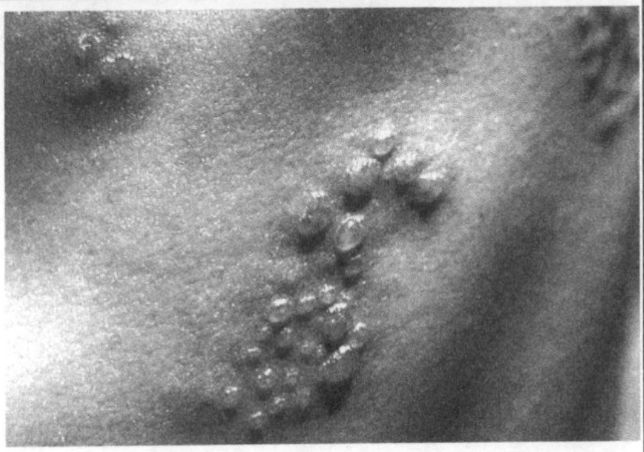 A cluster of fluid-filled blisters, often in a band around one side of the waist or on one side of the forehead, or around an eye or on the neck (less commonly anywhere else on the body).

Handwritten notes (left margin):

Zorivax® ① acyclovir 800 mg po 5x/day x 7-10 d
Valtrex® ② valacyclovir 1,000mg po TID x 7 d
Famvir® ③ famciclovir 500mg po TID x 7 d

Cytomegalovirus (CMV)

- Double stranded DNA virus within the herpes virus family (HHV-5)

- Occurs in patients with advanced immunocompromised states (e.g., HIV-AIDS, transplant recipients)

- Most commonly causes retinitis, colitis or esophagitis

- *(Cytovene® IV)* *(Valcyte®)* Ganciclovir 5 mg/kg IV Q12H or valganciclovir 900 mg PO Q12H x 21 days is the treatment choice for CMV. Valganciclovir *(Valcyte)* is a prodrug of ganciclovir that results in higher concentrations than oral ganciclovir. In general, 5 mg/kg IV ganciclovir = 900 mg PO valganciclovir.

- *(Foscavir®)* *(Vistide®)* Foscarnet and cidofovir should be reserved for refractory cases of CMV infection and/or when the CMV strain is found to be resistant to (val)ganciclovir.

West Nile Virus

- Transmitted via mosquitos

- Most patients do not get very sick; only ~20% show symptoms of fever, headache, or other flu-like symptoms but < 1% can develop encephalitis or meningitis

- Antivirals do not really work and the best medicine is prevention:

  - Use mosquito repellant with DEET, picaridin, oil of lemon eucalyptus (CDC recommended-products only) or IR3535

  - Wear protective clothing (long sleeves and pants)

  - Avoid/eliminate standing or stagnant water which are breeding grounds for mosquitos

MALARIA

Refer to Travelers Medicine chapter for background; this chapter discusses prophylactic options. Check the CDC website for updated resistance patterns.

DRUG	DOSING	SAFETY/SIDE EFFECTS/MONITORING

Areas with chloroquine-resistant *Plasmodium falciparum*

DRUG	DOSING	SAFETY/SIDE EFFECTS/MONITORING
Atovaquone/ proguanil (Malarone)	**Adult Prophylaxis Dose** 250/100 mg PO once daily **Initiation (Pre-Travel)** 1-2 days **Discontinue (Post-Travel)** 7 days	**CONTRAINDICATIONS** Prophylaxis use when CrCl < 30 mL/min **SIDE EFFECTS** GI upset (abdominal pain, N/V), ↑ LFTs, headache, dizziness **MONITORING** LFTs, renal function (SCr, BUN) **NOTES** Must be taken with food or milk. If patient vomits within 1 hour of administration, repeat the dose. For patients who have difficulty swallowing the tablets, they can be crushed and mixed with condensed milk just prior to administration.
Mefloquine	**Adult Prophylaxis Dose** 250 mg PO once weekly **Initiation (Pre-Travel)** 1-3 weeks **Discontinue (Post-Travel)** 4 weeks Check for resistance	**BOXED WARNINGS** Do not use for prophylaxis in patients with major psychiatric disorders. Neuropsychiatric effects, which can require drug discontinuation: ■ Psychiatric symptoms can include anxiety, paranoia, depression, hallucinations, and psychosis. ■ Neurologic symptoms of dizziness or vertigo, tinnitus, and loss of balance may occur and may be permanent. **CONTRAINDICATIONS** Hypersensitivity to mefloquine or related compounds (e.g., quinine and quinidine), prophylactic use in patients with a history of seizures or psychiatric disorder (including active or recent history of depression, generalized anxiety disorder, psychosis, schizophrenia, or other major psychiatric disorders) **SIDE EFFECTS** Loss of balance/dizziness, GI upset, chills, dizziness, fatigue, fever, headache, rash, tinnitus, psychiatric side effects (see warning above) **NOTES** Take with food and with at least 8 oz of water. If patient vomits within 30 minutes after the dose, repeat the full dose; if 30-60 minutes after dose, an additional half dose should be given. Tablets may be crushed and suspended in a small amount of liquid. Acceptable for use in pregnancy (Pregnancy Category B) and children.
Doxycycline (Vibramycin)	**Adult Prophylaxis Dose** 100 mg PO daily **Initiation (Pre-Travel)** 1-2 days **Discontinue (Post-Travel)** 4 weeks	See details under tetracycline section earlier in this chapter.

Malaria Continued

DRUG	DOSING	SAFETY/SIDE EFFECTS/MONITORING
Quinine (Qualaquin)	**Adult Prophylaxis Dose** 648 mg PO Q8H x 3-7 days – should be given with tetracycline, doxycycline or clindamycin ↓ BG	**BOXED WARNINGS** Quinine is not recommended for the prevention/treatment of nocturnal leg cramps due to the potential for severe and/or life-threatening side effects (e.g., cardiac arrhythmias, thrombocytopenia, and HUS/TTP, severe hypersensitivity reactions). **CONTRAINDICATIONS** Hypersensitivity to quinine or related compounds (e.g., mefloquine and quinidine); prolonged QT interval; myasthenia gravis; optic neuritis; G6PD deficiency **SIDE EFFECTS** GI upset (abdominal pain, N/V/D), visual changes (including blindess), hypersensitivity reactions including SJS/TEN, hypoglycemia, QT prolongation, photosensitivity, positive Coombs test

Areas with chloroquine-sensitive *Plasmodium falciparum*

| Chloroquine (Aralen) | **Adult Prophylaxis Dose** 500 mg PO once weekly **Initiation (Pre-Travel)** 1-2 weeks **Discontinue (Post-Travel)** 4 weeks | **CONTRAINDICATIONS** Hypersensitivity to 4-aminoquinoline compounds (e.g., chloroquine, hydroxychloroquine); retinal or visual field changes **WARNINGS** Retinopathy (dose and duration-related) and may be reversible if detected early. Rare hematologic reactions including agranulocytosis, aplastic anemia, and thrombocytopenia; monitoring (CBC) is recommended in prolonged therapy. May cause ECG changes, AV block, and cardiomyopathy (rare). Generally these are dose and/or duration dependent. May cause QT prolongation. G6PD deficiency – use caution **SIDE EFFECTS** GI upset (abdominal pain, N/V/D), visual disturbances (blurred vision, difficulty of focusing or accommodation), photosensitivity, alopecia and bleaching of hair pigment, skeletal muscle myopathy or neuromyopathy leading to progressive weakness and atrophy, exacerbation of psoriasis **NOTES** May be taken with meals to decrease GI upset. Drug has bitter taste. |

Areas with *Plasmodium vivax* and *P. ovale* with or without *P. falciparum*

| Primaquine | **Adult Prophylaxis Dose** 30 mg PO daily **Initiation (Pre-Travel)** 1-2 days G6PD screening required **Discontinue (Post-Travel)** 7 days Effective for *P. vivax* | **CONTRAINDICATIONS** Concurrent use with other medications causing hemolytic anemia or myeloid bone marrow suppression **SIDE EFFECTS** GI upset (abdominal cramps, dyspepsia, N/V), agranulocytosis, anemia, hemolytic anemia (in patients with G6PD deficiency) **NOTES** Take with meals to decrease adverse GI effects. Drug has a bitter taste. CDC requires screening for G6PD deficiency prior to initiating treatment. |

PRACTICE CASE

MJ is a 43 y/o black female who presents to the urgent care clinic with complaints of fever, runny nose, congestion, productive cough and body aches. She reports that she has been feeling this way for the past 36 hours and she needs to get better quickly to return to work. She noticed a lot of people coughing on the bus this week and figures that is where she picked this up. Her past medical history is significant for GERD and depression.

Allergies: Sulfa (extreme rash and hives)

Medications:
Prozac 20 mg PO daily
Zantac 150 mg PO BID
Tums 1-2 tabs PRN heartburn

Vitals:
Height: 5'6" Weight: 192 pounds BMI: 31
BP: 164/81 mmHg HR: 114 BPM RR: 24 BPM Temp: 102.3°F Pain: 2/10

Labs:

Na (mEq/L) = 142 (135 - 145)
K (mEq/L) = 3.5 (3.5 - 5)
Cl (mEq/L) = 97 (95 - 103)
HCO_3 (mEq/L) = 27 (24 - 30)
BUN (mg/dL) = 13 (7 - 20)
SCr (mg/dL) = 1.1 (0.6 - 1.3)
Glucose (mg/dL) = 129 (100 - 125)
Ca (mg/dL) = 10.1 (8.5 - 10.5)
Mg (mEq/L) = 2.0 (1.3 - 2.1)
PO_4 (mg/dL) = 4.2 (2.3 - 4.7)

WBC (cells/mm³) = 15.3 (4 - 11 x 10^3)
Hgb (g/dL) = 13.3 (13.5 - 18 male, 12 - 16 female)
Hct (%) = 42 (38 - 50 male, 36 - 46 female)
Plt (cells/mm³) = 315 (150 - 450 x 10^3)
PMNs (%) = 90 (45 - 73)
Bands (%) = 7 (3 - 5)
Eosinophils (%) = 2 (0 - 5)
Basophils (%) = 0 (0 - 1)
Lymphocytes (%) = 37 (20 - 40)
Monocytes (%) = 3 (2 - 8)

Tests:

Chest x-ray: left middle lobe infiltrate

CAP confirmed by chest x-ray. Start antibiotic and have patient stay home from work for 2 days.

Questions

1. The doctor confirms by chest X-ray that MJ has community-acquired pneumonia. What is the most appropriate therapy for MJ?

   a. *Zithromax* 500 mg PO x 1, then 250 mg PO daily x days 2-5
   b. *Avelox* 400 mg IV daily x 5-7 days
   c. *Levaquin* 500 mg PO x 1, then 250 mg PO daily x 5-7 days
   d. *Ceftin* 500 mg PO Q12H x 5-7 days
   e. *Bactrim* 1 DS tab PO Q12H x 5-7 days

2. MJ has accidentally lost the prescription and she cannot afford another office visit. She decides to tough it out and goes back to work. Two days later, MJ is admitted to the hospital due to worsening symptoms. What is the best agent(s) to treat her community-acquired pneumonia in the inpatient setting?

   a. Ciprofloxacin 500 mg PO daily
   b. Ceftriaxone 1 gram IV daily
   c. Ceftriaxone 1 gram IV daily + azithromycin 500 mg IV daily
   d. Vancomycin 1 gram IV Q12H + imipenem 500 mg Q6H
   e. Gemifloxacin 320 mg PO daily + clarithromycin 500 mg PO Q12H

3. While in the hospital, MJ develops a *Pseudomonal* infection in her lungs as well. Which of the following antibiotics would be an appropriate choice for coverage of *Pseudomonas*?

   a. Ampicillin
   b. *Cubicin*
   c. *Invanz*
   d. *Doribax* [doripenem]
   e. *Tygacil*

4. MJ's condition is (not) improving. She was placed on vancomycin a few days ago and now she has developed vancomycin-resistant *Enterococcus faecium*. The medical team puts her on linezolid. Which of the following statements regarding linezolid is correct?

   a. It is in a new class called cyclic lipopeptides.
   b. It is a MAO inhibitor and should be avoided with serotonergic agents.

   c. It is a combination product consisting of quinupristin and dalfopristin.
   d. It needs to be dose adjusted in patients with renal impairment.
   e. It is not effective for treating infections in the lung.

5. MJ has now been in the hospital for a month. She is still febrile, has an increased WBC count, and remains unable to wean off the ventilator. She has been on many intravenous antibacterial agents. The team decided to re-culture her and now they find *C. albicans* in the blood. They tried treating with fluconazole with no improvement. The team decides to treat with anidulafungin. Which of the following is correct regarding anidulafungin? [echinos good for azole-resistant Candida]

   a. This medication should be taken with meals for best absorption.
   b. This medication can cause an increase in liver transaminases.
   c. This medication is not effective for the treatment of candidemia.
   d. This medication needs to be dose adjusted in renal impairment.
   e. The brand name is *Cancidas*. [Eraxis © ↓ caspofungin]

6. MJ has turned the corner and was discharged home a few weeks later. After about 3-4 months, she returns to the doctor complaining of intense burning on urination, dysuria, and frequent bathroom visits. The doctor confirms that she has a urinary tract infection caused by *E. coli*, which is sensitive to all antibiotics tested. Which of the following is the best choice to treat MJ's UTI?

   a. *Bactrim* SS 1 tab PO BID x 3 days
   b. *Bactrim* DS 1 tab PO BID x 3 days
   c. Nitrofurantoin 100 mg PO BID x 3 days
   d. Nitrofurantoin 100 mg PO BID x 5 days
   e. Phenazopyridine 200 mg TID x 2 days

Questions 7-18 do not apply to the case

7. Which of the following statements regarding the intravenous formulation of *Bactrim* is/are correct? (Select **ALL** that apply.)

   (handwritten note: • infuse over 60-90 min • light protect)

   a. *Bactrim* IV should be protected from light.
   b. *Bactrim* IV should be refrigerated.
   c. *Bactrim* IV is compatible with NS. *(handwritten: dilute w/ D5W)*
   d. *Bactrim* IV needs to be dose adjusted in patients with significant renal impairment.
   e. *Bactrim* IV can be converted to *Bactrim* PO in a 1:1 fashion.

8. You are working in the ER when an intern comes to you and asks how to treat the patient in room 4 who has a gonorrheal STD infection. What is the best recommendation to treat this patient?

   a. Levofloxacin 750 mg PO x 1
   b. Doxycycline 100 mg PO BID x 7 days
   c. Benzathine penicillin G 2.4 million units IM x 1
   d. Metronidazole 2 grams PO x 1
   e. Ceftriaxone 250 mg IM x 1 + azithromycin 1 gram PO x 1

9. The intern is back. This time to ask you about herpes simplex virus and *Valtrex*. Which of the following statements is correct regarding *Valtrex*? *(handwritten: valacyclovir)*

   a. *Valtrex* is a prodrug of acyclovir and can be used as suppressive therapy in patients with herpes simplex virus.
   b. *Valtrex* is a prodrug of penciclovir and should not be used as suppressive therapy in patients with herpes simplex virus.
   c. *Valtrex* should only be used for herpes zoster virus. *(handwritten: also for herpes simplex)*
   d. *Valtrex* needs to be taken with a fatty meal for best absorption.
   e. *Valtrex* is contraindicated in patients with a CrCl < 30 mL/min.

10. Tommy is taking isoniazid (INH) as part of his tuberculosis treatment. Which of the following is/are correct regarding INH? (Select **ALL** that apply.)

    a. INH should be taken 1 hour before or 2 hours after a meal on an empty stomach.
    b. INH is a potent enzyme inducer. *(handwritten: inhib)*
    c. INH is contraindicated in acute gout. *(handwritten: pyrazinamide)*
    d. INH can be used alone to treat latent TB. *(handwritten: susceptible? continuation phase?)*
    e. INH requires dose adjustments in renal impairment.

11. Which of the following medications will help prevent peripheral neuropathies in patients taking isoniazid?

    a. Pyrazinamide
    b. Pyridoxine
    c. *Pyridium*
    d. Pyridostigmine
    e. Pyrimethamine

12. A patient taking amphotericin B is at risk for which electrolyte abnormalities assuming no evidence of nephrotoxicity?

    a. Hypocalcemia and hypomagnesemia
    b. Hyponatremia and hypokalemia
    c. Hypernatremia and hyperkalemia
    d. Hypokalemia and hypernatremia
    e. Hypokalemia and hypomagnesemia

13. A patient comes into your clinic. She is 5 months pregnant and has a UTI. She is allergic to cephalexin. Which of the following regimens would be the best choice for her?

    a. *Bactrim* 1 DS tab BID x 3 days
    b. *Cipro ER* 500 mg PO daily x 7 days
    c. Nitrofurantoin 100 mg PO BID x 7 days
    d. Cefpodoxime 100 mg PO Q12H x 7 days
    e. Do not treat since she is pregnant.

    (handwritten: or fosfomycin)

14. Which of the following statements is/are correct regarding *VFEND*? (Select **ALL** that apply.)

    a. *VFEND* can cause visual changes and patients should be instructed not to operate heavy machinery while taking the medication.

    b. *VFEND* must be taken on an empty stomach.

    c. *VFEND* oral tablets should not be used in patients with poor renal function.

    d. *VFEND* oral suspension should be refrigerated.

    e. *VFEND* is a preferred agent for *Aspergillosis* infections.

15. Which one of the following antibiotics does not require dose adjustment in renal impairment?

    a. Gentamicin
    b. Clarithromycin *only macrolide that requires renal adj. (CrCl < 30 ⇒ ↓ dose 50%)*
    c. Cefixime
    d. Tigecycline
    e. Daptomycin

16. Which one of the following antibiotics should be refrigerated?

    a. *Cipro*
    b. *Keflex*
    c. *Levaquin*
    d. *Septra*
    e. *Zithromax*

17. You should counsel a patient to use sunscreen when taking which of the following medication(s)? (Select **ALL** that apply.)

    a. *Cleocin* *clinda*
    b. *Biaxin* *clarithro*
    c. *Avelox* *moxi*
    d. *VFEND*
    e. *Tamiflu*

18. Which one of the following antimicrobials in the IV formulation is stable in and preferred to be reconstituted in normal saline (NS)?

    a. Quinupristin/dalfopristin
    b. Amphotericin B
    c. Ampicillin
    d. SMX/TMP
    e. Acyclovir

Answers

1-a, 2-c, 3-d, 4-b, 5-b, 6-d, 7-a,d,e, 8-e, 9-a, 10-a,d, 11-b, 12-e, 13-c, 14-a,b,e, 15-d, 16-b, 17-c,d, 18-c

27

HUMAN IMMUNODEFICIENCY VIRUS (HIV)

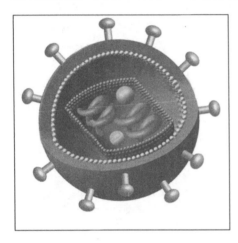

We gratefully acknowledge the assistance of Nancy N. Nguyen, PharmD, BCPS, AAHIVP, Associate Clinical Professor at the University of the Pacific Thomas J. Long School of Pharmacy and Health Sciences, in preparing this chapter.

BACKGROUND

Since the first cases of the Human Immunodeficiency Virus (HIV)/Acquired Immunodeficiency Syndrome (AIDS) were reported in 1981, the Centers for Disease Control now estimates that there are 1.2 million people in the United States living with HIV. HIV is a RNA retrovirus that attacks the immune system, mainly the CD4+ T-helper cells, causing a progressive decrease in the CD4+ T cell count. Once CD4+ cell counts fall below a critical level, the person becomes more susceptible to opportunistic infections due to the loss of cell-mediated immunity. CD4+ counts are the major laboratory indicator of immune function in patients infected with HIV and serve as a key factor in determining both the urgency of antiretroviral therapy

GUIDELINES

Panel on Antiretroviral Guidelines for Adults and Adolescents. Guidelines for the use of antiretroviral agents in HIV-1-infected adults and adolescents. Department of Health and Human Services. Available at: http://aidsinfo.nih.gov/contentfiles/lvguidelines/adultandadolescentgl.pdf. Accessed 2014 November 16.

Panel of Treatment of HIV-Infected Pregnant Women and Prevention of Perinatal Transmission. Recommendations for Use of Antiretroviral Drugs in Pregnant HIV-1-Infected Women for Maternal Health and interventions to Reduce Perinatal HIV Transmission in the United States. Available at: http://aidsinfo.nih.gov/contentfiles/lvguidelines/perinatalgl.pdf. Accessed 2014 October 15.

Panel on Opportunistic Infections in HIV-Infected Adults and Adolescents. Guidelines for the prevention and treatment of opportunistic infections in HIV-infected adults and adolescents: recommendations from the Centers for Disease Control and Prevention, the National Institutes of Health, and the HIV Medicine Association of the Infectious Diseases Society of America. Available at: http://aidsinfo.nih.gov/contentfiles/lvguidelines/adult_oi.pdf. Accessed 2014 October 18.

Addtl guidelines included with the video files (RxPrep Online).

(ART) initiation and the need for prophylaxis against opportunistic infections (OIs). Plasma HIV-1 RNA (viral load) should be measured in all HIV-1 infected patients at baseline and on a regular basis thereafter, especially in patients who are on treatment, because viral load is the most important indicator of response to antiretroviral therapy. The viral load quantifies the degree of viremia by measuring the amount of HIV RNA in the blood and is used to assess response to drug therapy, disease progression (along with CD4+ count) and possible medication adherence problems or drug resistance.

TRANSMISSION

HIV may be spread through infected blood, semen, and vaginal secretions. Unprotected intercourse and sharing needles with HIV-infected individuals are the two most common means of HIV transmission. The entry of the virus via sexual exposure may be facilitated through the presence of sores or cuts in the vagina, penis, rectum, or mouth. Vertical transmission (from mother to child) may also occur, either during pregnancy, at birth, or through breastfeeding.

DIAGNOSIS

Acute HIV infection is the phase in which there is an initial burst of viremia immediately following contraction of the infection in newly-infected patients. Persons with acute HIV infection may experience non-specific flu-like symptoms, such as fever, fatigue/malaise, myalgias/arthralgias, lymphadenopathy, and rash, although many persons may not recognize that they have developed an acute HIV infection since symptoms, if present, are self-limiting. Anti-HIV antibodies (HIV Ab) are undetectable at this time however HIV RNA and HIV p24 antigen will be present. Following this acute phase of the infection, HIV Ab test will usually become positive about 4-8 weeks from contracting the disease; for some individuals, it may take up to 3-6 months for HIV Ab to be detected. Recent infection is generally considered the phase up to 6 months after the onset of the infection during which HIV Ab are detectable.

Diagnosis of HIV is initially performed using the HIV immunoassay (often referred to as HIV ELISA) screening test. A positive HIV screening test may not always represent true infection (due to rare chance of false-positive tests) and therefore all positive screening tests must be followed by a second supplemental test. Diagnosis of HIV is confirmed when both the HIV screening and supplemental tests are positive. As of June 2014, the CDC recommends the following HIV testing algorithm:

- Initial HIV screening should be conducted using a FDA-approved combination HIV Ab and HIV p24 antigen immunoassay.

- If the initial screening test is reactive (positive), then a supplemental testing with a secondary HIV Ab immunoassay should be performed.

- If the initial test is reactive but the secondary test is non-reactive or indeterminate, then a third test should be conducted using the HIV-1 nucleic acid test.

HIV rapid tests are HIV Ab screening tests which can provide results within 20 to 60 minutes using either a fingerstick blood or an oral swab sample. These tests are available for point of

(handwritten margin notes)
(+) ELISA → do Western Blot

(+) ELISA (−) Western Blot → do HIV-1 nucleic acid test (3rd test)

care testing and as in-home test kits (see Over-the-Counter HIV Testing below). Of note, the CDC testing recommendations do not include HIV rapid test in the testing algorithm. Therefore, all patients with positive HIV rapid tests should undergo further HIV testing using the recommended testing algorithm.

The CDC recommends routine HIV screening for patients aged 13 – 64 years old in all healthcare settings (unless the patient declines testing). Additionally, pregnant women and patients initiating treatment for tuberculosis or sexually transmitted diseases (STDs) should also be tested for HIV. Persons at high risk for HIV (e.g. injection drug users, persons with high-risk sexual behaviors) should be tested for HIV at least annually. Persons with positive HIV tests should be referred for HIV medical care and receive initial evaluation, including testing for CD4+ counts and HIV viral load.

Over-the-Counter HIV Testing

There are 2 over-the-counter HIV tests that patients can do in their home. *Express HIV-1 Test System* is a blood test where the patient collects the sample of blood from a fingerstick, ships the sample in a pre-paid overnight envelope, and obtains results the next day (excluding weekends and holidays). The *OraQuick* test is an oral swab test where results are obtained in 20-40 minutes. Individuals who get a positive result do need to get a confirmatory HIV Ab test at their physician's office. These are HIV Ab tests, meaning they detect the presence of HIV Ab which may take up to 3 months after onset of infection to

HOW TO TAKE THE *ORAQUICK* TEST

- Do not eat, drink, or use oral care products at least 30 min before taking the test. Remove dental products such as dentures that cover your gums.

- Tear open the packet labeled "Test Tube". There is liquid in this tube so be careful upon opening not to spill out the liquid. POP off the cap – do NOT twist.

- Open the packet labeled "Test Stick". Do not touch the pad with your fingers. Gently swipe the pad along your upper gums once and your lower gums once. You may use either side on the flat pad. Make sure you swipe each gum only once or your results could be wrong (do not swab the roof of the mouth, inside of the cheek, or the tongue).

- Insert the test stick into the test tube which contains liquid at the bottom. Write down your start time. Then add 20 minutes and write down this number, which is your read time.

- Read the results after 20 minutes but not later than 40 minutes. Do not remove the test stick from the liquid while the test is running.

- If there is one line next to "C" and no line next to "T", your test result is negative. If there are 2 lines, one next to "C" and any line next to "T" (even a faint one), your test result is positive for HIV Ab; consult with your healthcare provider for a confirmatory test. The test is considered invalid if no line appears next to "C" or no lines appear at all.

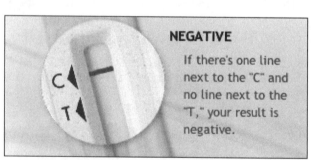

NEGATIVE

If there's one line next to the "C" and no line next to the "T," your result is negative.

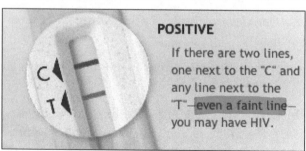

POSITIVE

If there are two lines, one next to the "C" and any line next to the "T"—even a faint line— you may have HIV.

develop. Patients should wait at least 3 months after the risk event to test as testing sooner than 3 months can lead to a false negative reading.

Initial Evaluation and Monitoring

Initial evaluation of newly infected patients should include a discussion on the benefits of ART for the patient's health and to prevent transmission. It is recommended that the following laboratory parameters be measured for all HIV-infected individuals:

dz progression
→ response, resistance

- CD4+ count and HIV viral load (an increase in viral load generally indicates inadequate treatment response and/or drug resistance while a decrease in the CD4+ count is a predictor of disease progression) – prior to ART initiation or modification, 2-8 weeks post initiation, then every 3-6 months thereafter

1) before tx start or Δ
2) 2-8 wks after tx start
3) q3-6 mo after

- Drug resistance testing – at entry into care regardless of ART initiation, at ART initiation and at ART modification

- Comprehensive metabolic panel (includes LFTs, SCr, and glucose), CBC with differential, and lipid panel – prior to ART initiation or modification and every 6-12 months thereafter

ANTIRETROVIRAL THERAPY

Treatment for HIV requires combination antiretroviral therapy ART. ART has dramatically reduced HIV-associated morbidity and mortality and has transformed HIV disease into a chronic, manageable condition. Without treatment, the vast majority of HIV-infected individuals will eventually develop progressive immunosuppression (as evident by low CD4+ count), leading to AIDS-defining illnesses and premature death. The primary goals of ART are to: restore and preserve the immune system, suppress HIV viral load to undetectable levels, reduce HIV-associated morbidity, prolong survival, and prevent HIV transmission.

hep B or C coinfection is a compelling indication to start ART

ART is recommended in ALL HIV-infected individuals but the strength of the recommendation varies depending on the patient's baseline CD4+ count and/or presence of certain comorbid conditions. Conditions that favor more rapid initiation of therapy are pregnancy, low CD4+ counts, acute OIs, history of an AIDS-defining illness [such as HIV-associated dementia or HIV-associated nephropathy (HIVAN)], hepatitis B virus (HBV) and/or hepatitis C virus (HCV) co-infection, and acute/recent HIV infection. ART is also recommended for HIV-infected individuals for the prevention of HIV transmission to non-HIV-infected sexual partners.

95% adherence required for long-term efficacy
(≤ 1 missed dose/month for someone on qd regimen)

Patients starting ART should be willing and able to commit to treatment and should understand the benefits and risks of therapy and the importance of adherence. Patients may choose to postpone therapy, and providers, on a case-by-case basis, may elect to defer therapy on the basis of clinical and/or psychosocial factors. Patients need to be advised that they need to have an adherence rate of 95% or higher in order for their ART regimen to be effective long-term. An example of 95% or higher adherence is no more than 1 missed dose per month for a patient who is taking a once daily regimen.

To the right is a diagram of the <u>HIV life cycle. It is very important to understand the steps involved in viral replication and know where each drug class works.</u>

HIV Replication Cycle Steps and the Sites of Action of Antiretrovirals

1. HIV attaches to the CD4 receptor and a co-receptor (either CCR5 or CXCR4) on the surface of the CD4+ host cell (antiretroviral: CCR5 antagonist).

attachment

fusion

2. Fusion of the HIV envelope with the CD4+ host cell surface allows HIV to enter the host cell, where uncoating of the virus releases HIV RNA and viral protein/enzymes needed for HIV replication into the host cell's cytoplasm (antiretroviral: Fusion inhibitor).

HIV Life Cycle

Stage 1: Binding (also called attachment)

Stage 2: Fusion

CD4 Receptors

Co-receptors (CCR5 or CXCR4)

CD4 cell membrane

HIV RNA

Reverse transcriptase

HIV DNA

Membrane of CD4 cell nucleus

Stage 3: Reverse Transcription

Integrase

Stage 4: Integration

HIV DNA

Integrase

Stage 5: Transcription & Translation

Protease

Stage 6: Assembly

Stage 7: Budding

RNA → DNA

3. HIV RNA is then converted to HIV DNA by reverse transcriptase (antiretrovirals: NRTIs and NNRTIs).

DNA → DNA

4. HIV DNA is transported across the host cell nuclear membrane and is integrated into the host DNA (antiretroviral: Integrase Strand Transfer Inhibitors (INSTIs).

DNA → mRNA → proteins (nonfunctional)

5. HIV DNA is transcribed and translated into new HIV RNA and viral proteins.

cleavage into final proteins & assembly

6. New HIV RNA and long-chain (non-functional) viral proteins move to the host cell surface to begin forming new HIV virus. Protease cleaves the long-chain viral proteins into smaller, functional proteins which become the active viral proteins/enzymes in new viruses (antiretroviral: PIs).

budding reinfection

7. Newly formed HIV cell buds off from the host cell and matures into new, infectious virus.

INITIAL COMBINATION REGIMENS FOR ANTIRETROVIRAL-NAÏVE HIV PATIENTS

Selection of an ART regimen should be individualized based on efficacy, toxicity, pill burden, dosing frequency, drug interaction potential, resistance test results, and comorbid conditions.

REGIMENS	COMMENTS

Preferred Regimens – Regimens with optimal and durable efficacy, favorable tolerability and toxicity profile, and ease of use.

REGIMENS	COMMENTS
NNRTI-BASED REGIMEN Efavirenz/tenofovir/emtricitabine (Atripla®)	Tenofovir should be used with caution in patients with renal insufficiency. Atazanavir should not be used in patients who require > 20 mg omeprazole equivalent per day. Elvitegravir/cobicistat/tenofovir/emtricitabine should only be initiated in patients with CrCL ≥ 70 mL/min and should not be used with other ART or with other nephrotoxic drugs. Abacavir should **not** be used in patients who test positive for HLA-B*5701. When combined with dolutegravir + lamivudine, abacavir can be used in patients with pre-treatment HIV viral load > 100,000 copies/mL.
PI-BASED REGIMENS Atazanavir + ritonavir + tenofovir/emtricitabine Darunavir + ritonavir + tenofovir/emtricitabine	
INSTI-BASED REGIMEN Dolutegravir + abacavir/lamivudine Dolutegravir + tenofovir/emtricitabine Elvitegravir/cobicistat/tenofovir/emtricitabine (Stribild®) Raltegravir + tenofovir/emtricitabine	

Handwritten annotations: "reclassified to alternative", "preferred 6/9/15", "gd", "dolutegravir + Epzicom® or Truvada®"

Additional Preferred Regimens, but ONLY IF Pre-treatment HIV Viral Load < 100,000 copies/mL

REGIMENS	COMMENTS
Atazanavir + ritonavir + abacavir/lamivudine	Rilpivirine is not recommended if CD4+ < 200 cells/mm³. Use of proton pump inhibitors is contraindicated with rilpivirine.
Efavirenz + abacavir/lamivudine	
Rilpivirine/tenofovir/emtricitabine (Complera®)	

Preferred Regimens for HIV-infected Pregnant Women

REGIMENS	COMMENTS
PREFERRED TWO-NRTI BACKBONE To be combined with either PI or NNRTI Abacavir/lamivudine (Epzicom®) Tenofovir/emtricitabine (or lamivudine) Zidovudine/lamivudine (Combivir®)	Abacavir should not be used in patients who test positive for HLA-B*5701. Tenofovir should be used with caution in patients with renal insufficiency. Zidovudine/lamivudine is the combination with the most experience for use in pregnancy. Requires twice daily administration and has increased risk for causing anemia.
PI-BASED REGIMENS Atazanavir + ritonavir + a preferred two-NRTI Backbone Lopinavir + ritonavir + a preferred two-NRTI Backbone	A PI-based regimen is preferred for women who may stop ART during the post-partum period. Once daily lopinavir + ritonavir is not recommended in pregnant women. Always use twice daily dosing regimen.

Preferred Regimens for HIV-infected Pregnant Women Continued

REGIMENS	COMMENTS
NNRTI-BASED REGIMENS Efavirenz + a preferred two-NRTI Backbone	Preferred regimen in women requiring co-administration of drugs with significant drug interactions with PIs.
	Efavirenz is not recommended for women who are planning or at risk of becoming pregnant (due to concerns of birth defects seen in primate studies; Pregnancy Category D). However, efavirenz may be initiated after the first 8 weeks of pregnancy.
	Since risk of neural tube defects is during the first 5-6 weeks of pregnancy, and pregnancy is rarely recognized before 4-6 weeks of pregnancy, pregnant women presenting for first trimester prenatal care may be continued on their efavirenz-based regimen as along as the HIV viral load is undetectable.

NUCLEOSIDE/TIDE REVERSE TRANSCRIPTASE INHIBITORS (NRTIs)

NRTIs are structurally similar to naturally occurring nucelosides/nucleotides needed to synthesize viral DNA. NRTIs compete for binding at the catalytic site of reverse transcriptase, interfering with HIV viral RNA-dependent DNA polymerase which results in DNA chain termination and halts further viral DNA synthesis (see Step #3 in the HIV life cycle diagram). All NRTIs have a boxed warning for lactic acidosis and severe hepatomegaly with steatosis, sometimes fatal (especially didanosine, stavudine and zidovudine). If the patient is suspected to have lactic acidosis or hepatotoxicity, stop treatment with NRTIs.

[Handwritten margin note: BBW lactic acidosis severe hepatomegaly w/steatosis]

DRUG	DOSING	SAFETY/SIDE EFFECTS/MONITORING
Abacavir, ABC (*Ziagen*) Tablet, oral solution (20 mg/mL) **+ lamivudine (*Epzicom*)** + lamivudine and zidovudine (*Trizivir*) + lamivudine and dolutegravir (*Triumeq*)	300 mg BID or 600 mg daily No renal dose adjustments required 1 tab daily (for *Epzicom*) 1 tab BID (for *Trizivir*) 1 tab daily (for *Triumeq*) Take without regards to food	**BOXED WARNING** Serious, sometimes fatal, hypersensitivity reaction – look for fever, skin rash, respiratory symptoms (dyspnea, cough), fatigue, malaise, and/or GI symptoms (N/V/D, abdominal pain); discontinue drug and do not re-challenge. Must screen for the HLA-B*5701 allele prior to starting abacavir therapy – if positive, ↑ risk for hypersensitivity reaction so do not use. Record as abacavir allergy in patient record. **WARNINGS** Some cohort studies have found ↑ risk of MI in patients taking abacavir. Absolute risk appears to be highest in patients with underlying CVD risks. **SIDE EFFECTS** N/V, headache, rash, ↑LFTs, hypersensitivity reaction, hyperlipidemia **MONITORING** LFTs, signs and symptoms of hypersensitivity **NOTES** Caution with alcohol (↑ abacavir AUC) MedGuide required with each prescription (for abacavir alone and abacavir combination pills).

*[Handwritten note at bottom: ALL NRTIs * monitor LFTs + renal, EXCEPT abacavir ↳ → renal adj (only monitor LFTs)]*

Nucleoside Reverse Transcriptase Inhibitors (NRTIs) Continued

DRUG	DOSING	SAFETY/SIDE EFFECTS/MONITORING
Didanosine, ddI **(Videx, Videx EC)** Caspule, solution (10 mg/mL)	≥ 60 kg: 400 mg daily < 60 kg: 250 mg daily **Take on an empty stomach** (at least 30 minutes before or 2 hours after a meal) ↓ dose when CrCl < 60 mL/min Oral soln: Stable for 30 days if refrigerated	**BOXED WARNINGS** Pancreatitis (sometimes fatal) **CONTRAINDICATIONS** Concurrent use with allopurinol or ribavirin **SIDE EFFECTS** Peripheral neuropathy, N/V/D, ↑ LFTs, ↑ amylase, insulin resistance/diabetes, non-cirrhotic portal HTN, retinal changes and optic neuritis (rare) **MONITORING** LFTs, eye exam, CBC, blood chemistry, renal function, amylase and lipase (with pancreatitis) **NOTES** Avoid didanosine and stavudine combination due to increased risk of pancreatitis, peripheral neuropathy, and hyperlactatemia. Avoid use with tenofovir due to resistance and virologic failure as well as increased didanosine concentrations. MedGuide required.
Emtricitabine, FTC **(Emtriva)** Capsule, oral solution (10 mg/mL) **+ tenofovir (Truvada)** **+ efavirenz and tenofovir (Atripla)** **+ tenofovir and rilpivirine (Complera)** **+ tenofovir and elvitegravir and cobicistat (Stribild)**	Cap: 200 mg daily Soln: 240 mg daily (stable for 3 months at room temp) Take without regards to food ↓ dose when CrCl < 50 mL/min 1 tab daily for *Truvada, Atripla, Complera* and *Stribild*. Take *Truvada* without regards to food. Take *Atripla* on an empty stomach, preferably at bedtime. Take *Complera* with a meal. Take *Stribild* with food.	**BOXED WARNING** May exacerbate Hepatitis B once drug is discontinued or when HBV resistance develops **SIDE EFFECTS** Hyperpigmentation primarily of palms and/or soles (mainly in children), N/V/D, rash, dizziness, HA, ↑ CPK, ↑ LFTs **MONITORING** LFTs, renal function **NOTES** Avoid combining with lamivudine (no benefit) as both are cytosine analogs: FTC and 3TC). Capsule and oral solution are not bioequivalent. *Atripla, Complera, Truvada, Stribild:* keep in original container (contains desiccant to protect from moisture) MedGuide required (for *Truvada*).
LamiVUDine, 3TC **(Epivir)** Tablet, oral solution (10 mg/mL) **+ zidovudine (Combivir)** **+ abacavir (Epzicom)** **+ abacavir and zidovudine (Trizivir)** **+ abacavir and dolutegravir (Triumeq)**	150 mg BID or 300 mg daily ↓ dose when CrCl < 50 mL/min Caution with solution in diabetic patients 1 tab daily for *Epzicom* and *Triumeq* 1 tab BID for *Combivir* and *Trizivir* Take without regards to food	**BOXED WARNINGS (2)** Do not use *Epivir-HBV* for treatment of HIV (contains lower dose of lamivudine) May exacerbate HBV once drug is discontinued or when HBV resistance develops **SIDE EFFECTS** Headache, N/V/D, fatigue, insomnia, myalgias, ↑ LFTs, rash **MONITORING** LFTs, renal function **NOTES** Avoid combining with emtricitabine (no benefit) as both are cytosine analogs: FTC and 3TC).

Handwritten annotations:

- like stavudine
- ↑ liver failure
- ③ → pancreatitis
- AVOID
  - ① didanosine + stavudine
    - ↑ pancreatitis
    - ↑ peripheral neuropathy
    - ↑ hyperlactatemia
  - ② didanosine + tenofovir
    - resistance/virol. failure
    - ↑ [did]
- Atripla® empty stomach ghs
- Complera® & Stribild® w/ food
- AVOID combo = benefit

Nucleoside Reverse Transcriptase Inhibitors (NRTIs) Continued

DRUG	DOSING	SAFETY/SIDE EFFECTS/MONITORING
Stavudine, d4T (Zerit) Capsule, oral solution (1 mg/mL)	≥ 60 kg: 40 mg Q12H < 60 kg: 30 mg Q12H ↓ dose when CrCl < 50 mL/min Oral soln: Stable for 30 days in refrigerator Take without regards to food	**BOXED WARNING** Pancreatitis (sometimes fatal) has occurred during combinations with didanosine **SIDE EFFECTS** Peripheral neuropathy, ↑ LFTs, lipoatrophy, insulin resistance/diabetes, hyperlipidemia, pancreatitis **MONITORING** LFTs, renal function, signs and symptoms of peripheral neuropathy, lipids **NOTES** Avoid stavudine and didanosine combination due to ↑ risk of peripheral neuropathy, pancreatitis, and hyperlactatemia. Do not combine with zidovudine (antagonist effect on HIV as both are thymidine analogs: d4T and AZT). MedGuide required.
Tenofovir, TDF (Viread) Tablet, oral powder (40 mg/g) + emtricitabine (Truvada) + emtricitabine and efavirenz (Atripla) + emtricitabine and rilpivirine (Complera) + emtricitabine and elvitegravir and cobicistat (Stribild)	300 mg daily ↓ dose when CrCl < 50 mL/min 1 tab daily for Truvada, Atripla, Complera and Stribild. Take tenofovir and Truvada without regards to food. Take Atripla on an empty stomach, preferably at bedtime. Take Complera with a meal. Take Stribild with food. Dispense in original container.	**BOXED WARNING** May exacerbate HBV once drug is discontinued or when HBV resistance develops **SIDE EFFECTS** Renal insufficiency, Fanconi's syndrome, osteomalacia and ↓ bone density, GI upset (N/V/D), flatulence, gas/bloating, ↑ LFTs, ↑ CPK **MONITORING** LFTs, CBC, renal function, phosphorus, urinalysis, CPK, bone density (long term) **NOTES** Avoid use with didanosine due to resistance and virologic failure as well as increased didanosine concentrations. Powder should be mixed with 2-4 oz of soft food (applesauce, yogurt) to avoid bitter taste. Do not mix powder with liquid. Consider vitamin D and calcium supplementation. MedGuide required for Truvada.

Handwritten annotations:

like didanosine

AVOID
① stavudine + [didanosine]
  • ↑ pancreatitis
  • ↑ peripheral neuropathy
  • ↑ hyperlactatemia
② stavudine + [zidovudine]
  • antagonist effect on HIV

AVOID
tenofovir + [didanosine]
  • resistance/virol. failure
  • ↑ [did]

Atripla®
empty stomach
qhs

Complera®
& Stribild®
w/ food

3 NRTIs that can exacerbate hep B
① emtricitabine
② lamivudine
③ tenofovir

Nucleoside Reverse Transcriptase Inhibitors (NRTIs) Continued

DRUG	DOSING	SAFETY/SIDE EFFECTS/MONITORING
Zidovudine, ZDV or AZT *(Retrovir)* Capsule, tablet, oral solution (10 mg/mL), injection + lamivudine *(Combivir)* + abacavir and lamivudine *(Trizivir)*	300 mg BID ↓ dose when CrCl < 15 mL/min 1 tab BID for *Combivir* and *Trizivir* Take without regards to food (although generally better tolerated when taken with food).	**BOXED WARNINGS (2)** ↗ ≠ w/ ribavirin Hematologic toxicities (neutropenia and anemia) especially in advanced HIV Prolonged use has been associated with symptomatic myopathy and myositis **SIDE EFFECTS** N/V, skin/nail hyperpigmentation (blue), HA, insomnia, malaise, myopathy, lipoatrophy, ↑ LFTs, insulin resistance/diabetes, hyperlipidemia, myelosuppression, macrocytic anemia **MONITORING** CBC, LFTs, mean corpuscular volume (MCV), CPK, lipids, glucose **NOTES** Avoid combining with stavudine (antagonist effect on HIV as both are thymidine analogs: d4T and AZT); Erythropoietin is indicated to manage ZDV-induced anemia. IV zidovudine should be administered in the setting of labor for HIV-infected pregnant women, unless viral load is < 1,000 copies/mL.

Handwritten note: AVOID — zidovudine + stavudine • antagonistic effect on HIV

Nucleoside/Tide Reverse Transcriptase Inhibitor Drug Interactions

NRTIs do not undergo hepatic transformations via the CYP metabolic pathway, therefore, they have fewer significant drug interactions compared to PIs and NNRTIs. Some NRTIs have other mechanisms of drug interactions. Here are a few notable drug interactions:

- Ribavirin may ↑ levels of all NRTIs (combo ↑ risk lactic acidosis and ↑ LFTs). Avoid concurrent use of ribavirin with didanosine (↑ risk liver failure, pancreatitis), and ribavirin with zidovudine (significantly ↑ risk and severity of anemia)

- Avoid didanosine (ddI) and stavudine (d4T) combination due to ↑ risk of peripheral neuropathy, hyperlactatemia and pancreatitis.

- Avoid didanosine and tenofovir combination due to resistance and virologic failure as well as increased didanosine concentrations.

- Allopurinol can ↑ didanosine levels. Avoid combination.

- Avoid emtricitabine and lamivudine combination (no benefit as both cytosine analogs: FTC and 3TC).

- Avoid zidovudine and stavudine (antagonist effect on HIV-1 as both are thymidine analogs: d4T and AZT).

- Methadone can ↑ zidovudine levels. Monitor for zidovudine toxicity.

ALL 3A4 SUB ! (handwritten)

NON-NUCLEOSIDE REVERSE TRANSCRIPTASE INHIBITORS (NNRTIs)

• rash (SJS/TEN) (handwritten margin note)
• hepato tox (handwritten margin note)

NNRTIs work by non-competitive binding to reverse transcriptase and blocking the RNA-dependent and DNA-dependent DNA polymerase activities including HIV-1 replication (see Step #3 in the HIV life cycle diagram). All NNRTIs can cause rash including SJS/TEN (monitor for erythema, facial edema, skin necrosis, blisters, tongue swelling) and hepatotoxicity.

DRUG	DOSING	SAFETY/SIDE EFFECTS/MONITORING
Delavirdine, DLV (*Rescriptor*) Tablet	400 mg TID Patients with achlorhydria should take with acidic beverage; separate dose from antacids by 1 hour Take without regards to food	**CONTRAINDICATIONS** Concurrent use of alprazolam, ergot alkaloids, midazolam, rifampin, triazolam, others **SIDE EFFECTS** Nausea, headache, depression, fever, rash, ↑ LFTs **NOTES** Rarely used due to TID dosing, drug interactions, and suboptimal response (compared to other antiretrovirals).
Efavirenz, EFV *(Sustiva)* Capsule, tablet **+ emtricitabine and tenofovir (*Atripla*)**	600 mg daily 1 tab daily for *Atripla* Take on an empty stomach, preferably at bedtime *Atripla:* keep in original container (contains desiccant to protect from moisture)	**CONTRAINDICATIONS** Concurrent use of ergot alkaloids, midazolam, pimozide, triazolam, voriconazole, and St. John's wort **SIDE EFFECTS** CNS (impaired concentration, somnolence, vivid dreams – usually resolve within 2-4 weeks) and psychiatric symptoms (depression, paranoia, mania, suicide), rash, hyperlipidemia, ↑ LFTs **MONITORING** Lipids, psychiatric effects, LFTs **NOTES** Pregnancy Category D – use other ART agents in women of childbearing potential who are planning to become pregnant or who are sexually active and not using effective contraception. For women who present in the first trimester already on an efavirenz-containing regimen and who have adequate viral suppression, efavirenz may be continued as changing regimens may lead to loss of viral control and increase the risk of perinatal transmission. Capsule contents may be sprinkled onto 1-2 teaspoons of food. May cause false positive cannabinoid and benzodiazepine on drug screening tests.

moderate 3A4 inducer + inhibitor (handwritten note)

↓ [methadone] ⇒ w/d (handwritten note)

Non-Nucleoside Reverse Transcriptase Inhibitors (NNRTIs) Continued

DRUG	DOSING	SAFETY/SIDE EFFECTS/MONITORING
Etravirine, ETR *(Intelence)* Tablet *moderate 3A4 inducer*	200 mg BID after meals	**CONTRAINDICATIONS** Concurrent use of rifampin, St. John's wort, unboosted PIs, carbamazepine, phenytoin, phenobarbital, clopidogrel **✗✗** **SIDE EFFECTS** Rash, nausea, ↑ cholesterol, ↑ LDL, hyperglycemia and peripheral neuropathy **MONITORING** LFTs, lipids, glucose **NOTES** Tablets may be dispersed in water to ease administration. Protect from moisture.
Nevirapine, NVP *(Viramune, Viramune XR)* Tablet, oral suspension (10 mg/mL) *≠ post-exp proph regimens* *hep impairment* *strong 3A4 inducer* *↓ [methadone] ⇒ w/d*	200 mg daily x 14 days; then 200 mg BID *(Viramune)* or 400 mg daily *(Viramune XR)* Need 14 day lead-in period Take without regards to food	**BOXED WARNINGS (2)** Severe hepatotoxic reactions may occur (liver failure, death) – risk highest during the first 6 weeks of therapy but may be seen out to 18 weeks (or more); more common in women and with higher CD4+ counts as noted below Severe, life-threatening skin reactions (SJS/TEN) – risk highest during the first 18 weeks of therapy **CONTRAINDICATIONS** Moderate-to-severe hepatic impairment, post-exposure prophylaxis regimens; concurrent use of St. John's wort, atazanavir, dolutegravir, ketoconazole **SIDE EFFECTS** !! GI (nausea, diarrhea), ↑ LFTs, rash (more common with this agent) **MONITORING** CBC, LFTs, rash **NOTES** Do not initiate therapy in women with CD4+ counts > 250 cells/mm³ and in men with CD4+ counts > 400 cells/mm³ due to ↑ risk of hepatotoxicity. MedGuide required.

Non-Nucleoside Reverse Transcriptase Inhibitors (NNRTIs) Continued

DRUG	DOSING	SAFETY/SIDE EFFECTS/MONITORING
Rilpivirine, RPV (*Edurant*) Tablet **+ emtricitabine and tenofovir (*Complera*)**	25 mg daily with a meal Keep in original container; protect from light 1 tab daily with a meal (*Complera*); meal should be normal to high-calorie (~500+ calories) to optimize absorption	**CONTRAINDICATIONS** All PPIs; concurrent use of rifabutin, rifampin, rifapentine, dexamethasone, carbamazepine, oxcarbazepine, phenobarbital, phenytoin, St. John's wort **SIDE EFFECTS** CNS (depression, mood changes, suicidal ideation, insomnia), headache, rash, ↑ LFTs **MONITORING** LFTs, rash, lipids **NOTES** Higher rates of failure have been seen in patients with HIV-viral load > 100,000 copies/mL at treatment initiation. H$_2$RAs should be administered at least 12 hours before or 4 hours after rilpivirine. Antacids should be given at least 2 hours before or 4 hours after rilpivirine.

Handwritten notes in left column:

≠ PPIs

	before	after
H₂ antag	12 hrs	4 hrs
antacids	2 hrs	4 hrs

use ONLY if pre-tx viral load < 100,000

≠ strong 3A4 inducers

Non-Nucleoside Reverse Transcriptase Inhibitor Drug Interactions

All NNRTIs are cleared non-renally and metabolized in the liver via the CYP 450 system and have MANY drug interactions. They are all 3A4 substrates and may also be an inducer (nevirapine and etravirine), inhibitor (delavirdine) or both inducer and inhibitor (efavirenz). Many of the NNRTIs inhibit other isoenzymes. You should always run a drug interaction check on all patients receiving NNRTIs. Below are some notable drug interactions:

- Delavirdine: Strong inhibitor of 2C9, 2C19, 2D6 and 3A4 and major 3A4 substrate.

- Efavirenz: Moderate inhibitor of 2C9, 2C19 and 3A4 and moderate inducer of 3A4 and a major substrate of 3A4. Do not co-administer with ergot alkaloids, midazolam, pimozide, triazolam, and St. John's wort.

- Etravirine: Moderate inhibitor of 2C9, 2C19, and p-glycoprotein and moderate inducer of 3A4 and major substrate of 3A4, 2C9, and 2C19. Do not co-administer with clopidogrel, carbamazepine, oxcarbazepine, phenobarbital, phenytoin, rifampin, and St. John's wort.

- Nevirapine: Strong 3A4 inducer and major 3A4 substrate. Avoid concurrent use of St. John's wort, atazanavir, dolutegravir, ketoconazole.

- Rilpivirine: Major substrate of 3A4. Contraindicated with strong 3A4 inducers (carbamazepine, oxcarbazepine, phenobarbital, phenytoin, rifampin, rifabutin, St. John's wort, dexamethasone) and PPIs. Use of H$_2$RAs should only be administered at least 12 hours before or 4 hours after rilpivirine. Antacids should be given at least 2 hours before or 4 hours after rilpivirine.

- Methadone levels can be decreased by efavirenz and nevirapine. Monitor for signs and symptoms of possible methadone withdrawal.

- Hormonal contraceptive levels may be decreased by efavirenz and nevirapine and result in unintended pregnancy. Patients should be counseled to use alternative or additional contraception.

ALL 3A4 SUB (MOST 34A INHIB)

PROTEASE INHIBITORS (PIs)

PIs work by inhibiting HIV-1 protease and rendering the enzyme incapable of cleaving the Gag-Pol polyprotein, resulting in non-functional viral proteins which lead to the production of immature, noninfectious virions (see Step #6 in the HIV life cycle diagram). To the right is a text box listing important PI drug class side effects.

PI SIDE EFFECTS

Hyperglycemia, insulin resistance, new-onset diabetes (highest risk with indinavir, lopinavir/ritonavir)

Fat maldistribution: lipohypertrophy

Hyperlipidemia (lowest risk with atazanavir and darunavir; increased TG highest with lopinavir/ritonavir and fosamprenavir)

Hepatitis and hepatic decompensation (highest risk with tipranavir)

Bleeding events (in patients with hemophilia)

Increased CVD risk (lowest with atazanavir and darunavir)

EKG changes (especially with saquinavir, lopinavir/ritonavir, and atazanavir)

DRUG	DOSING	SAFETY/SIDE EFFECTS/MONITORING
Atazanavir, ATV (Reyataz) Capsule *asymptomatic jaundice* *↑PR*	300 mg + 100 mg ritonavir daily 400 mg daily if therapy-naïve, not on tenofovir, and unable to tolerate ritonavir Take with food and water (better absorption)	**SIDE EFFECTS** *→ like lacosamide (Vimpat®)* PR interval prolongation, indirect hyperbilirubinemia (leading to jaundice or scleral icterus – think "bananavir"), rash, nephrolithiasis, cholelithiasis, ↑ CPK *kidney stones* **MONITORING** ECG in at-risk patients, LFTs (including bilirubin) **NOTES** Compared to other PIs, less like to cause lipodystrophy or affect affect blood glucose and lipids Caution with acid-suppressive agents as they can reduce the absorption (and blood levels) of atazanavir **With H₂RAs** Atazanavir alone (unboosted): take at least 2 hours before or 10 hours after H₂RA Atazanavir with ritonavir: take together or at least 10 hours after H₂RA **With Antacids** Atazanavir should be taken at least 2 hours before or 1 hour after antacids **With PPIs** Atazanavir with ritonavir: take at least 12 hours after PPIs. The dose should not be > 20 mg of omeprazole (or equivalent) per day (PPIs are not recommended if atazanavir unboosted or in treatment-experienced patients)

Handwritten notes:

	before	after	
antacids	2 hrs	1 hr	
H₂ antag	2 hrs	10 hrs	unboosted
	together	10 hrs	w/riton.
PPIs	—	12 hrs	w/riton.

* omeprazole ≤ 20 mg max/d
* do not use PPIs if:
  - unboosted ATV
  or - tx-experienced

Protease Inhibitors (PIs) Continued

DRUG	DOSING	SAFETY/SIDE EFFECTS/MONITORING
Darunavir, DRV (Prezista) Tablet, oral suspension (100 mg/mL)	Treatment naïve: 800 mg + 100 mg ritonavir daily Treatment-experienced: 600 mg + 100 mg ritonavir BID Take with food. Swallow whole. Must be given with ritonavir.	**WARNINGS** Use caution in patients with a sulfa allergy **SIDE EFFECTS** Nausea, diarrhea, rash (including SJS/TEN), ↑LFTs, HA **MONITORING** LFTs, rash
Fosamprenavir, FPV (Lexiva) Tablet, oral suspension (50 mg/mL) *PRODRUG* *boosted w/ food*	Treatment naïve: 1,400 mg ± 100-200 mg ritonavir daily or 700 mg + 100 mg ritonavir BID Treatment-experienced: 700 mg + 100 mg ritonavir BID Oral suspension: take without food (adults) Tablets: Take without regards to meals (unboosted); Take with food (boosted with ritonavir)	**WARNING** Use caution in patients with a sulfa allergy **SIDE EFFECTS** N/V/D, rash (including SJS/TEN), HA, nephrolithiasis **MONITORING** LFTs, GI symptoms, glucose　　*↑TG* **NOTES** Prodrug of amprenavir Caution when dispensing: potential for medication error among *Lexiva*, *Lexapro*, and *Levitra*
Indinavir, IDV (Crixivan) Capsule *⊘ high fat/calorie meal*	Without ritonavir: 800 mg every 8 hours. Take on empty stomach (1 hour before or 2 hours after a meal) With ritonavir: 800 mg BID + 100-200 mg ritonavir BID. Take without regards to food (although better tolerated with food) Swallow whole, do not break, crush, or chew	**SIDE EFFECTS** Nausea, nephrolithiasis [taking with 48 oz (1.5 L) of water may reduce risk], indirect hyperbilirubinemia, ↑LFTs, HA, rash, metallic taste, abdominal pain, alopecia　　*kidney stones* **MONITORING** LFTs (including bilirubin), UA　　*↑BG* **NOTES** Must dispense in the original container with the desiccant to protect from moisture. Avoid high fat/high calorie meal as indinavir absorption is decreased.
Lopinavir + Ritonavir, LPV/r (Kaletra) Tablet, oral solution (80 mg lopinavir + 20 mg ritonavir/mL) *↑PR, QT*	Treatment naïve: 800 mg lopinavir/200 mg ritonavir daily or 400/100 mg BID Treatment-experienced: 400/100 mg BID Take oral soln with food. Take tablets without regard to meals. Solution: Refrigerate. Good for 2 months if left at room temperature. Contains 42% alcohol. Tablets: Store at room temperature; swallow whole, do not break, crush, or chew.	**SIDE EFFECTS** N/V/D, pancreatitis, asthenia, abdominal pain, prolongation of PR and QT interval, ↑LFTs, rash, URTIs **NOTES** Avoid once daily dosing with carbamazepine, phenytoin, phenobarbital and in pregnant women. MedGuide required. *⊘ QD dosing* *• pregnancy* *• w/ CBZ* *PHT* *phenobarb* *↑TG* *↑BG*

≠ sulfa allergy
① darunavir (Prezista®)
② fosamprenavir (Lexiva®)
③ tipranavir (Aptivus®)

Protease Inhibitors (PIs) Continued

DRUG	DOSING	SAFETY/SIDE EFFECTS/MONITORING
Nelfinavir, NFV *(Viracept)* Tablet, oral powder	750 mg TID or 1,250 mg BID Take with food	**SIDE EFFECTS** Diarrhea (up to 20% in adults), flatulence, nausea, rash, ↑LFTs **NOTES** Boosting with ritonavir not recommended (high enough absorption on its own) Do not use with PPIs
Ritonavir, RTV *(Norvir)* Capsule, tablet, oral solution (80 mg/mL) Primarily used as a booster agent and not as a sole PI	100-400 mg/day – booster dose, given in 1 to 2 divided doses Take with food Capsules: Keep refrigerated; can be left at room temperature if used within 30 days Tablets: store at room temp; should be swallowed whole; do not break, crush, or chew Solution: contains 43% alcohol; do not refrigerate Keep in original container	**BOXED WARNING** Ritonavir may interact with many medications, including antiarrhythmics, ergot alkaloids, and sedatives/hypnotics, resulting in potentially serious and/or life-threatening adverse events **SIDE EFFECTS** N/V/D, paresthesias, asthenia, altered taste, PR prolongation, flushing, arthralgias, cough, oropharyngeal pain, ↑ CPK
Saquinavir, SQV *(Invirase)* Capsule, tablet	1,000 mg + ritonavir 100 mg BID Take with food (or within 2 hours of a full meal) Must be given with ritonavir	**CONTRAINDICATIONS** Severe hepatic impairment, prolonged QT interval, and refractory hypokalemia or hypomagnesemia **SIDE EFFECTS** N/V/D, HA, PR and QT interval prolongation (avoid use if QT > 450 msec) **MONITORING** ECG (baseline and ongoing) ,electrolytes (esp K⁺, Mg²⁺) **NOTES** MedGuide required
Tipranavir, TPV *(Aptivus)* Capsule, oral solution (100 mg/mL)	500 mg + ritonavir 200 mg BID Caps: Refrigerate. Can store at room temp up to 60 days; need to discard 60 days after opening bottle Solution: Store at room temperature (do not refrigerate); need to discard 60 days after opening bottle Take with food Swallow whole, do not break, crush, or chew Must be given with ritonavir	**BOXED WARNINGS (2)** In combination with ritonavir, can cause hepatitis (sometimes fatal) and intracranial hemorrhage **CONTRAINDICATIONS** Moderate or severe hepatic impairment **WARNING** Use caution in patients with a sulfa allergy **SIDE EFFECTS** Diarrhea, rash, ↑ CPK

Handwritten annotations:

Next to Nelfinavir: ≠ boost w/ ritonavir ; ≠ PPIs

Next to Ritonavir: ↑PR ; ↓ [methadone] ⇒ w/d

Next to Saquinavir: ↑PR, QT

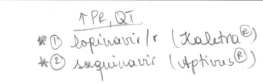

↑PR
* ① atazanavir (Reyataz®)
  ② ritonavir (Norvir®)

↑PR, QT
* ① lopinavir/r (Kaletra®)
* ② saquinavir (Aptivus®)

Protease Inhibitor Drug Interactions

All PIs are metabolized in the liver via the CYP 450 system and have many drug interactions. All PIs are 3A4 substrates and most are strong inhibitors of 3A4. Ritonavir is a potent 3A4 inhibitor used at low doses to increase, or boost, the level of other PIs. The drug interaction list below highlights the most important interactions and contraindications and is not all-inclusive.

- The following drugs are contraindicated with all PIs: alfuzosin, amiodarone, cisapride, ergot derivatives, flecainide, lovastatin, midazolam (oral), pimozide, propafenone, quinidine, sildenafil (when used for the treatment of pulmonary arterial hypertension), simvastatin, St John's wort, triazolam, and voriconazole (when ritonavir ≥ 800 mg/day). Many of the PIs should not be used with boceprevir, telaprevir, or simeprevir.

- Caution with the use of 3A4 inducers as they can lower the concentration of PIs. Avoid concurrent use with rifampin.

- PIs can alter the INR (mainly ↓) in patients taking warfarin due to 2C9 induction; the INR should be closely monitored.

- PIs increase the levels of trazodone and many tricyclic antidepressants. Start with low doses and then titrate anti-depressant doses based upon clinical response.

- Atazanavir: caution with the use of acid-suppressive agents. See chart above.

- Nelfinavir cannot be used with PPIs.

- Phosphodiesterase-5 inhibitors (PDE-5 inhibitors): PIs can increase levels of PDE-5 inhibitors and ↑ risk of toxicity. PDE-5 inhibitors should be initiated at lowest dose and the dosing interval should be extended.

- Hormonal contraceptives (especially those containing ethinyl estradiol and norethindrone): Ritonavir may ↓ levels via CYP induction. Patients should be counseled to use additional/alternative contraceptive methods.

- Methadone: Levels may be ↓ by ritonavir (via CYP induction). Monitor for possible methadone withdrawal.

- Statins: PIs can ↑ statin levels. Concurrent use of lovastatin or simvastatin with PIs is contraindicated. Start statin therapy with a low dose and titrate to response. Monitor closely for statin toxicity. Darunavir can significantly ↑ pravastatin levels, therefore consider alternative statin.

FUSION INHIBITORS

Fusion inhibitors block the fusion of the HIV-1 virus with the CD4+ cells by blocking the conformational change in gp41 required for membrane fusion and entry into CD4+ cells (see Step #2 in the HIV life cycle diagram). The currently available fusion inhibitor, enfuvirtide, is not metabolized through CYP and, therefore, has no significant drug interactions.

Sub Q

DRUG	DOSING	SAFETY/SIDE EFFECTS/MONITORING
Enfuvirtide, T20 *(Fuzeon)* *gp41* Powder for injection	90 mg SC BID	**SIDE EFFECTS** Local injection site reactions in almost 100% of patients (pain, erythema, induration, nodules and cysts, pruritus, ecchymosis); ↑ risk of bacterial pneumonia, hypersensitivity reaction (rare) **NOTES** Reconstituted solution should be refrigerated and used within 24 hours No significant drug interactions Patient should be counseled regarding proper reconstitution and injection technique and to rotate injection sites

no drug interaxns

CCR5 ANTAGONIST

CCR5 inhibitors bind to the CCR5 co-receptor on the CD4+ cells and prevent HIV cell entry (see Step #1 in the HIV life cycle diagram). Unlike the other antiretroviral drug classes, CCR5 inhibitors do not directly target the HIV cell but rather blocks the human host cell receptor.

DRUG	DOSING	SAFETY/SIDE EFFECTS/MONITORING
Maraviroc, MVC *(Selzentry)* Tablet *CCR5 antag*	300 mg BID Take without regard to meals ↓ dose when CrCl < 30 mL/min Dose adjust if concurrent CYP 3A4 inhibitor or inducer *≠ CrCl < 30 + on potent 3A4 ind/inhib*	**BOXED WARNING** Hepatotoxicity with allergic type features **CONTRAINDICATIONS** Patients with severe renal impairment (CrCl < 30 mL/min) taking potent 3A4 inhibitors/inducers **SIDE EFFECTS** URTIs, fever, rash (including SJS), cough, abdominal pain, musculoskeletal symptoms, hepatotoxicity, dizziness, orthostatic hypotension (especially in renal impairment) **MONITORING** Prior to starting therapy, patients must undergo a screening test (Trofile), to determine the tropism of the HIV since this agent will only work for patients with CCR5-tropic disease **NOTES** Swallow tablets whole. Do not chew, break, or crush MedGuide required

CCR5 Antagonist Drug Interactions

Maraviroc is a P-gp and major 3A4 substrate. Maraviroc concentrations can be significantly increased in the presence of strong 3A4 inhibitors and reduced with 3A4 inducers, and maraviroc dosage may need to be adjusted. Avoid use with St. John's wort.

INTEGRASE STRAND TRANSFER INHIBITORS (INSTIs)

INSTIs block the integrase enzyme needed for viral DNA to integrate with the host cell DNA/human genome (see Step #4 in the HIV life cycle diagram).

DRUG	DOSING	SAFETY/SIDE EFFECTS/MONITORING
Dolutegravir, DTG **(Tivicay)** Tablet	50 mg PO daily (not indicated for weight < 40 kg) 50 mg PO BID (for treatment-experienced patients or those with known RAL resistance) Take without regard to meals	**CONTRAINDICATION** Coadministration with dofetilide due to risk for significantly increased dofetilide concentration resulting in increased toxicity **SIDE EFFECTS** Insomnia, headache, diarrhea, rash, ↑ CPK, ↓ LFTs among Hep B/C patients, ↑ SCr without affecting GFR **MONITORING** CPK, LFTs (especially in Hep B/C patients)
Elvitegravir (EVG), cobicistat (COB), emtricitabine, tenofovir **(Stribild)** Elvitegravir *(Vitekta)* and Cobicistat *(Tybost)* Tablet	1 tablet daily with food Do not initiate if CrCl < 70 mL/min; discontinue when CrCl < 50 mL/min Keep in original container	**BOXED WARNINGS (2)** *tenofovir BBW* Lactic acidosis with severe hepatomegaly with steatosis and acute exacerbation of HBV in patients who are co-infected (specific for emtricitabine and tenofovir) **CONTRAINDICATIONS** *same as PIs* Concurrent use of alfuzosin, cisapride, ergot derivatives, lovastatin, midazolam (oral), pimozide, rifampin, sildenafil (when used for pulmonary arterial hypertension), simvastatin, St. John's wort and triazolam **WARNINGS** New onset or worsening renal impairment, decrease in bone density (likely due to tenofovir) **SIDE EFFECTS** Proteinuria, nausea and diarrhea, hyperlipidemia, insomnia, ↑ SCr (without effect on GFR – cobicistat; with effect on GFR – tenofovir) **MONITORING** CPK, SCr, UA, phosphate **NOTES** Cobicistat is a booster similar to ritonavir *protease inhibitor booster* Elvitegravir *(Vitekta)* and cobicistat *(Tybost)* were approved in Sept. 2014 as single agents. Clinical use of these individual agents is still being established.
Raltegravir, RAL **(Isentress)** Tablet (including chewable), powder packet for oral suspension	400 mg BID Take without regard to meals Chewable tablets – keep in original container	**SIDE EFFECTS** Nausea, diarrhea, headache, insomnia, pyrexia, ↑ CPK, myopathy and rhabdomyolysis, rash (including SJS) **MONITORING** CPK (if symptomatic)

Stribild®
abrupt d/c in pts w/ hep B
⇒ hep B worsening !

⟶ phenylketonuria

no dose separation w/ CaCO₃

Integrase Strand Transfer Inhibitor Drug Interactions

- INSTIs: Should be taken 2 hours before or 6 hours after taking cation-containing antacids or laxatives, sucralfate, iron supplements, calcium supplements or buffered medications. Exception for raltegravir and calcium carbonate: no dose separation needed. H_2RAs and PPIs do not pose an interaction with INSTIs.

- Raltegravir: Metabolized by the UGT1A1-mediated glucuronidation pathway. Rifampin, a strong inducer of UGT1A1, will ↓ levels of raltegravir. When given concurrently with rifampin, use raltegravir 800 mg BID. PPIs can ↑ levels of raltegravir although dosage adjustment is not needed.

- *Stribild:* Cobicistat, a component of *Stribild*, is a strong inhibitor of 3A4, 2D6 and P-gp. Cobicistat interactions are very similar to ritonavir interactions. Elvitegravir is a major 3A4 substrate and a modest inducer of 2C9 and may decrease the plasma concentrations of 2C9 substrates. *Stribild* should not be co-administered with any other ART.

COMBINATION PRODUCTS

GENERIC NAME	BRAND NAME	DOSE
Abacavir 600 mg + lamivudine 300 mg	Epzicom	1 tab daily
Emtricitabine 200 mg + tenofovir 300 mg	Truvada	1 tab daily
Lamivudine 150 mg + zidovudine 300 mg	Combivir	1 tab BID
Abacavir 300 mg + lamivudine 150 mg + zidovudine 300 mg	Trizivir	1 tab BID
Efavirenz 600 mg + emtricitabine 200 mg + tenofovir 300 mg	Atripla	1 tab daily on empty stomach
Emtricitabine 200 mg + rilpivirine 25 mg + tenofovir 300 mg	Complera	1 tab daily with food
Elvitegravir 150 mg + cobicistat 150 mg + emtricitabine 200 mg + tenofovir 300 mg	Stribild	1 tab daily with food
Abacavir 600 mg + dolutegravir 50 mg + lamivudine 300 mg	Triumeq	1 tab daily

Some Common Complications of ART

maily NRTI's & elvitegr.

Lactic acidosis and severe hepatomegaly with steatosis: suspend treatment in any patient who develops clinical or laboratory findings suggestive of lactic acidosis or hepatotoxicity (transaminase elevation may/may not accompany hepatomegaly and steatosis). Most commonly associated with NRTIs.

Immune reconstitution inflammatory syndrome (IRIS): A paradoxical worsening of a preexisting OI or malignancy when ART is initiated. Since ART leads to an improvement in immune function, an inflammatory reaction may occur at the site of the preexisting infection. Patients at highest risk for IRIS are those with low CD4+ counts and high viral loads. IRIS generally develops between 1-3 months of ART initiation. Commonly found pathogens associated with IRIS include *M. tuberculosis*, *M. avium*, *Pneumocystis jiroveci* pneumonia (PCP), herpes simplex virus (HSV), herpes zoster, cytomegalovirus (CMV), *Cryptococcus*, and HBV.

IRIS
1. TB
2. MAC
3. PCP
4. HBV
5. Cryptococcus
6. CMV
7. herpes simplex
8. herpes zoster (shingles)

Management of IRIS

- Start or continue therapy for the underlying opportunistic pathogen or malignancy.

- Continue ART if the patient is currently receiving ART. Among patients newly diagnosed with HIV with an opportunistic infection (OI), ART may be intentionally delayed while treating the OI to minimize risk for IRIS. However, ART should always be started within 2 weeks of OI treatment initiation for PCP and generally for *M. tuberculosis* secondary to mortality benefits.

- In select circumstances, the addition of corticosteroids may be appropriate.

Lipodystrophy is the term used to describe changes in fat distribution in the body, and is further subcategorized as: lipoatrophy (fat loss or wasting) and lipohypertrophy (fat accumulation).

Lipoatrophy: Loss of subcutaneous fat in the face, arms, legs, and buttocks. This is most commonly associated with the NRTIs, specifically with stavudine (and zidovudine to a lesser extent).

Lipohypertrophy: Fat accumulation in the upper back and neck ("buffalo hump"), abdominal area, and breast area in both men and women. This is most commonly associated with PIs. Breast enlargement with efavirenz has been reported.

Diarrhea: Diarrhea is a common side effect of ART. All ARTs have been associated with GI toxicity, however PIs are generally the most problematic: especially nelfinavir and lopinavir/ritonavir.

Adjunct Therapies in HIV Management

DRUG AND INDICATION	DOSING	SAFETY/SIDE EFFECTS/MONITORING
Poly-L-Lactic Acid (Sculptra) Lipoatrophy (facial)	About 20 injections (given intradermal or SC) per cheek Typical treatment course can require 3-6 treatments. Treatments should be separated by ≥ 2 weeks.	**SIDE EFFECTS** Injection site reactions (bleeding, bruising, erythema, edema, inflammation), photosensitivity, hematoma, discomfort
Calcium hydroxylapatite (Radiesse) Lipoatrophy (facial)	SC injection (considered a medical device – implant) Typical treatment course may require 1-3 treatments. In clinical trials, multiple treatments were separated by at least 1 month.	**SIDE EFFECTS** Injection site reactions (e.g. bruising, erythema, edema), pain, pruritus, nodules
Tesamorelin (Egrifta) HIV-associated lipodystrophy (specifically reduction of excess abdominal fat)	2 mg SC daily	**SIDE EFFECTS** Injection site reactions (pruritus, erythema, bruising, pain), rash, peripheral edema, hyperglycemia, arthralgias, development of IgG antibodies **NOTES** This medication is a growth hormone releasing factor

Adjunct Therapies in HIV Management Continued

DRUG AND INDICATION	DOSING	SAFETY/SIDE EFFECTS/MONITORING
Crofelemer *(Fulyzaq)* Non-infectious diarrhea due to ART	125 mg PO BID	**SIDE EFFECTS** URTIs, bronchitis, cough, flatulence and ↑ bilirubin and LFTs **NOTES** Due to cost, first consider trial of loperamide *(Imodium)* or diphenoxylate/atropine *(Lomotil)*
Megestrol *(Megace, Megace ES)* *Megace* 40 mg/mL, *Megace ES* 625 mg/5 mL Anorexia or cachexia associated with AIDS	400 – 800 mg suspension PO daily	**SIDE EFFECTS** Hyperglycemia, adrenal suppression, hypertension, headache, rash, N/V/D **NOTES** Medication is available as oral suspension (used in HIV-associated anorexia/cachexia) and tablets (used in cancer treatment) – dispense correct strength and formulation. Pregnancy Category X (suspension)/D (tablets)
Dronabinol *(Marinol)* C-III AIDS-related anorexia	2.5 mg PO BID (before lunch and dinner), max 20 mg/day	**SIDE EFFECTS** CNS effects (e.g. euphoria, somnolence, abnormal thinking, confusion), dizziness, abdominal pain, paranoia, N/V **NOTES** Causes positive cannabinoid drug test. Caution in patients with underlying cardiac or liver disease, or seizure disorders. Swallow capsule whole. Do not chew, break, or crush.

[handwritten margin note: synthetic deriv of progesterone]

PRIMARY PROPHYLAXIS OF OPPORTUNISTIC INFECTIONS IN PATIENTS WITH HIV

HIV-infected patients not taking ART are at risk for developing OIs as a result of uncontrolled HIV infection and progressive immunosuppression. Patients are at higher risk for specific OIs as CD4+ counts decline. The table below outlines select OIs, CD4+ count when patient becomes most at risk for the infection, and the primary prophylaxis regimen that should be initiated to prevent the first episode of the infection. Of note, patients with very low CD4+ counts should also receive the prophylactic regimens as recommended for patients with higher CD4+ counts (e.g. in a patient with CD4+ < 50 cells/mm³, the patient should receive prophylactic medications for MAC, *T. gondii*, and PCP).

[handwritten margin note: initiate < 200 or thrush]

[handwritten margin note: d/c > 200 x 3 mo on ART]

PATHOGEN	INDICATION	PRIMARY PROPHYLAXIS REGIMEN	CRITERIA FOR DISCONTINUING PRIMARY PROPHYLAXIS
Pneumocystis pneumonia (PCP)	CD4+ count < 200 cells/mm³ or oropharyngeal candidiasis	Preferred: TMP/SMX 1 DS tab PO daily or 1 SS PO daily Alternative: TMP/SMX 1 DS PO TIW or dapsone 100 mg PO daily or 50 mg PO BID, or (dapsone + pyrimethamine + leucovorin), or aerosolized pentamidine, or atovaquone	CD4+ count > 200 cells/mm³ for > 3 months on ART

Primary Prophylaxis Of Opportunistic Infections In Patients With HIV Continued

PATHOGEN	INDICATION	PRIMARY PROPHYLAXIS REGIMEN	CRITERIA FOR DISCONTINUING PRIMARY PROPHYLAXIS
Toxoplasma gondii	Toxoplasma IgG positive patients with CD4+ count < 100 cells/mm³	Preferred: TMP/SMX 1 DS tab PO daily Alternative: TMP/SMX 1 DS PO TIW or 1 SS PO daily or (dapsone 50 mg PO daily + pyrimethamine 50 mg PO weekly + leucovorin 25 mg PO weekly)	CD4+ count > 200 cells/mm³ for > 3 months on ART
Mycobacterium avium complex (MAC)	CD4+ count < 50 cells/mm³ after ruling out active disseminated MAC disease	Preferred: azithromycin 1,200 mg PO weekly or clarithromycin 500 mg PO BID or azithromycin 600 mg PO twice weekly	CD4+ count ≥ 100 cells/mm³ for ≥ 3 months on ART

Handwritten margin notes: "< 100", "< 50" (left margin); "d/c > 200 × 3 mo on ART", "≥ 100 × 3 mo on ART" (right margin)

TREATMENT OF OPPORTUNISTIC INFECTIONS

In patients who develop OIs, antimicrobial treatment for the infection should be initiated. In patients newly diagnosed with HIV and an OI, they should be monitored closely for IRIS when ART is started (see section on Some Common Complications of ART). The table below lists select OIs and the recommended treatments. Secondary prophylaxis should be given to prevent future episodes/recurrence of the infection, and should be started after the patient has completed the initial treatment for the infection.

PATHOGEN	FIRST LINE TREATMENT	ALTERNATIVE TREATMENT	SECONDARY PROPHYLAXIS
Cryptococcal Meningitis	Liposomal amphotericin B + flucytosine	Amphotericin B deoxycholate + flucytosine or fluconazole + flucytosine or fluconazole alone	Fluconazole (low dose)
Cytomegalovirus (CMV) retinitis	Valganciclovir or ganciclovir	Foscarnet or cidofovir	Continue same agent at reduced dose (usually valganciclovir)
Mycobacterium avium complex infection	Clarithromycin or azithromycin + ethambutol ± rifabutin	Add a 3rd or 4th agent using amikacin, streptomycin, moxifloxacin, or levofloxacin	Same agents at same doses
Pneumocystis pneumonia (PCP)	TMP/SMX ± corticosteroids	Atovaquone or (clindamycin + primaquine) or pentamidine IV or (dapsone + trimethoprim)*	TMP/SMX or dapsone or (dapsone + pyrimethamine**) or atovaquone or inhaled pentamidine
Toxoplasmosis meningoencephalitis	Pyrimethamine** + sulfadiazine	TMP/SMX, (pyrimethamine** + clindamycin or azithromycin), (atovaquone alone, or with sulfadiazine or with pyrimethamine**)	Same agents at reduced dose

* Selection of alternative therapy for PCP is dependent on severity of illness and patient specific factors (allergies and G6PD deficiency). For example, atovaquone, clindamycin + primaquine or pentamidine are all potential options in the setting of sulfa allergy, however only atovaquone (mild-to-moderate disease) and pentamadine (moderate-severe disease) are available options in the setting of G6PD deficiency.

** Leucovorin added as rescue therapy to reduce risk for myelosuppression associated with pyrimethamine.

PRE-EXPOSURE PROPHYLAXIS (PrEP)

PrEP is a new HIV prevention method in which people who do not have HIV take emtricitabine/tenofovir *(Truvada)* 1 tab PO daily, in combination with safer sex/behavior risk reduction practices, to reduce their risk of becoming infected. PrEP is recommended for both homosexual and heterosexual individuals who are at very high risk for sexual exposure to HIV as well as for active intravenous drug users.

Before Initiating PrEP

- Confirm HIV negative status through HIV antibody test
- Confirm CrCl ≥ 60 mL/min
- Confirm patient very high risk for acquiring HIV
- Screen for Hep B and STDs

Once PrEP is initiated, follow-up visits are needed at least every 3 months with the following recommendations during EACH visit:

- HIV test and document negative result
- Provide no more than 90-day supply at a time (renew Rx only once HIV negative status is confirmed)
- Pregnancy test (for non-HIV-infected women taking PrEP)
- Counseling on PrEP adherence and safe sex/behavior risk reduction practices
- Every 6 months, check SCr and calculate CrCl, and test for bacterial STDs (regardless of symptoms)

ADMINISTRATION	
With food	**Without food**
Atazanavir	*Atripla*
Complera (500+ calories)	Didanosine
Darunavir	Efavirenz (small amount of food ok)
Etravirine (after meals)	Fosamprenavir (oral suspension)
Indinavir – boosted	Indinavir – unboosted
Kaletra oral soln ↳ refrigerate	
Nelfinavir	
Rilpivirine (500+ calories)	
Ritonavir	
Saquinavir	
Stribild	
Tipranavir	
Tenofovir powder (to avoid bitter taste)	

NONOCCUPATIONAL POSTEXPOSURE PROPHYLAXIS (nPEP)

Nonoccupational exposure is the use of ART prophylaxis after sexual, injection drug use, or some other nonoccupational exposure to HIV. Regardless of whether or not nPEP is pre-

nPEP
→ HIV Ab test
  ① @ baseline
  ② 4-6 wks   } after event
  ③ 3 months
  ④ 6 months

scribed, the exposed patient should be tested for HIV Ab at baseline, 4-6 weeks, 3 months, and 6 months after the exposure event.

Nonoccupational Postexposure Prophylaxis (nPEP) Recommendations

PREFERRED REGIMENS	CRITERIA TO QUALIFY	DURATION
NNRTI-BASED Efavirenz + (Lamivudine or emtricitabine) + (Zidovudine or tenofovir) **PI-BASED** Lopinavir/ritonavir + (Lamivudine or emtricitabine) + Zidovudine	≤ 72 hours since exposure Known HIV (+) status of source (If HIV status unknown, then case-by-case determination) Exposed patient is HIV (-) or being tested for HIV Type of exposure is also factored into decision to initiate nPEP	28 days

OCCUPATIONAL POSTEXPOSURE PROPHYLAXIS RECOMMENDATIONS (PEP)

Occupational exposure typically refers to exposure of health care personnel to blood or body fluids that may potentially be contaminated with HIV. ART prophylaxis for occupational exposure is generally only recommended if the source of contaminated blood or body fluid is known to be HIV positive. If the source patient's HIV status is unknown, the HIV status should be determined, if possible, to guide need for HIV PEP. Therapy should be started right away, ideally within 72 hours, when treatment is indicated. Per the 2013 updated guidelines a three drug regimen including raltegravir + tenofovir/emtricitibine *(Truvada)* for a 4-week course is the preferred regimen. The exposed health care personnel should be tested for HIV Ab at baseline, 4-6 weeks, 3 months, and 6

STRATEGIES TO IMPROVE ADHERENCE TO ANTIRETROVIRAL THERAPY

Utilize a multidisciplinary team approach (e.g. nurses, social workers, pharmacists, psychologists, physicians)

Provide an accessible, non-judgmental health care team and establish a trusting relationship with patient

Evaluate patient's knowledge of HIV disease, prevention and treatment, and provide information as needed; establish patient readiness to start ART and involve patient in ART regimen selection

Identify potential barriers to adherence (e.g. psychosocial or cognitive issues, substance abuse, low literacy, busy daily schedule, lack of prescription coverage and/or social support)

Assess adherence at every clinic visit, and simplify ART regimen when possible; provide positive reinforcement to foster adherence success

Identify non-adherence and reasons for non-adherence (e.g. adverse effects from medications, complex regimen, difficulty swallowing large pills, forgetfulness, pill fatigue, food requirements, stigma)

Provide resources for patient (e.g. referrals for mental health and/or substance abuse treatment, prescription drug assistance programs, pillboxes, reminder tools, medication lists or calendars)

months after the exposure event. If PEP is initiated, then CBC, renal and liver function should be tested at baseline and repeated at 2 weeks post-exposure.

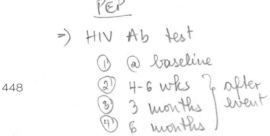

PEP
=> HIV Ab test
① @ baseline
② 4-6 wks ⎱ after
③ 3 months ⎰ event
④ 6 months

after PEP initiation
=> check CBC ⎱ @ baseline
renal ⎰ + q 2 wks
hepatic

PATIENT COUNSELING

All HIV Medications

- This medication is not a cure for HIV and, when used alone, does not prevent the spread of HIV to others through sexual contact or blood contamination (such as sharing used needles).

- It is very important to continue taking this medication (and other HIV medications in your regimen) exactly as prescribed by your doctor. Do not skip any doses or stop taking your HIV medication regimen even for a short time unless directed to do so by your doctor. Skipping or stopping your medication, or taking only some but not all of the HIV medications in your full regimen, may cause the amount of HIV virus to increase and make the infection more difficult to treat (resistant). Refill your medications before you run out.

- If you are taking HIV medications for the first time, you may experience symptoms of an old infection. This may happen as your immune system begins to work better. Contact your doctor immediately if you notice any of the following symptoms: new cough, trouble breathing, fever, new vision problems, new headaches or new skin problems.

NRTIs Patient Counseling

- This medication can cause changes in your body fat. You may notice loss of fat from the legs, arms and face although if these do occur, it's usually only after you have been on the medication for a long time.

- Rarely, this medication can cause severe liver problems. Tell your doctor immediately if you develop symptoms such as persistent nausea/vomiting, loss of appetite, stomach/abdominal pain, pale stools, dark urine, yellowing eyes/skin, or unusual tiredness.

- Rarely, this medication can cause a build-up of acid in your blood; report any symptoms such as stomach pain, nausea, vomiting, troubled breathing, weakness or muscle pain.

- If you have Hepatitis B and are taking lamivudine, emtricitabine, or tenofovir, your hepatitis symptoms may get worse or become very serious if you stop taking any of these medications. Talk with your doctor before stopping this medication. Tell your doctor immediately if you develop symptoms of worsening liver problems.

For Emtricitabine

- Rarely, this medication can cause darkening skin color on the palms of hands and on the soles of feet. Notify your doctor if this is problematic to you.

- This medication may cause rash in some people who take it. If you develop a rash, notify your healthcare provider as soon as possible.

- You can take this medication with or without food.

For Tenofovir

- Tell your doctor immediately if any of these rare but serious side effects occur: signs of kidney problems such as a change in the amount of urine, unusual thirst, muscle cramps/weakness, bone pain, or easily broken bones.

- Tenofovir tablets (or *Truvada*): You can take this medication with or without food.

- Tenofovir powder: This medication comes with a dosing scoop; use only the dosing scoop to measure the oral powder. Mix the oral powder with soft foods that can be swallowed without chewing (e.g., applesauce, baby food or yogurt). Do not mix with liquid as the powder may float to the top even after stirring. Give the entire dose right away after mixing to avoid a bad taste.

NNRTIs Patient Counseling

- Rarely, this medication can cause severe liver problems. Tell your doctor immediately if you develop symptoms such as persistent nausea/vomiting, loss of appetite, stomach/abdominal pain, pale stools, dark urine, yellowing eyes/skin, or unusual tiredness.

- This medication may cause a rash in some people who take it. If you develop a rash, notify your healthcare provider right away. If the rash is very severe, accompanied with a fever, or you develop skin blistering, seek care immediately.

- This medication may interact with many other medications. Tell your healthcare provider about all the medications you are taking, including any over-the-counter medications and herbal supplements. Do not start, stop, or change the dosage of any medication before checking with your doctor or pharmacist first.

For Efavirenz

- Take this medication by mouth on an empty stomach, usually once daily at bedtime or as directed by your doctor. Taking efavirenz with food especially fatty foods, can increase the blood level of this medication, which may increase your risk of certain side effects.

- Headache, nausea, vomiting, and diarrhea may occur.

- Dizziness, drowsiness, unusual/vivid dreams/nightmares, trouble sleeping, tiredness/fatigue, and trouble concentrating may occur. These side effects may begin 1-2 days after starting this medication and usually go away in 2-4 weeks. They are also reduced by taking efavirenz on an empty stomach at bedtime. If any of these effects persist or worsen, tell your healthcare provider promptly.

- Because efavirenz may impair your thinking or reactions, be careful if you drive or do anything that requires you to be awake and alert. Avoid drinking alcohol.

- Infrequently, serious psychiatric symptoms may occur during efavirenz treatment, especially in people who have mental health conditions. Tell your healthcare provider immediately if any of these unlikely but serious side effects occur: mental/mood changes such as depression, thoughts of suicide, nervousness, angry behavior, or hallucinations.

- This medication may decrease the effectiveness of hormonal birth control pills, patch, or ring, and may result in pregnancy. To reduce the risk of unintended pregnancy, and also the risk of spreading HIV to others, use barrier protection during all sexual activity.

- This medication can cause harm to an unborn baby. Do not use efavirenz without your doctor's consent if you are pregnant or planning to get pregnant. Use two forms of birth control, including a barrier form (such as a condom and diaphragm with spermicide gel) while you are taking efavirenz, and for at least 12 weeks after your treatment ends. Tell your doctor if you become pregnant during treatment.

For Rilpivirine (including Complera®)

- This medication may cause depression in some patients. If you noticed changes in your mood, such as feeling more sad than you usually do, contact your healthcare provider.

- It is very important to take this medication with a full meal as this helps ensure that your body is absorbing enough of the medication to work against the virus. Ideally, your meal should be at least 500 calories.

- Medications that reduce stomach acid can significantly affect the absorption of this medication and result in failure of your HIV treatment. Talk with your doctor or pharmacist before starting any acid suppressant medications.

PI Patient Counseling

- Diarrhea, nausea, vomiting, heartburn, stomach pain, loss of appetite, headache, dizziness, drowsiness, fatigue, weakness, or changes in taste may occur. If any of these effects persist or worsen, tell your doctor or pharmacist promptly.

- A mild rash (redness and itching) may occur within the first few weeks after the medicine is started and usually goes away within 2 weeks with no change in treatment. If a severe rash develops with symptoms of fever, body or muscle aches, mouth sores, shortness of breath, or swelling of the face, contact your doctor immediately.

- Tell your doctor immediately if any of these unlikely but serious side effects occur: persistent nausea/vomiting, stomach/abdominal pain, dark urine, yellowing eyes/skin, mental/mood changes (such as depression or anxiety), joint pain, muscle weakness/cramps/aches, increased urination (especially at night), or increased thirst.

- Before using this medication, tell your doctor or pharmacist your medical history, especially of: diabetes, heart problems (coronary artery disease, heart attack), hemophilia, high cholesterol/triglycerides, gout/high uric acid in the blood, liver problems (such as hepatitis B or hepatitis C), kidney problems, and/or pancreatitis. → lopinavir/r (Kaletra®)

- This medication may increase your blood sugar levels. If you have diabetes, check your blood sugar levels regularly as directed by your doctor. Tell your doctor immediately if you have symptoms of high blood sugar, such as increased thirst, increased urination, confusion, drowsiness, flushing, rapid breathing, or fruity breath odor.

- Changes in body fat may occur while you are taking this medication (such as increased fat in the upper back and neck, breasts, and belly areas). Discuss the risks and benefits of treatment with your doctor, as well as the possible use of exercise to reduce this side effect.

- This medication interacts with many other medications. Tell your healthcare provider about all the medications you are taking, including any over-the-counter medications and herbal supplements. Do not start, stop or change the dosage of any medicine before checking with your doctor or pharmacist first.

- Seek immediate medical attention if any of these rare but serious side effects occur: symptoms of a heart attack (such as chest/jaw/left arm pain, shortness of breath or profuse sweating), change in heart rhythm, dizziness, lightheadedness, severe nausea or vomiting, severe stomach pain, extreme weakness or trouble breathing.

For Atazanavir

- Take this medication once daily with food. If you are also prescribed ritonavir, make sure to take both atazanavir and ritonavir at the same time.

- Although rare, some patients have developed kidney stones while on this medication. Take this medication with plenty of water to reduce chances of developing kidney stones. Seek immediate medical attention if you notice signs of a kidney stone (e.g., pain in side/back/abdomen, painful urination or blood in the urine).

- Acid-lowering medications for indigestion, heartburn, or ulcers (e.g., prescription or over-the-counter medications such as antacids, famotidine or omeprazole) can significantly affect the absorption of atazanavir and result in failure of your HIV treatment. Ask your doctor or pharmacist how to use these medications together with atazanavir safely.

- May cause your skin or the whites of your eyes to turn yellow. This is usually not a dangerous side effect, however, if this becomes bothersome, talk with you doctor. If you develop yellowing of skin/ eyes along with severe abdominal pain and/or nausea/vomiting, contact your healthcare provider immediately as these could be signs of liver problems.

For Darunavir

- Take darunavir with ritonavir at the same time(s) each day with food.

- This medication may cause rash in some people, which is usually mild and will resolve on its own over time. If you develop a severe, bothersome rash, contact your healthcare provider immediately. If you have a sulfonamide allergy, tell your doctor or pharmacist right away.

INSTI Patient Counseling

- This medication can interact with antacids, multivitamins, iron and other supplements. Talk with your healthcare provider before taking these two medications together. Generally, you should separate this HIV medication at least 2 hours before or 6 hours after the antacids.

- May cause rash in some people. Notify your healthcare provider if it becomes bothersome. If you develop severe rash, accompanied with fever and/or difficulty breathing, seek medical attention immediately.

- May cause muscle pain or tenderness, or weakness. Inform your healthcare provider if you notice these symptoms, especially if you develop these out of proportion to your actual level of activity.

- May cause headache or difficulty sleeping.

- Rarely, may cause kidney or liver problems. Your healthcare provider will be checking your labs from time to time to monitor your kidney and liver functions.

For *Dolutegravir*

- You can take this medication with or without food.

- Follow the dosing instructions as prescribed by your doctor (once vs. twice a day).

- Do not take this medication if you are also taking dofetilide. Contact your healthcare provider to discuss alternative HIV therapy options.

For *Raltegravir*

- This medication is generally tolerated by most people who take it.

- Take with or without food. This medication is to be taken twice a day.

- The chewable tablets should not be taken by patients with phenylketonuria (PKU). Talk to your healthcare provider about alternative options if you have been diagnosed with PKU.

For *Stribild* (also see emtricitabine and tenofovir counseling points)

- This medication contains 4 medications in one pill: elvitegravir, cobicistat, emtricitabine, and tenofovir.

- Take this medication once a day with food.

- If you have Hepatitis B, it's very important that you do not suddenly stop this medication unless instructed to do so by your healthcare provider. Abruptly stopping this medication may result in worsening of your hepatitis symptoms.

- This medication interacts with many medications. Tell your doctor and pharmacist about all the medications you are taking, including any over-the-counter medications and herbal supplements. Do not start, stop, or change the dosage of any medication before checking with your doctor or pharmacist first.

DIABETES

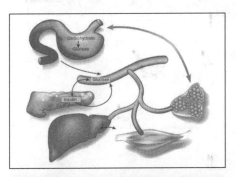

We gratefully acknowledge the assistance of Nathan Painter, PharmD, CDE, Associate Professor, University of California San Diego Skaggs School of Pharmacy and Pharmaceutical Sciences, in preparing this chapter.

GUIDELINES

American Diabetes Association (ADA) Position Statement. Standards of Medical Care in Diabetes – 2014. *Diabetes Care.* 2014; 37: Supplement 1. S14 - S80.

American Association of Clinical Endocrinologists (AACE)/American College of Endocrinology Consensus Panel on Type 2 Diabetes Mellitus: An Algorithm for Glycemic Control. *Endocr Pract.* 2013; 19:327-336.

BACKGROUND

Diabetes is the most common endocrine disorder in the United States, affecting 9.3% of the population. Diabetes is characterized by high blood glucose, or hyperglycemia. Glucose is the body's main source of energy. High blood glucose indicates that the glucose cannot get into the cell or cannot be properly stored. Insulin is a hormone that moves glucose into muscle and other tissue cells. In diabetes, there is ↓ insulin secretion, ↓ insulin sensitivity, or both. Continued hyperglycemia leads to many complications including organ and nerve damage. Acutely, hypoglycemia puts patients at risk for injury and death. In addition to type 1 and 2 diabetes, hypoglycemia could be due to genetic defects in β-cell function, genetic defects in insulin sensitivity, diseases of the exocrine pancreas (such as cystic fibrosis) or drugs from HIV/AIDS treatment or after organ transplantation. Gestational diabetes mellitus (GDM, described later in the chapter) may or may not continue after pregnancy.

DIAGNOSIS/DEFINITIONS

Prediabetes

Testing for type 2 diabetes and prediabetes should be considered in adults of any age who are overweight or obese (BMI ≥ 25 kg/m²) and have one or more additional risk factors for diabetes (see risk factors for type 2 diabetes on the following page). In patients without risk factors, testing should start at 45 years of age. If tests are normal, repeat testing at least every 3 years. Patients with prediabetes should be referred to a support program targeting 7% body weight loss and increasing physical activity to at least 150 min/week of moderate activity such as walking. Dietary strategies include reducing calories, limiting or avoiding sugar-sweetened beverages and consuming dietary fiber (14 g fiber/1,000 kcal) and foods containing whole grains. Metformin for prevention may be considered in patients with prediabetes, especially for those with a BMI > 35 kg/m², age < 60 years and in women with a history of GDM. Annual monitoring for development of diabetes in those with prediabetes and treatment of modifiable CVD risk factors is recommended.

Type 1 Diabetes

Type 1 diabetes affects ~5% of patients with diabetes and is caused by a cellular-mediated autoimmune destruction of the beta cells in the pancreas, leading to absolute insulin deficiency. Family history is less of a risk factor than with type 2 diabetes. Patients may initially present with diabetic ketoacidosis (DKA), which is a life-threatening condition. This type of diabetes usually presents in younger, thinner patients. Therapy must include insulin replacement.

Type 2 Diabetes

Type 2 diabetes accounts for ~95% of patients diagnosed with diabetes and is characterized by a combination of insulin resistance and relative insulin deficiency, with progressively lower insulin secretion over time. Type 2 diabetes may be managed with lifestyle modifications, oral medications, and/or injections, including insulin. Type 2 diabetes is strongly associated with obesity, physical inactivity, and a family history of diabetes. See risk factors in box.

DIAGNOSIS OF PREDIABETES AND DIABETES

Criteria for the Diagnosis of Prediabetes
- Fasting plasma glucose (FPG) 100-125 mg/dL
  or
- 2-hr plasma glucose in the 75-g oral glucose tolerance test (OGTT) of 140-199 mg/dL
  or
- A1C 5.7-6.4%

Criteria for the Diagnosis of Diabetes
- Classic symptoms of hyperglycemia (polyuria, polydipsia and unexplained weight loss) or hyperglycemic crisis AND a random plasma glucose ≥ 200 mg/dL
  or
- FPG ≥ 126 mg/dL – fasting is defined as no caloric intake for at least 8 hours*
  or
- 2-hr plasma glucose of ≥ 200 mg/dL during a 75 g oral glucose tolerance test (OGTT)*
  or
- A1C ≥ 6.5%*

* In the absence of unequivocal hyperglycemia, result should be confirmed by repeat testing

---

RISK FACTORS FOR TYPE 2 DIABETES

First-degree relative with diabetes

High-risk race/ethnicity (Native American, African American, Asian American, Latino, Pacific Islander) *anything but white*

Overweight (BMI ≥ 25 kg/m²)

Physical inactivity

Hypertension (≥ 140/90 mmHg or on medications for hypertension)

HDL < 35 mg/dL and/or TG > 250 mg/dL

History of CVD

A1C ≥ 5.7%, IGT or IFG on previous testing

Women who delivered a baby weighing > 9 pounds or had GDM

Women with polycystic ovary syndrome

Severe obesity

Acanthosis nigricans

LONG-TERM COMPLICATIONS OF DIABETES

Long-term complications of diabetes are classified as microvascular and macrovascular.

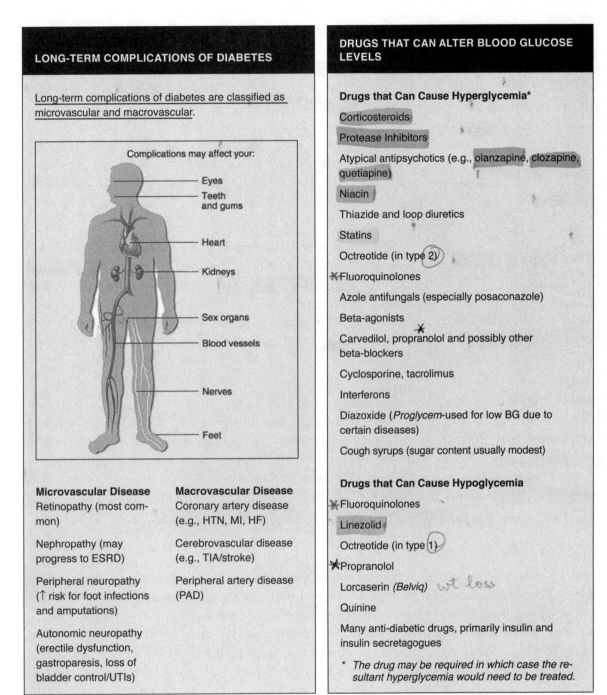

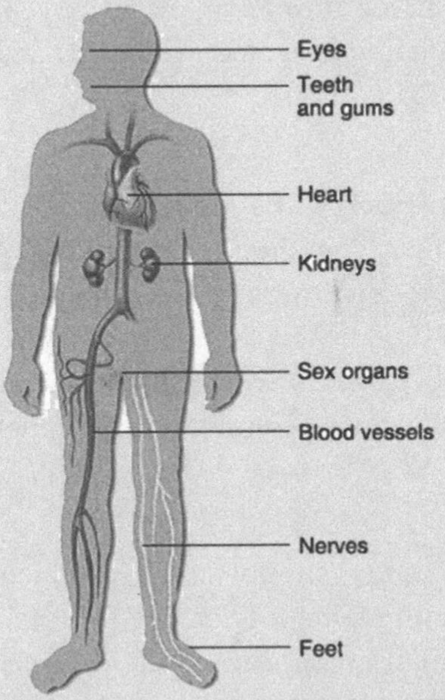
Complications may affect your:
Eyes
Teeth and gums
Heart
Kidneys
Sex organs
Blood vessels
Nerves
Feet

Microvascular Disease	Macrovascular Disease
Retinopathy (most common)	Coronary artery disease (e.g., HTN, MI, HF)
Nephropathy (may progress to ESRD)	Cerebrovascular disease (e.g., TIA/stroke)
Peripheral neuropathy (↑ risk for foot infections and amputations)	Peripheral artery disease (PAD)
Autonomic neuropathy (erectile dysfunction, gastroparesis, loss of bladder control/UTIs)	

DRUGS THAT CAN ALTER BLOOD GLUCOSE LEVELS

Drugs that Can Cause Hyperglycemia*

Corticosteroids

Protease Inhibitors

Atypical antipsychotics (e.g., olanzapine, clozapine, quetiapine)

Niacin

Thiazide and loop diuretics

Statins

Octreotide (in type 2)

Fluoroquinolones

Azole antifungals (especially posaconazole)

Beta-agonists

Carvedilol, propranolol and possibly other beta-blockers

Cyclosporine, tacrolimus

Interferons

Diazoxide (*Proglycem*-used for low BG due to certain diseases)

Cough syrups (sugar content usually modest)

Drugs that Can Cause Hypoglycemia

Fluoroquinolones

Linezolid

Octreotide (in type 1)

Propranolol

Lorcaserin (*Belviq*)

Quinine

Many anti-diabetic drugs, primarily insulin and insulin secretagogues

* *The drug may be required in which case the resultant hyperglycemia would need to be treated.*

Clinical Signs and Symptoms

Hyperglycemia commonly results in polyuria, polyphagia, polydipsia, blurred vision, and fatigue. Type 1 patients may also present with weight loss. In type 2 patients, symptoms of hyperglycemia will worsen and often are mistaken for symptoms due to other causes such as environmental changes or older age.

GDM MATERNAL CAPILLARY GOALS
Preprandial: ≤ 95 mg/dL
1 hour post-meal: ≤ 140 mg/dL
2 hours post-meal: ≤ 120 mg/dL
If patient has diabetes and becomes pregnant, goals are stricter: A1C: < 6%
Premeal, bedtime, and overnight: 60-99 mg/dL
Peak postprandial: 100-129 mg/dL

GESTATIONAL DIABETES MELLITUS (GDM)

GDM (diabetes of pregnancy) increases the risk for adverse maternal, fetal and neonatal outcomes. Treatment goals for GDM are stricter (see box). Nutritional therapy is the standard of care for both the needs of the pregnancy and to maintain proper blood glucose levels. SMBG must be done regularly to see if the changes in diet are adequate. If not, insulin is often used, but some pregnant women may take oral anti-diabetic medications. *SMBG = self-monitoring of BG*

NON-DRUG (LIFESTYLE) TREATMENT

Lifestyle modifications should be used in combination with medication therapy for all patients with diabetes. Some patients may be able to control their blood glucose using lifestyle modifications alone which can slow disease progression. All patients who smoke should receive cessation counseling and other forms of treatment as a routine component of diabetes care.

Weight Loss

Overweight or obese patients with diabetes or prediabetes should be encouraged to lose weight through reducing energy intake while maintaining a healthy eating pattern. Modest weight loss may provide clincal benefit (improved blood sugar, lower blood pressure and decreased cholesterol) especially those early in the disease process. Intensive lifestyle interventions (nutrition therapy, physical activity and behavior change) are recommended. A deficit of 3,500 kcal will produce a weight loss of 1 pound. Patients should also maintain a waist circumference < 35 inches for females and < 40 inches for males.

Diet

Patients with prediabetes and diabetes should receive individualized medical nutrition therapy by a registered dietitian. Patients with type 1 diabetes should have intensive insulin education using the carbohydrate-counting meal planning approach to improve glycemic control. No ideal percentage of calories from macronutrients (carbs, protein, fats) has been established. Carbohydrates should come from healthy sources such as legumes, whole grains, and vegetables. Fiber (14 g/1,000 kcal) and whole grains are encouraged. A variety of eating patterns have been shown to be effective in managing diabetes including a Mediterranean-style, monounsaturated fatty acids (MUFA)-rich diet and others. EPA and DHA (from fatty fish) is recommended to prevent heart disease. Sodium consumption should be < 2,300 mg/day.

Carbohydrates and Postprandial Levels

Monitoring carbohydrate intake has been used to maintain glycemic control, and many patients with diabetes match the prandial (meal-time) insulin dose to the carbohydrate intake. A carbohydrate serving is measured as 15 grams. A serving is approximately one small piece of fruit, 1 slice of bread, ⅓ cup of cooked rice/pasta, or ½ cup of oatmeal.

1 carb serving (15 g) = 1 small fruit, 1 slice bread, ⅓ cup cooked rice/pasta, ½ cup oatmeal

Fat Intake

The ADA recommends limiting saturated fat intake to < 7% of total calories to reduce cardio-vascular risk. Reducing intake of *trans* fat ↓ LDL cholesterol and ↑ HDL; therefore, intake of *trans* fat should be minimized. These recommendations are different from the obesity guideline recommendations (see Weight Loss chapter for more information).

Exercise

[handwritten: ≤ 150]

Aerobic exercise of moderate-intensity should be performed at least 50 minutes/week, spread over at least 3 days/week with no more than 2 consecutive days without exercise. Patients should be encouraged to perform resistance training at least twice per week.

COMPREHENSIVE CARE

[handwritten: DM + 10-yr CV risk > 10% ⟹ ♂ > 50 y/o, ♀ > 60 y/o + 1 risk factor · 1 family hx CVD · HTN · smoking · dyslipidemia · albuminuria]

Primary Prevention of Cardiovascular Disease

[handwritten left margin: 1° prevention = have NOT yet had a CV event]

Aspirin should be considered for primary prevention in patients with type 1 and type 2 diabetes at ↑ CV risk (10-year risk > 10%). This includes men > 50 years of age or women > 60 years of age who have at least one additional major risk factor (family history of CVD, HTN, smoking, dyslipidemia, or albuminuria). The dose of aspirin should be 75-162 mg daily (usually 81 mg EC) if there is no contraindication such as aspirin allergy or bleeding. If the patient has an aspirin allergy, other antiplatelet agents may be considered.

Nephropathy Screening/Treatment

[handwritten left margin: ACEI or ARB for 1° prevention in DM w/ normal bp + albumin-uria]

Diabetic nephropathy is the leading cause of end-stage renal disease (ESRD). An annual urine test to quantitate urine albumin excretion is recommended. Either an ACE inhibitor or an ARB (but not both in combination) should be started in diabetes patients with a urinary albumin excretion of ≥ 30 mg/24 hours. Optimizing glycemic and blood pressure control helps to slow the progression of diabetic nephropathy.

Retinopathy Screening

Diabetic retinopathy is the leading cause of blindness in adults. An annual dilated, comprehensive eye exam is recommended in patients with diabetes. If the patient has one or more normal eye exams and their blood sugar is well controlled, screening can be done every 2 years. The comprehensive eye exam should be performed by an ophthalmologist or optometrist. More frequent exams may be advised if retinopathy is progressing.

DIABETES SCREENING
Nephropathy
Looking for the presence of albuminuria (urine albumin excretion of ≥ 30 mg/day)
Type 1 diabetes: Annual testing starting 5 years after diagnosis in patients ≥ 10 years old
Type 2 diabetes: Annual testing starting at the time of diagnosis
Retinopathy
Type 1 diabetes: Annual testing beginning within 5 years of diagnosis in patients ≥ 10 years old
Type 2 diabetes: Annual testing beginning soon after diagnosis

Foot Care

All adult patients with diabetes should have a comprehensive foot exam, performed by a podiatrist, at least once per year. The podiatrist examines the skin of the feet for dryness/cracking and for signs of infection, ulcers, bunions, calluses, and any deformities such as claw toes.

Pedal pulses are assessed to look for signs of peripheral arterial disease. The 10-gram mono-filament test is performed to assess loss of sensation and presence of peripheral neuropathy.

All patients with diabetes should inspect their feet daily (or have a family member do so if they are unable). Patients should have their feet inspected at every physician visit as well. Daily self-care of the feet include:

- Wash feet daily and inspect them for any changes (red spots, cuts, blisters, and cracks). Be sure to look between the toes. Use a mirror, if needed, to inspect the bottom of the feet.
- Dry feet completely, particularly in between the toes. Rub a thin coat of skin lotion over to the tops and bottoms of dry feet, but not between toes due to ↑ risk of tinea pedis.
- Trim toe nails carefully – straight across – and file any sharp edges with an emery board to the contour of the toe.
- Callouses may be filed with a pumice stone or emery board. Patients should never use any instruments to cut hardened skin on the feet.
- Avoid walking barefoot.
- Use soft cotton or synthetic blend socks to absorb moisture.
- Wear properly fitting, comfortable, supportive shoes (with orthotics if needed). Use cau- tion when breaking in new shoes. Use extra-wide shoes to accommodate any deformities such as bunions or hammertoes.
- Inspect shoes for foreign objects before inserting feet.
- Keep the blood flowing to feet. Put feet up when sitting. Wiggle toes and move ankles up and down for 5 minutes, 2-3 times/day. Do not cross your legs for long periods of time.
- Remove socks and shoes at each physician visit to allow for visual inspection.
- Keep feet away from items that may cause burning such as fireplaces, electric blankets, or heating pads. Use another part of the body to test shower temperature.

Vaccinations for Adults with Diabetes

Do not share insulin pens (even if needle is changed) due to risk of hepatitis transmission, and other conditions. Multi-dose vials should be labeled for one patient only.

Required

- Hepatitis B: If 19-59 years of age and have never completed series. Consider vaccinating to unvac-cinated diabetes patients ≥ 60 years of age.

inactivated (shot)

- Influenza: annually for all diabetic patients ≥ 6 months of age. [*live flu vaccine not for pts w/ chronic dz*] *Flumist©*
- PPSV23 (Pneumovax): At 2-64 years of age and again at 65 years if > 5 years since previ- ous vac-cination.
- Tetanus, diphtheria, pertussis (TdaP): Once a lifetime then, Td booster every 10 years (more fre-quent if deep or dirty wound).

Possibly Required

- May require if at risk or at recommended age (see Immunizations chapter): Hepatitis A, PCV13 (Pre-vnar), Varicella, Zoster, Meningococcal, MMR, HPV

Durable Medical Equipment (DME)

DME covered by CMS under the Part B medical benefit includes glucose monitors, test strips, control solution, lancet devices and lancets, and diabetic shoes or inserts. Medicare has an anti-switching rule that prohibits suppliers from encouraging patients to switch glucose meters or test strips. If the supplier does not have the test strip that the meter requires the patient can ask about alternative brands, but the supplier cannot initiate the discussion. CMS does (not) cover continuous glucose monitoring (CGM) devices. Part B covers some other diabetes services, including self-management training, annual eye exam, foot exam every 6 months, glaucoma tests and nutrition therapy.

ADA TREATMENT GUIDELINES FOR TYPE 2 DIABETES

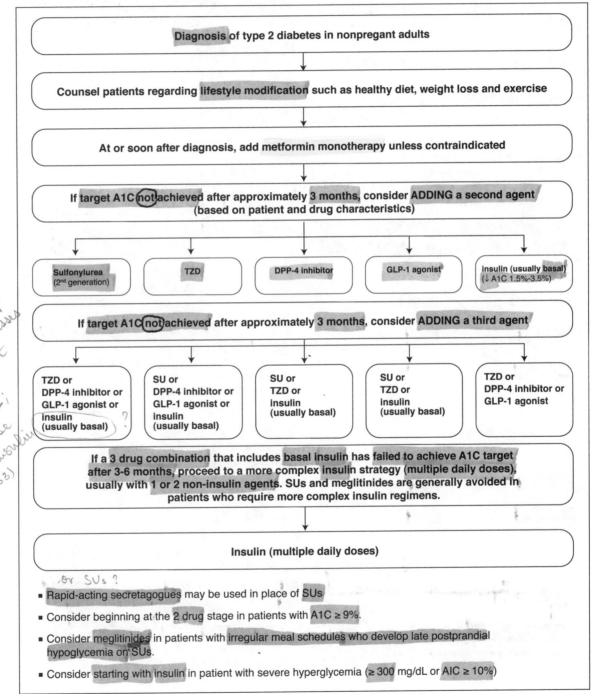

Handwritten note (left margin): metformin + any 2 of above classes BUT don't use DPP4 w/ GLP-1; don't use SU w/ insulin (top P. 463)

Flowchart:

Diagnosis of type 2 diabetes in nonpregnant adults

↓

Counsel patients regarding lifestyle modification such as healthy diet, weight loss and exercise

↓

At or soon after diagnosis, add metformin monotherapy unless contraindicated

↓

If target A1C (not) achieved after approximately 3 months, consider ADDING a second agent (based on patient and drug characteristics)

| Sulfonylurea (2nd generation) | TZD | DPP-4 inhibitor | GLP-1 agonist | insulin (usually basal) (↓A1C 1.5%-3.5%) |

↓

If target A1C (not) achieved after approximately 3 months, consider ADDING a third agent

| TZD or DPP-4 inhibitor or GLP-1 agonist or insulin (usually basal) | SU or DPP-4 inhibitor or GLP-1 agonist or insulin (usually basal) | SU or TZD or insulin (usually basal) | SU or TZD or insulin (usually basal) | TZD or DPP-4 inhibitor or GLP-1 agonist |

↓

If a 3 drug combination that includes basal insulin has failed to achieve A1C target after 3-6 months, proceed to a more complex insulin strategy (multiple daily doses), usually with 1 or 2 non-insulin agents. SUs and meglitinides are generally avoided in patients who require more complex insulin regimens.

↓

Insulin (multiple daily doses)

- Rapid-acting secretagogues may be used in place of SUs
- Consider beginning at the 2 drug stage in patients with A1C ≥ 9%.
- Consider meglitinides in patients with irregular meal schedules who develop late postprandial hypoglycemia on SUs.
- Consider starting with insulin in patient with severe hyperglycemia (≥ 300 mg/dL or A1C ≥ 10%)

TREATMENT GOALS FOR NON-PREGNANT ADULTS WITH DIABETES – THE ABC'S OF DIABETES

A – A1C

While a glucometer measures the blood glucose at that given moment, the A1C measures the average blood glucose over the past 2-3 months. The AIC should be measured:

- At least quarterly in patients not well controlled (at goal)
- Twice per year if at goal and have stable control

Use of Point of Care (POC) testing allows timely treatment changes.

Estimated average glucose (eAG) refers to the mean plasma glucose concentrations over 2-3 months, and may be easier for patients to understand over A1C. The eAG goal is < 154 mg/dL per the ADA guidelines.

MEASUREMENT	TARGET

ADA Treatment Guidelines

A1C	< 7.0%*
Preprandial capillary plasma glucose	70-130 mg/dL
Postprandial capillary plasma glucose (1-2 hours after the start of a meal)	< 180 mg/dL

AACE Treatment Guidelines

A1C	≤ 6.5%*
Preprandial capillary plasma glucose	< 110 mg/dL
Postprandial capillary plasma glucose	< 140 mg/dL

* *Must individualize target goals. Per the ADA, a more stringent A1C goal (such as < 6.5%) may be appropriate for younger adult patients not experiencing hypoglycemia, those with long life expectancy and no significant CVD. A less stringent A1C goal (such as < 8%) may be appropriate for patients with a history of severe hypoglycemia, limited life expectancy, extensive comorbid conditions, advanced complications, or longstanding diabetes where the goal is difficult to attain despite optimal efforts.*

Correlation of A1C with Average Glucose (estimated)

A1C (%)	MEAN PLASMA GLUCOSE (MG/DL)
6	126
7	154
8	183
9	212
10	240
11	269
12	298

B – Blood Pressure

Goal blood pressure for patients with diabetes is < 140/80 mmHg. A lower systolic target (such as < 130 mmHg) may be appropriate for certain individuals such as younger patients, if it can be reached without undue treatment burden, or in patients at high risk of stroke. A regimen consisting of an ACE inhibitor or ARB should be chosen first-line due to reduction of CVD outcomes and progression of diabetic nephropathy in patients with albuminuria. One or more antihypertensive medications should be given at bedtime. Most patients with diabetes will require 2 or more medications to control their blood pressure. Choice of additional agents will depend on the patient's comorbidities. Thiazide-like diuretics and dihydropyridine calcium channel blockers are generally used for additional BP control in most patients.

C – Cholesterol

Lifestyle modification should focus on reducing saturated fat, *trans* fat and cholesterol. Statin therapy should be added to lifestyle therapy, regardless of lipid levels, in patients

- with overt CVD
- without CVD and > 40 years and have 1 or more risk factors (family history of CVD, HTN, smoking, dyslipidemia, or albuminuria).

LDL cholesterol goal is < 100 mg/dL in patients without CVD. In patients with overt CVD, a LDL goal < 70 mg/dL is an option. Triglycerides < 150 mg/dL. HDL > 40 mg/dL in men and > 50 mg/dL in women are desirable. Note the ACC/AHA lipid guidelines have different recommendations on the use of statin therapy.

Handwritten notes:

bp goal
140/80
(or < 130 systolic in younger pts or at ↑ risk of stroke)

JNC - 8
- 18-59 y/o or DM or CKD ⇒ 140/90
- ≥ 60 y/o ⇒ 150/90

A1c < 6.5% — younger adults w/o hypoBG, long life expectancy w/o CV dz

A1c < 8% — hx of severe hypoBG, limited life expectancy, extensive comorbidities, advanced compx

longstanding / uncontrolled DM

lipid goals
- LDL < 100 (no CVD)
  < 70 (overt CVD)
- TG < 150
- HDL > 40 (♂)
  > 50 (♀)

The AACE guidelines agree with the ADA in recommending metformin as initial therapy (unless insulin is required or the patient cannot use metformin) – but they differ in 2nd line treatment options. The ADA lists sulfonylureas (SUs) as a second-line option whereas AACE does not favor SUs due to the risks of hypoglycemia, weight gain, and loss of efficacy over time. The AACE treatment algorithm recommends evaluating the initial A1C and, based on the value, initiating single, double or triple drug therapy. The AACE goal for A1C is ≤ 6.5% for healthy patients without concurrent illness and at a low hypoglycemic risk.

BIGUANIDE   *indicated for children 10 - 16 y/o*

Metformin works primarily by ↓ hepatic glucose production, ↓ intestinal absorption of glucose and ↑ insulin sensitivity.   *inhibits lipolysis in adipose tissue*

w/ meals
IR → BID dosing
max daily
2550 mg

ER - w/ dinner
max daily
2000 - 2500 mg

DRUG	DOSING	SAFETY/SIDE EFFECTS/MONITORING
MetFORMIN (Glucophage, Glucophage XR, Fortamet, Glumetza, *ER!* **Riomet)** Immediate release: 500, 850, 1,000 mg Extended release 500, 750, 1,000 mg *Riomet liquid (500 mg/5 mL)* + glipizide (Metaglip) **+ glyburide (Glucovance)** + pioglitazone (Actoplus Met, Actoplus Met XR) + rosiglitazone (Avandamet) **+ sitagliptin (Janumet, Janumet XR)** + saxagliptin (Kombiglyze XR) + linagliptin (Jentadueto) + repaglinide (PrandiMet) + alogliptin (Kazano) + canagliflozin (Invokamet) + dapagliflozin (Xigduo XR)	Start IR 500 mg BID or 850 mg daily Start ER 500-1,000 mg with dinner Titrate to 1.5-2 g daily, although higher doses are sometimes used. Max daily dose: 2,550 mg (IR), 2,000-2,500 mg (ER) First line therapy for type 2 treatment, and may be used for prevention. Extended release: Swallow whole; do not crush, break, or chew.	**BOXED WARNING** Lactic acidosis, ↑ risk in acute HF, dehydration, excessive alcohol intake, hepatic/renal impairment or sepsis *due to metformin accumulation* → *nonspecific sx @ onset (myalgia, malaise, resp. distress somnolence, abdominal distress)* **CONTRAINDICATIONS** Contraindicated with SCr ≥ 1.5 mg/dL (males) or ≥ 1.4 mg/dL (females) or abnormal creatinine clearance, metabolic acidosis. Temporarily discontinue in patients receiving intravascular iodinated contrast media. → *CrCl < 60* **WARNINGS** Metformin should be stopped in any case of hypoxia, such as decompensated heart failure, respiratory failure, acute MI or sepsis. Avoid in patients with renal/hepatic impairment due to ↑ risk for lactic acidosis. **SIDE EFFECTS** → *take w/ food to ↓ stomach upset* Diarrhea, nausea, vomiting, flatulence, long term vitamin B12 deficiency. Weight neutral (few patients may lose weight), little-to-no risk of hypoglycemia (when used as monotherapy). **MONITORING** FBG, A1C, SCr, BUN **NOTES** ↓ A1C 1-2% Pregnancy Category B *empty shell* The ER formulations may appear in the stool. See counseling section. *Glucophage XR, Fortamet, Glumetza*

Metformin Drug Interactions

- Alcohol can ↑ risk for lactic acidosis especially with renal impairment and advanced heart disease.

- Iodinated contrast dye ↑ risk of lactic acidosis – hold prior to procedure and wait 48 hours after and restart only once renal function has been confirmed as normal.

- Metformin can ↓ vitamin B-12 absorption (and possibly folic acid), leading to megaloblastic anemia. Consider vitamin supplementation. Separate metformin ER from colesevelam.

Metformin Counseling

- Some people have developed a very rare, life-threatening condition called lactic acidosis while taking metformin. Seek emergency medical help if you have any of these symptoms of lactic acidosis: weakness, ↑ somnolence, slow heart rate, shivers, muscle pain, shortness of breath, stomach pain, lightheadedness, and/or fainting.

  myalgia   *resp. distress*   *Sx @ onset nonspecific*
  labs: ↓ pH, ↑ anion gap, ↑ blood lactate

- If you need to have any type of X-ray or CT scan using contrast dye that is injected into your vein, you may need to temporarily stop taking metformin. Be sure to notify your healthcare provider ahead of time that you are taking metformin.

- Do not crush, chew, or break an extended-release tablet. Swallow the pill whole. It is specially made to release medicine slowly in the body. Breaking the pill would cause too much of the drug to be released at one time.

- Diarrhea, nausea, vomiting, abdominal discomfort, and flatulence may occur and often goes away with time. If taking the immediate release formulation, it should be given twice daily with meals. Taking with food will help ↓ stomach upset. You may find relief with the extended release formulation which is taken with dinner.   *GI SE*

- If using *Glumetza, Fortamet,* or *Glucophage XR*, you may see a shell of the medicine in the stool. This is normal, the medicine is in your body and the tablet is empty.

SULFONYLUREAS (SUs)

Sulfonylureas work by stimulating insulin secretion from the pancreatic beta cells. Do not use with meglitinides due to similar MOA.

DRUG	DOSING	SAFETY/SIDE EFFECTS/MONITORING
ChlorproPAMIDE (Diabenese) TOLAZamide TOLBUTamide	These older, first-generation agents should not be used *due to long lasting hypoBG*	**CONTRAINDICATIONS** Type 1 diabetes mellitus, diabetic ketoacidosis, concurrent use with bosentan (glyburide) *→ ↑↑ LFTs* *endothelin receptor antag for PAH*
GlipiZIDE (Glucotrol, Glucotrol XL, GlipiZIDE XL) + metformin (Metaglip)	IR: 5-10 mg daily-BID, max 40 mg/day *30 min before breakfast ± dinner* XL: 5-10 mg daily, max 20 mg daily *qd w/ 1st meal*	**WARNING** Sulfa allergy (not likely to cross-react – please see cautionary statement in Drug Allergies chapter)
Glimepiride (Amaryl) + pioglitazone (Duetact) + rosiglitazone (Avandaryl)	1-2 mg daily, max 8 daily *qd w/ 1st meal*	**SIDE EFFECTS** Hypoglycemia, weight gain **MONITORING** FBG, A1C
GlyBURIDE (DiaBeta) Micronized glyburide (Glynase) *↑ absorption* + metformin (Glucovance)	DiaBeta: 2.5-5 mg daily, max 20 mg daily Glynase: 1.5-3 mg daily, max 12 mg daily	**NOTES** ↓ A1C 1-2% Pregnancy Category C ↓ efficacy after long-term use First generation agents (chlorpropamide, tolazamide, tolbutamide) can cause long-lasting hypoglycemia. Glyburide has a partially active metabolite that is renally cleared and should be avoided in renal impairment. Glyburide is not a preferred agent. Glyburide regular tablets cannot be used interchangeably with micronized tablet formulations. Micronized glyburide has better absorption than glyburide (3 mg micronized glyburide = 5 mg of glyburide).

+ bosentan ← not preferred

partially active metab renally cleared ⇒ avoid in renal imp.

3 mg micronized = 5 mg regular

Sulfonylurea Drug Interactions

- Primary interaction is with insulin because both can cause hypoglycemia; sulfonylureas should be discontinued when insulin is initiated, per AACE.

- Use caution with drugs that can cause hypoglycemia, see table at the beginning of the chapter.

- Sulfonylurea dose reduction may be required when a TZD, GLP-1 agonist, DPP-4 inhibitor, or SGLT2 inhibitor is initiated.

- These agents are CYP 2C9 substrates, use caution with drugs that are 2C9 inducers or inhibitors.

Sulfonylurea Counseling

- Do not crush, chew, or break an extended-release tablet. Swallow the pill whole. It is specially made to release medicine slowly in the body. Breaking the pill would cause too much of the drug to be released at one time.

- Keep away from children, even 1 tablet can be dangerous.

- Glipizide XR is taken with the first meal of the day, the IR is either 30 minutes before breakfast and dinner, or if once daily 30 minutes before first meal. Glimepiride is once daily, with the first meal.

- If the patient is made NPO or plans to reduce caloric intake, may need to hold the dose.

- This medicine can cause low blood sugar. Be able to recognize the symptoms of low blood sugar including shakiness, irritability, hunger, headache, confusion, somnolence, weakness, dizziness, sweating, and fast heartbeat. Very low blood sugar can cause seizures (convulsions), fainting, or coma. Always keep a source of sugar available in case you have symptoms of low blood sugar.

MEGLITINIDES   *insulin secretagogues?*

Meglitinides work by stimulating insulin secretion from the pancreatic beta cells. Do not use with sulfonylureas due to similar MOA.

both TID dosing

DRUG	DOSING	SAFETY/SIDE EFFECTS/MONITORING
Repaglinide (Prandin) + metformin (PrandiMet)	A1C < 8%: 0.5 mg before each meal (TID) A1C ≥ 8%: 1-2 mg before each meal (TID), max 16 mg daily Take 15-30 minutes before meals	**CONTRAINDICATIONS** Type 1 diabetes, diabetic ketoacidosis, concurrent gemfibrozil therapy (repaglinide) → ↑↑ *myopathy, rhabdo* **SIDE EFFECTS** Hypoglycemia, mild weight gain, upper respiratory tract infection **MONITORING** FBG, A1C
Nateglinide (Starlix)	60 mg before each meal (TID) if near goal A1C, otherwise 120 mg before each meal (TID) Take 1-30 minutes before meals *< effective than repaglinide*	**NOTES** ↓A1C 0.5-1.5%; ↓postprandial BG Pregnancy Category C Nateglinide is slightly less effective than repaglinide

≠ gemfibrozil / 15-30 min before meals / 1-30 min before meals

Meglitinides Drug Interactions

- Primary interaction is with insulin because both can cause hypoglycemia.

- Meglitinide dose reduction may be required when a TZD, GLP-1 agonist, DPP-4 inhibitor, or SGLT2 inhibitor is initiated.

- Gemfibrozil can ↑ repaglinide concentrations and can ↓ BG, recommend fenofibrate instead.

- Use caution with drugs that can cause hypoglycemia, see table at the beginning of the chapter.

Meglitinides Counseling

1-30 min nateg
15-30 min repag

- Take 1-30 minutes prior to meals. If you forget to take a dose until after eating, skip that dose and take only your next regularly scheduled dose, before a meal.

- If you plan to skip a meal, skip the dose for that meal. Some patients will be told to increase dose if they eat significantly more food at a meal.

- This medicine can cause low blood sugar. Be able to recognize the symptoms of low blood sugar including shakiness, irritability, hunger, headache, confusion, somnolence, weak- ness, dizziness, sweating, and fast heartbeat. Very low blood sugar can cause seizures (convulsions), fainting, or coma. Always keep a source of sugar available in case you have symptoms of low blood sugar.

- Keep away from children, even ingesting 1 tablet can be dangerous.

THIAZOLIDINEDIONES (TZDs)

Thiazolidinediones are peroxisome proliferator-activated receptor gamma (PPARγ) agonists causing ↑ peripheral insulin sensitivity (↑ uptake and utilization of glucose by the peripheral tissues; insulin sensitizers).

muscle

DRUG	DOSING	SAFETY/SIDE EFFECTS/MONITORING
Pioglitazone (Actos) + metformin (Actoplus Met, Actoplus Met XR) + glimepiride (Duetact) + alogliptin (Oseni)	15-30 mg daily, max 45 mg daily *use > 1 yr => ↑ risk for bladder cancer* *↑HDL* *↓TG* *↓ total cholesterol*	**BOXED WARNING** May cause or exacerbate heart failure in some patients **CONTRAINDICATIONS** NYHA Class III/IV heart failure **WARNINGS** Avoid pioglitazone in patients with active bladder cancer **SIDE EFFECTS** Peripheral edema, weight gain, URTIs, macular edema, HF, ↑ fracture risk, ↑ LFTs, pioglitazone has ↑ risk of bladder cancer when used > 1 year; desirable side effects include ↑ HDL, ↓ TGs and ↓ total cholesterol (pioglitazone)
Rosiglitazone (Avandia) + metformin (Avandamet) + glimepiride (Avandaryl)	4-8 mg daily, max 8 mg daily	**MONITORING** LFTs, FBG, A1C, and signs and symptoms of heart failure **NOTES** ↓ A1C 0.5-1.4% Pregnancy Category C

both q d ± food

fracture risk in women > men (upper arm, hand, foot)

may take several weeks to have full effect

Glitazone Drug Interactions

- These agents can reduce the amount of insulin or insulin secretagogue required. Monitor blood glucose closely after initiation of therapy.

- These agents are CYP 2C8 substrates; use caution with drugs that are 2C8 inducers (e.g., rifampin) or inhibitors (e.g., gemfibrozil).

Glitazone Counseling

- May take several weeks for the drug to lower blood sugar, monitor your levels carefully.

- Take once daily, with or without food.

- Contact your healthcare provider right away if you are passing dark-colored urine, have pale stools, feel more tired than usual or if your skin and/or whites of your eyes become yellow. These may be signs of liver damage.

- This drug can cause water retention and can cause your ankles to swell. You may develop trouble breathing. If this happens, inform your healthcare provider right away.

- Women may be more likely than men to have bone fractures in the upper arm, hand, or foot while taking this medication. Talk with your healthcare provider if you are concerned about this possibility.

- Tell your healthcare provider if you have heart failure or heart disease or liver problems. For pioglitazone, tell your healthcare provider if you have or have had bladder cancer.

ALPHA-GLUCOSIDASE INHIBITORS

These agents reversibly inhibit membrane-bound intestinal alpha-glucosidases which hydrolyze oligosaccharides and disaccharides to glucose and other monosaccharides in the brush border of the small intestine. In patients with diabetes, this enzyme inhibition results in delayed glucose absorption and lowering of postprandial hyperglycemia.

DRUG	DOSING	SAFETY/SIDE EFFECTS/MONITORING
Acarbose (Precose) Miglitol (Glyset)	Both acarbose and miglitol are started at 25 mg with the first bite of each main meal; ↑ by 25 mg every 1-2 months, max 300 mg/day in divided doses. CrCl < 25 mL/min: not recommended Start low and titrate slow to ↓ GI effects	**CONTRAINDICATIONS** Inflammatory bowel disease (IBD), colonic ulceration, partial or complete intestinal obstruction, cirrhosis (acarbose) **SIDE EFFECTS** GI effects (flatulence, diarrhea, abdominal pain), ↑ LFTs (acarbose) Weight neutral **MONITORING** Postprandial BG, A1C, LFTs every 3 months during 1st year (acarbose) **NOTES** ↓ A1C 0.5-0.8%; ↓ postprandial BG Pregnancy Category B

[handwritten margin notes: take both w/ 1st bite; ≠ cirrhosis?; monitor LFTs q 3 mo × 1st yr]

Alpha-Glucosidase Inhibitor Counseling

- Take with a full glass of water with the first bite of food (the medicine needs to be in the stomach with your food). If you plan to skip a meal, skip the dose for that meal.

- This medicine can cause flatulence (gas), diarrhea and abdominal pain, but this usually goes away with time. The dose may be increased as you get over these side effects.

- These agents, by themselves, do not cause low blood sugar. If you get low blood sugar af- ter taking acarbose or miglitol, you cannot treat it with sucrose (present in fruit juice) or table sugar or candy. If you are using this agent with a drug that causes low blood sugar (such as insulin, a sulfonylurea or a meglitinide), you will need to purchase glucose tablets or gel to have on-hand to treat any hy- poglycemic episode.

- This medicine does not cause weight gain.

DIPEPTIDYL PEPTIDASE 4 INHIBITORS

Dipeptidyl peptidase IV (DPP-4) inhibitors prevent the enzyme DPP-4 from breaking down incretin hormones, glucagon-like peptide-1 (GLP-1) and glucose-dependent insulinotropic polypeptide (GIP). These hormones help to regulate blood glucose levels by ↑ insulin release from the pancreatic beta cells and ↓ glucagon secretion from pancreatic alpha cells. A reduc- tion in glucagon results in ↓ hepatic glucose production. These are incretin enhancers.

DRUG	DOSING	SAFETY/SIDE EFFECTS/MONITORING
SitaGLIPtin (Januvia)	100 mg daily	**SIDE EFFECTS**
+ metformin (Janumet, Janumet XR)	CrCl 30-49 mL/min: 50 mg daily	Nasopharyngitis, upper respiratory tract infections, UTIs, peripheral edema, rash
	CrCl < 30 mL/min: 25 mg daily	and hypoglycemia. Rarely can cause acute pancreatitis.
Saxagliptin (Onglyza)	2.5-5 mg daily	Weight neutral
+ metformin (Kombiglyze XR)	CrCl < 50 mL/min or with strong	
	CYP 3A4 inhibitors: 2.5 mg daily	**MONITORING**
	Kombiglyze XR is given daily with evening meal	FBG, A1C, renal function
Linagliptin (Tradjenta)	5 mg daily	
+ metformin (Jentadueto)	No renal dose adjustment	**NOTES**
Alogliptin (Nesina)	25 mg daily	↓ A1C 0.5-0.8%; ↓ postprandial BG
+ metformin (Kazano)	CrCl 30-59 mL/min: 12.5 mg daily	Pregnancy Category B
+ pioglitazone (Oseni)	CrCl < 30 mL/min: 6.25 mg daily	

DPP-4 Inhibitor Drug Interactions

- These agents can reduce the amount of insulin or insulin secretagogue required. Monitor blood glucose closely after initiation of therapy.

- Saxagliptin (Onglyza) is a major 3A4 and P-glycoprotein substrate. Use the lower 2.5 mg dose with strong CYP 3A4 inhibitors including ketoconazole, atazanavir, clarithromycin, indinavir, itraconazole, nefazodone, nelfinavir, ritonavir, saquinavir and telithromycin.

- Linagliptin (Tradjenta) is a major 3A4 and P-glycoprotein substrate. Linagliptin levels are ↓ by strong inducers (carbamazepine, efavirenz, phenytoin, rifampin, St. John's wort).

DPP-4 inhibitor Counseling

- Take once daily in the morning, with or without food.

- If you have trouble breathing, or any kind of rash, see your healthcare provider at once.

- Contact your healthcare provider right away if you develop symptoms of pancreatitis, which in- clude severe stomach pain that does not go away, with or without vomiting. The pain can radiate from the abdomen through to the back.

SODIUM GLUCOSE CO-TRANSPORTER-2 (SGLT2) INHIBITORS

Sodium glucose co-transporter-2 (SGLT2), expressed in the proximal renal tubules, is responsible for the majority of the reabsorption of filtered glucose from the tubular lumen. By inhibiting SGLT2, these agents reduce reabsorption of filtered glucose and lowers the renal threshold for glucose, which ↑ urinary glucose excretion.

all dosed qd

DRUG	DOSING	SAFETY/SIDE EFFECTS/MONITORING
Canagliflozin (Invokana) + metformin (Invokamet) *SE: ↑ K+*	100 mg daily prior to first meal of the day; can ↑ to 300 mg daily CrCl 45-60 mL/min: 100 mg max dose CrCl < 45 mL/min: do (not) use	**CONTRAINDICATIONS** Severe renal impairment (CrCl < 30 mL/min), ESRD, or on dialysis **WARNINGS** Genital mycotic infections, symptomatic hypotension due to intravascular volume depletion, ↑ LDL, urinary tract infections, renal insufficiency, ↑ risk of bladder cancer (dapagliflozin)
Dapagliflozin (Farxiga) + metformin (Xigduo XR) *do not use in active bladder cancer (CAUTION in pts w/ hx)*	5 mg daily in the morning; can ↑ to 10 mg daily CrCl < 60 mL/min: do (not) use	**SIDE EFFECTS** Genital mycotic infections, UTIs, hypoglycemia, ↑ LDL, ↑ urination, hypotension, ↑ thirst, ↓ weight (4-7 pounds), ↑ K+ with canagliflozin
Empagliflozin (Jardiance)	10 mg daily, in the morning; can ↑ to 25 mg daily CrCl < 45 mL/min: do (not) use	**MONITORING** Renal function, blood glucose, A1C, LDL, blood pressure **NOTES** ↓ A1C 0.7-1% Pregnancy Category C Consider a lower dose of insulin or insulin secretagogue when used in combo with SGLT2 inhibitors to reduce risk of hypoglycemia

SGLT2 Drug Interactions

- These agents can reduce the amount of insulin or insulin secretagogue required. Monitor blood glucose closely after initiation of therapy.

- UGT inducers (e.g., rifampin) can ↓ level of canagliflozin, consider ↑ dose to 300 mg.

- Monitor digoxin levels if taking digoxin concurrently due to ↑ AUC of digoxin.

GLUCAGON-LIKE PEPTIDE-1 (GLP-1) AGONISTS

These agents are analogs of glucagon-like peptide-1 (GLP-1) which ↑ insulin secretion, ↓ glucagon secretion, slow gastric emptying, improve satiety, and may result in weight loss. These are incretin mimetics.

all subQ in abdomen, thigh or back of upper arm **

DRUG	DOSING	SAFETY/SIDE EFFECTS/MONITORING
Exenatide (Byetta) 5 mcg, 10 mcg multidose pen	Start at 5 mcg SC BID for 1 month; then 10 mcg SC BID Should be given within 60 minutes before the morning and evening meal Can be stored at room temperature for up to 30 days	**BOXED WARNING** **For All Except _Byetta_** Thyroid C-cell carcinomas seen in rats – unknown if this could happen in humans. Contraindicated in patients with a personal or family history of medullary thyroid carcinoma (MTC) or patients with Multiple Endocrine Neoplasia syndrome type 2 (MEN2)
Exenatide extended release (Bydureon) 2 mg single-dose vial and pen	2 mg SC once every 7 days May inject without regard to meals Can be stored at room temperature for up to 28 days	**WARNINGS** Pancreatitis (fatal and usually in patients with risk factors: history of pancreatitis, gallstones, alcoholism, or ↑ TGs) Use caution with moderate renal impairment, not recommended in severe impairment (CrCl < 30 mL/min) (Byetta, Bydureon) Not recommended in severe GI disease
Liraglutide (Victoza) 18 mg/3 mL multidose pen _Saxenda_ – for weight loss	Start with 0.6 mg SC daily x 1 week, then 1.2 mg SC daily x 1 week. Can ↑ to 1.8 mg SC daily, if needed. Given without regard to meals Can be stored at room temperature for up to 30 days	**SIDE EFFECTS** Nausea (primary side effect), vomiting, diarrhea, constipation, antibodies, hypoglycemia, weight loss (2-6 pounds) **MONITORING** FBG, A1C, renal function
Dulaglutide (Trulicity) 0.75 mg/0.5 mL, 1.5 mg/0.5 mL single-dose pen	Start 0.75 mg SC once weekly. Can ↑ to 1.5 mg SC once weekly Given without regard to meals Can be stored at room temperature for up to 14 days	**NOTES** ↓ A1C 0.5-1.1%; ↓ postprandial BG Pregnancy Category C Exenatide is a synthetic version of exendin, a substance found in Gila monster saliva.
Albiglutide (Tanzeum) 30 mg/0.5 mL, 50 mg/0.5 mL single-dose pen	Start 30 mg SC once weekly Can ↑ to 50 mg SC once weekly Given without regard to meals Can be stored at room temperature for up to 4 weeks Use within 8 hours of reconstitution	Can be used as mono- or combination therapy only in type 2 diabetes. Abdomen is preferred SC injection site, but can use thigh or upper arm. Count to 5 before withdrawing syringe. MedGuide required.

Handwritten margin notes (left side):
BID
60 min before AM/PM meals
6 hrs apart
CAUTION in renal imp (≠ CrCl < 30)

qwk
1x vial/pen

qd

qwk
1x pen — dula Truli

qwk
1x pen — قلم التنزيوم

wait 15 min after mixing for med to dissolve then inject

GLP-1 Agonist Drug Interactions

- These agents can reduce the amount of insulin or insulin secretagogue required. Monitor blood glucose closely after initiation of therapy.

- These drugs slow gastric emptying and can reduce the extent and rate of absorption of orally administered drugs. Caution is warranted.

Byetta

- Oral contraceptive levels may be ↓ in patients taking _Byetta_. Patients should be advised to take oral contraceptives at least 1 hour before _Byetta_ injection.

- May enhance the anticoagulant effects of warfarin, monitor INR.

GLP-1 Agonist Counseling

- Pancreatitis, or inflammation of the pancreas, can rarely happen with the use of this drug. Seek immediate medical care if you develop stomach pain that does not go away, with or without vomiting. The pain can radiate from the abdomen through to the back. Alcohol consumption should be limited.
- If you develop nausea, which is common when starting therapy, be sure to drink enough water. If you are vomiting or have diarrhea, take fluid replacement drinks and contact your healthcare provider. Nausea generally decreases over time.
- Administer (using a fresh needle) by SC injection in stomach area (preferred), upper leg (thigh), or the back of the upper arm. Count to 5 before withdrawing the syringe.
- Store in the refrigerator, most GLP-1 agonists are stable at room temperature for up to 30 days (Trulicity is stable at room temperature for up to 14 days). Never freeze.
- Keep pens and needles out of the reach of children.
- Do not store your pen with the needle attached. If the needle is left on, medication may leak from the pen and air bubbles may form in the cartridge.
- GLP-1 agonists should not be used after the expiration date printed on the pen label.

Byetta

- Inject two times each day, within 60 minutes before the morning and evening meals (or before the 2 main meals of the day, at least 6 hours apart).
- Never inject after a meal due to the risk of hypoglycemia.
- After the first month, if the nausea is manageable, the dose will be increased from 5 mcg twice daily to a more concentrated pen that provides a 10 mcg dose twice daily.
- After 30 days of use, throw away the Byetta pen, even if it is not completely empty. Mark the date when you first used your pen and the date 30 days later.

Bydureon, Victoza, Trulicity, Tanzeum

- Do not take this medication if you or any family members have had thyroid cancer, especially medullary thyroid cancer.
- While taking this medication, tell your healthcare provider if you get a lump or swelling in your neck, hoarseness, trouble swallowing, or shortness of breath. These may be symptoms of thyroid cancer.
- Victoza is taken once daily. If a dose is missed, skip the dose and resume at the next scheduled dose.
- Bydureon: Must be injected right after it is mixed when using the single dose vial.
- Bydureon, Trulicity and Tanzeum are taken once weekly. If a dose is missed, it should be taken as soon as remembered, provided the next regularly scheduled dose is at least 3 days later. Each prefilled pen comes with 1 dose of medication and should be disposed of after a single use.
- Tanzeum: Must wait 15 minutes after mixing for the medicine to dissolve before injecting.

PRAMLINTIDE

Pramlintide is a synthetic analog of the human neuroendocrine hormone, amylin. Amylin is produced by pancreatic beta cells to assist in postprandial glucose control. Amylin helps slow gastric emptying, prevents ↑ serum glucagon following a meal, and ↑ satiety. This is an amylinomimetic agent.

(handwritten, left margin): only inject prior to meals (≥ 250 kcal or ≥ 30 g of carb)

DRUG	DOSING	SAFETY/SIDE EFFECTS/MONITORING
Pramlintide *(Symlin Pen 60, SymlinPen 120)* Can use in both Types 1 and 2 DM: ↓ rapid-acting, short-acting, and fixed mix insulins by 50% when starting this drug.	Type 1: Start at 15 mcg immediately prior to meals – titrate at 15 mcg increments every 3 days up to 60 mcg if no significant nausea. Type 2: Start at 60 mcg prior to meals – can ↑ to 120 mcg if no significant nausea. Administered SC in abdomen or thigh prior to each meal (≥ 250 kcal or ≥ 30 grams of carbohydrates, if consuming less than the above quantity, skip dose). Refrigerate pens not in use. Can be stored at room temperature for up to 30 days.	**BOXED WARNING** Co-administration with insulin may induce severe hypoglycemia (usually within 3 hours following administration) **CONTRAINDICATIONS** Gastroparesis, hypoglycemia unawareness **SIDE EFFECTS** Hypoglycemia (when starting therapy, reduce meal-time insulins by 50% to ↓ risk of hypoglycemia), nausea (30%), anorexia (15%), weight loss **MONITORING** FBG, A1C **NOTES** ↓ A1C 0.5-1% Pregnancy Category C MedGuide required

Pramlintide Drug Interactions

These drugs slow gastric emptying and can reduce the extent and rate of absorption of orally administered drugs. Caution is warranted.

(handwritten left):

drugs that ↓ postprandial BG
1. meglitinides
2. α-glucosidase inhibitors
3. DPP-4 inhibitors
4. GLP-1 agonists
5. pramlinitide

(handwritten right):

A1c lowering

① metformin / sulfonylureas } ↓ 1-2%

② meglitinides / TZDs } ~ ↓ 0.5-1.5%

④ α-glucosidase / DPP-4 } ↓ 0.5-0.8%

⑤ colesevelam / bromocriptine } ↓ 0.5%

③ GLP-1 agonists - ↓ 0.5-1.1%
pramlinitide - ↓ 0.5-1%

SGLT2 inhibitors - ↓ 0.7-1%

BILE ACID BINDING RESINS

Resins work by binding bile, blocking reabsorption. Bile is produced from cholesterol and cholesterol levels decrease. The mechanism by which colesevelam improves glycemic control in unknown.

DRUG	DOSING	SAFETY/SIDE EFFECTS/MONITORING
Colesevelam *(Welchol)* 625 mg tabs or 3.75 gram and 1.875 gram packets for oral suspension Also approved for hyperlipidemia	*Welchol* is taken as a 3.75 gram daily dose: 6 tablets daily or 3 tablets BID or 3.75 gram packet daily or 1.875 gram packet BID Tablets need to be taken with a meal and liquid Powder packets need to be dissolved in 4-8 oz of liquid and taken with a meal	**CONTRAINDICATIONS** History of bowel obstruction, TG > 500 mg/dL, history hypertriglyceridemia-induced pancreatitis **SIDE EFFECTS** Constipation (> 10%), dyspepsia, nausea, bloating. Can ↑ TGs (~5%) **MONITORING** FBG, A1C, LDL, TG **NOTES** ↓ A1C 0.5% Pregnancy Category B ↓ absorption of other drugs; see below *Welchol* has less GI SEs than the other agents in this class that are used for lipid-lowering

Handwritten note: take w/ food! qd or BID dosing

Colesevelam Drug Interactions

- The following medications should be taken 4 hours prior to colesevelam: cyclosporine, glimepiride, glipizide, glyburide, levothyroxine, olmesartan, phenytoin and oral contraceptives containing ethinyl estradiol + norethindrone.

- Colesevelam ↑ levels of metformin when coadministered with metformin extended release.

- With warfarin, monitor INR frequently during initiation and after dose change.

Colesevelam Counseling

- This drug may cause you to feel constipated. Talk to your pharmacist to see if you need a laxative (senna) or stool softener (docusate). Be sure to drink enough water while taking this medication.

- Take this medication at a different time than your multivitamin because *Welchol* may ↓ absorption of vitamins A, D, E, and K.

BROMOCRIPTINE

Bromocriptine is indicated as an adjunct to diet and exercise to improve glycemic control in adults with type 2 diabetes. It is a dopamine agonist but it improves glycemic control by working in the CNS to ↓ insulin resistance.

DRUG	DOSING	SAFETY/SIDE EFFECTS/MONITORING
Bromocriptine (*Cycloset*) *Parlodel* (higher dose) is indicated for hyperprolactinemia, Acromegaly, Parkinson Disease	Start 0.8 mg daily within 2 hours of waking, take with food to ↓ nausea. Titrate in 0.8 mg increments weekly to usual dose of 1.6-4.8 mg daily. If a dose is missed, skip it and take at next scheduled dose.	**CONTRAINDICATIONS** Syncopal migraines, breastfeeding (*Cycloset*), uncontrolled hypertension, pregnancy, postpartum women with hx of CAD or other severe CVD conditions (*Parlodel*) **SIDE EFFECTS** Nausea, dizziness due to orthostasis (requires slow dose titration), fatigue, headache, vomiting, rhinitis, psychiatric effects, ↓ prolactin levels **MONITORING** FBG, A1C **NOTES** ↓ A1C by 0.5% Pregnancy Category B

Bromocriptine Drug Interactions

- Bromocriptine is major CYP 3A4 substrate, inducers or inhibitors of 3A4 can lower or raise the bromocriptine concentration.
- Do not use with other ergot medications. May ↑ ergot-related side effects or reduce ergot effectiveness for migraines if co-administered within 6 hours of ergot-related drug.
- Monitor for hypoglycemia if patient is using a sulfonylurea – may need dose adjustment.

U-500 INSULIN
Currently, all insulins have a concentration of 100 units/mL, except *Humulin R* U-500 which has a concentration of 500 units/mL. This concentration of insulin is for patients requiring a large volume of insulin (≥ 200 units/day). *Humulin R* U-500 has an onset of action of 30 minutes, has a peak similar to U-100 regular insulin, and has a relatively long duration of action (up to 24 hours after a single dose) compared to U-100 regular insulin. The prescribed dose of *Humulin R* U-500 should be expressed in actual units of *Humulin R* U-500 along with corresponding markings on the syringe the patient is using [e.g., 200 units (0.4 mL)]. ISMP recommends the use of tuberculin syringes when administering *Humulin R* U-500 insulin. *Humulin R* U-500 is available in 20 mL vials.

INSULIN

Insulin is a hormone that muscle and adipose tissue require for glucose uptake. Insulin also has a role in regulating fat storage and inhibits the breakdown of fat for energy. Commercially available insulins differ in their onset and duration of action. All insulins have a concentration of 100 units/mL, except *Humulin R* U-500 (see box). There are no U-500 syringes therefore patients must measure the dose with a tuberculin syringe (preferred) or a U-100 syringe. Patients should convert the dose in "syringe units". A conversion chart should always be used when administering U-500 with the syringe type the patient is using.

Rapid-acting Insulin — *best for controlling postprandial BG*

Aspart *(NovoLOG, NovoLOG FlexPen)*, **Glulisine** *(Apidra, Apidra SoloStar)*, **Lispro** *(HumaLOG, HumaLOG KwikPen)*

Rapid-acting insulins are administered 15 minutes prior, just before, or right after a meal. They are designed to last for an entire meal (3-5 hours). In some patients they last an hour or two longer. The duration of action is shorter than regular insulin.

Rapid-acting insulin is dosed for the amount of carbohydrates in a meal, or is given on a fixed regimen for typical-sized meals. These insulins are clear in appearance and can be mixed with NPH insulin, but are usually given by itself with meals or in mixes with a longer-acting insulin. Rapid acting (and short-acting) insulins come in pre-filled injection syringe pens and in 10 mL vials, and are used in insulin pumps and sliding scales in hospitals.

Regular or Short-acting Insulin

Regular insulin *(HumuLIN R, NovoLIN R)* – Injectable

Regular insulin should be injected 30 minutes before a meal. The onset of action is at least 30 minutes. Regular insulin lasts around 6-10 hours. Regular insulin is clear, comes in pens and vials, and in mixes with intermediate acting insulin (N, NPH).

Regular insulin *(Afrezza)* – Inhaled

Afrezza is a regular insulin formulated for inhalation. It is available as 4 units or 8 units single-use cartridges and has onset within 15 minutes and a duration of action of 3-5 hours. *Afrezza* comes in a small inhaler with doses in a cartridge. Patients who smoke or have lung disease (COPD/asthma) should not use this medication (boxed warning). Pulmonary function (FEV1) should be assessed at baseline, after 6 months of therapy, and annually. Side effects include hypoglycemia, cough and throat pain or irritation.

Baseline, Basal or Intermediate Insulin

NPH insulin or Intermediate insulin *(HumuLIN N, NovoLIN N)*

NPH insulin is typically given once or twice daily. The onset of action is 1-2 hours, with a peak of 4-8 hours, and a duration of up to 24 hours. The variable pharmacokinetics of NPH insulin between patients make it more difficult to predict glycemic response, and the insulin usually peaks during mid-afternoon (when dosed in the morning) and early morning hours (when dosed in the evening) when the patient is not eating. It is not a good match for physiological insulin, but is used by some patients because it can be mixed with regular insulin (thus minimizing the injections needed per day) and is less costly. NPH insulin is cloudy, and all mixed insulin preparations containing protamine are cloudy. It comes in pens, vials, and in mixes.

Long-acting Insulin

clear! controls FPG, not prandial!

Insulin Detemir *(Levemir, Levemir FlexTouch)*, **Insulin Glargine** *(Lantus, Lantus SoloStar)*

The baseline insulins are dosed once or twice daily. The onset and duration is patient specific, but generally is ~1-2 hours. Glargine has a duration of action of ~24 hours while detemir lasts 12-24 hours. These insulins do not peak, therefore there is less risk of hypoglycemia. If hypoglycemia occurs, it can last a long time and may require retreatment. Detemir and glargine should not be mixed with other insulins in the same syringe.

Insulin Side Effects

Injectable insulins may cause hypoglycemia, weight gain, lipodystrophy, and local skin reactions (to avoid, rotate the injection site). Insulin glargine *(Lantus)* may sting a little when injecting. Inhaled insulin may cause hypoglycemia, cough and throat pain or irritation. Insulin will ↓ K⁺ and is used acutely to manage hyperkalemia.

Mixing Insulins & Insulin Mixes

NPH can be mixed with regular and rapid acting insulins. Some patients mix their own insulins to provide specific doses. This is done by first drawing up the clear insulin into a syringe (regular or rapid-acting insulin) and then drawing up the cloudy insulin (NPH). It may be helpful to remember that "clear before cloudy" is alphabetical. There are some commercial preparations of pre-mixed insulins as well. These include either NPH with regular, or aspart protamine or lispro protamine with the rapid-action insulin. The pre-mixed insulins are also cloudy because they contain protamine, which prolongs the duration of action. They come in varying proportions, including 70/30, 75/25 and 50/50. In a mix, the first number is the percentage of the longer-acting intermediate insulin (N, also written as NPH, or aspart protamine or lispro protamine), followed by the percentage of the shorter-acting insulin (R, for regular, or rapid-acting aspart or lispro). *Humulin* 70/30 contains 70% NPH and 30% regular insulin. They are named after the regular or rapid-acting insulin (example: *Novolog* 70/30 contains 70% insulin aspart protamine and 30% insulin aspart). Pre-mixed insulins are available in vials and pens.

Insulin Vials, Pens, and Pumps

Most insulin vials contain 10 mL. *Humulin R* U-100 insulin comes in both 3 mL and 10 mL vials. *Humulin R* U-500 insulin comes in a 20 mL vial. Most insulin pen cartridges contain 3 mL. In general, pens are easier to use and cause fewer dosing errors if used correctly. They are easier to use for patients with hand tremor, arthritis or vision difficulty. Insulin pumps are devices that consist of a pump, insulin reservoir, tubing, and cannula. The devices can be programmed to mimic the insulin secretion of the pancreas. Insulin pumps infuse a basal rate of insulin throughout the day, and boluses of insulin are taken when the patient eats. The pumps are very small devices (about the size of a deck of cards or smaller) and can use regular or rapid-acting insulins. Pumps are most often used by type 1 patients but are increasingly used by type 2 patients. Candidates for insulin pumps must be receiving multiple daily doses of insulin, be experienced in carbohydrate counting, be highly motivated and understand how to operate the pump and will test their blood sugar frequently throughout the day. Insulin pumps are not appropriate for newly diagnosed patients.

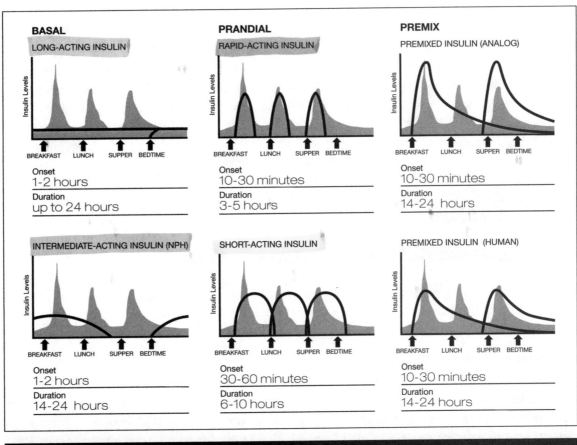

INSULIN	ONSET	PEAK	DURATION
Rapid-acting Insulin _ANALOGS_			
Insulin aspart (*NovoLOG, NovoLOG FlexPen*) **Insulin glulisine** (*Apidra, Apidra SoloStar*) **Insulin lispro** (*HumaLOG, HumaLOG KwikPen*)	10-30 minutes	0.5-2.5 hours	3-5 hours
Short-acting Insulin (OTC) _no Rx required_			
Regular (*HumuLIN R, NovoLIN R*) _Afrezza_	30-60 minutes ~ 15 min	1-3.5 hours	6-10 hours 3-5 hrs
Intermediate-acting Insulin (OTC) _no Rx required_			
NPH (*HumuLIN N, NovoLIN N*)	1-2 hours	4-8 hours	14-24 hours
Insulin NPH/insulin regular (*HumuLIN 70/30, NovoLIN 70/30*)	30 minutes	2-12 hours	14-24 hours
Long-acting Insulin _ANALOGS_			_12-24 hrs (p. 474 top)?_
Insulin detemir (*Levemir, Levemir FlexTouch*)	1-2 hours	–	14-24 hours
Insulin glargine (*Lantus, Lantus SoloStar*)	1-2 hours	–	24 hours

Handwritten margin notes:
- admin 15 min prior, just before or right after meal
- 30 min before meal (AM / PM – BID)

INSULIN DOSING

Initiating Insulin Therapy for Patients with Type 1 Diabetes

Most people with type 1 diabetes should be treated with pumps or multiple daily injections of insulin (3-4 injections/day of basal and prandial insulin). Patients should be educated on matching the prandial insulin dose to carbohydrate intake, premeal blood glucose and anticipated activity. Insulin analogs are preferred to reduce hypoglycemia risk and mimic the physiologic pattern of the insulin made by our body. Insulin analogs include rapid-acting and basal insulins. Patients with type 1 diabetes should be screened for other autoimmune disorders (thyroid disorders, vitamin B12 deficiency, celiac disease). Insulin should be started at a total daily dose (TDD) of 0.6 units/kg/day. If using rapid-acting and basal insulins, known as a basal-bolus strategy (preferred as these are insulin analogs), 50% of the TDD is used as the basal insulin dose and 50% of the TDD is used as the rapid-acting (bolus) insulin. The bolus insulin is divided evenly among the 3 meals (or can give more for a larger meal or less for a smaller meal). If using NPH and regular insulins, take ⅔ of the TDD as the intermediate-acting (NPH) dose and ⅓ as the regular insulin dose. These are generally dosed twice daily, 30 minutes prior to breakfast and dinner (evening meal).

Insulin-to-Carbohydrate Ratio (ICR)

Patients taking meal time insulin may be counting carbohydrates to better adjust the insulin dose for that meal and every person responds differently to insulin (some are more sensitive and some are less sensitive to insulin's effects). An insulin-to-carbohydrate ratio (ICR) is patient specific and can be calculated by the Rule of 500 (for rapid-acting insulins) or Rule of 450 (for regular insulin):

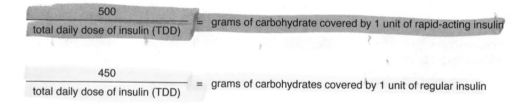

$$\frac{500}{\text{total daily dose of insulin (TDD)}} = \text{grams of carbohydrate covered by 1 unit of rapid-acting insulin}$$

$$\frac{450}{\text{total daily dose of insulin (TDD)}} = \text{grams of carbohydrates covered by 1 unit of regular insulin}$$

Correction Factor and Correction Dose

Patients with diabetes should know how to calculate their correction dose, which is the amount of additional insulin needed to keep their blood glucose in range. For example, a patient is going to a wedding and wants to enjoy a piece of cake. Knowing how to calculate a correction dose will allow the patient to accurately dose the "additional" insulin needed for the extra carbohydrate load. The amount of insulin would be added to the dose they would normally take for that meal.

Correction Factor – 1,800 Rule (Rapid-acting Insulin)

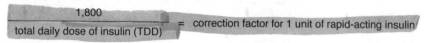

$$\frac{1,800}{\text{total daily dose of insulin (TDD)}} = \text{correction factor for 1 unit of rapid-acting insulin}$$

Correction Factor – 1,500 Rule (Regular Insulin)

$$\frac{1,500}{\text{total daily dose of insulin (TDD)}} = \text{correction factor for 1 unit of regular insulin}$$

Correction Dose

$$\frac{(\text{Blood glucose now}) - (\text{target blood glucose})}{\text{correction factor}} = \text{correction dose}$$

Initiation and Adjustment of Insulin for Patients with Type 2 Diabetes

ghs NPH
PM or AM Lantus
OR *Levemir*
10 units or 0.2 units/kg

✓ FPG qd
↑ by 2 units q3d
(if FPG > 180,
may ↑ by 4 units
q3d)

Start with bedtime intermediate-acting insulin or bedtime or morning long-acting insulin (can initiate with 10 units or 0.2 units per kg)

Check fasting glucose (fingerstick), usually daily, and increase dose as needed, typically by 2 units every 3 days until fasting levels are consistently in target range (70-130 mg/dL). Can increase dose in larger increments, e.g., by 4 units every 3 days, if fasting glucose is > 180 mg/dL

A1C ≥ 7% after 2-3 months

No / **Yes**

If hypoglycemia occurs, or fasting glucose level < 70 mg/dL, reduce bedtime dose by 4 units or 10% – whichever is greater

If fasting BG is in target range (70-130 mg/dL), check BG before lunch, dinner, and bed. Depending on BG results, add second injection as below. Can usually begin with ~4 units and adjust by 2 units every 3 days until BG is in range

Continue regimen. Check A1C every 3 months

Pre-lunch BG out of range: add rapid-acting insulin at breakfast

Pre-dinner BG out of range: add NPH insulin at breakfast or rapid-acting at lunch

Pre-bed BG out of range: add rapid acting insulin at dinner

A1C ≥ 7% after 3 months

Yes

Recheck pre-meal BG levels and if out of range, may need to add another injection. If A1C continues to be out of range, check 2 hour postprandial levels and adjust preprandial rapid-acting insulin

Insulin Conversions*

INSULIN TYPE	CONVERSION
NPH daily to glargine	1:1
NPH BID to glargine	Reduce daily dose by 20%
NPH to detemir	1:1
Glargine to detemir (or vice versa)	1:1
Regular to rapid (or vice versa)	1:1
Premixed to premixed	1:1 if the percent mixture is same/similar (e.g. 70/30 to 75/25 or 50/50 to 50/50)

* adjustment if BG is under good control (otherwise, may increase dose if warranted)

Insulin Stability

For all insulins: Discard insulin if it is frozen, discolored, or contains particulates. If needle is attached for use, discard used needle after use. Do not store under direct sunlight or heat. All insulins should be refrigerated when not in-use. If refrigerated and unopened, the insulin is stable until the expiration date on label. Stability of the different insulins at room temperature, once in-use, is listed in the box.

SLIDING SCALE EXAMPLE	
Blood Sugar Reading (mg/dL)	**Instruction**
BS < 60	Hold insulin; contact MD
150-200	Give 2 units of insulin
201-250	Give 4 units of insulin
251-300	Give 6 units of insulin
301-350	Give 8 units of insulin
351-400	Give 10 units of insulin
401-450	Call MD

STABILITY AT ROOM TEMP WHEN IN USE

Rapid-Acting Insulin

Apidra, Humalog, Novolog (vials and pens)	28 days

Regular Insulin

Humulin R (U-100, U-500 vial)	31 days
Novolin R (U-100 vial)	42 days

NPH Insulin

Humulin N (vial)	31 days
Humulin N and Novolin N (pens)	14 days
Novolin N (vial)	42 days

Mixed Insulin

Humalog 50/50, 75/25, Novolog 70/30 (vials)	28 days
Humulin 70/30 (vial)	31 days
Humalog 50/50, 75/25 and Humulin 70/30 (pens)	10 days
Novolin 70/30 (vial)	42 days
Novolog 70/30 (pen)	14 days

Long-Acting Insulin and Other Injectables

Lantus (vials and pens)	28 days
Levemir (vials and pens)	42 days
Byetta	30 days
Bydureon (vials) (pen should be refrigerated until 15 minutes before injection)	28 days
Victoza	30 days
Symlin (pen)	30 days
Trulicity (pen)	14 days
Tanzeum (pen)	4 weeks

[handwritten note: all Novolin products 42 days + Levemir]

Hospitalized Patients

Hospitalized patients on insulin should have the BG maintained between 140-180 mg/dL. More stringent goals may be appropriate for select patients. Instead of a sliding scale to control the BG, the correction dose is meant to "fine tune" the insulin regimen. A more physiological insulin regimen including basal, prandial and correctional insulin is preferred over sliding scales, however many hospitals currently use sliding scales as the sole method to control BG. This is against AACE and ADA recommendations.

Insulin Administration

- Keep unused vials or cartridges in the refrigerator. Vials or pens in current use are good at room temperature for a limited time. Please see stability information above.

- Wash hands and lay out all supplies.

- Check insulin for any discoloration, crystals, or lumps.

- If insulin is a suspension, roll bottle gently between hands (do not shake). If it is a pen, invert 4-5 times.

- Clean injection site area of the skin and wipe the top of the insulin vial with an alcohol swab.

- Inject an equal volume of air into the vial that is going to be taken out so not to create negative pressure in the vial. Make sure to limit the bubbles in the syringe.

- The abdomen is the preferred injection site. For alternate sites, see the diagram on the following page. Inject at least two fingers away from the belly button.

- Alternate injection sites around the abdomen regularly to prevent inflammation and atrophy.

- To inject subcutaneously, gently pinch a 2 inch portion of skin and fat between your thumb and first finger and insert the needle all the way at a 90 degree (or 45 degree if patient is thin). If using a syringe, inject insulin and remove needle slowly. If using an insulin pen, inject insulin and count 5 - 10 seconds before removing the needle.

- Properly dispose needles or entire syringes in a sharps container. These containers can be brought to any proper disposal site (e.g., public health clinic or local needle exchange). Ask the local health department for guidelines or check out the website www.safeneedledisposal.org.

Choosing the correct syringe is important. Choose the smallest syringe that will hold the dose. The smaller the syringe barrel, the easier it is to read the scale markings in order to draw up an accurate dose. This is also helpful for diabetes patients with vision problems. If the patient's largest dose is close to the maximum syringe capacity, choose the next syringe size up.

[lower gauge (thicker needle) ⇒↑pain] (or thinner)
insulin syringes have thin needles 25 or 29 G

Syringe size/volume

- If injecting < 30 units of insulin, use a 0.3 mL syringe (markings in 1 unit increments)

- If injecting 30-49 units of insulin, use a 0.5 mL syringe (markings in 1 unit increments)

- If injecting ≥ 50 units of insulin, use a 1 mL syringe (markings in 2 unit increments; holds up to 100 units)

Needle Length

- ½" (12.7 mm), ⁵⁄₁₆" (8 mm), ³⁄₁₆" (5 mm), ⁵⁄₃₂" (4 mm)

- Use longer needles for obese patients and if back leakage of insulin is a problem.

- Many users feel that shorter needles are more comfortable. Use ½" needles for obese patients and if back leakage of insulin is a problem.

Insulin Injection Sites

Insulin absorption is fastest and most predictable when injected into the abdomen followed by the posterior upper arm, superior buttocks area, and lateral thigh area. Because of these variations, the injections should be rotated within a specific region to limit fluctuations in blood glucose.

* abdomen > outer upper arm > upper buttocks > lateral thigh
* rotate WITHIN specific region to ↓ fluctuations

Hypoglycemia

Normal fasting blood glucose in a person without diabetes is 70-99 mg/dL. Hypoglycemia occurs when blood glucose falls below this level, or < 70 mg/dL. The lower the level, the more symptomatic the patient. At a blood glucose < 20 mg/dL, seizures, coma and death can occur.

Diabetes Drugs That Cause Hypoglycemia

Insulin is the #1 drug that can cause hypoglycemia. Drugs that make the body secrete more insulin such as sulfonylureas and meglitinides (insulin secretagogues) are also high-risk for causing hypoglycemia. Pramlintide is high risk since it is used concurrently (but injected separately) with insulin at mealtimes. Hypoglycemia is a serious risk, especially if meal-time insulin is not reduced appropriately. Look at the patient case for combination products which may be contain a sulfonylurea such as *Glucovance* (metformin + glyburide).

The GLP-1 agonists, DPP-4 inhibitors, thiazolidinediones and SGLT2 inhibitors can ↑ the risk of hypoglycemia, primarily in patients using a hypoglycemic agent (insulin or an insulin secretagogue). Concurrent use may necessitate a dose reduction due to hypoglycemic risk. Other drugs may list hypoglycemia as possible, but it is generally due to the medical condition rather than the agent. These are isolated cases.

Hypoglycemic Symptoms

Hypoglycemic symptoms include dizziness, headache, anxiety, shakiness, diaphoresis (sweating), excessive hunger, confusion, clumsy or jerky movements, tremors, palpitations or fast heart rate, and blurred vision.

Beta-blockers can mask the symptoms of shakiness, palpitations, and anxiety. However, sweating or hunger is not masked. That is why the beta-blocker propranolol is used for stage fright. This is most notable with the non-cardioselective agents such as carteolol, carvedilol, propranolol and others. The cardioselective beta-blockers (atenolol, metoprolol) are used more commonly.

Hypoglycemia Treatment

Recommended treatment of hypoglycemia in a conscious individual is 15-20 g of glucose, although any form of carbohydrate that contains glucose may be used including: ½ cup (4 oz) of any juice or regular (non-diet) soda, 1 cup (8 oz) milk, 1 tablespoon of sugar or honey, 2 tablespoons of raisins, 4-5 saltine crackers, 3 or 4 glucose tabs, or 1 serving of glucose gel. The blood glucose should be retested 15 minutes after treatment to see if it has reached a safe level. If the level still shows continued hypoglycemia, the treatment should be repeated. Once the blood glucose returns to normal, the patient should eat a meal (if close to meal-time), or a reasonable snack, to prevent recurrence. Patients often overeat when the blood glucose is low, which causes unnecessary weight gain

[handwritten margin note:] 15-20g glucose / ½ cup (4oz) juice / regular soda / 1 cup (8oz) milk / 1 tbs sugar/honey / 2 tbs raisins / 4-5 crackers / 3-4 glucose tabs / 1 serving glu gel

Glucagon *[handwritten:] secreted by α cells of pancreas (β cells ⇒ insulin, amylin)*

Glucagon should be prescribed for all patients at significant risk of severe hypoglycemia, and caregivers and family members should be instructed on its administration. Glucagon administration is not limited to health care professionals. Glucagon *(GlucaGen)* is only used

[handwritten:] inject into buttock, arm or thigh / can be readministered

if the patient is unconscious or not conscious enough to self-treat the hypoglycemia. If using glucagon, place patient in lateral recumbent position (on side) to protect airway and prevent choking when consciousness returns. A fast infusion rate will increase nausea. Once conscious, administer carbohydrate source. Glucagon 1 mg is given by SC, IM, or IV injection, or glucose can be given intravenously (Dextrose 25%, Dextrose 50%). The patient does not need to be unconscious to receive glucose intravenously.

After treating the low blood glucose, check the BG in 15 minutes. If the BG < 70 mg/dL or if the patient is still symptomatic, repeat the treatment and check the BG again in 15 minutes. All episodes of hypoglycemia are dangerous and should be reported to the physician. Hypoglycemia unawareness or one or more episodes of severe hypoglycemia should trigger re-evaluation of the treatment regimen.

Self-Monitoring Blood Glucose (SMBG)

This is important to prevent hypo- and hyperglycemia, and complications. Patients on multiple-dose insulin (MDI) or insulin pump therapy should do SMBG at least prior to meals and snacks, occasionally post-prandial, at bedtime, prior to exercise, when they suspect low

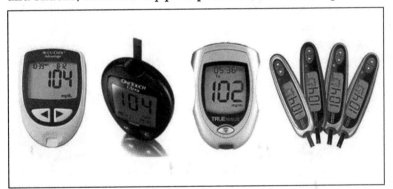

blood sugar, after treating low blood sugar until they are normoglycemic, and prior to critical tasks such as driving. For patients using less frequent insulin injections, non-insulin therapies or medical nutrition therapy, SMBG may be useful as a guide to the success of therapy.

Various Glucose Meters

Preparing to Test

- Some machines require calibration before first use, if a new package of strips is opened, machine is left in extreme conditions, machine is dropped, or if the level does not match how the patient is feeling.
- Read the test strip packaging to make sure the strips are compatible with the glucose meter.
- Do not use test strips from a damaged or expired bottle.
- Enter in the correct calibration code, if required.
- Thoroughly wash hands vigorously with warm water and mild soap to clean the site and increase circulation at the fingertip.
- Dry hands thoroughly since water can affect the blood sample and create an error or false reading.
- Allow arm to hang down at the side of the body for 30 seconds so blood can pool into the fingertips.

Testing Blood Glucose

- In order to minimize pain, lance the finger on the side where there are fewer nerves, instead of on the finger pads. Keep hand below the level of the heart.

- Make sure there is a large enough drop of blood as directed by the meter. Allow the blood to flow freely and do (not) squeeze the finger.

- Use a whole test strip for each test.

- Insert test strip completely into the glucose meter.

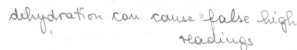

dehydration can cause false high readings

Maintaining Blood Glucose Meter

- Clean meter regularly.

- Test meter regularly with control solution.

- Store meter and supplies properly, away from heat and humidity.

- Keep extra batteries charged and ready.

- Close the lid of the strips container after every use, as air and moisture can destroy the strips and affect results.

best used for fasting readings ??

Notes on Alternative Site Testing

- Select meters are approved for testing on other areas, such as the upper arm, forearm, base of thumb, or thigh. *Calves*

- With regards to testing from alternate areas, measurements may be different, such as after meals when blood glucose levels are changing rapidly. A finger may have faster blood flow than other areas.

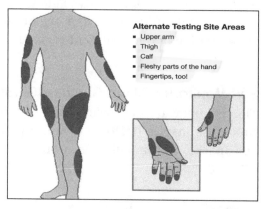

Alternate Testing Site Areas
- Upper arm
- Thigh
- Calf
- Fleshy parts of the hand
- Fingertips, too!

Alternative Glucose Testing Sites

Diabetic Ketoacidosis (DKA) & Hyperglycemia Hyperosmolar State (HHS)

DKA   *TG and a.a. used for → free fatty acids insulin→ no ketones (HHS) glucagon→ ketones (DKA)*

Diabetic ketoacidosis (DKA) is a hyperglycemic crisis most commonly presenting in type 1 and rarely in type 2 diabetes. DKA occurs due to insulin non-compliance (ran out, lost/homeless, refused to take), sub-therapeutic insulin dose (due to a stressor, such as infection, MI or trauma), or as the initial presentation in a type 1 patient. Ketones are present because triglycerides and amino acids are used for energy, which produces free fatty acids (FFAs). Glucagon converts the FFAs into ketones. Normally, insulin prevents this conversion but, in DKA, insulin is absent.

- DKA Symptoms: BG > 250 mg/dL, ketones (on lab report, or picked up as "fruity" breath), with an anion gap metabolic acidosis (arterial pH < 7.35, anion gap > 12).

- DKA Treatment: NS, followed by ½ NS, potassium replacement, insulin and occasionally sodium bicarbonate.   *1. NS 2. ½ NS + sometimes bicarb 3. K+ replacement 4. insulin*

HHS

Hyperglycemia hyperosmolar state (HHS) is a hyperglycemic crisis that most often occurs in type 2 and is due to some type of severe stress. Serum ketones would be negligible or not present because the type 2 patient has enough insulin to suppress ketogenesis. The blood glucose is usually much higher at presentation because acidosis is (not) present and the patient can endure the symptoms longer.

- Symptoms: BG > 600 mg/dL, high serum osmolality > 320 mOsm/L, extreme dehydration, altered consciousness (confusion, dizziness), pH > 7.3, elevated bicarbonate > 18 mEq/L, risk of seizures.

- Treatment: NS and insulin.   *1. NS 2. insulin*

PRACTICE CASE

IB is a 44 y/o Hispanic female who is a new patient to the Family Medicine Clinic. She has a past medical history of dyslipidemia, depression and type 2 diabetes. Her mother, father and brother all have diabetes. Her father is on dialysis due to diabetes and uncontrolled hypertension. IB is very concerned about her family history and wants to "control my sugars better." She has attended a diabetes education class, met with a dietitian, and joined a local exercise club. She has been to a podiatrist in the last month to have her feet checked. She has lost some sensation in both feet, but does not have any open cracks or wounds. Her annual vision exam was normal. Her only surgical history involved a caesarean section, with sterilization procedure, after the birth of her third child. She does not smoke or drink.

Allergies: NKDA

Medications:
Glumetza 1000 mg x 2 PO daily with dinner
Zocor 20 mg PO QHS
Niaspan 1000 mg x 2 PO QHS
Cymbalta 30 mg PO BID
Zoloft 100 mg PO daily
Multivitamin 1 daily

Vitals:
Visit Date: Dec. 1, 2014:
BP: 134/74 mmHg HR: 89 BPM RR: 15 BPM Temp: 98.8°F Pain: 0/10

Visit Date: Jan. 15, 2015:
Height: 5'3" Weight: 172 pounds BMI: 30
BP: 136/78 mmHg HR: 85 BPM RR: 14 BPM Temp: 98.2°F Pain: 1/10

Labs:

Na (mEq/L) = 139 (135 - 145)	WBC (cells/mm^3) = 9.1 (4 - 11 x 10^3)
K (mEq/L) = 4.2 (3.5 - 5)	Hgb (g/dL) = 13.1 (13.5 - 18 male, 12 - 16 female)
Cl (mEq/L) = 101 (95 - 103)	
HCO$_3$ (mEq/L) = 28 (24 - 30)	Hct (%) = 40 (38 - 50 male, 36 - 46 female)
BUN (mg/dL) = 12 (7 - 20)	
SCr (mg/dL) = 0.8 (0.6 - 1.3)	Plt (cells/mm^3) = 410 (150 - 450 x 10^3)
Glucose (mg/dL) = 143 (100 - 125)	AST (IU/L) = 22 (8 - 48)
Ca (mg/dL) = 9.5 (8.5 - 10.5)	ALT (IU/L) = 16 (7 - 55)
Mg (mEq/L) = 1.8 (1.3 - 2.1)	Albumin (g/dL) = 4.1 (3.5 - 5)
PO$_4$ (mg/dL) = 3.2 (2.3 - 4.7)	A1C (%) = 8.2

Lipid panel* (mg/dL): TC = 150, HDL = 55, LDL = 68, TG = 131
*Clinicians should refer to guidelines for goals of dyslipidemia management.

Tests:
Urinalysis: negative for albumin and ketones
Adjust/optimize pharmacotherapy and lifestyle to achieve A1C and glucose goals.

Questions

1. Based on the patient's current A1C, choose the correct statement:

    a. The A1C is elevated; it should be less than 7%, according to the ADA guidelines.

    b. The A1C is elevated; it should be less than 5%, according to the ADA guidelines.

    c. The A1C is well-controlled.

    d. The A1C is a little high, but is acceptable due to her age.

    e. None of the above.

2. Which of the following risk factors for diabetes are present in this patient? (Select **ALL** That Apply.)

    a. Ethnicity

    b. Obese

    c. Family history

    d. Low physical activity

    e. Number of births

3. Which lifestyle modification still needs to be discussed with IB?

    a. Exercise

    b. Weight loss

    c. Smoking cessation

    d. A and C

    e. None of the above

4. Which microvascular complication of diabetes is present in this patient?

    a. Retinopathy

    b. Nephropathy

    c. Peripheral neuropathy

    d. A and B only

    e. All of the above

5. IB has brought her fasting blood glucose recordings into the clinic. In the morning before breakfast, she has recorded a range of 135-143 mg/dL. Her postprandial blood glucose (after lunch) recordings have a range of 190-236 mg/dL. Using the American Diabetes Association (ADA) recommendations for blood glucose control, choose the correct statement:

    a. Her morning fasting blood glucose levels are controlled.

    b. Her morning fasting blood glucose levels are not controlled.

    c. Her lunch time postprandial blood glucose levels are not controlled.

    d. A and C

    e. B and C

6. According to the ADA guidelines, which of the following medications should be started for the patient's blood pressure?

    a. Enalapril

    b. Furosemide

    c. Losartan

    d. A or C

    e. No medication is necessary

7. What immunizations should IB receive?

    a. Influenza

    b. Hepatitis A

    c. Pneumococcal

    d. A and C

    e. A, B and C

8. Per the ADA guidelines, which therapy should be added to treat IB's diabetes?

    a. Bromocriptine

    b. Pramlintide

    c. Glimepiride

    d. Acarbose

    e. Cholestyramine

9. Which mechanism of action describes IB's current diabetes therapy?

    a. Increases pancreatic insulin secretion

    b. Decreases hepatic glucose output

    c. Replaces endogenous insulin

    d. Enhances the action of incretins

    e. Alpha glucosidase inhibitor

preprandial 70-130

postprandial < 180

Questions 10-13 do not apply to the case.

10. A patient currently uses 30 units of *Lantus* daily and 10 units of *Humalog* with breakfast, lunch, and dinner. She is going to be started on pramlinitide and needs to be counseled on how to adjust her dose of insulin. Select the correct adjustments.

    a. Reduce *Lantus* to 15 units and *Humalog* to 5 units with meals
    b. Reduce *Lantus* to 10 units and *Humalog* to 5 units with meals
    c. Reduce *Lantus* to 15 units and keep *Humalog* at 10 units with meals
    d. Do not adjust *Lantus* and reduce *Humalog* to 5 units with meals
    e. Do not adjust *Lantus* or *Humalog*

11. A patient is taking *Novolog Mix* 70/30, 10 units twice a day. How many units of insulin aspart does the patient inject in the morning?

    a. 20 units
    b. 10 units
    c. 7 units
    d. 6 units
    e. 3 units

12. Which of the following insulins has the shortest duration?

    a. Glulisine
    b. Detemir
    c. Regular
    d. Glargine
    e. NPH

13. A patient is prescribed *Glucovance*. What are the individual components?

    a. Metformin/glyburide
    b. Metformin/pioglitazone
    c. Metformin/sitagliptin
    d. Metformin/repaglinide
    e. Metformin/glipizide

Answers

1-a, 2-a,b,c,d, 3-b, 4-c, 5-e, 6-e, 7-d, 8-c, 9-b, 10-d, 11-e, 12-a, 13-a.

AUTOIMMUNE CONDITIONS:
RA, SLE, MS, RAYNAUD'S, CELIAC DISEASE, SJÖGREN'S SYNDROME & PSORIASIS

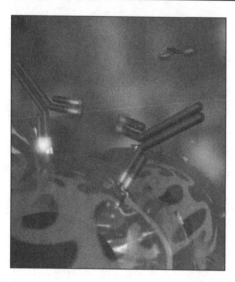

BACKGROUND

Autoimmune diseases are illnesses that occur when the body's tissues are attacked by the person's own immune system. The immune system is a complex organization of cells and antibodies designed to "seek and destroy" invaders of the body, particularly infections.

Rheumatoid arthritis (RA), systemic lupus erythematosus (SLE), multiple sclerosis (MS), celiac disease, Sjögren's syndrome, Raynaud's and psoriasis are discussed in this chapter. Other autoimmune diseases covered elsewhere in the book include type 1 diabetes (discussed in the Diabetes chapter), Hashimoto's thyroiditis and Graves disease (discussed in the Thyroid chapter).

Vaccination in Autoimmune Disease

Patients can be immune (or immuno-) compromised due to any one of the following:

- Disease states which destroy key components of the immune response (primarily, HIV patients with a CD4 T lymphocyte count < 200 cells/microliter);

- Steroids (oral or injectable only) taken 14 days or longer at a dose of either 2 mg/kg/day or 20 mg prednisone, or prednisone-equivalent dose;

- Oncology treatments that destroy white blood cells;

- Transplant drugs that depress the immune system;

- Asplenia (lack of a functioning spleen) increases the risk for certain types of infections;

- And, the use of the strong immune suppressants.

LABS THAT MAY BE ELEVATED WITH AUTOIMMUNE DISEASE

C-reactive protein (CRP)

Erythrocyte sedimentation rate (ESR)

Rheumatoid factor (RF)

Anti-nuclear antibodies (ANA)

These labs can be elevated by a number of diseases, both autoimmune and not; therefore, an abnormality of one or more of these is not enough to make the diagnosis of a specific autoimmune disease; each condition requires a certain number of criteria.

Most of the drugs in this chapter suppress or dampen the immune response; this is necessary with autoimmune disease, but the use of strong immune-suppressants (primarily, the biologics – these are the stronger agents and are used when others are not sufficient) will increase the risk of certain conditions due to the strong depression of the immune system. These conditions include:

- Tuberculosis and hepatitis B (if present) re-activation; testing (and treatment if needed) must be done prior to the start of immunosuppressive agents.

- Viruses; if the virus can be prevented by a live vaccine, the vaccine must be given prior to the start of immunosuppressive treatment.

- Lymphomas and certain skin cancers: these cancer types are normally suppressed by a competent immune system.

- Infections of various types (e.g., bacterial, fungal); this requires CBC monitoring, symptom monitoring (by the patient) and may require infection control mechanisms.

Vaccines for Immune-Compromised Patients

Live vaccines: If needed these must be given prior to the start of immunosuppressive drugs. Live vaccines include measles, rubella, varicella and zoster. Zoster should be given (if age appropriate) prior to the start of strong immunosuppressive drugs. Yellow fever vaccine is live, and may be requested for travel, but cannot be given to anyone with severe immune suppression; advise these patients to avoid travel to endemic regions.

Patients with any of the conditions in this chapter should get an annual influenza vaccine (inactivated shot). A one-time dose of Tdap should be substituted for the Td booster followed by the Td booster every 10 years. Pneumococcal vaccine (both PCV13 and PPSV23 in those who have not been vaccinated, see Immunization chapter for schedule) and the HPV vaccine for men and women up to the age of 26 years are recommended. Patients with asplenia or terminal complement deficiency require the meningococcal vaccine (either MPSV4 or MCV4) and those with asplenia or post-hematopoietic stem cell transplant should receive vaccination for haemophilus influenza type b (Hib). Those who desire protection or with certain indications may be vaccinated against hepatitis A and B (see the Immunization chapter).

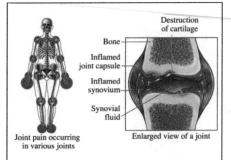

RHEUMATOID ARTHRITIS (RA)

RA causes inflammation of the joints and other organs in the body, including the kidneys, eyes, heart and lungs. This is a chronic, symmetrical, systemic and progressive disease – although the disease course is variable and some have much more aggressive disease than others. RA typically presents first in the hands and feet. Macrophages, cytotoxins, and free oxygen radicals promote cellular damage and inflammation. The inflammation leads to cartilage and bone destruction, resulting in the classic symptoms of RA: joint swelling, stiffness, pain and eventually, bone deformity.

GUIDELINES

Singh JA, Furst DE, Bharat A, et al. 2012 update of the 2008 American College of Rheumatology recommendations for the use of disease-modifying antirheumatic drugs and biologic agents in the treatment of rheumatoid arthritis. *Arthrit Care Res.* 2012; 64(5):625-639.

DIAGNOSIS

Criteria 1-4 must be present for ≥ 6 weeks and 4 or more criteria must be present.

Diagnostic Criteria

1. Morning stiffness around joints lasting > 1 hour

2. Soft tissue swelling (arthritis) in 3 or more joints

3. Swelling (arthritis) of hand, foot, or wrist joints

4. Symmetric involvement

5. Rheumatoid nodules

6. Positive serum rheumatoid factor (present in ~ 70% of patients)

7. Radiographic erosions or periarticular osteopenia in hand or wrist joints

Clinical Presentation

The disease process is highly variable, progressing rapidly in some and slow in others. Many are constitutional (general physical) symptoms, such as morning fatigue, fever, weakness, loss of appetite, and joint and muscle pain. Patients experience articular (affecting the joints) manifestations that are almost always polyarticular and symmetrical. Any synovial joint can be involved, but the finger joints of the hand are most often affected. The wrists, knees and toe joints are also frequently involved. Morning stiffness, swelling, redness, edema, pain, decreased range of motion, muscle atrophy, weakness, and deformity are typical articular symptoms of RA. Morning stiffness is a clue for RA and may last for up to 2 hours. Osteoarthritis (OA) does not cause prolonged stiffness.

Patients may also experience extra-articular manifestations (outside of the joints), including firm lumps, called rheumatoid nodules, which are subcutaneous nodules in places such as the elbow or hands. Other extra-articular symptoms may include vasculitis, pulmonary complications (fibrosis, effusions, nodules), lymphadenopathy, splenomegaly, eye inflammation, dry eyes and/or mouth from a related condition (Sjögren's syndrome), pericarditis/myocarditis, and atherosclerosis.

Non-Drug Treatment

Non-drug treatments include rest, physical therapy, occupational therapy, exercise, diet and weight control, and surgical intervention (e.g., a joint replacement).

Drug Treatment

The goal is to have the patient on a Disease-Modifying Antirheumatic Drug (DMARD) within 3 months of diagnosis. DMARDs work via various mechanisms to slow down the disease process and help prevent further joint damage. Patients may require bridging therapy (short-term) or, in some cases, long-term use of anti-inflammatory medications such as NSAIDs or steroids. NSAIDs and steroids have significant health risks when used long-term. NSAIDs are discussed in the Pain chapter; steroids are discussed in the Asthma chapter.

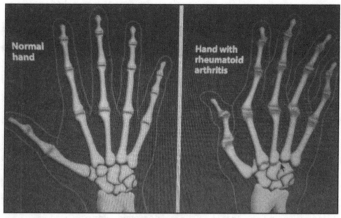

Degenerative joint damage with nodules

Patients with milder symptoms may be able to live acceptably on non-biologic DMARDs including methotrexate, hydroxychloroquine, leflunomide, sulfasalazine, and minocycline. Methotrexate is used most commonly, alone or in combination.

For patients with more severe disease, treatment can include newer biologic agents that antagonize tumor necrosis factor (TNF) or work via other mechanisms.

Agents Used for Pain and Inflammation

DRUG	DOSING

Non-Selective NSAIDs – for more information, see Pain chapter

Ibuprofen *(Motrin, Advil* and others)	**Rx** 800 mg Q6-8H; max 3,200 mg/day Need higher doses for anti-inflammatory effects

COX-2 Selective Inhibitor – for more information, see Pain chapter

Celecoxib *(CeleBREX)*	100-200 mg BID

Steroids, using prednisone as an example–for more information, see Asthma chapter

PredniSONE *[PredniSONE Intensol* (solution), *Rayos* (delayed release tablet), generics-oral]	Initial dose 5-60 mg daily, some use Alternate Day Therapy (ADT) dosing in which twice the usual daily dose is given every other day to ↓ adrenal supression/reduced toxic effects. Indicated for acute inflammation/pain and as bridge therapy while waiting for DMARDs to take effect. Steroids should not be used long-term. However, some patients may use chronically (≤ 10 mg daily) due to disease severity.

Disease-Modifying Anti-Rheumatic Drugs (DMARDs)

DRUG	DOSING	SAFETY/SIDE EFFECTS/MONITORING
Methotrexate **(Rheumatrex, Trexall,** *Otrexup, Rasuvo)* *Otrexup* and *Rasuvo* are SC auto-injectors used weekly	7.5-25 mg once weekly Low weekly doses are used for RA (the weekly dose can be split into 2-3 doses given 12 hrs apart); never dose daily for RA If patient is not using the *Rheumatrex* dose-pack, counsel the patient to take weekly. Numerous incidences of adverse events (mouth sores, intestinal bleeding, etc.) have occurred due to patients taking daily.	**BOXED WARNINGS** Hepatotoxicity, acute renal failure, pneumonitis, bone marrow suppression, mucositis/stomatitis, dermatologic reactions, malignant lymphomas, others – renal and lung toxicity more likely when using oncology doses. **CONTRAINDICATIONS** Pregnancy, alcoholism, chronic liver disease, blood dyscrasias, immunodeficiency syndrome **SIDE EFFECTS** Nausea, vomiting, diarrhea ↑ LFTs, stomatitis, alopecia, photosensitivity **MONITORING** LFTs, CBC, SCr (baseline and every 2-4 weeks for first 3 months, then less frequently). At baseline: chest X-ray, hepatitis B and C. Pulmonary function tests if lung-related symptoms. **NOTES** Pregnancy Category X Folic acid can be given to ↓ side effects associated with methotrexate–commonly given 5 mg PO weekly on the day following methotrexate administration
Hydroxychloroquine **(Plaquenil)**	400-600 mg/day initially, then 200-400 mg/day for maintenance dose Take with food or milk	**CONTRAINDICATIONS** Retinopathy and hypersensitivity to 4-aminoquinoline compounds **WARNINGS** May cause neuromuscular weakness and hematologic reactions with prolonged use **SIDE EFFECTS** Nausea, vomiting, diarrhea, abdominal pain, rash, pruritus, headache, vision changes (dose-related), pigmentation changes of the skin and hair (rare) **MONITORING** CBC at baseline and periodically, LFTs. Eye exam at baseline and every 3 months during prolonged therapy. **NOTES** Pregnancy Category C

Disease-Modifying Anti-Rheumatic Drugs (DMARDs) Continued

DRUG	DOSING	SAFETY/SIDE EFFECTS/MONITORING
SulfaSALAzine *(Azulfidine, Azulfidine EN-tabs, Sulfazine, Sulfazine EC)*	500-1,000 mg BID (max 3 grams/day) Take with food and 8 oz. of water to prevent crystalluria	**CONTRAINDICATIONS** Patients with a sulfa or salicylate allergy, GI or GU obstruction, porphyria **SIDE EFFECTS** Headache, rash, anorexia, dyspepsia, GI upset (N/V/D), oligospermia (reversible) (all > 10%); folate deficiency, arthalgias, crystalluria **WARNINGS** Caution in patients with blood dyscrasias, renal or hepatic impairment and G6PD deficiency; potential for severe skin reactions (SJS/TEN), pulmonary fibrosis **MONITORING** CBC with differential and LFTs (every other week x 3 months), urinalysis, SCr, hypersensitivity **NOTES** Can cause yellow-orange coloration of skin/urine Impairs folate absorption, may give 1 mg/day folate supplement
Minocycline *(Minocin, Solodyn)*	100 mg BID Take with 8 oz water to minimize GI irritation Stay upright for 30 minutes after taking	**WARNINGS** Children ≤ 8 years of age, pregnancy (suppresses bone growth and skeletal development, permanently discolors teeth) **SIDE EFFECTS** GI upset (nausea/vomiting/diarrhea), photosensitivity, rash **NOTES** Pregnancy Category D See Infectious Diseases chapter for more information
Leflunomide *(Arava)*	100 mg PO x 3 days, then 20 mg PO daily (may omit loading dose if at higher risk of liver or hematologic toxicity) Must have negative pregnancy test before starting this medication and use 2 forms of birth control. If pregnancy is desired, must wait 2 years after discontinuation or give cholestyramine to eliminate drug. Taken +/- methotrexate	**BOXED WARNINGS (2)** Women of childbearing potential should not receive leflunomide until pregnancy has been excluded, hepatotoxicity **CONTRAINDICATION** Pregnancy **SIDE EFFECTS** Hepatotoxicity, diarrhea, upper respiratory tract infections (URTIs), alopecia, rash, hypertension, blood dyscrasias **MONITORING** LFTs and CBC at baseline and monthly for first 6 months, BP at baseline and regularly. Screen for TB and pregnancy prior to starting therapy. **NOTES** Pregnancy Category X

Disease-Modifying Anti-Rheumatic Drugs (DMARDs) Continued

DRUG	DOSING	SAFETY/SIDE EFFECTS/MONITORING
Tofacitinib *(Xeljanz)*	5 mg PO BID Dose Adjustments: With strong CYP450 3A4 inducers: avoid use; with strong 3A4 inhibitors: 5 mg daily; with concomitant moderate 3A4 inhibitors and strong 2C19 inhibitors: 5 mg daily Can be used as monotherapy or with non-biologic DMARDs <u>Do not use</u> with biologic DMARDs or potent immunosuppressants	**BOXED WARNINGS (2)** Increased risk for serious infections (including active tuberculosis, fungal, viral, bacterial, or opportunistic infections). Screen for latent TB and treat before starting therapy Increased risk for lymphomas and other malignancies. **WARNINGS** GI perforation, not recommended in severe hepatic impairment, and should not be given concurrently with live vaccines. **SIDE EFFECTS** Bone marrow suppression, infections (URTIs), diarrhea, headache, ↑ lipids **MONITORING** CBC (dose adjustments for lymphopenia, neutropenia and anemia), LFTs, lipids, signs of infection **NOTES** Pregnancy Category C MedGuide required

Methotrexate Drug Interactions

- <u>Methotrexate should not be taken with alcohol</u>; this combination ↑ the risk of liver toxicity.

- Active transport renal elimination is ↓ by aspirin, beta-lactams, probenecid and NSAIDs, resulting in toxicity. Avoid concurrent use.

- Sulfonamides and topical tacrolimus ↑ adverse effects of methotrexate. Avoid concurrent use.

- Methotrexate can ↓ effectiveness of loop diuretics; loop diuretics can ↑ the methotrexate concentration. Use caution if using these agents concomitantly.

- Methotrexate and cyclosporine concentrations will both ↑ when used concomitantly, leading to toxicity; avoid this combination.

Methotrexate Counseling

- Patients should be encouraged to read the patient instruction sheet within the dose pack.

- If you are receiving this medicine for rheumatoid arthritis or psoriasis, the dosage is usually given <u>once weekly</u>. Some patients are told to divide the once weekly dose in half and take it over two days per week. <u>Do not use this medicine daily</u> or double-up on doses. Serious side effects could occur if it is used more frequently than directed. Choose a day of the week to take your medicine that you can remember.

- Methotrexate has caused birth defects and death in unborn babies (Pregnancy Category X). <u>If you are pregnant or have a chance of becoming pregnant, you should not use this medicine</u>. Use an effective form of birth control, whether you are a man or a woman. Tell your healthcare provider if you or your sexual partner become pregnant during treatment.

- Do not use methotrexate if you are breastfeeding.

- If you have kidney problems or excess body water (ascites, pleural effusion), you must be closely monitored and your dose may be adjusted or stopped by your healthcare provider.

- Your healthcare provider will perform periodic blood tests to measure your liver function to ensure it stays healthy.

- Methotrexate (usually at high dosages) has rarely caused severe (sometimes fatal) bone marrow suppression (decreasing your body's ability to fight infections) and stomach/intestinal disease (e.g., bleeding) when used at the same time as non-steroidal anti-inflammatory drugs (NSAIDs). Therefore, NSAIDs should not be used with high-dose methotrexate. Caution is advised if you also take aspirin. If you are using low-dose aspirin (81-325 milligrams per day) for heart attack or stroke prevention, continue to take it unless directed otherwise.

- Methotrexate use has rarely resulted in serious (sometimes fatal) side effects, such as lung problems, lung infections *(Pneumocystis* pneumonia), skin reactions, diarrhea, and mouth sores.

- Tell your healthcare provider right away if you develop any new or worsening symptoms, including black, tarry stools or symptoms of liver damage (unusual tiredness or weakness, yellow skin or eyes or darkened urine, stomach upset or pain).

- For *Rasuvo* and *Otrexup* auto-injectors: Inspect syringe. Liquid should be clear and yellow *(Otrexup)* to yellow-brown *(Rasuvo)*. Discard if cloudy or containing particles. Select an injection site on the abdomen (2 inches from navel) or upper thigh only. Swab with alcohol pad and allow to dry – do not fan or blow on the area. For *Otrexup*, twist cap to break seal and remove the safety clip. For *Rasuvo* pull the yellow cap directly off without twisting. Pinch the skin and inject at a 90 angle. Press firmly until you hear a click. Hold 3 seconds for *Otrexup* and 5 seconds for *Rasuvo*. Check the viewing window to be sure the medicine was given. Dispose of the used injector in a sharps container. Store at room temperature.

Biologic Agents
Tumor Necrosis Factor (TNFα) Inhibitors (Anti-TNF biologics)

TNF inhibitor dosing is provided for RA. Recommended dosing for psoriatic arthritis, plaque psoriasis, Crohn's disease, ulcerative colitis, and other indications may vary.

DRUG	DOSING	SAFETY/SIDE EFFECTS/MONITORING
Etanercept *(Enbrel, Enbrel SureClick)*	50 mg SC weekly, or 25 mg SC twice/week (separated by 72-96 hours)	**BOXED WARNINGS (2)** Risk for serious infections – some fatal (including active TB, fungal, viral, bacterial or opportunistic infections); lymphomas and other malignancies; discontinue therapy if a serious infection develops; screen for latent TB and treat before starting therapy **CONTRAINDICATIONS** Active systemic infection, dose > 5 mg/kg in mod-severe heart failure (infliximab), sepsis (etanercept)
Adalimumab *(Humira, Humira Pen)*	40 mg SC every other week (if not taking methotrexate, can ↑ dose to 40 mg SC weekly)	**WARNINGS** TNF inhibitors can cause demyelinating disease, hepatitis B reactivation, heart failure, hepatotoxicity, lupus-like syndrome, and severe infections. Do not use with other TNF inhibitors or immunosuppressive biologics, or live vaccines. **SIDE EFFECTS** Infections and injection site reactions (redness, rash, swelling, itching, or bruising), positive anti-nuclear antibodies, headache, nausea, ↑ CPK (adalimumab)
InFLIXimab *(Remicade)* – given only in combination with methotrexate in RA	3 mg/kg IV at weeks 0, 2, and 6, and then every 8 weeks (can ↑ dose to 10 mg/kg based on need but ↑ infection risk) IV infliximab requires a filter and is stable in NS only Infusion reactions: hypotension, fever, chills, pruritus (may pre-treat with acetaminophen, antihistamine, steroids) Delayed hypersensitivity reaction 3-10 days after administration (fever, rash, myalgia, HA, sore throat)	**MONITORING** TB test (prior to administration and annually), signs and symptoms of infection, CBC, LFTs, HBV (prior to initiation), HF, malignancies **NOTES** Do not shake. Requires refrigeration (biologics will denature if hot). Do not freeze. Etanercept may be stored at room temperature for a maximum of 14 days. Allow to reach room temperature before injecting (15-30 min). Usually, methotrexate is used 1st-line and these agents are add-on therapy. However, if the initial presentation is severe, these can be started as initial therapy.
Certolizumab pegol *(Cimzia, Cimzia* Prefilled)	400 mg SC at weeks 0, 2, and 4. Then, 200 mg SC every other week (may consider 400 mg every 4 weeks)	Do not use more than one biologic concurrently. Do not use live vaccines if using these drugs. Antibody induction can occur and will ↓ usefulness of drug. **MedGuide Required** All TNF inhibitors carry a boxed warning for risk of serious infections, including tuberculosis, invasive fungal and other opportunistic infections. All patients should be evaluated for TB before starting these drugs. Patients with latent TB should start prophylactic treatment. Retest for TB annually.
Golimumab *(Simponi, Simponi Aria)* – given only in combination with methotrexate in RA	50 mg SC monthly *(Simponi)* 2 mg/kg IV at weeks 0, 2, and 4. Then, 2 mg/kg IV every 8 weeks *(Simponi Aria)* IV golimumab requires a filter	

Other Biologics (Also known as Non-TNF Biologics)

Rituximab

<u>Depletes CD20 B cells</u>. B cells are believed to have a role in RA development and progression.

DRUG	DOSING	SAFETY/SIDE EFFECTS/MONITORING
RiTUXimab **(Rituxan)** – given with methotrexate in RA	1 gram IV on day 1 and 15 in combination with methotrexate for 2 doses. Can repeat treatment if needed. Need to pre-medicate with a steroid, acetaminophen, and an antihistamine Start infusion at 50 mg/hr; can ↑ by 50 mg/hr every 30 min if no reaction (max 400 mg/hr)	**BOXED WARNINGS (4)** Severe and fatal infusion-related reactions, usually with the first infusion Fatal progressive multifocal leukoencephalopathy (PML) due to JC virus infection Hepatitis B virus (HBV) reactivation; some cases resulting in fulminant hepatitis, hepatic failure and death Severe and fatal mucocutaneous reaction (e.g., SJS, TEN) **WARNINGS** Can cause serious infections, discontinue if a serious infection develops. <u>Screen for latent TB and HBV</u> prior to initiating therapy. Do not give with other biologics or live vaccines. **SIDE EFFECTS** In patients treated for RA: infusion-related reactions (fever, chills, pruritis, rash), URTIs, UTIs, nasopharyngitis, bronchitis (all > 10%), nausea, diarrhea, peripheral edema, hypertension, HA, angioedema, weight gain, fever, insomnia, pain **MONITORING** Cardiac monitoring during and after infusion, vital signs, infusion reactions, CBC, CD20+ cells, renal function **NOTES** MedGuide required Do not shake

Anakinra

IL-1 receptor antagonist. IL-1 mediates immunologic reactions in RA (degrades cartilage, increases bone resorption).

DRUG	DOSING	SAFETY/SIDE EFFECTS/MONITORING
Anakinra *(Kineret)*	100 mg SC daily (administer at same time daily)	**WARNINGS** Can cause serious infections, discontinue if a serious infection develops. <u>Screen for latent TB</u> prior to initiating therapy. Do not give with other biologics or live vaccines. **SIDE EFFECTS** Headache, fever, injection site reactions, infections, myelosuppression, arthralgia, nasopharyngitis **MONITORING** CBC, SCr, signs of infection **NOTES** Do not shake

Abatacept

Selective T cell costimulator; inhibits T cell activation by binding to CD80 and CD86 on cells that present these antigens (activated cells are detected in the synovium of RA joints).

DRUG	DOSING	SAFETY/SIDE EFFECTS/MONITORING
Abatacept *(Orencia)*	IV: 500-1,000 mg (based on body weight) IV at 0, 2, and 4 weeks, then every 4 weeks thereafter. Infuse over 30 min SC: 125 mg SC weekly SC w/IV loading dose: give first IV dose as above, followed by 125 mg SC within 24 hours, then 125 mg SC weekly	**WARNINGS** Increased risk for serious infections, discontinue if a serious infection develops. Screen for latent TB and HBV prior to initiating therapy. Do not give with other biologics or live vaccines. **SIDE EFFECTS** Headache, nausea, injection site reactions, infections, nasopharyngitis, antibody development **MONITORING** Signs of infection, CBC, hypersensitivity **NOTES** Stable in NS only. Requires a filter and light protection during administration; do not shake Caution in those with COPD– may worsen symptoms

Tocilizumab

IL-6 receptor antagonist. IL-6 mediates immunologic reactions in RA.

DRUG	DOSING	SAFETY/SIDE EFFECTS/MONITORING
Tocilizumab *(Actemra)*	IV: 4 mg/kg IV every 4 weeks given over 60 min (may ↑ to 8 mg/kg based on clinical response). Max 800 mg SC: if < 100 kg, 162 mg SC every other week (may ↑ to weekly based on response) If ≥ 100 kg, 162 mg SC weekly	**BOXED WARNING** Risk of serious infections; screen for latent TB prior to initiating therapy **WARNINGS** Increased risk for serious infections, discontinue if a serious infection develops. GI perforation, hypersensitivity reactions, do not give with other biologics or live vaccines. Do not start if ALT or AST is > 1.5 times ULN, ANC < 2,000 cells/mm^3, or platelets < 100,000 cell/mm^3 **SIDE EFFECTS** ↑ LFTs, infections, myelosuppression, GI perforation, ↑ LDL and total cholesterol **MONITORING** LFTs (baseline, at 2nd infusion and every 2-4 weeks), CBC, lipid panel, signs of infection **NOTES** MedGuide required Dose adjustments recommended for neutropenia, thrombocytopenia, and liver function abnormalities on therapy Do not shake

Pointers for All Immune Modulators

If hypersensitivity to a drug develops, further use is contraindicated (this is true for other drugs as well but these drugs cause more hypersensitivity). Consider varicella vaccination prior to the start of treatment. Patients should monitor for infections and for liver damage (see the counseling section). If dispensing a self-injectable, counseling must include how to store the medication, reconstitute (if a powder), and where to inject (these medications should be injected into the upper middle thigh or abdomen). All above SC biologics are to be kept refrigerated (except etanercept, which may be stored at room temperature for up to 14 days) and the patient should wait until the drug is at room temperature before injecting (cold injections are painful). Tell patients not to use external heat sources for warming the product; holding the medication or slowly rolling it in the hand is acceptable (except for go-limumab, which should simply be left sitting at room temperature). Do not shake.

Patient Counseling

Biologic Agents

- Read the medication guide that comes with this medicine.

- People taking this medicine should not get live vaccines. Make sure your vaccines are up-to-date before starting this medicine. You can continue to take the annual influenza shot (but not the nasal mist vaccine, since this is a live vaccine).

- Because this medicine works by blocking the immune system, it lowers your ability to fight infections. This may make you more likely to get a serious (rarely fatal) infection or can make any infection you have worse. You should be tested for tuberculosis (TB skin test or chest X-ray) before and during treatment with this medicine. Tell your healthcare provider immediately if you have any signs of infection such as a fever of 100.5°F (38°C) or higher, chills, very bad sore throat, ear or sinus pain, a cough or more sputum or a change in the color of sputum.

- This medicine has a possibility of causing liver damage. Call your healthcare provider right away if you have any of these symptoms: feel very tired, skin or eyes look yellow, poor appetite or vomiting, pain on the right side of your stomach (abdomen).

- This medicine may worsen heart failure (HF). Notify your healthcare provider if you experience sudden weight gain or shortness of breath.

- Common side effects include injection site reactions such as redness, swelling, itching, or pain. These symptoms usually go away within 3 to 5 days. If you have pain, redness or swelling around the injection site that does not go away or gets worse, call your healthcare provider.

- Other side effects can include upper respiratory infections (sinus infections), headache, dizziness or coughing.

- This medicine is injected subcutaneously (SC) under the skin of the thigh, abdomen, or upper arm, exactly as prescribed by your healthcare provider (once weekly for etanercept, every 2 weeks for adalimumab, every 2 or 4 weeks for certolizumab, monthly for golimumab).

- Store the medication (single-use syringes or multiple-use vials) in the refrigerator (etanercept may be stored at room temperature for a maximum of 14 days). Allow the medicine to warm to room temperature before injecting (takes 15-30 minutes). Do not shake the medicine. Before using, check for particles or discoloration. If either is present, do not use the medicine. Injectors require protection from light prior to administration.

- Before injecting each dose, clean the injection site with rubbing alcohol. It is important to change the location of the injection site each time you use this drug to prevent problems under the skin. New injections should be given at least 1 inch (2.5 centimeters) from the last injection site. Do not inject into areas of the skin that are sore, bruised, red, or hard.

- For adalimumab (Humira): Inject into abdomen, thigh, or upper arm. A loud click is heard when the plum-colored activator button is pressed. Continue to hold injector against the skin until the yellow marker fully appears in the window view and stops moving (may take 10 seconds).

- For etanercept *(Enbrel)* syringe or auto-injector: Inject into abdomen, thigh, or upper arm. A loud click is heard when injection begins, continue to hold autoinjector against skin for 15 seconds. You may hear a second click as the purple button pops back up, indicating all of the medicine has been injected.

- For entanercept *(Enbrel)* vials for reconstitution: When reconstituting *Enbrel* powder from the multidose vial, some foaming is normal. The final solution should be clear and colorless, with no particulate matter.

- For golimumab *(Simponi)*: Do not warm to room temperature any other way than letting the product sit at room temperature outside the carton for 30 minutes. Inject into abdomen, thigh, or upper arm. A loud click is heard when the injection begins, continue to hold autoinjector against skin until second click is heard (3-15 seconds).

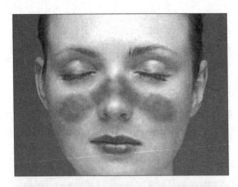

GUIDELINE

Hahn BH, McMahon MA, Wilkinson A, et al. American College of Rheumatology guidelines for screening, treatment, and management of lupus nephritis. *Arthritis Care Res.* 2012; 64(6):797-808.

SYSTEMIC LUPUS ERYTHEMATOSUS (SLE)

Background

SLE, or lupus, is a multisystem autoimmune disease that affects roughly 250,000 Americans, with a female-to-male ratio of 10:1. The disease predominantly occurs in persons 15-45 years of age, and it is more common in women of African-American and Asian descent. Patients experience flare-ups to varying degrees as well as periods of disease remission. As the disease progresses, symptoms may be present in almost every organ system, with the heart, lungs, kidneys, and brain being most affected. The hallmark of SLE is the development of auto-antibodies by B cells to cellular components that leads to chronic inflammation and tissue damage.

Clinical Presentation

The most common symptoms include fatigue, fever, anorexia, weight loss, muscle aches, arthritis, rash (butterfly rash), photosensitivity, and joint pain and stiffness. Over half of the people with SLE develop a characteristic red, flat facial rash over the bridge of their nose and cheeks. Because of its shape, it is frequently referred to as the SLE "butterfly rash." The rash is painless and does not itch. The facial rash, along with inflammation in other organs, can be precipitated or worsened by exposure to sunlight. Arthritis and cutaneous manifestations are most common, but renal, hematologic and neurologic manifestations contribute largely to morbidity and mortality. Lupus nephritis (kidney disease) develops in over 50% of patients with SLE.

DRUGS MOST COMMONLY ASSOCIATED WITH DRUG-INDUCED LUPUS ERYTHEMATOSUS (DILE)		
Procainamide	Quinidine	Minocycline
Hydralazine (alone, and in BiDil)	Methyldopa	Terbinafine
	Propylthiouracil	Anti-TNF agents
Isoniazid	Methimazole	

NON-DRUG AND DRUG TREATMENT

Non-drug treatment consists of rest and proper exercise to manage the fatigue. Smoking cessation is encouraged since tobacco smoke can be a trigger for disease flare. Photosensitivity is common with the condition and the treatment; sunscreens and sun protection/avoidance is required. Drug treatment for SLE consists of immunosuppressants, cytotoxic agents, and/or anti-inflammatory agents. Treatment approaches emphasize using a combination of drugs to minimize chronic exposure to corticosteroids.

Patients with mild disease may do well on an NSAID (dosed at anti-inflammatory doses) but use caution since the doses are high and these patients are more sensitive to the GI and renal side effects. Concurrent use with a PPI is generally recommended to reduce GI side effects of NSAIDs. Other agents are discussed below.

Agents Used in SLE

DRUG	DOSING	SAFETY/SIDE EFFECTS/MONITORING

Antimalarial agents – impair complement-dependent antigen-antibody reactions

DRUG	DOSING	SAFETY/SIDE EFFECTS/MONITORING
Hydroxychloroquine (Plaquenil)	200-400 mg daily	Hydroxychloroquine is safer (preferred); takes 6 months to see maximal effect
Chloroquine (Aralen)	250-500 mg daily	Effective for cutaneous symptoms and arthralgias, fatigue and fever – used for mild disease; chronic (not acute) therapy See more information in RA section

Corticosteroids

DRUG	DOSING	SAFETY/SIDE EFFECTS/MONITORING
PredniSONE (or **methylPREDNISolone** IV if life-threatening disease)	1-2 mg/kg/day PO; then taper 500-1,000 mg/day IV for 3-6 days (acute flare)	Used acutely to control flares at higher doses; taper to lower doses for chronic, suppressive therapy More complete information in the Asthma chapter.

Cytotoxic agents – used in severe disease

DRUG	DOSING	SAFETY/SIDE EFFECTS/MONITORING
Cyclophosphamide	500-1,000 mg/m² IV monthly for 6 months, then every 3 months for 2 years; or 1-3 mg/kg daily if using PO	**SIDE EFFECTS** Myelosuppression, infections, hemorrhagic cystitis (give mesna therapy and keep patient well hydrated), malignancy, sterility, and teratogenesis **MONITORING** CBC and urinalysis monthly **NOTES** Pregnancy Category D Can use IV or oral therapy; used for flares as induction therapy; very toxic for chronic therapy

DRUG	DOSING	SAFETY/SIDE EFFECTS/MONITORING
AzaTHIOprine (Azasan, Imuran)	2 mg/kg PO daily	**BOXED WARNINGS (2)** Chronic immunosuppression can ↑ risk of neoplasia (especially lymphomas) Hematologic toxicities (leukopenia, thrombocytopenia) and mutagenic potential **WARNINGS** GI (severe N/V/D), hematologic (leukopenia, thrombocytopenia, anemia) abnormalities and hepatotoxicity; patients with genetic deficiency of thiopurine methyltransferase (TPMT) are at ↑ risk for myelosuppression and may require lower dose. **SIDE EFFECTS** GI upset (N/V), rash, ↑ LFTs, myelosuppression **MONITORING** LFTs, CBC, renal function **NOTES** Pregnancy Category D
Mycophenolate mofetil (CellCept)	1-3 grams PO daily, can be divided BID	See Transplant chapter.
CycloSPORINE (Gengraf, Neoral, SandIMMUNE)	Initial Oral Dose: 2.5 mg/kg/day, divided twice daily Dose may be increased by 0.5-0.75 mg/kg/day after 8 and/or 12 weeks, up to a maximum of 4 mg/kg/day.	See Transplant chapter.

IgG1-lambda monoclonal antibody that prevents the survival of B lymphocytes by blocking the binding of soluble human B lymphocyte stimulator protein (BLyS) to receptors on B lymphocytes. This reduces the activity of B-cell mediated immunity and the autoimmune response.

| Belimumab (Benlysta) | 10 mg/kg IV at 2 week intervals for the first 3 doses, then 4 week intervals thereafter, infuse over 1 hour

Consider giving pre-medication for infusion reactions and hypersensitivity reactions | **WARNINGS**
Risk of serious (sometimes fatal) infections including progressive multifocal leukoencephalopathy (PML), acute hypersensitivity reactions, malignancy, psychiatric events (anxiety, depression, insomnia)

SIDE EFFECTS
Infection, hypersensitivity and infusion reactions, nausea, diarrhea

NOTES
Live vaccines should not be given 30 days prior or concurrently with therapy.

During reconstitution, direct diluent to sides of vial to minimize foaming. Swirl vial every 5 minutes, do not shake. Reconstitution may take up to 30 minutes. Protect from light. Stable in NS only.

MedGuide required. |

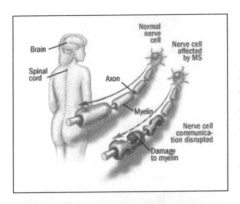

GUIDELINE

Goodin DS, Frohman EM, Garmany GP, et al. Disease modifying therapies in multiple sclerosis: report of the TTA/AAN/MS council for practice guidelines. *Neurology.* 2002; 58:169-78.

MULTIPLE SCLEROSIS (MS)

Background

MS is a chronic, progressive autoimmune disease in which the patient's immune system attacks the myelin peptide antigens, destroying the fatty myelin sheaths that surround the axons in the brain and spinal cord (CNS). As demyelination progresses, the symptoms worsen because the nerves can no longer properly conduct electrical transmission. Similar to other autoimmune conditions, most patients experience periods of disease activity followed by intervals of remission. The presentation is highly variable with some patients having a much more aggressive course while others have occasional discrete attacks.

Early symptoms include weakness, tingling, numbness and blurred vision. As the condition worsens, a variety of physical and psychological issues can make life very challenging, including deterioration of cognitive function, fatigue, muscle spasms, pain, incontinence, depression, heat sensitivity, sexual dysfunction, difficulty walking and gait instability, weakness and visual disturbances. If left untreated, about 30% of patients will develop significant physical disability. Up to 10% of patients have a milder phenotype in which no significant physical disability develops, although these patients may develop mild cognitive dysfunction. Male patients with primary progressive MS generally have the worst prognosis. Symptoms are characterized as primary (due to demyelination, such as muscle weakness), secondary (which result from primary symptoms, such as incontinence due to muscle impairment) and tertiary, which involve psychological and social concerns, such as depression.

MS occurs in both men and women, but (also similar to other autoimmune conditions) is more common in women. The typical age of onset is between 20 to 40 years old. Regretfully this is not an uncommon condition; MS is one of the most frequent neurologic disorders in young adults. Over two million people suffer with MS around the world, with about 500,000 cases in the U.S. In addition to the personal suffering caused by this condition, MS inflicts a heavy financial burden on individuals and society. A primary goal of therapy must be prevention of disease progression; what is lost in neuronal function cannot be regained. The agents that can modify disease progression are costly. The beta interferons cost about $40,000/year. The newer oral immune modulator fingolimod costs about $48,000/year. The newest agent, dimethyl fumarate, costs about $60,000/year.

Drug Treatment

Mitoxantrone is a chemotherapeutic agent that is sometimes used for MS and is approved for this condition; a review of mitoxantrone can be found in the Oncology chapter. Steroids are used to help with exacerbations. In addition to using disease-modifying drugs to prevent disease progression, the clinician must be focused on symptom control. The drugs used for various related symptoms are summarized at the end of this chapter, and detailed information on these agents can be found in other chapters of this text.

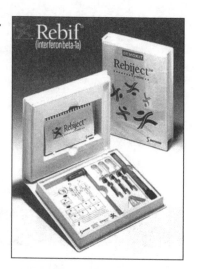

Disease Modifying Drugs

Interferon beta formulations (*Betaseron, Avonex, Rebif, Extavia, Plegridy*) and glatiramer acetate *(Copaxone)* have been the mainstay of treatment for patients with relapsing forms of MS. Fingolimod (*Gilenya*) and teriflunomide *(Aubagio)* were the first oral disease-modifying agents to be approved for MS. In 2013, a third oral agent, dimethyl fumarate *(Tecfidera)* was approved. Pegylated interferon beta *(Plegridy)* was approved in 2014. It allows for more convenient SC dosing every 14 days. If these are not effective the monoclonal antibodies or chemotherapy drugs can be tried; these have significant toxicities and are used in refractive cases.

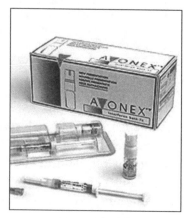

If the drug is a powder that is reconstituted, the drug powder may be required to be refrigerated or be kept at room temperature (they vary). If a drug is reconstituted, it has to be used right away (at most within a few hours; a few reconstituted injections permit short storage in the refrigerator; others do not). Some of the powders that are reconstituted contain albumin and some patients will not wish to or cannot use albumin-containing products.

DRUG	DOSING	SAFETY/SIDE EFFECTS/MONITORING

Glatiramer acetate is an immune modulator, mechanism not well-defined.

| Glatiramer acetate *(Copaxone)* Pre-filled syringes (20 and 40 mg/mL) | 20 mg SC daily or 40 mg SC 3 times per week (at least 48 hours apart) | **SIDE EFFECTS** Injection site reactions (inflammation, erythema, pain, pruritus, residual mass), infection, pain, flushing, diaphoresis, chest pain, weakness, anxiety, rash, nausea, vasodilation, lipoatrophy and skin necrosis at injection site **NOTES** Pregnancy Category B. Check solution for discoloration; if present, discard. Can be kept at room temperature for up to one month, or in the refrigerator (preferred). If cold, let stand to room temp prior to injecting. |

Multiple Sclerosis Drugs Continued

DRUG	DOSING	SAFETY/SIDE EFFECTS/MONITORING

Interferons have antiviral and antiproliferative effects. They reduce antigen presentation and T-cell proliferation, alter cytokine and matrix metalloproteinase (MMP) expression, and restore suppressor function.

DRUG	DOSING	SAFETY/SIDE EFFECTS/MONITORING
Interferon beta-1a *(Avonex, Avonex Pen, Rebif, Rebif Rebidose)* Powder (for reconstitution), pre-filled syringes and pens	**Target Dose** **Avonex** IM: 30 mcg <u>weekly</u> **Rebif** SC: 22 mcg or 44 mcg <u>three times per week</u> (at least 48 hours apart)	**WARNINGS** Depression/suicide, injection site necrosis, myelosuppression, ↑ LFTs, thyroid dysfunction, infections, anaphylaxis, worsening cardiovascular disease, seizure risk **SIDE EFFECTS** Flu-like symptoms following administration (lasting minutes to hours and ↓ with continued treatment - can use acetaminophen or NSAIDs prior to injection) <u>Injection site reactions</u>: range from mild erythema to severe skin necrosis.
Interferon beta-1b *(Betaseron, Extavia)* Powder (for reconstitution)	**Target Dose** SC: 0.25 mg <u>every other day</u>.	**MONITORING** LFTs, CBC (at 1, 3 and 6 months, then periodically); thyroid function every 6 months (in patients with pre-existing abnormalities and/or clinical indications)
Peginterferon beta-1a *(Plegridy, Plegridy Starter Pack)* Pre-filled syringes and pens	**Target Dose** SC: 63 mcg on Day 1, 94 mcg on Day 15, then 125 mcg <u>every 14 days</u> starting on Day 29	**NOTES** Pregnancy Category C Refrigerate all except *Betaseron* and *Extavia* (which can be stored at room temperature). <u>If refrigerated, let stand to room temp prior to injection. Do not expel small air bubble in pre-filled syringes due to loss of dose.</u> Do not shake *Avonex, Betaseron* or *Extavia*. Some formulations contain albumin – risk of Creutzfeldt-Jakob disease transmission (rare); avoid in albumin-sensitive patients. MedGuide required.

Oral Immune Modulators

DRUG	DOSING	SAFETY/SIDE EFFECTS/MONITORING
Teriflunomide *(Aubagio)* Active metabolite of leflunomide	7 mg or 14 mg PO daily	**BOXED WARNINGS (2)** Severe liver toxicity and teratogenicity **CONTRAINDICATIONS** Severe hepatic impairment, pregnancy, current leflunomide treatment **SIDE EFFECTS** ↑ LFTs, alopecia, diarrhea, influenza, nausea, paresthesia, hypophosphatemia, headache, neutropenia Rare: renal impairment, hyperkalemia, peripheral neuropathy **MONITORING** LFTs and bilirubin (within 6 months of starting and monthly for 6 months), SCr, BUN, K+, BP, CBC **NOTES** Pregnancy Category X. MedGuide required.

Multiple Sclerosis Drugs Continued

DRUG	DOSING	SAFETY/SIDE EFFECTS/MONITORING
Fingolimod (*Gilenya*)	0.5 mg capsule daily	**CONTRAINDICATIONS** Recent (within the last 6 months) MI, unstable angina, stroke, TIA, HF requiring hospitalization, or NYHA Class III/IV HF; history of 2nd or 3rd degree heart block or sick sinus syndrome (without a functional pacemaker), QT interval ≥ 500 msec, concurrent use of Class Ia or III anti-arrhythmics **WARNINGS** Decrease in heart rate (must monitor), BP, macular edema, infections, ↓ pulmonary function tests, ↑ LFTs **SIDE EFFECTS** Headache, diarrhea, flu-like syndrome, back pain, ↑ LFTs, cough, hypertension, posterior reversible encephalopthy syndrome (PRES - rare but can cause stroke/hemorrhage) **MONITORING** CBC (baseline and periodically thereafter); ECG (baseline; repeat after initial dose observation period); heart rate, blood pressure and signs and symptoms of bradycardia; if pre-existing cardiac condition, perform continuous ECG monitoring overnight after first dose. Eye exam at baseline and 3-4 months after initiation of treatment **NOTES** Pregnancy Category C. Avoid live vaccines until 2 months after stopping treatment. Blister packs; protect from moisture. Caution when used with drugs that slow heart rate, monitor continuous ECG overnight after first dose if concomitant use is necessary. MedGuide required.
Dimethyl fumarate (*Tecfidera*)	120 mg PO BID for 7 days, then 240 mg BID	**WARNINGS** Risk of fatal progressive multifocal leukoencephalopathy (PML) GI events (e.g., nausea, vomiting, diarrhea, abdominal pain, dyspepsia) commonly occur with use **SIDE EFFECTS** Flushing, abdominal pain, diarrhea, nausea, infection, ↓ WBC **MONITORING** CBC **NOTES** Can give aspirin 30 minutes prior to prevent flushing. Do not crush, chew, or sprinkle capsule contents on food. Pregnancy Category C.

Multiple Sclerosis Drugs Continued

DRUG	DOSING	SAFETY/SIDE EFFECTS/MONITORING

***Ampyra:* Potassium channel blocker, may increase nerve signal conduction.**

Dalfampridine (*Ampyra*)	10 mg BID, extended-release tablets	**CONTRAINDICATIONS** History of seizures, CrCl < 50 mL/min **WARNINGS** Can cause seizures (especially with higher doses), anaphylaxis **SIDE EFFECTS** Urinary tract infections, insomnia, dizziness, headache, nausea, weakness, back pain **NOTES** Pregnancy Category C. Take tablets whole; do not crush, chew, divide, or dissolve. Most do not respond; monitor for improvement, takes up to 6 weeks, if effective, it primarily improves walking. MedGuide required.

Monoclonal Antibodies

Natalizumab (*Tysabri*) Integrin receptor antagonist	300 mg IV given over 1 hour, <u>every 4 weeks</u>	**BOXED WARNING** <u>Risk for progressive multifocal leukoencephalopathy (PML)</u> – monitor mental status changes. Risk factors for PML include: anti-JC virus antibodies, ↑ treatment duration and prior immunosuppressant use. **CONTRAINDICATIONS** History of PML **SIDE EFFECTS** <u>Infusion reactions, headache, fatigue</u>, nausea, respiratory infections, rash, hepatotoxicity (rare) **NOTES** REMS: Only available through the TOUCH prescribing program; requires patient, physician and pharmacist registration. MedGuide required. Pregnancy Category C. Do not shake. Stable in NS only. Requires protection from light during administration.

Multiple Sclerosis Drugs Continued

DRUG	DOSING	SAFETY/SIDE EFFECTS/MONITORING

Recombinant humanized monoclonal antibody

Alemtuzumab *(Lemtrada)* CD52-directed cytolytic monoclonal antibody	First course: 12 mg IV (over 4 hours) daily x 5 days Second course: 12 mg IV daily x 3 days <u>12 months after first course</u>	**BOXED WARNINGS (4)** Serious (sometimes fatal) autoimmune conditions (ITP), infusion reactions, and malignancies. Available only through the *Lemtrada* REMS. **CONTRAINDICATIONS** HIV (causes prolonged ↓ CD4 count) **SIDE EFFECTS** Infections (<u>herpes viral infections</u>, fungal, URTIs, UTIs), <u>thyroid gland disorders</u>, rash, headache, fever, nausea, fatigue, insomnia, urticaria, pruritus, arthralgia, pain, diarrhea, paresthesia, dizziness, flushing, vomiting **NOTES** Indicated for those with inadequate response to ≥ 2 MS drugs. Complete all vaccinations 6 weeks before therapy. Pre-medicate with <u>1 gram methylprednisolone</u> (or equivalent) immediately prior to the infusion and for the first 3 days. Start <u>antiviral prophylaxis</u> on first day of each course and continue for 2 months or until CD4 count ≥ 200 (whichever is later). MedGuide required. Do not shake.

Glatiramer *(Copaxone)* Counseling

- This medication is given by injection under the skin as directed by your doctor. This medication is available in 2 different doses. Depending on your dose, this medication is injected daily or 3 times a week at least 48 hours apart.

- Common side effects include redness, warmth and itchy skin where you inject. Other common side effects include sweating, chest pain, weakness and anxiety. These should be mild; if they are not, contact your healthcare provider.

- The syringes can be kept at room temperature for up to one month. If it has been in the refrigerator keep the syringe at room temperature for 20 minutes. Do not inject the medication cold because this will be painful. This liquid in the syringe should be clear and colorless to slightly yellow. If particles or discoloration are present, do not use it.

- Change the injection site daily to prevent skin problems. Keep track of your injections and do not inject into the same site for at least 1 week.

- After pulling out the needle, apply gentle pressure on the injection site. Do not rub the area. Discard any unused portion after a single use and put the used syringe into a sharps container.

Fingolimod *(Gilenya)* Counseling

- An electrocardiogram (ECG) is performed before your first dose; once you take the medication, your pulse and blood pressure will be checked frequently and the ECG will be repeated 6 hours later. This is to check your heart rate to make sure it does not go too low.

- It is important not to take other drugs that lower your heart rate with this medication; discuss any questions about other drugs with your pharmacist.

- If you miss a dose, take it as soon as you remember but skip it if it is getting close to the next dose.

- Keep the capsules in the original container. This medication needs to be kept away from moisture. Do not store in the bathroom.

- Contact your healthcare provider right away if you are passing brown or dark-colored urine, have pale stools, feel more tired than usual or if your skin and/or whites of your eyes become yellow. These may be symptoms of liver damage.

- This drug has a risk of causing vision problems, including blurry vision, eye pain, increased sensitivity to light, or having a blind spot or shadows in the center of your vision (vision problems may occur 3 to 4 months after you start taking fingolimod). If you develop any vision problems tell your healthcare provider right away.

Drugs Used for Symptom Control

Patients with MS may use a variety of medications for symptom control. The individual agents used can be found in the different chapters in this book. Commonly used symptom-control agents for MS include anticholinergics for incontinence, laxatives for constipation (or loperamide if diarrhea), skeletal muscle relaxants for muscle spasms/spasticity, or various pain agents for muscle spasms and pain. For localized pain and spasms botulinum toxin (*Botox*) injections can provide relief for up to three months. Propranolol can help with tremor. For depression many antidepressants are used; if an SNRI is chosen these may help both neuropathic pain and depression. Fatigue is often treated with modafinil or similar agents, or stimulants used for ADHD, such as methylphenidate. Meclizine and scopolamine are used for dizziness and vertigo. Acetylcholinesterase inhibitors, including donepezil, are used to help cognitive function. Erectile dysfunction can be treated with the phosphodiesterase inhibitors.

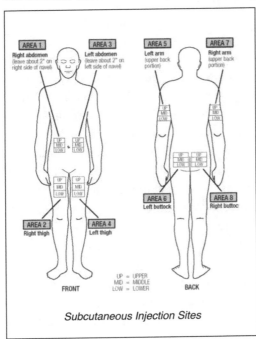

Subcutaneous Injection Sites

Notice that the drugs used for symptom control can worsen other symptoms. For example, anticholinergics can mildly worsen cognitive function (not all of them do, and this is patient-specific), but it happens. The vertigo agents can worsen cognitive function. Propranolol can worsen cognitive function, depression and cause problems with sexual performance. The SSRI and SNRI antidepressants can worsen sexual concerns. Opioids, if used for pain, will worsen constipation, can decrease cognition and have dependence concerns. Managing the various medications used for MS requires competent pharmacists.

RAYNAUD'S PHENOMENON

Raynaud's is a common condition which does not have drug tables discussed separately because the drugs used for treatment are common and are used for several other conditions. It is useful to know the presentation and which drugs are used for symptom relief. Raynaud's is triggered by exposure to cold and/or stress, which causes vasospasm in the extremities (most commonly in the fingers and/or toes). Laboratory findings that can signify other autoimmune conditions are generally absent. The vasospasm causes the skin to turn white and then blue, which is followed by painful swelling when the affected areas warm. The calcium channel blocker (CCB) <u>nifedipine</u> is commonly used for prevention – other CCBs can be used. Additional agents used for vasodilation include iloprost, topical nitroglycerin and the phosphodiesterase-5 inhibitors. Various other classes are used less commonly.

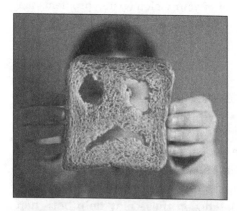

GUIDELINES

Rubio-Tapia, A, Hill ID, Kelly CP, et al. ACG clinical guidelines: diagnosis and management of celiac disease. *Am J Gastroenterol*. 2013; 108(5):656-76

King, AR. Gluten content of the top 200 medications: follow up to the influence of gluten on a patient's medication choices. *Hosp Pharm*. 2013; 48(9):736-43.

Gluten Free Drugs. www.gluten-freedrugs.com (accessed 2014 Nov 4).

CELIAC DISEASE

Background

Celiac disease (celiac sprue) is an immune response to eating <u>gluten, a protein found in wheat, barley and rye.</u> <u>The primary and effective treatment is to avoid gluten entirely</u>. Gluten is present in <u>many foods</u>, food additives <u>and in many drug excipients</u>. Pharmacists assist patients in avoiding gluten-containing drugs completely; <u>even a small exposure will trigger a reaction</u>. To emphasize this point, the FDA permits food products to be labeled "gluten-free' only if the food contains less gluten than 20 parts per million.

The <u>common symptoms</u> of celiac disease are <u>diarrhea, abdominal pain, bloating</u> and <u>weight loss</u>. Constipation (rather than diarrhea) can be present, and is more common in children. Symptoms can be atypical and sublime and diagnosis might occur only after a secondary problem is identified, such as growth problems in children or iron-deficiency anemia at any age. Vitamin deficiencies are common due to decreased absorption in the small intestine. Other complications include nutritional deficiencies (primarily anemia and osteoporosis), small bowel ulcers, amenorrhea and infertility, and increased risk of cancer (primarily lymphomas). Ninety-five percent of cases will respond well to dietary changes, although avoiding gluten entirely is not a simple task.

Dermatitis herpetiformis is an extremely itchy, blistery skin rash with chronic eruptions that is present in 20-25% of celiac patients, and occurs more often in males. The rash can be present with or without overt intestinal symptoms. The rash is often mistaken for eczema or psoriasis – which leads to a delay in diagnosis and treatment.

Non-Drug Treatment

The problem with identifying gluten content in drugs is due to the fact that while the FDA has strict regulations regarding the active ingredients in drugs they provide little oversight for the excipients. <u>Drugs themselves are gluten-free; it is the excipients that may be a problem</u>. And, it is not safe to assume that the generic formulations will contain the same excipients as the brand; there is no legal requirement to match the excipients.

The first place to look for excipient content is the <u>package insert</u>, which <u>may, or may not</u>, contain the <u>excipient components</u>. The key word to look for is "<u>starch</u>" which will be either <u>corn, potato, tapioca or wheat</u>. <u>If the package insert lists "starch" alone then the manufacturer must be consulted to find out if the starch is wheat</u>. The manufacturer may report that they do not use gluten in the manufacturing process, but they cannot state whether the excipients purchased from outside vendors are gluten-free; there may be cross-contamination. The risk of cross-contamination is low, but not absent, and this information should be provided to the patient who ultimately must decide, hopefully in consult with the prescriber, whether to take the drug or not.

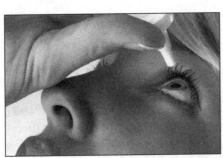

SJÖGREN'S SYNDROME

Sjögren's syndrome is an autoimmune disease, most often characterized by severe dry eyes and dry mouth. Many other symptoms can be associated with Sjögren's, including thyroiditis, Raynaud's phenomenon, neuropathy, and lymphadenopathy. Sjögren's syndrome can be primary or secondary, associated with another autoimmune disease such as RA or SLE. Dry mouth and dry eyes are a source of significant morbidity for these patients and can lead to complications such as dental caries, corneal ulceration and chronic oral infections. There is no known cure for Sjögren's; therefore, treatment focuses on reducing the symptoms of dry eyes and dry mouth.

Dry Eyes

The use of artificial teardrops is the primary treatment for dry eye. Popular OTC artificial teardrops available are *Systane, Refresh, Clear Eyes* and *Liquifilm*.

It may be necessary to try a couple of different OTC eye drops before finding one that provides the most comfort. If the preservative is irritating (likely benzoyl peroxide) most artificial tear drops come in individual use containers that are preservative-free. If the eyes dry out while sleeping an ointment is preferable.

Cyclosporine eye drops *(Restasis)* can be used in patients who do not get satisfactory relief from other measures, including ductal occlusion (lacrimal duct plugs). *Restasis* provides benefit for a small percentage of users and is expensive – patients should be instructed to monitor a reduction in symptoms and a reduction in the use of OTC eye drops and to <u>use properly to avoid infection</u>, which is more likely due to the dry eye state. Counsel patients that it may take up to 3-6 months to notice an increase in tear production.

Cyclosporine Emulsion Eye Drops

DRUG	DOSING	SAFETY/SIDE EFFECTS/MONITORING
CycloSPORINE Emulsion Eye Drops (*Restasis*)	1 drop to each eye twice daily (~12 hours apart)	**SIDE EFFECTS** Burning, stinging, redness, pain, blurred vision, foreign body sensation, discharge, itching eye **NOTES** One single-use vial is to be used immediately after opening on one or both eyes, and the remaining contents should be discarded immediately after administration. Do not allow the tip of the vial to touch the eye or any surface, as this can contaminate the emulsion. Remove contact lenses prior to administration, re-insert 15 min afterwards. Separate from artificial tears by 15 minutes.

Dry Mouth

Non-drug treatment for dry mouth includes salivary stimulation, using sugar-free chewing gum (with xylitol) and lozenges, and daily rinses with antimicrobial mouthwash. Salivary substitutes are available in lozenges, rinses, sprays, and swabs *(Plax, Oralube, Salivart)*. These contain carboxymethylcellulose or glycerin. If OTC treatments do not provide sufficient relief, prescription muscarinic agonists such as pilocarpine or cevimeline *(Evoxac)* can be used. Glycopyrrolate is used to decrease excessive salivation; this may be used in a few conditions, such as myasthenia gravis. Check that the dry mouth is not due to inappropriate use of this drug.

Muscarinic Agonists Used for Dry Mouth

DRUG	DOSING	SAFETY/SIDE EFFECTS/MONITORING
Pilocarpine *(Salagen)* Pilocarpine ophthalmic *(Isopto Carpine, Pilopine HS)* is used for glaucoma	5 mg four times daily Avoid taking with a high-fat meal	**CONTRANDICATIONS** Uncontrolled asthma, narrow-angle glaucoma, severe hepatic impairment **SIDE EFFECTS** Diaphoresis, flushing, nausea, urinary frequency, chills, weakness, rhinitis, dizziness
Cevimeline *(Evoxac)*	30 mg three times daily	**CONTRAINDICATIONS** Uncontrolled asthma, narrow-angle glaucoma, acute iritis **SIDE EFFECTS** Diaphoresis, nausea, URTIs (sinusitis, rhinitis)

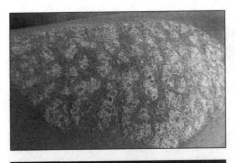

GUIDELINES

Menter A, Gottlieb A, Feldman SR, et al. Guidelines of care for the management of psoriasis and psoriatic arthritis. Section 1: overview of psoriasis and guidelines of care for the treatment of psoriasis with biologics. *J Am Acad Dermatol.* 2008; 58:826-50.

Additional guidelines included with the video files (RxPrep Online).

PSORIASIS

Psoriasis is a chronic, autoimmune disease that appears on the skin. There are several types of psoriasis. The most common is plaque psoriasis, which appears as raised, red patches covered with a silvery white buildup of dead skin cells, on any part of the body. Treatments can be divided into three main types: topical, light therapy, and systemic medications. Most psoriasis is treated with topicals and UV light therapy. Soaking helps loosen and remove the plaques.

Non-Drug Treatment

Ultraviolet (UV) light exposure causes activated T cells in the skin to die. This slows skin turnover and ↓ scaling and inflammation. Brief, daily exposures to small amounts of sunlight can improve psoriasis, but intense sun exposure can worsen symptoms and cause skin damage. UVB phototherapy, in controlled doses from an artificial source, can improve mild to moderate psoriasis symptoms. Other non-drug treatments include photochemotherapy (ultraviolet A light with psoralen, a light sensitizer), and laser light therapy.

Drug Treatment

There are many topical options for treating psoriasis including steroids, vitamin D analogues (calcipotriene), anthralin, topical retinoids (some of the same drugs used for acne), salicylic acid (primarily in medicated shampoo), coal tar and moisturizers. If these fail, calcineurin inhibitor topicals *(Protopic, Elidel)* can be tried. Treatment for more severe symptoms may require immune suppressing agents, including methotrexate, cyclosporine, hydroxyurea and the immunomodulators, such as etanercept and infliximab. Newer systemic agents approved for plaque psoriasis include *Stelara* and *Otezla*.

DRUG	DOSING	SAFETY/SIDE EFFECTS/MONITORING
Topical Steroids	Monotherapy: 1-2 times daily (product dependent)	Use high-potency steroids only short-term due to risk of side effects. Can be used with other therapies See Common Skin Conditions chapter
Retinoids		See Common Skin Conditions chapter
Coal tar, in many products, including *Neutrogena T, Denorex, Psoriasin, MG217 Psoriasis* Topical (cream, foam, emulsion, ointment, oil, shampoo), bath products (topicals, bar soap) + salicylic acid (*Sebutone, Tarsum,* others)	Body: Apply 1-4 times per day, usually at bedtime Scalp psoriasis: Apply sparingly to lesions 3-12 hours before each shampoo	Coal tar products are messy, time consuming and can stain clothing and bedding. Some patients get relief at a reasonable cost. Also used for dandruff and dermatitis Do not use salicylic acid products with other salicylates, systemic absorption can occur **SIDE EFFECTS** Skin irritation, photosensitivity

Psoriasis Drugs Continued

DRUG	DOSING	SAFETY/SIDE EFFECTS/MONITORING
Anthralin (*Zithranol*, others)	Body: once daily or as directed	Keratolyic with irritant potential, ↑ contact time as tolerated
Calcipotriene (*Dovonex, Calcitrene, Sorilux*) Cream, foam, ointment, solution + betamethasone (*Taclonex ointment, Taclonex scalp suspension*)	Plaque psoriasis: Cream, foam, solution: Apply BID Ointment: Apply daily-BID *Taclonex*: Apply once daily for up to 4 weeks Do not use > 100 g ointment weekly or use on > 30% of BSA	**CONTRAINDICATIONS** Avoid in hypercalcemia or vitamin D toxicity, do not use on face **NOTES** Vitamin D analog If suspension shake well Do not apply to face, axillae or groin
Acitretin (*Soriatane*) Tablet	25-50 mg daily with main meal of the day (lower doses ↓ side effects)	Used only in severe cases due to numerous contraindications and side effects Pregnancy Category X MedGuide required
Ustekinumab (*Stelara*) Injection Monoclonal antibody (see others in Rheumatoid Arthritis section of chapter)	Plaque psoriasis ≤ 100 kg: 45 mg at 0 and 4 weeks, then every 12 weeks thereafter > 100 kg: 90 mg at 0 and 4 weeks, then every 12 weeks thereafter	**WARNINGS** Risk for serious infections (including active TB, fungal, viral, bacterial or opportunistic infections), lymphomas and other malignancies. Discontinue therapy if a serious infection develops, screen for latent TB and treat before starting therapy, no live vaccines **SIDE EFFECTS** Infection, hypersensitivity reaction, neurotoxicity (rare) **NOTES** Indicated only for plaque psoriasis and psoriatic arthritis. Avoid injecting into areas where psoriasis is present. Do not shake. Requires protection from light prior to administration.
Apremilast (*Otezla*) Tablet Phosphodiesterase 4 inhibitor	Plaque psoriasis 10 mg daily in the morning, titrate daily to 30 mg BID ↓ dose in severe renal impairment	**SIDE EFFECTS** Weight loss, diarrhea, depression & suicidal ideation (rare) **NOTES** Indicated only for plaque psoriasis and psoriatic arthritis.

Apremilast Drug Interactions

- Apremilast is a major CYP450 3A4 substrate. Strong 3A4 inducers should be avoided concomitantly.

PRACTICE CASE

PATIENT PROFILE

Patient Name	Gina Campos				
Address	1954 Milton Drive, San Gabriel				
Age	44	**Sex** Female	**Race** Hispanic	**Height** 5'3"	**Weight** 140 lbs
Allergies	None known				

DIAGNOSES

Rheumatoid Arthritis	Poor exercise tolerance
Hypertension	
Depression	
Chronic fatigue	

MEDICATIONS

Date	No.	Prescriber	Drug & Strength	Quantity	Sig	Refills
4/20/13	55287	Casey	Lisinopril 20 mg	30	1 PO daily	11
4/20/13	55288	Casey	Methotrexate 7.5 mg	8	2 tabs weekly	3
4/20/13	55289	Casey	Prednisone 10 mg	45	1 PO daily	3
4/20/13	55292	Casey	Alendronate 70 mg	4	1 PO weekly	3
		(OTC)	Calcium 500+ D 400 IU		1 tab Q AM	

LAB/DIAGNOSTIC TESTS

Test	Normal Value	Results Date 5/12/13	Date	Date
Rheum Fact	< 40 IU/mL	88 IU/mL		
ESR	≤ 30 mm/hr	81.1 mm/hr		
Alk Phos	33-115 u/L			
AST	10-35 IU/L	48 IU/L		
ALT	6-40 IU/L	76 IU/L		
GLU	65-99 mg/dL			
Na	135-146 mEq/L			
K	3.5-5.3 mEq/L			
Cl	98-110 mEq/L			
HCO3-	22-28 mEq/L			
BUN	7-25 mg/dL			
Creatinine	0.6-1.2 mg/dL			
Calcium	8.6-10.2 mg/dL			
WBC	4-11 cells/mm³	5.8 cells/mm³		
TB test, PPD		Negative		

ADDITIONAL INFORMATION

Date	Notes
7/31/13	BP 122/78 mmHg. Patient reports morning stiffness for past 2 months which improves as the day progresses. Reports that wrists, arms and leg joints are swollen and tender. States she is physically exhausted. No chest pain, breathing problems.

Questions

1. The prescriber is deciding whether to change the dose of methotrexate to daily therapy or begin etanercept. Choose the correct response:

    a. The methotrexate can be increased safely to 50 mg daily for rheumatoid arthritis.
    b. The methotrexate can be increased safely to 100 mg daily for rheumatoid arthritis.
    c. The methotrexate can be increased safely to 150 mg daily for rheumatoid arthritis.
    d. The methotrexate can be increased safely to 200 mg daily for rheumatoid arthritis.
    e. Methotrexate is not given daily for this condition.

2. The pharmacist will counsel the patient on her methotrexate therapy. She should include the following counseling points: (Select **ALL** that apply.)

    a. Common side effects include GI upset, nausea and diarrhea.
    b. She should not get pregnant while using this medication.
    c. Her liver will need to be checked periodically with a blood test.
    d. Choose a day of the week that you will remember to take the medicine.
    e. She should be taking leucovorin as well.

3. The patient is using prednisone 10 mg daily and weekly bisphosphonate therapy. Choose the correct statement:

    a. She does not need supplemental calcium and vitamin D with the alendronate.
    b. The prednisone may improve her blood pressure control.
    c. If she is able, her healthcare provider should try and help her decrease the prednisone dose.
    d. Prednisone is not bad for bones; in fact, it builds strong bones.
    e. A, B and C.

4. The physician decides to begin etanercept therapy. Choose the correct administration route for this medication:

    a. Oral tablets
    b. Suppository
    c. Subcutaneous injection
    d. Intramuscular injection
    e. Intravenous infusion

5. The pharmacist will counsel the patient on the etanercept therapy. She should include the following counseling points: (Select **ALL** that apply.)

    a. Store the medication at room temperature.
    b. Inject subcutaneously in the deltoid muscle.
    c. This medication can activate latent tuberculosis; you will need to have a TB test prior to starting therapy.
    d. This medication does not cause increased risk of infections, except for tuberculosis.
    e. You can receive live vaccines, but not the annual influenza vaccine.

6. A physician has written a prescription for *Humira*. Choose the appropriate therapeutic interchange:

    a. Adalimumab
    b. Etanercept
    c. Rituximab
    d. Anakinra
    e. Infliximab

7. A physician has written a prescription for *Remicade*. Choose the appropriate therapeutic interchange:

    a. Adalimumab
    b. Etanercept
    c. Rituximab
    d. Anakinra
    e. Infliximab

Answers

1-e, 2-a,b,c,d, 3-c, 4-c, 5-c, 6-a, 7-e

THYROID DISORDERS

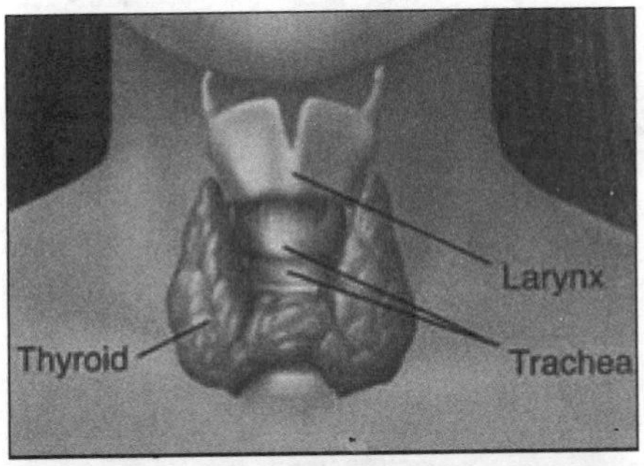
Larynx
Thyroid
Trachea

GUIDELINES

American Thyroid Association task force on thyroid hormone replacement. Guidelines for the treatment of hypothyroidism. http://www.thyroid.org/wp-content/uploads/publications/guidelines/thy.2014.0028.pdf (accessed 2014 Nov 6).

Garber JR, Cobin RH, Gharib H, et al. Clinical practice guidelines for hypothyroidism in adults: cosponsored by the American Association of Clinical Endocrinologists and the American Thyroid Association. *Endocr Pract.* 2012; 18(6):988-1028.

Bahn RS, Burch HB, Cooper DS, et al. Hyperthyroidism and other causes of thyrotoxicosis: management guidelines of the American Thyroid Association and American Association of Clinical Endocrinologists. *Thyroid.* 2011; 21(6):593-646.

Additional guidelines included with the video files (RxPrep Online).

BACKGROUND

The thyroid gland is a butterfly-shaped organ composed of two symmetrical lobes, one on each side of the windpipe, connected by the isthmus. The thyroid gland synthesizes and releases thyroid hormones. Thyroid hormones affect metabolism, brain development, respiration, cardiac and nervous system functions, body temperature, muscle strength, skin dryness, menstrual cycles, body weight, and cholesterol levels. The thyroid gland is one of the largest organs within the body's endocrine system and is the only organ which contains cells that have the ability to absorb iodine. Hyperthyroidism (overactive thyroid) and hypothyroidism (underactive thyroid) are the most common problems of the thyroid gland. Hypothyroidism occurs more commonly in women, and its incidence increases with age.

I_2 + tyrosine { T_3 = iodothyronine; T_4 = thyroxine

PATHOPHYSIOLOGY

The thyroid gland produces two thyroid hormones, triiodothyronine (T_3) and thyroxine (T_4). Iodine and tyrosine are used to form both T_3 and T_4. Less than 20% of T_3 is produced by the thyroid gland; T_3 is primarily formed from the breakdown of T_4 by peripheral tissues. T_3 is more potent than T_4 but has a much shorter half-life. Thyroid hormone production is regulated by thyroid-stimulating hormone (TSH or thyrotropin), which is made by the pituitary gland in the brain. Elevations in T_4 levels will inhibit the secretion of TSH, and create a negative feedback loop. Since T_3 and T_4 are transported in the blood and bound by proteins, it is important to measure the free T_4 (FT_4) levels as this is the active form. In hypothyroidism, there is a deficiency in T_4, and consequently an elevation

TSH = thyrotropin made by pituitary
↑T_4 ⇒ ↓TSH

- < 20% T_3 ⇒ made by thyroid
- (80%) T_3 primarily formed by T_4 → T_3 in periphery
- T_3 more potent than T_4, shorter $t_{1/2}$

free T_4 ⇒ ACTIVE form ⇒ measure!

hypothyroidism ⇒ ↓T_4, ↑TSH
hyperthyroidism ⇒ ↑T_4, ↓TSH

in TSH. In hyperthyroidism, there is over-secretion of T_4, and consequently a low level of TSH.

HYPOTHYROIDISM

In hypothyroidism, the decrease in thyroid hormone causes the body to slow down and the classic symptoms of low metabolism appear (fatigue, weight gain). The most common cause of hypothyroidism is Hashimoto's disease, an autoimmune condition in which a patient's antibodies attack their own thyroid gland. Screening for hypothyroidism should be considered for patients > 60 years old. Drugs can also cause hypothyroidism (listed in the chart to the right) and may require monitoring of thyroid function tests. When hypothyroidism decompensates or goes untreated for a long period, myxedema coma can result. Myxedema coma is a life-threatening emergency characterized by poor circulation, hypothermia and hypometabolism. Due to unpredictable absorption of oral thyroid hormone from the gastrointestinal tract, intravenous thyroid hormone products should be administered.

myxedema
↓ bp
↓ circulation
↓ metab
⇒ give IV thyroid hormone

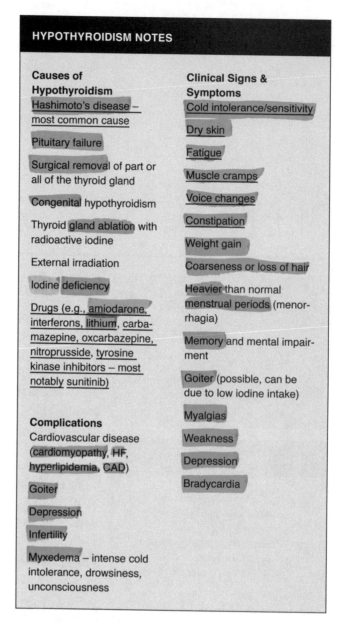

HYPOTHYROIDISM NOTES

Causes of Hypothyroidism
Hashimoto's disease – most common cause

Pituitary failure

Surgical removal of part or all of the thyroid gland

Congenital hypothyroidism

Thyroid gland ablation with radioactive iodine

External irradiation

Iodine deficiency

Drugs (e.g., amiodarone, interferons, lithium, carbamazepine, oxcarbazepine, nitroprusside, tyrosine kinase inhibitors – most notably sunitinib)

Complications
Cardiovascular disease (cardiomyopathy, HF, hyperlipidemia, CAD)

Goiter

Depression

Infertility

Myxedema – intense cold intolerance, drowsiness, unconsciousness

Clinical Signs & Symptoms
Cold intolerance/sensitivity

Dry skin

Fatigue

Muscle cramps

Voice changes

Constipation

Weight gain

Coarseness or loss of hair

Heavier than normal menstrual periods (menorrhagia)

Memory and mental impairment

Goiter (possible, can be due to low iodine intake)

Myalgias

Weakness

Depression

Bradycardia

Diagnosis

Low free thyroxine (↓ FT_4) (normal range 0.9 - 2.3 ng/dL)

High thyroid stimulating hormone (↑ TSH) (normal range 0.3 – 3.0 mIU/L)

Monitoring Parameters

TSH is the primary screening test for thyroid function and it is the most reliable therapeutic endpoint for treatment. Check TSH levels (rarely serum free T_4) and clinical symptoms every 4-6 weeks until levels are normal, then 4-6 months later, then yearly. It is important to monitor as the person ages; they may need a dose reduction. Over-dosing levothyroxine in elderly patents leads to atrial fibrillation and fractures. Serum free T_4 is monitored, in addition to TSH, in central hypothyroidism (rare) because the defect is pituitary production of TSH.

- √ TSH + sx q 4-6 wks until normal levels
  then 4-6 mo later
  then yearly

- ↑ levo dose in elderly
  → a fib, fractures

- monitor free T4 in CENTRAL HYPOTHYROIDISM!!
  (defect in pituitary, TSH production)

Pregnancy and Hypothyroidism

Levothyroxine is FDA pregnancy category A. Pregnant women with thyroid hormone deficiency or TSH elevation during pregnancy may have children at risk of impairment in their intellectual function and motor skills, unless properly treated. Pregnant women being treated with thyroid hormone replacement will require a 30-50% increase in the levothyroxine dose throughout the course of their pregnancy. The mother will need an elevated dose for several months after giving birth. In 2011 new guidelines called for more aggressive control of hypothyroidism in pregnancy. Preferably, treatment should start prior to pregnancy.

Drug Treatment

The goals of therapy are to resolve signs and symptoms of hypothyroidism, normalize serum TSH, and avoid overtreatment (causing hyperthyroidism). Counsel the patient regarding clinical symptoms for both hypo- and hyperthyroidism as the dose will be titrated to the individual's needs. Per the guidelines, levothyroxine (T_4) is the drug of choice and current recommendations encourage the use of a consistent preparation for the patient to minimize variability from refill to refill. There are patients who state they just do not "feel right" on T_4 alone, and may be supplementing with other formulations, such as liothyronine (T_3, *Cytomel* and *Triostat*) or desiccated thyroid (T_3 and T_4, *Armour Thyroid*). Desiccated thyroid is not favored since the preparations can contain variable amounts, although newer formulations have become standardized. This is called "natural thyroid" and it is dosed in "grains." Some patients choose to use these alternatives alone.

Levothyroxine should be taken with water consistently 60 minutes before breakfast or at bedtime 3 hours after the last meal. It should be stored properly per product insert and not taken with substances or medications that interfere with its absorption.

Iodine supplementation, including kelp or other iodine-containing functional foods, is not recommended in the management of hypothyroidism in iodine-sufficient areas.

Potassium Iodide Use After Exposure to Radiation

Potassium iodide (KI) blocks the accumulation of radioactive iodine in the thyroid gland; thus preventing thyroid cancer. Potassium iodide should be taken as soon as possible after radiation exposure, at the right dose, but not with an over-dose. The doses below are for 24 hours. If the radiation exposure is longer, refer to the CDC website for repeat-dose instructions. Iodized salt and foods do not contain enough iodine to block radioactive iodine and are not recommended.

doses for 24 hrs only (refer to CDC if radiation x > 24 hrs)

- Birth – 1 month: 16 mg KI

- Infants and children between 1 month–3 years: 32 mg KI

- Children 3 -18 years: 65 mg KI

- Adults and children > 68 kg: 130 mg KI

levothyroxine dosing:
① *1.6 ug/kg/day (IBW) – full replacement dose*
   * adults < 50 y/o
② *25-50 ug/day (or 0.5 ug/kg/day) – partial replacement dose*
   * elderly, mild dz or comorbidities
③ *12.5 – 25 ug/day – known CAD*

Hypothyroid Treatment

DRUG	DOSING	SAFETY/SIDE EFFECTS/MONITORING
Levothyroxine (T₄) *(Synthroid, Levothroid, Levoxyl, Unithroid, Tirosint)* Check AB-rating of a generic to a brand. Not all generic levothyroxine formulations are AB-rated to various brands. If you change formulations, check signs and symptoms and levels in 4-6 weeks. Capsule, tablet, inj.	13, 25, 50, 75, 88, 100, 112, 125, 137, 150, 175, 200, 300 mcg Full replacement dose = 1.6 mcg/kg/day (IBW) Can start with full replacement dose in otherwise healthy, young and middle age patients with markedly ↑ TSH. Can start with partial replacement dose (25-50 mcg daily) in the elderly, milder hypothyroidism, and those with comorbidities. If known CAD, start with 12.5-25 mcg daily. **Usual Dose** 0.5 mcg/kg/day for elderly; see above 1.6 mcg/kg/day in younger patients (< 50 years of age) **TABLETS** 25 mcg – orange 50 mcg – white (no dye) 75 mcg – violet 88 mcg – olive 100 mcg – yellow 112 mcg – rose 125 mcg – brown 137 mcg – turquoise 150 mcg – blue 175 mcg – lilac 200 mcg – pink 300 mcg – green	**BOXED WARNING** Thyroid supplements are ineffective and potentially toxic when used for the treatment of obesity or for weight reduction, especially in euthyroid patients. High doses may produce serious or even life-threatening toxic effects particularly when used with some anorectic drugs (e.g., sympathomimetic amines). **CONTRAINDICATIONS** Acute MI, thyrotoxicosis, uncorrected adrenal insufficiency **WARNINGS** Use with caution and reduce dosage in patients with cardiovascular disease; chronic hypothyroidism predisposes patients to coronary artery disease **SIDE EFFECTS** If patient is euthyroid, no side effects should exist. If dose is too high, patient will experience hyperthyroid symptoms such as ↑ HR, palpitations, sweating, weight loss, arrhythmias, irritability, others. **MONITORING** Check TSH levels (rarely free T₄) and clinical symptoms every 4-6 weeks until levels are normal, then 4-6 months later, then yearly. It is important to monitor as the person ages; they may need a dose reduction. Over-dosing levothyroxine in elderly patents leads to atrial fibrillation and fracture. Assessment of serum free T₄, in addition to TSH, can be used selectively in some patients. **NOTES** Pregnancy Category A Highly protein bound (> 99%) Levothyroxine is the drug of choice due to chemical stability, once-daily dosing, inexpensiveness, free of antigenicity and has more uniform potency. **Levothyroxine IV** Must be given upon reconstitution. Requires protection from light during administration. IV to PO ratio is 0.75:1
Thyroid, Desiccated USP (T₃ and T₄) *(Armour Thyroid, Nature-Throid, Westhroid, NP Thyroid, WP Thyroid)* Tablet	Start 15-30 mg daily (15 mg in cardiac disease and elderly); titrate in 15 mg increments. Usual dose is 60-120 mg daily	**Thyroid USP** Natural porcine-derived thyroid that contains both T₃ and T₄; less predictable potency and stability (Not preferred, but some feel better using it
Liothyronine (T₃) *(Cytomel, Triostat)* Tablet, inj.	Start 25 mcg daily; titrate in 12.5-25 mcg increments. Usual dose is 25-75 mcg daily	**Liothyronine** Shorter t ½ leading to fluctuations in T₃ levels
Liotrix (T₃ and T₄ in 1:4 ratio) *(Thyrolar)* Tablet	Start 25 mcg levothyroxine/6.25 mcg liothyronine – usual dose is 50-100 mcg levothyroxine/12.5-25 mcg liothyronine.	

(margin notes)

1st → line in guidelines

IBW

IV
- *give upon recon*
- *light protect during admin*
- $\dfrac{IV}{PO} = \dfrac{0.75}{1}$

levo has long t½ ~ 7 days

shorter t½ [T₃] ⇒ fluctuations

$\dfrac{T_3}{T_4} = \dfrac{1}{4}$

(handwritten top margin)
can ↓ thy roid {• Al⁻, Ca⁺⁺, Mg⁺⁺, Fe, orlistat, sevelamer – separate by ④ hrs
• lanthanum – separate by ② hrs
– β-blockers, amiodarone, steroids, PTU – ↓ $T_4 \to T_3$ conversion

Drug Interactions

Drugs that Decrease Thyroid Hormone Levels

- Aluminum (antacids), calcium, cholestyr-amine, iron, magnesium, multivitamins (containing ADEK, folate, iron), orlistat *(Xenical, Alli)*, sevelamer, sodium polystyrene *(Kayexa-late)*, sucralfate: all ↓ absorption; separate doses by 4 hours

  used to ↓[phosphate] in renal dz

- Separate doses of lanthanum by 2 hours from thyroid replacement therapy

- Estrogen and hepatic inducers (e.g., carbam-azepine, phenobarbital, phenytoin, rifampin, others): ↓ thyroid hormone levels

↓ $T_4 \to T_3$ (efficacy) - Beta-blockers, amiodarone, glucocorticoids, and PTU may decrease the effectiveness of levothyroxine by decreasing the conversion of T_4 to T_3

↓ [thyroid] - SSRIs can decrease thyroid levels

- Thyroid hormone is highly-protein bound (>99%). Drugs that may cause protein-binding site displacement include salicylates (> 2 g/day), heparin, phenytoin, NSAIDs, others.

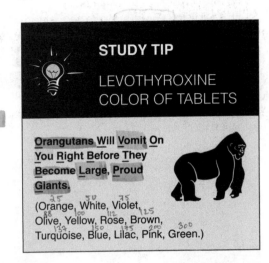

(handwritten numbers near colors: 25, 50, 75, 88, 100, 112, 125, 137, 150, 175, 200, 300)

Thyroid hormone can change concentrations/effects of these drugs:

- ↑ effect of anticoagulants (e.g., increased PT/INR with warfarin)

- ↓ digoxin levels

- ↓ theophylline levels

- ↓ effect of antidiabetic agents

(handwritten) ↑ anticoag effect (↑INR)
↓ [digoxin, theophylline, antiDM]

Patient Counseling for Levothyroxine

- Levothyroxine is a replacement for a hormone that is normally produced by your body to regulate your energy and metabolism. Levothyroxine is given when the thyroid does not produce enough of this hormone on its own.

- There are many medicines that can alter levothyroxine effects; tell the pharmacist about all medications you are taking. This includes over-the-counter vitamins, supplements and heartburn medications.

- Different brands of levothyroxine may not work the same. If you get a prescription refill and your new pills look different, ask the pharmacist.

- This medicine is safe to use while you are pregnant. It is also safe to use while you are breast-feeding a baby. It does pass into breast milk, but it is not harmful to a nursing infant.

(handwritten) ↑ 30-50% - Tell your healthcare provider if you become pregnant during treatment; it is likely that your dose will need to be increased during pregnancy or if you plan to breast-feed.

- Take this medication with water 60 minutes before breakfast or at bedtime, 3 hours after your last meal.

(handwritten) can cause insomnia if taken hs

- If you are taking other medicines on an empty stomach first thing in the morning, discuss the best dosing with your pharmacist. Medications for your bones (osteoporosis) like Actonel or Fosamax will need to separated from your thyroid medicine.

- Some patients will notice a slight reduction in symptoms within 1 to 2 weeks, but the full effect from therapy is often delayed for a month or two before people start to feel normal.

- Even if you feel well, you still need to take this medicine every day for the rest of your life to replace the thyroid hormone your body cannot produce.

- To be sure the dose being used is optimal for you, your blood will need to be tested on a regular basis (at least annually).

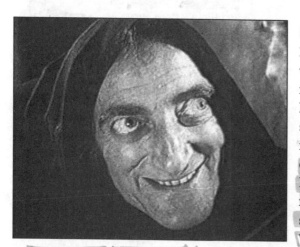

HYPERTHYROIDISM (THYROTOXICOSIS)

Hyperthyroidism (overactive thyroid) occurs when there is over-production of thyroid hormones. Instead of low FT_4 and high TSH, you have high FT_4 and low TSH and nearly opposite symptoms as compared to hypothyroidism. Hyperthyroidism can significantly accelerate the metabolism, causing sudden weight loss, a rapid or irregular heartbeat, sweating, nervousness, irritability, diarrhea and insomnia. Goiter and exophthalmos can occur. Without treatment, hyperthyroidism can lead to tachycardia, arrhythmias, heart failure and osteoporosis. No one should be using thyroid hormone to lose weight – they will be irritable and can end up with severe cardiac complications. Interestingly, older cats often get hyperthyroidism (more frequently than dogs) and pharmacists occasionally fill scripts for patients with names like Kitty.

HYPERTHYRODISM NOTES

Causes of Hyperthyroidism	Clinical Signs and Symptoms	
Graves' disease – most common cause	Heat intolerance or increased sweating	Insomnia
Toxic multinodular goiter	Weight loss (or gain)	Light or absent menstrual periods
Toxic adenoma	Agitation, nervousness, irritability, anxiety	Goiter (possible)
Thyroiditis		Thinning hair
Drugs (e.g., iodine, amiodarone, interferons, too much thyroid hormone)	Palpitations and tachycardia	Tremor
	Fatigue and muscle weakness	Exophthalmos (exophthalmia), diplopia
	Frequent bowel movements or diarrhea	

Causes

The most common cause of hyperthyroidism is Graves' disease, which tends to occur in females in their 30's and 40's. Graves' disease is an autoimmune disorder (like Hashimoto's) but instead of destroying the gland, the antibodies stimulate the thyroid to produce too much T_4. Less commonly, a single nodule is responsible for the excess hormone secretion. Thyroiditis (inflammation of the thyroid) can also cause hyperthyroidism. Drugs that can cause hyperthyroidism include iodine, amiodarone and interferons. Hyperthyroidism can also occur in patients who take excessive doses of any of the available forms of thyroid hormone.

do not give in pregnancy

Treatment involves anti-thyroid medications, destroying part of the gland via radioactive iodine (RAI-131) or surgery. RAI-131 is the treatment of choice in Graves' disease. With any option, the patient can be treated with beta blockers first for symptom control (to reduce palpitations, tremors and tachycardia). PTU or methimazole can be used as a temporary measure until surgery is complete. Initially, when treating with drugs, it takes 1-3 months at higher doses to control symptoms, at which point the dose is reduced to prevent hypothyroidism from occurring.

Hyperthyroid Treatment

DRUG	DOSING	SAFETY/SIDE EFFECTS/MONITORING

Thionamides – inhibit synthesis of thyroid hormones by blocking the oxidation of iodine in the thyroid gland; PTU also inhibits peripheral conversion of T_4 to T_3

DRUG	DOSING	SAFETY/SIDE EFFECTS/MONITORING
Propylthiouracil (PTU)	50-150 mg Q8H initially (or higher) until euthyroid, followed by dose reduction	**BOXED WARNING** Severe liver injury and acute liver failure (with PTU) *can occur suddenly even after long term use* **SIDE EFFECTS** GI upset, headache, rash, pruritus, fever, constipation, loss of taste/taste perversion, drug-induced lupus erythematosus (DILE), lymphadenopathy Hepatitis, agranulocytosis (rare): see MD at once for yellow skin, abdominal pain, high fever, or severe sore throat. *leukopenia (↓ WBC, esp. neutrophils) ⇒ monitor for signs of infxn* **MONITORING** CBC, LFTs, PT and thyroid function tests (TSH, FT_4, total T_3) every 4-6 weeks until euthyroid
Methimazole (*Tapazole*)	Mild hyperthyroidism: 15 mg Q8H initially until euthyroid (↑ doses for more severe hyperthyroidism), then 5-15 mg daily	**NOTES** Pregnancy Category D – PTU preferred in 1st trimester – change to methimazole for 2nd and 3rd trimesters due to increased risk of liver toxicity from PTU PTU is preferred in thyroid storm Take with food to reduce GI upset Patient must monitor for liver toxicity (abdominal pain, yellow skin/eyes, dark urine, nausea, weakness) PTU is not a first line treatment for hyperthyroidism except in patients who cannot tolerate other options or conditions where other antithyroid therapies are contraindicated.

Handwritten notes:
- MOA: both inhibit thyroid hormone synthesis by blocking oxidation of I_2 in thyroid gland
- MOA: $T_4 \nrightarrow T_3$ in periphery
- BBW: ① severe liver injury ② acute liver failure
- preferred in 1st trimester ONLY due to ↑ hepatotox
- can ↓ anticoag effect of warfarin
- use in 2nd & 3rd trimesters
- take both w/ food
- both dosed TID

Hyperthyroid Treatment Continued

DRUG	DOSING	SAFETY/SIDE EFFECTS/MONITORING

Iodides – temporarily inhibit secretion of thyroid hormones; T_4 and T_3 levels will be reduced for several weeks but effect will **not** be maintained

b/c thyroid gland then starts to use this I_2 to make thyroid hormone — *2 weeks – 2 mo*

DRUG	DOSING	SAFETY/SIDE EFFECTS/MONITORING
Potassium Iodide and Iodine solution (*Lugol's solution*) Off label	4-8 drops Q8H	**CONTRAINDICATIONS** Hypersensitivity to iodide or iodine; dermatitis herpetiformis; hypocomplementemic vasculitis, nodular thyroid condition with heart disease **SIDE EFFECTS** Rash, metallic taste, sore throat/gums, GI upset, urticaria, hypo/hyperthyroidism with prolonged use
Saturated solution of potassium iodide (*SSKI, ThyroShield*) *inorganic*	1-2 drops Q8H	**MONITORING** Thyroid function tests, signs and symptoms of hyperthyroidism **NOTES** Pregnancy Category D Dilute in a glassful of water, juice, or milk. Take with food or milk to reduce GI upset

w/ thionamides may ↓ INR dosed TID

Drug Interactions with Thionamides

- May decrease the anticoagulant effect of warfarin; monitor.

THYROID STORM

Thyroid storm is a life-threatening medical emergency characterized by decompensated hyperthyroidism that can be precipitated by infection, trauma, surgery, radio-active iodine treatment or non-adherence to antithyroid medication. The following treatment measures mentioned below must be implemented promptly.

Treatments

- ① Antithyroid drug therapy (PTU is preferred; 900-1,200 mg PO daily – divided every 4-6 hrs) PLUS
  - Can crush tablets and administer through NG-tube if needed
  - Given 1 hour before iodide to block synthesis of thyroid hormone

- + ② Inorganic iodide therapy such as SSKI 3-5 drops PO Q8H or Lugol's solution 5-10 drops PO Q8H PLUS

- + ③ Beta-adrenergic blockade (e.g., propranolol 40-80 mg PO Q6H) PLUS

- + ④ Corticosteroid therapy (e.g., dexamethasone 2-4 mg PO Q6H) PLUS

- + ⑤ Aggressive cooling with acetaminophen and cooling blankets and other supportive treatments (e.g., antiarrhythmics, insulin, fluids, electrolytes, etc.)

1) antiarrhythmics
2) insulin
3) fluids
4) electrolytes

THYROID STORM SIGNS & SYMPTOMS
Fever (> 103°F)
Tachycardia
Tachypnea
Dehydration
Profuse sweating
Agitation
Delirium
Psychosis
Coma

PRACTICE CASE

MT is a 45 y/o white female who comes to the clinic complaining of more fatigue than normal and constipation. On exam, the patient has some dry skin patches and looks a bit depressed. Her past medical history is significant for GERD.

Allergies: NKDA

Medications:
Dexilant 30 mg PO daily
Maalox 2 tablespoonfuls PRN heartburn

Vitals:
Height: 5'4" Weight: 122 lbs
BP: 139/82 mmHg HR: 62 BPM RR: 15 BPM Temp: 38°C Pain: 0/10

Labs:
Na (mEq/L) = 138 (135 - 145)
K (mEq/L) = 4.5 (3.5 - 5)
Cl (mEq/L) = 98 (95 - 103)
HCO_3 (mEq/L) = 29 (24 - 30)
BUN (mg/dL) = 11 (7 - 20)
SCr (mg/dL) = 0.9 (0.6 - 1.3)
Glucose (mg/dL) = 87 (100 - 125)
Ca (mg/dL) = 10.1 (8.5 - 10.5)
Mg (mEq/L) = 1.8 (1.3 - 2.1)
PO_4 (mg/dL) = 3.0 (2.3 - 4.7)
TSH (mIU/L) = 44 (0.3 - 3)
Free T_4 (ng/dL) = 0.5 (0.9 - 2.3)

Initiate therapy for new diagnosis of hypothyroidism and educate patient.

Questions

1. The physician is considering starting thyroid medication for MT. Which of the following options is considered <u>most</u> appropriate for <u>initial</u> therapy?

    a. Levoxyl
    b. Armour Thyroid
    c. Thyrolar
    d. RAI 131
    e. Propranolol

2. What is the full replacement starting dose of *Synthroid* for MT?

    a. 12.5 mcg daily
    b. 25 mg daily
    c. 75 mg daily
    d. 88 mcg daily
    e. 125 mg daily

3. Which of the following medications can decrease the levels of levothyroxine?

    a. Magnesium – Aluminum hydroxide (Maalox)
    b. Iron
    c. Warfarin
    d. A and B only
    e. A, B, and C

4. Propylthiouracil is associated with which of the following serious adverse effects?

    a. Pregnancy
    b. Liver failure
    c. Renal failure
    d. Rhabdomyolysis
    e. Priapism

5. What is the most common cause of hypo-thyroidism?

    a. Graves' disease
    b. Hashimoto's disease
    c. Surgery
    d. Amiodarone
    e. Lithium

6. A patient is beginning levothyroxine therapy. Patient counseling points should include the following:

    a. You should feel all better by this afternoon or tomorrow morning.
    b. Your doctor will need to recheck your thyroid hormone levels in 4-6 weeks.
    c. If you get pregnant, stop using this medicine.
    d. A and C only
    e. All of the above

7. Which of the following are symptoms of hypothyroidism?

    a. Fatigue
    b. Weight gain or increased difficulty losing weight
    c. Diarrhea
    d. A and B only
    e. All of the above

8. The pharmacist should instruct the patient to take levothyroxine in this manner:

    a. The first thing in the morning, with food
    b. The first thing in the morning, about 60 minutes before food or other medicines
    c. With the largest meal to reduce nausea
    d. With dinner since levothyroxine is sedating
    e. At bedtime

9. A pregnant female is being started on levo-thyroxine therapy. Levothyroxine has the following pregnancy rating:

    a. Pregnancy Category A
    b. Pregnancy Category B
    c. Pregnancy Category C
    d. Pregnancy Category D
    e. Pregnancy Category X

10. What is the most common cause of hyper-thyroidism?

    a. Hashimoto's disease
    b. Pituitary failure
    c. Lithium
    d. Amiodarone
    e. Graves' disease

Answers

1-a, 2-d, 3-d, 4-b, 5-b, 6-b, 7-d, 8-b, 9-a, 10-e

TRANSPLANT/ IMMUNOSUPPRESSION

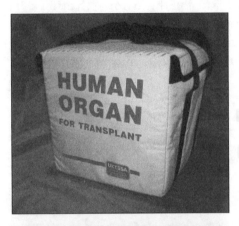

GUIDELINES

Resources available at: http://www.kidney.org/professionals/(accessed 2014 Dec 2).

Kasiske BL, Zeier MG, Chapman JR et al. KDIGO clinical practice guideline for the care of kidney transplant recipients: a summary. *Am J Transplant*. 2009; 9(Suppl 3):S1-155.

BACKGROUND

Transplantation medicine is one of the most challenging and complex areas of modern medicine. Some of the key areas for medical management are the problems of transplant rejection, during which the body has an immune response to the transplanted organ, possibly leading to transplant failure and the need to immediately remove the organ from the recipient. Although other organs can be transplanted (primarily kidney, liver, heart, lung, and pancreas), the majority of transplant cases are kidney (1st) and liver (2nd). Prior to any transplant, tissue typing or crossmatching is performed to assess donor-recipient compatibility for human leukocyte antigen (HLA) and ABO blood group. A mismatch in either would lead to a fast, acute rejection. This is followed by a Panel Reactive Antibody (PRA) test that is taken to gauge the degree to which the recipient is "sensitized" to foreign (or "non-self") proteins. A high score correlates with the likelihood of graft rejection and could necessitate some type of desensitization protocol prior to the transplant.

AVOIDING AN "ABO MISMATCH" OR INCOMPATIBILITY REACTION

Type A blood will react against type B or type AB blood.

Type B blood will react against type A or type AB blood.

Type O blood will react against type A, type B, or type AB blood.

Type AB blood will not react against type A, type B, or type AB blood.

Type O blood does not cause an immune response when it is received by people with type A, type B, or type AB blood. This is why type O blood cells can be given to patients of any blood type. People with type O blood are called "universal donors."

However, type O can only receive type O blood.

An allograft is the transplant of an organ or tissue from one individual to another of the same species with a different genotype. This can also be called an allogenic transplant or homograft. A transplanted organ from a genetically identical donor (such as an identical twin) is called an isograft. An autograft is when a tissue is a transplant from one site to another on the same patient, also termed autologous transplant (or autologous stem cell transplant). Hyperacute rejection occurs in the operating room within hours of the transplant and is due to some type of mismatch; no treatment exists, and the transplanted organ will be removed.

Induction immunosuppressant therapy is given before or at the time of transplant to prevent acute rejection during the early post-transplant period by providing a high degree of immune suppression. It mostly consists of a short course of very effective intravenous (IV) agents using either a biological drug or monoclonal antibody (these end in -mab). The most commonly used induction agent is basiliximab, an interleukin-2 (IL-2) receptor antagonist. The IL-2 receptor is expressed on activated T lymphocytes and is a critical pathway for activating cell-mediated allograft rejection. Higher risk patients will receive (in addition) the lymphocyte-depleting agent rabbit antithymocyte globulin. In some cases induction can be achieved with higher doses of the same drugs used for maintenance. Induction agents may not be required if the transplant is from an identical twin.

Maintenance immunosuppressant therapy is generally provided by the combination of:

- A CNI (tacrolimus is the 1st line CNI) plus

- An antiproliferative agent (mycophenolate is 1st line in most protocols), or everolimus, sirolimus, belatacept or azathioprine.

- ± steroids (typically prednisone).

If the patient is low immunological risk the steroids will be discontinued; otherwise, they are not and the long-term adverse effects will need to be considered. Attacking the immune system via multiple mechanisms through different drug classes is designed to both lower toxicity risk and to reduce the risk of graft rejection.

Cardiovascular Disease (CVD): The Common Cause of Death in Transplant Patients

A concerted effort must be made to reduce risk factors for CVD. This is challenging considering that the patient is using transplant-rejection drugs that cause metabolic syndrome. Nonetheless, these patients are among the highest risk for CVD and blood pressure, blood glucose, cholesterol and weight must be tightly controlled. In a renal transplant patient the blood pressure must be well-controlled with goals provided by the transplant center. Blood glucose is managed to the ADA guidelines and cholesterol to the NCEP guidelines. Weight is measured at each visit, with reduction programs used as-needed. Refer to the individual chapters.

Cancer: Higher Risk in Transplant Patients

Cancer risk is higher compared to the general population. Some cancer types are viral-mediated and related to immune suppression, which causes increased cancer incidence similar to that seen with the use of the stronger agents used for autoimmune conditions. Screening for common cancers should be routine, along with lifestyle measures to reduce risk. Skin cancer is common with transplant and sunscreen must be used routinely, along with sun avoidance or sun protection with clothing. In addition, CNIs cause photosensitivity. The skin should be assessed professionally at least annually.

Monitoring by the Patient & Health Care Team is Essential

In addition to drug toxicity symptoms, patients will need to monitor for symptoms of organ rejection. Common symptoms of an acute rejection include flu-like symptoms, such as chills, body aches, nausea, cough, and shortness of breath and organ-specific symptoms (for example, heart failure symptoms with a heart transplant rejection or a decrease in urine output/fluid retention/edema/blood pressure elevation with a kidney transplant rejection).

All immunosuppressive agents require careful monitoring (including drug trough levels) to minimize toxicities and decrease the incidence of rejection. Keep in mind which maintenance agents have the highest nephrotoxicity (tacrolimus, cyclosporine), the most likely to worsen diabetes or cause new-onset diabetes (tacrolimus, steroids, cyclosporine, and the mTOR inhibitors everolimus and sirolimus), which are the most likely to worsen lipid parameters (mTOR inhibitors, steroids, cyclosporine) and which are the highest risk for blood pressure elevations (steroids, cyclosporine, tacrolimus).

TRANSPLANT DRUGS: WHAT'S USED, WHEN

Induction Drugs, to avoid acute early rejection are either:
Basilixumab is an interleukin-2 (IL-2) receptor antagonist and is the primary induction agent.

Patients at highest risk of rejection may be receiving antithymocyte globulin.

Or, the maintenance drugs at higher doses.

Primary Immunosuppressive Drugs
The calcineurin inhibitors (CNIs), which are tacrolimus (primarily) or cyclosporine.

Adjuvant Agents (given with the primary drugs), also called Antiproliferative or Antimetabolite Agents
Given with the CNI (to enable lower doses of the CNI to reduce nephrotoxicity risk), and include steroids, azathioprine or mycophenolate mofetil (*CellCept*). The majority of transplant patients use a CNI ± steroids + *CellCept*. Or, patients may be using one of the drugs that bind to the mTOR protein (such as everolimus) to reduce the CNI nephrotoxicity risk. This class may act synergistically with the CNIs. *mTOR inhib + CNI → SYNERGY*

With the use of adjuvants, adequate immunosuppression can be achieved while decreasing the dose and toxicity of the individual agents.

Infection Risk Reduction
There are others; these are infections in which prophylaxis or treatment is available. Vaccines discussed in a separate sidebar.

Candida: Oral and esophageal prophylaxis with oral clotrimazole lozenges, nystatin or fluconazole used commonly 1-3 months post-transplant.

Cytomegalovirus: valganciclovir (pro-drug of ganciclovir) is the usual drug of choice for prophylaxis, which may be required.

Herpes simplex: prophylaxis or treatment with acyclovir, valacyclovir or famciclovir.

Varicella zoster (vaccine prior to transplant): if shingles appear, it is treated with IV or oral acyclovir or valacyclovir.

Pneumocystis jirovecii pneumonia: Daily sulfamethoxazole/trimethoprim for 3-6 months post-transplant.

Tuberculosis: if positive, same prophylaxis as general population.

All patients using strong immunosuppressants or with any condition that suppresses the immune system should self-monitor for symptoms of infection: fever of 100.5°F (38°C) or higher (or lower if elderly), chills, sore throat, ear or sinus pain, cough, more sputum or change in color of sputum, pain with passing urine, mouth sores, wound that will not heal, or anal itching or pain.

COMMON TOXICITIES OF MAINT. DRUGS

nephrotox
* tacrolimus
* cyclosporine

cause/worsen DM
* tacrolimus
* steroids
* cyclosporine
  everolimus } mTOR
  sirolimus } inhib

lipid
* mTOR inhib
  steroids
  cyclosporine

↑ bp
* steroids
* cyclosporine
  tacrolimus

Reducing Infection Risk

The use of potent drugs has made solid organ transplant widely available and successful. However, the use of these agents is interrelated to the development of infection. The majority of infections that occur in organ transplant recipients are opportunistic and are a major cause of death in the immunocompromised patient. Opportunistic infections are caused by organisms that are ubiquitous in the environment, but rarely cause disease in the immunocompetent host. Infection prophylaxis is essential; review the basics in the sidebar. Infection control must include reducing risk from transmission, such as proper hand-washing techniques (see Medication Safety chapter), air filtration systems, keeping the mouth clean, and keeping away from dusty, crowded areas and sick people. One of the sidebars discusses drugs used for common infections. Often the prophylaxis drugs are the same used for treatment, in larger doses and possibly given IV. Or, other drugs or a combination is required for treatment. Vaccine-preventable illness is an important consideration pre-transplant since live vaccines cannot be given post-transplant.

VACCINE-PREVENTABLE ILLNESS

Required vaccines should be given pre-transplant if the recipient is not current. The inactivated vaccines can be given post-transplant if needed; live vaccines cannot be given post-transplant. Influenza (inactivated, not live) annually (recurring, each October-November) should be given when the vaccine is available.

Pneumococcal vaccine in adults ≥ 19 years who are immunocompromised receive PCV13 first, followed by PPSV23 at least 8 weeks later. Subsequent doses of PPSV23 should follow current PPSV23 recommendations for adults at high risk (5 years after the first PPSV23 dose). Some of the transplant centers recommend PPSV23 every 5 years.

Transplant patients are at high risk for serious varicella infections, with a very high risk of disseminated disease with a primary infection. The best protection is to vaccinate the close contacts (in addition to the recipient pre-transplant). Although there is a small risk that transmission could occur (from the vaccine recipient to the transplant recipient) ACIP states "the benefits of vaccinating susceptible household contacts of immunocompromised persons outweigh the potential risk for transmission of vaccine virus to immunocompromised contacts."

If the vaccinated household contact develops a rash post-vaccine they should avoid contact with the transplant recipient; they are contagious – and should report to their physician. If the transplant patient develops a rash they will need to be seen right away.

INDUCTION AGENTS

DRUG	SAFETY/SIDE EFFECTS/MONITORING

Antibodies – reverse rejection by binding to antigens on T-lymphocytes (killer cells) and interfering with their function

Antithymocyte Globulin *(Atgam-Equine)* *(Thymocyte-Rabbit)*	**BOXED WARNING** Should be administered under the supervision of a physician experienced in immunosuppressive therapy. Adequate laboratory and supportive medical resources must be readily available (e.g., epinephrine). **SIDE EFFECTS** Anaphylaxis (intradermal skin testing recommended prior to 1st dose), fever, chills, pruritus, rash, leukopenia, chest pain, hypertension, edema and others **MONITORING** Lymphocyte profile (T-cell count), CBC with differential, vital signs during administration **NOTES** May need to pre-medicate (diphenhydramine, acetaminophen and steroids). Epinephrine and resuscitative equipment should be nearby.

Interleukin 2 (IL-2) receptor antagonist – Chimeric (murine/human) monoclonal antibody that inhibits the IL-2 receptor on the surface of activated T-lymphocytes preventing cell-mediated allograft rejection

Basiliximab *(Simulect)*	**BOXED WARNING** Should only be used by physicians experienced in immunosuppressive therapy. **SIDE EFFECTS** Hypertension, fever, weakness, stomach upset/nausea/vomiting/cramping, peripheral edema, dyspnea/upper respiratory irritation/infection, cough, tremor, painful urination; side effects listed are rated as severe and >10%, others are >10% and rated less severe **MONITORING** Signs and symptoms of hypersensitivity and infection

MAINTENANCE MEDICATIONS

DRUG	DOSING	SAFETY/SIDE EFFECTS/MONITORING

Corticosteroids – naturally occurring hormones that prevent or suppress inflammation and humoral immune responses

PredniSONE, others	2-5-5 mg PO daily, or on alternate days	**SHORT-TERM SIDE EFFECTS** Fluid retention, stomach upset, emotional instability (euphoria, mood swings, irritability), insomnia, ↑ appetite, weight gain, acute rise in blood glucose and blood pressure with high dose **LONG-TERM SIDE EFFECTS** Adrenal suppression/Cushing's syndrome, impaired wound healing, hypertension. See Asthma chapter for further information on chronic steroid use.

Maintenance Medications Continued

DRUG	DOSING	SAFETY/SIDE EFFECTS/MONITORING

Antiproliferative Agents – inhibit T-lymphocyte proliferation by altering purine synthesis

DRUG	DOSING	SAFETY/SIDE EFFECTS/MONITORING
Mycophenolate Mofetil (*CellCept*) **Mycophenolic Acid (*Myfortic*)**	1-1.5 g PO BID, depending on transplant type	**BOXED WARNINGS (4)** ↑ risk of infection; ↑ development of lymphoma and skin malignancies; ↑ risk of congenital malformations and spontaneous abortions when used during pregnancy, should only be prescribed by health care providers experienced in immunosuppressive therapy. **SIDE EFFECTS** Diarrhea, GI upset, vomiting, hyper- and hypotension, edema, tachycardia, pain, hyperglycemia, hypo/hyperkalemia hypomagnesemia, hypocalcemia, hypercholesterolemia, tremor, acne, infections **MONITORING** CBC, renal, liver, signs of infection **NOTES** *CellCept* and *Myfortic* should not be used interchangeably due to differences in absorption. *Myfortic* is enteric coated which helps to ↓ diarrhea. Protect tablets from moisture and light. *CellCept IV* is stable in D5W only. Do not use IV if allergy to polysorbate 80. Should be taken on an empty stomach to avoid variability in absorption. Pregnancy Category D, and decreases efficacy oral contraceptives.
AzaTHIOprine (*Azasan, Imuran*)	1-3 mg/kg PO daily, for maintenance	**BOXED WARNINGS (2)** Chronic immunosuppression can ↑ risk of neoplasia (esp. lymphomas) Hematologic toxicities (leukopenia, thrombocytopenia) and mutagenic potential **WARNINGS** GI (severe N/V/D), hematologic (leukopenia, thrombocytopenia, anemia) and hepatotoxicity; patients with genetic deficiency of thiopurine methyltransferase (TPMT) are at ↑ risk for myelosuppression and may require lower dose. **SIDE EFFECTS** GI upset (N/V), rash, ↑ LFTs, bone marrow suppression **MONITORING** LFTs, CBC, renal function **NOTES** Pregnancy Category D

Maintenance Medications Continued

DRUG	DOSING	SAFETY/SIDE EFFECTS/MONITORING

Calcineurin inhibitors – suppresses cellular immunity by inhibiting T-lymphocyte activation

DRUG	DOSING	SAFETY/SIDE EFFECTS/MONITORING
Tacrolimus *(Prograf, Astagraf XL, Hecoria)* *Protopic* – topical for eczema	Initial: 0.1-0.2 mg/kg/day (depending on transplant type) in 2 divided doses, given every 12 hours Trough level varies, dependent on: 1. Transplant type 2. Number of months since transplant 3. Concurrent medications Example: trough level with mycophenolate and IL-2 receptor antagonist at months 1-12: 4-11 ng/mL	**BOXED WARNINGS (4)** ↑ susceptibility to infection; possible development of lymphoma; not recommended in liver transplantation; should be administered under the supervision of a physician experienced in organ transplantation in a facility appropriate for monitoring and managing therapy; extended release tacrolimus associated with increased mortality in female liver transplant recipients **SIDE EFFECTS** Hypertension, nephrotoxicity, hyperglycemia, tremor, hyperkalemia, hypomagnesemia, edema, chest pain, headache, insomnia, generalized pain, dizziness, rash/pruritus, diarrhea, abdominal pain, nausea, dyspepsia, anorexia, constipation, urinary tract infection, anemia, leukopenia, leukocytosis, thrombocytopenia, elevated liver enzymes, paresthesia, arthralgia, hypophosphatemia, hyperlipidemia, QT prolongation **MONITORING** Trough levels, serum electrolytes, renal function, hepatic function if liver transplant, blood pressure, blood glucose, electrolytes (especially potassium), lipid profile **NOTES** Should be taken on an empty stomach to avoid variability in absorption. If taking with food, take consistently. (Higher fat food decreases absorption the most.) Do not interchange XL to immediate release. Conversion IV to PO IR is 1:4. Start oral dosing 8-12 hours after last IV dose. Most drugs will affect the tacrolimus level; this is a CYP 450 3A4 and P-gp substrate. Avoid alcohol.
CycloSPORINE *(Neoral, Gengraf, SandIMMUNE)* *Restasis* – for dry eyes	Dose depends on transplant type and formulation Cyclosporine (modified): Renal: 9 ± 3 mg/kg/day, divided twice daily Liver: 8 ± 4 mg/kg/day, divided twice daily Heart: 7 ± 3 mg/kg/day, divided twice daily Cyclosporine (non-modified): 3-10 mg/kg/day for maintenance Conversion to cyclosporine (modified) from cyclosporine (non-modified): Start with daily dose previously used and adjust to obtain pre-conversion cyclosporine trough concentration; monitor every 4-7 days and dose adjust as necessary Trough 100-400 ng/mL (nephrotoxicity can occur at any level)	**BOXED WARNINGS (7)** Renal impairment (with high doses), ↑ risk of lymphoma and other malignancies, ↑ risk of skin cancer, ↑ risk of infection, may cause hypertension, dose adjustments should only be made under the direct supervision of an experienced physician, cyclosporine (modified – *Gengraf/Neoral*) has ↑ bioavailability compared to cyclosporine (non-modified – *Sandimmune*) and cannot be used interchangeably. **SIDE EFFECTS** Hypertension, nephropathy, hyperkalemia, hirsutism, gingival hyperplasia, edema, hyperglycemia, headache, paresthesia, abdominal discomfort/nausea/diarrhea, hypertrichosis, photosensitivity, increased triglycerides, urinary tract infection, viral infections, tremor, QT prolongation **MONITORING** Trough levels, serum electrolytes, renal function, hepatic function if liver transplant, blood pressure, blood glucose, electrolytes (especially potassium), lipid profile **NOTES** Most drugs will affect the cyclosporine level; this is a CYP 450 3A4 and P-gp substrate. Avoid alcohol.

Maintenance Medications Continued

DRUG	DOSING	SAFETY/SIDE EFFECTS/MONITORING

Mammalian target of rapamycin (mTOR) kinase inhibitor which inhibits T-lymphocyte activation and proliferation; may be synergistic with CNIs

DRUG	DOSING	SAFETY/SIDE EFFECTS/MONITORING
Everolimus *(Zortress, Afinitor)* Tablets *(Afinitor, Zortress)* and tablets for oral suspension *(Afinitor Disperz)* are not interchangeable; *Afinitor Disperz* is only indicated for the treatment of subependymal giant cell astrocytoma (SEGA)	Initial: 0.75-1 mg PO twice daily; adjust maintenance dose if needed to reach serum level of 3-8 ng/mL	**BOXED WARNINGS (5)** ↑ risk of infection; ↑ risk of lymphoma and skin cancer; reduced doses of cyclosporine are recommended when used concomitantly; ↑ risk of renal thrombosis may result in graft loss; not recommended in heart transplant **SIDE EFFECTS** Peripheral edema, constipation, hypertension, hyperglycemia, hyperlipidemia, delayed wound healing, pneumonitis, fatigue, fever, headache, seizures, behavioral changes (anxiety/aggression), insomnia, dizziness, rash/pruritus, cellulitis, xeroderma, acne, onychoclasis (nail disease), hyperglycemia/new onset diabetes, hypertriglyceridemia, decreased serum bicarbonate, hypophosphatemia, hypocalcemia, decreased serum albumin, hypoglycemia, hypo/hyperkalemia, hyponatremia, hypomagnesemia, abdominal discomfort, nausea, stomatitis, diarrhea, amenorrhea, dysgeusia, weight loss, dry mouth, dysuria, anemia, prolonged PTT, lymphocytopenia, thrombocytopenia **MONITORING** Trough levels, renal function, liver function, lipids, blood glucose, BP, CBC, signs of infection **NOTES** *Afinitor* bottle contains desiccant; keep in original container to protect from moisture.
Sirolimus *(Rapamune)*	Usually 2-5 mg/day Serum drug concentrations should be determined 3-4 days after loading doses and 7-14 days after dosage adjustments; approximate range 4-12 ng/mL, level dependent on concurrent drug use, including potent inhibitors or inducers of CYP3A4 or P-gp.	**BOXED WARNINGS (4)** ↑ risk of infection; ↑ risk of lymphoma; not recommended for use in liver transplantation; not recommended for use in lung transplantation **SIDE EFFECTS** Delayed wound healing, pneumonitis/bronchitis, cough, hyperglycemia, hyperlipidemia, peripheral edema, hypertension, headache, pain, insomnia, acne, constipation, abdominal pain, diarrhea, nausea, urinary tract infection, anemia, thrombocytopenia, arthralgia, nephrotoxicity **MONITORING** Trough levels, liver function, renal function, blood glucose, lipids, BP, CBC **NOTES** Tablets and oral solution are not bioequivalent due to differences in absorption.

Maintenance Medications Continued

DRUG	DOSING	SAFETY/SIDE EFFECTS/MONITORING

Mammalian target of rapamycin (mTOR) kinase inhibitor which inhibits T-lymphocyte activation and proliferation

DRUG	DOSING	SAFETY/SIDE EFFECTS/MONITORING
Belatacept *(Nulojix)* Administer with silicone-free disposable syringe (comes with drug)	Initial: 10 mg/kg/day Maintenance: 5 mg/kg/day Round doses to the nearest 12.5 mg, dose using TBW	**BOXED WARNINGS (5)** Increased risk post-transplant lymphoproliferative disorder (PTLD), recipients without immunity to Epstein-Barr Virus (EBV) are at highest risk, use in EBV seropositive patients only. Increased susceptibility to infection and malignancies. Avoid use in liver transplant patients due to risk of transplant rejection and death. Should be administered under the supervision of a physician experienced in immunosuppressive therapy. **WARNINGS** Increased risk opportunistic infections, sepsis, and/or fatal infections. Increased risk tuberculosis (TB); test patients for latent TB prior to initiation, and treat latent TB infection prior to use **SIDE EFFECTS** Headache, anemia, leukopenia, constipation, diarrhea, nausea, peripheral edema, hypertension, cough, photosensitivity, insomnia, urinary tract infection, pyrexia, hypo/hyperkalemia **MONITORING** New-onset or worsening neurological, cognitive, or behavioral signs/symptoms; signs/symptoms of infection, TB screening prior to therapy initiation, EBV seropositive verification prior to therapy initiation

Drug Interactions

Transplant drugs affect the levels of each other and the following interactions must be considered: Cyclosporine will ↓ mycophenolate and ↑ sirolimus and everolimus (and will increase some of the statins, which transplant patients are usually taking) and the mTOR inhibitors (sirolimus and everolimus) are enzyme inhibitors and increase cyclosporine levels. Both cyclosporine and tacrolimus are CYP 450 3A4 and P-gp substrates. Inducers of either enzyme will decrease the CNI concentration, and inhibitors will increase the CNI concentration. Both will interact with the majority of drugs. Consistency is essential; the drug dose will be adjusted to the trough level. Tacrolimus absorption is decreased by food; take with or without, but consistently.

- Azathioprine – allopurinol, aspirin, ACE Is and sulfamethoxazole/trimethoprim may ↑ levels of azathioprine.

- Mycophenolate – can ↓ levels of hormonal contraception; mycophenolate levels can be ↓ by antacids and multivitamins, cyclosporine, metronidazole, PPIs, fluoroquinolones, sevelamer, bile acid resins, and rifampin and derivatives. Acyclovir, valganciclovir and ganciclovir will ↑ mycophenolate.

- Avoid grapefruit juice and St. John's wort with either CNI.

- Caution with additive drugs that are nephrotoxic with tacrolimus and cyclosporine.

- Caution with additive drugs that raise blood glucose with tacrolimus, steroids, cyclosporine and the mTOR inhibitors (everolimus/sirolimus).

- Caution with additive drugs that worsen lipids with the mTOR inhibitors, steroids and cyclosporine.

- Caution with additive drugs that raise blood pressure with steroids, cyclosporine and tacrolimus.

Patient Counseling for All Immunosuppressants

- Take the medication exactly as prescribed by your healthcare provider. It is important that you take your medication at the same time every day. Also, stay consistent on how you take your medication.

- Never change or skip a dose of medication. Remember, if you stop taking your immunosuppressive medications, your body will reject your transplanted organ.

- Monitor your health at home and keep daily records of your temperature, weight, blood pressure, and glucose (if diabetes is present).

- Do not take any NSAIDs (e.g., Advil, Naprosyn, Aleve) as these drugs could cause harm to your kidneys.

- Do not take any over-the-counter, herbal, or alternative medications without consulting with your health care provider.

- Protect and cover your skin from the sun. Be sure to use sunscreen with a SPF of 30 or higher. Avoid using tanning beds or sunlamps. People who take immunosuppressive agents have a higher risk of getting skin cancer.

- Do not get immunizations/vaccinations without the consent of your healthcare provider. The use of live vaccines should definitely be avoided. Avoid contact with people who have recently received oral polio vaccine or nasal flu vaccine.

- Patients are vulnerable to developing infections (severe infections) due to their suppressed immune system. Avoid contact with people who have the flu or other contagious illness. Practice infection control techniques such as good hand washing.

- Chronic immunosuppression has been associated with an increased risk of cancer, particularly lymphoma and skin cancer.

- If getting a blood test to measure the drug level, take your medication after you had your blood drawn (not before). It is important to measure the lowest (trough) level of drug in your blood.

Patient Counseling for Mycophenolate

- Take exactly as prescribed, every 12 hours (8 AM and 8 PM). It is important that you take your medication at the same time every day.

- If you miss a dose and it is less than 4 hours after the scheduled dose, take the missed dose and continue on your regular schedule. If you miss a dose and it is more than 4 hours after your scheduled dose, skip the missed dose, and return to your regular dosing schedule. Never take 2 doses at the same time. Record any missed doses.

- Take capsules, tablets and oral suspension on an empty stomach, either 1 hour before or 2 hours after a meal.

- Do not open or crush tablets or capsules. If you are not able to swallow tablets or capsules, your healthcare provider may prescribe an oral suspension. Your pharmacist will mix the medicine before giving it to you.

- Do not mix the oral suspension with any other medicine.

- This medication can cause <u>diarrhea</u>. Call your healthcare provider right away if you have diarrhea. Do not stop the medication without first talking with your healthcare provider. Other side effects include nausea, vomiting, abdominal pain/cramping, headache, and decreased white blood cells and platelets.

- Do not get pregnant while taking this medication. Women who take this medication during pregnancy have a higher risk of losing a pregnancy (miscarriage) during the first 3 months (first trimester), and a higher risk that their baby will be born with birth defects. Birth control pills do not work as well with this drug.

- <u>Do not take with antacids or multivitamins concurrently. Separate the doses by 2 hours. Avoid use with bile acid resins.</u>

- <u>Limit the amount of time you spend in sunlight.</u> Avoid using tanning beds or sunlamps. Use sunscreen with a SPF of 30 or higher. People who take this medicine have a higher risk of getting skin cancer.

- <u>Mycophenolic acid *(Myfortic)* and mycophenolate mofetil *(CellCept)* are not interchangeable. Do not switch between products unless directed by your healthcare provider. These medicines are absorbed differently. This may affect the amount of medicine in your blood.</u>

Patient Counseling for Tacrolimus

- Take this medication as directed by your healthcare provider, usually every 12 hours. It is best to take on an empty stomach for best absorption. However it is taken, you must be consistent (with food or without food) and take this medication the same way every day so that your body always absorbs the same amount of drug.

- It is important to take all doses on time to keep the amount of medicine in your body at a constant level. Remember to take it at the same times each day. Patients should be informed of the need for repeated appropriate laboratory tests while receiving tacrolimus. They should be given complete dosage instructions, advised of the potential risks during pregnancy, and informed of the increased risk of neoplasia. Patients should be informed that changes in dosage should not be undertaken without first consulting their healthcare provider.

- If you miss a dose and it is <u>less than 4 hours after the scheduled dose, take the missed dose</u> and continue on your regular schedule. If you miss a dose and it is <u>more than 4 hours after your scheduled dose, skip the missed dose</u>, and return to your regular dosing schedule. Never take 2 doses at the same time. Record any missed doses.

- As with other immunosuppressive agents, owing to the potential risk of malignant skin changes, exposure to sunlight and ultraviolet (UV) light should be limited by wearing protective clothing and using a sunscreen with a SPF of 30 or higher.

- <u>Avoid eating grapefruit or drinking grapefruit juice</u> while being treated with tacrolimus. Grapefruit can increase the amount of tacrolimus in your bloodstream.

- Tacrolimus may cause your blood pressure to increase. You may be required to check your blood pressure periodically and/or take another medication to control your blood pressure.

- Side effects of tacrolimus also include tremors/shaking, headache, diarrhea, nausea/vomiting, upset stomach, loss of appetite, tingling of the hands/feet, increased blood pressure, increased cholesterol, increased blood sugar, and increase in potassium levels.

- <u>Tacrolimus may cause diabetes.</u> Tell your healthcare provider if you experience any of the following symptoms of high blood sugar: increased thirst/hunger or frequent urination.

- Tacrolimus may cause a condition that affects the heart rhythm (QT prolongation). QT prolongation can infrequently result in serious fast/irregular heartbeat and other symptoms (such as severe dizziness, fainting) that require immediate medical attention. The risk of QT prolongation may be increased if you have certain medical conditions or are taking other drugs that may affect the heart rhythm. Before using tacrolimus, tell your healthcare provider if you have any of the following conditions: certain heart problems (heart failure, slow heartbeat, QT prolongation in the ECG), family history of certain heart problems (QT prolongation or sudden cardiac death).

- High (or low) levels of potassium or magnesium in the blood may also increase your risk of QT prolongation. This risk may increase if you use certain drugs (such as diuretics/"water pills") or if you have conditions such as severe sweating, diarrhea, or vomiting. This drug may increase your potassium levels.

Patient Counseling for Cyclosporine (using *Neoral* as an example)

- Because different brands deliver different amounts of medication, do not switch brands of cyclosporine without your doctor's permission and directions.

- Patients should be advised to take *Neoral* on a consistent schedule with regard to time of day and relation to meals. Grapefruit and grapefruit juice affect metabolism, increasing blood concentration of cyclosporine, thus should be avoided.

- If you miss a dose and it is less than 4 hours after the scheduled dose, take the missed dose and continue on your regular schedule. If you miss a dose and it is more than 4 hours after your scheduled dose, skip the missed dose, and return to your regular dosing schedule. Never take 2 doses at the same time. Record any missed doses.

- Patients should be informed of the necessity of repeated laboratory tests while they are receiving cyclosporine. Laboratory tests (e.g., kidney function tests, blood tests) may be performed to monitor your progress. If getting a blood test to measure the drug level, take your medication after you had your blood drawn.

- Patients should be given careful dosage instructions. *Neoral* Oral Solution (cyclosporine oral solution, USP) Modified should be diluted, preferably with orange or apple juice that is at room temperature. Do not administer oral liquid from plastic or styrofoam cup. The combination of *Neoral* Oral Solution (cyclosporine oral solution, USP) Modified with milk can be unpalatable. *(Sandimmune* may be diluted with milk, chocolate milk, or orange juice). Avoid changing diluents frequently. Mix thoroughly and drink at once. Use syringe provided to measure dose, mix in glass container and rinse container with more diluent to ensure total dose was taken.

- Cyclosporine can also cause high blood pressure and kidney problems. The risk of both problems increases with higher doses and longer treatment with this drug.

- Side effects of cyclosporine also include increased cholesterol, headache, nausea, vomiting, diarrhea, stomach upset, increased hair growth on the face/body, tremor, swollen/red/painful gums, and acne. If any of these effects persist or worsen, notify your healthcare provider promptly.

- This drug may increase your risk for developing skin cancer. Avoid prolonged sun exposure, tanning booths and sunlamps. Use a sunscreen, SPF 30 or higher, and wear protective clothing when outdoors.

- This medication may cause swelling and growth of the gums (gingival hyperplasia). Brush your teeth and floss daily to minimize this problem. See your dentist regularly.

CONTRACEPTION & INFERTILITY

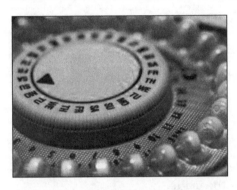

BACKGROUND

There are 62 million U.S. women in their childbearing years. Seven in 10 women of reproductive age (43 million) are sexually active and do not want to become pregnant, but could become pregnant if they or their partner fails to use a contraceptive method. The typical U.S. woman wants only two children. To achieve this goal, she must use contraceptives for roughly three decades. (source: Guttmacher Institute)

Among the 43 million women who do not want to become pregnant, 89% are practicing contraception. Sixty-three percent of reproductive-age women who practice contraception use nonpermanent methods, including hormonal methods (such as the pill, patch, implant, injectable and vaginal ring), the IUD and condoms. The remaining women rely on female or male sterilization.

Contraceptive choices vary markedly with age. For women younger than 30 years old, the pill is the leading method. Among women aged 30 and older, more rely on sterilization, which is often performed post-partum. Male contraception options are limited. Presently, vasectomy is the only option. A long-acting, nonhormonal contraceptive injection is in development.

Many women are not aware that birth control pills provide health benefits, including decreased blood loss and a lower incidence of iron-deficiency anemia, reduced cramps, ovarian cysts, ectopic pregnancy, less noncancerous breast cysts/lumps, less acute pelvic inflammatory disease and a decreased risk of endometrial and ovarian cancer. The combination pill also protects against bone loss.

MENSTRUAL CYCLE PHASES/TEST KITS

A normal menstrual cycle ranges from 23-35 days (average 28 days). Menstruation starts on day 1 and typically lasts a few days.

Ovulation

The mid-cycle luteinizing hormone (LH) surge results in release of the oocyte (egg) from the ovary into the fallopian tube.

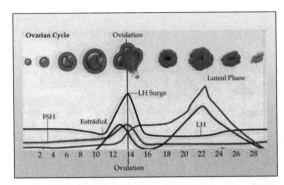

If the oocyte is not fertilized, it is washed out through menstruation. <u>Ovulation kits test for LH and are positive if LH is present.</u> They predict the best time for a patient to have intercourse in order to try to conceive (get pregnant).

Pregnancy

A female has the highest chance to become pregnant on days 8-16 of her cycle, although pregnancy can occur during any time – no time is considered 100% "safe". <u>Pregnancy test kits are positive if hCG (human chorionic gonadotropin) is in the urine.</u>

If a case indicates hCG+, the patient is pregnant and teratogenic drugs should be discontinued, if possible. <u>Well-known teratogens</u> include alcohol, ACE inhibitors, angiotensin receptor blockers, benzodiazepines, carbamazepine, ergot-derivatives, isotretinoin, leflunomide, lithium, methimazole, nafarelin, NSAIDs, paroxetine, phenytoin, phenobarbital, propylthiouracil, quinolones, ribavirin, tazarotene, tetracyclines, topiramate, valproic acid, misoprostol, methotrexate, statins, dutasteride, finasteride, warfarin, lenalidomide and thalidomide. Refer to the Drug Use in Pregnancy chapter for a further discussion of teratogenic drugs.

Any woman planning to conceive (and all women of child-bearing age) should be taking a <u>folic acid supplement (400-800 mcg/day)</u> to help prevent birth defects of the brain and spinal cord (neural tube defects). Folic acid should be taken at least one month <u>before pregnancy</u>, since it takes time to build up adequate body stores. Folic acid is in many healthy foods, including fortified cereals, dried beans, leafy green vegetables and orange juice. A couple of the newer pill formulations contain folic acid – see chart of formulations later in this chapter.

HORMONAL CONTRACEPTIVES

These contain progestin only (pill or injectable) or estrogen/progestin combinations (in pills, a patch, and a ring).

Progestin-only pill (POPs): The use of POPs as a contraceptive method is mostly recommended for lactating (breastfeeding) women, because estrogen reduces the milk production. They are sometimes used for women who cannot tolerate or have a contraindication to estrogen, however they must be taken on a tight schedule and are less "forgiving" if a pill is late or forgotten; it is easier to get pregnant accidentally on a POP if the woman is not lactating.

Estrogen and progestin combination oral contraceptives (COCs) inhibit the production of both follicle stimulating hormone (FSH) and LH, which prevents ovulation. Contraceptives also may prevent pregnancy by altering the endometrial lining, altering cervical mucus, interfering with fertilization or transport of an egg, or preventing implantation. COCs are used for various indications, including dysmenorrhea, PMS, perimenopausal symptoms (hot flashes, night sweats, as well as pregnancy protection), anemia due to excessive period-related blood loss, and acne (in females). They are sometimes used for reduction in premenstrual migraine (a common migraine in women). The POPs are useful for this purpose, and are safest for migraines with aura (in this type of migraine estrogen should not be used due to stroke risk). Polycystic ovary syndrome (PCOS) is a common condition (~15% of women) with a typical presentation of infrequent or prolonged menstrual periods, hirsutism, acne and excessive weight, often with insulin resistance. The use of COCs to induce regular menses is first-line treatment. Other drugs used for PCOS (such as spironolactone for hirsutism, metformin for prediabetes) are used off-label.

BIRTH CONTROL PILLS: WHAT'S IN A NAME?

0.5/35 (or similar)
Monophasic formulation (progestin/estrogen)

Tri or 7/7/7 or Cycl-
Triphasic formulation

Lo
Low estrogen < 35 mcg

Fe
Contains iron

Progestin only
Often have "nor" in name-for norethindrone (in HRT products "pro" means containing a progestin)

DO NOT USE ANY FORM OF ESTROGEN WITH THESE CONDITIONS

History of blood clot disorders (DVT, PE)

History of stroke or heart attack

Heart valve disease with complications

Severe hypertension

Diabetes that causes blood vessel problems

Poorly controlled diabetes

Severe headaches (for example, migraines – some forms helpful)

Recent major surgery with prolonged bed rest

Breast cancer

Liver cancer or disease

Uterine cancer or other known or suspected estrogen-dependent cancers

Unexplained abnormal bleeding from the uterus

Jaundice during pregnancy or jaundice with prior hormonal contraceptive use

Known or possible pregnancy

Boxed Warning
Do not use if > 35 years and smoke due to cardiovascular risk (contraindicated)

CLOTTING RISK! WATCH FOR HIGH RISK PATIENTS

3 things to keep in mind (in addition to the patient's risk factors):

- Higher estrogen dose, higher clotting risk.

- FDA Safety Announcement [4-10-2012] Drospirenone-containing birth control pills may be associated with a higher risk for blood clots than other progestin-containing pills.

- *Ortho Evra* patch: higher systemic estrogen exposure than most COC pills.

Adverse Effects Due to Estrogen

Estrogen can cause nausea, breast tenderness/fullness, bloating, weight gain or elevated blood pressure. If low-dose estrogen pills are used, or if there is insufficient estrogen (the patient may be a fast metabolizer, or be using an enzyme inducer), then early or mid-cycle breakthrough bleeding can occur and may require a higher estrogen dose. The general practice is to wait three monthly cycles prior to changing the dose to see if spotting dissipates.

FORMULATION CONSIDERATIONS

Breastfeeding
Choose progestin only pill.

Elevated Clotting Risk
Avoid drospirenone-containing COCs.

Avoid the *Ortho Evra* patch.

Use lower dose estrogen content.

Choose progestin-only pill.

Estrogen contraindication, including clotting risk
Choose progestin-only pill.

Estrogenic side effects
Use low estrogen formulation.

Spotting/"breakthrough bleeding"
(This is more common with *Seasonale, Seasonique* and *Amethyst.*) When starting the conventional formulations, wait for three cycles before switching. If early or mid-cycle spotting the estrogen dose may be too low. If later in the cycle the progestin dose may need to be increased.

Avoiding monthly cycle
Use 91-day or continuous formulations.

Migraine
Choose among various formulations, if with aura choose POP.

Fluid retention/bloating
Choose a product containing drospirenone, if low clotting risk. Progestin component helps reduce water retention.

The progestin component is a mild diuretic. It retains potassium, and is contraindicated with renal or liver disease. Check potassium, renal function and use of other potassium-retaining agents.

Premenstrual dysphoric disorder
Choose *Yaz* or sertraline or fluoxetine (*Sarafem*) – see Depression chapter.

Nausea
Take at night, take with food, can consider decreasing estrogen dose (if after 3 months, if no spotting). The ring has less nausea than pills.

Acne
Can use most formulations; COCs are likely to be chosen if contraception is also required.

Heavy Menstrual Bleeding
Any oral contraceptive will decrease monthly blood loss. The COC *Natazia* is indicated for this condition (menorrhagia). Tranexamic acid (*Lysteda*), which slows clot breakdown, is indicated for menorrhagia. It is not more effective than COC's, and has clotting risk – do not use with estrogen-containing products. Used for up to 5 days when bleeding. Visual changes could be due to clotting in retina – counsel. The bleeding loss is slight with the injectables, implants and IUDs.

Serious adverse effects are rare but can include thrombogenic disorders, including heart attack, stroke, DVT/PE. The risk for clotting disorders increases as the woman ages, if she smokes, if she has diabetes or hypertension, if she requires prolonged bed rest, and if she is overweight. (See table on contraindications to estrogen use.) The progestin drospirenone, as well as the *Ortho Evra* patch (due to a higher systemic estrogen level) are linked to a higher risk of blood clots and are best avoided in at-risk women. Higher dose estrogen formulations have higher risk. Birth control pills do not provide protection from sexually transmitted infections (STIs). Condoms provide some protection. The best protection from STIs (and pregnancy) is abstinence.

Adverse Effects Due to Progestin

Progestin can cause breast tenderness, headache, fatigue or changes in mood. If late cycle breakthrough bleeding occurs a higher progestin dose may be required.

ORAL CONTRACEPTIVE TYPES (REPRESENTATIVE LIST)

Monophasic COCs
all active pills contain the same level of the hormones throughout the 3 active weeks
Alesse, Loestrin, Ortho-Cyclen, Yaz

Biphasic or Triphasic (also called Multiphasic), where the dose of the hormones changes over the course of 21 days;
including biphasic forms:
Kariva, Mircette
and triphasic forms:
Cyclessa, Ortho-Novum 7/7/7. Ortho Tri-Cyclen Lo, Tri Lo Sprintec, Nortrel 7/7/7, Enpresse

1 formulation is four-phasic
(Natazia), with four phases of estradiol valerate and the progestin dienogest

Low-dose pills are popular and chosen since less withdrawal symptoms (emotional/physical) and less estrogen side effects, including lower clotting risk; these contain 20-35 mcg estrogen (compared to 50 mcg)
Kariva, Mircette, Cyclessa, Ortho-Novum 7/7/7. Ortho Tri-Cyclen Lo, Tri Lo Sprintec, Nortrel 7/7/7, Enpresse

Drospirenone-containing formulations (see following page on issues with this progestin)
Yasmin, Yaz, Gianvi, Loryna, Ocella, Zarah, Daylette, Angeliq, Nikki, Safyral, Syeda, Vestura, Beyaz (Safyral & Beyaz contain folate*)*

Progestin Only Mini-Pills (POPs) with
Norethindrone 35 mcg *(Camila, Errin, Heather, Jolivette, Micronor, Nor-QD, Nora-BE* – some names include "nor")

EXTENDED CYCLE COCs
Placebo days are < 1 week (or none at all), either containing norethindrone, drospirenone or levonorgestrel (LNG) with ethinyl estradiol (EE)

24 days active tx + 4 days ferrous fumarate 75 mg (the iron takes the place of the placebo for the 4-days hormone-free)
Loestrin 24 Fe, Minastrin 24 Fe (chewable), Lomedia 24 Fe

26 days active tx, 24 days are the same as above followed by 2 days with EE 10 mcg followed by 2 days ferrous fumarate 75 mg
Lo Loestrin Fe, Lo Minastrin Fe

3 months (91 days total) with 84 days of EE 30 mcg/LNG 0.15 mg + 7 days of EE 10 mcg (low dose EE in "placebo" week)
Seasonique, Amethia

Similar to above but the doses are lower: EE 20 mcg/LNG 0.1 mg in the 84 days, with the same EE 10 mcg in the placebo week
LoSeasonique, Amethia Lo

Continuous EE 20 mcg/LNG 0.09 mg with no placebo. The packets look like regular pill packets; they contain 28 tablets each, all the same – when done, go straight to the next packet, no placebo
Amethyst

Drug Interactions that can Decrease Efficacy of Hormonal Contraceptives

Use back-up while taking the antibiotics listed (with rifampin, use other form of birth control since the induction will last – if switching back, a back-up method needs to be used for 1½ months after rifampin is stopped). Rifapentine and rifabutin are also strong inducers. A strong inducer, used long-term, will require an alternate form of birth control, such as condoms/spermicide, an IUD or the *Depo-Provera* injection. *Depo-Provera* does not have drug interactions (although it does lower bone density and should be avoided in women at risk for osteoporosis.)

Decreases Hormone Efficacy

- Antibiotics (rifampin, rifapentine, rifabutin)

- Anticonvulsants (barbiturates, carbamazepine, oxcarbazepine, phenytoin, topiramate and felbamate)

- St John's wort

- Several protease inhibitors (PIs) and non-nucleoside reverse transcriptase inhibitors (NNRTIs) – ↑ or ↓ contraceptives

- Bosentan *(Tracleer)*, Mycophenolate *(CellCept, Myfortic)*

- Separate from colesevelam. Take at least 1 hour prior to *Byetta* injection.

- Smoking

- Check the package insert for new drugs that are being dispensed to a patient on birth control pills since it is important not to miss counseling on an interaction that could decrease the pill's efficacy.

POP Start Day Options

- Start at any time. Use another method of birth control for the first 48 hours of progestin-pill use – protection begins after two days. All come in 28-day packs and all pills are active.

- POPs need to take exactly around the same time of day everyday; if 3 hours have elapsed from the regular scheduled time, back up is needed for 48 hours after taking the late pill. If a dose is missed, patient could be pregnant and EC may be suitable.

COC Start Day Options

- Start on the Sunday following the onset of menses (will menstruate during the week – most common start is a Sunday start.)

- Start on 1st day of menses – if COCs are started within five days after the start of the period, no back up method of birth control is needed; protection is immediate. If not within 5 days, use back-up for first week of use.

Missed COC Pills – Instructions for Typical Formulations

Missed pills (particularly if the seven-day hormone-free interval is extended on either end) are a common cause of contraceptive failure. Accidental pregnancies are often due to picking up the refill late. Check the package insert of the formulation dispensed; the instructions vary.

PILLS MISSED	NOTES
Single Pill Missed	If a single pill is missed anywhere in the packet, the forgotten pill needs to be taken when noticed and the next pill is taken when it is due, which may mean taking two pills on the same day. No additional contraception is required.
2+ Pills Missed	Back-up contraception is generally needed if two or more consecutive hormonal pills are missed.
	Women should take one of the missed active (hormonal) pills as soon as possible and then continue taking one pill each day as prescribed. Depending on when she remembers her missed pill, she may take two pills on the same day.
	If the two or more pills are missed in the first week of the cycle and unprotected intercourse occurs during this week, use of emergency contraception could decrease the risk of pregnancy.
	If pills were missed in the last week of hormone pills, days 15 to 21 of a 28-day pack, omit the hormone-free week by finishing the hormone pills in current pack and start a new pack the next day. If unable to start a new pack, use back-up until hormonal pills from a new pack are taken for seven consecutive days.

Select Different Formulation Overview, Start Day, Gap in Treatment

Seasonale (and generics, several), *Seasonique (Amethia), Lo Seasonique (Amethia Lo)* contain 91-pills:

- These all contain a 91-day pill regimen with 84 active pills. The difference is the placebo week: *Seasonale* has 7 days of placebo, and the *Seasonique*-type formulations (see above) have 7 days of low dose estrogen. This is not the only formulation where the placebo week has been replaced with low dose estrogen, to ↓ symptoms and bleeding.

- These are started on the Sunday after the period starts, even if the patient is still bleeding. If the period began on Sunday, they should start that same day.

- They must use another method of birth control (such as condom or spermicide) as a back-up method if they have sex anytime from the Sunday they start until the next Sunday (the first 7 days). These formulations require that the pill be taken at the same time each day.

Continuous Pills With No Monthly Cycle *(Amethyst)*

- *Amethyst* comes in 28 day packets of all active (yellow) pills, with no placebo pills; the packets are taken continously. When empty, start the next pack.

- With this formulation, it can be difficult to tell if a woman is pregnant.

- It is important to take at the same time each day. Have the patient pick the time of day preferred.

- There is a higher discontinuation rate with the continuous formulations than with other COCs, due to spotting; counsel patients that the spotting should decrease over time.

- <u>Beginning</u>: If no previous contraception, begin on the first day of menstrual cycle. If previously taking a 21-day or 28-day combination hormonal contraceptive: Begin on day 1 of the withdrawal bleed (at the latest, 7 days after the last active tablet). If on POP, begin next day after stopping. Back up is needed for 7-days only after switching from a POP or from an implant or injection.

- <u>Missed doses</u>: If one missed, take as soon as remembered then continue (2 tablets in 1 day). If more than two missed, see package insert. Any missed pills requires back up for 7 days and may require EC.

Drospirenone Formulations: *Yasmin, Yaz, Gianvi, Loryna, Ocella, Zarah, Daylette, Angeliq, Nikki, Safyral, Syeda, Vestura, Beyaz (Safyral & Beyaz* contain folate)

These are popular COCs, since they <u>decrease</u> bloating, PMS symptoms and weight gain. This is due to the progestin drospirenone, which is a potassium-sparing diuretic.

- Drospirenone-containing formulations have a risk of increased K^+ and caution must be used with K^+-sparing agents, including aldosterone antagonists, potassium supplements, salt substitutes (KCl), ACE inhibitors, angiotensin receptor blockers, heparin, canaglifozin and calcineurin inhibitors.

- <u>Avoid use if kidney, liver, or adrenal gland disease</u>. On a case, <u>check the potassium level</u>. It should be in the safe range of 3.5-5 mEq/L.

- This type of progestin puts the patients at a <u>slightly higher risk of clotting</u>, and should be avoided in women with clotting risk.

Ortho Evra COC Contraceptive Patch

- Thin, beige, plastic patch placed on clean, dry skin of buttocks, stomach, upper arm, or upper torso <u>once a week for 21 out of 28 days</u>. Do not apply to breasts.

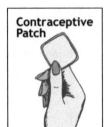

Contraceptive Patch

- Start on either Day 1 (no back-up needed) or Sunday (back-up 7-days if not day 1).

- If patch becomes loose or falls off $\geq$ 24 hours during the 3 weeks of use or if > 7 days have passed during the 4th week where no patch is required, there is a risk of pregnancy; thus a back-up method should be used for 1 week while a new patch is put in place.

- Has the same side effects, contraindications and drug interactions as the pills except that the patch causes a <u>higher systemic estrogen exposure</u>; avoid carefully in anyone with clotting risk factors.

- <u>Less effective in women > 198 pounds</u>. Do not use if smoker and over 35 years old.

NuvaRing Vaginal Contraceptive Ring

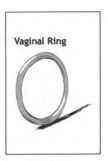

Vaginal Ring

- Small flexible ring inserted into the vagina <u>once a month</u>.

- Similar to OCs in that the ring is inserted <u>in place for 3 weeks</u> and taken out for 1 week before replacement with a new ring.

- For starting: insert the ring between day 1 and day 5 of menses.

- Exact position of ring in vagina does not matter.

- If ring is out > 3 hours during week 1, rinse with cool to luke-warm water and reinsert; use back-up method for 1 week while the ring is in place, consider EC if intercourse within last 5 days.

- If ring is out < 3 hours during week 2 or 3, rinse and re-insert ring.

- If ring is out > 3 hours during week 2 or 3, rinse and re-insert ring and use back-up for 7 days.

- If starting 1st cycle of birth control, use back-up method for the 1st week.

- Has the same side effects, contraindications and drug interactions as the pills.

- Patient can store for up to 4 months at room temperature – refrigerated at pharmacy.

Combination Oral Contraceptives Patient Counseling

- Forgetting to take pills considerably increases the chances of pregnancy.

- The FDA requires that the Patient Package Insert (PPI) be dispensed with oral contraceptives – they are in the product packaging. Tell the patient that the PPI has important safety information and instructions how to use them properly and what to do if pills are missed.

- For the majority of women, oral contraceptives can be taken safely. But there are some women who are at high risk of developing certain serious diseases that can be life-threatening or may cause temporary or permanent disability or death. The risks associated with taking oral contraceptives increase significantly if you:

  - Have or have had clotting disorders, heart attack, stroke, angina pectoris, cancer of the breast or sex organs, jaundice, or malignant or benign liver tumors.

- You should not take the pill if you suspect you are pregnant or have unexplained vaginal bleeding.

- Cigarette smoking increases the risk of serious adverse effects on the heart and blood vessels from oral contraceptive use. This risk increases with age and with heavy smoking and is quite marked in women over 35 years of age. Women who use oral contraceptives should not smoke.

- Most side effects of the pill are not serious. The most common such effects are nausea, vomiting, bleeding between menstrual periods, weight gain, and breast tenderness. These side effects, especially nausea and vomiting may subside within the first three months of use. Many women have nausea, and some have spotting or light bleeding, during the 1st three months. Nausea can be reduced by taking with food or at night.

- For any estrogen containing product and for any containing the progestin drospirenone, counsel to watch for severe pain in leg/calf, severe abdominal pain, chest pain/shortness of breath/cough, blurred or loss of vision – all due to clotting risk. Clotting is rare with current dosages; look at the preceeding table for women at highest risk (overweight, on bed rest, smokers) Any previous clotting history means that estrogen, in any form, is contraindicated.

- Make sure to discuss with your pharmacist if you start any new medicines, including over-the-counter products, or antibiotics for illness.

- Your pharmacist will also discuss whether to start your pill on the 1st Sunday following your period (which is done most commonly) or on a different day.

ADDITIONAL METHODS OF BIRTH CONTROL AND "SAFE" OR "SAFER SEX"

Abstinence is the only 100% way to prevent pregnancy and STIs. Safer sex recommendations:

- Alcohol and other drugs can make people forget safer sex; avoid use when in high-risk situations.

- Condoms form a barrier between the penis and anus, vagina or mouth. The barrier keeps one partner's fluids from getting into or on the other. Latex (not natural) condoms must be used.

- Oral sex is safer than vaginal or anal sex to reduce HIV risk, but will still put the person at risk for herpes, syphilis, hepatitis B, gonorrhea, and HPV. The *Sheer Glyde* dam is FDA-approved for safer sex; it blocks passage of infectious organisms during oral contact.

- Lubricant is important for safer sex because it makes condoms and dams slippery and less likely to break, and reduces dry friction. Never recommend oil-based lubricant (called "lube") with a latex or non-latex rubber condom; only recommend water or silicone-based lubricants. These products are discussed in the Hormone Therapy chapter.

Condoms

- Male condoms are a thin latex or plastic sheath worn on the penis. Female condoms are inserted into the vagina. Both are OTC and are used with spermicide for contraception, or as a back-up method.

- Condoms help protect against many STIs (only if latex condoms, not "natural").

- To increase the efficacy for contraception, use with nonoxynol-9 spermicide.

- Do not use spermicide with anal sex. It is irritating and can increase the risk of STIs. Some of the condoms are lubricated with nonoxynol-9.

OTC contraceptive methods (and some condoms) all contain the spermicide <u>nonoxynol-9.</u>

■ Available as foams, film, creams, suppositories, and jellies.

■ Place deep into the vagina right before intercourse where they melt (except for foam, which bubbles).

Diaphragm, Caps & Shields

These 3 options are soft latex or silicone barriers that cover the cervix and prevent sperm passage.

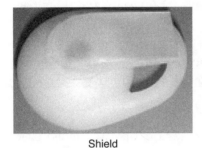
Shield

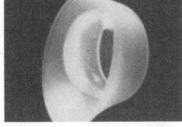
Cap

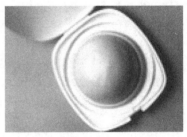
Diaphragm

Diaphragm Directions for Use

■ Wash hands thoroughly.

■ Place 1 tablespoon of spermicide in the diaphragm and disperse inside and to rim.

■ Pinch the ends of the cup and insert the pinched end into the vagina.

■ Diaphragms should not be in place greater than 24 hours.

■ Leave in for six hours after intercourse.

■ Reapply spermicide if intercourse is repeated, by inserting jelly with applicator.

■ Wash with mild soap and warm water after removal, air dry.

■ Needs refitting after a greater than 20% weight change and after pregnancy.

Other Forms of Contraception not Dispensed by Pharmacists

■ Intrauterine device *(Mirena, Skyla)* are both hormonal IUDs. These cause light bleeding and minor or no cramping. *Mirena* lasts up to 5 years and *Skyla* up to 3 years. The copper-T IUD *(ParaGard)* can be used for EC, and lasts up to 10 years, but has more bleeding and cramping.

■ Subdermal rod *(Implanon, Nexplanon)* – contains the progestin etonogestrel.

■ Injection *(Depo-Provera, Depo-subQ Provera)* – medroxyprogesterone acetate, a progesterone given by IM or SC injection every 3 months. These contribute to bone loss; some of the bone loss may be irreversible.

Emergency Contraception (EC)

<u>Emergency contraception (the "morning after pill") is a form of contraception that prevents pregnancy up to 72 hours (3 days) for levonorgestrel EC and up to 120 hours (5 days) after sexual intercourse for *Ella*. Another option to prevent pregnancy is the copper IUD insertion *(ParaGard)*.</u>

Higher-than-normal doses of regular daily oral contraceptives can be used, but are not preferred and are used when the recommended EC products are not available, such as 5 tablets of *Aviane* or *Alesse* x 2 doses, taken 12 hours apart. A reference list of common contraceptive pill brands and the numbers needed to prevent pregnancy is available at http://ec.princeton.edu/questions/dose.html#dose

The two common formulations are *Plan B One Step* and generics, which come as one 1.5 mg tab or two separate 0.75 mg tabs of levonorgesterol. This formulation of EC reduces the risk of pregnancy by 89 percent when started within 72 hours after unprotected intercourse. The sooner it is started, the higher the efficacy. EC has been available for 30 years and there have been no reports of serious complications or birth defects.

EC can be an important resource after unprotected sex, such as from missed pills, a condom breaking during intercourse, a diaphragm or cap that moved out of place during intercourse, or if a woman may have been sexually assaulted.

[Note that EC is not the same as abortion; abortion is used to interrupt an established pregnancy while EC is used to prevent one. This follows the FDA definition of pregnancy as a fertilized egg implanted in the uterine wall. If a person believes that pregnancy occurs at the point of conception (from the time of sexual intercourse) they may not want to use EC. Some pharmacists and patients do not wish to dispense, or use, the EC formulation ulipristal (*Ella*), which is a chemical cousin to misoprostol (*Mifeprex*), one of the components in the "abortion pill" RU-486. They are not the same drugs and are used differently. In RU-486, misoprostol is used to expel the uterine contents (which is why it is pregnancy category X because it causes uterine contractions). In EC, ulipristal is used at a lower dose to delay or inhibit ovulation. It may also prevent implantation and this is a cause of concern for some. All forms of EC, whether ulipristal or levonorgestrel, do not interfere with the fertilized egg after implantation.]

If sexual assault has occurred the woman may require STI treatment, including HIV prevention. Pharmacists should have referrals for other providers available to suggest to patients. Referrals may be needed for regular contraception care.

If a patient vomits within 2 hours of taking the pill/s, they should consider repeating the dose. If easily nauseated, recommend an OTC antiemetic (1 hour prior to use, and caution if driving home due to sedation).

Occasionally women may be using EC after sex as a means of birth control; this may be done when a woman has occasional (not regular) sexual activity. This is not preferred due to a lower efficacy than regular birth control pills and changes in the menstrual cycle due to the high, intermittent levonorgestrel doses. Depending on insurance coverage, it may also be more expensive.

Levonorgestrel EC

Plan B One-Step and generics *(Take Action, Next Choice One-Dose, My Way)* are over-the-counter with no age or other restrictions. The pharmacy does not need to be open to sell this product. Per the FDA, these should be placed in the OTC aisles with the other family-planning products, such as condoms and spermicides. The generics cost $35-$45, about $10 less than the brand. Two-pill generics (levonorgestrel 0.75 mg tablets) are still available only behind the counter without a prescription for ages 17 or older; ages 16 and under still need a prescription. Both sexes require proof of age if getting behind the counter OTC. There is no reason to use a prescription with the formulations available OTC (unless someone wanted the 2 pill formulation) except to use insurance coverage.

If the EC is coming from behind the counter, there is no requirement for purchasers to sign a registry. They can receive multiple packets and ACOG recommends an additional packet for future use, if needed, since EC is more effective the sooner it is used.

Levonorgestrel Formulations

- Mechanism of action: similar to other hormonal contraceptives. All of them act by one or more of the following mechanisms: altering the endometrial lining, altering cervical mucus, interfering with fertilization or transport of an egg, or preventing implantation. There is evidence that levonorgestrel primarily works by preventing or delaying ovulation, but other mechanisms may be involved.

- This type of EC is indicated for up to 3 days (the sooner, the better) after unprotected intercourse (and is used longer off-label).

- Take 1.5 mg as a single dose *(Plan B One Step)*, or in two divided doses (0.75 mg) separated by 12 hours.

- Primary side effect is nausea, which occurs in 23% of women, and 6% have vomiting. If the women is easily nauseated OTC anti-emetics should be recommended to avoid losing the dose.

- If the period is more than a week late, a pregnancy test should be taken. If they have severe abdominal pain, they may have an ectopic pregnancy (outside of the uterus) and need immediate medical attention.

Ulipristal *(Ella)*

- Requires a prescription or ordered through an online site for $59, which includes next-day shipping.

- Works primarily by delaying ovulation. May also prevent implantation in the uterus – this mechanism is more controversial than levonorgestrel.

- Indicated for up to 5 days after unprotected intercourse.

- Primary side effects are headache, nausea and abdominal pain. Some women have changes in their menstrual cycle, but all should get their period within a week. If the period is more than a week late, they should get a pregnancy test. If they have severe abdominal pain, they may have an ectopic pregnancy (outside of the uterus) and need immediate medical attention.

- Use contraception the rest of the cycle as ovulation may occur later than normal.

Resuming Contraception after EC

Regular hormonal contraceptives (OCs, the shot, the ring, or the patch), should be started on the following day after completing the last EC dose. The patch and the ring can also be started on the first day of menses.

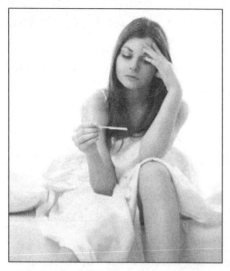

INFERTILITY

Infertility affects 10-15% of persons trying to conceive, or over 2 million American couples annually. One in sixteen babies are now conceived by women using fertility medications. From a business perspective, the sale of infertility medications is profitable. Detailed knowledge of this topic is a "specialty" area; this section provides "basic competency" knowledge.

The chance of pregnancy in couples attempting pregnancy is about 25% per month, and most will become pregnant within a year. If pregnancy has not occurred at one year's time, the couple should be referred for medical consultation. Infertility can be due to either the male or female. Males can be contributory due to various problems with sperm production. Females could have one or more contributory factors, including congenital defects, infectious pathogens (including damage from chlamydia or trichomoniasis), abdominal conditions, ectopic pregnancy, scarring from previous surgeries, hypothyroidism or polycystic ovary syndrome (PCOS).

In the beginning part of this chapter there is a brief description of ovulation kits; these are a reasonable place to start, prior to outside referral. Ovulation kits test for <u>luteinizing hormone</u> (LH), which is present in the urine and surges 24-48 hours prior to ovulation. The LH surge triggers the release of an egg from an ovary (ovulation). Ovulation is the most fertile time of the cycle. <u>The three days immediately from the positive result is the highest chance for pregnancy</u>. The kits are simple to use and require either running the test stick under the urine stream, or collecting the urine in a small container and dipping the test strip.

There are other more complex ways to assess ovulation, including testing body temperature, cervical mucus, and using fertility monitors. Any women trying to conceive should have possible teratogens discontinued, if possible. The pharmacist should check the woman's OTC and Rx medication use and consult with the prescriber. It may also be necessary to eliminate medications from the male partners regimen. Possible teratogens are discussed in more detail in the Drug Use in Pregnancy chapter.

Patient-Specific Infertility Treatment Goals

- Address any underlying medical condition.

- Increase quantity of quality sperm

- Increase number of eggs

- In-vitro fertilization (IVF)

If medications are used they are either oral or injectable. The table below provides a summary of the common fertility medications.

DRUG	DOSING	SAFETY/SIDE EFFECTS/MONITORING

Oral

DRUG	DOSING	SAFETY/SIDE EFFECTS/MONITORING
Clomiphene (Clomid, Serophene) GnRH → ↑ FSH & ↑ LH, to ↑ ovulation Selective Estrogen Receptor Modulator (SERM)	50 mg x 5 days, taken on days 3, 4 or 5 after period starts. Can increase to 150 mg, 5 days/cycle.	**CONTRAINDICATIONS** Liver disease, pregnancy, uncontrolled adrenal or thyroid disorders **SIDE EFFECTS** Hot flashes, ovarian enlargement, abdominal bloating/discomfort, blurred vision, headache, fluid retention. Can ↑chance of multiple births (but less than injectables), ovarian enlargement, thrombosis risk

Injectable

DRUG	DOSING	SAFETY/SIDE EFFECTS/MONITORING
Human Chorionic Gonadotropin (hCG) (Ovidrel), SC (Pregnyl, Novarel), IM **Gonadotropins** Follitropin Beta (Follistim AQ), IM, SC **Urofollitropin** (Bravelle), IM, SC **Follitropin Alpha** (Gonal-F), SC **Menotropins** (Menopur, Repronex), IM, SC **Gonadotropin Releasing Hormone Agonist (GnRH agonist)** Sometimes used: leuprolide (Lupron), Goserelin (Zoladex), Nafarelin (Synarel), IM, SC **Gonadotropin Releasing Hormone Antagonist (GnRH antagonist)** Cetrorelix (Cetrotide), SC	These come in either prefilled syringes, or as pens that may be preloaded, or pens with prefilled cartridges, or in ampules that are reconstituted, with supplied diluent. If reconstituting: insert syringe needle into vial, invert, slowly draw entire contents into syringe. Make sure tip of needle is not sticking through the solution or it will not be pulled into the syringe. Remove needle and syringe, replace syringe with injection needle. If air bubbles they can be tapped out. Some multiple dose pens require priming – these pens have dose counters on them and the instructions will designate the priming dose. The pen is primed when liquid appears at the tip. All SC injections: keep needle in skin for at least 5 seconds; some are longer, to avoid the drug "popping" out onto the skin. If multiple use, recap. Otherwise, discard entire device without recapping into appropriate container (sharps container, milk container, unbreakable plastic container).	**SIDE EFFECTS** Injection site pain, CNS (depression, fatigue, headache), ovarian hyperstimulation syndrome (ovaries become enlarged and tender, small risk multiple pregnancies). **NOTES** SC: abdomen is generally preferred due to a more even absorption, or other SC sites. Instructions will indicate either 45 or 90 degrees. See immunization chapter for more details: these are short needles (½" or less). For IM: Upper outer quadrant is often used, as marked in this picture. These are 1" or longer needles; more information on injections in the Immunization chapter. 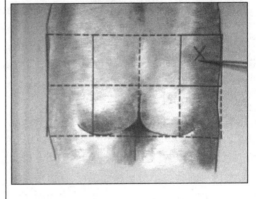

OSTEOPOROSIS & HORMONE THERAPY

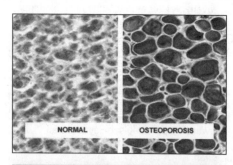

NORMAL   OSTEOPOROSIS

We gratefully acknowledge the assistance of Renu F. Singh, PharmD, BCACP, CDE, Clinical Professor, University of California San Diego Skaggs School of Pharmacy and Pharmaceutical Sciences, in preparing this chapter.

GUIDELINES

National Osteoporosis Foundation: Clinician's Guide to Prevention and Treatment of Osteoporosis, 2014. http://nof.org/hcp/clinicians-guide (accessed 2014 Sept 24).

American College of Obstetricians and Gynecologist's Practice Bulletin No. 141: Management of Menopausal Symptoms. 2014; 123(1):202-216.

Dandona, P. and Rosenberg, MT. A practical guide to male hypogonadism in the primary care setting. *Int J Clin Pract.* 2010; 64:6:682-696.

BACKGROUND

Osteoporosis, which means "porous bones," causes bones to become weak and brittle. It is estimated that half of all adults in the U.S. have osteoporosis or low bone mass. Half of all women and one in five men will have an osteoporotic-related fracture during their life. Falls are a common cause of fracture, but with extremely porous bones, coughing or rolling over in bed can cause fractures. The most common location of a fracture is the lower (lumbar) spine. These vertebrae turn over more rapidly (higher rate of cell turnover) than hip bones, and are holding the weight of the upper spine and head. Vertebral fractures can often occur without symptoms, with a gradual loss of height being the only clue to collapsing vertebrae.

Hip fractures occur with more severe disease (or bad falls) and can be debilitating. They are also more common after age 75. A hip fracture in a woman has a 25% risk of mortality at one year, with a higher risk of mortality in men, since men with osteoporosis are often using long-term steroids or androgen blockers and may be sicker at baseline. Hip fractures, if not fatal, can lead to loss of independence and/or chronic pain. Wrist fracture, which appears often in younger women, may be an early warning sign of poor bone health.

DIAGNOSIS/DEFINITIONS

<u>Osteoporosis (OP) is defined by a T-score equal to or < -2.5</u>. This indicates that the BMD is at least 2.5 standard deviations below that of an average BMD for young adults. Osteopenia, or low bone mass, is lower bone density than normal, but not as low as osteoporosis. <u>Osteopenia is defined by a T-score between -1 and -2.5</u>. Similarly, this indicates that the BMD is between 1 and 2.5 standard deviations below that of an average BMD for young adults.

Notice that the scores are negative; a T-score from -1 and higher indicates normal bone density. A higher number correlates with stronger (denser) bones, which are less likely to fracture. The T-score is calculated by comparing a person's bone mineral density (BMD) to the average peak BMD of a normal, young adult of the same gender. Z-scores are scored the same way as T-scores but they compare the patient's bone mineral density (BMD) to the mean BMD of an age, gender and ethnicity-matched population.

<u>Osteoblasts are the cells involved in bone formation</u>, and <u>osteoclasts break-down bone</u>; that is, they are involved in <u>resorption</u>. Bone is not "dead tissue"; it is living and constantly remodels, although some types of bone remodels very slowly, and others remodel at a faster rate. Some medications (bisphosphonates, raloxifene, estrogens, denosumab) slow down bone break-down, or resorption. Teriparatide (*Forteo*) does both – it helps prevent bone break-down and helps build bone. Teriparatide is a strong agent and is reserved for high-risk patients.

The gold standard to diagnose osteoporosis is a bone scan of the hip and spine performed by a dual energy x-ray absorptiometry (<u>DEXA, or DXA</u>) machine. Ultrasound devices are not optimal, yet they are less expensive, portable, and do not emit radiation.

RISK FACTORS FOR LOW BONE DENSITY

Genetic factors are most important, with Caucasian and Asian American women at highest risk

Advanced age

Low bone mineral density (usually evidenced by the T-score)

Previous fracture as an adult after age 50, not due to a traumatic injury

More than 2 alcoholic drinks per day

Oral or IM glucocorticoid use for ≥ 3 months at a daily dose of 5 mg prednisone equivalent, or greater

Excessive thinness

A decline in adult estrogen levels, from menopause, anorexia nervosa, lactation, hypogonadism

Rheumatoid arthritis and Lupus

Low level of physical activity and adequate nutrition – low over the life span

Calcium and vitamin D – low intake over life span

Smoking

DRUGS AND OSTEOPOROSIS RISK

Steroid use, long-term, is the major drug-contributing factor to poor bone health (≥ 5 mg/d of prednisone equivalent for ≥ 3 months). Other medications that lower bone density include:

Depot medroxyprogesterone acetate

Anticonvulsants (carbamazepine, fosphenytoin, phenobarbital, phenytoin, primidone, others)

Heparin

Lithium

Excess thyroid hormone

Loop diuretics

Aromatase inhibitors used for breast CA

Nafarelin (*Synarel*) – used for endometriosis

Androgen blockers used for prostate CA and some other chemotherapeutics

Proton pump inhibitors used chronically (↓ calcium absorption due to ↓ gastric pH)

Selective serotonin reuptake inhibitors

Thiazolidinediones (pioglitazone, rosiglitazone)

An ultrasound reading provides bone density in one location, such as the heel. An ultrasound reading, if low, should encourage the patient to get a DEXA scan. All women at age 65 and men at age 70 should receive a DEXA, and in women younger than 65 years or men between 50 – 69 years, bone density can be determined earlier if there is a history of a fragility fracture after age 50, medical or drug-induced bone loss, parental history of hip fracture, current smoker, alcoholism, rheumatoid arthritis, or other clinical risk factors. Since vertebral fractures are so common in older adults and usually lack symptoms, vertebral imaging may be done if height loss is observed or if BMD indicates osteopenia. In addition to monitoring the BMD over time, biochemical markers of bone turnover are also useful.

Fracture Risk Assessment Tool (FRAX)

The FRAX tool estimates the risk of fracture in the next 10 years (http://www.sheffield.ac.uk/FRAX/). It has been well-validated and its usefulness and limitations are outlined in the (NOF) guidelines. FRAX is a computer-aided program developed by the World Health Organization (WHO). The patient's age, sex, BMI, previous fragility fracture, parental hip fracture, femoral neck BMD, current smoking status, steroid use, alcohol intake and a few other measures are entered to assess the usefulness (risk/benefit) of drug therapy.

Phases of Bone Loss

Bone accumulates until approximately age 30. After that, bone loss occurs throughout life. Men lose bone at a rate of 0.2-0.5% per year, unless they use drugs that accelerate bone loss (such as long-term steroids) or prostate cancer agents. Women lose bone slowly after peak bone growth, and then at an increased rate in the 10 years from menopause (1-5% bone loss per year) and then at a slower rate thereafter.

Fall Risk/Fall Prevention Measures

If the bone density is low, care must be taken to avoid falls. Factors that put a patient at increased fall risk include the use of drugs that cause CNS depression or cause falls by another mechanism (such as SSRIs or initiation of anti-hypertensives), any condition that causes physical instability or poor coordination, impaired vision, dementia, poor health/frailty, low physical activity and a history of recent falls. A home safety assessment should ensure that lighting is appropriate, floors are safe (throw rugs/clutter/cords have been removed), storage is at reasonable heights, bathrooms have safety bars and nonskid floors, handrails are present on all stairs, and the stairs are well-lit with non-skid treads or carpet.

Additional "Lifestyle" Recommendations

In addition to the changes in the environment listed above, all patients with low bone density should be encouraged to perform weight-bearing exercise (such as walking, jogging, Tai-Chi) and muscle-strengthening exercise (weight training, yoga), taking adequate vitamin D and calcium, stopping smoking and avoiding secondhand smoke, reducing alcohol intake and adopting fall prevention strategies.

Preventing falls requires measures to improve muscle strength, balance and vision. Adequate corrective lenses, safe shoes and appropriate clothing (that will not cause falls) are required. If a disability is present, canes or walkers should be strongly recommended.

OSTEOPOROSIS IN MEN

Age-related bone loss occurs in men, not just women, and is frequently underdiagnosed. In addition, secondary bone loss can occur from drugs used for prostate cancer (androgen-blocking agents) or with COPD (receiving series of systemic steroids), with rheumatoid arthritis, or other bone-debilitating conditions. In these patients, fractures have high fatality as the patient is weak. Typically, bisphosphonates are used. It is still necessary to limit treatment duration (3-5 years), as is done with women. High-risk agents *(Forteo, Prolia)* are other options, depending on the risk and condition. Men, as with women, will require adequate calcium and vitamin D.

CALCIUM & VITAMIN D

All prescription medications for low bone density require adequate calcium and vitamin D taken concurrently. Dietary intake of calcium should be assessed first and is preferred, with supplements used if insufficient. Over half of the U.S. population has low calcium and vitamin D intake. Adequate calcium intake is required throughout life, and is critically important in children (who can build bone stores), in pregnancy (when the fetus can deplete the mother's stores if intake is insufficient) and during the years around menopause, when bone loss is rapid. Vitamin D is required for calcium absorption, and low levels contribute to various health conditions, including autoimmune conditions and cancer. Vitamin D deficiency in children causes rickets, and in adults causes osteomalacia (softening of the bone, with low levels of collagen and calcium). In 2010 and 2011 there were news reports that calcium supplementation with or without vitamin D, may increase heart attack risk; at present, recommend that patients obtain the recommended levels and ensure adequate intake of calcium with vitamin D.

NIH's Recommended Dietary Allowances (RDAs) for Calcium (2013)

AGE	MALE	FEMALE
0-6 months	200 mg	200 mg
7-12 months	260 mg	260 mg
1-3 years	700 mg	700 mg
4-8 years	1000 mg	1000 mg
9-13 years	1,300 mg	1,300 mg
14-18 years	1,300 mg	1,300 mg
19-50 years	1,000 mg	1,000 mg
51-70 years	1,000 mg	1,200 mg
71+ years	1,200 mg	1,200 mg

Notes on Calcium Selection & Absorption

- Calcium absorption is saturable; doses should be divided (maximum 500 – 600 mg of elemental calcium per dose).

- Dietary calcium is generally not sufficient; most women need an additional 600 – 900 mg/day (2 to 3 dairy portions) to reach recommended levels.

- Calcium requires vitamin D for absorption.

- Calcium citrate *(Citracal*, others) has better absorption and can be taken with or without food; usual tab has 315 mg of elemental calcium (21% elemental calcium). It may be preferable with little or no stomach acid – such as what occurs with elderly patients and/or with the use of PPIs, which have been shown to increase fracture risk due to impaired calcium carbonate absorption (including the dietary calcium).

- Calcium carbonate *(Oscal, Tums,* others) has acid-dependent absorption and should be taken with meals; usual tab is 500 – 600 mg of elemental calcium (40% elemental calcium).

- There is no known benefit of using more expensive formulations – recommend products made by reputable manufacturers, since lead may be present in untested products, especially those containing calcium from dolomite, oyster shell, or bone meal.

- Both forms come as chewables, liquids, and in food products.

Notes On Vitamin D Selection

- The NOF recommends an intake of 800 – 1,000 IU of vitamin D for adults age 50 years and older. The Institute of Medicine and NIH's recommended intake for vitamin D for people up to age 70 years is 600 IU daily, and 71+ years is 800 IU daily. However, these levels are currently controversial and many endocrinologists are recommending a higher intake of 800 – 2,000 IU daily. The Institute of Medicine and ACOG guidelines has a recommended upper intake of 4,000 IU daily for adolescents and adults. A few years ago vitamin D levels were not routinely ordered; this has become commonplace. A serum vitamin D level [25 (OH) D], should be measured and supplements given to reach a level of 30 mg/mL (75 nmol/L).

- The 50,000 unit vitamin D2 supplement (ergocalciferol; the green capsules) are used in renal disease or short-term in adults with deficiency to replenish stores. Cholecalciferol, or vitamin D3, is the preferred source, although vitamin D2 is often the type in supplements and will provide benefit. See Renal Disease & Dosing Considerations chapter for information on vitamin D analogs and calcitriol.

DRUG TREATMENT

Bisphosphonates are used first-line in most patients. They increase bone density, and except for ibandronate, reduce both vertebral and hip fracture risk. Patients with gastrointestinal problems with oral bisphosphonates may prefer an injectable bisphosphonate. Or, adherence issues may make a once monthly dose of oral risedronate or oral ibandronate, or an every 3 month injection of ibandronate or an annual infusion of zoledronic acid preferable.

Duration of bisphosphonate therapy: <u>Due to the rare risk of atypical</u> (or low trauma) <u>femur fracture and osteonecrosis of the jaw</u>, bisphosphonates can be stopped <u>after 3-5 years in patients</u> at low risk for fracture. A high risk patient can be continued indefinitely (sometimes after a one year drug holiday) or be switched to a completely different class of drug, such as denosumab, although atypical fractures and osteonecrosis of the jaw has also been reported with this drug class.

<u>Teriparatide injection</u> *(Forteo)* is used in patients with osteoporosis who are at <u>high risk</u> for having fractures, or who have already had an osteoporotic fracture while taking a bisphosphonate, or who have OP and need to take long-term steroids, or who cannot tolerate bisphosphonates. The newer agent denosumab *(Prolia)* is difficult to administer (it must be given in a doctor's office) and is expensive; it is also reserved for those with high risk.

Estrogen is no longer used first-line for osteoporosis treatment because of health risks. However, if used for menopausal symptoms, estrogen does increase bone density. Estrogen with or without a progestin <u>can be used for osteoporosis prevention in post-menopausal women</u>, primarily in women with <u>vasomotor symptoms of menopause</u>, and should be given at the <u>lowest possible dose and only for up to 2 years</u>. Conjugated estrogens/bazedoxifene *(Duavee)* <u>contains estrogen plus an</u> estrogen agonist/antagonist (bazedoxifene) which is also used for prevention of osteoporosis in post-menopausal women with a uterus. <u>Bazedoxifene</u> prevents endometrial hyperplasia in women with a uterus, <u>just like progestin</u>. Raloxifene can be used for treating or preventing osteoporosis and is used <u>most commonly in postmenopausal women who are at risk or have fear of breast cancer.</u> Calcitonin is used less often than in previous years since the evidence of benefit for bone density improvement is poor and in 2014 the FDA required new safety labeling on possible cancer risk.

Osteoporosis Prevention & Treatment Options

DRUG	DOSING	SAFETY/SIDE EFFECTS/MONITORING

Bisphosphonates work by inhibiting osteoclast activity. They are used for prevention (osteopenia), treatment (osteoporosis), Paget's disease, glucocorticoid-induced osteoporosis (and zoledronic acid is also used for hypercalcemia of malignancy).

Oral Bisphosphonates

DRUG	DOSING	SAFETY/SIDE EFFECTS/MONITORING
Alendronate *(Fosamax, Binosto)* Bisphosphonates are 1st line for most patients *[handwritten: effervescent (Binosto®)]*	**Prevention (post-menopausal women)** 5 mg PO daily, or 35 mg PO weekly **Treatment (post-menopausal women and men)** 10 mg PO daily, or 70 mg PO weekly alone, or with vitamin D3 2,800 or 5,600 IU (cholecalciferol), or 70 mg/75 mL solution – drink with at least 2 oz plain water (tablets need to be taken with 6-8 oz of plain water) **GIO-induced OP** 5 mg PO daily, or 10 mg PO daily if postmenopausal woman not on estrogen **Paget's Disease** 40 mg PO daily x 6 months	**CONTRAINDICATIONS** Inability to stand or sit upright for at least 30 minutes (60 minutes with once-monthly *Boniva*), difficulty swallowing, esophageal stricture, or at high risk for aspiration Hypocalcemia **WARNINGS** Rare risk of atypical femur fracture (AFF), esophageal cancer and osteonecrosis of the jaw (ONJ). Risk increases with dental surgery, poor dental hygiene, and with high doses used for hypercalcemia of malignancy. AFF and ONJ risk ↑ with duration of exposure. Bone, joint or muscle pain, which may be severe. Esophagitis, dysphagia, esophageal ulcers, esophageal erosions and esophageal stricture (rare). Hypocalcemia must be corrected prior to use. Ensure adequate calcium and vitamin D intake. Creatinine clearance < 35 mL/min (some are < 30 mL/min) **SIDE EFFECTS** Hypocalcemia (mild, transient), musculoskeletal pain, abdominal pain, dyspepsia, N/V, dysphagia, heartburn, esophagitis, skin rash, eye inflammation. **NOTES** *Binosto* (effervescent alendronate) contains 650 mg Na⁺. Avoid in sodium restricted patients, such as those with CHF or HTN. With *Atelvia*, no H$_2$RAs or PPIs. For all bisphosphonates, separate calcium, antacids, iron and magnesium supplements by at least 2 hours. Caution when using with aspirin or NSAIDs; will worsen gastric irritation. Due to risk of jaw decay/necrosis – dental work should be done prior to starting therapy. Due to transient hypocalcemia when initiating check calcium and vitamin D levels prior to starting therapy. Consider injectable bisphosphonate due to the risk of esophageal cancer risk if esophagitis is present, or with other GI issues, or with adherence issues. MedGuide required.
Risedronate *(Actonel, Atelvia)* *Actonel + Calcium:* 35 mg weekly and Ca²⁺ carb 500 mg x 6 days *Atelvia* is long-acting risedronate that is taken after breakfast, with 4 oz. plain water	**Prevention (post-menopausal women)** 5 mg PO daily, or 35 mg PO weekly **Treatment (post-menopausal women)** 5 mg PO daily, or 35 mg PO weekly, or 75 mg PO on two consecutive days/month, or 150 mg PO monthly **Treatment in men** 35 mg PO weekly **GIO-induced OP** 5 mg PO daily **Paget's Disease** 30 mg PO daily x 2 months	
Ibandronate *(Boniva)*	**Prevention or Treatment (post-menopausal women)** 150 mg PO monthly (on same date every month)	

Osteoporosis Treatment & Prevention Options Continued

DRUG	DOSING	SAFETY/SIDE EFFECTS/MONITORING

Injectable Bisphosphonates

DRUG	DOSING	SAFETY/SIDE EFFECTS/MONITORING
Ibandronate (*Boniva*)	**Treatment (post-menopausal women)** 3 mg IV every 3 months (in MD's office)	**CONTRAINDICATIONS** CrCl < 35 mL/minute and if evidence of acute renal impairment *(Reclast* only). **WARNINGS** Kidney injury and death can occur due to kidney failure. Monitor serum creatinine before every dose. Use with caution in dehydrated patients, elderly, other conditions/drugs that can predispose to kidney impairment. *Boniva* IV is NOT recommended for CrCl <30. **SIDE EFFECTS** No GI problems (bypasses gut), but can cause all others, and TPS (transient post-dose syndrome) in patients on days 2-3 post-injection: flu-like symptoms such as achiness, runny nose, headache, taking NSAIDs or APAP prior and afterwards can ↓ symptoms.
Zoledronic Acid *(Reclast)* *Zometa* – for hypercalcemia of malignancy	**Prevention (post-menopausal women)** 5 mg IV infusion once every 2 years **Treatment (post-menopausal women and men)** 5 mg IV infusion once yearly **GIO-induced OP** 5 mg IV once yearly **Paget's Disease** 5 mg IV once yearly	**NOTES** MedGuide required.

Raloxifene is an estrogen agonist/antagonist, also called a Selective Estrogen Receptor Modulator (SERM). It acts to ↓ bone resorption. Conjugated estrogens/bazedoxifene (*Duavee*) is an estrogen/SERM combination indicated for both osteoporosis prevention (in postmenopausal women with a uterus) and for vasomotor symptoms (raloxifene causes vasomotor symptoms).

DRUG	DOSING	SAFETY/SIDE EFFECTS/MONITORING
Raloxifene *(Evista)* Used often in women at risk (or have a fear of) breast CA	**Prevention and treatment of postmenopausal osteoporosis** 60 mg PO daily Favorable lipid effects (↓ CH and LDL; no effect on HDL)	**BOXED WARNINGS (2)** ↑ risk of thromboembolic events (DVT, PE, MI, stroke) The risk of death due to stroke may be increased in women with coronary heart disease or in women at risk for coronary events **SIDE EFFECTS** Hot flashes, peripheral edema, arthralgia, leg cramps/muscle spasms, flu-like syndrome, infection, amenorrhea, vaginal bleeding/discharge, skin changes **NOTES** Pregnancy Category X Separate raloxifene and levothyroxine by 12 hours. If on warfarin, monitor INR when starting or stopping raloxifene.

Osteoporosis Treatment & Prevention Options Continued

DRUG	DOSING	SAFETY/SIDE EFFECTS/MONITORING
Conjugated estrogens/bazedoxifene (*Duavee*) Osteoporosis prevention (in postmenopausal women with a uterus) & for vasomotor symptoms	One tablet (0.45/20 mg) PO daily	**BOXED WARNINGS (4)** Endometrial cancer risk (if used without a progestin in women with a uterus) Dementia risk in women ≥ 65 years of age taking estrogen alone. Women taking *Duavee* should not be taking additional estrogens. Do not use to prevent cardiovascular disease due to ↑ VTE risk in postmenopausal women 50-79 years of age. **WARNINGS** Breast cancer risk (from use of estrogen alone), patients with inherited thrombophilias at ↑ VTE risk, changes in CH values (↑ HDL, ↑ TGs, ↓ LDL), ↑ risk of ovarian cancer, ↑ risk of retinal vascular thrombosis **SIDE EFFECTS** Diarrhea, nausea, dyspepsia, abdominal pain, muscle spasms, oropharyngeal pain (all 7-9%) **NOTES** Pregnancy Category X

Calcitonin Nasal Spray and Injection – inhibits osteoclastic bone resorption

Calcitonin (*Miacalcin, Fortical*)	**Treatment of osteoporosis in women > 5 years post-menopausal** Inhale 1 spray (200 IU) in one nostril daily (alternate nostril daily) SC or IM: 100 IU daily	**CONTRAINDICATIONS** Allergy to calcitonin salmon **WARNINGS** May ↑ risk of cancer, and ↑ sediment in urine (reversible on discontinuation). Nasal spray may cause nasal ulceration; periodic nasal examinations are recommended. Hypocalcemia; monitor levels, supplement **SIDE EFFECTS** Rhinitis, back pain, muscle aches, headache. SC/IM formulation can cause local inflammation, nausea, flushing **NOTES** Keep unused bottles refrigerated. Possible antibody development to salmon that reduces efficacy. Not first-line. May have a role in elderly patients or short-term in patients with acute pain from vertebral fractures.

Osteoporosis Treatment & Prevention Options Continued

DRUG	DOSING	SAFETY/SIDE EFFECTS/MONITORING

Teriparatide Injection – stimulates new bone formation and depresses osteoclast activity; recombinant human PTH 1-34

Teriparatide *(Forteo)* For patients who are at very high risk for fracture, or who have already had a fracture due to osteoporosis, or for GIO, or if cannot take other medications	20 mcg SC daily for max of 2 years If bone pain with bisphosphonates it is less risky (although painful) than with teriparatide; bone pain from this drug could be bone cancer	**BOXED WARNING** Osteosarcoma (bone cancer) **WARNINGS** Orthostatic hypotension with initial doses, use cautiously if history or current urolithiasis (urinary stones) **SIDE EFFECTS** Hypercalcemia (transient, post-dose), arthralgias, pain, nausea, orthostasis/dizziness and ↑ HR **NOTES** 28-day pen, keep refrigerated and protect from light, inject in thigh or abdomen. Orthostasis/dizziness and ↑ HR mostly with the 1st few doses – caution when initiating drug. MedGuide required.

Denosumab – Monoclonal antibody that binds to nuclear factor-kappa ligand (RANKL) and prevents interaction between RANKL and RANK (a receptor on osteoclasts), preventing osteoclast formation; leads to ↓ bone resorption and ↑ bone mass

Denosumab *(Prolia)* *Xgeva* – for hypercalcemia of malignancy For high risk patients, or cannot use other agents	60 mg SC (in MD's office) every 6 months	**CONTRAINDICATIONS** Hypocalcemia – (must be corrected prior to using), pregnancy **WARNINGS** Osteonecrosis of the jaw (rare); risk ↑ with dental surgery or poor dental hygiene; serious infections, atypical femur fractures (rare), dermatitis/eczema/rash, severe bone/joint/muscle pain, anaphylaxis risk, hypocalcemia (monitor levels), use cautiously if hypoparathyroidism or thyroid surgery or infection **SIDE EFFECTS** Back pain, limb pain, dermatitis, eczema, rash, hypocalcemia, increased serum cholesterol. **NOTES** Pregnancy Category X (*Prolia*)/D (*Xgeva*). MedGuide required.

Bisphosphonate Patient Counseling

- Take first thing in the morning before you eat or drink anything, with 6-8 oz (1 cup) of plain water. If you are using formulations that are not once daily (such as weekly), choose the day of the week that is easy to remember (such as Sunday if you going to church, or bridge day, etc.)

- Take the medicine while you are sitting up or standing and stay upright for at least 30 minutes (60 minutes with monthly *Boniva)*. During this time, you cannot eat or drink anything else except more plain water. You cannot take any other medicines or vitamins. Nothing but plain water! If you plan to lie down again, you must first eat food.

- This medicine must be swallowed whole, and washed down with water. Do not crush or chew the tablet or keep it in your mouth to melt or dissolve.

- For effervescent tablets (*Binosto*), dissolve one tablet in 4 oz of room temperature water. Wait 5 minutes after effervescence is completed before stirring well and then drinking.

- For oral solution, administer in the morning with at least 2 oz (60 mL) of plain water.

- This medicine does not work well if you are not taking enough calcium and vitamin D. Some formulations contain calcium or vitamin D. Discuss with your pharmacist if you need to use calcium or vitamin D supplements.

- If you are using a proton pump inhibitor for heartburn, discuss with your pharmacist. These drugs may increase fracture risk. You may need to use a calcium citrate tablet, with adequate vitamin D.

- Your bone and muscle strength will improve faster if you are doing exercise. Your healthcare provider should discuss with you safe and healthy ways to exercise.

- Common side effects include GI upset, joint or muscle pain, back pain, dyspepsia or heartburn.

- Stop taking the medicine if you develop difficult or painful swallowing, have chest pain, have very bad heartburn that does not go away, or have severe pain in the bones, joints or muscles.

- Tell your healthcare provider right away if you develop thigh or groin pain while on this medication. Some patients have developed serious jaw-bone problems after using this medicine, which may include infection and slower healing after teeth are pulled. Tell your healthcare providers, including your dentist, right away if you have these symptoms. If you have dental work due now, you should have it done before starting the medicine.

- *Atelvia*: This is a long-acting form of risedronate. Take the medicine after breakfast. Sit or stand upright for 30 minutes or longer after taking. Do not use acid suppressing "heartburn" therapy with this medicine. Do not take calcium, iron, magnesium, antacids or multivitamin supplements until later in the day.

Bisphosphonate Missed Doses

- If on a weekly schedule and missed one dose, take the following morning (but not 2 doses on the same day).

- If on a daily schedule and missed one dose, skip that dose. Take the next dose at the regularly scheduled time.

- If on monthly *Boniva* and miss a dose, take it as soon as you remember (in the morning before eating) except if it is less than one week to the next dose, skip it (do not take 2 doses in the same week).

Raloxifene Patient Counseling

- This drug has a risk of dangerous blood clots. If any of the following occurs it could be due to a blood clot and you should get medical treatment quickly: any sudden leg pain, chest pain, shortness of breath, vision changes, an inability to speak or slurred speech, loss of movement on any side of your body.

- This drug can cause hot flashes during the day and can make you feel hot and sweaty during the night. If these occur and are bothersome discuss treatment options with your healthcare provider.

- Discontinue *Evista* at least 72 hours prior to and during prolonged immobilization, such as after a surgery or with prolonged bed rest.

Teriparatide Patient Counseling

- This medication is similar to a hormone made by the body called parathyroid hormone or PTH. This medication helps to form new bone, increase bone mineral density and bone strength.

- Please read the Medication Guide. During the drug testing process, *Forteo* caused some rats to develop a bone cancer called osteosarcoma. Osteosarcoma has been reported rarely in people who took *Forteo*. The warning states that it is not known if people who use *Forteo* have a higher chance of having osteosarcoma.

- <u>You may feel dizzy or have a fast heartbeat after the first few doses</u>. This usually happens within 4 hours of taking the medication and goes away within a few hours. <u>For the first few doses, inject this medication where you can sit or lie down right away if these symptoms occur</u>.

- Inform your healthcare provider if you develop bone or joint pain.

- The medicine comes in a prefilled injection pen that lasts 28 days. Each injection provides a 20-mcg dose. You should change the needle each day.

- The pen should be kept in the <u>refrigerator</u> and re-capped after each use. <u>After 28 days, the pen should be discarded</u> even if some medicine remains. There is a place at the end of the user manual to mark the date when the pen is started and the date (28 days later) when the pen should be thrown away.

- Inject one time each day in your <u>thigh or abdomen</u> (lower stomach area). The injection sites must be rotated.

- Do not transfer the medicine from the delivery device to a syringe. The injection pen is set at the right dose and does not require any dose adjustment.

- You can inject at any time of the day. Take it at about the same time each day.

- If you forget or cannot take the medicine at your usual time, take it as soon as you can on that day. Do not take more than one injection in the same day.

- <u>Do not exceed 2 years of use</u>.

- This medicine does not work well if you are not taking enough calcium and vitamin D. Discuss with your pharmacist if you need to use calcium or vitamin D supplements.

- If you are using a proton pump inhibitor for heartburn, discuss with your pharmacist. <u>These drugs may increase fracture risk</u>. You may need to use a calcium citrate tablet, with adequate vitamin D.

Calcitonin Nasal Spray Counseling

- This medicine is sprayed in one nostril daily. The other nostril is used the following day.

- Keep unused bottles in the refrigerator, but not the one being used. When a new bottle is removed it should be allowed to reach room temperature prior to priming. To prime the pump, hold the bottle upright and press the 2 white side arms toward the bottle until a faint spray is seen. Once the pump is primed, it does not have to be re-primed if the bottle is stored in an upright position.

- To use the nasal spray, remove the protective cap, keep head upright and insert the tip into a nostril. Press down firmly on the pump to deliver the medication. Use the other nostril the next day.

- After 30 doses, the pump may not deliver the correct amount of medicine with each spray and should be discarded.

- See your healthcare provider immediately if you any any allergic reaction (e.g. swelling of throat, trouble breathing). Some nose irritation may occur. However, see your healthcare provider if you get nasal crusting, dryness, redness or swelling, nose sores (ulcers) or nose bleeds.

- This medicine does not work well if you are not taking enough calcium and vitamin D. Some formulations contain calcium or vitamin D. Discuss with your pharmacist if you need to use calcium or vitamin D supplements.

- If you are using a proton pump inhibitor for heartburn, discuss with your pharmacist. These drugs may increase fracture risk. You may need to use a calcium citrate tablet, with adequate vitamin D.

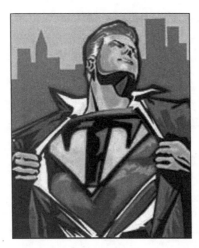

HORMONE THERAPY (HT)

HT is used for women who are in perimenopause, or what is commonly referred to as menopause (menopause technically means that menses has ceased for 12 months). Perimenopause normally occurs between the ages of 45 and 55. Many women experience <u>vasomotor symptoms as their ovaries produce less estrogen. A decrease in estrogen causes an increase in luteinizing hormone (LH), which can result in hot flashes and night sweats</u> (hot flashes that occur during sleep). Sleep can be disturbed, and mood changes may be present. Due to a decline in estrogen in the vaginal mucosa, vaginal dryness, burning and painful intercourse may be present.

Some women remain largely asymptomatic during menopause. In others the symptoms can be quite bothersome. Women who have had their ovaries removed, or are receiving anti-estrogen therapy for cancer may experience similar symptoms, but more acutely initially due to a sudden, rather than gradual, estrogen decline.

Estrogen-Progestin Use: Health Risks/Considerations For Use

The most effective therapy for vasomotor symptoms (hot flashes, night sweats) is <u>estrogen, which causes a decrease in LH, and, consequently, more stable temperature control</u>. Estrogen improves bone density and has historically been used to <u>prevent postmenopausal osteoporosis</u>.

<u>In women with a uterus, estrogen should not be given alone</u>. This will put the woman at elevated risk for endometrial cancer – the risk is 5 times higher if using estrogen alone for 3+ years. Progestins can cause mood disturbances in some women, and may be hard to tolerate. If given intermittently, such as with *Premphase*, spotting can be a nuisance. Progestins (norethindrone, levonorgestrel, norgestimate, drospirenone) are given in combination with the estrogen, or as a separate tablet (generally medroxyprogesterone, or MPA).

Several years ago the data from large trials on hormone therapy became available – these were the Women's Health Initiative (WHI) postmenopausal hormone therapy trials. At first, the news was scary and led to several boxed warnings on the use of HT, including warnings for increased risk of stroke, heart attacks and probable risk of dementia. As the data was reanalyzed, it became apparent that the majority of risk was highest in older women. Currently, the following considerations for use should be followed:

- Hormone therapy is safest around the time of menopause, and can be used in younger women, without contraindications, such as cancer or clotting history. The hormone therapy will likely be discontinued as the woman gets older and the risk for complications, such as thrombosis, increase.

- Bioidentical Hormone Replacement Therapy (BHRT, discussed below) may or may not be safer; the risk/benefit profile is unknown, at present.

Bioidentical Hormone Replacement Therapy (BHRT), other "Natural" Formulations

The warnings for HT therapy are based on the analysis of the WHI data and do not distinguish between hormone type. In the future, when more information is available, these warnings should be refined. At present it is safest to assume that known risk for one estrogen formulation applies to others. Some women will prefer to use compounded formulations.

In the WHI trial, the estrogen component was *Premarin*, or conjugated estrogens made from desiccated mare (horse) urine. Many clinicians (and patients) prefer to use "natural" hormones such as estradiol, a hormone made by human females. It is interesting to note that estradiol is made by pre-, rather than post-menopausal women.

The term "bioidentical" generally refers to compounds that have the same chemical and molecular structure as hormones that are produced in the human body. Many woman, physicians and compounding pharmacists believe that BHRT is safer, but keep in mind that there are no well-designed studies to confirm risk or benefit and compounded preparations are not regulated by the FDA. If a woman is using BHRT products and feels better, this is important. She should understand the risks that may be present [it is safest to assume risks known from available trial data (above) for any hormone therapy, until proven otherwise].

Natural Products Used for Vasomotor Symptoms

Natural products used for vasomotor symptoms include black cohosh, red clover, soy, flaxseed and evening primrose. The mild "plant estrogens," such as soy, are called phytoestrogens; phyto means plant. These natural products may help a little bit with mild symptoms, but would not provide the benefit of estrogen due to the strong feedback inhibition on LH.

Formulation Considerations

Topical formulations, given as a patch, gel or emulsion, bypass first pass metabolism, and lower doses can be used. Topical formulations usually cause less nausea, have little or no effect on cholesterol levels and may expose the woman to lower systemic estrogen. Estrogen use is generally well tolerated, but can cause nausea, dizziness, bloating and breast tenderness/fullness.

Topical products are preferred for patients who have vaginal symptoms only (vaginal dryness and/or painful intercourse). Any of the topicals included in this chapter (creams, vaginal tablets, vaginal rings) or OTC lubricants can be helpful. Common OTC lubricants include *Replens* and *Luvena*. A lubricant marketed specifically for dyspareunia (dry, painful intercourse) is *Astroglide*. Do not use oil-based lubricants with condoms – the condom can tear. *Astroglide* or silicon-based lubricants are safe to recommend with condoms. Ospemifene *(Osphena)* is a newer drug indicated for dyspareunia; see the warnings concerning this drug – it is not used lightly.

SSRI to ↓ Vasomotor Symptoms, SERM to ↓ Dyspareunia due to Vulvar/Vaginal Atrophy

Paroxetine (*Brisdelle*) is the first non-hormonal treatment indicated to reduce moderate-severe hot flashes associated with menopause. Women who are taking warfarin or tamoxifen should not use *Brisdelle*. As an SSRI, it will increase the risk of bleeding, and <u>as a CYP450 2D6 inhibitor, it will block the effectiveness of tamoxifen</u> and block the metabolism of warfarin, causing bleeding risk. Women in the perimenopause may have an accidental pregnancy as the menstrual cycle has become irregular; they should be counseled to use effective birth control. *Brisdelle* is <u>Pregnancy Category X</u> (other forms of <u>paroxetine are pregnancy category D, due to cardiovascular risk to the newborn)</u>, and with paroxetine specifically, a high risk of withdrawal effects in the newborn post-delivery. SNRIs (desvenlafaxine), clonidine and gabapentin also show effectiveness for treating vasomotor symptoms related to menopause, but these are not FDA approved for this indication.

Ospemifene (*Osphena*), is an oral SERM indicated for dyspareunia (painful intercourse). Topical vaginal products are safer for this purpose. One of the boxed warnings is for risk versus benefit; this drug has <u>VTE risk</u> and is <u>not indicated for mild symptoms</u>. It is only for a short treatment period for moderate-to-severe symptoms.

Testosterone in combination with HT has been used to improve sexual libido in postmenopausal women, but is not effective for treating vasomotor symptoms and has potential problems related to its androgenic side effects.

DRUG	DOSING	SAFETY/SIDE EFFECTS/MONITORING

SSRI to ↓ Vasomotor Symptoms

DRUG	DOSING	SAFETY/SIDE EFFECTS/MONITORING
PARoxetine *(Brisdelle)* *Paxil, Pexeva, Paxil CR*-for depression	7.5 mg PO QHS	**BOXED WARNING** Suicide risk; same as with other SSRIs **CONTRAINDICATIONS/WARNINGS** Same as with other SSRIs; see Depression chapter. **SIDE EFFECTS** Same sexual side effects (see Depression chapter), and in the *Brisdelle* trials > 10% incidence for sedation, insomnia, restlessness, tremor, dizziness/weakness, nausea, dry mouth, constipation, diaphoresis **NOTES** Lag time to effect (~4 weeks) <u>Pregnancy Category X</u> <u>Do not use with warfarin (↑ bleeding risk) or tamoxifen (↓ efficacy tamoxifen)</u>

SERM to ↓ Dyspareunia due to Vulvar/Vaginal Atrophy

DRUG	DOSING	SAFETY/SIDE EFFECTS/MONITORING
Ospemifene *(Osphena)*	60 mg PO daily Take with food	**BOXED WARNINGS (3)** Endometrial Cancer, CVD, Risk vs Benefit **CONTRAINDICATIONS** Undiagnosed abnormal vaginal bleeding, DVT or PE (current or history of), active or history of arterial thromboembolic disease (e.g., stroke, MI), estrogen-dependent tumor (known or suspected), women who are or may become pregnant **SIDE EFFECTS** Hot flashes, vaginal discharge, hyperhidrosis

Common HRT Products

Estradiol is used primarily for vasomotor symptoms, vaginal atrophy & osteoporosis prevention. The products below have one or more of these indications. Birth control pills contain ethinyl estradiol (primarily) and the estrogen dose is higher than with HRT.

COMPONENTS	FORMULATION	SAFETY/SIDE EFFECTS/MONITORING
Estradiol	Topical gel (*Divigel, Elestrin, EstroGel*) Topical spray (*Evamist*) Transdermal patch (*Alora, Climara, Minivelle, Vivelle-Dot, Menostar*) Vaginal ring (*Femring*)*	**BOXED WARNINGS (5), ESTROGEN** Endometrial cancer risk (if used without a progestin in women with a uterus). Dementia risk in women ≥ 65 years of age taking estrogen alone. Do not use to prevent cardiovascular disease due to ↑ VTE risk in postmenopausal women 50-79 years of age.
17-b-Estradiol	Vaginal cream (*Estrace*) Vaginal ring (*Estring*) Vaginal tablet (*Vagifem*)	Breast Cancer Hx, Risk vs Benefit (lowest effective doses and for the shortest duration consistent with treatment goals and risks).
Estradiol and Levonorgestrel	Transdermal patch (*ClimaraPro*)* *"Pro" indicates a progestin (+estrogen)	For *Evamist* only: Breast budding. breast masses (prepubertal females), gynecomastia, breast masses (prepubertal males) from unintentional secondary exposure; keep children away from
Estradiol and Norethindrone	Transdermal patch (*CombiPatch*) Oral tablet (*Activella, Mimvey*)	Evamist spray.
Estradiol and Norgestimate	Oral tablet (*Prefest*) – cyclic treatment, estradiol x 3 days, E+P x 3 days, repeat	**CONTRAINDICATIONS** Undiagnosed abnormal vaginal bleeding, any clotting incident or disorder (DVT, PE, MI, CVA, etc.), liver disease, pregnancy, any hormone-dependent cancer
Estradiol and drospirenone	Oral tablet (*Angeliq*)	
Conjugated Equine Estrogens (CEE)	Oral tablet (*Premarin*) – 0.3, 0.45, 0.625, 0.9, 1.25 mg Vaginal cream (*Premarin*) – 0.625 mg/gram Injection (*Premarin*)	**WARNINGS** Breast cancer risk (from use of estrogen alone), patients with inherited thrombophilias at ↑ VTE risk, changes in CH values (↑ HDL, ↑ TGs, ↓ LDL), ↑ risk of ovarian cancer, ↑ risk of retinal vascular thrombosis
CEE and MedroxyPROGESTERone (MPA)	Oral tablet (*Prempro*) – 0.3-0.625 conjugated E + 1.5-5 MPA Oral tablet (*Premphase*) – 0.625 mg CEE + 5 mg MPA days 15-28 (phasic dosing)	**SIDE EFFECTS** Nausea, dizziness, bloating, breast tenderness/fullness, ↑ triglycerides, ↑ HDL, and if patch, redness/irritation at the application site
MedroxyPROGESTERone (*Provera*)	2.5, 5, 10 mg oral tablets, suspension available	**NOTES** Some formulations come in patches – for all patches check if the patch must be removed before MRI.
Conjugated estrogens/bazedoxifene (CEE/SERM)	Oral tablet (*Duavee*)	Patch summary table in Drug Formulations chapter, *Vivelle-Dot, Alora, Minivelle* is applied twice weekly. *Climara* and *Menostar* patches are once weekly. *Evamist* spray: Each morning spray on inside of the forearm between the elbow and the wrist. Gels and *Evamist* spray are flammable. Gels: wash hands after application. Applied once daily: *Divigel* (upper thigh, alternate sides), *Elestrin* (upper arm/shoulder), *Estrogel* (arm).

Estrogen Counseling

- This product does not contain a progestin, which should be dispensed to a woman with a uterus. Estrogen increases the risk of cancer of the uterus.

- Report any unusual vaginal bleeding right away while you are taking estrogen. Vaginal bleeding after menopause may be a warning sign of cancer of the uterus (womb). Your healthcare provider should check any unusual vaginal bleeding to find out the cause.

- Do not use estrogens, with or without progestins, to prevent heart disease, heart attacks, or strokes.

- Using estrogens with or without progestins may increase your chances of heart attacks, strokes, breast cancer, and blood clots. Using estrogens may increase your risk of dementia. You and your healthcare provider should talk regularly about whether you still need treatment with this product.

- Estrogen use is primarily for menopausal symptoms, and should not be continued indefinitely. When you are ready to stop discuss with your healthcare provider the best way to stop the medicine – it will need to be decreased slowly.

- Estrogen can help keep your bones healthy. Ask your pharmacist for help in figuring out if you need to take calcium and vitamin D – these are important for healthy bones.

Vivelle-Dot Patch Application

- Your *Vivelle-Dot* (estradiol transdermal system) individual carton contains a calendar card printed on its inner flap. Mark the two-day schedule you plan to follow on your carton's inner flap.

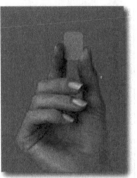

- If you forget to change your patch on the correct date, apply a new one as soon as you remember.

- Apply patch to lower abdomen, below the waistline. Avoid the waistline, since clothing may cause the patch to rub off.

- The area must be clean, dry, free of powder, oil or lotion. This applies to all patches. And never apply a patch to cut or irritated skin (unless it is a bandage!)

- Do not apply patch to breasts. (Never apply any estrogen patch to the breasts.)

- If any adhesive residue remains on your skin after removing the patch, allow the area to dry for 15 minutes. Then, gently rub the area with oil or lotion to remove the adhesive from your skin.

TESTOSTERONE THERAPY

Hypogonadism (low testosterone) is due to diseases, procedures, or a normal age-related decline in men. Treating opioid dependence with methadone lowers testosterone levels significantly. Other opioids may have an effect; the risk should be considered. Chemotherapy drugs used for prostate cancer, cimetidine and spironolactone can lower testosterone. The increases in testosterone use over the past few years is largely due to older males requesting testosterone therapy for improved sexual interest (↑ libido) and performance, increased muscle mass, increased bone density, sharpened memory and concentration, and increased energy. The use of testosterone replacement is controversial and a clear benefit between improved sexual function or quality of life has not been established. Many men feel that the testosterone product helps with their "Low T" symptoms. Recently, there have been reports of increased clotting risk in men using testosterone therapy, but the men with clotting may have had higher risk at baseline; at present, the link is unclear. Testosterone increases hematocrit, which can cause polycythemia and may increase clotting risk. Testosterone can cause non-cancerous prostate growth in men with benign prostatic hypertrophy (BPH). Testosterone replacement is restricted in men with severe BPH. (However, even with mild or moderate BPH, if dispensing a 5-α-reductase inhibitor for BPH that blocks the conversion of testosterone active form, it would not make sense to dispense another drug that provides testosterone directly.) Common side effects of testosterone include increased male pattern baldness, acne and gynecomastia.

Testosterone Formulations

Testosterone comes in intramuscular injections which are painful and require medical visits. Patients complain that they feel symptomatic when it is getting close to the time for the next dose. The injections may increase the hematocrit more than topical formulations. The injectable pellets in *Testopel* require medical visits. The pellets are a little smaller than Tic-Tacs and have the unfortunate tendency of popping out. *Striant* is a buccal form that is held inside the cheek twice daily; it has a high incidence of buccal irritation. The *Androderm* patch has a high incidence of skin irritation. In some cases it is tolerated with prior application of a topical steroid.

The gel formulations (*AndroGel* and other topical gels) are the most popular formulations and are relatively well-tolerated. *AndroGel* is the top-selling "Low-T" product and it is applied to the upper body. The man does not put his shirt on until the gel is dry; the biggest problem with the gel is when others touch the gel. Topical testosterone products require a MedGuide, primarily due to the risk of drug transfer from dad or grandpa to children. This causes "early virilization" and can affect both boys and girls. Depending on the dose received, the child could have enlarged genital organs, aggressive behavior and premature pubic hair growth. The risk of early virilization is a boxed warning. Pharmacists need to counsel men to wash their hands after each application and to be careful that no one touches the areas of application when wet.

There are new topical formulations that reduce accidental exposure risk: *Axiron* is applied to the underarms using an applicator that looks like deodorant, *Fortesta* is applied to the thighs with one finger (the amount is small) and *Natesto* is applied to the nostrils. Testosterone products are usually applied in the morning.

Testosterone Products: C-III

TESTOSTERONE	COUNSELING	SAFETY/SIDE EFFECTS/MONITORING
Topical Gels and Solutions		**BOXED WARNINGS (2)** Secondary exposure to testosterone in children and women can occur with use of testosterone. Cases of secondary exposure resulting in virilization of children have been reported. Women and children should avoid contact with any unwashed or unclothed application sites in men using testosterone gel.
AndroGel 1%, 1.62% Meter-dose pumps (# of pumps depends on dose) or foil packets of 2.5 g or 5 g gel *Vogelxo* meter-dose pump	*AndroGel* 1.62% is applied to the area of the upper arms and shoulders, but not the abdomen; with the 1% the abdomen can be used.	Injection only: Pulmonary oil microembolism (POME) reactions. **CONTRAINDICATIONS** Breast or prostate cancer.
Testosterone gel *(Vogelxo)*	Applied to upper arms and shoulders once daily	**WARNINGS** Patients with benign prostatic hyperplasia (BPH) treated with androgens are at an increased risk for worsening signs and symptoms of BPH.
Testosterone solution *(Axiron)*	Applied to underams once daily	
Testosterone gel *(Fortesta)*	Applied to thighs once daily	↑ risk of thromboembolic events (DVT, PE). The FDA is evaluating risk of stroke, MI, and death with testosterone products.
Testim gel 1%	Applied to arms and shoulders, not abdomen, once daily	Never apply to breast or genitals.
Testosterone nasal gel *(Natesto)*	1 actuation per nostril TID	**SIDE EFFECTS** ↑ appetite, ↑ SCr, sensitive nipples, acne, gynecomastia, dyslipidemia, edema, ↑ PSA, ↑ risk of hepatotoxicity, reduced sperm count, sleep apnea
Vogelxo gel 1%	Applied to arms and shoulders, not abdomen, once daily	
Alternative Formulations		**Additional Issues By Formulation Type** Patch: skin irritation
Androderm patch	2 mg, 4 mg patch Apply to back, abdomen, thighs or upper arms once daily. Skin irritation, but minimal exposure risk	Buccal tabs: buccal irritation Nasal gel: nasal irritation
Striant buccal tabs	30 mg to the gum region BID	**MONITORING** Testosterone levels, PSA, liver function, cholesterol, some products recommend checking hematocrit
Testopel pellets	SC every 3-6 months	
Testosterone undecanoate *(Aveed)* injection	IM every 10+ weeks	**NOTES** Remove patches before MRI; will burn skin.
Testosterone cypionate *(Depo-Testosterone)* injection	IM every 2-4 weeks	Gel is flammable until dry. Wash hands after application. Do not dress until skin dry.
Testosterone enanthate injection	IM every 2-4 weeks	
First-Testosterone ointment/cream	Apply daily, as directed	

AndroGel Patient Counseling

Pump

- Before using the pump for the first time, you will need to prime the pump. To prime *AndroGel*, fully push down on the pump 3 times. Do not use any *AndroGel* that came out while priming. Wash it down the sink or throw it in the trash to avoid accidental exposure to others.

- Your healthcare provider will tell you the number of times to press the pump for each dose.

Packets

- Tear open the packet completely at the dotted line.
- Squeeze all of the *AndroGel* out of the packet into the palm of your hand. Squeeze from the bottom of the packet to the top.

For Both

- This medication should not be used by women or children. Testosterone can cause birth defects in unborn babies. A pregnant woman should avoid coming into contact with testosterone topical gel, or with a man's skin areas where a testosterone topical patch has been worn or the gel has been applied. If contact does occur, wash with soap and water right away.
- Topical testosterone is absorbed through the skin and can cause side effects or symptoms of male features in a child or woman who comes into contact with the medication. Contact with the medication can cause enlarged genitals, premature pubic hair, increased libido, aggressive behavior, male-pattern baldness, excessive body hair growth, increased acne, irregular menstrual periods, or any signs of male characteristics.
- The testosterone transdermal patch may burn your skin if you wear the patch during an MRI (magnetic resonance imaging). Remove the patch before undergoing such a test.

How to apply (1+ push from pump/day or 1 packet/day), or topical gels

- Apply the medication as directed to clean, dry skin of the shoulders/upper arms and/or abdomen (1% only to abdomen) once daily in the morning. Apply only to areas that would be covered if you were to wear a short sleeve t-shirt. Avoid applying this medication to broken, irritated skin. Do not apply to genitals (penis or scrotum). Do not let others apply this medication to your body.
- After applying, wash your hands thoroughly with soap and water to reduce the risk of accidentally spreading it from your hands to other people. Before dressing, wait a few minutes for the application site to dry completely. Be sure to always wear clothing (such as a t-shirt) to cover the application site until you wash the areas well with soap and water.
- If you expect to have skin-to-skin contact with another person, first wash the application area well with soap and water.
- For best effect, wait at least 2 to 6 hours after applying the medication before showering or swimming.
- This medication is <u>flammable</u> until dry. Let the gel dry before smoking or going near an open flame.
- *Axiron* gel (applied to underarms): Apply deodorant first.
- *Fortesta* (applied to the front and inner thighs with one finger), *Natesto* (prime pump 10x first, insert actuator into nostril, depress slowly, remove from nose, wipe tip to transfer gel to lateral side of nostril then press on the nose and lightly massage. Try not to blow nose or sniff for one hour.)

pain

→ nociceptive

physical trauma to organ

→ somatic

from skin, muscles, bones, joints, ligaments

→ visceral

from internal organs (e.g. ♡, lung)

→ neuropathic

damage to nerve / CNS
- uncontrolled DM
- neurotoxic chemotx

⟹ antidepressants (NE)
AED
↳ gabapentin
↳ pregabalin
CBZ
[may need opioids for severe cases]

PAIN

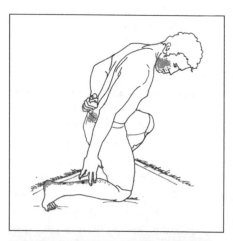

We gratefully acknowledge the assistance of Jeffrey Fudin, BS, PharmD, FCCP, DAAPM, Adjunct Associate Professor, Western New England University College of Pharmacy and Adjunct Assistant Professor of Pharmacy Practice, University of Connecticut School of Pharmacy, in preparing this chapter.

BACKGROUND

Pain is the physical suffering or discomfort caused by illness or injury. Pain originating from the same source can be both acute and chronic.

Chronic pain can be the result of an acute injury or secondary to various diseases such as osteoarthritis or rheumatoid diseases, or various neuropathies associated with poor glucose control in diabetes or from viruses such as HIV or herpes zoster. Pharmacists and prescribers should be concerned about inadequate pain treatment, but must often balance this against the potential abuse and misuse of opioid therapy. Drug interactions and side effects are always a concern.

Joint Commission standards require that pain be treated in the same manner as vital signs, making it compulsory for health care professionals in accredited facilities to inquire about, measure, and treat pain as they would blood pressure, pulse or respiratory rate. Pain is considered to be the "fifth vital sign."

GUIDELINES

Many resources, including guidelines, at the American Pain Society Website: www.ampainsoc.org. Selected resources include:

Common Elements in Guidelines for Prescribing Opioids for Chronic Pain. http://www.cdc.gov/homeandrecreationalsafety/overdose/guidelines.html (accessed 2014 Sept 10).

American Pain Society's Principles of Analgesic Use in the Treatment of Acute Pain and Cancer Pain, 6th Edition, 2008.

Addtl guidelines included with the video files (RxPrep Online).

TREATMENT PRINCIPLES

Pain is subjective, and thus, the primary measurement for assessing pain is the patient's own report, along with behavioral observations. Patients should be taught to monitor and document their pain. This will enable the clinician to adjust

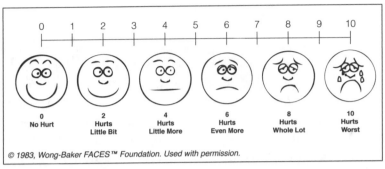

© 1983, Wong-Baker FACES™ Foundation. Used with permission.

medications more precisely. Pain scales (as shown here) can be used as guides to assess pain severity. The patient should record the pain level or severity, pain type or quality (using words such as burning, shooting, stabbing, aching, etc.) and the time of day that pain is better or worse. Timing is important; the frequency of breakthrough or "end-of-dose" pain can indicate the need for continuous scheduled extended release (ER) pain medication.

It is preferable to treat severe pain at initial onset since delays may require a higher total analgesic dose. The lowest dose that adequately reduces the pain is considered to be the appropriate dose. Using medicines with multiple mechanisms of action (termed "multimodal" pain control) can produce better responses via additive effects or synergism. Opioid agents in particular can be difficult to manage even for the patient who needs them, and an appropriate goal may be to try and reduce or avoid the use of opioids altogether. The addition of non-opioids to a regimen can often reduce the total opioid dose required while providing superior analgesia. This has been shown to be true in both the ambulatory setting and in acute medical-surgical settings. Additionally, access to non-medication techniques and modalities, such as physical therapy, heat/cold, massage therapy and directed exercise, is essential.

In recent years there has been an increased concern over the incorrect use of chronic opioids. Headache (described in the Migraine chapter) and low back pain are treated commonly. For low back pain, non-drug measures are useful: medium-firm mattress, active lifestyle with exercise, smoking cessation (smokers rate pain higher), weight loss and other modalities. If medications are used, acetaminophen or NSAIDs are helpful. Many patients find benefit with chronic use of amitriptyline or duloxetine (a SNRI). SSRIs have not been found to be beneficial. If severe, tramadol or opioids (lowest effective dose, shortest time required) can be tried next. Steroids have not been found to be helpful. In some cases skeletal muscle relaxants are used.

OPIOID TERMINOLOGY

Patients taking opioids chronically will often develop physiological adaptation ("physical dependence") and ultimately may live "dose to dose." Such patients will suffer withdrawal symptoms including anxiety, tachycardia, shakiness, shortness of breath or GI symptoms if a dose is missed or late.

It is important to distinguish between physiological adaptation and addiction. All patients, including addicts, become physiologically adapted to opioids after repeated exposure. By contrast, addiction involves a strong desire or compulsion to take the drug despite harm, and is manifested by drug-seeking behavior (exaggerated physical problems) or criminal activity (prescription forgery or theft).

Occasionally, patients exhibit "pseudo-addiction." The patient is anxious about running out of drug and may have used up the medication too quickly – signs which can be mistaken for addiction, but may actually be due to poorly controlled pain. The response to this type of patient is not to scold – but to determine which aspects of their pain are inadequately controlled, and counsel them to return to their pain management provider for reassessment and additional help in developing a tailored pain management regimen. Frequently, the reason for "pseudo-addiction" is the over-reliance on a short-acting agent such as a hydrocodone/acetaminophen combination. In such cases, if continuation of opioids is appropriate, consideration of conversion to an ER agent is warranted. Over-use of combination agents could put the patient at risk of hepatotoxicity with combination acetaminophen products or nephrotoxicity with NSAID combinations.

Tolerance to opioids develops over time and necessitates a higher dose to produce the same analgesic response. It is important to distinguish whether the condition causing the pain has worsened (e.g., cancer), or there is a decrease in effectiveness of the medication, or both. It has been proposed that opioid agonists have no maximum upper dose (no ceiling effect) but as the dose increases, a different opioid may be considered. Different pain types may be treated better with alternative agents such as NSAIDs for bone and connective tissue pain and SNRIs and anticonvulsants for neuropathic pain. In some patients chronic opioid use can worsen pain sensitivity, a phenomenon known as opioid hyperalgesia. In cases where this is suspected it is prudent to switch patients to a different opioid, or to consider weaning off opioids and using other types of analgesics.

"Break-through" pain (BTP), also called end of dose pain, is acute pain that occurs despite use of an ER or scheduled opioid. It is treated with an immediate release (IR) opioid. If repeat doses of BTP medication are required, then the baseline opioid dose should be increased or substituted with a different opioid. New or adjusted baseline opioids should be dispensed with a BTP medication until the dose of the scheduled opioid is stabilized. In the surgical setting, this can be done with the use of patient controlled analgesia (PCA): the infusion pump provides a continuous basal rate infusion and/or a patient controlled bolus.

Constipation prophylaxis is an essential component of a chronic opioid regimen. Inpatients on intravenous opioids must be monitored for sedation; sedation is the most important predictor of respiratory depression, the usual cause of fatality with an opioid overdose.

DRUG THERAPY

Choosing the correct analgesic requires that the pain be characterized correctly. Pain is either nociceptive (physical trauma to an organ) or neuropathic (due to damage to a nerve or damage in the CNS).

Nociceptive pain is one of two types: somatic (from the skin, muscles, bones, joints and ligaments – this is commonly called musculoskeletal pain) or visceral (from the internal organs, such as the heart or lungs). Neuropathic pain is associated with injury to a nerve or the central nervous system. Common causes of neuropathic pain are uncontrolled diabetes and neurotoxic chemotherapy.

Neuropathic pain often responds best to antidepressants that affect norepinephrine reuptake and/or anticonvulsants (gabapentin, pregabalin, carbamazepine). In severe cases, other classes of agents are used, including opioids. There are situations where both types are present at the same time. An example is the patient with an acute herniated disc (somatic pain from the disc rupture and neuropathic pain from nerve inflammation). Both nociceptive and somatic pain can present as mild, moderate or severe. The level of pain is considered when the type of analgesic is chosen. Mild somatic pain can be self-treated with OTC topicals and oral medications. The OTC topical capsaicin can be helpful for somatic and neuropathic pain. Most mild pain responds to acetaminophen, NSAIDs, or combinations of analgesics with antihistamines to relax muscle tension. Moderate somatic pain is treated with tramadol or combination agents, such as hydrocodone, oxycodone, or tramadol with acetaminophen or ibuprofen. Adjuvants and non-opioid analgesics can reduce the total daily dose of opioids required to control the pain.

MILD PAIN AGENTS, AVAILABLE RX AND OTC: ACETAMINOPHEN AND NSAIDs

Acetaminophen

⊖ anti-inflammation
⊖ effect on PLTs

Acetaminophen reduces pain (analgesia) and reduces fever (antipyretic) but does not provide a significant anti-inflammatory effect nor does it inhibit thromboxane and therefore, has no effect on platelets. The mechanism of action is not well defined but is thought to involve several pathways in combination. The primary mechanism may involve inhibition of cyclooxygenase (COX) enzymes which prevents the metabolism of arachidonic acid, which in turn reduces prostaglandin (PG) formation. Other mechanisms may include the endogenous cannabinoid system and inhibition of N-methyl-D-aspartate (NMDA) receptors.

Acetaminophen

DRUG	DOSING	SAFETY/SIDE EFFECTS/MONITORING
Acetaminophen *(Tylenol, most "Non-Aspirin" pain relievers, others)* **+ hydrocodone** *(Vicodin, Norco, Lortab)* **+ oxycodone** *(Percocet, Endocet)* **+ codeine**: *(Tylenol #2, 3, 4)* **+ traMADol** *(Ultracet)* … and many OTC combos **+ diphenhydramine** *(Tylenol PM)* And in multiple cough cold products Acetaminophen rectal supp *(FeverAll)* **IV Acetaminophen** *(Ofirmev)* – used inpatient to enable lower opioid doses, and can be used when oral routes are not available	**Adults** Keep below 4,000 mg/day and max of 325 mg per prescription dosing unit, per the FDA. OTC dosing ranges depend on the hrs, formulation, or are weight-based: 325 mg, max 2 tabs Q4-6H, NTE 10 tabs per 24 hr (3,250 mg) 500 mg, max 2 tabs Q6H, NTE 6 tabs per 24 hr (3,000 mg) 650 ER, max 2 tabs Q8H, NTE 6 tabs per 24 hr (3,900 mg) rectal supp: 650 mg Q4-6H, NTE 6 supp per 24 hr (3,900 mg) ≥ 50 kg: 650 mg Q4H or 1000 mg Q6H, max dose 4 g/day **Pediatrics (< 12 yrs)** 10-15 mg/kg Q4-6H, max 5 doses/d or use weight and age based dosing table on container rectal supp: 80, 120, 325 mg Infant drops are now the same concentration as the children's suspension (160 mg/5 mL) to ↓ dosing confusion and thus ↓ toxicity risk **Safety Considerations** Use dosing syringe or cup provided with the medicine. Caution with dosing IV acetaminophen: Solution is 10 mg/mL, in 100 mL vials. Use caution that doses ordered in mg are not dispensed as mL (for example, a 75 mg dose is not 75 mL, it is 7.5 mL). Do not permit nurses to prepare doses in the units. All IV acetaminophen doses should be prepared in the pharmacy.	**BOXED WARNING** Acetaminophen may cause severe hepatotoxicity, potentially requiring liver transplant or resulting in death; hepatotoxicity is usually associated with excessive acetaminophen intake (> 4 g/day), high risk of dosing errors with injection. **SIDE EFFECTS** Hepatotoxicity (with high, acute doses - can be fatal), nephrotoxicity (with chronic overdose), rash (Rare) but cases of severe skin rash: SJS, TEN, AGEP. Stop drug, seek immediate medical help. Nephrotoxicity: rare renal damage but generally safer than NSAIDs in renal disease **Antidote for Overdose** N- Acetylcysteine (NAC) MOA: Restores intracellular glutathione (acts as a glutathione substitute) NAC should be administered immediately, even before the results of APAP level are obtained; within 8 hours of ingestion. Oral loading dose is 140 mg/kg PO, followed by 70 mg/kg Q4H x 17 doses, unless the APAP level is non-toxic. Has an odor of rotten eggs and often causes N/V. IV form *(Acetadote)* can be used as an alternative, but is more costly. **NOTES** Pregnancy Category C; often used for mild pain in pregnancy. Do not use "APAP" on labels so that patients understand that they are getting acetaminophen.

Acetaminophen Drug Interactions

- May be used with warfarin; however, if used chronically, can alter INR – monitor accordingly.

- Avoid or limit alcohol use due to the risk of hepatotoxicity – see counseling section.

Acetaminophen Counseling

- Contact your healthcare provider right away for any condition that is being self-treated if the condition worsens, if it lasts for more than two days, if there is a high fever (> 102.5°F), or with rash, nausea, vomiting or blood in the stool. These are true also for children. Infants should be seen by the pediatrician.

H₁
(allergies)

H₂
(GERD)

- Many products contain acetaminophen, including prescription pain medicines and over-the-counter pain and cough-and-cold products. The name may be written as acetaminophen, *Tylenol*, APAP, non-aspirin pain reliever, etc. The total daily dose of all products should not exceed the limits above.

- Too much acetaminophen can cause kidney damage, and can permanently harm the liver. This can be exacerbated by the use of too much alcohol. Women should not exceed more than 1 drink per day, and men should not exceed more than 2 drinks per day.

Non-Steroidal Antiinflammatory Drugs (NSAIDs), Salicylates

NSAIDs include the traditional (non-selective) NSAIDs such as ibuprofen, the salicylates, which includes aspirin, and the COX-2 inhibitors. The cyclooxygenase 1 and 2 (COX) enzymes catalyze the conversion of prostaglandins (PGs) and thromboxane A2 (TXA2) from arachidonic acid. The nonselective NSAIDs block the synthesis of both COX enzymes. The COX-2 selective agents block the synthesis of COX-2 only – this ↓ GI risk because COX-1 protects the gut layer. Both groups ↓ the formation of the PGs that are involved in ↓ inflammation, ↓ pain and ↓ fever. Blocking COX-1 ↓ the synthesis of PG-H2, which ↓ the formation of TXA2. TXA2 is required for both platelet activation and aggregation and blocking TXA2 ↓ clotting and provides the cardiovascular benefit. Aspirin is a more effective antiplatelet agent than other non-selective NSAIDs because aspirin inhibits COX-1 irreversibly (with a covalent, irreversible bond). The other non-selective NSAIDs bind to COX-1 reversibly.

** NSAID BBW
1) serious GI - bleeding, ulceration, perforation of stomach/intestine
2) serious CV thrombotic events - MI, stroke
3) peri-operative pain mgt - CABG

NSAIDs, Salicylates

DRUG	DOSING	SAFETY/SIDE EFFECTS/MONITORING
Aspirin – Acetylsalicylic Acid primarily used for cardioprotection (81-162 mg) *Bayer, Bayer "Advanced" Aspirin* (dissolves slightly faster), *Ascriptin, Bufferin* (↓ stomach upset), *Ecotrin, Excedrin* (Aspirin + Acetaminophen + Caffeine) Enteric-coated (EC) and buffered products ↓ nausea NSAIDs, Non-acetylated salicylates	Analgesic dosing: 325-650 mg All NSAIDs: known risk factors for GI bleeding: Elderly, previous bleed, chronic or high dose use, hypoxic gut – check for dark, tarry stool, stomach upset, weakness, coffee-ground emesis (indicates a more serious, fast GI bleed) Also increases GI risk: concomitant anticoagulants or steroids, SSRIs/SNRIs, smoking, "poor health" Ibuprofen and naproxen have relatively lower risk for GI complications, but have risk, especially if high doses taken chronically; counsel against chronic use (including OTC) if avoidable	**BOXED WARNINGS** See preceeding page **CONTRAINDICATIONS** Pregnancy Category: most are C/D (avoid, esp 3rd trimester) Avoid with NSAID hypersensitivity (past reaction with trouble breathing), nasal polyps, asthma Avoid aspirin (not other NSAIDs) in children (< 16 y/o) with any viral infection due to potential risk Reye's syndrome (symptoms include somnolence, N/V, lethargy, confusion) **SIDE EFFECTS** Dyspepsia, heartburn (more common with aspirin – EC or buffered products can reduce symptoms) – take NSAIDs with food to ↓ nausea Blood pressure may increase (monitor) GI irritation/bleeding, renal impairment, CNS effects (fatigue, confusion, dizziness), photosensitivity, fluid retention/edema Patient-specific: CNS effects (confusion/dizziness), hyperkalemia (in renal impairment/with potassium-retaining agents), blurred vision (Rare) but cases of severe skin rash: SJS, TEN. Stop drug, seek immediate medical help. **NOTES** Not a contraindication, but NSAIDs (except aspirin) are unsafe after a heart attack; try to avoid use. Avoid with heart failure. Due to antiplatelet effects, stop all NSAIDs at least a week prior to elective surgery. Patients may be using PPIs to protect the gut with chronic NSAID use. If done, consider the risk from chronic PPIs (decreased bone density, increased infection risk).

(Handwritten left margin: take 1 hr before or 8 hrs after ibuprofen)

(Handwritten note: * EC – does not ↓ GI bleed risk ⇒ systemic effect: depletion of gut-protective PG ↑ bleed risk)

NSAIDs, Non-Acetylated Salicylates

DRUG	DOSING	SAFETY/SIDE EFFECTS/MONITORING
Salsalate	Up to 3 grams/day, divided BID-TID	
Magnesium Salicylate (*Doans, Doans ES, Momentum, Keygesic*)	ES: 500 mg/caplet 2 caplets Q6H, max 8 caplets/day	**NOTES, SALICYLATE-SPECIFIC** Salicylate overdose can cause tinnitus. Take with food or water or milk to minimize GI upset. All NSAIDs are taken with food; note that the salicylates usually cause more nausea & this counseling is important. Methyl salicylate is a popular OTC topical; most stores carry their own formulation. Brands include *Bengay, Icy Hot, Flexal, Thera-Gesic*. Do not cover with tight bandage or apply heat source. *(Handwritten: ± camphor, menthol)*
Choline Magnesium Trisalicylate	500 mg-1.5 g 2-3 times/day or 3 g at bedtime	
Diflunisal	500 mg-1.5 g 2-3 times/day or 3 g at bedtime	
Salicylate salts (*Arthropan, Asproject, Magan, Mobidin, Rexolate, Tusal*)	No longer commonly used	

NSAIDs, Others

DRUG	DOSING	SAFETY/SIDE EFFECTS/MONITORING
Ibuprofen *(Motrin, Advil)* **IV** *Caldolor*, also for mild-mod pain, can ↓ opioid dose, and can be used when oral routes are not available; must be diluted	**Adult** OTC: 200-400 mg Q4-6H, max 1.2 g/day, limit self-t x to 10 days or less OTC is for mild-mod pain, fever, dysmenorrhea Rx: 400-800 mg Q6-8H, max 3.2 g/day Rx is moderate pain or inflammation **Pediatric** <u>5–10 mg/kg/dose</u> (as an antipyretic), max daily dose 40 mg/kg/day	**BOXED WARNINGS** See preceeding page All NSAIDs, even OTC written on a prescription, require a MedGuide for warnings above. Other issues are similar to aspirin except for the risk of Reye's in children is not present (ibuprofen is used in pediatrics), tinnitus is not as likely with overdose and, since aspirin is a topical acid, the NSAIDs do not cause as much nausea as aspirin, but they do cause some and are best taken with food.
Naproxen *(Aleve-*OTC, *Naprelan & Anaprox*-Rx) *Treximet* (Sumatriptan-Naproxen 85-500 mg) *Vimovo* (Naproxen-Esomeprazole) – <u>the PPI is used to protect the gut from damage caused by the NSAID</u>	<u>All given BID</u> **OTC** Typical pain, OTC: 500 mg, then 250 mg (or 220 mg, if naproxen Na$^+$) Q6-8H; max 1,250 mg (day 1), subsequent doses 1,000 mg/day naproxen base **Rx** Inflammation, mild-mod pain, Rx: 500-1,000 mg/day in 2 divided doses; may increase to 1.5 g/day of naproxen base	Prescribers and patients sometimes prefer naproxen since it is BID dosing.

Other NSAIDs

Diclofenac *(Cataflam, Voltaren-XR, Zorvolex* "nano" formulation, *Zipsor, Cambia* – oral solution) *Arthrotec* (50 mg-200 mcg misoprostol) *Voltaren, Solaraze* gel *Flector* patch, *Pennsaid* topical solution	50-75 mg BID	**BOXED WARNING** Same as other NSAIDs, plus: *Arthrotec:* not to be used in women of childbearing potential <u>unless woman is capable of complying with effective contraceptive measures.</u> **NOTES** In addition to increasing uterine contractions (which can terminate pregnancy), misoprostol component causes cramping and diarrhea. Misoprostol is used to replace the gut-protective prostaglandin to reduce the risk of GI damage from the NSAID. This used to be a more popular agent before the advent of PPIs. Topical forms of diclofenac for mild pain, possible risk GI/renal issues; *Zorvolex* is lower dosing.
Indomethacin *(Indocin, Tivorbex)* Oral solution, rectal suppository, injection	IR 25-50 mg BID-TID CR 75 mg daily-BID The IR formulation is an older NSAID approved for gout; others can be used	High risk for CNS SEs (avoid in psych conditions) and GI toxicity
Piroxicam *(Feldene)*	10-20 mg daily	High risk for GI toxicity and severe skin reactions, including SJS/TEN Use for inflammatory conditions if failed other NSAIDs, and may need agent to protect gut (PPI, misoprostol)

Handwritten margin notes:
- *lasts a little longer ?? than APAP*
- *DOA: 6-8 hrs (vs 4-6 hrs for APAP)*
- *≠ ♀ childbearing → ↑ uterine contractions cramping diarrhea (↓ GI damage by ↑ gut-protective PGs) — PG analog*
- *HIGH RISK TOX*
- *oxaprozin (Daypro®) - same CAUTION*

NSAIDs, Salicylates Continued

DRUG	DOSING	SAFETY/SIDE EFFECTS/MONITORING
Ketorolac *(Sprix NS)* Toradol®	10-20 mg (oral) Always start IV, IM or nasal spray and continue with oral, if necessary. Not to be used in any situation with increased bleeding risk. 5 days total max treatment.	Can cause severe adverse effects including GI bleeding and perforation, post-op bleeding, acute renal failure, liver failure and anaphylactic shock. For short-term moderate to severe acute pain (max 5 days in adults), usually in post-op setting and never pre-op.
Sulindac	150 – 200 mg BID	Sulindac is sometimes used with reduced renal function, and in patients on lithium who require an NSAID.
Other less-commonly used NSAIDs include: meclofenamate, mefenamic acid *(Ponstel)*, ketoprofen, fenoprofen *(Nalfon)*, Flurbiprofen *(Ansaid)*, oxaprozin *(Daypro* – caution similar to piroxicam – higher risk side effects).		

COX-2 Selective – Lower risk for GI complications (but still present), ↑ risk MI/stroke (avoid with CVD risk – which is dose related, do not use higher doses in CVD-risk patients), same risk for renal complications

Celecoxib *(CeleBREX)* ≠ sulfa	50-400 mg OA: 100 BID or 200 daily RA: 100-200 BID Indications: OA, RA, juvenile RA, acute pain, primary dysmenorrhea, ankylosing spondylitis	Highest COX-2 selectivity Contraindicated with sulfonamide allergy Same Boxed Warnings as other NSAIDs Pregnancy Category C prior to 30 weeks gestation; Category D starting at ≥ 30 weeks gestation
Meloxicam *(Mobic)*	7.5-15 mg/day	Agents that have some COX-2 selectivity.
Etodolac Lodine®	300-500 mg Q6-8H	
Nabumetone Relafen®	1,000-2,000 mg daily (can be divided BID)	

NSAID Drug Interactions

■ Caution for additive bleeding risk with the use of concurrent agents with antiplatelet activity, such as aspirin, clopidogrel *(Plavix)*, prasugrel *(Effient)*, ticagrelor *(Brilinta)*, dipyridamole *(Persantine)* and with warfarin, dabigatran, rivaroxaban, ginkgo biloba, and others.

■ Do not use NSAIDs with steroids due to very high risk GI bleeding with concurrent use.

■ There is no reason to use two different NSAIDs concurrently (exception: low dose aspirin for cardioprotection but the cardioprotective effects may be blocked by ibuprofen and other NSAIDs). If using aspirin for cardioprotection and ibuprofen for pain, take aspirin one hour before or eight hours after ibuprofen.

■ NSAIDs can increase the level of lithium (avoid concurrent use) and methotrexate.

■ Caution with use of aspirin and other ototoxic agents (aminoglycosides, IV loop diuretics, etc.)

NSAID Patient Counseling

■ Take with food if this medicine upsets your stomach.

- This medicine may increase the chance of a heart attack or stroke that can lead to death. The risk increases in people who have heart disease. If you have heart disease, please discuss using this medicine with your healthcare provider.
- Do not use this medicine before any elective surgery.
- Do not use after coronary heart surgery, unless you have been instructed to do so by your healthcare provider.
- This medicine can cause ulcers and bleeding in the stomach and intestines at any time during treatment. The risk is highest if you use the drugs at higher doses, and when used long-term. To help reduce the risk, limit alcohol use while taking this medicine, and use the lowest possible dose for the shortest possible time. This medicine should not be used with medicines called steroids (such as prednisone) or anticoagulants (such as warfarin, *Pradaxa* or *Xarelto)*. [There are some exceptions in very high risk (clotting) patients who use both aspirin and warfarin. In general, using them together is not recommended.]
- The risk of bleeding with these medicines is also higher with many antidepressants, including SSRIs and SNRIs.
- Do not use this medicine if you have experienced breathing problems or allergic-type reactions after taking aspirin or other NSAIDs.
- This medicine can raise your blood pressure. If you have high blood pressure, you will need to check your blood pressure regularly. You may have to stop using this medicine if your blood pressure increases too much.
- This medicine can cause fluid and water to accumulate, particularly in your ankles. If you have heart disease, discuss the use of this medicine with your healthcare provider and monitor your weight.
- Photosensitivity: Limit sun exposure, including tanning booths, wear protective clothing, use sunscreen that blocks both UVA and UVB (this actually applies to some of the NSAIDs, but there is a class risk).
- Do not use this medicine if you are pregnant.

OPIOIDS

Opioid drugs interact in a variety of ways with the three primary types of opioid receptors: μ (mu), κ (kappa) and δ (delta). The primary mechanism for pain relief occurs when the opioid binds to the mu receptor in the CNS.

On July 9, 2012, the FDA approved a risk evaluation and mitigation strategy (REMS) for ER opioid medications-including *Nucynta ER*. Primary components of the REMS: Education for the prescribers, and requirement that the prescribers counsel the patients.

morphine allergy
→ choose:

fentanyl ..... meperidine
tapentadol   methadone
[tramadol] don't use in morphine allergy
(per package insert)

DRUG	DOSING	SAFETY/SIDE EFFECTS/MONITORING
Morphine (ER brands: *MS Contin, AVINza, Kadian, Oramorph SR, Roxanol*) C-II Injections: *Astramorph, Duramorph, Infumorph* + naltrexone (*Embeda*) **OPIOID AUX LABELS** Controlled substance: do not share with others. May cause dizziness or drowsiness. Do not operate machinery. Do not share: can be fatal to others. Keep away from children and animals. If ER: Do not crush or chew – swallow whole. Do not drink alcoholic beverages. Take with food or milk. The long-acting morphine formulations, including *Embeda*, are REMS drugs.	Common dosing IR: 10-30 mg Q4H PRN ER: 15, 30, 60, 100, 200 mg Q8-12H *Avinza* daily *Kadian* daily or BID Do not crush or chew any ER or CR opioids *Avinza*: No alcohol, can shorten extended release duration. Can sprinkle on applesauce, soft food. *Kadian*: can be opened and can sprinkle on applesauce, soft food. If renally impaired, start at a lower dose, or avoid morphine, oxycodone, tramadol or tapentadol which are all primarily renally cleared.	**BOXED WARNING** Fatal respiratory depression has occurred with administration with the highest risk at initiation and with dosage increases. Proper dosing and titration should be done by a healthcare professional who is knowledgeable in the use of potent opioids for chronic pain management. Instruct patient about proper administration to prevent rapid release and absorption of long-acting products. Crushing, dissolving, or chewing of the long acting products can cause the delivery of a potentially fatal dose. **SIDE EFFECTS** **GI effects** Constipation, nausea, vomiting (may need anti-emetics, such as prochlorperazine, ondansetron, etc.) **CNS effects** Somnolence, dizziness, changes in mood, confusion, delirium **Skin reactions** Flushing, pruritus, diaphoresis – may need antihistamine (more likely with IV dosing), impotence possible with chronic use **Respiratory depression** Caused by opioid overdose or combination with other sedatives and CNS depressants, and can be fatal (see opioid antagonist section that follows) **NOTES** **Constipation** Tolerance usually develops to opioid side effects except constipation. When opioids are ATC, constipation will likely require stimulant laxatives (senna, bisacodyl) or osmotic laxatives (e.g., MOM). Rarely, docusate alone may be enough, or docusate + stimulant laxative. Methylnaltrexone (*Relistor*) is a laxative for constipation due to opioids (it blocks gut opioid-receptors). The patient must have failed DSS + laxative (senna, bisacodyl). Administered SC every other day. Cost-effective alternative: oral naloxone solution. **Allergy Information** The following agents cross-react: morphine, oxymorphone, codeine, hydrocodone, hydromorphone, oxycodone, pentazocine – and less commonly used agents: nalbuphine, buprenorphine, butorphanol, levorphanol, naloxone, heroin (diacetyl-morphine). Tapentadol does not have an opioid-allergy contraindication in the US package labeling; tramadol does, however the two agents are structurally similar. Use caution if recommending in an opioid allergy; if allergy to tramadol an allergy to tapentadol is likely, and vice-versa. If morphine-group allergy, choose (if appropriate): fentanyl, meperidine, methadone, tramadol, tapentadol (meperidine and fentanyl cross react). Opioid Allergy Symptoms (rare, but dangerous if present): Difficulty breathing, severe drop in BP, serious rash, swelling of face, lips, tongue, larynx – use an agent in a different chemical class. Do not write MSO4 or MS for morphine or magnesium – due to risk of errors.

REMS

1st line stimulant senna ® (Ex-Lax®)

cross-react

morphine   pentazocine
codeine
hydro/oxycodone
hydro/oxymorphone
heroin (diacetyl morphine)
naloxone
tramadol
nalbuphine
buprenorphine
butor/levorphanol

CAUTION tapentadol

morphine
oxycodone
tramadol
tapentadol
} RENALLY CLEARED

Opioids Continued

DRUG	DOSING	SAFETY/SIDE EFFECTS/MONITORING
FentaNYL *(Duragesic)* C-II Fentanyl injection *Actiq SL lozenge* on a stick "lollipop": always start with 200 mcg, can titrate to 4 BTP episodes/day. Only for cancer BTP. *Abstral, Fentora SL* pills *Onsolis* SL film, *Subsys* SL spray *Lazanda* nasal spray -keep in child-resistant box. -empty unused drug into carbon lined pouch. Fentanyl transmucosal forms (all of them except patch and injection) are REMS drugs and pharmacies must be enrolled in REMS to dispense. These products are only for patients who need BTP control, who are on scheduled opioids, and who are the minimum age (16 or 18 years). Primarily for cancer BTP. **Similar Drugs, IV only** Alfentanil *(Alfenta)*, remifentanil *(Ultiva)*, sufentanil *(Sufenta)*	Patch: 12 (delivers 12.5 mcg/hr), 25, 50, 75, 100 mcg/h transdermal patch – change patch Q 3 days (occas. Δ Q48H – do not ↑ dose if pain is controlled but doesn't last long enough – in this case you shorten the interval, as you would do with any ER opioid. Otherwise, you risk overdose or higher degree of side effects.) Fentanyl, in any form, is for chronic pain management only: can transfer patient who has been using morphine 60 mg daily or equivalent for at least 7 days – not used PRN and not used as initial opioid agent PATCH Analgesic effect of patch can be seen 8-16 hrs after application – do not stop other analgesic at first (decrease dose 50% for the first 12 hrs). Do not apply > 1 patch each time and do not heat up patch or skin area before applying. Do not cover with heating pad or any bandage. Caution with fever (tell patient to call healthcare provider if they have a fever). Do not cover with heating pads.	**BOXED WARNINGS (2)** May cause potentially life-threatening hypoventilation, respiratory depression, and/or death; only for opioid-tolerant patients (not injection). Risk of respiratory depression increased in elderly patients, debilitated patients, and patients with conditions associated with hypoxia or hypercapnia; usually occurs after administration of initial dose in nontolerant patients or when given with other drugs that depress respiratory function. Use with strong or moderate CYP 3A4 inhibitors may result in increased effects and potentially fatal respiratory depression. **SIDE EFFECTS** Constipation, bradycardia, confusion, dizziness, somnolence, diaphoresis, dehydration, dry mouth, N/V, muscle rigidity, weakness, miosis, dyspnea ↳ pupil constriction **NOTES** Cannot use in opioid-naïve patients – especially the potent SL forms; these are for cancer-related BTP. The SL forms are REMS drugs (*Onsolis Focus* program, etc.) Cut off stick and flush unused/unneeded *Actiq*. Do not switch generic fentanyl patches – try to use the same one. Some patches need to be removed prior to MRI. Apply to hairless skin (cut short if necessary) on flat surface (chest, back, flank, upper arm) and change every 72 hrs. Press in place for 30 seconds. Do not use soap, alcohol, or other solvents to remove transdermal gel if it accidentally touches skin. Use large amount of water. Dispose patch in toilet or cut it up and put it in coffee grounds. Keep away from children and animals, including used patches. Alfentanil *(Alfenta)*, remifentanil *(Ultiva)*, sufentanil *(Sufenta)*: same chemical class, IV only.

Handwritten margin notes:

Sublimaze® inj

not absorbed po

3A4

not for opioid-naïve pts

cancer BTP

apply above waist

(cancer)
↓
⊝ place patch on skin that received radiation
⊝ shave before applying patch
⇒ irritation
⇒ cut hair w/ scissors instead

* most long-acting opioids (including fent. patch) require MedGuide

* if patch is covered, only use indicated coverings such as Tegaderm® that do not cause patch to overheat

* if applied skin moisturizer, wait 2 hrs before applying patch

Opioids Continued

DRUG	DOSING	SAFETY/SIDE EFFECTS/MONITORING
Hydrocodone C-II **+ acetaminophen** ***Lorcet, Lortab, Vicodin**, Zydone, Anexsia, Co-Gesic,* **Norco** (325 mg APAP – safer combo) + chlorpheniramine (Tussicaps) + chlorpheniramine and pseudoephedrine (Zutripro) + pseudoephedrine (Rezira) + homatropine (Tussagon) + ibuprofen *(Vicoprofen, Reprexain)*	2.5, 5, 7.5, 10 mg in combo with APAP	
Hydrocodone ER *(Zohydro)* C-II *Zohydro ER* is a REMS drug.	Start at 10 mg Q 12 (opioid-naïve) Range 10-50 mg	**BOXED WARNINGS (6)** Addiction potential, respiratory depression (do not crush/chew/dissolve), accidental exposure (especially children), neonatal opioid withdrawal syndrome, alcohol interaction (do not use concurrently), 3A4 drug interactions (inhibitors increase, can cause fatal respiratory depression, inducers decrease and if stopped suddenly will cause *Zohydro* to increase). **NOTES** Do not crush, chew or dissolve; swallow whole. Do not use alcohol. Substrate of 3A4 (major) & 2D6 (minor). Preferably avoid use if breast feeding. Use lower doses of *Zohydro* with 3A4 inhibitors.
Hydrocodone ER *(Hysingla ER)* C-II *Hysingla ER* is a REMS drug.	Start at 20 mg Q 24 (opioid naïve) Range 20-120 mg	**BOXED WARNINGS** New hydrocodone single entity formulation approved by FDA in November, 2014. This differs from *Zohydro ER* because it is once daily instead of twice daily dosing and it is approved as an abuse-deterrent formulation.
HYDROmorphone *(Dilaudid, Dilaudid-HP)* *Exalgo* (hydromorphone ER) C-II *Exalgo* is a REMS drug.	2, 4, 8 mg *Exalgo* contraindicated in opioid-naïve patients. 2 week washout required between *Exalgo* and MAO-Is. Potent, high risk for overdose May cause less nausea, pruritus	**BOXED WARNING** May cause potentially life-threatening respiratory depression even with therapeutic use, especially with initiation or dose increases; instruct patients on proper administration of extended-release tablets. The use of ethanol, other opioids, and other CNS depressants may increase the risk of adverse outcomes, including death. **NOTES** Opioid-naïve patients should start with no more than 2 to 4 mg orally or 1 to 2 mg by injection every four to six hours. *Exalgo* – crush and extraction resistant. *Dilaudid HP* is higher potency injection (10 mg/mL). Potent; start low, convert carefully. Caution with 3A4 Inhibitors, use lower doses initially.

Handwritten margin notes:
- 3A4 (next to Hydrocodone)
- BID (next to Hydrocodone ER Zohydro)
- 3A4 inducers ↓ [ ] – if stopped suddenly, ↑↑ [ ]
- QD abuse deterrent (next to Hysingla ER)
- 3A4 (next to HYDROmorphone)
- dosed q 4-6 hrs

Opioids Continued

DRUG	DOSING	SAFETY/SIDE EFFECTS/MONITORING
OxyCODONE **IR: OxyCODONE,** *Oxecta, Roxicodone* + naloxone *(Targiniq ER)* **CR:** *OxyCONTIN* **+ acetaminophen** *(Endocet, Percocet, Roxicet, Xartemis XR)* + ibuprofen + aspirin *(Percodan)* C-II – full opioids and oxycodone combos CR formulations are REMS drugs.	IR – 5-20 mg CR – 10-80 mg (60, 80 mg only for opioid-tolerant patients) Avoid high fat meals with higher doses Do not use or reduce with renal impairment. If ER cut dose by 1/2 - 1/3.	**BOXED WARNINGS (2)** Report abuse, misuse and diversion. Avoid use with 3A4 inhibitors – will increase oxycodone levels. **NOTES** *Oxecta, OxyContin* and *Targiniq ER* are abuse-deterrent formulations. Substrate of 3A4 (major) & 2D6 (minor). Preferably avoid use if breast feeding. Avoid high fat meals with higher doses (except reformulated *OxyContin*).
Oxymorphone *(Opana, Opana ER,* Opana Injectable)* C-II *Opana ER* is a REMS drug.	*Opana ER* 5-30 mg BID *Opana IR* 5-10 mg Q4-6H PRN Take on empty stomach (most other analgesics are with food to help avoid stomach upset) No alcohol with ER formulation	**BOXED WARNINGS (3)** *Opana ER* is an ER oral formulation of oxymorphone and is not suitable for use as an "as needed" analgesic. Tablets should not be broken, chewed, dissolved, or crushed; tablets should be swallowed whole. *Opana ER* is intended for use in long-term, continuous management of moderate-to-severe chronic pain. The coingestion of ethanol or ethanol-containing medications with *Opana ER* may result in accelerated release of drug from the dosage form, abruptly increasing plasma levels, which may have fatal consequences. Healthcare provider should be alert to problems of abuse, misuse, and diversion. **NOTES** Do not use with moderate-to-severe liver impairment. Use low doses in elderly, renal or mild liver impairment; there will be higher drug concentrations in these patients. *Opana* – crush and extraction resistant.
Methadone *(Dolophine)* *(Methadose* liquid) C-II Methadone is a REMS drug.	Start at 2.5-10 mg Q8-12H Methadone 40 mg is indicated for detox and maintenance treatment of opioid-addicted patients. Useful for detox because it relieves opioid craving and blocks euphoric effects of abusable opioids.	**BOXED WARNINGS (2)** QTc interval prolongation and serious arrhythmias (e.g., TdP) have occurred during treatment. Most cases involve patients being treated for pain with large, multiple daily doses. Fatal respiratory depression has occurred with the highest risk at initiation and with dosage increases. Should be prescribed by professionals who know requirements for safe use. **NOTES** Due to variable half-lives from 15-60 hrs and in some cases up to 100 hrs due to polymorphism. Methadone is hard to dose safely AND has a risk of QT prolongation (pro-arrhythmic) – which will be aggravated if dosed incorrectly. Can ↓ testosterone, contribute to sexual dysfunction (others can, this one noteable). In combo with other drugs, it is serotonergic and can raise risk of serotonin syndrome. Methadone also blocks reuptake of norepinephrine. Methadone is a major 3A4 substrate; avoid inhibitors concurrently or lower methadone dose.

Opioids Continued

DRUG	DOSING	SAFETY/SIDE EFFECTS/MONITORING
Meperidine *(Demerol)* C-II	50-150 mg Q3-4H PRN Short duration of action (pain control for max 3 hrs) Avoid as agent for chronic pain management and even short-term in elderly. Acceptable for short-term acute or single use (e.g., sutures in ER).	**WARNING** Renal impairment/elderly at risk for CNS toxicity **SIDE EFFECTS** Lightheadness, dizziness, somnolence, N/V, sweating **NOTES** Normeperidine (metabolite) is renally cleared and can accumulate and cause CNS toxicity, including seizures. In combo with other drugs, it is serotonergic and can raise risk of serotonin syndrome ISMP discourages use as analgesic – especially in elderly and renally impaired.
Codeine + acetaminophen *(Tylenol #2, 3, 4)* C-II: codeine C-III: combos (w/acetaminophen) C-V: used as antitussive (anti-cough) agent, codeine cough syrups	Usually 30 mg Q4-6H PRN, range 15-120 mg	**BOXED WARNING** Respiratory depression and death have occurred in children who received codeine following tonsillectomy and/or adenoidectomy and were found to have evidence of being ultra-rapid metabolizers of codeine due to a 2D6 polymorphism. Deaths have also occurred in nursing infants after being exposed to high concentrations of morphine because the mothers were ultra-rapid metabolizers. Use is contraindicated in the postoperative pain management of children who have undergone tonsillectomy and/or adenoidectomy. **SIDE EFFECTS** Codeine has a high degree of GI side effects: constipation, N/V/D.

Handwritten margin note: 2D6

Combination Opioid Agonists/Norepinephrine Reuptake Inhibitors – and Tramadol Also Inhibits 5HT Reuptake

DRUG	DOSING	SAFETY/SIDE EFFECTS/MONITORING
TraMADol *(Ultram, Ultram ER, Conzip IR/ER)* C-IV + acetaminophen *(Ultracet)*	50 mg, or with APAP 37.5-325 mg 50-100 mg Q4-6H, max 400 mg/d (300 mg/day for ER forms) Reduce if renal impairment, tramadol ER contraindicated if CrCl < 30 mL/min	**WARNING** ↑ seizure risk – avoid in patients with seizure history, head trauma **SIDE EFFECTS** Dizziness, nausea, constipation, loss of appetite, flushing, dry mouth, dyspepsia, pruritus, insomnia (some patients find tramadol sedating but for most it is not sedating; this can be an advantage over hydrocodone), possible headache, ataxia. Lower severity of GI side effects versus strong opioids. **NOTES** Respiratory depression (rare), like opioids, can cause physiological dependence. Serotonin syndrome risk if used in combination with others, such as SSRIs, etc. and is dose-dependent. ✱✱ Avoid tramadol with 2D6 Inhibitors (requires conversion) ✱✱

Handwritten margin notes: ADC; may ↑ INR w/ warfarin (monitor)

Combination Opioid Agonists/Norepinephrine Reuptake Inhibitors Continued

DRUG	DOSING	SAFETY/SIDE EFFECTS/MONITORING
Tapentadol *(Nucynta, Nucynta ER)* C-II *Nucynta ER* is a REMS drug.	IR: 50-100 mg Q4-6H PRN ER: 50-250 mg BID Use not recommended with CrCl < 30 mL/min (not studied). Use with severe renal insufficiency is CI in Canada.	**BOXED WARNINGS (2)** Respiratory depression, possibly fatal, may occur. Proper dosing, titration, and monitoring are essential. Extended release tablets must be swallowed whole and should NOT be split, crushed, broken, chewed, or dissolved in order to avoid rapid release and potential for fatal dose. No alcohol with ER formulation. **SIDE EFFECTS** Dizziness, somnolence, nausea but lower severity of GI side effects than stronger opioids **NOTES** Like opioids, can cause physiological dependence, risk 5HT additive toxicity. No alcohol with ER formulation; alcohol may increase tapentadol systemic exposure which may lead to possible fatal overdose. Use not recommended with CrCl < 30 mL/min (not studied). At this level is CI in Canada.

Opioid Drug Interactions

- Caution with use of concurrent CNS depressants: Additive somnolence, dizziness, confusion, increased risk of respiratory depression. These include alcohol, hypnotics, benzodiazepines, muscle relaxants, etc.

- Increased risk of hypoxemia with underlying respiratory disease (e.g., COPD) and sleep apnea.

- With methadone, caution with agents that worsen cardiac function or increase arrhythmia risk. Caution with other serotonergic agents.

- With meperidine, caution with agents that worsen renal function, elderly and those with seizure history. Caution with other serotonergic agents.

- With tramadol and tapentadol: caution with other agents that lower seizure threshold. Caution with other serotonergic agents. Avoid tramadol with 2D6 inhibitors (requires conversion). Possibility of increased INR with warfarin; monitor. Tapentadol may enhance the adverse/toxic effect of MAOIs; avoid concurrent use.

- *(handwritten: due to ↑ absorption → fatal [ ])* ✱ All opioids: No alcohol, special warning to avoid alcohol with *Opana ER, Nucynta ER* and *Avinza*.

Opioid Counseling

- Do not crush, chew, break, or open controlled-release forms. Breaking them would cause too much drug to be released into your blood at one time.

- *Avinza* and *Kadian* must be swallowed whole or may be opened and the entire bead contents sprinkled on a small amount of applesauce immediately prior to ingestion. The beads must NOT be chewed, crushed, or dissolved due to the risk of exposure to a potentially toxic dose of morphine. *Avinza* can be put down a G-tube.

- *Opana*: take on empty stomach (1 hr before, 2 hr after eating).

- ✱ All opioids, special warning for *Avinza, Kadian* and *Opana ER, Nucynta ER*: No alcohol.

- To ensure that you get a correct dose, measure liquid forms with a special dose-measuring spoon or cup, not with a regular tablespoon. If you do not have a dose-measuring device, ask your pharmacist.

- This medicine will cause drowsiness and fatigue. Avoid alcohol, sleeping pills, antihistamines, sedatives, and tranquilizers that may also make you drowsy, except under the supervision of your healthcare provider.

- Take with a full glass of water. Take with food or milk if it upsets your stomach.

- Do not stop taking suddenly if you have been taking it continuously for more than 5 to 7 days. If you want to stop, your healthcare provider will help you gradually reduce the dose.

- This medicine is constipating. Increase the amount of fiber and water (at least six to eight full glasses daily) in your diet to prevent constipation (if not fluid restricted due to heart failure). Your pharmacist or healthcare provider will recommend a stronger agent for constipation if this is not adequate. (If asked, recommend stool softener if hard stool, stimulants for most scheduled opioid patients.)

- Do not share this medication with anyone else.

- Never take more pain medicine than prescribed. If your pain is not being adequately treated, talk to your healthcare provider.

Opioid Dose Conversions

The correct dose is the lowest dose that provides effective pain relief. If the dose has been increased and the pain relief is not adequate or if the side effects are intolerable (patients react differently to different opioids) or if the drug is unaffordable or not included on formulary, then switch. Switch safely and always be on the watch for hyperalgesia, which should be suspected when opioids increase pain (rather than decreasing pain) due to a paradoxical situation. This happens occasionally, and if so, increasing the dose will not work. If switching to morphine and the patient has renal insufficiency, a 50% reduction in the total daily dose or similar would be wise; morphine has an active metabolite that is renally cleared, thus a lower dose is required. Always use breakthrough medication, as-needed, when converting.

For opioid conversions (not methadone) you can use ratio conversion. Make sure the units and route in the numerator match, and the units and route in the denominator match. You can technically convert with fentanyl (note no oral dose conversion as fentanyl is not absorbed orally) but it is sometimes done differently using a dosing table. Some clinicians use this estimation: morphine 60 mg total daily dose = 25 mcg/hr fentanyl patch. If converting fentanyl using the chart, remember that you are finding the total daily dose in mg, and will then need to convert it to mcg (multiply by 1,000) and then divide by 24 to get the patch dose; fentanyl is dosed in mcg per hour.

When converting one opioid to another, round down (do not round up) and use breakthrough doses for compensation. A patient may respond better to one agent than another (likely due to less tolerance) and estimating lower will reduce the risk of overdose.

* hydrocode and morphine *
* *
* ⇒ ≈ equivalent dosing *

* to start a pt on fentanyl upon d/c, they must've been using *
* morphine 60 mg/day or more (morphine equiv) x 7+ days *

DRUG	IV/IM (MG)	ORAL (MG)
Morphine	10	30
Hydromorphone	1.5	7.5
Oxycodone	–	20
Hydrocodone	–	30
Codeine	130	200
Fentanyl	0.1	–
Meperidine	75	300
Oxymorphone	1	10

! <u>If the medicine is effective, but runs out too fast, do not increase the dose.</u> This will cause a risk of respiratory depression. Rather, shorten the dosing interval.

To convert

- Calculate total 24 hr dose requirement of the current drug.

- Use ratio-conversion to calculate the dose of the new drug: make sure the numerators and denominators match in both drug and route of administration.

- Calculate 24 hr dose of new drug and <u>reduce dose at least 25%.</u> (If the problem on the exam does not specify to reduce it, but just to find the equivalent dose, then do not reduce it.)

- Divide to attain appropriate interval and dose for new drug.

- Always have breakthrough pain (BTP) medication available while making changes. Guideline recommendation for BTP dosing ranges from 5-17% of the total daily baseline opioid dose.

↓ dose b/c pt may have developed tolerance to previous opioid (→ pain not controlled anymore) → start new agent @ ↓ dose

Example of Opioid Conversion:

A hospice patient has been receiving 12 mg/day of IV hydromorphone. The pharmacist will convert the hydromorphone to morphine ER, to be given Q12H. The hospice policy for opioid conversion is to reduce the new dose by 50%, and to use 5-17% of the total daily dose for breakthrough pain.

The conversion factors (the left fraction) are taken from the above table. The right fraction has the patient's current total daily IV dose of hydromorphone in the denominator, and the total daily dose of morphine in the numerator:

$$\frac{30 \text{ mg oral morphine}}{1.5 \text{ mg IV hydromorphone}} = \frac{X \text{ mg oral morphine}}{12 \text{ mg IV hydromorphone}}$$

Multiply the top left numerator (30) by the bottom right denominator, and then divide by the left denominator. This will give a total daily dose of morphine (PO) of 240 mg. Reduce by 50%, as instructed. The correct dose of morphine ER would be 60 mg BID.

Morphine IR can be given for BTP as 10 mg Q4H PRN. Other agents commonly used for BTP include combo agents, such as hydrocodone/acetaminophen. In an inpatient setting, injections can be given – injections will have a faster onset and since BTP is typically severe, they may be preferable. However, if the patient does not have a port, the injection itself will cause discomfort. In real life, morphine IR may not be available. Hydrocodone/acetaminophen is often used for breakthrough pain. The hydrocodone dose is roughly the same as the morphine dose. If the patient is using acetaminophen alone for more mild pain, and the combination if moderate, the total daily acetaminophen intake will need to be counted. Keep in mind that any drug that requires oral absorption will take time; if the patient has cancer pain (in which case the breakthrough pain is likely to be quite severe) a sublingual form of fentanyl may be used, which has faster onset.

Example of Conversion to Fentanyl Patch using a Fentanyl Patch Conversion Table

MJ is a 52 year old male patient who has been using *OxyContin* 40 mg BID and *Endocet* 5-325 mg as-needed for breakthrough pain. He uses the breakthrough pain medication 2-3 times weekly. Using the *OxyContin* dose only select the fentanyl patch strength that should be chosen for this patient, using the following table.

OPIOID CONVERSION TO FENTANYL PATCH USING CHART IN THE DURAGESIC PACKAGE INSERT

Table 1[1]: DOSE CONVERSION TO DURAGESIC				
Current Analgesic	Daily Dosage (mg/day)			
Oral morphine	60–134	135–224	225–314	315–404
Intramuscular or Intravenous morphine	10–22	23–37	38–52	53–67
Oral oxycodone	30–67	67.5–112	112.5–157	157.5–202
Oral codeine	150–447			
Oral hydromorphone	8–17	17.1–28	28.1–39	39.1–51
Intravenous hydromorphone	1.5–3.4	3.5–5.6	5.7–7.9	8–10
Intramuscular meperidine	75–165	166–278	279–390	391–503
Oral methadone	20–44	45–74	75–104	105–134
	⇓	⇓	⇓	⇓
Recommended DURAGESIC Dose	25 mcg/hour	50 mcg/hour	75 mcg/hour	100 mcg/hour

Alternatively, for adult and pediatric patients taking opioids or doses not listed in Table 1, use the conversion methodology outlined above with Table 2.

[1] Table 1 should not be used to convert from DURAGESIC to other therapies because this conversion to DURAGESIC is conservative. Use of Table 1 for conversion to other analgesic therapies can overestimate the dose of the new agent. Overdosage of the new analgesic agent is possible *[see Dosage and Administration (2.3)]*.

SOLUTION

Oxycodone 80 mg daily is in the range of 67.5-112 mg daily which correlates to the 50 mcg/h patch.

Methadone Conversion: Not straight-forward; should be done by pain specialists

Methadone conversion from morphine ranges from 1-20:1; this is highly variable due to patient tolerance and duration of therapy. The half-life of methadone varies widely. There are separate conversion charts for pain specialists to estimate methadone dosing. This should be done only by specialists with experience in using methadone. In addition to the variable half-life, methadone is arrhythmogenic and has other safety issues. Methadone is used both for the treatment of opioid addiction and for chronic pain. When used for chronic pain syndromes, it is administered 2 to 3 times per day after the proper dose is determined by titration. It should be started at very low doses of no more than 2.5 mg PO BID or TID, and escalated slowly.

AGONIST   ANTAGONIST

Buprenorphine and Naloxone Formulations: For Pain, Addiction or Overdose.

Buprenorphine is an opioid agonist and naloxone is an opioid antagonist. Higher doses of buprenorphine are used to treat addiction, lower doses used to treat pain. Given by itself, naloxone is used for opioid overdose. As an opioid antagonist, it replaces the opioid on the mu receptor.

DRUG	DOSING	SAFETY/SIDE EFFECTS/MONITORING
Naloxone (*Evzio* auto-injector) Nalmefene Naltrexone is an opioid blocker normally used to help treat alcoholism; the IV form (*Vivitrol*) is used for alcohol and opioid dependence	Naloxone-Initially, 0.4 mg-2 mg Q 2-3 min or IV infusion at 100 mL/hr (0.4 mg/hr) Repeat dosing may be required (opioid may last longer than blocking agent); monitor the patient after administration Will cause an acute withdrawal syndrome (pain, anxiety, tachypnea) in patients physically dependent on opioids The *Evzio* auto-injector has voice directions-can be given by patients or friends for overdose emergency; give in thigh through clothing, hold for 5 seconds, if any doubt, inject, then call 911	**ACUTE OVERDOSE SIGNS AND SYMPTOMS** Somnolence, respiratory depression with shallow breathing, cold and clammy skin and constricted (pinpoint, miosis) pupils. Can lead to coma and death. **NOTES** Highest risk of respiratory depression in opioid-naïve patients (new users), if dose is ↑ too rapidly, and in illicit substance abuse (e.g., heroin). Due to low bioavailability, can be given orally to prevent opioid-induced constipation (off-label).
Buprenorphine **+ naloxone** (to block opioid if used) (*Bunavail* – buccal tablets, ***Suboxone*** – sublingual tablets) **Buprenorphine transdermal** (*Butrans*) – only for mod-severe pain in patients who need ATC opioid Buprenorphine (*Buprenex* Inj) C-III Buprenorphine formulations are REMS drugs	*Suboxone:* Used as alternative for methadone (so patients can get from a regular healthcare provider and filled at any pharmacy and can get over opioids since withdrawal Sx are reduced). Used daily for addiction. To prescribe *Suboxone:* Prescribers need Drug Addiction Treatment Act (DATA 2000) waiver. If they have it, the DEA number will start with X. **PATCH APPLICATION** Apply to upper outer arm, upper chest, side of chest, upper back. Change weekly. Do not use same site for at least 3 weeks. Disposal: Fold sticky sides together, flush or put in disposal unit that comes with drug.	***BUTRANS* BOXED WARNING (PATCH)** Do not exceed a one 20 mcg/hr patch due to risk of QT prolongation. **SIDE EFFECTS** Sedation, dizziness, headache, confusion, mental and physical impairment, diaphoresis QT prolongation, respiratory depression: dose-dependent Side effects from patch: nausea, headache, application site pruritis/rash, dizziness, constipation, somnolence, vomiting, application site erythema, dry mouth. **NOTES** Do not expose to patch to heat. Buprenorphine reduces patients' opioid cravings and withdrawal symptoms. In addition, buprenorphine may discourage use of nonprescribed opioids by binding to the mu receptor, thereby blocking other opioids' effects.

Handwritten notes:
- do not reverse completely → pt may experience acute pain
- short t½ → repeated dosing or drip
- Subutex® for pain & addiction
- WEEKLY PATCH

Buprenorphine Drug Interactions

- Caution with use of concurrent CNS depressants: Additive sedation (somnolence), dizziness, confusion. These include alcohol, hypnotics, benzodiazepines, skeletal muscle relaxants, etc.

- Prolongs the QT interval – do not use with other QT-prolonging agents or in patients at risk of arrhythmia.

MUSCLE RELAXANTS

Muscle relaxant mechanism: various; some work as sedatives (carisoprodol, chlorzoxazone, metaxalone, methocarbamol) and others via effects on spinal reflexes.

DRUG	DOSING	SAFETY/SIDE EFFECTS/MONITORING
Antispasmodics with analgesic effects		
Baclofen (Lioresal) **AUX LABELS** May cause drowsiness. Do not operate machinery….	5-20 mg TID-QID, PRN	**BOXED WARNING** Avoid abrupt withdrawal of the drug; abrupt withdrawal of intrathecal baclofen has resulted in severe sequelae (hyperpyrexia, obtundation, rebound/exaggerated spasticity, muscle rigidity, and rhabdomyolysis), leading to organ failure and some fatalities. **SIDE EFFECTS** For all muscle relaxants Excessive sedation, dizziness, confusion **NOTES** Do not overdose in elderly (e.g., start low, titrate carefully), watch for additive side effects.
Cyclobenzaprine (Fexmid, Amrix ER) *Flexeril®*	5-10 mg TID, PRN ER: 15-30 mg once daily	Dry mouth. May have efficacy with fibromyalgia Serotonergic; should not be combined with other serotonergic agents. May precipitate or exacerbate cardiac arrhythmias; caution in elderly or those with heart disease (similar to tricyclics)
TiZANidine (Zanaflex) *α-2 agonist*	2-4 mg Q6-8H, PRN (max 36 mg/d)	Central alpha-1 agonist: hypotension, dizziness, xerostomia, weakness, QT prolongation

 # cipro, fluvoxamine   *& like clonidine*

Drugs that exert their effects by sedation   *+ chlorzoxazone (Parafon®, Forte DSC)*

DRUG	DOSING	SAFETY/SIDE EFFECTS/MONITORING
Carisoprodol (Soma) C-IV (due to dependence, withdrawal symptoms, and diversion and abuse)	250-350 mg QID, PRN	Somnolence Poor 2C19 metabolizers will have higher carisoprodol concentrations (up to 4-fold)
Metaxalone (Skelaxin)	800 mg TID-QID, PRN	Decreased cognitive/sedative effects; hepatotoxic; monitor
Methocarbamol (Robaxin, Robaxin-750)	1,500-2,000 mg QID, PRN	Hypotension; monitor BP

Rarely used muscle relaxants include dantrolene (*Dantrium* – sometimes used for malignant hyperthermia), chlorzoxazone (*Parafon Forte DSC*), orphenadrine (*Norflex*)

Muscle Relaxant Drug Interactions

- Caution with use of concurrent agents that are CNS depressants: Additive somnolence, dizziness, confusion. These include alcohol, hypnotics, benzodiazepines, opioids, etc.

- Carisoprodol: Poor 2C19 metabolizers will have higher carisoprodol concentrations (up to 4-fold).

- Tizanidine: contraindicated with ciprofloxacin and fluvoxamine due to elevated tizanidine levels.

Muscle Relaxant Counseling

- This medicine will cause somnolence and fatigue and can impair your ability to perform mental and physical activities. Do not drive when using this medicine.

- Avoid alcohol, sleeping pills, antihistamines, sedatives, pain pills and tranquilizers that may also make you drowsy, except under the supervision of your healthcare provider.

Common Neuropathic Pain Agents

For a fuller discussion, see Epilepsy and Depression chapters.

DRUG	DOSING	SAFETY/SIDE EFFECTS/MONITORING
Pregabalin (Lyrica) Diabetic neuropathic pain, postherpetic neuralgia, fibromyalgia, spinal cord damage, adjunctive therapy for adult patients with partial onset seizures C-V Capsule, solution	Initial: 75 mg BID Maximum: 600 mg/day ↓ dose and ↑ interval if CrCl < 60 mL/min	**SIDE EFFECTS** Dizziness, somnolence, peripheral edema, weight gain, ataxia, diplopia, blurred vision, dry mouth, mild euphoria
DULoxetine (Cymbalta) Peripheral neuropathic pain Fibromyalgia Chronic musculoskeletal pain Depression Generalized Anxiety Disorder (GAD)	30-60 mg/day	**SIDE EFFECTS** **Common to all SNRIs** ↑ BP, HR, sexual side effects (20-50%) include ↓ libido, ejaculation difficulties, anorgasmia, increased sweating (hyperhydrosis), restless leg (see if began when therapy was started) Possibility of mood changes – requires MedGuide and monitoring **Duloxetine-Specific Side Effects** Nausea, dry mouth; somnolence, fatigue, ↓ appetite
Gabapentin (Neurontin) *Gralise* – indicated for postherpetic neuralgia *Horizant* – indicated for postherpetic neuralgia and restless leg syndrome Capsule, tablet, solution	Initial: 300 mg TID Maximum: 3,600 mg/day ↓ dose and ↑ interval if CrCl < 60 mL/min	**SIDE EFFECTS** Dizziness, somnolence, ataxia, peripheral edema, weight gain, diplopia, blurred vision, xerostomia **NOTES** Used more often for off-labeled uses such as fibromyalgia, pain, headache, peripheral neuropathy, drug abuse, alcohol withdrawal. Take ER formulation with food.
Amitriptyline (Elavil)	10-50 mg QHS, sometimes higher	**SIDE EFFECTS** Are uncommon with low doses used for pain, but could include: **Cardiotoxicity** (QT-prolongation) with overdose – can be used for suicide- counsel carefully Orthostatic hypotension, tachycardia, anticholinergic – dry mouth, blurred vision, urinary retention, constipation, delirium in elderly

Fibromyalgia Agents

DRUG	DOSING/INDICATIONS	SAFETY/SIDE EFFECTS/MONITORING
Milnacipran *(Savella)* Serotonin-Norepinephrine Reuptake Inhibitor (SNRI)	Day 1: 12.5 mg daily Days 2-3: 12.5 mg BID Days 4-7: 25 mg BID Then 50 mg BID (CrCl < 30 mL/min, max dose is 25 mg BID)	**BOXED WARNINGS** Milnacipran is a SNRI similar to SNRIs used to treat depression and other psychiatric disorders. Antidepressants increase the risk of suicidal thinking and behavior in children, adolescents, and young adults (18-24 years of age) with major depressive disorder (MDD) and other psychiatric disorders (not approved for depression). **CONTRAINDICATIONS** Concomitant use or within 2 weeks of MAOIs; uncontrolled narrow-angle glaucoma **SIDE EFFECTS** Nausea, headache, constipation, dizziness, insomnia, hot flashes **DRUG INTERACTIONS** Digoxin: Milnacipran may enhance the adverse/toxic effect of digoxin. The risk of postural hypotension and tachycardia may be increased, particularly with IV digoxin. Do not use IV digoxin in patients receiving milnacipran. Do not use with IV methylene blue or linezolid. Increased bleeding risk with anticoagulants or antiplatelets.
Pregabalin *(Lyrica)*	See above neuropathic pain section	
DULoxetine *(Cymbalta)*	See above neuropathic pain section	

Topical Pain Agents, For Localized Pain

DRUG	DOSING/NOTES	SAFETY/SIDE EFFECTS/MONITORING
Lidocaine 5% patches *(Lidoderm)* Lidocaine viscous gel (Rx) *LidoPatch*, OTC, 3.99%	Apply to affected area 1-3 patches/day for up to 12 hrs/day (5% patch) Approved for postherpetic neuralgia (shingles)	**SIDE EFFECTS** Minor topical burning, pruritus, rash **NOTES** Can cut into smaller pieces (before removing backing). Do not apply more than 3 patches at one time. Caution with used patches; can harm children and pets; fold patch in half and discard safely. Do not cover with heating pads/electric blankets.
Capsaicin 0.025% and 0.075% *(Zostrix, Zostrix HP)* *Qutenza 8%* – Rx capsaicin patch	Apply to affected area TID-QID ↓ TRPV1-expressing nociceptive nerve endings (↓ substance P)	**SIDE EFFECTS** Topical burning, which dissipates with continued use **NOTES** *Qutenza* is given in the healthcare provider's office only – it causes topical burning and requires pre-treatment with lidocaine – applied for 1 hour and lasts for months – works in ~ 40% of patients to reduce pain, indicated for post-herpetic neuralgia (PHN) pain.

12 hrs on 12 hrs off

Topical Pain Agents Continued

DRUG	DOSING/NOTES	SAFETY/SIDE EFFECTS/MONITORING
Diclofenac topical *Voltaren* gel *Flector* patch	Apply to affected area TID-QID NSAIDs, for OA	**NOTES** *Flector* patch: apply to most painful area, twice daily. Remove if bathing/showering. Remove for MRI.
Methyl salicylate topical OTCs (*BenGay, Icy Hot, Precise, SalonPas, Thera-Gesic*, store brands) Methyl salicylate plus other ingredients	Patches, creams	**NOTES** OTC counseling: contact healthcare provider if rash, pruritus, or excessive skin irritation occurs, or symptoms persist for > 7 days. Do not apply over wounds or damaged skin. Occasionally the topicals have caused first to third-degree burns, mostly in patients with neuropathic damage: Discontinue use and seek medical attention if signs of skin injury (pain, swelling, or blistering) occur following application.

Lidoderm Patient Counseling

- Patches may be cut into smaller sizes with scissors before removal of the release (plastic) liner.
- Safely discard unused portions of cut patches where children and pets cannot get to them.
- Apply up to three (3) patches at one time to cover the most painful area. Apply patches only once for up to 12 hr in a 24-hr period (12 hr on and 12 hr off).
- Remove patch if skin irritation occurs.
- Fold used patches so that the adhesive side sticks to itself and safely discard used patches or pieces of cut patches where children and pets cannot get to them. Even a used patch contains enough medicine to harm a child or pet.
- Do not use on broken, abraded, severely burned or skin with open lesions (can significantly increase amount absorbed).

Capsaicin Patient Counseling

- Apply a thin film of cream to the affected area and gently rub in until fully absorbed.
- Apply 3 to 4 times daily.
- Best results typically occur after 2 to 4 weeks of continuous use. Do not use as-needed, since frequent, long-term use is required for benefit.
- Unless treating hand pain, wash hands thoroughly with soap and water immediately after use.
- If treating hands, leave on for 30 minutes, then wash hands as above.
- Do not touch genitals, nasal area, mouth or eyes with the medicine; it will burn the sensitive skin.
- The burning pain should dissipate with continual use; starting at the lower strength will help.
- Never cover with bandages or a heating pad; serious burning could result.

PRACTICE CASE

PATIENT PROFILE

Patient Name	Gene Schneider
Address	11188 Countryclub Drive

Age 50	**Sex** Male	**Race** White	**Height** 5'6"	**Weight** 239lbs

Allergies SULFA

DIAGNOSES

Hypertension

Osteoarthritis

MEDICATIONS

Date	No.	Prescriber	Drug & Strength	Quantity	Sig	Refills
12/13	57643	Suhlbach	Atenolol 100 mg	30	1 PO daily	11
12/13	57647	Suhlbach	Amlodipine 5 mg	30	1 PO daily	11
12/13	57648	Suhlbach	HCTZ 25 mg	30	1 PO daily	11
OTC			Acetaminophen 500 mg		1-2 PO prn, 4-5x daily	
OTC			Capsaicin cream 0.025%		Apply QID	

LAB/DIAGNOSTIC TESTS

Test	Normal Value	Results Date 12/11/2013	Date	Date
GLU	65-99 mg/dL	118		
Na	135-146 mEq/L	130		
K	3.5-5.3 mEq/L	3.7		
Cl	98-110 mEq/L	104		
C02	21-33 mmHg	28		
BUN	7-25 mg/dL	26		
Creatinine	0.6-1.2 mg/dL	1.5		

ADDITIONAL INFORMATION

Date	Notes
12/15/2013	BP today 152/92, Pt reports pain at 5-7 throughout day, describes knee as "grating." Capsaicin and APAP used regularly; asking for stronger pain medicine.

Questions

1. Gene's wife asks if OTC ibuprofen would be useful when the pain is not relieved with acetaminophen. The pharmacist counsels Gene and his wife that this may be unsafe due to the following reasons. (Select **ALL** that apply).

    a. It could cause acute kidney problems.
    b. It could cause his blood pressure to increase.
    c. It could cause an interaction with the acetaminophen.
    d. Ibuprofen is contraindicated with a sulfa allergy.
    e. Ibuprofen is not safe to use with concurrent capsaicin.

2. Gene's physician prescribes *Ultracet*. This drug contains the following ingredients:

    a. Tramadol-acetaminophen
    b. Tramadol-ibuprofen
    c. Hydrocodone-acetaminophen
    d. Hydrocodone-ibuprofen
    e. Codeine-acetaminophen

3. Gene's wife uses *Percocet*, and she suggests that this might help Gene. Which of the following statements is correct?

    a. This drug contains an NSAID.
    b. It is no more effective for pain than aspirin and can be dangerous.
    c. There are no significant side effects.
    d. It is more effective for pain than acetaminophen alone.
    e. It may raise blood pressure.

4. Gene fills a prescription for *Ultracet*, and finds that the pain relief is satisfactory for about one year. After this time, the physician tries *MS Contin*, and eventually switches Gene over to the *Duragesic* patch. Choose the correct statement:

    a. *Duragesic* is the brand name for hydromorphone.
    b. This is a poor choice due to his degree of renal insufficiency.
    c. This medication can only be used in patients who have dysphagia.
    d. The starting application frequency is one patch Q 48 hours.
    e. The starting application frequency is one patch Q 72 hours.

Questions 5-11 are NOT based on the above case.

5. Tramadol is not a safe choice in a patients with this condition in their profiles:

    a. Muscle spasticity
    b. Aspirin allergy
    c. Seizures
    d. Peptic ulcer disease
    e. Gout

6. A physician has called the pharmacist. He has a patient on morphine sulfate extended-release who is having difficulty with regular bowel movements. The patient is using docusate sodium 100 mg BID. The patient reports that his stools are difficult to expel, although they are not particularly hard or condensed. Which of the following recommendation is most appropriate to prevent the constipation?

    a. Senna
    b. Bismuth subsalicylate
    c. *Relistor*
    d. Mineral oil
    e. Phosphate soda

7. A patient with cancer is using the fentanyl patch along with the *Actiq* transmucosal formulation for breakthrough pain. Which statement is correct?

   a. *Actiq* contains hydromorphone for sublingual absorption.

   b. No more than 4 BTP episodes per day should be treated with *Actiq*; if more are required, the patient should consult with his/her physician.

   c. A patient who is not taking an extended-release version of an opioid may still use *Actiq* for occasional, breakthrough cancer pain.

   d. *Actiq* contains oxymorphone for sublingual absorption.

   e. This drug is contraindicated in patients older than 65 years of age.

8. Which of the following brand-generic combinations is correct? *meloxicam*

   a. Celecoxib *(Mobic)* Celebrex ℮

   b. Naproxen *(Motrin)* Aleve

   c. Morphine *(Opana)*

   d. Hydromorphone *(Dilaudid)*

   e. Methadone *(Demerol)* Dolophine ℮

9. Choose the correct statement regarding the pain medication *Celebrex*:

   a. This may be a safer option for patients with GI bleeding risk.

   b. This may be a safer option for patients with reduced renal function.

   c. This is a non-selective NSAID, and has a better safety profile.

   d. This drug is safe to use in patients with any type of sulfonamide allergy.

   e. The maximum dose for inflammatory conditions, such as RA, is 200 mg daily.

	IV/IM	PO
hydro	–	30
morphine	10	30

$$\frac{30 \text{ mg po hydro}}{30 \text{ mg po Avinza}} = \frac{80 \text{ mg po hydro}}{x \text{ mg po Avinza}} \Rightarrow x = 80 \text{ mg}$$

$$0.75 \times 80 \text{ mg} = 60 \text{ mg Avinza}$$

10. A pain patient with poor control has been taking hydrocodone-acetaminophen 10 mg-500 mg 8 tablets daily. The physician will convert the patient to *Avinza* to provide adequate pain relief and to reduce the risk of acetaminophen toxicity. Using the hydrocodone component only, calculate the total daily dose of *Avinza* that is equivalent to the hydrocodone dose, and then reduce the dose by 25% (to lessen the possibility of excessive side effects from the initial conversion). The final daily dose of *Avinza* is:

    a. 10 mg *Avinza*

    b. 40 mg *Avinza*

    c. 60 mg *Avinza*

    d. 80 mg *Avinza*

    e. 110 mg *Avinza*

11. Which is the correct antidote for acetaminophen toxicity?

    a. Flumazenil

    b. N- Acetylcysteine

    c. Pyridoxine

    d. Physostigmine

    e. Atropine

Answers

1-a,b, 2-a, 3-d, 4-e, 5-c, 6-a, 7-b, 8-d, 9-a, 10-c, 11-b

MIGRAINE

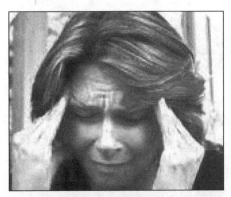

GUIDELINES

Evidence-Based Guidelines for Migraine Headache in the Primary Care Setting: Pharmacologic Management for Prevention of Migraine, American Academy of Neurology. http://tools.aan.com/professionals/practice/pdfs/gl0087.pdf (accessed 2015 Nov 26).

ICSI Health Care Guideline: Diagnosis and Treatment of Headache, 2013. https://www.icsi.org/_asset/qwrznq/Headache.pdf (accessed 2014 Nov 25).

BACKGROUND

Headache treatment is a common concern in the community pharmacy, one of the most common patient complaints in neurologists' offices and the most common pain complaint seen in family practice. Most headaches are migraine and tension-type headaches.

Migraines are chronic headaches that can cause significant pain for hours or days. In addition to severe pain, most migraines cause nausea, vomiting, and sensitivity to light and sound. Some migraines are preceded or accompanied by sensory warning symptoms or signs (auras), such as flashes of light, blind spots or tingling in the arms or legs. Most migraines do not have an aura.

Rarely, a migraine could be occurring with a serious cardiovascular, cerebrovascular or infectious event. Patients should be seen at once if the headache is accompanied with fever, stiff neck, rash, mental confusion, seizures, double vision, weakness, numbness, chest pain, trouble breathing or trouble speaking.

Children get migraines and may ask the pharmacist for advice. OTC agents, usually ibuprofen, are used first. Triptans are used in children.

MIGRAINE CAUSES

Migraines may be caused by changes in the trigeminal nerve and imbalances in neurotransmitters, including serotonin, which decreases during a migraine causing a chemical release of neuropeptides that trigger vasodilation in cranial blood vessels. Triptan drugs are serotonin-receptor agonists and cause vasoconstriction of cranial blood vessels.

The cause of migraines is not well-understood but "trigger" identification can be useful to help the patient avoid triggers and reduce migraine incidence. A common type of migraine is a menstrual-associated migraine in women. These may be treated with oral contraceptives or the estradiol patch or creams to decrease migraine frequency. Women who have migraine with aura are at higher risk for stroke and should not use estrogen-containing contraceptives.

NATURAL PRODUCTS
Feverfew, willow bark (a salicylate), butterbur, magnesium, and riboflavin may be helpful, alone or in combination.

NON-DRUG TREATMENT
Non-pharmacologic interventions involve avoiding triggers, mental relaxation, stress management, or applying cold compresses to the head.

DRUG TREATMENT
Migraine treatment is divided into acute drugs (for a headache that is present) and prophylactic drugs (to reduce headache frequency).

Drug options are many, including OTC options: acetaminophen, *Advil Migraine*, (which is plain ibuprofen), *Excedrin migraine* (aspirin, acetamin-

COMMON MIGRAINE TRIGGERS

Hormonal Changes in Women
Fluctuations in estrogen trigger headaches in many women. Some women will use monophasic birth control pill formulations to keep estrogen levels more constant and help reduce pre-menstrual migraines, the most common type of female migraine. ACOG recommends progestin-only bcp's for women with migraine with aura, due to stroke risk with estrogen-containing contraceptives.

→ *Nora-Be®, Nor-QD®, Camila®*

Foods
Common offending agents include alcohol, especially beer and red wine, aged cheeses, chocolate, aspartame, overuse of caffeine, monosodium glutamate (MSG), salty foods and processed foods.

Stress
Stress is a major instigator of migraines.

Sensory Stimuli
Bright lights, sun glare, loud sounds and scents (which may be pleasant or unpleasant odors).

Changes in Wake-Sleep Pattern
Either missing sleep or getting too much sleep (including jet lag).

Changes in the environment
A change of weather or barometric pressure.

ophen and caffeine) or other agents, including store brands of these options. OTC agents can be tried for migraines that are mild to moderate. Some patients get more relief from OTC products, some from triptans and others need to use combinations of both OTC and prescription agents. Triptans are considered first-line for acute treatment. In patients who are contraindicated to triptans or do not find benefit with a triptan, ergotamine is generally used next.s *Fiorinal* and *Fioricet*, although commonly used for migraines, contain butalbital, which can cause physical dependence and has abuse potential. These are not as effective as the first-line migraine treatments and are not recommended. Tramadol, tapentadol and opioids are not recommended agents (for the same reasons). However, if other agents have failed, these are used in select cases.

If a patient uses acute treatments more than twice per week, or if the migraines decrease their quality of life, or it the patient desires to try an agent to decrease migraine frequency (with any incidence) a prophylactic agent can be used to decrease migraine occurrence.

prophylaxis may be used if:
1. pt uses acute tx > 2x/wk
2. migraines ↓ pt's QoL
3. regardless of migraine frequency, pt wants to try agent to ↓ frequency

(handwritten top margin:)
prophylactic agents
1. antidepressants   3. vit/natural products — • feverfew • Mg++
2. AEDs   • willow bark • riboflavin

These agents can be antidepressants, anticonvulsants, vitamins or natural products. These should be started at a low dose and titrated to a therapeutic dose (to minimize side effects) and maintained at target dose for an 8-12 week trial period. All prophylactic agents can ↓ frequency by 50%, but a patient may need to try several options before finding an agent (or combination of agents) that works for them. Do not recommend valproic acid any longer for migraine prophylaxis due to safety concerns (see Epilepsy chapter). Valproic acid is Pregnancy Category X when used for migraine prophylaxis.

Natural Products

Feverfew, willow bark (a salicylate), butterbur, magnesium, and riboflavin may be helpful, alone or in combination. The ICSI guidelines mention that acupuncture can be helpful for reducing migraines.

DRUG	DOSING	SAFETY/SIDE EFFECTS/MONITORING
Naratriptan (Amerge)	1 and 2.5 mg, can repeat x 1 after 4 hr Max 5 mg/day	**CONTRAINDICATIONS** Serious but rare cerebrovascular events; contraindicated in patients with cerebrovascular disease or uncontrolled hypertension.
Almotriptan (Axert)	6.25 and 12.5 mg, can repeat x 1 after 2 hr Max 25 mg/day	A few are contraindicated with MAO Is (see below). All must be used with caution with concurrent use of other serotonergic drugs.
\triptan (Frova) *frovatriptan*	2.5 mg, can repeat x 1 after 2 hr Max 7.5 mg/day $t_{1/2} = 26$ hrs	**SIDE EFFECTS** Somnolence, nausea, paresthesias (tingling/numbness), throat/neck pressure, dizziness, hot/cold sensations, chest pain/tightness Triptan sensations include pressure in the chest or heaviness or pressure in the neck region and usually dissipate after administration.
SUMAtriptan (Imitrex, Alsuma) *pre-filled auto-injector* (Sumavel DosePro- 6 mg – injection by air pressure – may hurt) **Imitrex STATdose SC injection** **Imitrex** nasal spray SUMAtriptan + naproxen 85-500 mg (Treximet) • Zecuity transdermal	PO: 25, 50 and 100 mg, can repeat x 1 after 2 hr Max 200 mg/day Nasal Spray: 5, 10, 20 mg in one nostril can repeat x 1 after 2 hr Max 40 mg/day SC inj: 4, 6 mg, can repeat x 1 after 1 hr Max 12 mg/day Treximet max 2 tabs/24 hr	**NOTES** ODTs are useful if nausea is present. No water is required. Nasal sprays and injections are useful if nausea and are faster. Sumatriptan has a nasal spray and a SC injection – fast onset for migraines that come on quickly, and avoids oral route. Zolmitriptan has an intranasal spray (and the disintegrating tablet).
Rizatriptan (Maxalt, Maxalt-MLT disint tabs)	5 mg and 10 mg, can repeat x 1 after 2 hr Maxalt MLT 5 mg, no water needed Max 30 mg/day	**Duration of Action** The longest-acting triptans (longer acting, but slower onset) are frovatriptan (the longest – has 26 hr t½ – and naratriptan. Choose if HA recurs after dosing, lasts a long time. Can use agents with shorter durations of action if fast onset required. The ones with a shorter half-life have a faster onset: almotriptan, eletriptan, rizatriptan, sumatriptan and zolmitriptan.
Eletriptan (Relpax)	20 mg and 40 mg, can repeat after 2 hr Max 80 mg/day	Study: eletriptan (Relpax) 40 mg was more effective than sumatriptan (Imitrex) 100 mg in relieving pain.
ZOLMItriptan (Zomig, Zomig-ZMT disint tabs) Zomig nasal spray	PO: 2.5 and 5 mg, can repeat after 2 hr NS: 5 mg, can repeat after 2 hr Max 10 mg/day (PO, NS, ODT)	Treximet: keep in original container (contains dessicant).

(handwritten left margin:)
≠ cerebro-vascular dz ≠ uncontrolled HTN
• longer acting • slower onset ⇒ good for recurrent b/a after dosing that lasts long
≠ MAOIs
≠ MAOIs
≠ strong 3A4 inhib
≠ MAOIs

(handwritten bottom:)
long acting triptans (slow onset):
1. naratriptan (Amerge®)
2. frovatriptan (Frova®)

Triptans: are 5HT$_1$ receptor agonists. Blood vessels in the brain become dilated during a migraine attack and the triptans, by binding to 5HT$_1$-receptors, causes cranial vessel constriction, inhibiting neuropeptide release and ↓ pain transmission.

Triptan Drug Interactions

- FDA warning about combining triptans with serotonergic drugs such as SSRIs and SNRIs. Counsel patients on both medications to report restlessness, sweating, poor coordination, confusion, hallucinations. However, many patients take both types together. It may present a problem when another serotonergic agent is added to the combination.

- *Imitrex, Maxalt* and *Zomig* are contraindicated with MAO-Is, the others are not.

- Eletriptan *(Relpax)* is contraindicated with strong CYP 3A4 inhibitors.

Patient Counseling for Triptans

- Side effects that you may experience include sleepiness, nausea, numbness, throat or neck pressure, dizziness, hot or cold sensations, and a heaviness or pressure in the chest or neck region. These usually occur after the drug is taken and go away shortly.

- If nausea prevents you from swallowing or holding down your medicine, your healthcare provider can prescribe a tablet that dissolves in your mouth or an injection or nasal spray.

- If you have migraines that come on very quickly, a nasal spray or SC injection will provide faster relief.

- Serious, but rare, side effects such as heart attacks and strokes have occurred in people who have used this type of medicine; because of this, triptans cannot be used in patients who have had a stroke, have heart disease or have blood pressure that is not well-controlled. If any of this applies to you, please inform your healthcare provider.

- With *Imitrex, Maxalt* and *Zomig*: There is a chance of serotonin syndrome when using this drug with some drugs for low mood (depression) or weight loss. The syndrome is caused by too much serotonin in the body. Signs include agitation, changes in blood pressure, loose stools, a fast heartbeat, hallucinations, upset stomach and throwing up, change in balance, and change in thinking clearly and with logic. [MAOIs]

- Take the medicine with or without food, at the first sign of a migraine. The migraine treatment will not work as well if you wait to use it.

- If you use the orally disintegrating tablets *(Maxalt-MLT* and *Zomig-ZMT)*, peel open the blister pack and place the orally disintegrating tablet on your tongue, where it will dissolve and be swallowed with saliva. You do not need to use water with the medicine. These formulations should not be used in patients with phenylketonuria, due to the sweetener.

- If your symptoms are only partly relieved, or if your headache comes back, you may take a second dose in the time period explained to you by the pharmacist.

- If you use migraine treatments more than twice a week or if they are severe, you should be using a daily medicine to help reduce the number of migraines. Please discuss using a "prophylaxis" medicine with your healthcare provider if you are not using one.

Imitrex Injection Counseling using the STATdose system [→ upper outside arm]

Imitrex injections can be administered by prefilled SC syringe, or commonly using the STAT-dose injection device. *Alsuma* is a pre-filled auto injector. Protect all from light.

- Inject the medication just below the skin (always SC, never IM or IV) as soon as the symptoms of your migraine appear.

- Use the STATdose system to administer your injection. This system includes a carrying case and two syringes which will assist you in taking your subcutaneous shot. The shot is relatively mild as it is not a large needle.

- Clean the area of skin, usually in the upper outside arm, with rubbing alcohol prior to administering the injection.

- Open the *Imitrex* injection carrying case and pull off the tamper-proof packaging from one of the cartridge packs. Open the lid of the cartridge. Pull the unused STATdose cartridge from the carrying case.

- Load the STATdose pen by inserting it into the cartridge and turning it clockwise. The cartridge is loaded when you are no longer able to turn the pen clockwise.

- Gently pull the loaded pen out of the carrying case. The blue button on the side triggers the injection. There is a safety feature that does not allow the injection to be triggered unless it is against your skin

- Hold the loaded pen to the area that you have cleaned to receive the shot. Push the blue button on the side of the pen. To make sure you receive all of the medicine, you must hold the pen still for 5 seconds.

- Follow safety procedures and return the used injection needle to the cartridge. Insert the pen once again into the cartridge. This time turn it counterclockwise to loosen the needle. Remove the empty STATdose pen from the cartridge and store it in the carrying case.

- Replace the cartridge pack after both doses of have been used. Discard the pack and insert a new refill.

or front of thigh

Zomig Nasal Spray Counseling

- Blow your nose gently before use.

- Remove the protective cap.

- Hold the nasal sprayer device gently with your fingers and thumb as shown in the picture to the right.

- There is only one dose in the nasal sprayer. Do not try to prime (test) the nasal sprayer or you will lose the dose.

- Do not press the plunger until you have put the tip into your nostril or you will lose the dose. Insert into nose about a half an inch, close your mouth, press the plunger, keep head level for 10-20 seconds, gently breathe in through your mouth.

upper arm or thigh

Zecuity Transdermal Patch Counseling

- This is a transdermal patch that runs on lithium batteries. The red light indicates the drug is being released. Use on upper arm or thigh (dry, clean, relatively hair-free). Remove for MRI. Most common side effect is application site irritation.

Ergotamine Drugs

Used primarily in patents who are contraindicated to or do not respond to triptans. Stimulates cerebral vasoconstriction and has some effect on serotonin.

DRUG	DOSING	SAFETY/SIDE EFFECTS/MONITORING
Dihydroergotamine *(DHE 45, Migranal)* ⇒ may repeat twice (×2) (max 3 doses/day total) ≠ 3A4 inhib MAOIs (past 2 wks) vasoconstrictors/pressor agents ergot/5HT deriv pregnancy (X) ↳ like valproic acid	IM/SubQ: 1 mg at first sign of headache; repeat hourly to a maximum dose of 3 mg/day, maximum 6 mg/week Intranasal: 1 spray (0.5 mg) into each nostril; if needed, repeat after 15 minutes, up to a total of 4 sprays (2 mg)	**BOXED WARNING** Serious and life-threatening peripheral ischemia have been associated with the coadministration of DHE with potent CYP3A4 inhibitors including protease inhibitors and macrolide antibiotics. Because CYP3A4 inhibition elevates the serum levels of DHE, the risk for vasospasm leading to cerebral ischemia and ischemia of the extremities is increased. Hence, concomitant use of these medications is contraindicated. **WARNINGS** Cardiac valvular fibrosis: Ergot alkaloids have been associated with fibrotic valve thickening (aortic, mitral, tricuspid), usually with long-term, chronic use. Cardiovascular effects: Vasospasm or vasoconstriction risk. Do not use in any patient with baseline risk. Cerebrovascular events have occurred after injection. Ergotism (intense vasoconstriction) resulting in peripheral vascular ischemia and possible gangrene can occur with over-dosage or prolonged chronic use; do not exceed dosing limits. Pleural/retroperitoneal fibrosis: Rare cases of pleural and/or retroperitoneal fibrosis have been reported with prolonged daily use. **SIDE EFFECTS** Nasal spray: rhinitis, dysgeusia, nausea, dizziness **NOTES** Nasal spray: prime by pumping 4 times. Do not inhale deeply (to let drug absorb into skin in nose). Use at first sign of attack, but can be used at any time during migraine. Pregnancy Category X, do not use in pregnancy or lactation. Many drug interactions; see boxed warning. Contraindicated with many drugs including ergot/5-HT derivatives within last 24 hours, pressor/vasconstrictive medications. Avoid during or within 2 weeks of discontinuing MAO Is.

OTC MIGRAINE AGENTS

If recommending an OTC product, any OTC NSAID such as *Advil Migraine* (ibuprofen only, or generics), or *Excedrin Migraine* (acetaminophen/aspirin/caffeine) are reasonable options. Aspirin would not be a good choice due to nausea. Always ask the patient what they have tried in the past, and if it was useful.

Advil Migraine® - ibuprofen
Excedrin Migraine® - APAP/ASA/caffeine

* APAP - DOC (OTC) for pain in pregnancy
* NPX - dosed q12 hrs (less frequently than other NSAIDs)

Less Commonly Used Acute Migraine Medications

Acetaminophen/butalbital/caffeine (*Fioricet*), also comes as *Fioricet* with codeine, C-III, *Fiorinal* is aspirin/butalbital/caffeine.

- Neither are recommended agents for this purpose due to abuse/dependence issues and lower efficacy.

- *Fioricet* generic is popular drug. It contains a barbiturate and if using regular, and long-term, must taper off or patient will get worsening of headache, tremors, and be put at risk of delirium and seizures.

- If using codeine formulation, counsel on possible nausea, constipation.

- Do not mix with alcohol.

- Do not exceed safe doses of acetaminophen.

Can also use hydrocodone/APAP combinations *(Vicodin* etc), or other opioid combo products.

mixed agonist antagonist (K)

Butorphanol *(Stadol NS)*, C-IV, intranasal spray may provide fast and effective relief of migraine. Onset in 15 mins.

Migraine Prophylaxis

Consider using a prophylactic if the patient requests it, if they use acute treatments more than twice per week, or if the migraines decrease their quality of life. This is an agent taken daily. Typically, the reduction in migraines is ~50%, but a patient may have to try more than one agent to find one that works well for them. A full trial, at a reasonable dose, should be 2-6 months. Topiramate is being used commonly since it has a better side effect profile than most of the other agents, and causes weight loss. The efficacy data is similar; choose the prophylactic agent based on the patient and the side effect profile. If hypertension, using a beta-blocker may be the most practical. If weight loss is desirable, topiramate may be chosen. Valproic acid is useful in some patients, but has safety concerns. It should not be recommended in women who might become pregnant.

First-line therapies for migraine prophylaxis in adults include:

- Beta-blockers: best evidence with propranolol *(Inderal)*, timolol *(Blocadren)*, metoprolol, valproic acid, and topiramate *(Topamax)*. Extended-cycle oral contraceptives if pre-menstrual migraine, or start NSAIDs or triptan 2 days prior to menses, continue for 5-7 days.

Second-line therapy for migraine prophylaxis include:

- Other beta-blockers, ACE Inhibitors, antidepressants, natural products (see introduction section), birth control pills (for premenstrual migraine) and botulinum toxin type A *(Botox)* injections – *Botox* is for CHRONIC migraines only (lasts 15 or more days/month.) Amitriptyline is a lower dose than for depression. This is why venlafaxine is often used first, but amitriptiline can be added on as a low dose QHS for migraine if the patient is using an SSRI.

First-line Agents for Migraine Prophylaxis

DRUG	TYPICAL DOSING RANGE	COMMENTS/SIDE EFFECTS
Beta-blockers		
Propranolol (*Inderal*)	40-120 mg, divided BID	Fatigue, ↓ HR, possible depression with propranolol (most lipophilic); complete discussion in Hypertension chapter.
Timolol (*Blocadren*)	10-15 mg twice daily	Both propranolol and timolol are non-selective beta-blockers; do not use in COPD, emphysema, complete discussion in Hypertension chapter.
Metoprolol (*Lopressor*, if long acting: *Toprol XL*)	100-200 mg daily	Metoprolol is beta-1 selective. Caution with all beta-blockers if low HR (they will ↓ HR), monitor for hypotension, dizziness; complete discussion in Hypertension chapter.
Anticonvulsants		
Divalproex (*Depakote*), Valproic acid (*Depakene*) Preg X (migraine prophylaxis)/D (other indications): Avoid in women of childbearing age	250-500 mg twice daily	Liver toxicity, pancreatitis, sedation, weight gain, tremor, teratogenicity, thrombocytopenia, alopecia, nausea (less with divalproex), polycystic ovarian syndrome; complete discussion in Epilepsy chapter.
Topiramate (*Topamax*) Preg D: Avoid in women of childbearing age	Start 25 mg QHS, titrate to 50 mg BID	Nephrolithiasis, open angle glaucoma, hypohydrosis (children), depression, metabolic acidosis, 6-13% weight loss, reduced efficacy of oral contraceptives, cognitive impairment; complete discussion in Epilepsy chapter.

(handwritten margin note: non selective)

Medication-overuse ("rebound") headaches

These result from overuse of most headache medicines: NSAIDs, opioids, the butalbital-containing drugs, any analgesic combination products, triptans, and ergotamines (except DHE). Pharmacists are in a position to see many patients who are chronically using headache medicines, and have daily headaches. It may be best to discuss this with a healthcare provider if the patient seems at risk or is unlikely to try and cut down analgesic use independently. To prevent medication-overuse headaches, educate patients to limit acute treatment medications to 2 or 3 times per week, at most. The most important thing is to stop the "over-used" medication. If the drug is an opioid or contains butalbital *(Fioricet, Fiorinal)* they will require a slow taper to discontinue.

GOUT

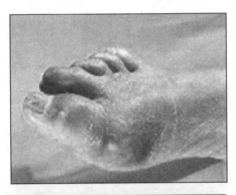

GUIDELINE

Khanna D, Fitzgerald JD, Khanna PP, et al. 2012 American College of Rheumatology Guidelines for Management of Gout. Arthritis Care and Research. 2012;64(10):1431-1461.

BACKGROUND

Gout is a type of arthritis caused by a buildup of uric acid crystals, primarily in the joints. Uric acid is a breakdown product of purines, which are one of the base pairs of DNA and are present in many foods. Gout attacks are sudden with severe pain, burning, and swelling. Gout typically occurs in one joint, which is most often the metatarsophalangeal joint (MTP, the big toe). If left untreated, the attacks can occur over and over, and will eventually damage the joints, tendons and other tissues.

CAUSES

Uric acid is produced as an end-product of purine metabolism (see following figure). Under normal conditions, uric acid is excreted ⅔ renally and ⅓ by the GI tract. When uric acid builds up in the blood, the patient may remain asymptomatic (many people with high uric acid, or hyperuricemia, never get gout) or the uric acid can crystallize in the joints, resulting in a severe, painful gout attack. Gout typically strikes after many years of persistent hyperuricemia.

Risk Factors

Risk factors for gout include male sex, obesity, excessive alcohol consumption (particularly beer), hypertension, chronic kidney disease, lead intoxication, advanced age and using medications that increase uric acid. To reduce the risk of recurrent gout attacks patients should avoid organ meats, high-fructose corn syrup and alcohol. Servings of fruit juices, table sugar, sweetened drinks and desserts, salt, beef, lamb, pork and seafood with high purine content (sardines, shellfish) should be limited. A healthy diet (including low fat dairy products and vegetables), hydration, weight control, smoking cessation and exercise are recommended in the guidelines to reduce the risk for gout attacks.

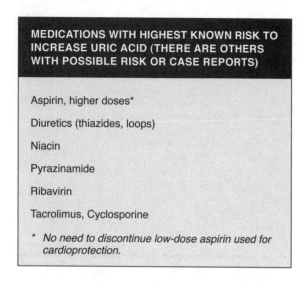

MEDICATIONS WITH HIGHEST KNOWN RISK TO INCREASE URIC ACID (THERE ARE OTHERS WITH POSSIBLE RISK OR CASE REPORTS)

Aspirin, higher doses*

Diuretics (thiazides, loops)

Niacin

Pyrazinamide

Ribavirin

Tacrolimus, Cyclosporine

* No need to discontinue low-dose aspirin used for cardioprotection.

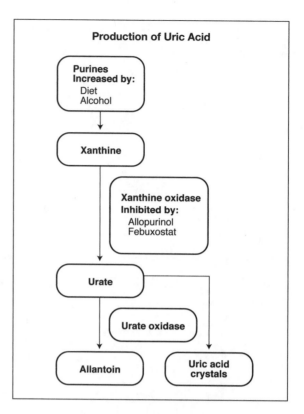

Laboratory Parameters

A normal serum uric acid (urate) level is ~2.0 – 7.2 mg/dL. Do not start treatment until gout has occurred; asymptomatic hyperuricemia is not treated. The treatment goal is a urate level < 6 mg/dL.

DRUG THERAPY

The goal of treatment is to treat acute attacks, prevent future flare-ups, and reduce UA levels. Note that the drugs used to treat an acute attack (colchicine, NSAIDs, steroids) are different than the drugs used to prevent attacks. Colchicine or NSAIDs, however, are recommended during the initiation of prophylactic therapy to reduce the risk of acute attacks which can occur when uric acid is lowered rapidly.

Acute Gout Attack Treatment

Gout attacks are painful and treatment should be started within 24 hours. Single agent treatment with an NSAID, systemic corticosteroid or oral colchicine is recommended for most cases. In more severe disease, combination therapy is suggested with colchicine and NSAIDs, oral corticosteroids and colchicine, or intra-articular steroids (injected into the joint) with one of the other options.

Any of these drugs can be supplemented with topical ice therapy as needed. If patients were taking chronic urate-lowering therapy (ULT) (allopurinol, febuxostat), they should continue the ULT without interruption.

Chronic Urate Lowering Therapy (ULT)

Chronic ULT (see following figure) should be started in all patients with gout who experience intermittent symptoms or tophi (uric acid crystals that can form under the skin in long-term gout). First-line agents for chronic prophylactic therapy are the XO inhibitors (allopurinol or febuxostat). These agents are titrated up (slowly for allopurinol) to lower the uric acid level to a target of < 6 mg/dL. Allopurinol is started at a lower dose with moderate or severe CKD. Patients who are at high risk of severe allopurinol hypersensitivity reaction (including certain Asian groups) should be screened for the HLA-B*5801 allele. Probenecid is a 2nd line agent and can be used if XO inhibitors are contraindicated or not tolerated or can be added when the uric acid level is not at goal despite maximal doses of XO inhibitors (but only in patients with adequate renal function). Pegloticase is reserved for severe, refractory disease. Due to the high rate of gout attacks when beginning ULT, colchicine at a dose of 0.6 mg once or twice daily or NSAIDs are used concurrently for the first 3 – 6 months.

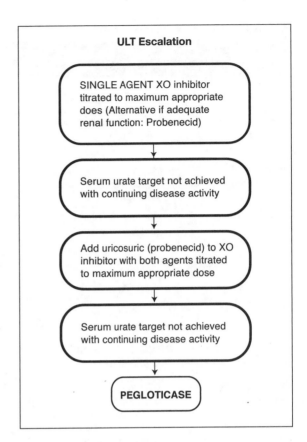

Acute Gout Attack Treatment

DRUG	DOSING	SAFETY/SIDE EFFECTS/MONITORING

Colchicine

| Colchicine (*Colcrys*) | **Treatment**
1.2 mg orally (this is two 0.6 mg tablets) followed by 0.6 mg in 1 hr (do not exceed a total of 1.8 mg)

Dose to be repeated no earlier than 3 days.

Prophylaxis
0.6 mg once or twice daily

In severe renal impairment the treatment dose is the same, but do not repeat treatment dose for 2 weeks. For prophylaxis use 0.3 mg/day. | **CONTRAINDICATIONS**
Concomitant use of a P-gp or strong CYP 3A4 inhibitor in the presence of renal or hepatic impairment

WARNINGS
Blood dyscrasias, gastrointestinal symptoms (reduce dose if anorexia, diarrhea, N/V), neuromuscular toxicity (including rhabdomyolysis); concomitant use of cyclosporine, diltiazem, verapamil, fibrates, and statins increases myopathy risk.

SIDE EFFECTS
Diarrhea, nausea, vomiting, ↓ vitamin B12

Myelosuppression, myopathy, neuropathy (dose-related)

NOTES
Recommended only when treatment is started within 36 hrs of onset of symptoms. |

Acute Gout Attack Treatment Continued

DRUG	DOSING	SAFETY/SIDE EFFECTS/MONITORING

NSAIDs

DRUG	DOSING	SAFETY/SIDE EFFECTS/MONITORING
Indomethacin *(Indocin)*	50 mg TID until attack resolved	See Pain chapter for more complete information. **NOTES** Avoid use in severe renal disease (uric acid is renally cleared and patients with gout may have renal insufficiency); consider risk of bleeding (however risk of GI bleeding is less due to short duration of therapy), CVD risk (most with celecoxib). Indomethacin was the 1st NSAID approved and is the traditional DOC; however, it is more toxic than ibuprofen (increased risk for GI toxicity) and has psychiatric side effects. Indomethacin, naproxen and sulindac are approved for gout; the guideline does not limit treatment to these NSAIDs and states that celecoxib is appropriate if other NSAIDs are not tolerated (and the patient has low CVD risk).
Naproxen *(Naprosyn, others)*	750 mg x 1, then reduce to 250 mg Q8H until attack resolved	
Sulindac *(Clinoril)*	300-400 mg daily until attack resolved	
Celecoxib *(CeleBREX)*	800 mg x 1, then 400 mg x 1 (later in day), then 400 mg BID x 1 week	

Steroids: Can be given PO, IM, IV, intra-articular or via ACTH (adrenocorticotropic hormone) which triggers endogenous glucocorticoid secretion.

DRUG	DOSING	SAFETY/SIDE EFFECTS/MONITORING
PredniSONE/ PredniSOLONE	0.5 mg/kg/day PO for 5-10 days (no taper) or 0.5 mg/kg/day for 2-5 days, then taper (reduce dose by 5 mg each day) over 7-10 days	See Asthma chapter for more complete information. **NOTES** Acute side effects of steroids (e.g., hyperglycemia, hypertension, nervousness, insomnia, increased appetite, edema).
MethylPREDNISolone *(Medrol, Solu-Medrol)*	Intra-articular: If 1-2 large joints involved Oral: Methylprednisolone dose pack	Systemic side effects with intraarticular steroid injections are infrequent. There may be mild pain at the injection site.
Triamcinolone	IM: Triamcinolone 60 mg, then start PO prednisone	Repeated injections can increase the risk of joint damage.

Colchicine Drug Interactions

- Colchicine is a substrate (major) of CYP 3A4 and the efflux transporter P-glycoprotein (P-gp). Fatal toxicity can occur if colchicine is combined with strong 3A4 inhibitors, such as clarithromycin or a strong inhibitor of P-gp, such as cyclosporine. Check for inhibitors prior to dispensing drug. If using a moderate 3A4 inhibitor, the maximum dose for acute treatment is 1.2 mg (2 tablets).

- Myopathy and rhabdomyolysis are higher risk with concomitant colchicine and cyclosporine, diltiazem, verapamil and statins; have patients monitor muscle pain/soreness.

Colchicine Counseling

- At the first sign of an attack, take 2 tablets. You can take 1 more tablet in one hour. Do not use more than this amount. Taking too much colchicine can lead to serious side effects.

- You should not take the 2nd dose if you have upset stomach, nausea or diarrhea.

- Report any serious nausea, vomiting, diarrhea, fatigue, unusual bleeding, tingling in your fingers or toes or muscle soreness to your healthcare provider right away.

- Wait at least 3 days before initiating another acute course of therapy.

Prophylaxis with Chronic Urate Lowering Therapy (ULT)

Allopurinol and febuxostat are <u>xanthine oxidase</u> inhibitors (<u>block UA production</u>). Probenecid inhibits reabsorption of uric acid in the proximal tubule of the nephron, thus promoting uric acid excretion. Pegloticase is a recombinant uricase enzyme, which converts uric acid to an inactive, water-soluble metabolite that can be easily excreted. With ULT: Use <u>colchicine 0.6 mg once or twice daily</u> or <u>NSAIDs</u> for 3-6 months <u>to reduce the risk of acute flares</u> when beginning ULT.

DRUG	DOSING	SAFETY/SIDE EFFECTS/MONITORING

Xanthine Oxidase Inhibitors

DRUG	DOSING	SAFETY/SIDE EFFECTS/MONITORING
Allopurinol (*Zyloprim, Aloprim, Lopurin*)	Start at 100 mg daily, then slowly titrate up until UA < 6 mg/dL (doses > 300 mg may be necessary and should be divided BID)	**WARNINGS** Hypersensitivity reactions can occur, including severe rash (SJS/TEN). Can test for HLA-B*5801 prior to starting treatment (consider testing in Koreans with stage 3 or worse CKD, and Han Chinese or Thai irrespective of renal function). Hepatotoxicity, caution in patients with liver impairment. **SIDE EFFECTS** Rash, acute gout attacks, nausea, diarrhea, ↑ LFTs **MONITORING** Uric acid level, goal < 6 mg/dL, CBC (for bone marrow suppression), liver enzymes, renal function **NOTES** Higher doses used for tumor lysis syndrome (in chemotherapy)
Febuxostat (*Uloric*)	40-80 mg daily	**CONTRAINDICATIONS** Concomitant use with azathioprine or mercaptopurine **WARNINGS** Hepatotoxicity, use with caution in patients with liver impairment and discontinue therapy if LFTs > 3x ULN Possible increase in thromboembolic events **SIDE EFFECTS** ↑ LFTs, rash **MONITORING** LFTs at 2 months, 4 months, then periodically **NOTES** Very expensive compared to allopurinol No dose reduction necessary in renal impairment Reduced risk for hypersensitivity reactions compared to allopurinol

Chronic UA – Lowering Therapy Continued

DRUG	DOSING	SAFETY/SIDE EFFECTS/MONITORING

Probenecid (a uricosuric) inhibits reabsorption of uric acid in the kidneys, which ↑ uric acid excretion. Competes with penicillins and cephalosporins in the kidneys, which ↓ the beta lactam excretion and ↑ the plasma levels.

Probenecid 2nd line agent	Start 250 mg BID, can increase to 2 g/day	**CONTRAINDICATIONS** Concomitant aspirin therapy; blood dyscrasias; uric acid kidney stones (nephrolithiasis); children < 2 years of age; initiation during an acute gout attack
Colchicine-Probenicid	0.5/500 mg daily for 1 week, then BID (for starting probenecid, to reduce risk acute attack)	**WARNINGS** Increased risk of hemolytic anemia in patients with G6PD deficiency **SIDE EFFECTS** Hypersensitivity reactions, hemolytic anemia **NOTES** Requires adequate renal function; not recommended as monotherapy in patients with CrCl < 50 mL/min; avoid use in patients with CrCl < 30 mL/min

Pegloticase is a pegylated form of uricase, an enzyme which converts uric acid to allantoin (an inactive and water soluble metabolite of uric acid); it does not block uric acid formation.

Pegloticase (*Krystexxa*) – injection, costly, refractory cases only	8 mg IV every 2 weeks	**BLACK BOX WARNING** Anaphylactic reactions can occur during infusion; patients should be monitored by healthcare personnel and premedicated with antihistamines and corticosteroids. Risk is highest if UA level is > 6 mg/dL. Consider discontinuing treatment if UA is > 6 mg/dL. **CONTRAINDICATIONS** G6PD deficiency **WARNINGS** Acute gout flares may occur upon initiation of therapy; an NSAID or colchicine should be given as prophylaxis (1 week prior to infusion; continue for at least 6 months) **SIDE EFFECTS** Antibody formation, gout flare, infusion reactions, nausea, bruising, urticaria, erythema, pruritus **NOTES** Very expensive (~$6,500/dose) Do not use in combination with allopurinol (increased risk of anaphylaxis)

Allopurinol Drug Interactions

■ Antacids ↓ the absorption of allopurinol.

■ Allopurinol ↑ the concentration of mercaptopurine, the active metabolite of azathioprine. Avoid concurrent use of either drug with allopurinol, or ↓ dose, and monitor for toxicity.

■ Avoid concurrent use with didanosine; allopurinol can ↑ didanosine levels.

Probenecid Drug Interactions

- Probenecid may decrease the renal clearance of other medications taken concurrently, including aspirin (do not use salicylates concurrently), methotrexate, penicillins, cephalosporins and carbapenems.

- Probenecid may be used with penicillins to ↑ the penicillin plasma concentrations; this will ↑ adverse reactions. Probenecid can decrease the efficacy of loop diuretics, but increases the loop's toxicity.

Allopurinol Counseling

- Take after a meal to reduce stomach upset (higher doses can be divided). Drink plenty of fluids.
- It may take up to several weeks for this medicine to have an effect and you may have more gout attacks for several months after starting this medicine while the body removes extra uric acid. If this happens, you can use different medicine to treat the gout and help with the pain.
- If you feel ill or get a rash, you should seek medical help quickly. The rash could become serious.

PRACTICE CASE

BK is a 62 y/o white male with hypertension. He presents to the clinic today with pain described as 10/10. He is trying to avoid putting weight on his right foot. Physical exam reveals a swollen, tender, enlarged big toe. His blood pressure has a daily range of 155-178/88-99 mmHg. The patient reports that he consumes low fat yogurt with berries or nuts for breakfast each day. He walks each night around the track at the neighborhood high school. He reports "weekend" alcohol use (3-4 beers on Saturday/Sunday). No past or present history of tobacco use.

Allergies: NKDA

Medications:
Norvasc 10 mg PO daily
Zestril 10 mg PO daily
Chlorthalidone 25 mg PO daily
Aspirin EC 81 mg daily
Fish oil capsule with dinner
Coenzyme Q10 with dinner

Vitals:
Height: 5'11" Weight: 255 pounds
BP: 177/95 mmHg HR: 89 BPM RR: 16 BPM Temp: 98.8°F Pain: 10/10

Labs: Na (mEq/L) = 142 (135 - 145)
K (mEq/L) = 4.8 (3.5 - 5)
Cl (mEq/L) = 100 (95 - 103)
HCO_3 (mEq/L) = 28 (24 - 30)
BUN (mg/dL) = 22 (7 - 20)
SCr (mg/dL) = 1.4 (0.6 - 1.3)
Glucose (mg/dL) = 119 (100 - 125)
Ca (mg/dL) = 10.2 (8.5 - 10.5)
Mg (mEq/L) = 1.8 (1.3 - 2.1)
PO_4 (mg/dL) = 4.2 (2.3 - 4.7)

AST (IU/L) = 12 (8 - 48)
ALT (IU/L) = 14 (7 - 55)
Albumin (g/dL) = 4.8 (3.5 - 5)
Uric Acid (mg/dL) = 18.3 (3.5 - 7.2 male, 2 - 6.5 female)

April 1st: 62 y/o male with first episode of acute gout in right great toe. Provide therapy for gout and optimize therapy for uncontrolled HTN. Prescription written for *Dilacor XR* 120 mg Q daily.

Questions

1. What is Brian's creatinine clearance (in mL/min), using the Cockcroft-Gault equation and his ideal body weight?

   a. 89
   b. 71
   c. 58
   d. 34
   e. 11

2. The physician is considering allopurinol to treat the acute attack. Choose the correct statement:

   a. This is not appropriate therapy for an acute attack.
   b. He should receive a starting dose of 50 mg daily.
   c. He should receive a starting dose of 75 mg daily.
   d. He should receive a starting dose of 100 mg daily.
   e. He should receive a starting dose of 150 mg daily.

3. Brian will receive a short-course of prednisone therapy, with taper, that will last less than 2 weeks. Which of the following side effects are possible and should be explained to Brian?

   a. Growth suppression
   b. Insomnia/spaciness
   c. Osteoporosis
   d. Cataracts
   e. Seizures

4. Choose the correct dosing regimen for colchicine for an acute gout attack:

   a. 1.2 mg followed by 0.6 mg every 2 hours, not to exceed 6 tablets/24 hours
   b. 1.2 mg followed by 0.6 mg every 2 hours, not to exceed 8 tablets/24 hours
   c. 1.2 mg followed by 0.6 mg in 2-4 hours (total 1.8 mg)
   d. 1.2 mg followed by 0.6 mg in 1 hours, then as-needed for 3 additional doses (total 3.6 mg)
   e. 1.2 mg followed by 0.6 mg in 1 hours (total 1.8 mg)

Questions 5 – 8 do not apply to the above case.

5. A pharmacist receives a prescription for *Zyloprim*. Which medication is an acceptable alternative?

   a. Probenecid
   b. Colchicine
   c. Allopurinol
   d. Naproxen
   e. Febuxostat

6. Which of the following are true regarding pegloticase? (Select **ALL** that apply.)

   a. The brand name is *Krystexxa*
   b. The recommended dose is 8 mg PO daily
   c. It should not be given in combination with allopurinol
   d. It is a first-line treatment for acute gout
   e. Patients must be monitored for anaphylactic reactions when receiving this agent

7. Which of the following side effects are likely to occur with colchicine therapy?

   a. Nausea, cramping, loose stools
   b. Xerostomia, xerophthalmia
   c. Mental confusion
   d. Skeletal bone loss
   e. Risk of severe rash/hypersensitivity reactions

8. A pharmacist has just attended an education program on the use of febuxostat. He wants to present the main points about this drug to his pharmacy colleagues. He should include the following points: (Select **ALL** that apply.)

   a. Febuxostat works by increasing the renal excretion of uric acid.
   b. Febuxostat appears to have lower risk of hypersensitivity reactions than allopurinol, including less of a risk of serious rash.
   c. Febuxostat costs much more than generic allopurinol and is reserved for refractory cases.
   d. The brand name of febuxostat is *Zyloprim*.
   e. Febuxostat is a xanthine oxidase inhibitor.

Answers

1-c, 2-a, 3-b, 4-e, 5-c, 6-a,c,e, 7-a, 8-b,c,e

HYPERTENSION

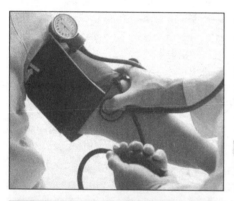

GUIDELINES

James PA, Oparil S, Carter BL, et al. 2014 evidence-based guideline for the management of high blood pressure in adults: report from the panel members appointed to the Eighth Joint National Committee (JNC8). *JAMA*. 2014; 311:507-520.

Eckel RH, Jakicic JM, Ard JD, et al. 2013 AHA/ACC guideline on lifestyle management to reduce cardiovascular risk: a report of the American College of Cardiology/American Heart Association Task Force on Practice Guidelines. *Circulation*. 2014; 129:S76-S99.

Hypertension in Pregnancy. Report of the American College of Obstetricians and Gynecologists' Task Force on Hypertension in Pregnancy. American College of Obstetricians and Gynecologists. 2013; 122(5):1122–1131.

BACKGROUND

One in three American adults have hypertension. It is one of the most common conditions seen in primary care. If left untreated, the patient is at increased risk of heart disease, stroke and kidney disease. Hypertension is largely asymptomatic, and is often untreated. Only when the blood pressure is very high (such as with hypertensive crisis) are symptoms such as throbbing headache, fatigue and shortness of breath likely to appear. Pharmacists should screen patients for hypertension and advise adherence to medication therapy and lifestyle management. One in four patients discontinue antihypertensive therapy within 6 months. Diuretics can increase urination, ACE inhibitors can cause cough and calcium channel blockers can cause edema, especially at higher doses. These side effects can each lead to discontinuation, but the major cause of non-adherence is a lack of understanding of the necessity for treatment and cost.

Counseling should include healthy lifestyle measures that can decrease blood pressure, such as a healthy diet, physical activity, maintaining a healthy weight, smoking cessation and sodium restriction. A home blood pressure monitoring device can help the patient get involved and improve motivation and success of therapy.

PATHOPHYSIOLOGY

Most patients have essential hypertension, which is not linked to a specific cause. Poor lifestyle and genetics can be contributory. Secondary hypertension is linked to a specific cause, such as renal disease, adrenal disease and/or drug-induced hypertension.

DRUGS THAT CAN CAUSE OR WORSEN HYPERTENSION

ACTH

Alcohol (excessive)

Amphetamines (e.g., ADHD drugs, cocaine)

Appetite suppressants

Caffeine

Calcineurin antagonists (cyclosporine, tacrolimus)

Corticosteroids

Decongestants (e.g., pseudoephedrine)

Erythropoiesis Stimulating Agents *Epogen®*

Estrogen

Herbals [bitter orange, ephedra (ma-huang), ginseng, guarana, St. John's wort]

Mirabegron *(Myrbetriq)*

NSAIDs

Certain oncology drugs

SNRIs, at higher doses

Thyroid hormone (if overdosed)

THE EIGHTH JOINT NATIONAL COMMITEE (JNC 8) GUIDELINE

JNC 8 has simplified the treatment of hypertension in adults. Treatment is based on age, and the presence of diabetes (DM) and/or chronic kidney disease (CKD). In the general non-black patient population, drug therapy for hypertension should be initiated using one or more agents from 4 medication classes – angiotension converting enzyme inhibitors (ACE inhibitors), angiotensin receptor blockers (ARBs), calcium channel blockers (CCBs), or thiazide-type diuretics. Black patients have been separated out for 2 reasons: this group is at high risk for stroke, and BP reduction is not as great with ACE inhibitors or ARBs compared with other drug classes. In black hypertensive patients, initial therapy should include a CCB and/or thiazide-type diuretic unless they have CKD and proteinuria. Patients with CKD should be started on an ACE inhibitor or ARB. If patients do not reach the blood pressure (BP) goal, add another drug from the 4 recommended drug classes, but do not combine an ACE inhibitor with an ARB. Note that beta blockers are not among the initial recommended drug classes for uncomplicated hypertension.

Key Points with the JNC 8 Guidelines

- Thiazides are no longer the preferred first-line drug class but are now one of four preferred first-line groups. If a thiazide is used, chlorthalidone or indapamide may have better evidence over hydrochlorothiazide (not all experts agree – if a patient is on hydrochlorothiazide and is doing well they do not need to switch).

- There are 3 ways to manage BP once a drug is chosen: titrate the first drug up to the maximum dose and then add a 2nd drug, or, start a 2nd drug before the 1st one is at the maximum dose, or, begin with 2 drugs at the same time. Two drugs will be needed if the systolic blood pressure (SBP) is > 20 mmHg or the diastolic blood pressure (DBP) is > 10 mmHg above goal.

- ACE inhibitors or ARBs or CCBs or thiazides can be used first-line in non-black patients with diabetes. Do not use ACE inhibitors and ARBs together.

- If CKD is present (± diabetes), ACE inhibitors or ARBs are used first-line.

- Black patients: Thiazides are more protective against stroke and CCBs also have better outcomes, including blood pressure reduction, in black patients. However, when CKD and proteinuria are present, an ACE inhibitor or ARB is recommended as initial therapy instead because of the higher likelihood of progression to ESRD (these drug classes help slow progression to kidney disease). Emphasize medication adherence and sodium reduction.

- Beta blockers are no longer among the initial recommended drug classes for uncomplicated hypertension.

- Once-daily regimens are preferred for increased patient compliance. Check BP 2-4 weeks after starting therapy and until goal BP is reached.

JNC 8: When to Treat*

TARGET GROUP	TARGET SBP (in mmHg)	TARGET DBP (in mmHg)
≥ 60 years	< 150	< 90
18-59 years or those with diabetes or CKD regardless of age	< 140	< 90

The ADA recommends a BP goal < 140/80 mmHg although the SBP can be targeted to < 130 mmHg in younger patients. If an exam question wanted the ADA goal versus JNC 8 it should specify.

JNC 8 Drug Therapy Recommendations

TARGET GROUP	JNC 8 RECOMMENDATION
Nonblack ± diabetes	Thiazide or CCB or ACE inhibitor or ARB
Black patients ± diabetes	Thiazide or CCB
CKD – all races	ACE inhibitor or ARB
All: if BP > 20/10 mmHg above goal	Consider initial therapy of 2 drugs
All: if BP remains elevated with current drugs	Encourage adherence, lifestyle, titrate dose to the maximum dose or add on another drug

Combination Blood Pressure Drugs – There are Many

The majority of patients require more than one drug to reach goal blood pressure. Many of the common (and a few not-so-common) drugs used together are available in combinations. One of the recommendations in the JNC 8 guideline is to use a combination before titrating one drug to the maximum dose; these may be used as the initial therapy, especially in patients with higher blood pressure. Or, lower doses are used as a combination to reduce side effects. Counseling includes each of the components, including any of the side effects or adverse reactions from either drug. Using a diuretic with any other agent requires caution for dizziness and risk of falls. The more commonly used agents are bolded. Notice that for many you can figure out the brand name: diuretic combinations often have part of the brand name at the front and HCT or -ide or -etic at the end.

COMBINATION BLOOD PRESSURE DRUGS

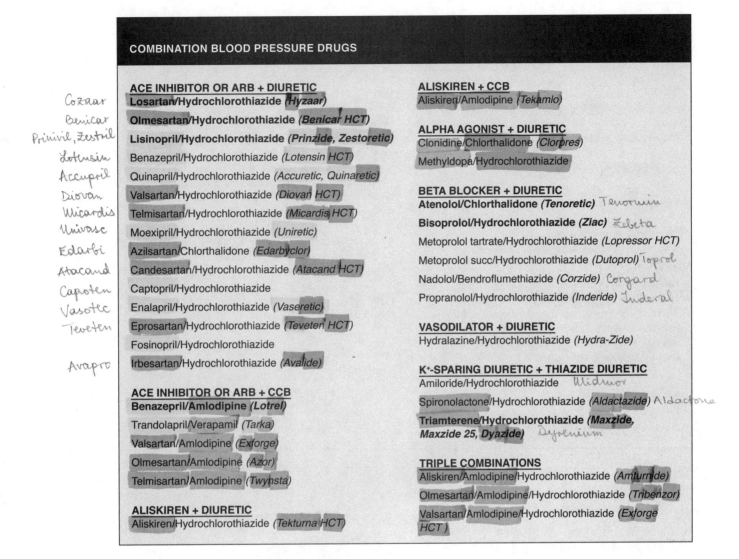

ACE INHIBITOR OR ARB + DIURETIC
Losartan/Hydrochlorothiazide (*Hyzaar*)
Olmesartan/Hydrochlorothiazide (*Benicar HCT*)
Lisinopril/Hydrochlorothiazide (*Prinzide, Zestoretic*)
Benazepril/Hydrochlorothiazide (*Lotensin HCT*)
Quinapril/Hydrochlorothiazide (*Accuretic, Quinaretic*)
Valsartan/Hydrochlorothiazide (*Diovan HCT*)
Telmisartan/Hydrochlorothiazide (*Micardis HCT*)
Moexipril/Hydrochlorothiazide (*Uniretic*)
Azilsartan/Chlorthalidone (*Edarbyclor*)
Candesartan/Hydrochlorothiazide (*Atacand HCT*)
Captopril/Hydrochlorothiazide
Enalapril/Hydrochlorothiazide (*Vaseretic*)
Eprosartan/Hydrochlorothiazide (*Teveten HCT*)
Fosinopril/Hydrochlorothiazide
Irbesartan/Hydrochlorothiazide (*Avalide*)

ACE INHIBITOR OR ARB + CCB
Benazepril/Amlodipine (*Lotrel*)
Trandolapril/Verapamil (*Tarka*)
Valsartan/Amlodipine (*Exforge*)
Olmesartan/Amlodipine (*Azor*)
Telmisartan/Amlodipine (*Twynsta*)

ALISKIREN + DIURETIC
Aliskiren/Hydrochlorothiazide (*Tekturna HCT*)

ALISKIREN + CCB
Aliskiren/Amlodipine (*Tekamlo*)

ALPHA AGONIST + DIURETIC
Clonidine/Chlorthalidone (*Clorpres*)
Methyldopa/Hydrochlorothiazide

BETA BLOCKER + DIURETIC
Atenolol/Chlorthalidone (*Tenoretic*) *Tenormin*
Bisoprolol/Hydrochlorothiazide (*Ziac*) *Zebeta*
Metoprolol tartrate/Hydrochlorothiazide (*Lopressor HCT*)
Metoprolol succ/Hydrochlorothiazide (*Dutoprol*) *Toprol*
Nadolol/Bendroflumethiazide (*Corzide*) *Corgard*
Propranolol/Hydrochlorothiazide (*Inderide*) *Inderal*

VASODILATOR + DIURETIC
Hydralazine/Hydrochlorothiazide (*Hydra-Zide*)

K⁺-SPARING DIURETIC + THIAZIDE DIURETIC
Amiloride/Hydrochlorothiazide *Midmor*
Spironolactone/Hydrochlorothiazide (*Aldactazide*) *Aldactone*
Triamterene/Hydrochlorothiazide (*Maxzide, Maxzide 25, Dyazide*) *Dyrenium*

TRIPLE COMBINATIONS
Aliskiren/Amlodipine/Hydrochlorothiazide (*Amturnide*)
Olmesartan/Amlodipine/Hydrochlorothiazide (*Tribenzor*)
Valsartan/Amlodipine/Hydrochlorothiazide (*Exforge HCT*)

Handwritten left margin notes:
Cozaar, Benicar, Prinivil, Zestril, Lotensin, Accupril, Diovan, Micardis, Univasc, Edarbi, Atacand, Capoten, Vasotec, Teveten, Avapro

PREGNANCY AND HYPERTENSION

Planning for pregnancy includes the discontinuation of teratogenic drugs that could cause fetal harm. If pregnancy is detected, ACE inhibitors, ARBs and the direct renin inhibitor aliskiren should be discontinued immediately. It must first be confirmed that the elevated BP is not preeclampsia as this condition would be managed differently than hypertension in pregnancy. Preeclampsia includes elevated blood pressure and proteinuria in the majority of cases. Preeclampsia occurs after week 20 of pregnancy and is more common in women who are overweight, and/or have hypertension, renal disease or diabetes. Antihypertensive therapy is recommended in pregnant patients with a SBP ≥ 160 mmHg or DBP ≥ 105 mmHg. First-line recommended agents include labetalol, nifedipine extended-release and methyldopa. BP should be maintained between 120-160 mmHg systolic and 80-105 mmHg diastolic.

Handwritten notes:
tx recommended if systolic ≥ 160 or diastolic ≥ 105
bp goal 120-160 / 80-105
1st line ① labetalol ② nifedipine XR ③ methyldopa
hCG+ ⇓ d/c ACEI/ARB aliskerin

LIFESTYLE MANAGEMENT

Weight
Maintain normal BMI and waist circumference.

Moderate Alcohol Consumption
Alcohol should be limited to 1 drink/day (most women) and 2 drinks/day (most men).

Increase Physical Activity
Engage in regular aerobic physical activity: 3-4 sessions per week, lasting 40 minutes on average per session and involving moderate-to-vigorous intensity.

Reduce Sodium Intake
Limit sodium to ≤ 2,400 mg/day; further reduction to 1,500 mg/day is associated with ever greater BP reduction (however this is currently being debated in the medical community and very low Na⁺ diets have been linked to increased CV events).

Smoking Cessation
Pharmacists should be able to recommend how to quit and assist with therapy (see Smoking Cessation chapter).

Diet
Consume a dietary pattern that emphasizes intake of vegetables, fruits and whole grains; includes low-fat dairy products, poultry, fish, legumes, nontropical vegetable oils and nuts; and limits intake of sweets, sugar-sweetened beverages and red meats. Adapt this dietary pattern to appropriate calorie requirements, personal and cultural food preferences and nutrition therapy for other medical conditions (such as diabetes mellitus). Achieve this pattern by following plans such as the DASH dietary pattern, the USDA Food Pattern or the AHA Diet. Aim for 5-6% of calories from saturated fat and reduce *trans* fat.

Control Blood Glucose And Lipids To Reduce Cardiovascular Disease Risk!

THIAZIDE-TYPE DIURETICS

Thiazide-type diuretics are inexpensive, effective and have mild side effects. Thiazides are one of the 4 recommended treatment groups for treating hypertension. Loop diuretics are used primarily in heart failure (see Heart Failure chapter).

Thiazides and thiazide-type diuretics inhibit Na⁺ reabsorption in the distal convoluted tubules of the nephron causing ↑ excretion of Na⁺ and water as well as K⁺ and H⁺ ions.

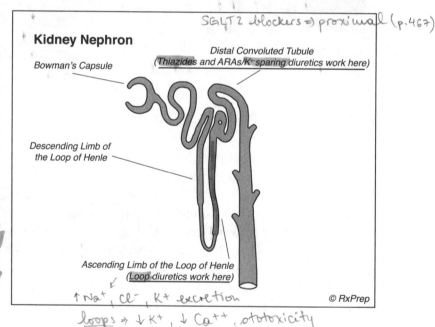

SG4T2 blockers ⇒ proximal (p.467)

Kidney Nephron

Bowman's Capsule

Distal Convoluted Tubule
(Thiazides and ARAs/K⁺ sparing diuretics work here)

Descending Limb of the Loop of Henle

Ascending Limb of the Loop of Henle
(Loop diuretics work here)

↑ Na⁺, Cl⁻, K⁺ excretion

loops ⇒ ↓ K⁺, ↓ Ca⁺⁺, ototoxicity

© RxPrep

* ethacrynic acid is safe in pts w/ sulfa allergy (vs. loops, thiazides)

* metolazone has some effects on PCT (additional benefit vs. other thiazides only work on DCT) ⇒ used in hosp in pts w/ diuretic resistance

K+ rich foods to counteract K+ - lowering effect of thiazides: bananas, avocados, oranges

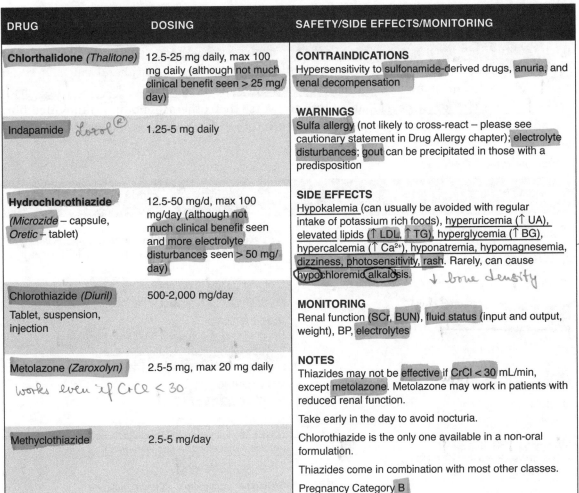

DRUG	DOSING	SAFETY/SIDE EFFECTS/MONITORING
Chlorthalidone (*Thalitone*)	12.5-25 mg daily, max 100 mg daily (although not much clinical benefit seen > 25 mg/day)	**CONTRAINDICATIONS** Hypersensitivity to sulfonamide-derived drugs, anuria, and renal decompensation
Indapamide *Lozol®*	1.25-5 mg daily	**WARNINGS** Sulfa allergy (not likely to cross-react – please see cautionary statement in Drug Allergy chapter); electrolyte disturbances; gout can be precipitated in those with a predisposition
Hydrochlorothiazide (*Microzide* – capsule, *Oretic* – tablet)	12.5-50 mg/d, max 100 mg/day (although not much clinical benefit seen and more electrolyte disturbances seen > 50 mg/day)	**SIDE EFFECTS** Hypokalemia (can usually be avoided with regular intake of potassium rich foods), hyperuricemia ($\uparrow$ UA), elevated lipids ($\uparrow$ LDL, $\uparrow$ TG), hyperglycemia ($\uparrow$ BG), hypercalcemia ($\uparrow$ Ca^{2+}), hyponatremia, hypomagnesemia, dizziness, photosensitivity, rash. Rarely, can cause hypochloremic alkalosis.
Chlorothiazide (*Diuril*) Tablet, suspension, injection	500-2,000 mg/day	**MONITORING** Renal function (SCr, BUN), fluid status (input and output, weight), BP, electrolytes
Metolazone (*Zaroxolyn*) *works even if CrCl < 30*	2.5-5 mg, max 20 mg daily	**NOTES** Thiazides may not be effective if CrCl < 30 mL/min, except metolazone. Metolazone may work in patients with reduced renal function. Take early in the day to avoid nocturia. Chlorothiazide is the only one available in a non-oral formulation. Thiazides come in combination with most other classes. Pregnancy Category B
Methyclothiazide	2.5-5 mg/day	

better evidence over other thiazides

only thiazide that comes in non-po

↓ bone density

↓ K+
↓ Na+
↓ Mg++

↑ Ca++
↑ UA
↑ LDL, TG
↑ BG

Thiazide-Type Diuretic Drug Interactions

- All antihypertensives can potentiate the therapeutic effect of other blood pressure lowering drugs; always carefully monitor BP when adding on therapy.

- Diuretics may $\downarrow$ lithium's renal clearance and $\uparrow$ risk of lithium toxicity.

- Patients with hypertension should not be routinely using agents that can cause Na^+ and H_2O retention, such as NSAIDs, COX-2 inhibitors or corticosteroids. These agents can lower the effectiveness of antihypertensive medications.

- Thiazide-type diuretics can $\uparrow$ dofetilide concentration leading to $\uparrow$ risk of QT prolongation; concurrent use is contraindicated.

CALCIUM CHANNEL BLOCKERS (CCBs)

There are 2 types of CCBs: dihydropyridines and non-dihydropyridines. With CCBs, be careful to check the Orange Book since there are many long-acting formulations of nifedipine and diltiazem; choose a generic that is AB-rated to the brand.

Dihydropyridine CCBs

The dihydropyridines which end in (-pine) are used for HTN and Prinzmetal's angina. These agents inhibit Ca²⁺ ions from entering the "slow" channels or voltage-sensitive areas of vascular smooth muscle, causing peripheral arterial vasodilation and ↓ peripheral vascular resistance and ↓ blood pressure. The peripheral vasodilation leads to reflex tachycardia, headache, flushing, and peripheral edema. Some agents are worse than others; amlodipine and nifedipine extended release formulations are used often since they do not commonly cause these effects.

Dihydropyridine CCBs

DRUG	DOSING	SAFETY/SIDE EFFECTS/MONITORING
AmLODIPine (Norvasc)	2.5-10 mg daily	**WARNINGS**
Felodipine (Plendil)	2.5-10 mg daily	Increased angina and/or MI has occurred with initiation or dosage titration of dihydropyridine calcium channel blockers
Isradapine	2.5-10 mg BID	Use with caution in patients with aortic stenosis; may reduce coronary perfusion resulting in ischemia
NIFEdipine ER (Adalat CC, Afeditab CR, Nifediac CC, Nifedical XL, Procardia XL), NIFEdipine IR (Procardia)	30-90 mg/day	**SIDE EFFECTS** Peripheral edema, fatigue, dizziness, headache, palpitations, flushing, tachycardia/reflex tachycardia, hypotension, gingival hyperplasia
Nisoldipine ER (Sular)	8.5-34 mg/day	**MONITORING** BP, HR, peripheral edema
Nisoldipine ER (original formulation)	10-60 mg/day	**NOTES** Do not use immediate release nifedipine for acute BP reduction (not effective and is harmful)
NiCARdipine ER (Cardene SR) NiCARdipine IR (Cardene) is TID **NiCARdipine IV (Cardene IV)** Capsule, Injection	30-60 mg BID 20-40 mg TID	Pregnancy Category C Nifedipine: protect from light and moisture Covera HS, Adalat CC, and Sular have capsular shells that can be seen in feces (ghost shells) Adalat CC, Afeditab CR and Nifediac CC should be taken on an empty stomach Amlodipine is considered the safest CCB in patients with HF Cardene IV: requires light protection during administration
Clevidipine (Cleviprex) Injection	1-21 mg/hr	**CONTRAINDICATIONS** Do not use in soy or egg allergy, acute pancreatitis, severe aortic stenosis, lipoid nephrosis **SIDE EFFECTS** Headache, nausea/vomiting. Rare: hypertriglyceridemia, infections **MONITORING** BP, HR **NOTES** Pregnancy Category C In a lipid emulsion (provides 2 kcal/mL); it is milky-white in color. Risk of infection and hypertriglyceridemia. Use strict aseptic technique upon administration. Maximum hang-time per vial/bottle is 12 hours.

Handwritten annotations:
- Safest in HF (cardiac neutral)
- ghost — EMPTY STOMACH
- IR not for acute ↓ bp
- light/moisture
- ghost
- protect from light during admin
- lipid emulsion 2 kcal/ml (↑TG)
- ① soy/egg allergy
- ② acute pancreatitis (↑TG)
- ③ severe aortic stenosis
- ④ lipid nephrosis
- SE: N/V, ↑TG (rare), infxns ↳ requires strict aseptic technique during admin [max hang time per vial/bottle: 12 hrs]
- * sublingual nifedipine ⇒ uncontrollable ↓ bp ⇒ MI, other ischemic compx

Non-dihydropyridine CCBs *DO NOT USE IN HF !*

The non-dihydropyridines consist of verapamil and diltiazem and are used primarily for arrhythmias to control/slow HR, and sometimes for HTN and angina. Diltiazem and verapamil are negative inotropes (↓ contraction force) and negative chronotropes (↓ HR). The dihydropyridines do not have these properties. These agents inhibit Ca^{2+} ions from entering the "slow" channels or voltage-sensitive areas of vascular smooth muscle and myocardium during depolarization, resulting in coronary vasodilation.

DRUG	DOSING	SAFETY/SIDE EFFECTS/MONITORING
Diltiazem *(Cardizem, Cardizem CD, Cardizem LA, Cartia XT, Dilacor XR, Dilt-CD, Dilt-XR, Diltzac, Tiazac, Taztia XT)* Tablet, Capsule, Injection	60-360 mg in 1-2 divided doses; max 480-540 mg daily	**CONTRAINDICATIONS** Severe hypotension (SBP < 90 mmHg), 2nd or 3rd degree heart block, sick sinus syndrome (unless the patient has a functioning artificial ventricular pacemaker), cardiogenic shock, pulmonary congestion and HF
Verapamil *(Calan, Calan SR, Covera HS, Verelan, Verelan PM)* ↳ *ghost* Tablet, Capsule, Injection	240-480 mg in 1-3 divided doses	**SIDE EFFECTS** Edema, headache, dizziness, AV block, bradycardia, hypotension, arrhythmias, HF, constipation (more with verapamil), gingival hyperplasia **MONITORING** BP, HR, ECG, LFTs **NOTES** Pregnancy Category C Verapamil: requires light protection during administration

constipation

protect from light during admin

Calcium Channel Blocker Drug Interactions

- Diltiazem and verapamil are both major CYP 3A4 substrates and moderate 3A4 inhibitors. They will raise the concentration of many other drugs, and 3A4 inducers and inhibitors will affect their concentration; check for interactions prior to dispensing. Avoid grapefruit juice.

ACEI
ARB ⟍
aliskiren ✓
!

RENIN-ANGIOTENSIN ALDOSTERONE SYSTEM (RAAS) INHIBITORS

- RAAS inhibitors reduce vasoconstriction, ↓ aldosterone release, and some agents have shown benefit in renal protection and heart failure. The use of 2 RAAS inhibitors (ACE inhibitor ± ARB ± aliskiren) is never recommended due to poor clinical outcomes.

- Angioedema is more common in black patients. Although angioedema is more likely with ACE inhibitors than ARBs or aliskiren, if a patient has had angioedema with these classes of agents, all others are contraindicated since angioedema can become fatal. Counsel patients to report any swelling of lips, mouth, tongue, face, or neck immediately.

- RAAS inhibitors ↑ potassium; patients on these medicines should be careful with salt substitutes that contain potassium chloride (instead of sodium chloride).

[handwritten top margin: ang I →ACE I→ ang II ↳ potent vasoconstrictor → efferent arteriole constriction ≫ afferent ⇒ ↑ perfusion pressure, damage]

Angiotensin-Converting Enzyme Inhibitors (ACE Inhibitors)

These agents inhibit the angiotensin converting enzyme (ACE), preventing the conversion of angiotensin I (Ang I) to angiotensin II (Ang II), a potent vasoconstrictor. Angiotensin II constricts the efferent arterioles to a greater extent than the afferent arterioles within the kidney causing increased perfusion pressure in the glomeruli resulting in kidney damage over time. Therefore, blocking Ang II formation will cause vasodilation and reduce BP. ACE inhibitors have been shown to slow progression of renal disease in patients with diabetes and/or hypertension who have albuminuria; they also slow progression of heart failure.

[handwritten left margin: SE: taste ∆ ↓ taste]

DRUG	DOSING	SAFETY/SIDE EFFECTS/MONITORING
Benazepril *(Lotensin)*	10-40 mg in 1-2 divided doses	**BOXED WARNING** Can cause injury and death to developing fetus; discontinue as soon as pregnancy is detected.
Captopril *(Capoten)*	50-100 mg BID-TID Take 1 hour before meals (empty stomach)	**CONTRAINDICATIONS** Angioedema. Do not use in bilateral renal artery stenosis since renal function will worsen. Do not use concurrently with aliskiren in patients with diabetes.
Enalapril, Enalaprilat IV injection *(Vasotec, Epaned)* Tablet, Solution, Injection	10-40 mg in 1-2 divided doses	**WARNINGS** Angioedema (if occurs, do not use); avoid concomitant use with an ARB or aliskiren due to increased risk of hypotension, hyperkalemia, and renal dysfunction; avoid concomitant use with aliskiren in patients with GFR < 60 mL/min; renal impairment; hypotension can occur upon initiation in patients who are salt- or volume-depleted (e.g., those treated with high-dose diuretics) – correct volume depletion prior to administration; rare: cholestatic jaundice and hepatic failure.
Fosinopril	10-40 mg daily	
Lisinopril *(Prinivil, Zestril)*	5-40 mg daily	
Moexipril *(Univasc)*	3.75-30 mg in 1-2 divided doses Take on an empty stomach	**SIDE EFFECTS** Cough, hyperkalemia, hypotension, dizziness and headache. Captopril has more SEs (taste perversion, rash).
Perindopril *(Aceon)*	4-8 mg daily in 1-2 divided doses	**MONITORING** BP, K+, SCr, BUN
Quinapril *(Accupril)*	10-40 mg daily	**NOTES** Pregnancy Category D
Ramipril *(Altace)*	2.5-20 mg daily	Patients inadequately treated with once daily dosing may be treated with twice daily dosing.
Trandolapril *(Mavik)*	2-8 mg daily	

Angiotensin Receptor Blockers (ARBs)

ARBs block angiotensin II from binding to the angiotensin II type-1 (AT₁) receptor on vascular smooth muscle, preventing vasoconstriction. ARBs have been shown to slow progression of renal disease in patients with diabetes and/or hypertension who have albuminuria; they also slow progression of heart failure.

[handwritten box at bottom: ✱ Sodium polystyrene sulfonate (Kayexalate®) – for tx of hyper K+]

DRUG	DOSING	SAFETY/SIDE EFFECTS/MONITORING
Valsartan *(Diovan)*	80-320 mg daily	**BOXED WARNING** Can cause injury and death to developing fetus; discontinue as soon as pregnancy is detected.
Losartan *(Cozaar)*	25-100 mg in 1-2 divided doses	**CONTRAINDICATIONS** Angioedema. Do not use in bilateral renal artery stenosis since renal function will worsen. Do not use concurrently with aliskiren in patients with diabetes.
Irbesartan *(Avapro)*	150-300 mg daily	**WARNINGS** Angioedema (if occurs, do not use); avoid concomitant use with an ACE inhibitor or aliskiren due to increased risk of hypotension, hyperkalemia, and renal dysfunction; avoid concomitant use with
Candesartan *(Atacand)*	8-32 mg daily	aliskiren in patients with GFR < 60 mL/min; renal impairment; hypotension can occur upon initiation in patients who are salt- or volume-depleted (e.g., those treated with high-dose diuretics) – correct volume depletion prior to administration.
Olmesartan *(Benicar)*	20-40 mg daily	Olmesartan only: Sprue-like enteropathy – severe, chronic diarrhea with substantial weight loss has been reported in patients taking olmesartan months to years after drug initiation.
Telmisartan *(Micardis)*	40-80 mg daily	**SIDE EFFECTS** Hyperkalemia, hypotension, dizziness and headache
Eprosartan *(Teveten)*	400-800 mg in 1-2 divided doses	**MONITORING** BP, K+, SCr, BUN
Azilsartan *(Edarbi)*	40-80 mg daily	**NOTES** Pregnancy Category D Azilsartan: keep in original container

(handwritten note next to Olmesartan: Sprue-like enteropathy →)

(handwritten note under Azilsartan: keep in original container)

RAAS Inhibitor Drug Interactions

- All RAAS inhibitors ↑ the risk of hyperkalemia. Monitor K+ and renal function frequently.

- Dual inhibition of the renin-angiotensin system leads to increased risks of renal impairment, hypotension, and hyperkalemia; avoid.

- Patients with hypertension should not routinely use agents that can cause Na+ and H$_2$O retention, such as NSAIDs, COX-2 inhibitors or corticosteroids.

- RAAS inhibitors can ↓ lithium's renal clearance and ↑ the risk of toxicity.

ALTERNATIVE AGENTS FOR TREATING HYPERTENSION

Potassium-Sparing Diuretics

Potassium-sparing diuretics are not as effective and are not used as monotherapy for reducing BP, however, they are commonly used in combination with HCTZ *(Maxzide/Dyazide)* to counter thiazide's mild potassium loss and help (a little) with BP. If any potassium-retaining agent is used, there will be a risk of hyperkalemia, especially with reduced renal function. Spironolactone and eplerenone are used for HF (and HTN) and ↑ K+ is a considerable risk with these agents.

Spironolactone is a non-selective aldosterone receptor blocker (also blocks androgen). Eplerenone is a selective aldosterone receptor blocker and does not exhibit the endocrine side effects. These agents compete with aldosterone at the receptor sites in the distal convoluted tubule and collecting ducts of the nephron, increasing Na+ and water excretion while conserving K+ and H+ ions.

(handwritten left margin: both used for HF & HTN • compete w/ aldost. in DCT and coll. ducts ⇒ Na+/H₂O excretion; K+/H+ retention)

DRUG	DOSING	SAFETY/SIDE EFFECTS/MONITORING
AMILoride (Midamor)	5-20 mg daily	**BOXED WARNINGS** Tumor risk with spironolactone; tumorigenic in chronic rat toxicity studies. Avoid unnecessary use. **CONTRAINDICATIONS** Anuria, significant renal impairment, hyperkalemia (Addison's disease or other conditions that ↑ K+), concomitant use with K+-sparing diuretics.
Triamterene (Dyrenium) + HCTZ (Maxzide, Maxzide-25, Dyazide) *(handwritten: 75/50 mg)*	37.5 mg/25 mg daily – BID *(handwritten: ↳ HCTZ component above usual effective max → ↓↓K+, ↑↑BG, UA)* *(handwritten: 37.5/25 mg)*	For eplerenone: concomitant use of strong 3A4 inhibitors, type 2 diabetes with microalbuminuria, SCr > 2 mg/dL in males, SCr > 1.8 mg/dL in females, CrCl < 50 mL/min
Spironolactone (Aldactone) *(handwritten: nonselective)*	HF: 12.5-25 mg daily, max 50 mg daily HTN: 25-100 mg in 1-2 divided doses	**SIDE EFFECTS** Hyperkalemia, ↑ serum creatinine, dizziness. For eplerenone, ↑ TGs. For spironolactone: gynecomastia, breast tenderness, impotence, irregular menses, amenorrhea. Rare for all: hyperchloremic metabolic acidosis.
Eplerenone (Inspra) *(handwritten: selective)*	HF: 25-50 mg daily *(handwritten: SE:)* HTN: 50-100 mg daily *(handwritten: ↑TG)*	**MONITORING** Pregnancy Category C Check K+ before starting and frequently thereafter; BP, electrolytes, SCr/BUN, fluid status (input and output, weight)

(handwritten below table: # ① strong 3A4 inhib ② DM2 + microalbuminuria ③ SrCr > 2 ♂ > 1.8 ♀   ④ CrCl <50) ②-④ specific for HTN)

K+-Sparing Diuretic Drug Interactions

- Eplerenone is a CYP 3A4 substrate; use with strong 3A4 inhibitors is contraindicated.

- Potassium-sparing diuretics have a risk of hyperkalemia. Monitor K+ and renal function frequently and be careful of other medications that can increase potassium (see Drug Interactions chapter).

Beta Blocking Agents

Beta blockers are no longer recommended as first-line agents for uncomplicated hypertension unless the patient has a condition where these agents are recommended first-line (e.g., S/P MI, HF, others). Beta blockers inhibit the effects of catecholamines (especially norepinephrine) at the beta-1 and beta-2 adrenergic receptors, causing BP and HR reduction. Beta blockers with intrinsic sympathomimetic activity (ISA) partially stimulate beta receptors while blocking against additional stimulation and are contraindicated in S/P MI patients. These agents are carteolol, acebutolol, penbutolol, and pindolol (CAPP).

(handwritten: !SA ① carteolol ② acebutolol ③ penbutolol ④ pindolol   CART - ACE   PEN - PIND)

DRUG	DOSING	SAFETY/SIDE EFFECTS/MONITORING

Beta-1 Selective Blockers

DRUG	DOSING	SAFETY/SIDE EFFECTS/MONITORING
Acebutolol (Sectral) preg B	200-600 mg in 1-2 divided doses	**BOXED WARNING** Beta blockers should not be withdrawn abruptly (particularly in patients with CAD), gradually taper over 1-2 weeks to avoid acute tachycardia, HTN, and/or ischemia. **CONTRAINDICATIONS** Sinus bradycardia, 2nd or 3rd degree heart block, sick sinus syndrome (unless patient has a functioning artificial pacemaker) or cardiogenic shock. Do not initiate in patients with active asthma exacerbation.
Esmolol (Brevibloc) Injection	0.5-1 mg/kg bolus followed by 50-150 mcg/kg/min infusion, titrate as needed	
Atenolol (Tenormin) preg D	25-100 mg daily	**WARNINGS** Caution in patients with diabetes particularly with recurrent hypoglycemia, asthma, severe COPD or peripheral vascular disease and Raynaud's disease. May mask signs of hyperthyroidism; may aggravate psychiatric conditions
Betaxolol	5-20 mg daily	**SIDE EFFECTS** ↓ HR, hypotension, fatigue, dizziness, depression, ↓ libido, impotence, hyperglycemia (non-selective agents can ↓ insulin secretion in type 2 diabetes), hypoglycemia (more common with non-selective agents), hypertriglyceridemia, ↓ HDL
Bisoprolol (Zebeta)	2.5-20 mg daily	**MONITORING** HR, BP, titrate every 2 weeks (as tolerated); ↓ dose if HR < 55 **NOTES** Avoid abrupt discontinuation – must taper
Metoprolol tartrate (Lopressor), Metoprolol succinate extended release (Toprol XL) Tablet, Injection	IR: 100-450 mg in 2-3 divided doses XL: 25-100 mg daily; max dose 400 mg daily HF: Start 12.5-25 mg extended release daily (target 200 mg XL daily)	Take metoprolol immediate-release tablets with food. Metoprolol extended-release tablets are taken without regard to meals. Pregnancy Category B (acebutolol)/C/D (atenolol) Caution: Metoprolol IV is not equivalent to oral doses (IV:PO ratio is 1:2.5) Beta-1 selective agents – AMEBBA – Atenolol, Metoprolol, Esmolol, Bisoprolol, Betaxolol, Acebutolol

(handwritten margin notes: IR - w/ food, XL - w/o food, Lopressor (p.663) $\frac{IV}{PO} = \frac{1}{2.5}$*)*

Beta-1 Blocker and Produces Nitric Oxide-Dependent Vasodilation

DRUG	DOSING	SAFETY/SIDE EFFECTS/MONITORING
Nebivolol (Bystolic)	5-10 mg daily; max 40 mg daily With a CrCl < 30 mL/min or moderate liver impairment, start at 2.5 mg daily	**CONTRAINDICATIONS** Same as above plus severe liver impairment **WARNINGS** Same as above **SIDE EFFECTS** Headache, fatigue, dizziness, diarrhea, nausea, bradycardia, hypertriglyceridemia, ↓ HDL **NOTES** Nitric oxide causes peripheral vasodilation; clinical benefit unclear Pregnancy Category C

(handwritten margin note: CAUTION w/ 2D6 inhibitors!*)*

Beta Blockers Continued

DRUG	DOSING	SAFETY/SIDE EFFECTS/MONITORING

Beta-1 and Beta-2 Blockers (non-selective)

DRUG	DOSING	SAFETY/SIDE EFFECTS/MONITORING
Nadolol *(Corgard)*	40-320 mg daily	**NOTES** Propranolol has high lipid solubility (lipophilic); therefore, it is associated with more CNS side effects since it crosses the blood brain barrier. CNS side effects include sedation, depression, cognitive effects and others.
Penbutolol *(Levatol)*	10-80 mg daily	
Pindolol	10-60 mg/day	Pregnancy Category C
Propranolol *(Inderal LA, InnoPran XL)*	40-640 mg/day	
Capsule, Tablet, Solution, Injection		
Timolol	10-60 mg/day	

used for migraine prophylaxis, stage fright, essential tremor

Alpha-1 and Non-selective Beta Blocker

DRUG	DOSING	SAFETY/SIDE EFFECTS/MONITORING
Labetalol *(Trandate)* Tablet, Injection	100-1,200 mg BID	Used commonly in the hospital setting Pregnancy Category C

α₁

Non-selective Alpha- and Beta-Blockers

DRUG	DOSING	SAFETY/SIDE EFFECTS/MONITORING
Carvedilol *(Coreg, Coreg CR)* Tablet, Capsule (XR)	HTN: Start IR 6.25 mg BID (max: 25 mg BID) or CR 20 mg daily (max: 80 mg daily) HF: Start IR 3.125 mg BID (max 50 mg BID if > 85 kg; 25 mg BID if ≤ 85 kg) or CR 10 mg/day (max 80 mg)	**CONTRAINDICATIONS** Same as above **SIDE EFFECTS** Same plus weight gain and edema **NOTES** Take all forms of carvedilol with food Pregnancy Category C Carvedilol CR has less bioavailability than carvedilol IR, therefore, dose conversions are not 1:1. Dosing conversion from *Coreg* to *Coreg CR*: *Coreg* 3.125 mg BID = *Coreg CR* 10 mg daily *Coreg* 6.25 mg BID = *Coreg CR* 20 mg daily *Coreg* 12.5 mg BID = *Coreg CR* 40 mg daily *Coreg* 25 mg BID = *Coreg CR* 80 mg daily

w/ food

2D6!
(rifampin ↓ [carvedilol])

↑ [digoxin, CsA]
=) dose adjust!

to ↓ absorption =) ↓ dizziness

Beta Blocker Drug Interactions

- Beta blockers can enhance the hypoglycemic effects of insulin and sulfonylureas. Non-selective beta blockers can ↓ insulin secretion in type 2 diabetes. Monitor blood glucose in patients with diabetes.

- Beta blockers, particularly the non-selective agents, can mask the symptoms of hypoglycemia (e.g., shakiness, palpitations, anxiety). Sweating and hunger are symptoms that are not masked.

Sx of hypo BG
masked ← → NOT masked
shakiness   sweating
palpitations   hunger
anxiety

- Use caution when administering other drugs that slow HR; see Drug Interactions chapter.

- Carvedilol is a substrate of CYP 2D6; 2D6 inhibitors may increase carvedilol levels and rifampin may decrease carvedilol levels.

- Carvedilol can ↑ digoxin and cyclosporine levels; may require dose adjustments.

- Nebivolol should be used with caution in patients taking 2D6 inhibitors.

angiotensinogen renin → ang I ⇒ ↓ ang II

Direct Renin Inhibitor (DRI)

Aliskiren directly inhibits renin which is responsible for the conversion of angiotensinogen to angiotensin I (Ang I). A decrease in the formation of Ang I results in a decrease in the formation of Ang II, a potent vasoconstrictor.

DRUG	DOSING	SAFETY/SIDE EFFECTS/MONITORING
Aliskiren *(Tekturna)*	150-300 mg daily Avoid high fat foods (reduces absorption) Take with or without food and take the same way each day. Protect from moisture.	**BOXED WARNING** Can cause injury and death to developing fetus; discontinue as soon as pregnancy is detected. **CONTRAINDICATIONS** Angioedema. Do not use in bilateral renal artery stenosis since renal function will worsen. Do not use concurrently with ACE inhibitors or ARBs in patients with diabetes. **WARNINGS** Angioedema (if occurs, do not use); avoid concomitant use with ACE inhibitors or ARBs in patients with GFR < 60 mL/min due to ↑ risk of renal failure and hyperkalemia; hypotension can occur upon initiation in patients who are salt- or volume-depleted (e.g., those treated with high-dose diuretics) – correct volume depletion prior to administration. **SIDE EFFECTS** ↑ SCr and BUN, hyperkalemia, diarrhea, hypotension. **MONITORING** BP, K⁺, SCr, BUN **NOTES** Pregnancy Category D

3A4 inhibitors
CsA
itraconazole } ↑ [aliskiren]

aliskiren ↓ [furosemide]

Direct Renin Inhibitor Drug Interactions

- Aliskiren is metabolized by CYP 3A4; concentration is affected by 3A4 inducers and inhibitors. Do not use with cyclosporine or itraconazole due to increased aliskiren levels.

- Aliskiren ↓ the level of furosemide; monitor effectiveness.

Centrally-Acting Alpha-2 Adrenergic Agonists

These agents stimulate alpha-2 adrenergic receptors in the brain which results in reduced sympathetic outflow from the CNS. Clonidine is used commonly for resistant hypertension and in patients who can not swallow (due to dysphagia, dementia) since it comes as a patch formulation. Since the patch is changed weekly, it can help with adherence.

[handwritten left margin: resistant HTN]

DRUG	DOSING	SAFETY/SIDE EFFECTS/MONITORING
CloNIDine *(Catapres, Catapres-TTS patch, Duraclon inj)* Kapvay – for ADHD Tablet, Patch, Injection *[handwritten: used in dysphagia/dementia]*	0.1-0.3 mg BID *[handwritten: BUT q wk patch]* Catapres-TTS-1 = 0.1 mg/24 hr Catapres-TTS-2 = 0.2 mg/24 hr Catapres-TTS-3 = 0.3 mg/24 hr	**CONTRAINDICATIONS – Methyldopa only** Active liver disease, concurrent use with MAO-I **SIDE EFFECTS** Dry mouth, somnolence, headache, fatigue, dizziness, constipation, bradycardia, hypotension, depression, behavioral changes, sexual dysfunction; skin rash, pruritus, erythema, contact dermatitis – with patch
GuanFACINE *(Tenex)* Intuniv – for ADHD	0.5-2 mg daily	For methyldopa: same side effects as above plus hypersensitivity reactions, hepatitis, myocarditis, positive Coombs test (risk for hemolytic anemia), drug-induced fever, drug-induced lupus erythematosus (DILE) and can ↑ prolactin levels. **MONITORING** BP, HR, mental status
Methyldopa Tablet, Injection *[handwritten: SE: ① hypersens. rxns ② hepatitis ③ myocarditis ④ + Coombs test (risk for hemolytic anemia) ⑤ drug-induced fever ⑥ " " lupus ⑦ ↑ prolactin]*	250 mg BID-TID; max 3 grams/day	**NOTES** Clonidine patch is applied weekly. Apply patch to a hairless area on upper, outer arm or on upper chest. Place white round adhesive cover over patch to hold it in place. Rotate application site. Remove patch before MRI. Dispose of safely, away from children and pets. Rebound hypertension (with sweating/anxiety/tremors), if stopped abruptly (less likely with the patches). Do not stop abruptly, must taper. Pregnancy Category B (methyldopa oral, guanfacine)/C (methyldopa injectable, clonidine)

Direct Vasodilators

Cause direct vasodilation of arterioles with little effect on veins causing a decrease in systemic vascular resistance and a reduction in BP.

DRUG	DOSING	SAFETY/SIDE EFFECTS/MONITORING
HydrALAZINE Tablet, Injection	10-50 mg PO QID (max 300 mg/day) 10-20 mg IV Q4-6H PRN	**WARNING** Drug-induced lupus erythematosus (DILE – dose and duration related) **SIDE EFFECTS** Headache, reflex tachycardia, palpitations **MONITORING** HR, BP
Minoxidil *Rogaine* – OTC topical for hair growth	2.5-10 mg/day	**SIDE EFFECTS** Fluid retention, tachycardia, aggravation of angina, pericardial effusion, hair growth

Alpha Blockers

Alpha blockers bind to alpha-1 adrenergic receptors which results in vasodilation of arterioles and veins; not first-line therapy for HTN.

DRUG	DOSING	SAFETY/SIDE EFFECTS/MONITORING
Prazosin (Minipress)	1-5 mg BID-TID	**WARNINGS** Can cause significant orthostatic hypotension and syncope, especially with the first dose, restarting the dose, rapidly ↑ the dose, or initiation with another antihypertensive agent or PDE-5 inhibitor
Terazosin (Hytrin)	1-2 mg QHS	Intraoperative floppy iris syndrome has occurred in cataract surgery patients who were on or were previously treated with an alpha-1 blocker
Doxazosin (Cardura, Cardura XL)	1-2 mg daily	Priapism **SIDE EFFECTS** Dizziness, fatigue, headache, fluid retention

Hypertensive Urgencies and Emergencies

	URGENCY: NOT LIFE-THREATENING	EMERGENCY: POTENTIALLY LIFE-THREATENING
Definition	BP (generally ≥ 180/110-120) without acute target organ damage	BP (generally ≥ 180/110-120) with acute target organ damage (such as encephalopathy, MI, unstable angina, pulmonary edema, eclampsia, stroke, aortic dissection, etc).
Treatment	Any oral medication with an onset of action within 15-30 minutes; reduce BP gradually over 24-48 hrs.	Reduce MAP or BP by no more than 25% (within the first hour), then if stable, to 160/100-110 mmHg within the next 2-6 hours. Use IV medications such as hydralazine, labetalol, sodium nitroprusside, nicardipine, or others.

[handwritten left margin] ≥ 180 / 110-120 - organ damage

[handwritten right margin] ≥ 180 / 110-120 + organ damage · ↓ bp to 160 / 100-110 over 2-6 hrs

[handwritten note] DOC: IV nitroglycerin ↓ effective antiHTN + anti-ischemic more rapid ↓bp ⇒ ischemia (organ damage)

Patient Counseling

All Hypertension Medications

- Hypertension often has no symptoms, so you may not even feel that you have high blood pressure. Continue using this medicine as directed, even if you feel well. You may need to use blood pressure medication for the rest of your life to prevent complications such as kidney damage, stroke and heart attack.

- To be sure this medication is helping your condition, your blood pressure will need to be checked on a regular basis. It is important that you do not miss any scheduled visits to your healthcare provider.

- This medicine is only part of a complete program of treatment for hypertension that also includes diet, exercise, and weight control. Follow your diet, medication, and exercise routines very closely.

- You may have been instructed to check your blood pressure at home. Record the measurements in a notebook for your provider to see.

Diuretics

- This medication will cause you to urinate more throughout the day. This is expected from your medication. If you require 2 doses per day, be sure to take your 2nd dose no later than 4 P.M. to avoid getting up at night to urinate.

- This medicine may make you feel dizzy and lightheaded when getting up from a sitting or lying position. Get up slowly. Let your feet hang over the bed for a few minutes before getting up. Hang on to the bed or nearby dresser when standing from a sitting position.

[handwritten bottom] * nitroprusside - cyanide and thiocyanate toxicity

- Be sure that all objects are off the floor as you make your way to the bathroom. It is best to have a clear path to prevent falls.

- Potassium supplements may be needed while you are on this medication to ensure you have enough potassium for your heart. (Do not include if counseling on potassium-sparing diuretics.)

- If you have diabetes, your blood sugar may have to be monitored more frequently in the beginning as this medication can affect your blood sugar.

ACE Inhibitors, ARBs, and Aliskiren

- Do not use this medicine without telling your healthcare provider if you are pregnant or planning a pregnancy. This medicine could cause birth defects if you take the medication during pregnancy. Use an effective form of birth control. Stop using this medication and tell your healthcare provider right away if you become pregnant during treatment.

- Take the missed dose as soon as you remember. If it is almost time for your next dose, skip the missed dose and take the medicine at the next regularly scheduled time. Do not take extra medicine to make up the missed dose.

- Do not use salt substitutes or potassium supplements while taking this medication, unless your healthcare provider has told you to do so. Be careful of your potassium intake.

- Get emergency medical help if you have any of these signs of an allergic reaction: hives; difficulty breathing; swelling of your face, lips, tongue, or throat.

- Tell your healthcare provider if you develop a bothersome, dry occasional cough while taking this medicine (with ACE inhibitors only).

Beta Blockers

- Remember to take at the same time every day.

- This medication can cause a few side effects, including dizziness and fatigue, and can rarely cause sexual problems. If the side effects bother you, please let your healthcare provider know.

- Do not skip doses. If you miss a dose, take the missed dose as soon as you remember. If it is almost time for your next dose, skip the missed dose and take the medicine at the next regularly scheduled time. Do not take extra medicine to make up the missed dose.

TAPER!
- Do not discontinue your medication without consulting your physician. Stopping this medicine suddenly may make your condition worse.

- Contact your healthcare provider if you experience any difficulty in breathing (for non-selective beta-blockers).

- If taking carvediolol (Coreg/Coreg CR), take with food.

- If taking immediate-release metoprolol (Lopressor), take with food.

Calcium Channel Blockers

↓ risk of stroke, MI

- This medication relaxes your blood vessels and helps lower your blood pressure. This will decrease your risk of having a stroke or heart attack.

- This medication can cause a few side effects, including swelling of the ankles, tiredness, dizziness, headache, hot or warm feeling in your face, and irregular or fast heart beat.

- Do not start any new prescription or non-prescription medicines or supplements unless you check with your healthcare provider first.

- Adalat CC, Afeditab CR and Nifediac CC should be taken on an empty stomach.

- Avoid grapefruit and grapefruit juice while taking this medication.

Clonidine

- Do not stop clonidine suddenly; this can cause your blood pressure to become dangerously high. Make sure you do not run out of medicine.

- Clonidine can cause a variety of side effects, including sedation, dizziness, fatigue, dry mouth, and can aggravate depression and contribute to sexual dysfunction. If the side effects bother you, please let your healthcare provider know.

- The clonidine patch (Catapres-TTS) is changed weekly: Apply the patch to a hairless area of the skin on the upper outer arm or chest every 7 days. Do not use on broken or irritated skin. After 7 days, remove the used patch and apply a new patch to a different area than the previous site to avoid skin irritation.

- This patch will need to be removed before a MRI.

- When removing the patch, be sure to discard of safely, away from the reach of any children or pets.

PRACTICE CASE

FP is a 58 y/o black male at the clinic today for a routine follow-up visit. His past medical history includes hypertension and chronic lower back pain. He states that he feels fine except for his back pain and does not understand why he has to take any other medications. His diet consists of mostly processed and pre-packaged foods. He is a non-smoker and does not drink alcohol.

Allergies: NKDA

Medications:
Lortab 1-2 tabs PRN pain NTE 8 tabs/day
Prinzide 20/25 mg 1 tab daily

Vitals:
BP: 162/95 mmHg   HR: 88 BPM   RR: 18 BPM   Temp: 38°C   Pain: 3/10

Labs: Na (mEq/L) = 141 (135 - 145)
K (mEq/L) = 3.8 (3.5 - 5)
Cl (mEq/L) = 100 (95 - 103)
HCO_3 (mEq/L) = 27 (24 - 30)
BUN (mg/dL) = 35 (7 - 20)
SCr (mg/dL) = 1.2 (0.6 - 1.3)
Glucose (mg/dL) = 180 (100 - 125)
Ca (mg/dL) = 9.1 (8.5 - 10.5)
Mg (mEq/L) = 1.7 (1.3 - 2.1)
PO_4 (mg/dL) = 4.1 (2.3 - 4.7)

Reinforce disease state education and adjust medication.

Questions

18-59 y/o or DM or CKD ⇒ goal < 140/90

* 1. Which of the following medication combinations is *Prinzide*?

    a. Benazepril and hydrochlorothiazide
    b. Enalapril and hydrochlorothiazide
    c. Irbesartan and hydrochlorothiazide
    d. Lisinopril and hydrochlorothiazide
    e. Triamterene and hydrochlorothiazide

2. FP has a risk factor for developing angioedema. Which of the following increases his risk of angioedema?

    a. Age
    b. Gender
    c. Ethnicity
    d. Concurrent medications
    e. Electrolyte profile

3. FP needs better BP control. Which of the following medications would be the best recommendation to add to his profile?

    a. *Lasix* furosemide
    b. *Zaroxolyn* metolazone
    c. *Hytrin* terazosin
    d. *Avalide* irbesartan / HCTZ
    e. *Norvasc*

Questions 4-9 do not apply to the above case.

4. What is the mechanism of action for *Bystolic*? (Select **ALL** that apply.)

    a. Beta-2 selective blocker
    b. Beta-1 selective blocker
    c. Increases nitric oxide production
    d. Alpha-1 selective blocker
    e. Alpha-2 agonist

5. Choose the correct statement(s) concerning *Coreg CR*: (Select **ALL** that apply.)

    a. The generic name is nebivolol.
    b. The starting dose for hypertension is 12.5 mg BID. 6.25 mg BID
    c. The drug is a non-selective beta and alpha blocker.
    d. The drug decreases heart rate.
    e. The drug should be taken without food.

6. Shantal is a 62 year old black female who comes to the clinic for a regular check up. She has chronic kidney disease with proteinuria and is taking *Accupril* 20 mg daily. Her 3 BP readings on this visit are 143/93, 149/91 and 146/95. What would be the best recommendation to make at this time?

    a. Discontinue her *Accupril* and start *Norvasc*.
    b. Add on *Diovan*.
    c. Add on hydrochlorothiazide
    d. Discontinue her *Accupril* and start *Trandate*
    e. No additional medication is needed at this time.

7. A patient comes in with a new prescription for *Exforge*. Which of the following medications are the correct match for this prescription?

    a. Aliskiren and hydrochlorothiazide
    b. Aliskiren and valsartan
    c. Amlodipine and benazepril
    d. Valsartan, amlodipine, and hydrochlorothiazide
    e. Amlodipine and valsartan

8. A patient develops angioedema while taking *Altace*. Which of the following medications would be a safe, alternative agent to use for BP control?

    a. *Maxzide*
    b. *Atacand*
    c. *Lotrel* ⎫ benazepril
    d. *Lotensin* ⎭
    e. *Tekturna*

9. Which one of the following beta-blockers has intrinsic sympathomimetic activity (ISA)?

    a. Atenolol   carteolol
    b. Acebutolol acebutolol
    c. Carvedilol pindolol
    d. Timolol   penbutolol
    e. Nadolol

Answers
1-d, 2-c, 3-e, 4-b,c, 5-c,d, 6-c, 7-e, 8-a, 9-b

DYSLIPIDEMIA

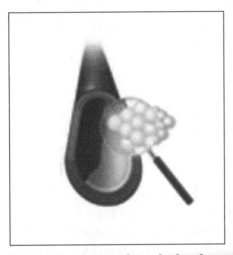

We gratefully acknowledge the assistance of Joel C. Marrs, PharmD, FCCP, FNLA, BCPS-AQ Cardiology, BCACP, CLS, Associate Professor at the University of Colorado Skaggs School of Pharmacy and Pharmaceutical Sciences and Eric Gupta, PharmD, FNLA, BCPS, CLS, Associate Professor at Western University of Health Sciences, in preparing this chapter.

BACKGROUND

Cholesterol is needed for cell membrane formation and function, hormone synthesis, and fat soluble vitamin production. Production of cholesterol occurs in the liver, intestines, adrenal glands, and reproductive organs and it is absorbed from certain foods including dairy products (whole milk), eggs, meat, and many types of prepared food. Cholesterol is recycled; the liver excretes cholesterol in a non-esterified form (via bile) in the digestive tract, of which 50% gets reabsorbed back into the bloodstream. Lipids, being water immiscible, are not present in the free form in the plasma, but rather circulate as lipoproteins. Abnormalities of plasma lipoproteins can result in a predisposition to coronary, cerebrovascular, and peripheral arterial and are a major risk factor for the development of

GUIDELINES/REFERENCES

Stone NJ, Robinson JG, Lichtenstein AH, et al. 2013 ACC/AHA Guideline on the Treatment of Blood Cholesterol to Reduce Atherosclerotic Cardiovascular Risk in Adults: A Report of the American College of Cardiology/ American Heart Association Task Force on Practice Guidelines. *Circulation.* 2014; 129:S1-S45.

Eckel RH, Jakicic JM, Ard JD, et al. 2013 AHA/ACC guideline on lifestyle management to reduce cardiovascular risk: a report of the American College of Cardiol-

ogy/American Heart Association Task Force on Practice Guidelines. *Circulation.* 2014; 129 (25 Suppl 2):S76-99.

Jacoboson TA, Ito MK, Maki KC, et al. National Lipid Association Recommendations for Patient-Centered Management of Dyslipidemia: Part 1 - Executive Summary. *J Clin Lipidol.* 2014; 8(5):473-488.

Goff Jr DC, Lloyd-Jones DM, Bennett G, et al. 2013 ACC/AHA Guideline on the Assessment of Cardiovascular Risk. JACC, doi:10.1016/j.jacc.2013.11.005.

inflammation → thrombus formation → MI, CV events

coronary heart disease (CHD). Premature coronary atherosclerosis, leading to the manifestations of ischemic heart disease, is the most common and significant consequence of dyslipidemia. Other dyslipidemias can exist, including elevated triglycerides, which can cause acute pancreatitis.

CLASSIFICATION OF DYSLIPIDEMIA

↑total ↑TG
↑LDL ↓HDL

non HDL = total - HDL

Dyslipidemia refers to any lipoprotein disorder including ↑ total cholesterol (TC), ↑ low-density lipoprotein cholesterol (LDL-C), ↑ triglycerides (TGs) and/or ↓ high-density lipoprotein cholesterol (HDL-C). Non-high-density lipoprotein cholesterol (non-HDL-C) has emerged as a stronger predictor of atherosclerotic cardiovascular disease (ASCVD) than LDL-C and can be calculated from the values obtained in a traditional lipid panel. Non-HDL-C compromises cholesterol carried by all atherogenic particles, including LDL, intermediate density lipoproteins (IDL), very low-density lipoproteins (VLDL), chylomicron remnants and lipoprotein (a). Non-HDL-C = TC - HDL-C. Apolipoprotein B (apoB), present on all atherogenic particles, is another marker that may be used to assess atherogenic risk, after non-HDL-C and LDL-C.

Primary (or Familial)

- Familial dyslipidemias are classified according to the Fredrickson classification. Familial hypercholesterolemias (FH) are genetic defects resulting in severe cholesterol elevations and increased risk of premature ASCVD.

LDL = 200 - 300 (heterozygous)
LDL = 300 - 500 (homozygous, rare)

Secondary (or Acquired)

- Acquired dyslipidemias mimic primary forms of dyslipidemia and can have similar consequences. Some common causes of secondary dyslipidemia are listed in the table below. Secondary causes of severe elevations of LDL-C ≥ 190 mg/dL and triglycerides ≥ 500 mg/dL often contribute to the magnitude of the dyslipidemia and should be evaluated and treated appropriately.

Secondary Causes of Dyslipidemia

SECONDARY CAUSE	↑ LDL	↑ TRIGLYCERIDES
Diet	Saturated or *trans* fats, weight gain, anorexia	Weight gain, very low-fat diets, high intake of refined carbohydrate, excessive alcohol intake
Drugs	Diuretics, cyclosporine, tacrolimus, glucocorticoids, amiodarone, some progestins, danazol, isotretinoin, thiazolidinediones, anabolic steroids, sodium-glucose cotransporter 2 inhibitors, fibric acids (with ↑ TGs), cyclosporine, protease inhibitors, atypical antipsychotics	Oral estrogen, glucocorticoids, bile acid sequestrants, protease inhibitors, retinoids, anabolic steroids, sirolimus, cyclosporine, tacrolimus, raloxifene, tamoxifen, beta blockers (not carvedilol), thiazides, atypical antipsychotics, alpha interferons, propofol
Diseases	Biliary obstruction, nephrotic syndrome	Nephrotic syndrome, chronic renal failure, lipodystrophies
Disorders and altered states of metabolism	Hypothyroidism, obesity, pregnancy, polycystic ovary syndrome	Diabetes (poorly controlled), hypothyroidism, obesity, pregnancy

acute pancreatitis

↑LDL and TG
1. cyclosporine
2. glucocorticoids
3. protease inhibitors
4. anabolic steroids
5. tacrolimus
6. atypical antipsych

Handwritten margin notes:
- 9-12 hr fast
- $LDL = total - HDL - \frac{TG}{5}$ DO NOT USE WHEN TG > 400 !!
- and LDL falsely ↓
- lovastatin

Cholesterol (Lipoprotein) Types and Normal Values

Many clinicians will recommend checking lipoprotein levels after a 9-12 hour fast (if patient did not fast, the TG level may be falsely elevated). LDL may need to be calculated if it is not given using the Friedewald equation: $LDL\text{-}C = TC - HDL\text{-}C - (TG/5)$. This formula can not be used when the TGs are > 400 mg/dL. Non-HDL-C and apo-B do not require fasting for accurate assessment.

Natural Products

Red yeast rice is the product of yeast grown on rice that contains naturally occurring HMG-CoA reductase inhibitors (statins) and is commercially available in capsules. The amount of statin in each product can vary. Both myalgias and myopathy have been reported with the use of the red yeast rice and it would be prudent to apply the same precautions, interactions and monitoring parameters that are recommended for statins. Garlic may have a very small beneficial effect on cholesterol. Over-the-counter fish oils (can be used to ↓ TGs in patients with TG ≥ 500 mg/dL) and plant sterols/stanols may provide additional benefit.

TREATING DYSLIPIDEMIAS ACCORDING TO ACC/AHA GUIDELINES

In November 2013, new national guidelines for the treatment of high cholesterol were released. While the previous ATP III guidelines focused on specific LDL and non-HDL cholesterol target goals, the new guidelines identify <u>four</u> key patient groups who should consider statin initiation with appropriate intensity to obtain relative reductions in LDL-C. The recommendations aim to simplify treatment guidelines based on evidence from large randomized controlled trials. Of note, <u>nonstatin therapies are not recommended unless statins are not tolerated</u>, and treating to specific LDL-C goals is no longer recommended.

CLASSIFICATIONS OF CHOLESTEROL & TRIGLYCERIDE LEVELS IN MG/DL

Non-HDL-C*

< 130	Desirable
130-159	Above desirable
160-189	Borderiine high
190-219	High
≥ 220	Very high

LDL-C

< 100	Desirable
100-129	Above desirable
130-159	Borderiine high
160-189	High
≥ 190	Very high

HDL-C

< 40 (men)	Low
< 50 (women)	Low

Triglycerides

< 150	Normal
150-199	Borderiine high
200-499	High
≥ 500	Very high†

HDL-C, high-density lipoprotein cholesterol; LDL-C, low-density lipoprotein cholesterol; non -HDL-C, non-high-density lipoprotein cholesterol

* Non-HDL-C = total cholesterol minus HDL-C.

† Severe hypertriglyceridemia is another term used for very high triglycerides in pharmaceutical product labeling.

clinical ASCVD (3 buckets):
① CHD : ACS, MI, angina, coronary revascularization * balloon angioplasty or stenting
② cerebral vascular dz : stroke, TIA
③ PAD

Identification of 4 Statin Benefit Groups

The following 4 groups of patients should be initiated on statin therapy:

1. Clinical atherosclerotic cardiovascular disease (ASCVD), including coronary heart disease (ACS, S/P MI, stable or unstable angina, coronary or other arterial revascularization), stroke, TIA, or peripheral arterial disease thought to be of atherosclerotic origin

2. Primary elevations of LDL-C ≥ 190 mg/dL

3. Diabetes and 40-75 years of age with LDL-C between 70-189 mg/dL

4. 40-75 years of age with LDL between 70-189 mg/dL and estimated 10-year ASCVD risk of ≥ 7.5% (using the Global Risk Assessment Tool)

Global Risk Assessment Tool

use do not ASCVD calculator in Hispanics

The race- and gender-specific Pooled Cohort Equations to predict 10-year risk for a first hard ASCVD event should be used in non-Hispanic African Americans and non-Hispanic whites, 40-79 years of age (other populations may be considered as well). This tool assesses the risk of an initial cardiovascular event in patients without ASCVD. The clinician inputs information on gender, age, race, total cholesterol, HDL-C, systolic blood pressure, whether antihypertensive treatment is used, presence of diabetes, and smoking status. A 10-year ASCVD score of ≥ 7.5% is an indication to start statin therapy in individuals between the age of 40-75 years of age. This risk assessment should be repeated every 4-6 years in persons who are found to be at low 10-year risk (< 7.5%). The tool can be downloaded and completed at: http://my.americanheart.org/cvriskcalculator.

KEY POINT

The new ACC/AHA guidelines state that there is no evidence to support continued use of specific LDL-C treatment targets. Statins (primarily), dosed at the appropriate intensity, are used in patients with ASCVD and patients at risk for ASCVD.

ADDITIONAL FACTORS* PER ACC/AHA GUIDELINES

If after quantitative risk assessment, a risk-based treatment decision is uncertain, additional factors may be considered to assist with decision making. These factors include:

- LDL ≥ 160 mg/dL or other evidence of genetic hyperlipidemia

- Family history of premature ASCVD with onset < 55 years in a first degree male relative or < 65 years in a first degree female relative

- High-sensitivity C-reactive protein ≥ 2 mg/L

- Coronary Artery Calcium score ≥ 300 Agatston units or ≥ 75 percentile for age, sex and ethnicity

- Ankle Brachial Index < 0.9

* These factors support revising risk assessment upward

---

video   desirable levels ?? [15:00]

atherogenic cholesterol
{ LDL < 100
non-HDL < 130 (always 30 points > LDL)
TG < 150

↓ contain apo B (measurable marker)

HDL > 40 ♂ normal } HDL has
      > 50 ♀ normal } apo A on surface

Determining Appropriate Statin Treatment Intensity Based on Patient Risk

PREVENTION LEVEL	STATIN TREATMENT

Primary Prevention

Primary elevation of LDL ≥ 190 mg/dL	High-intensity*
Diabetes and 40-75 years with LDL between 70-189 mg/dL with estimated 10-year ASCVD risk < 7.5%	Moderate-intensity
Diabetes and 40-75 years with LDL between 70-189 mg/dL with estimated 10-year ASCVD risk ≥ 7.5%	High-intensity*
Ages 40-75 years with LDL between 70-189 mg/dL with estimated 10-year ASCVD risk < 7.5%	Consider risk benefit
Ages 40-75 years with LDL between 70-189 mg/dL with estimated 10-year ASCVD risk ≥ 7.5%	Moderate-to-high intensity

Secondary Prevention

Clinical atherosclerotic cardiovascular disease (ASCVD) ≤ 75 years	High-intensity*
Clinical atherosclerotic cardiovascular disease (ASCVD) > 75 years	Moderate-intensity

Use moderate-intensity statin if not candidate for high-intensity

Statin Therapy Intensity Definitions and Selection Options

HIGH-INTENSITY	MODERATE-INTENSITY	LOW-INTENSITY
DAILY DOSE ↓ LDL ≥ 50% Atorvastatin 40-80 mg daily	**DAILY DOSE ↓ LDL 30%-49%** Atorvastatin 10-20 mg daily	**DAILY DOSE ↓ LDL < 30%** Simvastatin 10 mg daily
Rosuvastatin 20-40 mg daily	Rosuvastatin 5-10 mg daily	Pravastatin 10-20 mg daily
	Simvastatin 20-40 mg daily	Lovastatin 20 mg daily
	Pravastatin 40-80 mg daily	Fluvastatin 20-40 mg daily
	Lovastatin 40 mg daily	Pitavastatin 1 mg daily
	Fluvastatin XL 80 mg daily	
	Fluvastatin 40 mg BID	
	Pitavastatin 2-4 mg daily	

(handwritten annotations:)

• MIRACL
• PROVE-IT
  TIM 22

high-intensity statin tx initiated w/in 96 hrs of hospitalization for ACS ⇒ ↓ recurrent ischemia
⇒ atorvastatin 80mg

Treating Dyslipidemias with the 2014 NLA Expert Panel Recommendations

In October 2014, the National Lipid Association (NLA) released their own cholesterol recommendations which reinstituted treating atherogenic cholesterol to predetermined goals. The focus was shifted from targeting to LDL cholesterol goals to non-HDL and LDL cholesterol as primary targets. The NLA recommendations are structured similarly to the ATP III guidelines with changes in the way risk for future ASCVD is determined. In general, statin therapy should be increased to the maximally tolerated dose before starting nonstatin therapies.

(handwritten annotations:)

statin potency (Robertson)

long t½

1. rosuvastatin (Crestor®)
2. atorvastatin (Lipitor®)
3. pitavastatin (Livalo®)
4. simvastatin (Zocor®)
5. pravastatin (Pravachol®) - minimal P450 interaxns

6. lovastatin (Mevacor®)
7. fluvastatin (Lescol®)

NON-DRUG THERAPY

Lifestyle modifications are an important part of dyslipidemia management. These recommendations apply to adults < 80 years old with and without ASCVD and should be emphasized, monitored and reinforced.

- Follow a healthy diet (such as DASH, USDA Food Pattern, or AHA) which emphasizes intake of vegetables, fruits, whole grains, low-fat dairy products, poultry, fish, legumes, nontropical vegetable oils and nuts while limiting intake of sweets, sugar-sweetened beverages and red meats. Modify diet as needed for appropriate calorie requirements, personal preferences and nutritional therapy for other medical conditions.

- Aim for 5-6% of calories from saturated fat; reduce % of calories from *trans* fat.

- Engage in aerobic physical activity 3-4 sessions per week, lasting 40 minutes/session and involving moderate-to-vigorous intensity (can reduce LDL-C 3-6 mg/dL).

- Maintain a healthy weight (BMI 18.5-24.9 kg/m²).

- Avoid tobacco products.

Please note these recommendations are different from the obesity guideline recommendations (see Weight Loss chapter for more information).

> ### MANAGEMENT OF MILD-TO-MODERATE MUSCLE SYMPTOMS ASSOCIATED WITH STATIN USE
>
> Discontinue the statin and evaluate symptoms
>
> Evaluate patient for other conditions that may increase the risk for muscle damage
>
> If muscle symptoms resolve, and if no contraindication, restart same statin at the same or lower dose
>
> If myalgias return, discontinue original statin. Once muscle symptoms resolve, use a low dose of a different statin
>
> If low dose of a different statin is tolerated, gradually increase the dose as tolerated

DRUG THERAPY

Statins are the drugs of choice in treating elevated non-HDL and LDL cholesterol and reducing ASCVD risk due to strong evidence from several randomized controlled trials. According to the ACC/AHA guidelines, the appropriate statin intensity is based on the patient's level of risk. The NLA recommendations use the same statin intensity concept as outlined in the ACC/AHA guidelines. In individuals who are candidates for statin therapy but are completely statin intolerant, it is reasonable to use nonstatin cholesterol-lowering drugs that have been shown to reduce ASCVD events in randomized controlled trials. Many of the drug classes used for cholesterol management are potentially hepatotoxic (statins, niacin, potentially fibrates and ezetimibe). Liver enzymes should be monitored and the drug stopped if AST (10 - 40 units/L) or ALT (10 - 40 units/L) become > 3 times the upper limit of normal. Increases in liver transaminases are similar to the general population; however, LFTs should be monitored at baseline and periodically thereafter. Newer agents, lomitapide and mipomersen, are effective in treating homozygous familial hypercholesterolemia (HoFH), which is a rare genetic disorder resulting in very high LDL-C levels. Although some of the statins are indicated for HoFH, they are only minimally effective and this condition usually requires additional lipid lowering therapies.

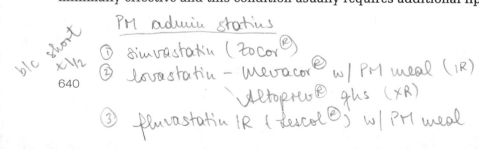

A new "lipid" drug not discussed in the drug tables is metreleptin (Myalept). This is a recombinant human leptin analog used as an adjunct to diet to treat the complications of leptin deficiency in patients with congenital or acquired generalized lipodystrophy. The drug may be a breakthrough for some patients with leptin deficiency, but due to safety issues (the development of antibodies to leptin and/or metreleptin and increased risk of lymphoma) metreleptin is not available outside of specialty pharmacies. It is obtained through a REMS distribution program.

[handwritten] pitavastatin - most potent on mg basis
[handwritten] rosuvastatin - most potent LDL reduction

STATINS

Statins inhibit the enzyme 3-hydroxy-3-methylglutaryl coenzyme A (HMG-CoA) reductase preventing the conversion of HMG-CoA to mevalonate (the rate-limiting step in cholesterol synthesis). Extensive evidence exists that the appropriate intensity of statin therapy be used to reduce ASCVD risk in those most likely to benefit.

DRUG	DOSING	SAFETY/SIDE EFFECTS/MONITORING
AtorvaSTATin (Lipitor) + amlodipine (Caduet) + ezetimibe (Liptruzet)	10-80 mg daily Equiv dose = 10 mg	**CONTRAINDICATIONS** Active liver disease (including any unexplained elevations in hepatic transaminases), pregnancy, breastfeeding; concurrent use of strong 3A4 inhibitors – with simvastatin and lovastatin; pitavastatin is contraindicated with cyclosporine use **WARNINGS**
Simvastatin (Zocor) + ezetimibe (Vytorin) + niacin (Simcor)	10-40 mg daily in the evening Equiv dose = 20 mg	Skeletal muscle effects (e.g., myopathy, rhabdomyolysis) – risk ↑ with higher doses and concomitant use of certain medicines. Predisposing factors include advanced age *[handwritten: due to ↓ metabolism?]* (≥ 65), female gender, uncontrolled hypothyroidism, vitamin D deficiency, and renal impairment. Patients should be advised to report promptly any unexplained and/or persistent muscle pain, tenderness, or weakness
Rosuvastatin (Crestor)	5-40 mg daily Equiv dose = 5 mg ✱ Most potent statin ✱	Immune-mediated necrotizing myopathy (IMNM) can occur in rare cases Diabetes – can ↑ A1C and fasting blood glucose; benefits of statin therapy far outweigh the risk of hyperglycemia
Pravastatin (Pravachol)	10-80 mg daily Equiv dose = 40 mg	Liver enzyme elevations in hepatic transaminases can occur (rare)
Lovastatin (Mevacor, Altoprev) + niacin (Advicor)	20-80 mg Mevacor (immediate release) is taken with evening meal Altoprev (extended release) is taken at bedtime Equiv dose = 40 mg	**SIDE EFFECTS** *[handwritten: check if pt develops sx of rhabdo]* Myalgias, arthralgias, myopathy, diarrhea, ↑ CPK, rhabdomyolysis (↑ risk with higher doses), cognitive impairment (memory loss, confusion – reversible), ↑ blood glucose, ↑ A1C, ↑ LFTs **MONITORING** LFTs at baseline and as clinically indicated thereafter; obtain a lipid panel 4-12 weeks after initiation or up titration of therapy to assess for medication adherence; then every 3-12 months thereafter *[handwritten: ✓ lipids 4-12 wks after start or ∆ then q3-12 mo]*
Fluvastatin (Lescol, Lescol XL)	20-80 mg Lescol is taken with evening meal Lescol XL is taken daily, anytime Equiv dose = 80 mg	**NOTES** Pregnancy Category X Can take Crestor, Lipitor, Livalo, Lescol XL and Pravachol at any time of day. Use lower doses if CrCl < 30 mL/min, except with Lipitor. With Livalo, use lower doses when CrCl < 60 mL/min. *[handwritten: any time admin Lipitor Crestor Livalo (pita) Pravachol Lescol XL (flu)]*
Pitavastatin (Livalo)	1-4 mg daily Equiv dose = 2 mg *[handwritten: ↓ dose if CrCl < 60]*	**Lipid Effects** ↓ LDL ~20-55%, ↑ HDL ~5-15%, ↓ TG ~10-30% *[handwritten: b/c long t½]*

[handwritten left margin notes:]
PM meal
IR - Mevacor® PM meal
XR - Altoprev® hs
Lescol® PM meal
Lescol® XL any time!
✗ w/ CsA

[handwritten bottom notes:]
equiv doses
PIT pitavastatin 2 mg
ROS rosuvastatin 5 mg
ATO atorvastatin 10 mg
SIM simvastatin 20 mg
PRA/LO oral lovastatin 40 mg
FLU fluvastatin 80 mg

PIT – ROS – ATO   SIM – PRA/LO – FLU
2   5   10   20   40   80mg

✱ lovastatin has 2 names
IR - Mevacor®
XR - Altoprev®

handwritten annotation: Statin + gemfibrozil / niacin ≥ 1 g / colchicine } ↑↑ myopathy, rhabdo

Statin Drug Interactions

All Statins

- Concomitant lipid-lowering therapies: use with fibrates (esp. gemfibrozil – which should be avoided with some statins including lovastatin, simvastatin, and rosuvastatin and used with caution with all other statins) and niacin products containing ≥ 1 gram ↑ the risk of myopathies.

- Cases of myopathy, including rhabdomyolysis, have been reported with statins coadministered with colchicine.

Simvastatin, Lovastatin & Atorvastatin

- *Simvastatin, *lovastatin and atorvastatin are major 3A4 substrates. Simvastatin and lovastatin undergo extensive first-pass metabolism by CYP 3A4. Atorvastatin undergoes less first-pass metabolism by 3A4; therefore, most 3A4 inhibitors cause a smaller ↑ in plasma concentration than with simvastatin and lovastatin.

- Simvastatin: do not initiate patients on simvastatin 80 mg/day due to ↑ risk of myopathy. Restrict use to patients already taking simvastatin 80 mg/day chronically (e.g., for 12 months or more) without evidence of muscle toxicity. Avoid with strong 3A4 inhibitors (see box). Do not exceed simvastatin 10 mg/day with verapamil, diltiazem or dronedarone. Do not exceed simvastatin 20 mg/day with amiodarone, amlodipine or ranolazine.

- Lovastatin: avoid with strong 3A4 inhibitors (see box). Do not exceed lovastatin 20 mg/day with danazol, diltiazem, dronedarone or verapamil. Do not exceed lovastatin 40 mg/day with amiodarone.

- Atorvastatin: avoid with cyclosporine, tipranavir plus ritonavir or telaprevir. Do not exceed atorvastatin 20 mg/day with clarithromycin, itraconazole, lopinavir + ritonavir, darunavir + ritonavir, fosamprenavir ± ritonavir, or saquinavir + ritonavir. Do not exceed atorvastatin 40 mg/day with nelfinavir and boceprevir.

- Digoxin levels may ↑ with these agents; monitor.

Rosuvastatin

- Rosuvastatin is a substrate of 2C9 (minor) and 3A4 (minor): may ↑ INR in patients taking warfarin; monitor PT/INR after initiation or dose change.

- Cyclosporine may ↑ rosuvastatin; do not exceed 5 mg/day of rosuvastatin.

- Ritonavir-boosted lopinavir or atazanavir: do not exceed 10 mg/day of rosuvastatin.

Pravastatin

- Cyclosporine can ↑ pravastatin; do not exceed pravastatin 20 mg/day.

STRONG 3A4 INHIBITORS – AVOID WITH SIMVASTATIN AND LOVASTATIN
Itraconazole
Ketoconazole
Posaconazole
Voriconazole
Erythromycin
Clarithromycin
Telithromycin
HIV protease inhibitors
Boceprevir
Telaprevir
Nefazodone
Cyclosporine
Gemfibrozil
Danazol (with simvastatin)
Grapefruit juice

- Clarithromycin can ↑ pravastatin; do not exceed pravastatin 40 mg/day.

Fluvastatin

- Fluvastatin inhibits 2C9 (moderate): may ↑ INR in patients taking warfarin; monitor.

- Cyclosporine and fluconazole can ↑ fluvastatin.

- Fluvastatin can enhance the levels of glyburide; monitor.

Pitavastatin

- Minimal CYP450 metabolism. Contraindicated with cyclosporine. Limit dose to 1 mg daily with erythromycin and 2 mg daily with rifampin. Monitor PT/INR after dose initiation or dose change of warfarin.

EZETIMIBE

Inhibits absorption of cholesterol at the brush border of the small intestine.

DRUG	DOSING	SAFETY/SIDE EFFECTS/MONITORING
Ezetimibe *(Zetia)* + simvastatin *(Vytorin)* + atorvastatin *(Liptruzet)*	10 mg daily If CrCl < 60 mL/min, do not exceed simvastatin 20 mg/day when using combination product *(Vytorin)*	**WARNINGS** Avoid use in moderate-or-severe hepatic impairment Skeletal muscle effects (e.g., myopathy, including risk of rhabdomyolysis), risk ↑ when combined with a statin **SIDE EFFECTS** URTIs, diarrhea, arthralgias, myalgias, pain in extremities, sinusitis **MONITORING** When used with a statin and/or fibrate, obtain LFTs at baseline and as clinically indicated thereafter **NOTES** Pregnancy Category C Clinical trials showed a ↓ in LDL, but no reduction in clinical outcomes **Lipid effects with ezetimibe monotherapy** ↓ LDL 18-23%, ↑ HDL 1-3%, ↓ TG 5-10%

rarely causes liver dysfxn on its own (↑ risk w/ statin)

Ezetimibe Drug Interactions

- When ezetimibe and cyclosporine are given together, the concentration of both can ↑; monitor levels of cyclosporine.

- Concomitant bile acid sequestrants ↓ ezetimibe; give ezetimibe 2 hours before or 4 hours after bile acid sequestrants.

- Can ↑ risk of cholelithiasis when used with fenofibrate; avoid use with gemfibrozil.

- If using warfarin, monitor INR/bleeding after dose initiation or dose change.

BILE ACID SEQUESTRANTS/BILE ACID BINDING RESINS

Binds bile acids in the intestine forming a complex that is excreted in the feces. This non-systemic action results in a partial removal of the bile acids from the enterohepatic circulation, preventing their reabsorption.

DRUG	DOSING	SAFETY/SIDE EFFECTS/MONITORING
Cholestyramine (*Questran, Questran Light, Prevalite*) Also approved for pruritus due to increased levels of bile acids, regression of arteriosclerosis 4 g powder packet	4 grams initially (max 24 g/day), divided BID with meals *pruritis associated w/ partial biliary obstruction*	**CONTRAINDICATIONS** Cholestyramine – Complete biliary obstruction Colesevelam – Bowel obstruction, TG > 500 mg/dL, history of hypertriglyceridemia-induced pancreatitis **SIDE EFFECTS** Constipation (may need dose reduction or laxative), dyspepsia, nausea, abdominal pain, cramping, gas, bloating, hypertriglyceridemia, esophageal obstruction, ↑ LFTs.
Colesevelam (*Welchol*) 625 mg tablet, 1.875 g and 3.75 g granule packet Also approved for DM Type 2 (↓ A1C~ 0.5%)	Tablets/granules: 3.75 grams daily or in divided doses with a meal and liquid	**NOTES** Pregnancy Category B (*Welchol*)/C (others) ACC/AHA guidelines do not recommend using these agents when TGs are ≥ 300 mg/dL. *b/c ↑ pancreatitis risk* Cholestyramine packet – Mix powder with 2-6 oz. water or non-carbonated liquid. Sipping or holding the resin suspension in the mouth for prolonged periods may lead to changes in the surface of the teeth resulting in discoloration, erosion of enamel or decay; good oral hygiene should be maintained.
Colestipol (*Colestid*) 1 g tablet, 5 g granule packet	Tablets: 2 g daily or BID (max 16 g/day) Granules: 5 g daily or BID (max 30 g/day)	Colesevelam packet – Empty 1 packet into a glass; add 4-8 oz. of water, fruit juice, or a diet soft drink and mix well. Colestipol packet - Empty 1 packet into at least 3 oz. of liquid and stir until completely mixed. **Lipid Effects** ↓ LDL ~10-30% ↑ HDL ~3-5% No change or ↑ TG (~5%)

Bile Acid Sequestrants Drug Interactions

- Colesevelam has less drug interactions than the other 2 bile acid sequestrants and is more commonly used. For cholestyramine or colestipol, separate all other drugs by 1-4 hours before or 4-6 hours after the bile acid sequestrants.

- The following medications should be taken 4 hours prior to colesevelam: cyclosporine, glimepiride, glipizide, glyburide, levothyroxine, olmesartan, phenytoin, and oral contraceptives containing ethinyl estradiol and norethindrone. Consider separation with other drugs as well. Colesevelam ↑ levels of metformin ER.

- With warfarin, monitor INR frequently during initiation and after dose change.

- Bile acid sequestrants may ↓ absorption of fat-soluble vitamins (A, D, E, K), folic acid and iron. Separate administration times with concurrent multivitamin use as noted above.

FIBRATES

Fibrates are peroxisome proliferator receptor alpha (PPARα) activators, which upregulate the expression of apolipoprotein CII and apoliporotein A-I. Apo CII ↑ lipoprotein lipase activity leading to ↑ catabolism of VLDL particles. This will ↓ TG significantly, but in the setting of high TG (increased VLDL particles) fibrate therapy may lead to an ↑ LDL particles and subsequently an ↑ LDL cholesterol. The ↓ TG may lead to an ↑ in HDL cholesterol. Also ↑ Apo A-I will lead to ↑ HDL since Apo A-I is the building blocks of HDL particles. The ACCORD Lipid Study showed no significant difference in experiencing a major cardiac event between patients treated with fenofibrate plus simvastatin compared with simvastatin alone.

DRUG	DOSING	SAFETY/SIDE EFFECTS/MONITORING
Fenofibrate, Fenofibric Acid (Antara, Fenoglide, Fibricor, Lipofen, Lofibra, **TriCor**, Triglide, **Trilipix**, generics)	*Antara* (micronized capsule): 43-130 mg daily *Fenoglide*: 40-120 mg daily with meals *Fibricor*: 35-105 mg daily *Lofibra* (micronized capsule): 67-200 mg daily with meals *Lofibra* (tablet): 54-160 mg daily *Lipofen*: 50-150 mg daily with meals *TriCor*: 48-145 mg daily *Triglide*: 50-160 mg daily *Trilipix*: 45-135 mg daily *[handwritten] only fibrate w/ indication for use w/ a "statin"* *[handwritten] NOT interchangeable!*	**CONTRAINDICATIONS** Severe liver disease including primary biliary cirrhosis Severe renal disease (CrCl < 30 mL/min) Gallbladder disease Nursing mothers (fenofibrate derivatives only) Concurrent use with repaglinide (gemfibrozil only) *[handwritten] Prandin®* **WARNINGS** Myopathy, ↑ risk when co-administered with a statin particularly in the elderly, diabetes, renal failure, or hypothyroidism *[handwritten] ↑ myopathy risk in elderly and diabetes* Cholelithiasis Reversible ↑ SCr (> 2 mg/dL); clinical significance unknown **SIDE EFFECTS** ↑ LFTs (dose related), abdominal pain, ↑ CPK, dyspepsia, URTIs **MONITORING** LFTs, renal function **NOTES** Pregnancy Category C Reduce dose if CrCl 30-80 mL/min with fenofibrates **Lipid Effects** ↓ TGs ~20-50% ↑ HDL ~15% ↓ LDL ~5-20% (but can ↑ LDL when TG are high)
Gemfibrozil (Lopid)	600 mg BID, 30 minutes before breakfast and dinner *[handwritten] AVOID W/ STATINS!*	

Fibrate Drug Interactions

- When used in combination with statins, fibrates can ↑ the risk of myopathies and rhabdomyolysis, especially with gemfibrozil. Only *Trilipix* has the indication for use with a statin although others (except gemfibrozil – avoid if on a statin) may have a similar safety profile. Monitor liver enzymes with all fibrates, statins, and when the 2 drug classes are used in combination.

- Fibrates may ↑ cholesterol excretion into the bile, leading to cholelithiasis.

- Colchicine can ↑ the risk of myopathy when coadministered with fenofibrate.

- Gemfibrozil is contraindicated with repaglinide [*Prandin®*] as it may ↑ hypoglycemic effects.

- Fibrates may increase the effects of sulfonylureas and warfarin.

NIACIN

Decreases the rate of hepatic synthesis of VLDL (↓ TGs) and LDL; may also ↑ rate of chylomicron TG removal from plasma. Alters the binding of HDL particles to scavenger receptor B-1 in the liver which removes the cholesterol inside but does not take up the HDL particle which leaves it free to return to the circulation for reverse cholesterol transport. Also known as nicotinic acid or vitamin B3, although doses for cholesterol reduction are much higher than doses found in multivitamin products.

[handwritten left margin: flushing occurs mostly at night → CAUTION if awakened (dizziness)]

[handwritten left margin: max dose 2000mg/ 40 mg per day]

DRUG	DOSING	SAFETY/SIDE EFFECTS/MONITORING
Immediate-Release (crystalline) niacin (*Niacor*) – OTC	250 mg with dinner; can ↑ every 4-7 days to max dose 6 g daily, divided in 2-3 doses	**CONTRAINDICATIONS** Active liver disease, active PUD, arterial bleeding, arterial hemorrhage **WARNINGS** Use with caution in patients with unstable angina or in the acute phase of an MI Hepatotoxicity
Extended-Release Niacin (*Niaspan*) **500, 750, 1,000 mg** + lovastatin (*Advicor*) + simvastatin (*Simcor*)	500 mg QHS x 4 weeks Can ↑ every 4 weeks to a max dose of 2 g daily *[handwritten: after low-fat snack]*	**SIDE EFFECTS** Flushing, pruritus (itching), N/V, diarrhea, GI distress, hyperglycemia, hyperuricemia (or gout), cough, hepatotoxicity, orthostatic hypotension, hypophosphatemia **MONITORING** Check LFTs at the start (baseline), every 6 to 12 weeks for the first year, and then ~ 6-months; blood glucose (if have diabetes); uric acid (if have gout); INR (if on warfarin) *[handwritten: ✓ LFTs – baseline then q 6-12 wks x 1st yr then q 6 mo]*
Controlled-(or sustained) Release Niacin (*Slo-Niacin*, OTC) 250, 500, 750 mg	250-750 mg daily	**NOTES** Pregnancy Category C Immediate-release niacin has poor tolerability due to flushing/itching. Extended-release forms (CR and SR) have less (but still significant) flushing but more hepatotoxicity. Therefore, the best clinical choice is *Niaspan* with less flushing and less hepatotoxicity – but it is the most expensive. Formulations of niacin (IR vs ER) are not interchangeable. Flush-free niacins (inositol hexaniacinate or hexanicotinate), niacinamide or nicotinamide are not effective. Take with food, avoid hot beverages and spicy food which can worsen flushing. **Lipid Effects** ↓ LDL 5-25%, ↑ HDL 15-35%, ↓ TG 20-50%

[handwritten bottom notes:]
(OTC) IR - Niacor® w/ dinner (↑ flushing)
646 (OTC) CR/SR - Slo-Niacin® (↑ LFTs, less flushing than IR)
XR - Niaspan® qhs ← BEST clinical choice! ⇒ less hepatotox flushing

Niacin Drug Interactions

- Monitor for other concurrent drugs that are potentially hepatotoxic. The combination drug lovastatin/niaspan *(Advicor)* has a max dose of 2,000/40 mg and simvastatin/niaspan *(Simcor)* has a max dose of 2,000/40 mg.

- Take niacin 4-6 hours after bile acid sequestrants.

FISH OILS

Not completely understood; may be due to reduction of hepatic synthesis of TGs. These are indicated as an adjunct to diet in patients with TGs ≥ 500 mg/dL. Also known as omega-3 fatty acids.

DRUG	DOSING	SAFETY/SIDE EFFECTS/MONITORING
Omega-3 Acid Ethyl Esters *(Lovaza)* 1 g capsule contains 465 mg EPA (eicosapentaenoic acid) and 375 mg DHA (docosahexaenoic acid)	4 capsules daily or 2 capsules BID	**WARNINGS** Use with caution in patients with known hypersensitivity to fish and/or shellfish. *Lovaza* and *Epanova* may ↑ levels of LDL; monitor. There is a possible association between *Lovaza* and more frequent recurrences of symptomatic atrial fibrillation or flutter in patients with paroxysmal or persistent atrial fibrillation, particularly within the first months of initiating therapy.
Icosapent ethyl *(Vascepa)* contains 1 gram of icosapent ethyl, an ethyl ester of omega-3 fatty acid eicosapentaenoic acid (EPA)	2 capsules BID with or following meals	**SIDE EFFECTS** Eructation (burping), dyspepsia, taste perversions *(Lovaza, Epanova)*; arthalgias *(Vascepa)* **MONITORING** LFTs (in patients with hepatic impairment) and LDL periodically during therapy
Omega-3-carboxylic acids *(Epanova)* 1 gram capsule contains omega-3-carboxylic acids with 850 mg of polyunsaturated fatty acids (mostly EPA+DHA)	2 capsules or 4 capsules daily	**NOTES** Pregnancy Category C There are many OTC omega-3 fatty acid products marketed as dietary supplements. Only prescription medications *Epanova, Lovaza, Omtryg* and *Vascepa* are FDA approved for TG lowering when TG ≥ 500 mg/dL in addition to diet. Stop prior to elective surgeries due to increased risk of bleeding.
Omega-3-acid ethyl esters A *(Omtryg)*	4 capsules daily or 2 capsules BID with meals	**Lipid Effects** ↓ TGs up to 45%, ↑ HDL ~9% Can ↑ LDL (up to 44% with *Lovaza*; 25% with *Omtryg*, and 15% with *Epanova*). No ↑ seen with *Vascepa*.

Handwritten margin notes:
- can ↑ LDL
- ↑ 44%
- no ↑ LDL
- ↑ 15%
- ↑ 25%
- taste alterations
- possible recurrence of sx a fib/flutter in pts w/ PAF
- arthralgias
- taste alterations

Fish Oil Drug Interactions

- Omega-3-acids may prolong bleeding time. Monitor INR if patients are taking warfarin at dose initiation or dose change. Caution with other medications that can ↑ bleeding risk.

Handwritten notes:
- omega 3 acid ethyl esters (Lovaza®) - EPA + DHA
- icosapent ethyl (Vascepa®) - pure EPA
- omega 3 carboxylic acids (Epanova®)
- omega 3 ethyl acids (Omtryg®)

AGENTS FOR HOMOZYGOUS FAMILIAL HYPERCHOLESTEROLEMIA (HoFH)

Lomitapide

Lomitapide binds to and inhibits microsomal triglyceride transfer protein (MTP) in the endo-plasmic reticulum. MTP inhibition prevents the assembly of apo-B containing lipoproteins in enterocytes and hepatocytes resulting in reduced production of chylomicrons and VLDL and subsequently reduced plasma LDL concentrations.

DRUG	DOSING	SAFETY/SIDE EFFECTS/MONITORING
Lomitapide (Juxtapid)	5-60 mg daily Initiate at 5 mg daily. If tolerated, increase after 2 weeks to 10 mg daily; double the dose at 4 week intervals to a max of 60 mg Take whole with water and without food, at least two hours after the evening meal	**BOXED WARNING** Hepatotoxicity **CONTRAINDICATIONS** Pregnancy; concomitant use with moderate or strong CYP3A4 inhibitors; moderate or severe hepatic impairment; active liver disease including unexplained persistent elevations of serum transaminases **WARNINGS** GI side effects occur in majority of patients and may affect absorption of concomitant oral medications **SIDE EFFECTS** Diarrhea, N/V, dyspepsia, abdominal pain, constipation, flatulence, ↑ LFTs, chest pain, back pain, fatigue **MONITORING** ALT, AST, alkaline phosphatase, total bilirubin and pregnancy test in females of reproductive potential at baseline; measure transaminases prior to any increase in dose or monthly (whichever occurs first) during the first year, and then every 3 months and prior to dosage increases **NOTES** Pregnancy Category X Due to the risk of hepatotoxicity, this agent is only available through a Juxtapid Risk Evaluation and Mitigation Strategy (REMS) program. MedGuide required.

(handwritten margin note: monitor transaminases q mo or w/ dose Δ x 1st yr then q 3mo or w/ dose Δ after)

Lomitapide Drug Interactions

- Strong and moderate CYP3A4 inhibitors are contraindicated with lomitapide. Refer to the Drug Interactions chapter for a complete list of moderate and strong 3A4 inhibitors.

- If using weak CYP3A4 inhibitors concomitantly, do not exceed 30 mg/day of lomitapide. See Drug Interactions chapter.

- Warfarin: ↑ INR; monitor after dose initiation or dose change.

- Simvastatin, lovastatin; concomitant use may increase risk of myopathy. Do not exceed simvastatin 20 mg/day (may use 40 mg/day if patients have previously tolerated simvastatin 80 mg/day for 12 months or more without evidence of muscle toxicity). Lovastatin dose should also be reduced when starting lomitapide concomitantly.

- Lomitapide is an inhibitor of P-glycoprotein, which may increase drugs that are P-glyco-protein substrates (See Drug Interactions chapter). Dose reduction of the P-glycoprotein substrates should be considered when used concomitantly.

- Monitor for other concurrent drugs that are potentially hepatotoxic. This includes isotret-inoin, amiodarone, high dose acetaminophen, methotrexate, tetracyclines, and tamoxifen.

- Lomitapide reduces absorption of fat soluble vitamins from the small intestine.

- Separate dosing from bile acid sequestrants by 4 hours.

Mipomersen

Mipomersen is an oligonucleotide inhibitor of apo B-100 synthesis. ApoB is the main compo-nent of LDL and very low density lipoprotein (VLDL), which is the precursor to LDL.

DRUG	DOSING	SAFETY/SIDE EFFECTS/MONITORING
Mipomersen (Kynamro)	200 mg SC once weekly	**BOXED WARNING** Hepatotoxicity
	Maximal LDL reduction seen after ~ 6 months	**CONTRAINDICATIONS** Liver disease (including unexplained elevations in hepatic transaminases), moderate or severe hepatic impairment
		WARNINGS Can cause hepatotoxicity, with elevations in transaminases and/or hepatic steatosis
		SIDE EFFECTS Injection site reactions, flu-like symptoms, nausea, headache, ↑ ALT, antibody formation, fatigue
		MONITORING ALT, AST, total bilirubin, alkaline phosphatase at baseline; then monthly for the first year of treatment, then every 3 months thereafter, lipids every 3 months for the first year
		NOTES Pregnancy Category B Due to the risk of hepatoxicity, this agent is only available through a *Kynamro* Risk Evaluation and Mitigation Strategy (REMS) program. MedGuide required.

Handwritten margin notes:
monitor
ALT
AST
total bili
alk phos
baseline
then q mo x 1st yr
then q 3 mo

monitor
lipids q 3 mo
x 1st yr

Mipomersen Drug Interactions

- Monitor for other concurrent drugs that are potentially hepatotoxic. This includes isotret-inoin, amiodarone, high dose acetaminophen, methotrexate, tetracyclines, and tamoxifen.

Patient Counseling

Statin

For <u>all</u> cholesterol medicines: Your healthcare provider should start you on lifestyle changes including a heart healthy food pattern and exercise.

- Contact your healthcare provider right away if you have muscle weakness, tenderness, aching, cramps, stiffness or pain that happens without a good reason, especially if you also have a fever or feel more tired than usual. These may be symptoms of muscle damage.

- Contact your healthcare provider right away if you are passing brown or dark-colored urine, have pale stools, feel more tired than usual or if your skin and/or whites of your eyes become yellow. These may be symptoms of liver damage.

- Grapefruit and grapefruit juice may interact with this medicine. This could lead to higher amounts of drugs in your body. Do not consume grapefruit products without discussing with your healthcare provider (for lovastatin, simvastatin, atorvastatin).

- Do not use if pregnant or nursing or if you think you may be pregnant. This drug may harm your unborn baby. If you become pregnant, stop statin therapy and call your healthcare provider right away.

Ezetimibe

- Contact your healthcare provider right away if you are passing brown or dark-colored urine, have pale stools, feel more tired than usual or if your skin and/or whites of your eyes become yellow. These may be symptoms of liver damage. Contact your healthcare provider right away if you have muscle weakness, tenderness, aching, cramps, stiffness or pain that happens without a good reason, especially if you also have a fever or feel more tired than usual. These may be symptoms of muscle damage.

- Take this medicine once daily, with or without food.

Fish Oil

- This medication is taken in addition to a healthy diet.

- *Lovaza* and *Omtryg* can be taken once daily, or split BID. *Epanova* is taken once daily.

- Take *Omtryg* and *Vascepa* with food. Take *Epanova* and *Lovaza* with or without food.

- Take whole; do not break, crush, dissolve, or chew.

- This medicine does not usually cause side effects, but may cause indigestion (stomach upset), burping, or a distorted sense of taste *(Lovaza)* or joint pain *(Vascepa)*.

Niacin

- *Niaspan*: Take at bedtime after a low-fat snack. Other niacins: Take with food.

- Do not crush or chew long-acting formulations.

- Contact your healthcare provider right away if you are passing brown or dark-colored urine, feel more tired than usual or if your skin and/or whites of your eyes become yellow. These may be symptoms of liver damage.

- Flushing (warmth, redness, itching and/or tingling of the skin) is a common side effect that may subside after several weeks of consistent use. Pretreatment with 325 mg aspirin (or 200 mg of ibuprofen) 30-60 minutes before the dose (for a few weeks) may help to ↓ flushing. With *Niaspan*, flushing will occur mostly at night; use caution if awakened due to possible dizziness.

- Avoid using alcohol or hot beverages or eating spicy foods around the time of taking this medicine to help reduce flushing.

- If you have diabetes, check your blood sugar when starting this medicine because there may be a mild increase.

Bile Acid Sequestrant

- See notes section in chart for instructions regarding food/fluid intake for specific agents.

- Take this medication at mealtime with plenty of water or other liquid. Never take dry.

- This medication may cause constipation, your pharmacist can recommend a laxative (senna) or stool softener (docusate). Drink plenty of water and eat food with fiber such as fruits, vegetables, and grains.

- Separate the dose of this medication from multivitamin dosing due to ↓ absorption of vitamins A, D, E and K (mostly K), folic acid and iron. You may need to take a multivitamin (esp. in women and children) while taking this medication.

Fibrate

- *Antara, Fibricor, TriCor, Triglide* and *Trilipix*: Take once daily, with or without food.

- *Fenoglide, Lofibra* (micronized capsules) *and Lipofen*: Take once daily, with food.

- *Lopid*: Take twice daily, 30 minutes before breakfast and dinner.

- Do not crush or chew. Contact your healthcare provider if you experience muscle aches.

- Contact your healthcare provider right away if you experience abdominal pain, nausea or vomiting. These may be signs of inflammation of the gallbladder or pancreas.

- Contact your healthcare provider right away if you are passing brown or dark-colored urine, feel more tired than usual or if your skin and/or whites of your eyes become yellow. These may be signs of liver damage.

* all drugs in this chapter ↑ LFTs, except ezetimibe
    * monitor LFTs w/ ezetimibe/simvastatin (Vytorin®)
        ezetimibe/atorvastatin (Liptruzet®)

* all drugs in this chapter - pregnancy C, except
    X { * statins
        * lomitapide (Juxtapid®)
    B { * colesevelam (Welchol®)
        * mipomersen (Kynamro®)

lovastatin
atorvastatin } + grapefruit — inhibits drug-metabolizing enzyme
simvastatin   (separating admin time does not
                                prevent interaxn)
    * other statins do not interact w/ grapefruit

PRACTICE CASE

PATIENT PROFILE

Patient Name David Armistead

Address 1882 Peekaborn

Age 57   **Sex** Male   **Race** White   **Height** 5'11"   **Weight** 246 lbs

Allergies NKDA

DIAGNOSES

Coronary Heart Disease, stent placement 7/14

Dyslipidemia

Hypertension

Diabetes Type 2

MEDICATIONS

Date	No.	Prescriber	Drug & Strength	Quantity	Sig	Refills
5/15/14	77328	Gallagher	*Actos* 45 mg	#30	1 PO daily	2
5/15/14	73768	Gallagher	Metformin 1000 mg	#60	1 PO BID	2
5/15/14	73554	Gallagher	Lisinopril-HCT 20-25 mg	#30	1 PO daily	2
			Fish oils 1000 mg cap		1 PO BID	
			Aspirin 81 mg EC		1 PO daily	
			Multivitamin		1 PO daily	

LAB/DIAGNOSTIC TESTS

Test	Normal Value	Results Date 5/12/14	Date	Date
Protein, T	6.2-8.3 g/dL			
Albumin	3.6-5.1 g/dL			
Alk Phos	33-115 units/L			
AST	10-35 units/L	32		
ALT	6-40 units/L	20		
CH, T	125-200 g/dL	224		
TG	<150 g/dL	248		
HDL	> 40 mg/dL	36		
LDL	< 100 mg/dL			
GLU	65-99 mg/dL	114		
Na	135-146 mEq/L	131		
K	3.5-5.3 mEq/L	3.8		
Cl	98-110 mEq/L	105		
HCO3-	22-28 mEq/L	25		
BUN	7-25 mg/dL	18		
Creatinine	0.6-1.2 mg/dL			
Calcium	8.6-10.2 mg/dL			
WBC	4-11 x 10^3 cells/mm^3	4.6		
RBC	3.8-5.1 x 10^6 mL/mm^3			
Hemoglobin	Male: 13.8- 17.2 g/dL Female: 12.1-15.1 g/dL	14.2		
Hematocrit	Male: 40.7-50.3% Female: 36.1- 44.3%	38		
MCHC	32-36 g/dL			
MCV	80-100 μm			
Platelet count	140-400 x 10^3/mm^3	210		
TSH	0.4-4.0 mIU/L	3.2		
FT4	4.5- 11.2 mcg/dL			
Hgb A1c	4-6%	7.2%		

ADDITIONAL INFORMATION

Date	Notes
11/11/14	Patient reports walking more since heart procedure. He has lost 13 lbs in last 5 months by decreasing "donuts and sugar." No EtOH, no tobacco use (past Hx smoking). Patient states he prefers not to take more pills, and is scared about his heart. BP today is 145/88.

Questions

1. What is David's calculated LDL?

   a. 188
   b. 176
   c. 138
   d. 105
   e. 99

   [handwritten: LDL = total - HDL - TG/5]
   [handwritten: = 224 - 36 - 248/5]

2. David needs to be placed on statin therapy. According to the ACC/AHA Treatment of Blood Cholesterol Guideline, which would be the most appropriate statin regimen for David?

   [handwritten margin: ASCVD 25.3%]

   a. Pravastatin 40 mg daily
   b. Rosuvastatin 20 mg daily
   c. Lovastatin 40 mg daily
   d. Atorvastatin 20 mg daily *[handwritten: 40-80]*
   e. Pitavastatin 4 mg daily

3. David returns to the clinic for follow up and complains of pain in his legs with occasional weakness. The statin therapy is stopped and the pain resolves. What is the best course of action to take for treatment of David's dyslipidemia according to the ACC/AHA Treatment of Blood Cholesterol Guideline?

   a. Restart the same statin at a lower dose
   b. Switch to a different statin
   c. Consider the patient unable to tolerate statin therapy and start a nonstatin cholesterol medication
   d. Recommend angiography to evaluate the leg for claudication
   e. Recommend a venous ultrasound to evaluate the leg for a DVT

Questions 4-8 do not relate to the case.

4. Which of the following cholesterol medicines should be taken with dinner?

   a. Niaspan *[handwritten: q hs]*
   b. Mevacor *[handwritten: - lova]*
   c. Zetia *[handwritten: +/- food]*
   d. Zocor *[handwritten: PM]*
   e. Altoprev *[handwritten: - lova]*

5. A patient is going to be started on *Niaspan* therapy. Which of the following statements is correct?

   a. *Niaspan* is immediate release niacin.
   b. *Niaspan* has a higher degree of hepatotoxicity than all the other niacin formulations.
   c. *Niaspan* must be taken on an empty stomach.
   d. *Niaspan* is taken with breakfast.
   e. *Niaspan* causes less flushing than immediate release niacin.

[handwritten: ✱] 6. A physician has called the pharmacist. He has a patient on phenytoin who cannot tolerate statins. He wishes to begin *Welchol*. Which of the following statements is correct?

   a. The phenytoin should be given 4 hours before *Welchol*.
   b. He cannot use this class of drugs with phenytoin.
   c. *Questran* would be a better option due to a lower risk of drug interactions.
   d. The dose of *Welchol* is 5 g twice daily, with food and water.
   e. There is no drug interaction between phenytoin and *Welchol*.

7. Which of the following drug classes can significantly reduce triglycerides by > 10%? (Select **ALL** that apply.)

   a. Fibrates *[handwritten: 20-50%]*
   b. Fish oils
   c. Bile Acid Resins *[handwritten: no Δ or ↑]*
   d. Ezetimibe *[handwritten: ↓ 5-10%]*
   e. Niacin *[handwritten: 20-50%]*

8. Which of the following generic/brand combinations is correct?

   a. Amlodipine/Atorvastatin (*Vytorin*) *[handwritten: Caduet Ⓐ]*
   b. Fenofibric Acid (*Trilipix*)
   c. Amlodipine/Rosuvastatin (*Caduet*) *[handwritten: no combo]*
   d. Fluvastatin (*Mevacor*) *[handwritten: Lescol Ⓔ]* *[handwritten: w/ rosu]*
   e. Pitavastatin (*Lescol*) *[handwritten: Livalo Ⓔ]*

Answers

1-c, 2-b, 3-a, 4-b, 5-e, 6-a, 7-a,b,e, 8-b

HF = inability of ♡ to supply enough O₂ to perfuse body

low-output
= ↓ ability of ♡ to eject blood

high-output
= blood flow ≠ metab needs due to ↑↑ requirements (acute medical condition, e.g. sepsis, thyrotoxicosis)

Systolic dysfxn (HFrEF)
• ↓↓EF (<40%)
b/c LV not **ejecting** enough blood

diastolic dysfxn (HFpEF)
• EF mildly ↓ or normal (preserved → >40-50%)
b/c impaired ability of LV to **fill** w/ blood ← no guidelines

HEART FAILURE (HF)

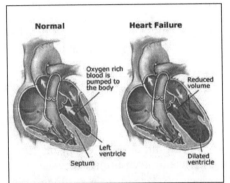

Normal   Heart Failure

Oxygen rich blood is pumped to the body   Reduced volume

Left ventricle   Dilated ventricle

Septum

We gratefully acknowledge the assistance of Tien Ng, PharmD, FCCP, BCPS (AQ-C), Associate Professor, University of Southern California School of Pharmacy, in preparing this chapter.

GUIDELINES

Yancy CW, Jessup M, Bozkurt B, et al. 2013 ACCF/AHA Guideline for the Management of Heart Failure: A Report of the American College of Cardiology Foundation/American Heart Association Task Force on Practice Guidelines. Circulation 2013;128:e240-e327.

Executive Summary: HFSA 2010 Comprehensive Heart Failure Practice Guideline. Journal of Cardiac Failure. June 2010;16(6):475-539.

BACKGROUND

Heart failure is a syndrome where the heart is not able to supply sufficient blood flow (↓ cardiac output) to provide adequate perfusion to the body. Most commonly, heart failure is caused by a reduced ability of the heart to eject blood, known as low-output heart failure. Low cardiac output commonly occurs because the left ventricle is not ejecting enough blood [systolic dysfunction; heart failure with a reduced ejection fraction (HFrEF)] or impaired ability of the left ventricle to fill with blood [diastolic dysfunction; heart failure with a preserved ejection fraction (HFpEF)]. Generally, systolic dysfunction (HFrEF) is characterized by a left ventricular ejection fraction < 40%, whereas diastolic dysfunction (HFpEF) patients have only mildly reduced (> 40 – 50%) or normal left ventricular ejection fraction. Many patients with low-output heart failure have components of both systolic and diastolic dysfunction. Less commonly, the reason for the mismatch in blood flow and metabolic need is caused by very high requirements due to an acute medical condition, such as sepsis or thyrotoxicosis. This is called "high output" heart failure. For the purposes of this chapter, the term "heart failure" will refer to systolic heart failure, or HFrEF.

Heart failure is characterized by frequent hospitalizations, a reduced quality of life, and ↑ mortality. Heart failure is a leading cause of hospitalizations in the elderly. Patients hospitalized for new-onset or worsening heart failure symptoms are referred to as having acute heart failure or acute decompensated heart failure, respectively. Although some hospitalizations are unavoidable due to disease progression or association with an acute cardiac event, <u>many are attributable to non-adherence to medications and/or lifestyle modifications</u>, such as <u>sodium and fluid</u> restriction. This is a major cause of increased health care costs. Studies have shown that pharmacists positively impact the outcome of heart failure patients by providing education on dietary and lifestyle measures, and optimizing the complex medication regimens. <u>Heart failure is one of the most important conditions to counsel on lifestyle modifications and medication adherence</u>.

DRUGS THAT CAUSE OR WORSEN HEART FAILURE

Some chemotherapeutic agents, particularly anthracyclines [doxorubicin *(Adriamycin, Doxil)*, daunorubicin *(Cerubidine, DaunoXome)*, etc.] and some tyrosine kinases inhibitors such as lapatinib *(Tykerb)* and sunitinib *(Sutent)*. Also, trastuzumab *(Herceptin)*, ado-trastuzumab *(Kadcyla)*, imatinib *(Gleevec)* and docetaxol *(Taxotere)* can cause fluid retention.

Amphetamines and other sympathomimetics.

Routine use of calcium channel blockers, particularly nondihydropyridines, in systolic HF.

Antiarrhythmic drugs (lower risk with amiodarone and dofetilide). Do NOT use class I antiarrhythmic agents (mexiletine, tocainide, procainamide, quinidine, disopyramide, flecainide and propafenone).

Avoid itraconazole for non-life threatening infections (such as onychomycosis).

[handwritten: BBW has (-) ionotropic effect]

Immunomodulators, including interferons, TNF inhibitors, rituximab and others.

NSAIDs, including celecoxib *(Celebrex)*.

Glucocorticoids can worsen heart failure.

Triptan migraine drugs (contraindicated with history of cardiovascular disease or uncontrolled hypertension).

Thiazolidinediones due to increased risk of edema.

Excessive alcohol use: modest use may have mild cardiovascular benefit, but excessive use does not.

CAUSES OF SYSTOLIC HEART FAILURE

The heart is a muscle, and cardiomyopathy means an enlarged and damaged heart muscle. Ischemia means lack of oxygen due to decreased blood flow. Heart failure etiology is commonly classified as either ischemic or non-ischemic cardiomyopathy. Ischemic cardiomyopathy is due to damage from a myocardial infarction (MI). The damage from the MI decreases the ability of the damaged ventricle to contract. Non-ischemic cardiomyopathy is less common and is mostly due to hypertension. Other less common causes include valvular disease, excessive alcohol intake or illicit drug use, congenital heart defects, viral infections, diabetes, and cardiotoxic drugs. <u>In the U.S. most HF cases are due to damage from a MI or from hypertension.</u>

PATHOPHYSIOLOGY

Cardiac output (CO) is the <u>volume of blood</u> (expressed in liters) <u>pumped in one minute</u>. It is a function of heart rate (HR) and stroke volume (SV, or the amount of blood ejected from the left ventricle during one cardiac cycle). The equation for cardiac output is CO = HR x SV. Stroke volume is determined by the <u>volume of blood in the ventricle</u> (preload), the <u>resistance to forward flow</u> in the arterial vessels (afterload), and <u>how hard the ventricle squeezes</u> during systole (contractility). Cardiac index (CI) is the cardiac output divided by the body surface area (BSA) of the patient:

$$CI = \frac{CO}{BSA}$$

Heart failure is progressive; over time, left ventricular systolic function will continue to decline resulting in a decrease in CO. To compensate, several acute adaptations occur, including structural changes in the shape and composition of the myocardium, and activation of neurohormonal systems. Activation of the sympathetic nervous system and the renin-angiotensin-aldosterone system [endothelin and vasopressin (anti-diuretic hormone) are also activated] results in vasoconstriction, or increased systemic vascular resistance (SVR). This vasoconstriction helps maintain blood pressure and perfusion to vital organs. Sympathetic (adrenergic) activation also increases heart rate and contractility, which augments cardiac output. Aldosterone increases sodium and water retention which ↑ preload in an attempt to ↑ stroke volume and cardiac output. The excess fluid causes the body to become "congested" and the classic symptoms of "congestive" heart failure appear, including dyspnea (shortness of breath), fatigue, and peripheral edema.

These changes ↑ CO in the short-term but damage the heart in the long-term. A vicious cycle of neurohormonal activation and reduced cardiac function ensues. The pathophysiology of heart failure also involves changes at the genetic and molecular level, including ↑ inflammation and oxidative stress. The drugs that slow the progressive decline in cardiac function and improve survival in heart failure patients antagonize these neurohormonal systems.

Clinical Presentation and Assessment

Symptoms of heart failure are generally a result of either congestion behind the failing ventricle or ↓ blood flow (hypoperfusion) due to the ↓ cardiac output. As the pressure in the left or right ventricle increases, the blood "backs up" in the circulatory system. This leads to signs and symptoms of congestion, which are categorized as right-sided or left-sided failure symptoms (see table). Hypoperfusion of essential organs may lead to end-organ damage, especially the kidney. Heart failure can lead to renal failure.

Heart failure patients are categorized by the presence or severity of symptoms. The American College of Cardiology and American Heart Association (ACC/AHA) recommends categorizing patients by heart failure stage (see table below). The staging system is used to guide treatment in order to slow the development of symptoms in asymptomatic patients (stages A and B) or slow the progression (stages C and D). Heart failure patients can also be classified by their level of physical functional limitation or New York Heart Association (NYHA) functional class (FC). The FC is an important prognostic indicator. With proper treatment, functional classification may improve.

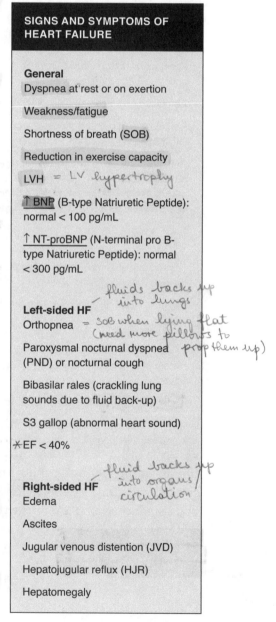

SIGNS AND SYMPTOMS OF HEART FAILURE

General
Dyspnea at rest or on exertion

Weakness/fatigue

Shortness of breath (SOB)

Reduction in exercise capacity

LVH = LV hypertrophy

↑ BNP (B-type Natriuretic Peptide): normal < 100 pg/mL

↑ NT-proBNP (N-terminal pro B-type Natriuretic Peptide): normal < 300 pg/mL

Left-sided HF — fluids backs up into lungs
Orthopnea = SOB when lying flat (need more pillows to prop them up)

Paroxysmal nocturnal dyspnea (PND) or nocturnal cough

Bibasilar rales (crackling lung sounds due to fluid back-up)

S3 gallop (abnormal heart sound)

＊EF < 40%

Right-sided HF — fluid backs up into organs/circulation
Edema

Ascites

Jugular venous distention (JVD)

Hepatojugular reflux (HJR)

Hepatomegaly

ACC/AHA STAGING SYSTEM		NYHA FUNCTIONAL CLASS	
A	At high risk for development of HF, but without structural heart disease or symptoms of HF (e.g., patients with HTN, CHD, DM, obesity, metabolic syndrome)		No corresponding category
B	Structural heart disease present, but without signs or symptoms of HF (e.g., LVH, low EF, valvular disease, previous MI)	I	No limitations of physical activity. Ordinary physical activity does not cause symptoms of HF (e.g., fatigue, palpitations, dyspnea).

Clinical Diagnosis of HF

C	Structural heart disease with prior or current symptoms of HF (e.g., patients with known structural heart disease, SOB and fatigue, reduced exercise tolerance)	I	No limitations of physical activity. Ordinary physical activity does not cause symptoms of HF (e.g., fatigue, palpitations, dyspnea).
		II	Slight limitation of physical activity. Comfortable at rest, but ordinary physical activity results in symptoms of HF.
		III	Marked limitation of physical activity. Comfortable at rest but minimal exertion (bathing, dressing) causes symptoms of HF
D	Advanced structural heart disease with symptoms of HF at rest despite maximal medical therapy (Refractory HF requiring specialized interventions)	IV	Unable to carry on any physical activity without symptoms of HF, or symptoms of HF at rest.

NON-DRUG (LIFESTYLE) TREATMENT

Patients with heart failure should be instructed to:

- Monitor and document body weight daily. This should be done in the morning before eating and after voiding.

- Notify their provider if heart failure symptoms worsen or when weight increases. These should be reported: weight gain of 2 – 4 pounds in 1 day, 3 – 5 pounds in 1 week, increased shortness of breath with activity, increased cough or wheezing, increased swelling in the feet/ankles/legs, increased number of pillows needed to sleep, needing to sleep in a chair, or feeling more tired than usual.

- Maintain sodium restriction of less than 1,500 mg/d for most patients with stage A and B HF (not enough evidence in stage C and D HF).

- Maintain fluid restriction (1.5 – 2 L/d) in stage D, especially in patients with hyponatremia, to reduce congestive symptoms.

- Stop smoking. Limit alcohol intake. Avoid illicit drug use.

- Obtain pneumococcal polysaccharide and annual influenza vaccination; may consider Tdap and zoster (60 years and older); other vaccines may be required in younger patients.

- Consider weight reduction to BMI < 30. Weight reduction is important to reduce workload on the failing heart.

- Exercise training (or regular physical activity) is recommended as safe and effective in patients with HF who are able to participate to improve functional status. Cardiac rehabilitation can be useful in stable HF patients.

OTC and Alternative Medications

↑ 1g/day

- *fish oil* Omega-3 polyunsaturated fatty acid (PUFA) supplementation is reasonable to use as adjunctive therapy in patients with NYHA class II – IV symptoms to ↓ mortality and cardiovascular hospitalizations.

- Avoid using products containing ephedra (ma huang) or ephedrine.

- Avoid NSAIDs (including COX-2 inhibitors) due to the risk of renal insufficiency and fluid retention.

- Hawthorn and coenzyme Q10 may improve heart failure symptoms based on small studies. Patients should consult with their provider before beginning these alternative medications.

DRUG THERAPY

The cornerstones of heart failure therapy are diuretics to control fluid volume, angiotensin antagonists [Angiotensin Converting Enzyme (ACE) inhibitors or Angiotensin Receptor Blockers (ARBs)] and beta blockers to delay or halt the progression of cardiac dysfunction and improve survival. These medications should be utilized in all heart failure patients who do not have a contraindication or intolerance to their use. ACE inhibitors are considered first line therapy over ARBs, however, ARBs are equivalent in terms of clinical benefit. As the syndrome progresses, additional therapies may provide added symptomatic (digoxin) and survival advantages [aldosterone receptor antagonists (ARAs) and/or hydralazine/nitrate].

Loop Diuretics

Loop diuretics are used to ↓ fluid volume to make it easier for the heart to pump. Loop diuretics block sodium and chloride reabsorption in the thick ascending limb of the loop of Henle, interfering with the chloride-binding co-transport system. They ↑ excretion of sodium, chloride, magnesium, calcium, and water. They are used to reduce congestive symptoms (reduction in preload) and restore euvolemia (or "dry" weight). Diuretics have not been shown to alter the survival of heart failure patients; therefore, the lowest effective dose should be used. Care must be taken not to over-diurese patients to avoid hypotension or worsen renal function. If the response to the loop is poor, a combination with thiazide-type diuretics, such as *Zaroxolyn®* metolazone, can be useful. Loops can be used for BP reduction in patients with renal impairment when other options are not adequate.

1st line agents
- *β-blockers ↓ mort*
- *ACEIs ↓ mort.*

2nd line
- *loop diuretics +/-*
- *ARBs*
- *aldosterone antag ↓ mort*
- *digoxin ↑QOL, ↓ hosp*
- *BiDil ↓ mort.*
- *hydralazine, nitrates*

loops **WASTE** Ca^{2+} ⇒ used for hyper Ca of malignancy
all have potential to cause ototox, ESPECIALLY ethacrynic acid

° IV ⇒ light sensitive (amber bottles)

° preg C ↑

$$\frac{IV}{po} = \frac{1}{2}$$

most potent

preg B ↙ ↑

ototox
- hearing loss
- tinnitus
- vertigo

DRUG	DOSING	SAFETY/SIDE EFFECTS/MONITORING
Furosemide *(Lasix)*	Oral: 20-40 mg daily or BID, max 600 mg/day. Oral loop dose equivalency = 40 mg	**BOXED WARNING** Can lead to profound diuresis resulting in fluid and electrolyte depletion
- Store IV @ room temp - do NOT use if solution is yellow		**CONTRAINDICATIONS** Anuria
Bumetanide	Oral: 0.5-1 mg daily or BID, max 10 mg/day Oral loop dose equivalency = 1 mg	**WARNINGS** Sulfa allergy (not likely to cross-react – please see cautionary statement in Drug Allergy chapter) – this warning does not apply to ethacrynic acid
		SIDE EFFECTS Hypokalemia, orthostatic hypotension, ↓ Na⁺, ↓ Mg²⁺, ↓ Cl⁻, ↓ Ca²⁺ (different than thiazides which ↑ Ca²⁺), ↑ HCO₃/metabolic alkalosis, hyperuricemia (↑ UA), hyperglycemia (↑ BG), ↑ TGs, ↑ total cholesterol, photosensitivity, ototoxicity (more with ethacrynic acid) including hearing loss, tinnitus and vertigo
Torsemide *(Demadex)*	Oral: 10-20 mg daily, max 200 mg/day Oral loop dose equivalency = 20 mg	**MONITORING** Renal function (SCr, BUN), fluid status (input and output, weight), BP, electrolytes, hearing with high doses or rapid IV administration
		NOTES IV formulations of furosemide and bumetanide are light-sensitive (in amber bottles). All available in IV and PO formulations.
Ethacrynic Acid *(Edecrin)*	Oral: 50-200 mg daily or divided, max 400 mg/day Oral loop dose equivalency = 50 mg	Furosemide IV:PO ratio is 1:2 (furosemide 20 mg IV = furosemide 40 mg PO). Store at room temp (refrigeration causes precipitation – warming may dissolve crystals). Do not use furosemide solutions if they are yellow in color; must be clear.
		Bumetanide, torsemide and ethacrynic acid IV:PO ratio is 1:1.
		Take early in the day to avoid nocturia.
		Pregnancy Category B (torsemide, ethacrynic acid)/C (furosemide, bumetanide).

Loop Diuretic Drug Interactions

- Can acutely ↓ blood pressure. Always carefully monitor BP when adding-on therapy.

- Loop diuretics can increase the ototoxic potential of other ototoxic drugs (see Drug Interactions chapter), especially with impaired renal function. This combination should be avoided if possible.

- Diuretics can ↓ lithium's renal clearance and ↑ risk of lithium toxicity.

- Do not use NSAIDs in patients with HF. NSAIDs ↑ sodium and water retention and ↓ the effect of the loop diuretics.

- The combination of a loop and a thiazide-type diuretic may ↑ diuretic response, however, electrolyte abnormalities are more likely and must be monitored closely.

★ loops & digoxin - only 2 that do not improve survival in HF (↓ morbidity/mortality) [no benefit in stable pts, benefit in ADHF]

ACE Inhibitors and Angiotensin Receptor Blockers

ACE inhibitors block the conversion of angiotensin I to angiotensin II by inhibiting the angiotensin converting enzyme. ACE inhibitors also prevent the degradation of bradykinin, which is thought to contribute to the vasodilatory effect (and the side effects of cough and angioedema). ARBs block the angiotensin II receptor, AT_1, which is responsible for the vasoconstrictive, aldosterone stimulating, and remodeling effects of angiotensin II. Overall, these agents decrease renin-angiotensin-aldosterone system (RAAS) activation, specifically ↓ the effects of angiotensin II and aldosterone. This results in a decrease in preload and afterload. They ↓ pathologic cardiac remodeling, improve left ventricular function, and reduce morbidity and mortality. The clinical benefits appear to be a drug class effect. The use of an ACE inhibitor (or ARB if intolerant to ACE inhibitors) is indicated for all heart failure patients regardless of symptoms (NYHA FC I – IV). Other important points include:

- The target doses for these agents are the doses used in clinical trials demonstrating their benefit or the maximum tolerated dose for a given patient. Titrate the drug to target doses, if possible. Titrate the dose to reduce symptoms, not BP.

- The combination of an ACE inhibitor and ARB has been shown to ↓ hospitalizations for HF, however, this is not frequently done as it is more common to combine with an aldosterone receptor antagonist (ARA). Triple combination of ACE inhibitor/ARB/ARA is not recommended due to a higher risk of hyperkalemia and increased of renal insufficiency.

- There is an increased incidence of angioedema in black patients. Angioedema is more likely with ACE inhibitors than ARBs, but if a person had angioedema with either class of agents (or aliskiren), these agents should not be used since angioedema can be fatal. Counsel to report any swelling of lips, mouth, tongue, face or neck immediately.

- ACE inhibitors and ARBs ↑ potassium; patients on these medicines should be careful using salt substitutes (which contain KCl rather than NaCl) or potassium supplements.

all except benazepril (Lotensin ®)
· benazepril (Lotensin ®)
· moexipril (Univasc ®)

shortest ★
t ½
among
ACEIs

even though clinical benefit appears to be class effect

DRUG	DOSING	SAFETY/SIDE EFFECTS/MONITORING

ACE Inhibitors – only those mentioned in the guidelines (see complete list in Hypertension chapter)

DRUG	DOSING	SAFETY/SIDE EFFECTS/MONITORING
Captopril (*Capoten*) *SE: taste perversion rash*	Start 6.25 mg TID, 1 hr before meals Target dose: 50 mg TID	**BOXED WARNING** Can cause injury and death to developing fetus; discontinue as soon as pregnancy is detected.
Enalapril (*Vasotec*)	Start 2.5 mg BID Target dose: 10-20 mg BID	**CONTRAINDICATIONS** Angioedema; Do not use in bilateral renal artery stenosis; renal function will worsen. Do not use concurrently with aliskiren in patients with diabetes.
Fosinopril	Start 5-10 mg daily Target dose: 40 mg daily	**WARNINGS** Angioedema (if occurs, do not use); avoid concomitant use
Lisinopril (*Prinivil, Zestril*)	Start 2.5-5 mg daily Target dose: 20-40 mg daily	with an ARB or aliskiren due to increased risk of hypotension, hyperkalemia and renal dysfunction; avoid concomitant use with aliskiren in patients with GFR < 60 mL/minute; renal impairment;
Quinapril (*Accupril*)	Start 5 mg BID Target dose: 20 mg BID	hypotension can occur particularly in salt- or volume-depleted patients.
Perindopril (*Aceon*)	Start 2 mg daily Target dose: 8-16 mg daily	Rare: cholestatic jaundice and hepatic failure. **SIDE EFFECTS** *prevent bradykinin degradation*
Ramipril (*Altace*)	Start 1.25-2.5 mg daily Target dose: 10 mg daily	Cough, hyperkalemia, hypotension, dizziness and headache. Captopril has more SEs (taste perversion, rash).
Trandolapril (*Mavik*)	Start 1 mg daily Target dose: 4 mg daily	**MONITORING** BP, K+, renal function; signs and symptoms of HF. **NOTES** Pregnancy Category D

Angiotensin Receptor Blockers (ARBs) – only those mentioned in the guidelines (See complete list in Hypertension chapter)

DRUG	DOSING	SAFETY/SIDE EFFECTS/MONITORING
Candesartan (*Atacand*)	Start 4-8 mg daily Target dose: 32 mg daily	**BOXED WARNING** Can cause injury and death to developing fetus; discontinue as soon as pregnancy is detected. **CONTRAINDICATIONS** Angioedema; Do not use in bilateral renal artery stenosis since renal function will worsen. Do not use concurrently with aliskiren in patients with diabetes.
Losartan (*Cozaar*) – benefit in clinical trials but no FDA indication	Start 25-50 mg daily Target dose: 50-150 mg daily	**WARNINGS** Angioedema (if occurs, do not use); avoid concomitant use of an ACE inhibitor or aliskiren due to increased risk of hypotension, hyperkalemia and renal dysfunction; avoid concomitant use with aliskiren in patients with GFR < 60 mL/minute; renal impairment; hypotension can occur in patient who are salt- or volume-depleted. **SIDE EFFECTS** Hyperkalemia, hypotension, dizziness and headache.
Valsartan (*Diovan*)	Start 20-40 mg BID Target dose: 160 mg BID	(Note: side effects same as for ACE inhibitors except lack of cough) **MONITORING** BP, K+, renal function; signs and symptoms of HF. **NOTES** Pregnancy Category D

ACE Inhibitor/ARB Drug Interactions

- All RAAS inhibitors ↑ the risk of hyperkalemia (most significant side effect). Monitor K⁺ and renal function frequently.

- Dual inhibition of the renin-angiotensin system with ACE inhibitors and ARBs leads to increased risks of renal impairment, hypotension, and hyperkalemia; avoid the combination.

- The triple combination of ACE inhibitor, ARB and ARA is <u>not</u> recommended due to a higher risk of hyperkalemia and increased renal insufficiency.

- ACE inhibitors or ARBs should not be used in combination with the renin inhibitor aliskiren in patients with diabetes.

- All RAAS inhibitors can have additive antihypertensive effects – monitor BP.

- RAAS inhibitors can ↓ lithium's renal clearance and ↑ risk of lithium toxicity.

Beta Blockers *NOT CLASS EFFECT !! (benefit in HF)*

FC II - IV

Beta-adrenergic receptor antagonists, or simply beta blockers, antagonize the effects of catecholamines (especially norepinephrine) at the beta-1 and beta-2 adrenergic receptors. Beta blockers ↓ vasoconstriction. Historically, beta blockers were avoided in HF because they are negative inotropes (↓ CO); however, they are used because studies demonstrated that beta blockers improve cardiac function when taken chronically and ↓ morbidity and mortality in HF. A beta blocker is recommended for all heart failure patients, especially those in NYHA FC II – IV. Unlike ACE inhibitors (or ARBs), the clinical benefits of beta blockers are not considered a class effect. Only carvedilol (IR and ER), metoprolol succinate extended-release and bisoprolol are recommended in the guidelines. The target doses for these agents are the doses used in clinical trials demonstrating their benefit or the maximum tolerated dose for a given patient. Beta blockers with intrinsic sympathomimetic activity (ISA) should be avoided.

* *amlodipine may be added to regimen if HTN not controlled on ACEI/ARB + β-blocker + loop + aldosterone antagonist*

- amlodipine ⇒ "cardiac neutral" safest CCB in HF

DRUG	DOSING	SAFETY/SIDE EFFECTS/MONITORING

Beta blockers – only those mentioned in the guidelines (see complete list in Hypertension chapter)

[handwritten margin note: both β-1 selective]

Bisoprolol *(Zebeta)* – benefit in clinical trials but no FDA indication *[handwritten: ō w/]*	Start 1.25 mg daily Target dose: 10 mg daily	**BOXED WARNING** Beta blockers should not be withdrawn abruptly (particularly in patients with CAD), gradually taper over 1-2 weeks to avoid acute tachycardia, HTN, and/or ischemia. **CONTRAINDICATIONS** Sinus bradycardia, 2nd or 3rd degree heart block, sick sinus syndrome (unless patient has a functioning artificial pacemaker) or cardiogenic shock; do not initiate in patients with active asthma exacerbation. **WARNING** Caution in patients with diabetes particularly with recurrent hypoglycemia, asthma, severe COPD or peripheral vascular disease and Raynaud's disease. May mask signs of hyperthyroidism; may aggravate psychiatric conditions. *[handwritten: hyperthyroidism]*
Metoprolol succinate extended-release *(Toprol XL)* [Metoprolol tartrate *(Lopressor)*] is not recommended by guidelines)	Start 12.5-25 mg/daily Target dose: 200 mg daily	**SIDE EFFECTS** ↓ HR, hypotension, fatigue, dizziness, depression, ↓ libido, impotence, hyperglycemia (non-selective agents can ↓ insulin secretion in type 2 diabetes), hypertriglyceridemia, ↓ HDL; weight gain and edema especially with carvedilol **MONITORING** HR, BP (titrate every 2 weeks as tolerated); ↓ dose if HR < 55 BPM; signs and symptoms of HF, renal function, liver function. **NOTES** Avoid abrupt discontinuation – must taper. Caution: Metoprolol tartrate IV dose is not equivalent to oral dose (IV:PO ratio is 1:2.5)

[handwritten: α₁]

Non-selective Alpha- and Beta Blocking Agent

[handwritten margin notes: target dose; IR { •<85 kg ⇒ 25 mg BID, •>85 kg ⇒ 50 mg BID }; CR • 80 mg/day]

Carvedilol *(Coreg, Coreg CR)*	Immediate release: Start 3.125 mg BID Target dose: <85 kg, 25 mg BID; >85 kg, 50 mg BID Controlled release: Start 10 mg daily Target dose: 80 mg daily	**NOTES** Same as above + *[handwritten: wt gain, edema]* Take all forms of carvedilol with food to decrease rate of absorption, thus minimizing risk of orthostatic hypotension Dosing conversion from *Coreg* to *Coreg CR:* *Coreg* 3.125 mg BID = *Coreg CR* 10 mg daily *Coreg* 6.25 mg BID = *Coreg CR* 20 mg daily *Coreg* 12.5 mg BID = *Coreg CR* 40 mg daily *Coreg* 25 mg BID = *Coreg CR* 80 mg daily *[handwritten: capsules can be opened (applesauce ONLY, not warm)]*

Beta Blocker Drug-Drug and Drug-Disease Interactions

- Beta blockers, particularly the non-selective agents, can mask the symptoms of hypoglycemia (shakiness, palpitations, anxiety). Sweating and hunger are not masked.

- Beta blockers can increase the effects of insulin and oral hypoglycemic agents such as sulfonylureas. Non-selective beta blockers can ↓ insulin secretion in type 2 diabetes. Monitor blood glucose in patients with diabetes.

- Use caution when administering other drugs that slow HR; see Drug Interactions chapter.

- Carvedilol is a substrate of CYP450 2D6; 2D6 inhibitors may increase carvedilol levels and rifampin may decrease carvedilol levels.

- Carvedilol can ↑ digoxin and cyclosporine levels; may require dose adjustments.

FC II – IV

Aldosterone Receptor Antagonists (ARAs)

Spironolactone is a non-selective aldosterone receptor blocker (also blocks androgen and weakly activates progesterone receptors). Eplerenone is a selective aldosterone blocker and does not exhibit the endocrine side effects. ARAs compete with aldosterone at the receptor sites in the distal convoluted tubule and collecting ducts, increasing Na^+ and H_2O excretion while conserving K^+ and H^+ ions. Aldosterone (mineralocorticoid) receptors are also located on other organ systems such as the heart, brain, vasculature, and adipose and immune cells. Clinically, these effects lead to a reduction in sodium and water retention, cardiac remodeling (especially myocardial fibrosis), and risk of sudden cardiac death. Overall, ARAs reduce morbidity and mortality. An ARA should be added to standard therapy in patients with NYHA FC II – IV.

DRUG	DOSING	SAFETY/SIDE EFFECTS/MONITORING

Aldosterone Receptor Antagonists

DRUG	DOSING	SAFETY/SIDE EFFECTS/MONITORING
Spironolactone (*Aldactone*)	Start 12.5-25 mg daily Target dose: 25 mg daily or BID	**BOXED WARNING** Tumor risk with spironolactone; tumorigenic in chronic rat toxicity studies. Avoid unnecessary use. **CONTRAINDICATIONS** Anuria, significant renal impairment (CrCl ≤ 30 mL/min), hyperkalemia (Addison's disease or other conditions that ↑ K^+); concomitant use of strong 3A4 inhibitors with eplerenone. **WARNINGS** Do not initiate therapy in heart failure patients with K^+ > 5.0 mEq/L; SCr > 2.0 mg/dL (females) or SCr > 2.5 mg/dL (males) **SIDE EFFECTS** Hyperkalemia, ↑ SCr, dizziness. For spironolactone: gynecomastia, breast tenderness, impotence, irregular menses
Eplerenone (*Inspra*)	Start 25 mg daily Target dose: 50 mg daily	Rare: hyperchloremic metabolic acidosis **MONITORING** Check K^+ before starting and frequently thereafter. BP, SCr/BUN; fluid status (input and output, weight), signs and symptoms of HF **NOTES** To minimize risk of hyperkalemia Avoid in ↓ renal function (CrCl ≤ 30 mL/min) Do not start if K^+ > 5 mEq/L Start with a low dose. Higher risk when concurrent ACE inhibitors or ARBs are used at higher doses. Do not use NSAIDs concurrently (which should be avoided in HF). Monitor frequently. Counsel patient about ↑ risk if dehydration occurs (due to vomiting, diarrhea or ↓ fluid intake).

Handwritten notes (left margin, Spironolactone):

nonselective
- also blocks androgen
- weakly activates progesterone antagonists

* BBW: tumor risk (rats)

Handwritten notes (left margin, Eplerenone):

selective
- ө endocrine SE

≠ strong 3A4 inhib (azoles)

do not exceed 25mg qd if on moderate 3A4 inhib (diltiazem)

Handwritten notes (bottom):

do not use:
- CrCl < 30
- SrCr > 2 (♀), 2.5 (♂)
- K > 5 or Addison's dz

ARA Drug Interactions

- Eplerenone is a CYP 3A4 substrate; use with strong 3A4 inhibitors is contraindicated.

- All RAAS inhibitors ↑ the risk of hyperkalemia (most significant side effect). Monitor K⁺ and renal function frequently.

- The triple combination of ACE inhibitor, ARB, and ARA is not recommended due to high risk of hyperkalemia and renal insufficiency.

- All RAAS inhibitors can have additive antihypertensive effects – monitor BP.

- RAAS inhibitors can ↓ lithium's renal clearance and ↑ risk of lithium toxicity.

Hydralazine/Nitrate

FC III-IV (handwritten)

Hydralazine is a direct arterial vasodilator which ↓ afterload. Nitrates are venous vasodilators and ↓ preload. The nitrate ↑ the availability of nitric oxide which causes vasodilation. Hydralazine decreases the development of nitrate tachyphylaxis (decrease in response/tolerance). The combination improves the survival of heart failure patients, although not as much as ACE inhibitors. Therefore, this combination is used as alternative therapy for patients who cannot tolerate ACE inhibitors or ARBs due to poor renal function, angioedema, or hyperkalemia. And, it can be added to standard therapy in black patients based on a study demonstrating improved survival. The combination product, *BiDil*, is indicated in self-identified black patients with NYHA FC III or IV who are symptomatic despite optimal therapy with ACE inhibitors and beta blockers. Hydralazine or oral nitrates may be used as monotherapy for other indications, however, they have not individually been shown to affect HF outcomes. Isosorbide dinitrate was the oral nitrate used in clinical trials – there are no data with isosorbide mononitrate although it is used in practice. As with ACE inhibitors or ARBs, the target doses are those shown to be beneficial in clinical trials.

DRUG	DOSING	SAFETY/SIDE EFFECTS/MONITORING
Isosorbide dinitrate/hydrALAZINE (BiDil)	Start 20/37.5 mg TID (1 tab TID) Target dose: 40/75 mg TID (2 tabs TID) No nitrate tolerance	**CONTRAINDICATIONS** CI with PDE-5 Inhibitors **WARNING** Drug-induced lupus erythematosus (DILE – dose and duration related – report fever, joint/muscle aches, fatigue) **SIDE EFFECTS** Headache, dizziness, hypotension, tachycardia, weakness **MONITORING** HR, BP; signs and symptoms of HF

⊕ nitrate-free interval (handwritten)

indicated in self-identified black pts w/ NYHA FC III-IV symptomatic despite optimal tx w/ β-blockers & ACEI (handwritten)

tx w/ APAP (handwritten)

studied as adjunct to triple regimen of β-blocker + ACEI + aldost. antag (handwritten)

for ALL races: if pt has angioedema on ACEI & ARB, start on hydralazine & dinitrate (handwritten)

Hydralazine/Nitrate Continued

DRUG	DOSING	SAFETY/SIDE EFFECTS/MONITORING
HydrALAZINE	Start 25-50 mg TID-QID Target dose: 7300 mg/day in divided doses	**CONTRAINDICATION** Mitral valve rheumatic heart disease **WARNING** Drug-induced lupus erythematosus (DILE – dose and duration related) **SIDE EFFECTS** Headache, reflex tachycardia, palpitations **MONITORING** HR, BP; signs and symptoms of HF, ANA titer
Isosorbide mononitrate (Monoket) Isosorbide dinitrate *(Isordil Titradose, Dilatrate SR)* Preferred for systolic HF	Start 20-30 mg TID-QID Target dose: 120 mg daily in divided doses	**CONTRAINDICATIONS** CI with PDE-5 Inhibitors **SIDE EFFECTS** Headache, dizziness, lightheadedness, flushing, hypotension, tachyphylaxis (need 10-12 hour nitrate free interval), syncope **MONITORING** HR, BP; signs and symptoms of HF

[handwritten note next to Isosorbide row: mono QD-BID]

Hydralazine/Nitrate Drug Interactions

- Must avoid nitrate administration within 12 hours of avanafil, within 24 hours of sildenafil or vardenafil and within 48 hours of tadalafil. Do not dispense nitrates to patients using PDE-5 inhibitors.

Digoxin

[handwritten: do not confuse w/ H⁺/K⁺ ATPase pump inhibitors (PPIs)]

Digoxin inhibits the Na^+/K^+ ATPase pump which results in a positive inotropic effect ($\uparrow$ in CO). It also exerts a parasympathetic effect which provides a negative chronotropic effect ($\downarrow$ HR). Digoxin is added in patients who remain symptomatic despite receiving standard therapy of an ACE inhibitor (or ARB) with a beta blocker. Digoxin improve symptoms, exercise tolerance, and quality of life (QOL). Overall, digoxin does not improve survival of heart failure patients, but it does reduce hospitalizations for heart failure. Dosing should take into account the patient's renal function, body size, age and gender (lower dose for renal insufficiency, smaller, older, female), with the majority of patients being on no more than 0.125 mg daily. Serum digoxin concentrations for HF should be kept < 1.0 ng/mL (range 0.5 – 0.9 ng/mL).

[handwritten margin note: > 1 ng/mL ⇒ ↑ mortality]

[handwritten notes:
MOA: ① inhibits Na⁺/K⁺ ATPase pump ⇒ (+) ionotrope (↑CO)
② parasympathetic effect ⇒ (-) chronotrope (↓HR)

* improves sx / exercise tolerance / quality of life
* ↓ HF-related hospitalizations
* does NOT improve survival]

tx range for a fib = 0.8 - 2 (b/c ↑ dose = ↑ HR reduction)
* dig used for a fib is used for its (–) chronotropic effect
(arrhythmias)

RxPrep Course Book | RxPrep © 2015

DRUG	DOSING	SAFETY/SIDE EFFECTS/MONITORING
Digoxin *(Digox, Lanoxin)* Tablet, solution, injection	Available as 0.0625, 0.125, 0.1875, 0.25 mg Typical dose: 0.125 mg daily Loading doses not used in HF Therapeutic range for HF = 0.5-0.9 ng/mL (higher range for AFib) When CrCl < 30 mL/min; ↓ dose or use less frequently ↓ 20-25% when going from PO to IV/IM. Antidote: *DigiFab*	**CONTRAINDICATIONS** Ventricular fibrillation **WARNINGS** Vesicant Avoid in 2nd or 3rd degree heart block with a functional pacemaker Avoid in Wolff-Parkinson-White syndrome (WPW) with AFib **SIDE EFFECTS** Dizziness, mental disturbances, headache, diarrhea, nausea, vomiting **MONITORING** HR, BP, electrolytes (K^+, Ca^{2+}, Mg^{2+}), renal function, ECG and drug level **TOXICITY** First signs of toxicity are nausea/vomiting, loss of appetite and bradycardia. Other signs of toxicity include blurred/double vision, altered color perception, greenish-yellow halos around lights or objects, abdominal pain, confusion, delirium, arrhythmia (prolonged PR interval, accelerated junctional rhythm, bidirectional ventricular tachycardia).

Handwritten margin notes:
- po → IV or IM ↓ 20-25%.
- toxicity
  - 1st signs :- N/V
    - appetite loss
    - brady ♡
  - other signs :- blurred/double vision
    - altered color perception/greenish-yellow halos
    - abdominal pain
    - confusion, delirium
    - arrhythmia ↳ PR prolongation
- ↑ risk w/
  - ↓ K⁺ < 3.5
  - ↓ Mg⁺⁺
  - ↑ Ca⁺⁺
- pt has to have tox sx

Digoxin Drug-Drug and Drug-Disease Interactions

- Use caution when administering other drugs that slow HR (such as beta blockers); see Drug Interactions chapter.

- Digoxin is mostly renally cleared and partially cleared hepatically. Decreased renal function requires a ↓ digoxin dose. In acute renal failure, digoxin is held. *(handwritten: ~85%)*

- Digoxin is a P-gp and 3A4 substrate (minor). Digoxin levels ↑ with amiodarone, dronedarone, quinidine, verapamil, erythromycin, clarithromycin, itraconazole, cyclosporine, propafenone, and many other drugs. Reduce digoxin dose by 50% if patient is on amiodarone or dronedarone. *(handwritten: ↓ 50% digoxin)*

- Hypokalemia ($K^+ < 3.5$ mEq/L), hypomagnesemia, and hypercalcemia ↑ risk of digoxin toxicity.

- Hypothyroidism can ↑ digoxin levels.

Potassium Oral Supplementation

Potassium supplementation is an important aspect of managing HF since loop diuretics cause ↓ K^+ while other HF drugs (RAAS, ARAs) ↑ K^+. Maintenance of potassium levels is essential to reduce the proarrhythmic risk of digoxin, especially as HF ↑ arrhythmia risk. There are different formulations (tablets, capsules and liquids) which also vary by salt form (acetate, bicarbonate, citrate, chloride, gluconate and phosphate). The salt used depends on patient factors including acid-base status and deficiency of other electrolytes such as phosphate. Potassium chloride is used most commonly.

↓ Mg++ ⟹ ↓ K+ ⟹ *potential dig tox* (handwritten annotation)

Potassium levels should be monitored with the frequency dependent on the stability of the renal function, medication regimen, and the clinical status. Check levels after any change in diuretic, ACE inhibitor, ARB or ARA dose. It should also be checked if the renal function changes. Magnesium deficiency aggravates hypokalemia. The magnesium level may need to be checked and should be corrected prior to correcting the potassium level.

The usual range of K+ is 3.5 – 5 mEq/L. Patients on digoxin should keep the level between 4 - 5 mEq/L. Supplementation may not be needed in patients who are able to supplement their intake of potassium through dietary sources (e.g., bananas, potatoes, orange juice, beans, dark leafy greens, apricots, peaches, avocados, white mushrooms, tomatoes, and some varieties of fish).

DRUG	DOSING	SAFETY/SIDE EFFECTS/MONITORING
Potassium chloride *(K-Tab, K-Vescent, Kaon-Cl, Klor-Con, Klor-Con 10, Klor-Con M10, Klor-Con M15, Klor-Con M20, Micro-K, others)*	Prevention of hypokalemia: 20-40 mEq/day in 1-2 divided doses Treatment of mild hypokalemia: Generally 40-100 mEq/day in 2-5 divided doses; adjust dose according to laboratory values No more than 20-25 mEq should be given as a single dose to avoid GI discomfort For infusions > 10 mEq K+/hour, central line and continuous ECG monitoring required	**CONTRAINDICATIONS (3)** Severe renal impairment, hyperkalemia Oral solid dosage forms are contraindicated in patients with delayed or obstructed passage through the GI tract. **WARNINGS** Caution in patients with mild-moderate renal impairment; patients with disorders that alter K+ (untreated Addison's disease, heat cramps, severe tissue trauma/burns), and in patients taking other medications that ↑ K+ **SIDE EFFECTS** Diarrhea, nausea, vomiting, abdominal pain, flatulence, hyperkalemia **MONITORING** Serum potassium, glucose, chloride, magnesium, pH, urine output **NOTES** Take with meals and a full glass of water or other liquid to minimize the risk of GI irritation. Caution when used in patients on ACE inhibitors, ARBs, ARAs or other medications that ↑ K+ (see Drug Interactions chapter). Caution if using potassium supplement and salt substitutes, as many salt substitutes contain potassium. *Micro-K:* capsules may be opened and contents sprinkled on a spoonful of applesauce or pudding and immediately swallowed without chewing. *K-Tab, Kaon-Cl, Klor-Con:* Swallow whole, do not crush, cut, chew, or suck on tablet. *Klor-Con M:* Swallow whole, do not crush, chew, or suck on tablet. Tablet may also be cut in half and swallowed separately, or can dissolve the whole tablet in 4 oz. of water – stir for 2 mins. and drink immediately.

Acute Decompensated Heart Failure (ADHF)

Heart failure patients may experience episodes of worsening symptoms such as sudden weight gain, inability to lie flat without becoming short of breath, decreasing functionality (e.g., unable to perform their daily routine), increasing shortness of breath and fatigue. Patients in ADHF are generally hospitalized.

(handwritten annotations:)

caps.

Sx: → *worsening congestion*
- ↑ jugular venous pulsation
- lower extremity/ pulmon. edema
- rales
- ascites

most pts

hypoperfusion
- cool extremities
- ↓ bp
- ↓ renal fxn
- impaired mental fxn

Clinical Presentation and Assessment

ADHF is due to the disease getting worse (disease progression), a cardiac event (MI, arrhythmias, valvular disease, uncontrolled hypertension or myocarditis) or a non-cardiac cause. Common non-cardiac causes include non-adherence with medications or dietary restrictions, worsening renal function, thyroid disease, infection, alcohol binging, illicit drug use and the use of drugs that can worsen cardiac function (e.g., initiation of negative inotropic drugs, sudden use of NSAIDs/COX-2 inhibitors, drugs which promote fluid retention, and direct cardiotoxic drugs).

Patients in ADHF present with either worsening congestion and/or hypoperfusion. Evidence of congestion includes elevated jugular venous pulsation, lower extremity or pulmonary edema, rales, and ascites. Evidence of hypoperfusion includes cool extremities, hypotension, decreased renal function, and impaired mental function. The majority of ADHF patients present with worsening congestion.

In all ADHF cases, counsel on the importance of medication adherence and optimize drug doses. Beta blockers should only be stopped if hypotension or hypoperfusion is present.

Treating Congestion   *DO NOT STOP β-BLOCKERS!*

Congestion is treated with diuretics and possibly IV vasodilators. Loop diuretics are initially given IV since congestion can ↓ absorption. If diuretic resistance develops, the dose can be increased or a thiazide-type diuretic (e.g., metolazone, chlorothiazide) can be added to the the loop diuretic. IV vasodilators include nitroglycerin, nitroprusside, and nesiritide. Frequent blood pressure monitoring is required (↓ dose if hypotensive or worsening renal function).

STOP β-BLOCKERS!

Treating Hypoperfusion   ** ionotrope of choice in HF w/ systolic < 90: DA **

In hypoperfusion or cardiogenic shock, IV vasodilators are contraindicated. In these patients, it may become necessary to initiate therapy with an IV inotropic drug (dobutamine, dopamine or milrinone). Dobutamine is a beta-1 and beta-2 adrenergic agonist which ↑ CO in a dose-dependent manner. Dobutamine has some vasodilatory effect (beta-2) and is used if SBP > 90 mmHg. Milrinone is a phosphodiesterase-3 inhibitor that ↑ CO in a dose-dependent manner. Milrinone also has profound vasodilatory effects and can only be used if blood pressure is adequate. Milrinone requires dose adjustment in renal insufficiency. Dopamine has dose-dependent effects (dopaminergic receptor agonist at low doses, beta$_1$ at moderate doses, alpha$_1$ at higher doses) and is used as an inotrope and vasopressor. Dopamine is the inotrope of choice in heart failure patients with SBP < 90 mmHg. Inotropes are associated with worse outcomes and should be discontinued once the patient is stabilized. See the IV Drugs and the Critical Care chapters.

milrinone (Primacor®) PDE-3 inhib

DA dose
low → DA
mod → β$_1$
high → α$_1$

dobutamine
β$_1$ → ↑ CO
β$_2$ → vasodilation

VASODILATORS

Vasodilators used in ADHF are nitroglycerin, nitroprusside, and nesiritide. With all three, blood pressure must be monitored closely.

milrinone dobutamine } vasodilatory effects → use only when systolic > 90

if systolic < 90 → use DA

Nitroglycerin is more of a venous vasodilator, particularly at low doses, but is an effective arterial vasodilator at higher doses. To achieve a desirable effect, the dose should be titrated up. Nitroglycerin may be preferred in ADHF with active myocardial ischemia or uncontrolled hypertension, but the effectiveness may be limited after 2-3 days.

Nitroprusside is an equal arterial and venous vasodilator at all doses. Nitroprusside has a greater effect on blood pressure than nitroglycerin, and unlike nitroglycerin, its use is discouraged in the setting of active myocardial ischemia as it can cause "coronary steal" or shunting of blood away from areas with diseased coronary arteries. Nitroprusside metabolism results in the formation of thiocyanate and cyanide, both of which can cause toxicity (especially in the setting of renal and hepatic insufficiency, respectively). Therefore, nitroprusside may be a desirable choice in patients with uncontrolled hypertension, but renal and hepatic function must be monitored closely. Although tachyphylaxis does not occur with nitroprusside, prolonged administration is discouraged due to increased risk of toxicity. Hydroxycobalamin can be administered to reduce the risk of thiocyanate toxicity, whereas, sodium thiosulfate may be used treat cyanide toxicity.

↓ anion gap metabolic acidosis

Nesiritide *(Natrecor)* is a recombinant B-type natriuretic peptide that binds to vascular smooth muscle, ↑ cGMP resulting in smooth muscle cell relaxation which causes vasodilation. Nesiritide provides both arterial and venous vasodilation which ↑ CO. Nesiritide has a longer half-life than nitroglycerin or nitroprusside. Nesiritide does not have an effect on mortality and does not ↓ hospitalizations compared to standard therapies. Therefore, it is not commonly used.

DRUG	DOSING	SAFETY/SIDE EFFECTS/MONITORING
Nesiritide (Natrecor) *recomb. B-type natriuretic peptide* *arterial + venous vasodilation* *LONG t½ !*	Draw bolus only from prepared (reconstituted) infusion bag: 2 mcg/kg IV bolus followed by a continuous infusion at 0.01 mcg/kg/min; max 0.03 mcg/kg/min.	**CONTRAINDICATIONS (2)** Persistent SBP < 100 mmHg prior to therapy, cardiogenic shock (when used as primary therapy) *⊖ effect on mortality* *⊖ ↓ hospitalizations* **SIDE EFFECTS** Hypotension, SCr *↑ SrCr* **MONITORING** BP, SCr, BUN, urine output **NOTES** Limited experience with infusions lasting longer than 96 hours.
Nitroglycerin *↓ doses venous vasodilation* *↑ doses arterial vasodilation*	Continuous IV infusion due to short t½. Prepare in glass bottles, PAB™, EXCEL™ (polyolefin) containers. Soft plastic-like PVC can cause adsorption of drug. Use administration sets intended for NTG.	**CONTRAINDICATIONS** SBP < 90 mmHg, concurrent use with PDE-5 Inhibitors, ↑ intracranial pressure **SIDE EFFECTS** Hypotension, headache, lightheadedness, tachycardia, tachyphylaxis **MONITORING** BP, HR • preferred in ADHF w/ active myocardial ischemia / uncontrolled HTN • ↓ effectiveness after 2-3 days (tachyphylaxis)

↓ only use non-PVC tubing

Vasodilators Continued

DRUG	DOSING	SAFETY/SIDE EFFECTS/MONITORING
Nitroprusside *(Nitropress)*	Requires light protection during administration. A blue-color solution indicates degradation to cyanide – do not use.	**BOXED WARNINGS (3)** Except when used briefly or at low (<2 mcg/kg/minute) infusion rates, nitroprusside gives rise to large cyanide quantities. Can cause excessive hypotension; continuous BP monitoring required Solution must be further diluted with D5W; do not give undiluted **CONTRAINDICATIONS** SBP < 90 mmHg, CI with PDE-5 Inhibitors, ↑ intracranial pressure **SIDE EFFECTS** Hypotension, headache, tachycardia, thiocyanate/cyanide toxicity (especially in renal and hepatic impairment) **MONITORING** BP, HR, SCr, BUN, urine output, thiocyanate/cyanide toxicity, acid-base status, venous oxygen concentration

Handwritten margin notes:
- > effect on bp than NTG
- arterial + venous vasodilation
- do not use in ♡ ischemia → coronary steal !
- → tachyphylaxis

Preventing Heart Failure Readmissions

Reducing readmissions is a priority for healthcare professionals. As the U.S. transitions from a fee-for-service model to an accountable care organization (ACO) model, providers and healthcare systems will become increasingly responsible for the costs associated with treating their patients. HF is one of the disease states that insurers are focusing on because it is a very high-cost condition. Medicare has started penalizing hospitals for excessive readmissions due to heart failure exacerbations. This has led most organizations to devote additional resources to preventing readmissions. Below are some of the ways pharmacists (and other healthcare professionals) are reducing readmissions in patients with HF:

- Use a transitional care nurse or pharmacist to help ensure a smooth transition between levels of care (e.g., inpatient to outpatient). This includes medication reconciliation.

- Educate patients about their disease. This includes identifying the signs/symptoms of worsening heart failure, recording daily weights, avoiding foods that can worsen their condition and the importance of medication adherence.

- Schedule regular medication management appointments with patients to reinforce counseling and answer medication-related questions.

- Ensure the appropriate, evidence-based medications are prescribed (ACE inhibitors or ARBs, beta blockers, loop diuretics, ARAs, hydralazine/nitrates).

- Ensure the dose of each agent is titrated to target dosing for heart failure.

- Reduce or eliminate medications that can worsen heart failure (e.g., NSAIDs, TZDs, diltiazem, verapamil).

Patient Counseling

All Heart Failure Patients

- Monitor body weight daily, in the morning before eating and after using the restroom. Weight should be recorded in a notebook.
- Call your doctor if your symptoms worsen or if you gain weight (2-4 pounds in one day or 3-5 pounds in one week).
- Follow a sodium restricted diet. Foods high in sodium include:
  - ❑ Prepared sauces and condiments (such as soy sauce, BBQ sauce, Worcestershire sauce or salsa)
  - ❑ Canned vegetables and soups
  - ❑ Frozen dinners
  - ❑ Deli meats (sandwich meats, bacon, ham, hot dogs, sausage or salami)
  - ❑ Salty foods (pickles, olives, cheese, nuts, chips or crackers)
- Take nutrition classes and learn to read nutrition labels. Choose "no sodium added" or "low sodium" options. Healthy ways of cooking include broiling, baking, poaching, and steaming without added salt.
- Stop smoking. Do not use any illegal drugs; they can badly damage the heart. Alcohol, including beer and wine, should be avoided or limited to 1 drink per day for females and 2 drinks per day for males.
- Avoid pain medicines like ibuprofen or *Celebrex* or other "NSAIDs" without checking with the pharmacist or cardiologist. Also, do not use nutritional supplements, vitamins or herbals for HF without discussing with the pharmacist if they are safe to use.
- Stay compliant with all medications – discuss with the pharmacist if medications are too expensive. Remind patients that non-compliance to medications and food restrictions often lead to worsening of HF and possible hospitalizations. Patients may need extra support during celebrations and holiday seasons.

Beta Blockers in HF

- Do not stop taking the medication unless your healthcare provider tells you to do so.
- If you miss a dose, take your dose as soon as you remember, unless it is time to take your next dose. Do not double the dose.
- This medication can cause you to feel dizzy, tired, or faint. Do not drive a car, use machinery, or do anything that requires you to be alert until you adjust to the medication and the symptoms subside.
- This medication may make you feel more tired and dizzy at first. These effects will go away in a few days. However, call your healthcare provider if the symptoms feel severe, or you have weight gain or increased shortness of breath.
- This medication can cover up some of the signs and symptoms of low blood sugar (hypoglycemia); make sure to test your blood sugar often, and take a fast-acting sugar source if needed.
- Medications used to treat severe allergic reactions may not work as well while taking this medication.

Toprol XL

- If you have been told to cut the *Toprol XL* or its generic equivalent tablet in half, you must use a pill cutter and cut only at the score line. Otherwise, the medicine will enter your body too quickly. Swallow the ½ tablet whole. The tablets cannot be crushed or chewed.

Coreg CR

- Take with food, to help reduce dizziness.
- Swallow *Coreg CR* capsules whole. Do not chew or crush the capsules. If you have trouble swallowing *Coreg CR* whole:
- The capsule may be carefully opened and the beads sprinkled over a spoonful of applesauce which should be taken right away. The applesauce should not be warm. Only use applesauce.

Digoxin

- This medicine helps make the heart beat stronger. Keep taking as directed, even if you feel well.
- Do not stop taking this medicine without talking to your healthcare provider. Stopping this medication suddenly may make your condition worse.
- Avoid becoming overheated or dehydrated as an overdose can easily occur if you are dehydrated.
- Symptoms of overdose include poor or no appetite, nausea, vomiting, diarrhea, vision changes (such as blurred or yellow/green vision), uneven heartbeats, and feeling like you might pass out. If any of these occur, see a healthcare provider right away.
- There are many medications that can interact with digoxin. Check with your physician or pharmacist before starting any new medicines, including over the counter, vitamin, and/or herbal products.
- To be sure that this medication is not causing harmful effects, your blood may need to be tested on a regular basis. Your kidney function will also need to be monitored.

PRACTICE CASE

Janice Fernandez: SOAP Note for 09/24/2014 Age on DOS: 74 yrs, DOB: 08/29/1940	**San Diego Medical Group** 35 La Jolla Drive Suite 100 San Diego, CA 92130 (444) 444-4444

seen by: Alison James
seen on: Wednesday 24 September 2014

VS

Height:	Weight:	BMI:	Blood Pressure:	Temp:	Pulse:	Resp Rate:
61.0 in	132.0 lb	24.9	105 / 75 mmHg	98.7 F	104 bpm	23 rpm

CC | "Shortness of breath and puffy legs"

S | **ADMISSION NOTE**
JF is a pleasant 74 y/o female accompanied by her husband.

HPI: Per her husband, JF was doing well with her heart failure regimen over the past several months. Over the Easter holiday, they visited family and ate ham, canned vegetables, and casseroles. Her shortness of breath symptoms started to get worse at that time and continued to worsen over the next 2 weeks. JF reports a 7 pound weight gain over < 2 weeks. Her appetite is normally good, but has decreased in the past week and she has experienced some mild nausea. She hoped the SOB would go away, but it hasn't. She used to be able to walk several blocks without getting SOB, but for the past week she gets SOB after only 1 block. Her legs and feet are puffy by noon. Her urine output is good, but the fluid is not going away. If she sits in a chair and does nothing, she does not have SOB. She states that she is compliant with her medications. Review of the prescription bottles and refill history support this statement.

Allergies: NKDA

O | **Past Medical History:**
HF (LVEF 35% documented by ECHO in 2012) / HTN / Type 2 DM (diet controlled) / Depression

Medications Prior to Admission:
Lasix 40 mg PO daily / Prinivil 40 mg PO daily / Digox 0.25 mg PO daily / Toprol XL 100 mg PO daily / Celexa 20 mg PO daily

Social History: No alcohol, drugs, or tobacco
Family History: Mother with HTN, dyslipidemia, and MI. Father with HTN. Both deceased. Sister with Type 2 DM.

Labs (reference range)
Na 142 (135 - 145 mEq/L)
K 4.7 (3.5 - 5.0 mEq/L)
Cl 101 (95 - 103 mEq/L)
HCO3 25 (24 - 30 mEq/L)
BUN 30 (7 - 20 mg/dL)
SCr 1.6 (0.6 - 1.3 mg/dL)
Glu 218 (70 - 110 mg/dL)
Digoxin 1.8 ng/mL (indication specific)
BNP 372 pg/mL (< 100 pg/mL)

Tests
ECG: sinus tachycardia, no ST or T wave changes
Chest xray: cardiomegaly, bilateral pleural effusions, and mild right-sided pulmonary edema

A | 1) Decompensated heart failure likely secondary to recent dietary indiscretion
2) Hypertension
3) Type 2 Diabetes
4) Depression

P | Admit JF for management of decompensated heart failure.

Questions

CrCl = 29 (<30) ⇒ ↓ dose/frequency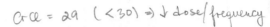

1. JF is taking *Digox* for her heart failure. What is the therapeutic range for this medication when used for heart failure?

   a. 0.8 – 2 mcg/mL
   b. < 1 mcg/mL
   c. 0.8 – 2 ng/mL
   d. 0.5 – 0.9 ng/mL
   e. < 2 mcg/mL

2. In assessing JF's clinical scenario, which of the following statements is correct?

   a. Sodium bicarbonate should be started to treat her metabolic acidosis.
   b. Stop the *Toprol XL*.
   c. *Prinivil* should be titrated to the target dose of 80 mg daily.
   d. Start an intravenous loop diuretic.
   e. Start dopamine at this time.

3. While in the hospital, JF is started on furosemide IV to remove some fluid that has accumulated around her lungs. Choose the correct statement concerning JF's furosemide therapy:

   a. If JF experiences ototoxicity, she should be switched to ethacrynic acid.
   b. Furosemide is not effective as a diuretic when the creatinine clearance is < 30 mL/min.
   c. The furosemide will increase her risk of hyperkalemia.
   d. The intravenous equivalent dose to her oral dose is 40 mg.
   e. None of the above.

4. JF is ready to be discharged home. She is restarted on all of her previous medications at the same doses before hospitalization. Which of the following counseling points are correct? (Select **ALL** that apply.)

   a. If you lose your appetite, become nauseated, have mental disturbances, and/ or lightheadedness, contact your doctor immediately as this may indicate that the digoxin level is too high.
   b. The dose of digoxin is too high for JF.
   c. Digoxin therapy can cause you to be more symptomatic at first, but this will resolve within a week.
   d. Digoxin therapy is best taken at night, after dinner.
   e. Taking digoxin can improve your symptoms and increase your quality of life.

5. Which of the following medications should JF generally avoid as they may worsen her heart failure? (Select **ALL** that apply.)

   a. Celecoxib
   b. Verapamil
   c. Amiodarone
   d. Pioglitazone
   e. Naproxen

6. JF has been home for 1 month and goes in for her first doctor's appointment since her hospitalization. She is taking all her medications which include lisinopril 40 mg daily, *Lasix* 40 mg daily and *Toprol XL* 100 mg daily. She is following a sodium restricted diet and monitoring her weight but she still gets fatigued quite easily. The doctor decides to increase her *Toprol XL* dose to 200 mg daily. Which of the following patient counseling points should be discussed with JF regarding this change? (Select **ALL** that apply.)

   a. The increase in medication may make you feel more tired and dizzy at first. These effects will likely improve in a few days – if they do not, contact the doctor.
   b. This increase in medication can cause a loss of appetite, blurred vision, light-headedness, and/or visual changes.
   c. This medication may be cut in half (if directed to do so) with a pill cutter, but do not crush or chew the tablets.
   d. This medication can be taken without regards to food.
   e. The increase in medication will cause an increase in your heart rate. Call your healthcare provider if you feel your heart racing.

Questions 7-10 do not pertain to the above case.

7. A 70 kg patient is beginning carvedilol therapy for heart failure. The starting dose is 3.125 mg BID. What should the target dose for carvedilol be in this patient?

   a. 6.25 mg BID
   b. 12.5 mg BID
   c. 25 mg BID
   d. 50 mg BID
   e. 100 mg BID

8. A 75 year-old patient comes to the emergency department with acute decompensated heart failure. He presents with pulmonary congestion, altered mental status and poor urine output. His vital signs are BP 80/57, HR 112, RR 24 and oxygen saturation of 93%. He is started on bumetanide 1mg IV Q12 hours. Which of the following medications is most appropriate to initiate in this patient at this time?

   a. Dopamine
   b. Nitroprusside
   c. Metolazone
   d. Nitroglycerin
   e. Milrinone

   b/c systolic < 90

9. What is the trade name for eplerenone?

   a. *Invega*
   b. *Invanz*
   c. *Invirase*
   d. *Isuprel*
   e. *Inspra*

10. The medical team will start a dobutamine drip on a 60 kg patient at 10 mcg/kg/min. The standard concentration of dobutamine in the pharmacy is a 250 mg/250 mL bag. Calculate how many hours the bag will last at the prescribed infusion rate.

    a. 3 hours
    b. 5 hours
    c. 7 hours
    d. 10 hours
    e. 15 hours

    $$\frac{10\ \mu g}{kg\ min} \cdot 60\ kg = 600\ \frac{\mu g}{min}$$

    $$600\ \mu g = 0.6\ mg \rightarrow 1\ min$$
    $$36\ mg? \leftarrow 1\ hr$$

    $$\frac{250\ mg}{36\ mg/hr} = 6.9\ hrs$$

Answers

1-d, 2-d, 3-e, 4-a,b,e, 5-a,b,d,e, 6-a,c,d, 7-c, 8-a, 9-e, 10-c

"lub" • P wave - atrial contraction
"dub" • QRS complex - ventricular contraction (depolarization)
• T wave - ventricular repolarization (filling up w/ blood)
  ↳ hypo K⁺ ⇒ flattened T wave
    hyper K⁺ ⇒ peaked

ANTIARRHYTHMICS

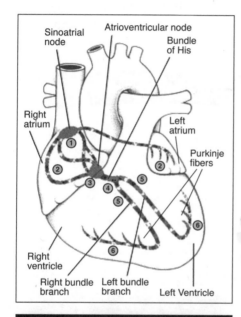

We gratefully acknowledge the assistance of Tien Ng, PharmD, FCCP, BCPS (AQ-C), Associate Professor at the University of Southern California School of Pharmacy, in preparing this chapter.

BACKGROUND

A normal heart beats in a regular, coordinated way because electrical impulses traveling down the cardiac conduction system trigger a sequence of organized contractions. Arrhythmias are caused by abnormalities in the formation and/or conduction of these electrical impulses. Heart rate describes the frequency of depolarization of the ventricles. Arrhythmias can result in the heart rate being slow (bradyarrhythmias) or fast (tachyarrhythmias). Normally the resting heart rate (HR) in adults is 60 to 100 beats per minute (BPM). An arrhythmia can be silent (asymptomatic) which may only be detected during a routine physical exam. However, most patients experience symptoms. The common complaints of patients experiencing an arrhythmia are: palpitations (feeling like there is fluttering or racing), dizziness, light-headedness, shortness of breath, chest pain, fatigue, and in severe cases can lead to syncope, heart failure, and death.

PATHOPHYSIOLOGY OF ARRHYTHMIAS

Activation of the heart in the normal sequence through the cardiac conduction system, and at the usual rate of 60 to 100 BPM, is called normal sinus rhythm (NSR). The diagram above traces the normal sequence of formation and conduction of an electrical impulse in the heart. The sinoatrial (SA) node (1) initiates an electrical im-

GUIDELINE

January CT, Wann LS, Alpert JS, et al. 2014 AHA/ACC/HRS Guideline for the Management of Patients With Atrial Fibrillation: A Report of the American College of Cardiology/American Heart Association Task Force on Practice Guidelines and the Heart Rhythm Society. *Journal of the American College of Cardiology.* 2014; doi:10.1016/j.jacc.2014.03.022.

pulse that spreads throughout the right and left atria (2), resulting in atrial contraction. The electrical impulse reaches the atrioventricular (AV) node (3), where its conduction is slowed. Once through the AV node, the impulse travels down the bundle of HIS (4), which divides into the right bundle branch for the right ventricle (5) and the left bundle branch for the left ventricle (5). The impulse then spreads through the ventricles via Purkinje fibers (6), resulting in a coordinated and rapid contraction of both ventricles. Any disruption in the normal sequence of impulse formation or conduction can result in an arrhythmia.

Na+
K+
Mg++
Ca++

Many factors can contribute to the development of arrhythmias. The most common cause of arrhythmias is myocardial ischemia or infarction. Other conditions resulting in damage to cardiac tissue, including heart valve disorders, hypertension and heart failure, can cause arrhythmias. Non-cardiac conditions can trigger or predispose a patient to arrhythmias. Electrolyte imbalances, especially those involving potassium, magnesium, sodium and calcium (since these are important to cardiac electrophysiology), can result in arrhythmias. Elevated sympathetic states, including hyperthyroidism and infection, can contribute. Drugs can cause or worsen arrhythmias; this includes the drugs used to treat arrhythmias. Many drugs can affect conduction and/or prolong repolarization through effects on ion currents in the heart. Drug-induced slowing of repolarization, as indicated by prolongation of the QT interval on an electrocardiogram, can result in a particularly dangerous ventricular tachyarrhythmia called Torsade de Pointes (TdP).

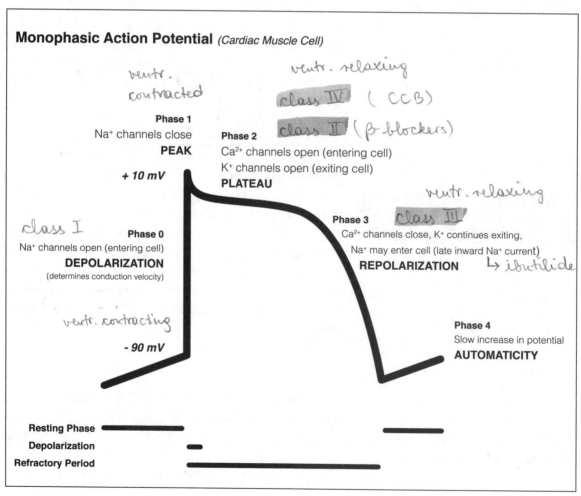

Monophasic Action Potential *(Cardiac Muscle Cell)*

ventr. contracted

ventr. relaxing
class IV (CCB)
class II (β-blockers)

Phase 1
Na+ channels close
PEAK
+ 10 mV

Phase 2
Ca²⁺ channels open (entering cell)
K⁺ channels open (exiting cell)
PLATEAU

ventr. relaxing
Phase 3 class III
Ca²⁺ channels close, K⁺ continues exiting,
Na⁺ may enter cell (late inward Na⁺ current)
REPOLARIZATION   ↳ ibutilide

class I
Phase 0
Na+ channels open (entering cell)
DEPOLARIZATION
(determines conduction velocity)

ventr. contracting
- 90 mV

Phase 4
Slow increase in potential
AUTOMATICITY

Resting Phase
Depolarization
Refractory Period

rhythm control in a fib

1) convert to NSR
** • direct current ♡version **
• amiodarone, dofetilide, ibutilide
• flecainide, propafenone

2) maintain NSR
• dofetilide, dronedarone, sotalol
• flecainide, propafenone

CLASSIFICATION OF ARRHYTHMIAS

Arrhythmias are generally classified based on their location of origin into two broad categories: supraventricular (originating above the atrioventricular node) or ventricular (originating below the atrioventricular node). Common supraventricular tachyarrhythmias include sinus tachycardia, atrial fibrillation, atrial flutter, focal atrial tachycardias, and supraventricular re-entrant tachycardias (formerly known as paroxysmal supraventricular tachycardias or PSVTs). Common ventricular arrhythmias include premature ventricular contractions (PVCs), ventricular tachycardia and ventricular fibrillation.

TYPE OF AFIB	DEFINITION
Paroxysmal	AFib that terminates spontaneously or with intervention within 7 days of onset; episodes may recur with variable frequency
Persistent	Continuous AFib that is sustained > 7 days
Longstanding Persistent	Continuous AFib of > 12 months duration
Permanent (⊖ rhythm control)	Permanent AFib is used when a joint decision has been made by clinician and patient to cease further attempts to restore and/or maintain NSR; this represents a therapeutic attitude rather than an inherent attribute of the AFib

Atrial fibrillation (AFib) is the most common type of arrhythmia. AFib results from multiple waves of electrical impulses in the atria, resulting in an irregular and usually rapid ventricular response. The rapid ventricular rate can result in hypotension, and worsen underlying ischemia and heart failure. Due to the disorganized depolarization of the atria, coordinated atrial contraction is impaired, which increases the risk of thromboembolism and stroke. Therefore, the management of atrial fibrillation usually involves anticoagulation (see Anticoagulation chapter), and antiarrhythmics to either slow the ventricular rate (rate-control) and/or terminate the atrial fibrillation to restore normal sinus rhythm (rhythm-control). Beta blockers (preferred) or nondihydropyridine calcium channel blockers are recommended for treatment in patients with AFib for controlling ventricular rate. Of note, patients with underlying heart failure should not receive a nondihydropyridine calcium channel blocker. Amiodarone and digoxin are not first-line agents for ventricular rate control, but may be considered for refractory patients. The goal resting HR is < 80 BPM in patients with symptomatic AFib; however, a more lenient rate-control strategy of < 110 BPM may be reasonable in patients who are asymptomatic and have preserved left ventricular function. Rhythm-control consists of 1) methods for conversion to NSR and 2) maintenance of NSR. Conversion to NSR is most effective with direct current cardioversion. Medications can be used as well and include amiodarone (oral and IV), dofetilide, flecainide, ibutilide and propafenone. For maintenance of NSR, dofetilide, dronedarone, flecainide, propafenone, or sotalol is recommended. Due to toxicities, amiodarone should only be used when other agents have failed or are contraindicated. Rhythm control antiarrhythmics should not be used when AF becomes permanent.

rate control

rhythm control

Atrial flutter is caused by one or more rapid circuits in the atrium. Atrial flutter is usually more organized and regular than atrial fibrillation. This arrhythmia occurs most often with heart disease, and in the first week after heart surgery. Atrial flutter often converts to AFib.

Premature ventricular contractions (PVCs) are among the most common arrhythmias and occur in people with and without heart disease. This is a "skipped heartbeat" that anyone

ventr. tachy & antiarrhythmics + pulse

ventr. tachy & medical - pulse ER !!

can experience. These electrical impulses are generated from within the ventricular tissue. In some people, it can be related to stress, too much caffeine or nicotine, or too much exercise. A series of PVCs in a row resulting in a heart rate of greater than 100 beats per minute is known as ventricular tachycardia. Ventricular tachycardia is further classified based on the presence or absence of a detectable peripheral pulse. Ventricular tachycardia with a pulse is treated with certain antiarrhythmics, whereas, ventricular tachycardia without a pulse is a medical emergency. Untreated ventricular tachycardia can degenerate into ventricular fibrillation (complete disorganized electrical activation of the ventricles) which is always a medical emergency.

↗ tx: IV Mg

QT Prolongation & Torsade De Pointes (TdP)

Prolongation of the QT interval is a risk factor for Torsade de Pointes, a particularly lethal ventricular tachyarrhythmia which is most commonly associated with drugs and can result in sudden cardiac death. The QT interval is measured from the beginning of the QRS complex to the end of the T wave. It reflects ventricular depolarization and repolarization. Drug-induced QT prolongation is dose-dependent (concentration-dependent). Combining different drugs that can cause QT prolongation can have additive effects, and the benefit-risk of using multiple QT prolonging medications must be evaluated carefully. Reduced drug clearance or drug interactions which result in increased concentrations of QT prolonging drugs will also accentuate the effect on the QT interval and increased risk for TdP. Therefore, if a patient is using low dose of amitriptyline for neuropathic pain, this may not be considered a particularly risky drug due to the low dose, although the risk may be additive with other drugs or if the elimination of amitriptyline is impaired.

Additive QT Prolongation

The following QT interval prolonging drugs must be used with caution in patients with any arrhythmia risk (including those with any pre-existing cardiac condition or history of arrhythmia, electrolyte abnormalities or those taking other proarrhythmic drugs).

proarrhythmic agents →

- Class I (Class Ia in particular) and Class III antiarrhythmics (amiodarone, disopyramide, dofetilide, dronedarone, ibutilide, procainamide, quinidine, sotalol), flecainide, lidocaine and mexiletine.

- Antibiotics including quinolones (*Avalox®* moxifloxacin, gemifloxacin, levofloxacin, ciprofloxacin, norfloxacin and ofloxacin), macrolides (azithromycin, erythromycin, clarithromycin), amantadine, bedaquiline, foscarnet, metronidazole, sulfamethoxazole/trimethoprim, telavancin, telithromycin and others.

- Azole antifungals (fluconazole, itraconazole, ketoconazole, posaconazole and voriconazole).

- Antidepressants including tricyclics (amitriptyline, doxepin, others), SSRIs (citalopram, escitalopram, others), SNRIs, mirtazapine and trazodone. Sertraline is preferred in cardiac patients.

- Antiemetic agents including the 5-HT$_3$-receptor antagonists (dolasetron, granisetron, ondansetron, palonosetron) and droperidol and phenothiazines.

- Antipsychotics (aripiprazole, asenapine, chlorpromazine, clozapine haloperidol, iloperidone, olanzapine, paliperidone, pimozide, quetiapine, risperidone, thioridazine, ziprasidone).

- Oncology agents (arsenic, bosutinib, crizotinib, dasatinib, nilotinib, *Tasigna®* pazopanib, sorafenib, sunitinib, others).

- Protease inhibitors (atazanavir, nefinavir, ritonavir, saquinavir) and rilpivirine. *Edurant®*

- Other agents: alfuzosin, apomorphine, buprenorphine, chloroquine, cyclosporine, dexmedetomidine, diphenhydramine, ezogabine, fingolimod, galantamine, methadone, mirabegron, pentamidine, quinine, ranolazine, sevoflurane, solifenacin, tacrolimus, tizanidine, others. *Precedex®*

DRUG THERAPY

Antiarrhythmic drugs are used for two main purposes in the treatment of cardiac arrhythmias. Some antiarrhythmic drugs are used to terminate the arrhythmia and restore and maintain normal sinus rhythm (class I and III antiarrhythmics). Other agents are used to slow the ventricular rate during a supraventricular arrhythmia (class II and IV antiarrhythmics, digoxin).

Antiarrhythmics work by affecting the electrical currents in the cells of the heart. By blocking the movement of ions in different phases of the cardiac action potential (see figure), select drugs can reduce conduction velocity and/or automaticity, or prolong the refractory period which can slow or terminate abnormal electrical activity which results in arrhythmias. They can also occasionally worsen the existing arrhythmia or cause other arrhythmias. All patients should be instructed to be seen if they suspect they have "worse heartbeat problems" or have an increase in their symptoms. Prior to starting any medication for a non life-threatening arrhythmia, be sure to always check the patient's electrolytes and run a toxicology screen.

class I & III
- *terminate arrhythmia*
- *restore/ maintain NSR*

⇓

[*RHYTHM*]

1) convert to NSR
- *amiodarone*
  dofetilide
  ibutilide

2) maintain NSR
- *dofetilide*
  dronedarone
  sotalol

- *flecainamide*
  propafenone

[*** direct current*
  ♡ *version ***]

both 1st line?   *not 1st line*

class II & IV, digoxin
(HR)
↓ ventricular rate during
supraventricular arrhythmia

* β-blockers ⇒ 1st line!

⇓

[*RATE*]

* no difference in efficacy
between rate control
and rhythm control
agents
BUT rate control agents
are safer
(rhythm control are
proarrhythmic!)

681

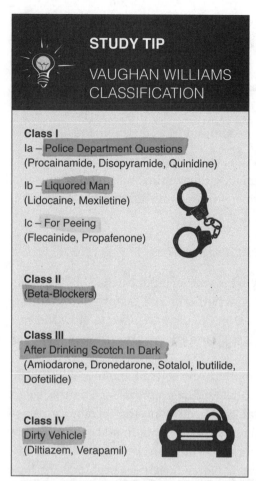

STUDY TIP

VAUGHAN WILLIAMS CLASSIFICATION

Class I
Ia – Police Department Questions
(Procainamide, Disopyramide, Quinidine)

Ib – Liquored Man
(Lidocaine, Mexiletine)

Ic – For Peeing
(Flecainide, Propafenone)

Class II
(Beta-Blockers)

Class III
After Drinking Scotch In Dark
(Amiodarone, Dronedarone, Sotalol, Ibutilide, Dofetilide)

Class IV
Dirty Vehicle
(Diltiazem, Verapamil)

Vaughan Williams Classification of Antiarrhythmics

The Vaughan Williams classification system is the most commonly used classification system for anti-arrhythmic drugs. Here the drugs are split into categories based on their dominant electrophysiological effect. It has the virtue of simplicity, although many drugs overlap into more than one category.

CLASS	DRUGS
Ia	Procainamide, Disopyramide, Quinidine
Ib	Lidocaine, Mexiletine, (Phenytoin)
Ic	Flecainide, Propafenone
II	Beta-blockers (e.g., esmolol, propranolol)
III	Amiodarone, Dronedarone, Sotalol, Ibutilide, Dofetilide
IV	Diltiazem, Verapamil

CLASS I ANTIARRHYTHMICS

Class I antiarrhythmics are sodium channel blockers. All sodium channel blockers have the potential to have negative inotropic effects. They are further sub-classified based on the duration of time they bind to the sodium channel. Class Ia are intermediate sodium channel blockers and they also block the potassium channels. Class Ib are fast sodium channel blockers. Class Ic are long sodium channel blockers.

The Cardiac Arrhythmia Suppression Trial (CAST) was a negative study in which patients with premature ventricular contractions (PVCs) after a MI were randomized to flecainide, encainide or placebo. Those taking flecainide or encainide had an increase in mortality compared to patients taking placebo. This led to a boxed warning on many of the Class I antiarrhythmics, particularly the Class Ic agents.

Class Ia Antiarrhythmics

Class Ia antiarrhythmics block both sodium channels and potassium channels. Quinidine and disopyramide also have strong anticholinergic effects. Procainamide is metabolized by acetylation to N-acetyl-procainamide (active metabolite). Class Ia antiarrhythmic drugs ↓ conduction velocity, ↑ refractory period, and ↓ automaticity.

DRUG	DOSING	SAFETY/SIDE EFFECTS/MONITORING
QuiNIDine Tablet, Injection	IR: 400 mg PO Q6H ER: 300-648 mg PO Q8-12H Take with food or milk to ↓ GI upset	**BOXED WARNING** Quinidine may ↑ mortality in treatment of AFib or flutter; control AV conduction before initiating. Antiarrhythmic drugs have not been shown to enhance survival in non-life-threatening ventricular arrhythmias and may increase mortality; the risk is greatest in patients with structural heart disease. **CONTRAINDICATIONS** Concurrent use of quinolones that prolong the QT interval, amprenavir, ritonavir; 2nd/3rd degree heart block or idioventricular conduction delays (unless patient has a functional artificial pacemaker), thrombocytopenia, thrombocytopenic purpura, myasthenia gravis **SIDE EFFECTS** Diarrhea (35%), stomach cramping (22%), lightheadedness, QT prolongation, nausea, vomiting, anorexia, cinchonism (tinnitus, hearing loss, blurred vision, headache, delirium), rash, positive Coombs test (risk for hemolytic anemia), hemolysis risk in G6PD positive patients, drug-induced lupus erythematosus (DILE) **MONITORING** ECG (QT interval, QRS duration), electrolytes (esp. K^+, Mg^{2+}), BP, CBC, LFTs, renal function **NOTES** Different salt forms are not interchangeable (267 mg of gluconate = 200 mg of sulfate form) Avoid changes in Na^+ intake. ↓ Na^+ intake can ↑ quinidine levels Alkaline foods may ↑ quinidine levels
Procainamide Injection	Active metabolite, N-acetyl procainamide (NAPA), is renally cleared; ↓ dose when CrCl < 50 mL/min **Therapeutic levels:** Procainamide: 4-10 mcg/mL NAPA: 15-25 mcg/mL Combined: 10-30 mcg/mL Draw levels 6-12 hours after IV infusion has started	**BOXED WARNINGS (3)** Potentially fatal blood dyscrasias (e.g., agranulocytosis) → monitor patient closely in the first 3 months of therapy and periodically thereafter. Long-term use leads to positive antibody (ANA) test in 50% of patients which may result in drug-induced lupus erythematosus (DILE) in 20-30% of patients. In the Cardiac Arrhythmia Suppression Trial (CAST), recent (> 6 days but < 2 years ago) myocardial infarction patients with asymptomatic, non-life-threatening ventricular arrhythmias did not benefit and may have been harmed by attempts to suppress the arrhythmia with flecainide or encainide. **CONTRAINDICATIONS** 2nd/3rd degree heart block (unless patient has a functional artificial pacemaker), SLE, torsade de pointes, procaine or other ester-type local anesthetics **SIDE EFFECTS** Hypotension, rash, lupus-like syndrome, QT prolongation **MONITORING** ECG (QT interval, QRS duration), electrolytes (esp. K^+, Mg^{2+}), BP, renal function, signs of lupus (butterfly rash, stabbing chest pain, joint pain), procainamide and NAPA levels, CBC

Handwritten annotations:

LUPUS

works on phase 0 of cardiac axn potential

"scrubbing butts"

cinchona tree (alkaloid)

antiACh effects

metabolized by acetylation

Class Ia Antiarrhythmic Agents Continued

DRUG	DOSING	SAFETY/SIDE EFFECTS/MONITORING
Disopyramide (*Norpace, Norpace CR*) Capsule	IR: 100-200 mg PO Q6H CR: 200-400 mg PO Q12H CrCl ≤ 40 mL/min: Decrease frequency of IR and do not use CR formulation Take on an empty stomach	**BOXED WARNING** In the Cardiac Arrhythmia Suppression Trial (CAST), recent (> 6 days but < 2 years ago) myocardial infarction patients with asymptomatic, non-life-threatening ventricular arrhythmias did not benefit and may have been harmed by attempts to suppress the arrhythmia with flecainide or encainide. **CONTRAINDICATIONS** 2nd/3rd degree heart block (unless patient has a functional artificial pacemaker), cardiogenic shock, congenital QT syndrome, sick sinus syndrome **WARNINGS** HF, BPH/urinary retention/narrow-angle glaucoma, myasthenia gravis (due to anticholinergic effects) **SIDE EFFECTS** Anticholinergic effects > 10% (dry mouth, constipation, urinary retention), hypotension, QT prolongation, HF **MONITORING** ECG (QT interval, QRS duration), electrolytes (esp. K^+, Mg^{2+}), BP, signs of HF

Class Ia Antiarrhythmic Drug Interactions

- Quinidine is a substrate of CYP450 3A4 (major), 2C9 (minor) and P-gp; inhibits 2D6 (strong), 2C9 (weak), 3A4 (weak) and P-gp. Some major drug interactions with quinidine include digoxin (↓ digoxin dose by 50%), warfarin (↑ INR), potent 3A4 inhibitors and others.

- Procainamide is a substrate of 2D6 (major). Moderate and strong 2D6 inhibitors will ↑ levels of procainamide.

- Disopyramide is a substrate of 3A4 (major). Inhibitors of 3A4 and drugs with anticholinergic side effects may ↑ risk of side effects; 3A4 inducers may ↓ the effects of disopyramide.

- All Class Ia antiarrhythmic agents can have additive QT prolongation with other agents that also prolong the QT interval.

Class Ib Antiarrhythmics

Class Ib antiarrhythmics are pure sodium channel blockers. They are only useful for ventricular arrhythmias (no efficacy for supraventricular arrhythmias such as atrial fibrillation). They cross the blood-brain-barrier and, therefore, can cause CNS adverse effects. Class Ib antiarrhythmic drugs have little effect on conduction velocity at normal heart rates but will have greater effects on ↓ conduction and automaticity at higher heart rates with little effect on ↓ refractory period.

only for ventr arrhythmias!!

DRUG	DOSING	SAFETY/SIDE EFFECTS/MONITORING
Lidocaine *(Xylocaine)* Injection	1-1.5 mg/kg IV bolus; can repeat bolus 0.5-0.75 mg/kg every 5-10 mins up to 3 mg/kg (cumulative dose); followed by 1-4 mg/min IV infusion. Can be given via endotracheal tube (need higher dose – 2-2.5x the IV dose)	**BOXED WARNING** In the Cardiac Arrhythmia Suppression Trial (CAST), recent (> 6 days but < 2 years ago) myocardial infarction patients with asymptomatic, non-life-threatening ventricular arrhythmias did not benefit and may have been harmed by attempts to suppress the arrhythmia with flecainide or encainide.
Mexiletine Capsule	200 mg PO Q8H; max 1.2 g/day Take with food.	**CONTRAINDICATIONS** $2^{nd}/3^{rd}$ degree heart block (unless patient has a functional artificial pacemaker). Lidocaine: Wolff-Parkinson-White syndrome, Adam-Stokes syndrome, allergy to corn or corn-related products or amide type anesthetic **WARNINGS** Caution in the elderly, in patients with hepatic impairment and in patients with HF **SIDE EFFECTS** Lightheadedness, dizziness, incoordination, nausea, vomiting, tremor, CNS (hallucinations, disorientation, confusion) **MONITORING** ECG, BP, LFTs, mental status, electrolytes (esp. K^+, Mg^{2+})

Class Ib Antiarrhythmic Drug Interactions

- Lidocaine is a substrate of 3A4 (major), 1A2 (major), and 2C9 (minor); inhibits 1A2 (weak). Amiodarone, beta-blockers, 3A4 inhibitors (e.g., diltiazem, verapamil, grapefruit juice, erythromycin, clarithromycin, itraconazole, ketoconazole, protease inhibitors) ↑ lidocaine levels.

- Mexiletine is a substrate of 1A2 (major) and 2D6 (major); inhibits 1A2 (strong).

Class Ic Antiarrhythmics

Class Ic antiarrhythmic agents are sodium channel blockers and exhibit negative inotropic properties. Propafenone also has significant beta-adrenergic receptor blocking effects. These drugs are absolutely contraindicated in patients with heart failure or with a recent myocardial infarction (due to negative inotropic properties). Class Ic antiarrhythmic drugs significantly ↓ conduction velocity and automaticity, but have little-to-no effect on refractory period.

DRUG	DOSING	SAFETY/SIDE EFFECTS/MONITORING
Flecainide Tablet	50 mg PO Q12H; max 400 mg/d CrCl ≤ 50 mL/min: ↓ dose by 50%	**BOXED WARNINGS (3)** When treating atrial flutter, 1:1 atrioventricular conduction may occur; pre-emptive negative chronotropic therapy (e.g., digoxin, beta-blockers) may lower the risk. Proarrhythmic effects – not recommended for patients with permanent atrial fibrillation. In the Cardiac Arrhythmia Suppression Trial (CAST), recent (> 6 days but < 2 years ago) myocardial infarction patients with asymptomatic, non-life-threatening ventricular arrhythmias did not benefit and may have been harmed by attempts to suppress the arrhythmia with flecainide or encainide. Do not use in patients with structural heart disease (HF, S/P MI) **CONTRAINDICATIONS** $2^{nd}/3^{rd}$ degree heart block (unless patient has a functional artificial pacemaker), cardiogenic shock, coronary artery disease (heart failure, myocardial infarction), concurrent use of amprenavir or ritonavir **SIDE EFFECTS** Dizziness, visual disturbances, headache, dyspnea, new or worsening arrhythmia **MONITORING** ECG, BP, HR, electrolytes (esp. K^+, Mg^{2+})
Propafenone *(Rythmol, Rythmol SR)* Capsule, tablet	IR: 150-300 mg PO Q8H SR: 225-425 mg PO Q12H	**BOXED WARNING** In the Cardiac Arrhythmia Suppression Trial (CAST), recent (> 6 days but < 2 years ago) myocardial infarction patients with asymptomatic, non-life-threatening ventricular arrhythmias did not benefit and may have been harmed by attempts to suppress the arrhythmia with flecainide or encainide. Do not use in patients with structural heart disease (HF, S/P MI). **CONTRAINDICATIONS** Sinoatrial and atrioventricular disorders (unless patient has a functional artificial pacemaker), sinus bradycardia, cardiogenic shock, HF, hypotension, bronchospastic disorders **SIDE EFFECTS** Taste disturbance (metallic), dizziness, visual disturbances, nausea, vomiting, new or worsening arrhythmia, bronchospasm, worsening HF **MONITORING** ECG, BP, HR, electrolytes (esp. K^+, Mg^{2+})

Class Ic Antiarrhythmics Drug Interactions

- Flecainide is a substrate of 2D6 (major) and 1A2 (minor); inhibits 2D6 (weak).

- Propafenone is a substrate of 2D6 (minor), 3A4 (minor) and 1A2 (minor); inhibits 1A2 and 2D6 (weak).

work on phase 2 of cardiac action potential

Class II Antiarrhythmic Agents

Class II antiarrhythmic drugs block beta receptors and indirectly block calcium channels in the SA and AV nodes, resulting in decreased automaticity and conduction velocity in the nodes. These drugs are used to slow the ventricular rate in supraventricular tachyarrhythmias. Please refer to the Hypertension chapter for review of the beta blockers.

DRUG	DOSING	SAFETY/SIDE EFFECTS/MONITORING
Esmolol *(Brevibloc)* Injection Beta-1 selective *vesicant!!! – monitor IV site*	0.5–1 mg/kg–followed by 50-150 mcg/kg/min; max 300 mcg/kg/min	**CONTRAINDICATIONS** 2nd/3rd degree heart block (unless patient has a functional artificial pacemaker), sinus bradycardia, sick sinus syndrome, cardiogenic shock, decompensated heart failure, bronchial asthma *↳ IF hypoperfusion ONLY!* **SIDE EFFECTS** Hypotension, bradycardia, hyperkalemia, hypo- and hyperglycemia **MONITORING** ECG, BP, HR, electrolytes (esp. K^+, Mg^{2+}) **NOTES** Esmolol is a vesicant; monitor IV site
Propranolol *(Inderal LA, InnoPran XL)* Injection, oral Non-selective beta-blocker	Dose varies Oral: 10-30 mg Q6-8H IV: 1 mg/min, may repeat every 2 mins up to 3 doses	

For drug interactions/counseling of beta blockers, refer to the Hypertension chapter.

work on phase 3 of cardiac axn potential

Class III Antiarrhythmic Agents

Class III antiarrhythmic drugs all significantly prolong the refractory period. Most drugs in this class act through blockade of potassium channels. Ibutilide is the exception, and works by activating the late inward sodium current which results in a significant ↑ in refractory period. Amiodarone and dronedarone also block alpha- and beta-adrenergic receptors, and calcium and sodium channels. Sotalol also has significant beta-adrenergic receptor blocking activity.

DRUG	DOSING	SAFETY/SIDE EFFECTS/MONITORING
Amiodarone (*Cordarone, Pacerone, Nexterone*) Tablet, Injection	**IV dosing** Pulseless VT/VF = 300 mg IV push x 1, may repeat 150 mg x 1 if needed VT with pulse = 150 mg IV bolus, 1 mg/min x 6 hours, then 0.5 mg/min x 18 hours or longer **Atrial fibrillation** 600-800 mg/d for a 10 gram loading dose, followed by 200 mg daily **Maintenance of NSR** 400-600 mg/d for 2-4 weeks; then 100-200 mg daily **Ventricular arrhythmias** 800-1,600 mg/d x 1-3 weeks, then 600-800 mg/d x 4 weeks, then 400 mg/d	**BOXED WARNINGS (4)** Only for life-threatening arrhythmias due to toxicity: patients should be hospitalized when therapy is initiated Pulmonary toxicity may occur without symptoms Liver toxicity Proarrhythmic: exacerbation of arrhythmias making them more difficult to tolerate or reverse **CONTRAINDICATIONS** Severe sinus-node dysfunction, 2nd/3rd degree heart block (unless patient has a functional artificial pacemaker), bradycardia causing syncope, cardiogenic shock, hypersensitivity to iodine **SIDE EFFECTS** > 10% Hypotension, bradycardia, corneal microdeposits, dizziness, ataxia, GI upset, constipaton, peripheral neuropathy, tremor, hypothyroidism/hyperthyroidism (more hypo), optic neuritis, pulmonary fibrosis, photosensitivity, ↑ LFTs, slate blue (blue-grayish) skin discoloration *skin exposed to sunlight* **MONITORING** Pulmonary (including chest X-ray), thyroid (amiodarone partially inhibits the peripheral conversion of T4 to T3), and liver function tests at baseline and periodically thereafter; ECG, BP, HR, electrolytes (esp. K+, Mg2+), regular ophthalmic exams **NOTES** Pregnancy Category D Infusions longer than 2 hours must be administered in a non-polyvinyl chloride (PVC) container such as polyolefin or glass. Premixed *Nexterone* comes in GALAXY containers which are non-PVC and non-DEHP and can be stored up to 24 months at room temperature. PVC tubing is fine to use. Use a 0.22 micron filter, incompatible with heparin (flush with saline). Administer IV according to protocol. Premixed IV bag advantages: longer stability, PVC bag not an issue, available in most commonly used concentrations. If hypotension or bradycardia occurs, slow infusion rate or discontinue. t½ = 40-60 days. Recommended as a drug of choice in patients with concomitant heart failure. MedGuide required.

Handwritten margin notes:

pre-mixed already in non-PVC, non DEHP => (GALAXY)

DOC IN ♡ FAILURE !

leeching - drug absorbed by PVC

- *↓ digoxin 50%*
- *↓ warfarin 30-50%*
- *simvastatin max 20 mg/day*
- *lovastatin max 40 mg/day*

* BBW x 4
1) pts hospitalized when iniating
2) pul tox
3) hepatotox
4) pro-arrhythmic

Class III Antiarrhythmic Agents Continued

DRUG	DOSING	SAFETY/SIDE EFFECTS/MONITORING
Dronedarone (Multaq) Tablet	400 mg PO BID with meals $t\frac{1}{2}$ = 13-19 hrs (less lipophilic than amiodarone)	**BOXED WARNINGS (2)** HF (NYHA Class IV or any class with a recent hospitalization) and in patients with permanent AFib. **CONTRAINDICATIONS** 2nd/3rd degree heart block (unless patient has a functional artificial pacemaker), symptomatic heart failure, HR < 50, concomitant use of strong 3A4 inhibitors, concomitant use of drugs that prolong the QT interval, QT ≥ 500 msec, PR interval > 280 msec, lung or liver toxicity related to previous amiodarone use, severe hepatic impairment, pregnancy, nursing mothers **WARNINGS** Hepatic failure (esp. in the first 6 months), lung disease (including pulmonary fibrosis and pneumonitis), marked ↑ SCr, prerenal azotemia and acute renal failure have been reported usually in the setting of heart failure or hypovolemia, hypokalemia or hypomagnesemia with concomitant administration of potassium-depleting diuretics **SIDE EFFECTS** QT prolongation, ↑ SCr, N/V, abdominal pain, diarrhea, bradycardia, dermatitis, asthenia **MONITORING** LFTs (especially in the first 6 months), ECG, BP, HR, electrolytes (esp. K^+, Mg^{2+}), SCr, BUN **NOTES** Pregnancy Category X Noniodinated derivative of amiodarone MedGuide required

Handwritten notes (left margin):

- ↓ digoxin 50%
- w/ warfarin → monitor INR

$t\frac{1}{2}$ = 13-19 hrs

Handwritten notes (bottom):

drug-induced lupus in this chapter
1. procainamide - 20-30% of pts
2. quinidine

monitor LFTs
1. amiodarone
2. dronedarone
   ↳ + SrCr, BUN
3. quinidine
4. class Ib (lido/mex)
5. CCB

monitor SrCr/BUN
1. procainamide
2. sotalol
3. dofetilide
4. dronedarone
   ↳ + LFTs
5. digoxin

class Ia } most potent
class III } QT prolonging
antiarrhythmics

Class III Antiarrhythmic Agents Continued

DRUG	DOSING	SAFETY/SIDE EFFECTS/MONITORING
Sotalol *(Betapace, Betapace AF, Sotylize, Sorine)* Tablet, Solution, Injection Non-selective beta-blocker	80 mg PO BID; can ↑ to 160 mg PO BID (monitor QT interval and renal function closely) CrCl ≤ 60 mL/min: ↓ frequency	**BOXED WARNINGS (3)** Sotalol can cause life-threatening ventricular tachycardia and QT prolongation. To minimize risk of arrhythmias, initiation (or reinitiation) and dosage increase should be done in a hospital with continuous monitoring and staff familiar with recognizing and treating life-threatening arrhythmias Adjust dosing interval based on creatinine clearance to decrease risk of proarrhythmia, QT prolongation is directly related to sotalol concentration *Betapace* should not be substituted with *Betapace AF* since *Betapace AF* is distributed with educational information specifically for patients with AFib/Atrial flutter. **CONTRAINDICATIONS** 2nd/3rd degree heart block (unless patient has a functional artificial pacemaker), congenital or acquired long QT syndrome, sinus bradycardia, uncontrolled HF, cardiogenic shock, asthma For *Betapace AF*: QT > 450 msec, bronchospastic conditions, CrCl < 40 mL/min, K^+ < 4 mEq/L, sick sinus syndrome **SIDE EFFECTS** Bradycardia, palpitations, chest pain, dizziness, fatigue, dyspnea, hypotension, nausea/vomiting, torsades, HF, bronchoconstriction **MONITORING** SCr, ECG, BP, HR, electrolytes (esp. K^+, Mg^{2+})
Ibutilide *(Corvert)* Injection	≥ 60 kg: 1 mg IV over 10 min, may repeat x 1 after 10 minutes <60 kg: 0.01 mg/kg over 10 min, may repeat x 1 after 10 minutes	**BOXED WARNINGS (2)** Potentially fatal arrhythmias can occur Patients with chronic AFib may not be the best candidates since they often revert back **SIDE EFFECTS** Ventricular tachycardias (e.g., torsades), headache, hypotension, increased QT interval
Dofetilide *(Tikosyn)* Capsule	500 mcg PO BID if CrCl > 60 mL/min; ↓ dose in renal impairment and/or if QT interval increases T.I.P.S. *(Tikosyn In Pharmacy System)* – designated to allow retail pharmacies to stock and dispense *Tikosyn*; must be enrolled and staff must be educated. Pharmacists must verify that the hospital/prescriber is a confirmed participant before drug is dispensed.	**BOXED WARNING** Must be initiated (or reinitiated) in a setting with continuous ECG monitoring for a minimum of 3 days or 12 hrs after cardioversion, whichever is greater **CONTRAINDICATIONS** Patients with congenital or acquired long QT syndromes, concurrent use of dolutegravir, HCTZ, itraconazole, ketoconazole, megestrol, prochlorperazine, trimethoprim, verapamil; HR < 50, CrCl < 20 mL/min, QT > 440 msec **SIDE EFFECTS** Headache, dizziness, ventricular tachycardias (e.g., torsades), increased QT interval **MONITORING** ECG, BP, HR, SCr, electrolytes (esp. K^+, Mg^{2+}). Then monitor QT interval and CrCl every 3 months (discontinue if QT > 500 msec) **NOTES** MedGuide required REMS program – available to prescribers and hospitals through *Tikosyn* Education Program. This program provides comprehensive education about the importance of in-hospital treatment initiation and individualized dosing.

Handwritten annotations:
- solution
- ↓ renal fxn = extend dosing interval
- Betapace – ventr. arrhythm
- Betapace AF – a fib
- CrCl > 60 ⇒ 500 mg BID
- CrCl = 40–60 ⇒ 250 mg BID
- CrCl = 20–40 ⇒ 125 mg BID
- CrCl < 20 ⇒ ∅

Class III Antiarrhythmic Drug Interactions

- All Class III antiarrhythmic agents can have additive QT prolongation with other agents that also prolong the QT interval.

- Use extreme caution with other negative chronotropes (e.g., beta blockers, verapamil, diltiazem) which can ↑ risk of bradycardia with sotalol, amiodarone, and dronederone.

- Electrolyte abnormalities (K^+, Na^+, Ca^{2+}, Mg^{2+}, etc.) should be corrected before any antiarrhythmic therapy is initiated or the risk of arrhythmia is increased (true for all antiarrhythmics).

- Do not use grapefruit juice/products. Avoid ephedra and St. John's wort (P-gp inducer).

Amiodarone Drug Interactions

- Amiodarone is an inhibitor of 2C9 (moderate), 2D6 (moderate), 3A4 (weak) and P-gp; major substrate of 3A4 and 2C8 and P-gp. Strong/moderate inhibitors of 3A4, 2C8 and P-gp will increase the levels of amiodarone and strong/moderate inducers of 3A4, 2C8 and P-gp will decrease the levels of amiodarone.

- When starting amiodarone, ↓ dose of digoxin by 50% and ↓ dose of warfarin by 30-50%. Do not exceed 20 mg/day of simvastatin or 40 mg/day of lovastatin in patients taking amiodarone.

both
3A4
subs

Dronedarone Drug Interactions

- Dronedarone is a moderate inhibitor of 2D6, 3A4, and P-gp; major substrate of 3A4. Avoid use with strong inhibitors and inducers of 3A4 and other other drugs that can prolong the QT interval. If using digoxin, reduce dose of digoxin by 50%. Caution with the use of statins at higher doses (see above under amiodarone).

- Monitor INR after initiating dronedarone in patients taking warfarin.

Dofetilide Drug Interactions

- Dofetilide is a minor 3A4 substrate. Avoid with other QT prolonging agents.

class	1° channel	phase of ♡ AP
I	Na^+	0
II	Ca^{++} (indirect)	2
III	K^+	3
IV	Ca^{++} (direct)	2

Class IV Antiarrhythmic Agents

Class IV antiarrhythmic drugs block L-type calcium channels, slowing SA and AV nodal conduction velocity. These drugs are used to slow the ventricular rate in supraventricular tachyarrhythmias. Nondihydropyridine calcium channel blockers should not be used in patients with LV systolic dysfunction and decompensated HF due to their negative inotropic effects, but they may be used in patients with HF with preserved LV systolic function.

DRUG	DOSING	SAFETY/SIDE EFFECTS/MONITORING
Diltiazem *(Cardizem, Cardizem CD, Cardizem LA, Cartia XT, Dilacor XR, Dilt-CD, Dilt-XR, Diltzac, Tiazac, Taztia XT)* Tablet, Capsule, Injection	120-360 mg PO daily	**CONTRAINDICATIONS** Severe hypotension (systolic < 90 mmHg), 2nd/3rd degree heart block, sick sinus syndrome (unless the patient has a functioning artificial pacemaker), severe hypotension, cardiogenic shock, acute MI and pulmonary congestion, systolic HF, Wolff-Parkinson-White syndrome (WPW) with AFib **SIDE EFFECTS** Edema, headache, dizziness, AV block, bradycardia, hypotension, arrhythmias, HF, constipation (more with verapamil), gingival hyperplasia
Verapamil *(Calan, Calan SR, Covera HS, Verelan, Verelan PM)* Tablet, Capsule, Injection	180-480 mg PO daily	**MONITORING** ECG, BP, HR, electrolytes (esp. K+, Mg2+), LFTs **NOTES** Only non-dihydropyridine CCBs are used as antiarrhythmics

Ø grape-fruit

constipation

For drug interactions/counseling of calcium channel blockers, please see Hypertension chapter.

Agents Not Included In Vaughan Williams Classification

- Adenosine slows conduction through the AV node via activation of adenosine-1 receptors. Adenosine is used to restore normal sinus rhythm (NSR) in supraventricular re-entrant tachyarrhythmias. ↳ by causing transient AV block

- Digoxin causes direct AV node suppression, ↑ refractory period and ↓ conduction velocity. Digoxin enhances vagal tone, resulting in decreased ventricular rate in supraventricular tachyarrhythmias. Digoxin reduces the resting heart rate but it is ineffective at controlling the ventricular response during exercise; therefore, it is not used first line for rate control.

DRUG	DOSING	SAFETY/SIDE EFFECTS/MONITORING
Adenosine *(Adenocard)* Injection	Used in paroxysmal supraventricular tachycardia (PSVTs) and not for converting AFib/Atrial flutter or ventricular tachycardia 6 mg IV push (may increase to 12 mg if not responding) t½: less than 10 sec 60 sec	**CONTRAINDICATIONS** 2nd/3rd degree heart block, sick sinus syndrome, symptomatic bradycardia (except in patients with a functional pacemaker), bronchospastic lung disease **SIDE EFFECTS** Transient new arrhythmia, facial flushing, chest pain/pressure, neck discomfort, dizziness, headache, GI distress, transient decrease in blood pressure, dyspnea

Class IV Antiarrhythmic Agents Continued

$t_{1/2} = 24\text{-}48\ hrs$ *(handwritten)*

DRUG	DOSING	SAFETY/SIDE EFFECTS/MONITORING
Digoxin *(Digox, Lanoxin)* Tablet, Solution, Injection	0.125-0.25 mg PO daily Loading dose [called total digitalizing dose (TDD)] is 0.5 -1 mg. Give ½ of the TDD as the initial dose, followed by ¼ of the TDD in 2 subsequent doses at 6-8 hour intervals. Alternatively, give 0.25 mg IV and repeat dosing to a max of 1.5 mg over 24 hours. Therapeutic range for AFib = 0.8 – 2 ng/mL (lower therapeutic range in heart failure) When CrCL < 50 mL/min, ↓ dose or ↓ frequency ↓ dose by 20-25% when going from oral to IV Antidote: *DigiFab*	**CONTRAINDICATIONS** Ventricular fibrillation **WARNINGS** 2nd/3rd degree heart block without a pacemaker, Wolff-Parkinson-White syndrome (WPW) with AFib **SIDE EFFECTS** Dizziness, mental disturbances, headache, diarrhea, nausea, vomiting **MONITORING** ECG, HR, BP, electrolytes (esp. K^+, Ca^{2+}, Mg^{2+}) SCr and drug level (optimally obtain a level 12 to 24 hours after a dose) **Toxicity** First signs of toxicity are nausea/vomiting, loss of appetite and bradycardia. Other signs of toxicity include blurred/double vision, altered color perception, greenish-yellow halos around lights or objects, abdominal pain, confusion, delirium, arrhythmia (prolonged PR interval, accelerated junctional rhythm, bidirectional ventricular tachycardia). **NOTES** Pregnancy Category C Digoxin is not given alone; used in combination with a beta blocker or CCB.

Handwritten margin notes:
hold in acute renal failure
po → IV or IM ↓ dose 20-25%
↑ tox risk
∘ ↓ $K^+ < 3.5$
∘ ↓ Mg^{2+}
∘ ↑ Ca^{2+}
use only if sx
(LD)
TDD = 0.5 - 1 mg
↦ ½ initially
↦ ¼ × 2 subsequent doses @ 6-8 hr intervals
OR 0.25 mg IV, repeat, max 1.5mg over 24 hrs

Digoxin Drug-Drug and Drug-Disease Interactions

- Use caution when administering other drugs that slow HR (such as beta blockers); see Drug Interactions chapter.

- Digoxin is mostly renally cleared and partially cleared hepatically. Decreased renal function requires a ↓ digoxin dose. In acute renal failure, digoxin is held.

- Digoxin is a P-gp and 3A4 substrate. Digoxin levels ↑ with amiodarone, dronedarone, quinidine, verapamil, erythromycin, clarithromycin, itraconazole, propafenone, and many other drugs. Reduce digoxin dose by 50% if patient is on amiodarone or dronedarone.

- Hypokalemia (K+ < 3.5 mEq/L), hypomagnesemia, and hypercalcemia ↑ the risk of digoxin toxicity.

- Hypothyroidism can ↑ digoxin levels.

Amiodarone Patient Counseling

- Dispense Medication Guide.

- This medication is used to treat certain types of serious (possibly fatal) irregular heartbeat problems called arrhythmias. It is used to restore and maintain the normal heart rhythm and keep a regular, steady heartbeat. Amiodarone works by blocking certain electrical signals in the heart that can cause an irregular heartbeat. This medication has not been shown to help people with these arrhythmias live longer. Treatment should be started in a hospital to monitor your condition.

- Take this medication by mouth, usually once or twice daily or as directed by your healthcare provider. If stomach upset occurs, take the medication with food.

- Severe (sometimes fatal) lung or liver problems have occurred in some rare instances with amiodarone use. Tell your doctor immediately if you experience any of these serious side effects: cough, fever, chills, chest pain, difficult or painful breathing, coughing up blood, severe stomach pain, nausea, vomiting, fatigue, yellowing eyes or skin, or dark-colored urine, and new shortness of breath. Your blood will need to be checked, and possibly a chest X-ray during treatment.

- Like other medications used to treat irregular heartbeats, amiodarone can infrequently cause them to become worse. Seek immediate medical attention if your heart continues to pound or skips a beat.

- This drug may infrequently cause serious vision changes. Tell your healthcare provider immediately if you develop any vision changes (such as seeing halos or blurred vision). You will need to have your eyes checked before and during the time you are taking amiodarone.

peripheral neuropathy

- You may develop "pins and needles" or numbness in your legs, hands and feet, or muscle weakness, or trouble walking. Discuss with your healthcare provider if this happens.

- This drug can change how your thyroid gland works, and may cause your metabolism to speed up or slow down. Tell your healthcare provider if you develop any symptoms of low or overactive thyroid including cold or heat intolerance, unexplained weight loss/gain, thinning hair, unusual sweating, nervousness, irritability, or restlessness. Please discuss this with your healthcare provider and tests can be ordered to check your thyroid function.

- This drug may cause your skin to be more sensitive to the sun. Stay out of the sun during the midday and use protective clothing and broad spectrum sunscreen (see Skin chapter). Infrequently, this medication has caused the skin to become a blue-gray color. This effect is not harmful and usually goes away months after the drug is stopped.

- Do not consume grapefruit or drink grapefruit juice while using this medication. Grapefruit juice can increase the amount of medication in your blood.

- This drug can interact with other medicines. Before starting a new medicine including any over-the-counter medications, discuss with your pharmacist if it is safe to use with amiodarone.

- If you miss a dose, do not take a double dose to make up for the dose you missed. Continue with your next regularly scheduled dose.

Digoxin Patient Counseling

- This medicine helps the heart beat with a more regular rate. Keep taking as directed, even if you feel well.

- Do not stop taking this medicine without talking to your healthcare provider. Stopping suddenly may make your condition worse.

- Avoid becoming overheated or dehydrated as an overdose can occur more easily if you are dehydrated.

- Symptoms of overdose may include nausea, vomiting, diarrhea, loss of appetite, vision changes (such as blurred or yellow/green vision), confusion and hallucinations, and feeling like you might pass out. If any of these occur, see your healthcare provider right away.

- There are many medications that can interact with digoxin. Check with your healthcare provider before starting any new medicines, including over the counter, vitamin, and/or herbal products.

- To be sure that this medication is not causing harmful effects, your blood may need to be tested on a regular basis. Your kidney function will also need to be monitored.

PRACTICE CASE

AH is a 57 y/o Hispanic male who had an appointment in the clinic this morning. He has asked to speak to the pharmacist at the clinic pharmacy. He tells you that he went to the clinic because he felt like his heart was racing and he felt dizzy. The doctor told him that he has atrial fibrillation. He is concerned that this will affect his life span. You are able to access his clinic records and learn that his past medical history includes heart failure (NYHA Class 3) and hypertension. He is a smoker.

Allergies: Sulfa

Medications:
Digox 0.25 mg PO daily
Lasix 40 mg PO daily
Spironolactone 12.5 mg PO daily
Coreg CR 20 mg PO daily
Lisinopril 40 mg PO daily

Vitals:
BP: 152/83 mmHg   HR: 84 BPM   RR: 15 BPM   Temp: 98.5°F

Labs: Na (mEq/L) = 137 (135 - 145)
K (mEq/L) = 5.2 (3.5 - 5)
Cl (mEq/L) = 99 (95 - 103)
HCO_3 (mEq/L) = 28 (24 - 30)
BUN (mg/dL) = 43 (7 - 20)
SCr (mg/dL) = 1.4 (0.6 - 1.3)
Glucose (mg/dL) = 112 (100 - 125)
Ca (mg/dL) = 9.5 (8.5 - 10.5)
Mg (mEq/L) = 1.8 (1.3 - 2.1)
PO_4 (mg/dL) = 3.8 (2.3 - 4.7)

The cardiologist has written a new prescription for amiodarone 200 mg PO daily that AH would like to have filled.

Questions

1. Before the prescription for amiodarone is filled, the pharmacist should call the doctor to decrease the dose of which of AH's medications?

   a. Digox
   b. Lasix
   c. Spironolactone
   d. Coreg CR
   e. Lisinopril

2. When counseling AH on the use of amiodarone, he should be told to expect periodic monitoring of these organ systems:

   a. Liver, kidney, and eyes
   b. Liver, colon, and kidney
   c. Kidney, gall bladder, and CNS
   d. Thyroid, kidney, and liver
   e. Thyroid, liver, and lungs

*amiodarone
→ NOT renally cleared!*

3. Which of the following are side effects of amiodarone? (Select **ALL** that apply.)

   a. Skin discoloration
   b. Corneal deposits
   c. Pulmonary fibrosis
   d. Taste perversions — *propafenone (Rythmol)*
   e. Hypothyroidism

4. AH develops thyroid dysfunction. His doctor switches him to *Multaq* to try and alleviate the problem. Choose the correct therapeutic equivalent for *Multaq*:

   a. Mexiletine
   b. Flecainide
   c. Lidocaine
   d. Dronedarone
   e. Dofetilide

Questions 5-10 do not apply to the above case.

5. What class of antiarrhythmic is disopyramide in the Vaughan Williams classification system?

   a. Ia
   b. Ib
   c. Ic
   d. III
   e. IV

6. A patient has a long QT interval. She is at risk for fatal arrhythmias. Which of the following medications will increase her risk of further QT prolongation? (Select **ALL** that apply.)

   a. Quinidine
   b. Ketorolac
   c. Docusate
   d. Amiodarone
   e. Sotalol

7. A patient is using digoxin. The doctor must make sure that the potassium level stays within a safe range. This safe range is defined as:

   a. 0.8-2 ng/mL
   b. 2.5-5 ng/dL
   c. 3.5-5 mEq/L
   d. 3.5-5 mEq/mL
   e. 7.8-10 mEq/mL

8. A patient is beginning digoxin 0.125 mg daily in addition to her *Lopressor* therapy. After a few weeks, the patient develops an infection with nausea and vomiting. She is weak and dehydrated and is admitted to the hospital. Her work up is significant for new onset acute renal failure, mental confusion, pneumonia and atrial fibrillation. She is started on levofloxacin for her pneumonia. Which of the following statements regarding this patient and her digoxin therapy is true? (Select **ALL** that apply.)

   a. The digoxin may have become toxic due to her decreased renal function.
   b. An elevated digoxin level can worsen nausea and vomiting.
   c. The digoxin level will increase due to the initiation of levofloxacin.
   d. Mental confusion may be due to an elevated digoxin level.
   e. The patient will need to stay on digoxin therapy regardless of the level.

9. Which of the following statement(s) are true regarding *Tikosyn*? (Select **ALL** that apply.)

   a. *Tikosyn* does not need to be dose-adjusted in renal impairment.
   b. *Tikosyn* comes orally and can be started at home. *must be initiated in hospital*
   c. The generic name is dronedarone.
   d. *Tikosyn* is considered first-line therapy for rate control in patients with atrial fibrillation.
   e. Monitoring of the QT interval and renal function is essential in patients receiving *Tikosyn*.

10. A patient is slightly bradycardic. The physician does not wish to further lower the heart rate. Choose the agent that will least likely cause the patient's heart rate to drop any lower:

    a. Verapamil
    b. Sotalol *nonselective β-blocker*
    c. Digoxin
    d. Amlodipine
    e. Diltiazem

Answers

1-a, 2-e, 3-a,b,c,e, 4-d, 5-a, 6-a,d,e, 7-c, 8-a,b,d, 9-e, 10-d

ANTICOAGULATION

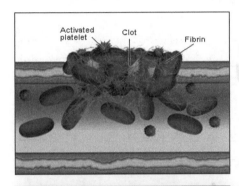

Activated platelet   Clot   Fibrin

GUIDELINES

January CT, Wann LS, Alpert JS, et al. 2014 AHA/ACC/HRS Guideline for the Management of Patients With Atrial Fibrillation: A Report of the American College of Cardiology/American Heart Association Task Force on Practice Guidelines and the Heart Rhythm Society. *Journal of the American College of Cardiology.* 2014; doi:10.1016/j. jacc.2014.03.022.

Executive Summary of Antithrombotic Therapy and Prevention of Thrombosis, 9th ed: American College of Chest Physicians Evidence-Based Clinical Practice Guidelines. *CHEST* 2012;141(2):7S-47S.

ISMP has many resources on safe use of anticoagulants available at www.ismp.org

BACKGROUND

Anticoagulants are used to prevent blood clots from forming and to keep existing clots from becoming larger or expanding. They do not break down existing clots (like thrombolytics such as tPA). Anticoagulants must be carefully monitored due to the risks involved with either clotting or bleeding. A deep vein thrombosis (DVT) is a blood clot (thrombus) in a vein. DVTs can occur anywhere in the body but are most frequently found in the deep veins of the legs, thighs, and pelvis. A blood clot which has traveled from its point of origin is called an embolus (plural emboli). When a clot forms in a deep vein, the clot or a piece of the clot can break off, travel to the heart and be pumped into the arteries of the lung. This can cause a pulmonary embolism (PE). Venous thromboembolism (VTE) refers to a DVT and/or a PE. Patients with atrial fibrillation or patent foramen ovale (PFO) can form clots in the heart which can travel to the brain causing a transient ischemic attack (TIA) or ischemic stroke. Anticoagulants are used for the prevention and treatment of venous thromboembolism (DVT/PE), for the prevention of stroke, and in the treatment of acute coronary syndrome (ACS).

CLOT FORMATION

Coagulation is the process by which blood clots form. A number of factors can lead to activation of the coagulation process such as blood vessel injury, blood stasis, and pro-thrombotic conditions. The coagulation process involves activation of platelets and the clotting cascade which leads to fibrin formation and a stable clot. All of the clotting factors have an inactive and an active form. Once ac-

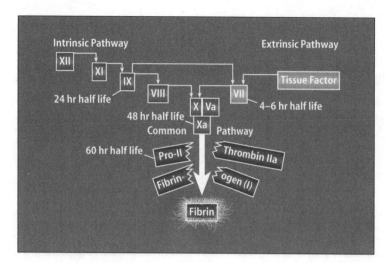

tivated, the clotting factor will serve to activate the next clotting factor in the sequence until fibrin is formed. The coagulation cascade has two pathways which leads to fibrin formation: the contact activation pathway (or the intrinsic pathway) and the tissue factor pathway (or the extrinsic pathway). Anticoagulants are used to inhibit the clotting cascade, thereby reducing clot formation.

DRUG TREATMENT

Anticoagulants work by various mechanisms. Unfractionated heparin, low molecular weight heparins (LMWHs), and ^Ifondaparinux work by binding to antithrombin (AT) causing a conformational change which increases ATs activity 1,000-fold. AT inactivates thrombin and other proteases involved in blood clotting, including factor Xa. LWMHs inhibit factor Xa more specifically than unfractionated heparin. Fondaparinux (Arixtra) is a synthetic pentasaccharide that requires AT binding to selectively inhibit Factor Xa.

Direct thrombin inhibitors (which block thrombin directly, as the name suggests) decrease the amount of fibrin available for clot formation. The intravenous direct thrombin inhibitors have been very important clinically since they do not cross-react with heparin-induced thrombocytopenia (HIT) antibodies. Once HIT develops in the hospital setting, the injectable direct thrombin inhibitor argatroban is the drug of choice. The oral direct thrombin inhibitor, dabigatran (Pradaxa), does not require blood tests to monitor for effectiveness, is not subject to food interactions and has few drug interactions; these are advantages over warfarin. It does, however, cause significant dyspepsia/gastritis and has an increased risk of GI bleeding compared to other oral anticoagulants.

Rivaroxaban (Xarelto) and apixaban (Eliquis) work by inhibiting Factor Xa. These oral agents are taken once or twice daily and require no laboratory monitoring for efficacy. Dabigatran, rivaroxaban and apixaban should not be used in patients with prosthetic heart valves. Warfarin interacts with many other drugs; these three anticoagulants have less problematic drug interactions.

Warfarin is a vitamin K antagonist. Vitamin K is required for the carboxylation of clotting factors II, VII, IX, and X. Without adequate vitamin K, the liver produces the factors – but they have reduced coagulant activity. Warfarin requires careful patient monitoring – with frequent blood tests to measure the INR (international normalized ratio), the test used to measure warfarin's safety and efficacy. Warfarin has a narrow therapeutic range and the INR is highly variable and is affected greatly by many drugs or changes in dietary vitamin K intake.

Safety Concerns & the Pharmacist's Role

All of the anticoagulants can cause significant bleeding and are classified as "High Alert" medications by the Institute for Safe Medication Practices (ISMP). Bleeding events associated with anticoagulants put the patient at risk for increased mortality, including higher risk for stroke and myocardial infarction. Ten percent of all adverse drug events treated in the emergency department are due to anticoagulants. The Joint Commission's National Patient Safety Goals require the implementation of policies and protocols to properly initiate and manage anticoagulant therapy. Patients receiving anticoagulants should receive individualized care through a defined process that includes standardized ordering, dispensing, administration, monitoring and patient/caregiver education (for treatment doses). When pharmacists are involved in managing anticoagulants, patient care and outcomes are improved and costs are decreased. Pharmacists are also involved with ensuring that patients who need anticoagulants for VTE prophylaxis – such as orthopedic and cardiac surgical patients – receive them.

VTE PROPHYLAXIS

The CHEST guidelines provide specific recommendations for the prevention of VTE depending on the level of risk. Risk factors for the development of VTE are found in the table (see left). Patients may have a contraindication to anticoagulants (bleeding) or have a high risk for bleeding and will need non-drug alternatives to prevent clotting. These options include intermittent pneumatic compression (IPC) devices or graduated compression stockings (GCS). For acutely ill hospitalized medical patients at increased risk for thrombosis, the recommended drugs and their respective regimens are listed below.

e.g. intra-cranial hemorrhage

RISK FACTORS FOR THE DEVELOPMENT OF VENOUS THROMBOEMBOLISM

- Surgery
- Major trauma or lower extremity injury
- Immobility
- Cancer or chemotherapy
- Venous compression (tumor, hematoma, arterial abnormality)
- Previous venous thromboembolism
- Increasing age
- Pregnancy and postpartum period
- Estrogen-containing medications or selective estrogen receptor modulators
- Erythropoiesis-stimulating agents
- Acute medical illness
- Inflammatory bowel disease
- Nephrotic syndrome
- Myeloproliferative disorders
- Paroxysmal nocturnal hemoglobinuria
- Obesity
- Central venous catheterization
- Inherited or acquired thrombophilia

Anticoagulant Recommendations for Acutely Ill Hospitalized Patients at Increased Risk of VTE

DRUG	DOSE
Unfractionated heparin (UFH)	5,000 units SC Q8-12H
Low Molecular Weight Heparin (LMWH)	Enoxaparin 30 mg SC BID or 40 mg SC daily (If CrCl < 30 mL/min, give 30 mg SC daily)
	Dalteparin 2,500-5,000 units SC daily
Factor Xa inhibitor	Fondaparinux 2.5 mg SC daily (do not use if CrCl < 30 mL/min or if patient weighs < 50 kg)
	Rivaroxaban 10 mg PO daily (do not use if CrCl < 30 mL/min)
	Apixaban 2.5 mg PO BID

For long distance travelers at risk for VTE (previous VTE, recent surgery or trauma, active malignancy, pregnancy, estrogen use, advanced age, limited mobility, severe obesity, or known thrombophilic disorder), the following recommendations will ↓ VTE risk: frequent ambulation, calf muscle exercise, sitting in an aisle seat and using graduated compression stockings with 15 - 30 mmHg of pressure at the ankle during travel. Aspirin or anticoagulants should not be used.

limit tx to 3 mo if bleeding ↑↑ risk ↑↑
- *VTE caused by surgery/transient risk factor ⇒ tx VTE x 3 mo*
- *VTE unprovoked ⇒ tx VTE x > 3 mo; bleeding risk: low-moderate*
- *2+ unprovoked VTEs ⇒ tx ∞*

VTE TREATMENT

Any VTE that is provoked (caused) either by surgery or a transient (reversible) risk factor should be treated for 3 months. If the cause of the VTE is unprovoked, extending therapy longer than 3 months is recommended, as long as the bleeding risk is low-to-moderate. If the risk of bleeding is high, limit the treatment to 3 months. When patients have 2 episodes of unprovoked VTE, long-term treatment may be warranted.

Heparin-Induced Thrombocytopenia (HIT) Overview

Heparin-induced thrombocytopenia is an immune-mediated IgG drug reaction that is associated with a high risk of venous and arterial thrombosis. The immune system forms antibodies against heparin when it binds to platelet factor 4 (PF 4). These IgG antibodies form a complex with heparin and PF 4. In HIT, this complex binds to the Fc receptors on platelets, which leads to further platelet activation, and causes a release of PF 4 and other pro-coagulant microparticles from platelet granules. If left untreated, HIT can lead to a pro-thrombotic state causing many complications including heparin-induced thrombocytopenia and thrombosis (HITT). HITT causes amputations, post-thrombotic syndrome, and/or death. The estimated incidence of HIT is ~3% of those patients exposed to heparin for more than four days. It is lower with a shorter duration of treatment. The typical onset of HIT occurs 5-14 days after the start of heparin or within hours if a patient has been exposed to heparin within the past 3 months. A diagnosis is made by a compatible clinical picture, a profound, unexplained drop in platelet count (defined as > 50% drop from baseline) and laboratory confirmation of antibodies or platelet activation by heparin. Although thrombocytopenia is the most common presenting feature of HIT, in up to 25% of patients with HIT, the development of thrombosis precedes the development of thrombocytopenia. Platelets are checked at baseline and monitored frequently.

HIT = ↓ by >50% PLTs from baseline + Ab/PLT activation

Management of HIT Complicated by Thrombosis (HITT) per the CHEST 2012 Guidelines

- If HIT is suspected/confirmed, stop all forms of heparin and LMWH [including heparin flushes (can use regional citrate) and heparin-coated catheters]. If the patient is on warfarin and diagnosed with HIT, the warfarin should be discontinued and vitamin K should be administered. Although the patient is at a high risk of thrombosis, warfarin use with a low platelet count has a high correlation with warfarin-induced limb gangrene and necrosis.

- In patients with HIT, nonheparin anticoagulants are recommended, in particular, argatroban, over the further use of heparin or LMWH or initiation/continuation of vitamin K antagonists. Argatroban is also favored in patients with renal impairment.

- Do not start warfarin therapy until the platelets have recovered to at least 150,000/mm³. Warfarin should be initiated at lower doses (5 mg maximum). Overlap warfarin with a nonheparin anticoagulant for a minimum of 5 days and until the INR is within target range for 24 hours.

- If urgent cardiac surgery or PCI is required, bivalirudin is the preferred anticoagulant.

Angiomax®

UNFRACTIONATED HEPARIN (UFH)

UFH binds to antithrombin (AT) and inactivates thrombin (Factor IIa) and Factor Xa (as well as factors IXa, XIa, XIIa, and plasmin) and prevents the conversion of fibrinogen to fibrin.

DRUG	DOSING	SAFETY/SIDE EFFECTS/MONITORING
Unfractionated Heparin Anticoagulation Treatment/ Prophylaxis Many strengths and volumes (ranging from 1 unit/mL to 20,000 units/mL), including total units of 5,000, 10,000, 12,500, 20,000, 25,000 & others. Usual infusion for treatment is 25,000 units in 250 mL (concentration: 100 units/ mL) in D5W, ½ NS or NS. Line Flush 10 units/mL, 100 units/mL syringes (in 1, 2, 2.5, 3, 5, 10, 30 mL) **SAFETY NOTE** Heparin lock-flushes (*HepFlush*) are used to keep IV lines open (patent), not used for anticoagulation. There have been fatal errors, especially in neonates, made by choosing the incorrect heparin strength. Heparin injection 10,000 units/ mL and heparin flushes 10 or 100 units/mL look and sound alike. Using a higher dose to flush a line could cause fatal hemorrhage. Refer to the Medication Safety chapter for safe use of antithrombotics.	**Prophylaxis of VTE** 5,000 units SC Q8-12H **Treatment of VTE** 80 units/kg IV bolus followed by 18 units/kg/hr infusion or a fixed dose of 5,000 units IV bolus followed by 1,000 units/hr infusion. If treating as an outpatient, give 333 units/kg x 1 dose SC, then 250 units/kg SC Q12H **Treatment of ACS/STEMI** 60 units/kg IV bolus (max 4,000 units); 12 units/kg/hr (max 1,000 units/hr) infusion Use actual body weight for dosing Onset – IV: immediate; SC: 20-30 min t½ = 1.5 hrs. Monitor for a ↓ in platelet count of > 50% from baseline. HIT has cross-sensitivity with LMWHs Antidote: Protamine – 1 mg protamine will reverse ~100 units of heparin; max dose 50 mg	**BOXED WARNING** Some products contain benzyl alcohol as a preservative, use of these products is contraindicated in neonates and infants. **CONTRAINDICATIONS** Uncontrolled active bleed, severe thrombocytopenia, ICH, history of HIT, hypersensitivity to pork products **WARNING** Do not give IM due to hematoma risk **SIDE EFFECTS** Bleeding (epistaxis, ecchymosis, gingival, GI), thrombocytopenia, heparin induced thrombocytopenia (HIT), hyperkalemia and osteoporosis (with long-term use) **MONITORING** Heparin is monitored via the aPTT (or anti-Xa level: 0.3-0.7 units/mL) aPTT is taken 6 hours after initiation, every 6 hours until therapeutic range of 1.5-2.5 x control (patient's baseline) is reached, then every 24 hours. Also check aPTT after every dosage change. Platelet count, Hgb, Hct at baseline and daily to monitor for thrombocytopenia and bleeding **NOTES** Pregnancy Category C Unpredictable anticoagulant response – has variable and extensive binding to plasma proteins and cells

↑K+

to ↓ med errors, outsource prep of heparin flushes, i.e. buy prefilled syringes

protamine 1mg = heparin ~ 100 units ↓ max 50 mg

do NOT use packaging color to verify dose!

normal aPTT = 22 - 38 sec (tx aPTT determined individually for each hospital / laboratory based on reagent)

* UFH, LMWHs, fondaparinux do NOT work in pts w/ antithrombin deficiency

Heparin Drug Interactions

- Most drug interactions are due to additive effects with other agents that can ↑ bleeding risk (other anticoagulants, antiplatelet drugs, some herbals, NSAIDs, SSRIs, SNRIs, thrombolytics, and possibly others). See the Drug Interactions chapter.

LOW MOLECULAR WEIGHT HEPARINS (LMWHs)

LMWHs work similar to heparin except that the inhibition is much greater for Factor Xa than Factor IIa.

DRUG	DOSING	SAFETY/SIDE EFFECTS/MONITORING
Enoxaparin (Lovenox) Comes in multidose vials (300 mg/3 mL) and prefilled syringes: 30 mg/0.3 mL, 40 mg/0.4 mL, 60 mg/0.6 mL, 80 mg/0.8 mL, 100 mg/mL, 120 mg/0.8 mL, 150 mg/mL 1 mg = 100 units Anti-Xa activity ↑ K+ ↑ LFTs	**Prophylaxis of VTE** 30 mg SC Q12H or 40 mg SC daily CrCl < 30 mL/min: 30 mg SC daily **Treatment of VTE and UA/NSTEMI** 1 mg/kg SC Q12H (or 1.5 mg/kg SC daily for VTE inpatient treatment only) CrCl < 30 mL/min: 1 mg/kg SC daily **Treatment for STEMI** In patients < 75 years: 30 mg IV bolus plus a 1 mg/kg SC dose followed by 1 mg/kg SC Q12H (max 100 mg for the first two doses only) CrCl < 30 mL/min: 30 mg IV bolus plus a 1 mg/kg SC dose, followed by 1 mg/kg SC daily In patients ≥ 75 years: 0.75 mg/kg SC Q12H (no bolus – max 75 mg for the first two doses only) CrCl < 30 mL/min: 1 mg/kg SC daily (no bolus) In patients managed with percutaneous coronary intervention (PCI): if the last SC dose was given 8-12 hours before balloon inflation, give 0.3 mg/kg IV bolus	**BOXED WARNING** Patients receiving neuraxial anesthesia (epidural, spinal) or undergoing spinal puncture are at risk of hematomas and subsequent paralysis. **CONTRAINDICATIONS** History of HIT, active major bleed, hypersensitivity to pork **SIDE EFFECTS** Bleeding, anemia, ↑ LFTs, thrombocytopenia, hyperkalemia, injection site reactions (bruising) **MONITORING** Anti-Xa levels can be used to monitor, but is not routine in the general patient population. Monitoring is recommended in pregnancy and in patients with mechanical heart valves. Monitoring may be done in obesity, low body weight, pediatrics, elderly or renal insufficiency. aPTT is not used. Obtain peak anti-Xa levels 4 hours post dose. VTE treatment using enoxaparin daily: 1-2 anti-Xa units/mL VTE treatment using enoxaparin Q12H: 0.6-1 anti-Xa units/mL Recurrent VTE prophylaxis in pregnancy: 0.2-0.6 anti-Xa units/mL Monitor platelet count, Hgb, Hct, stool occult blood tests, SCr **NOTES** Pregnancy Category B More predictable anticoagulant response compared to heparin and does not require anti-Xa level monitoring in most cases. This makes LMWH more cost effective even though the actual drug costs more than UFH. Do not expel air bubble from syringe prior to injection. Do not administer IM. ↳ may lose some medicine Store at room temperature. Largely neutralized by protamine.
Dalteparin (Fragmin)	**Prophylaxis of VTE** 2,500-5,000 units SC daily **Treatment of UA/NSTEMI** 120 units/kg (max 10,000 units) Q12H	

tinzaparin (Innohep®)
ardeparin (Normiflo®)

* LMWHs are recommended over warfarin in cancer pts!!

LMWH Drug Interactions

- Most drug interactions are due to additive effects with other agents that can ↑ bleeding risk (other anticoagulants, antiplatelet drugs, some herbals, NSAIDs, SSRIs, SNRIs, thrombolytics, and possibly others). See the Drug Interactions chapter.

FACTOR Xa INHIBITORS

Fondaparinux *(Arixtra)* is a synthetic pentasaccharide that selectively inhibits Factor Xa via antithrombin (AT). Therefore, it is an indirect inhibitor of Factor Xa. Rivaroxaban *(Xarelto)* and apixaban *(Eliquis)* are direct Factor Xa inhibitors and are available orally. Fondaparinux is often used off label in clinical practice for HIT.

DRUG	DOSING	SAFETY/SIDE EFFECTS/MONITORING

Injectable Indirect Factor Xa Inhibitor (SC)

DRUG	DOSING	SAFETY/SIDE EFFECTS/MONITORING
Fondaparinux *(Arixtra)* Comes in prefilled syringes: 2.5 mg/0.5 mL, 5 mg/0.4 mL, 7.5 mg/0.6 mL, 10 mg/0.8 mL ↓ K+ ↓ bp *not indicated for stroke prophylaxis in a fib*	**Prophylaxis of VTE** ≥ 50 kg: 2.5 mg SC daily < 50 kg: contraindicated **Treatment of VTE** < 50 kg: 5 mg SC daily 50-100 kg: 7.5 mg SC daily > 100 kg: 10 mg SC daily	**BOXED WARNING** Patients receiving neuraxial anesthesia (epidural, spinal) or undergoing spinal puncture are at risk of hematomas and subsequent paralysis. **CONTRAINDICATIONS** Severe renal impairment (CrCl < 30 mL/min), active major bleed, bacterial endocarditis, thrombocytopenia with positive test for anti-platelet antibodies in presence of ^lfondaparinux, or body weight < 50 kg (for prophylaxis only) **SIDE EFFECTS** Bleeding (epistaxis, ecchymosis, gingival, GI, etc.), anemia, local injection site reactions (rash, pruritus, bruising), thrombocytopenia, hypokalemia, hypotension **MONITORING** Anti-Xa levels, CBC, platelet count, Hgb, SCr, stool occult blood testing Anti-Xa levels should be obtained 3 hours post dose. **NOTES** Pregnancy Category B Do not expel air bubble from syringe prior to injection. No antidote. Do not administer IM. Store at room temperature.

$ 20.10

Factor Xa Inhibitors Continued

DRUG	DOSING	SAFETY/SIDE EFFECTS/MONITORING

Oral Direct Factor Xa Inhibitors

Rivaroxaban (Xarelto)

Conversions

Switching from warfarin to rivaroxaban: discontinue warfarin and start rivaroxaban when INR < 3

Switching from rivaroxaban to warfarin: stop rivaroxaban and begin a parenteral anticoagulant and warfarin when the next schedule dose of rivaroxaban would have been taken, discontinue the parenteral anticoagulant when INR reaches therapeutic range.

Switching from anticoagulants other than warfarin to rivaroxaban: start rivaroxaban ≤ 2 hrs before the next scheduled evening dose and discontinue other anticoagulant. For UFH given via continuous infusion, stop UFH and give rivaroxaban at the same time.

Missed Doses

Administer the dose as soon as possible on the same day as follows:
For patients receiving 15 mg twice daily: take rivaroxaban immediately to ensure intake of 30 mg rivaroxaban per day. In this particular instance, two 15 mg tablets may be taken at once. Then continue with the regular 15 mg twice daily intake as recommended on the following day.

For patients receiving 10, 15, or 20 mg once daily: take the missed rivaroxaban dose as soon as possible on the same day; otherwise skip.

Non-valvular AFib
CrCl > 50 mL/min: 20 mg PO daily with evening meal

CrCl 15-50 mL/min: 15 mg PO daily with evening meal

CrCl < 15 mL/min: avoid use

Treatment of DVT/PE
15 mg PO BID with food x 21 days, then 20 mg PO daily with food.

CrCL < 30 mL/min: avoid use

Prophylaxis for DVT (after knee/hip replacement)
10 mg PO daily – without regards to meals

Do not use in CrCl < 30 mL/min

First dose given 6-10 hours after surgery

Take for 35 days after hip replacement surgery; take for 12 days after knee replacement surgery

Reduction in the Risk of Recurrence of DVT and PE
20 mg PO daily with food

CrCL < 30 mL/min: avoid use

BOXED WARNINGS (2)
Patients receiving neuraxial anesthesia (epidural, spinal) or undergoing spinal puncture are at risk of hematomas and subsequent paralysis.

Premature discontinuation of rivaroxaban increases the risk of thrombotic events.

CONTRAINDICATIONS
Active major bleeding

WARNINGS
Avoid in patients with moderate to severe hepatic impairment or with any degree associated with coagulopathy.

Avoid use in severe renal impairment [DVT treatment and prophylaxis (CrCl < 30 mL/min) and AFib (CrCl < 15 mL/min)].

Use is not recommended with prosthetic heart valves.

SIDE EFFECTS
Bleeding, anemia

MONITORING
CBC with differential; renal function prior to initiation, when clinically indicated, and at least annually; hepatic function

NOTES
Pregnancy Category C

No antidote.

No monitoring of efficacy required.

Discontinue 24 hours prior to elective surgery.

Handwritten notes:

qd dosing (except tx for VTE tx → BID x 21d → then qd)

same for apixaban but INR > 2

| warfarin → rivaroxaban |
- d/c warfarin
- start Xarelto® when INR < 3

| rivaroxaban → warfarin |
- d/c Xarelto®
- start IV anticoag + warfarin @ next Xarelto® dose
- when INR tx, d/c IV anticoag

| other anticoag → rivaroxaban |
- start Xarelto® ≤ 2 hrs before next scheduled PM dose; d/c other anticoag

| UFH continuous infusion → Xarelto® |
- d/c UFH; start Xarelto® @ same time

704

Factor Xa Inhibitors Continued

(handwritten: BID dosing)

DRUG	DOSING	SAFETY/SIDE EFFECTS/MONITORING
Apixaban (Eliquis) **Conversions** Switching from warfarin to apixaban: discontinue warfarin and start apixaban when the INR < 2. Switching from apixaban to warfarin: stop apixaban and begin a parenteral anticoagulant and warfarin when the next schedule dose of apixaban would have been taken, discontinue the parenteral anticoagulant when INR reaches therapeutic range. Switching from apixaban to anticoagulants other than warfarin: Discontinue apixaban and start the other anticoagulant at the next scheduled dose. **Missed Doses** The dose should be taken as soon as possible on the same day and twice daily administration should be resumed. The dose should not be doubled to make up for a missed dose.	**Non-valvular AFib** 5 mg BID If have at least 2 of the following: age ≥ 80 years, body weight ≤ 60 kg, or SCr ≥ 1.5 mg/dL, give 2.5 mg BID **Treatment of DVT/PE** 10 mg PO BID x 7 days, then 5 mg PO BID **Prophylaxis for DVT (after knee/hip replacement)** 2.5 mg PO BID First dose given 12-24 hours after surgery Take for 35 days after hip replacement surgery; take for 12 days after knee replacement surgery **Reduction in the Risk of Recurrence of DVT and PE** 2.5 mg PO BID after at least 6 months of treatment for DVT or PE	**BOXED WARNINGS (2)** Patients receiving neuraxial anesthesia (epidural, spinal) or undergoing spinal puncture are at risk of hematomas and subsequent paralysis. Premature discontinuation of apixaban increases the risk of thrombotic events. **CONTRAINDICATIONS** Active pathological bleed **WARNINGS** Use is not recommended with prosthetic heart valves or severe hepatic impairment. **MONITORING** Renal function prior to initiation, when clinically indicated, and at least annually in all patients; hepatic function; signs of bleeding. **SIDE EFFECTS** Bleeding, anemia **NOTES** Pregnancy Category B No antidote. No monitoring of efficacy required. Discontinue 48 hours prior to elective surgery with moderate-high bleeding risk or 24 hours prior to elective surgery with a low bleeding risk.

Factor Xa Inhibitor Drug Interactions

- Rivaroxaban is a substrate of 3A4 (major) and P-gp. Avoid concomitant use with drugs that are combined P-gp and strong 3A4 inducers (e.g., carbamazepine, phenytoin, rifampin, St. John's wort) or strong 3A4 inhibitors (e.g., ketoconazole, itraconazole, lopinavir/ritonavir, ritonavir, indinavir, and conivaptan). The benefit must outweigh the potential risks in these situations: CrCl 15-80 mL/min who are receiving combined P-gp and moderate 3A4 inhibitors, and in patients with impaired renal function receiving erythromycin or clarithromycin.

- Apixaban is a substrate of 3A4 (major) and P-gp. Avoid concomitant use with strong dual inducers of 3A4 and P-gp (e.g., carbamazepine, phenytoin, rifampin, St. John's wort). For patients receiving doses > 2.5 mg BID, the dose of apixaban should be decreased by 50% when coadministered with drugs that are strong dual inhibitors of 3A4 and P-gp (e.g., clarithromycin, itraconazole, ketoconazole, or ritonavir). For patients taking 2.5 mg BID, avoid these strong dual inhibitors.

- See Drug Interactions chapter for drugs that can ↑ bleeding risk.

- Drugs that ↑ clotting risk (including estrogen and SERMs) should be discontinued.

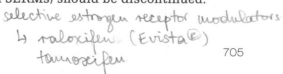
(handwritten: selective estrogen receptor modulators ↳ raloxifen (Evista®) tamoxifen)

DIRECT THROMBIN INHIBITORS

These agents directly inhibit thrombin (Factor IIa); they bind to the active thrombin site of free and clot-associated thrombin.

DRUG	DOSING	SAFETY/SIDE EFFECTS/MONITORING
Direct Thrombin Inhibitors (injectable; IV or SC)		
Argatroban Indicated for HIT and patients undergoing PCI who are at risk for HIT *light protect during admin*	**HIT** Initial: 2 mcg/kg/min – titrate to target aPTT. Max: 10 mcg/kg/min **PCI** Intravenous drugs given as a bolus followed by an infusion; all are weight-based Used in patients with a history of HIT	**CONTRAINDICATIONS** Active major bleeds **SIDE EFFECTS** Bleeding, anemia, hematoma **MONITORING** aPTT, and/or ACT (for bivalirudin); platelets, Hgb, Hct, SCr **NOTES** Pregnancy Category B No cross-reaction with HIT. No antidote.
Bivalirudin (Angiomax) Indicated for patients with ACS undergoing PCI and are at risk for HIT *monitor ACT*	Argatroban – ↓ dose in hepatic impairment Bivalirudin – ↓ dose when CrCl < 30 mL/min	Argatroban can increase the INR if starting on warfarin concurrently do not use a loading dose of warfarin; dose cautiously. Argatroban requires light protection during administration.
Desirudin (Iprivask) Indicated for VTE prevention after hip arthroplasty	15 mg SC Q12H ↓ dose when CrCl < 60 mL/min	**BOXED WARNING** Patients receiving neuraxial anesthesia (epidural, spinal) or undergoing spinal puncture are at risk of hematomas and subsequent paralysis. **MONITORING** aPTT, SCr, stool occult blood test, CBC **NOTES** Pregnancy Category C No antidote

---

(like apixaban)

warfarin → dabigatran
- d/c warfarin
- start Pradaxa® when INR < 2

dabigatran → IV anticoag
- wait 12 hrs (CrCl ≥ 30)
  OR 24 hrs (CrCl < 30)
  after last dose of Pradaxa®
- start IV anticoag

dabigatran → warfarin
- CrCl = 15-30 ⇒ start warfarin 1 day before d/c Pradaxa®
  = 30-50 ⇒   2
  ≥ 50 ⇒   3

Direct Thrombin Inhibitors Continued

DRUG	DOSING	SAFETY/SIDE EFFECTS/MONITORING

Direct Thrombin Inhibitor (oral)

Dabigatran *(Pradaxa)* 75, 150 mg capsules **Conversions** Switching from warfarin to dabigatran: discontinue warfarin and start dabigatran when INR < 2. Switching from UFH/ LMWHs to dabigatran: start dabigatran ≤ 2 hrs before the next scheduled dose of LMWH, or at the time of discontinuation of UFH infusion. Switching from dabigatran to parental anticoagulants: Wait 12 hrs (CrCl ≥ 30 mL/min) or 24 hrs (CrCl < 30 mL/min) after the last dose of dabigatran before starting therapy. Switching from dabigatran to warfarin: start warfarin 3 days before stopping dabigatran when CrCl ≥ 50 mL/min, start warfarin 2 days before stopping dabigatran when CrCl 30-50 mL/min, start warfarin 1 day before stopping dabigatran when CrCl 15-30 mL/min.	**Non-Valvular AFib** 150 mg BID; 75 mg BID if CrCl 15-30 mL/min **Treatment of DVT/PE and Reduction in the Risk of Recurrence of DVT and PE** 150 mg BID when CrCl > 30 mL/min; no recommendations when CrCl < 30 mL/min Swallow capsules whole. Do not break, chew, crush or open. Do not put in NG tube. Take missed dose ASAP unless it is within 6 hours of next scheduled dose; do not double up Keep in original container. Discard 4 months after opening the original container. Keep bottle tightly closed to protect from moisture. Blister packs are good until the date on the pack (usually 6-12 months)	**BOXED WARNINGS (2)** Discontinuing dabigatran puts patients at ↑ risk for thrombotic events. If dabigatran must be discontinued for reason(s) other than pathological bleeding, consider the use of another anticoagulant during the time of interruption. Patients receiving neuraxial anesthesia (epidural, spinal) or undergoing spinal puncture are at risk of hematomas and subsequent paralysis. **CONTRAINDICATIONS** Active pathological bleed and patients with mechanical prosthetic heart valve(s) **SIDE EFFECTS** Dyspepsia, gastritis-like symptoms, bleeding (including more GI bleeding) **MONITORING** Renal function at baseline and annually, CBC with differential **NOTES** Pregnancy Category C Causes increases aPTT, PT/INR. Dabigatran prevents 5 more strokes per 1,000 patients/year than warfarin (therefore preferred by CHEST guidelines for stroke prevention in non-valvular AFib). These guidelines came out before rivaroxaban and apixaban were approved. Discontinue if undergoing invasive surgery (1-2 days before if normal renal function, 3-5 days before if CrCl < 50 mL/min). No antidote. No monitoring of efficacy required. Store in a cool, dry place; not in bathrooms. Take with a full glass of water with or without food.

Dabigatran Drug Interactions

- Dabigatran is a substrate of P-gp. Avoid concomitant use with P-gp inducers including rifampin; rifampin will cause the dose to become subtherapeutic.

- In moderate renal impairment (CrCl 30-50 mL/min), reduce dose to 75 mg BID when given with the P-gp inhibitors dronedarone or systemic ketoconazole. In severe renal impairment (CrCl 15-30 mL/min), concomitant use of P-gp inhibitors should be avoided.

- The use of the P-gp inhibitors verapamil, amiodarone, quinidine, clarithromycin and ticagrelor does not require a dose adjustment of *Pradaxa*. Do not assume other P-gp inhibitors are similar.

- See Drug Interactions chapter for drugs that can ↑ bleeding risk.

- Drugs that ↑ clotting risk (including estrogen and SERMs) should be discontinued.

WARFARIN *(COUMADIN, JANTOVEN)*

Warfarin competitively inhibits the C1 subunit of the multi-unit vitamin K epoxide reductase (VKORC1) enzyme complex, thereby reducing the regeneration of vitamin K epoxide and causing depletion of active clotting factors II, VII, IX and X and proteins C and S.

DRUG	DOSING	SAFETY/SIDE EFFECTS/MONITORING
Warfarin *(Coumadin, Jantoven)* Racemic mixture of R- and S-enantiomers with the S- enantiomer being 2.7-3.8 times more potent.	Healthy outpatients should be started on warfarin 10 mg daily for first 2 days, then adjust dose per INR values. Doses of ≤ 5 mg may be an appropriate starting dose for those who are elderly, malnourished, taking drugs which can ↑ warfarin levels, liver disease, heart failure, or have a high risk of bleeding. 1 mg (pink) 2 mg (lavender) * 2.5 mg (green) 3 mg (tan) 4 mg (blue) 5 mg (peach) 6 mg (teal) * 7.5 mg (yellow) 10 mg (white) See Study Tip on the next page Highly protein bound (99%)	**BOXED WARNING** May cause major or fatal bleeding **CONTRAINDICATIONS** Hemorrhagic tendencies (cerebrovascular hemorrhage, bacterial endocarditis, pericarditis, pericardial effusions), blood dyscrasias, pregnancy, uncontrolled hypertension, anon-compliance, recent or potential surgery of the eye or CNS, major regional lumbar block anesthesia or traumatic surgery resulting in large, open surfaces, pericarditis or pericardial effusion, bacterial endocarditis, (pre-) eclampsia, threatened abortion, and pregnancy (except with mechanical heart valves at high risk for thromboembolism). **SIDE EFFECTS** Bleeding, skin necrosis, purple toe syndrome **MONITORING** INR target is 2.5, range 2-3, for most indications (DVT, AFib, bioprosthetic mitral valve, mechanical aortic valve, antiphospholipid syndrome) and should be 2.5-3.5 for some high-risk indications such as a mechanical mitral valve or 2 mechanical heart valves. INR monitoring to begin after the initial 2 or 3 doses, or if on a chronic, stable dose of warfarin, monitor at intervals up to 12 weeks. Hct, Hgb, signs of bleeding **NOTES** Pregnancy Category X/D (women with mechanical heart valves) Antidote: vitamin K Take at the same time each day. Missed doses – take the dose as soon as possible on the same day; do not double the dose the next day to make up for a missed dose. Dental cleanings and single tooth extraction do not generally require a change in warfarin dosing if INR is in therapeutic range.

[Handwritten margin notes, left: "↑ risk for purple toe syndrome in pts w/ atherosclerotic dz ⇒ d/c warfarin"]

[Handwritten notes, bottom left: "• healthy outpts start on 10mg/day × 2days, then adjust INR • elderly, malnourished, on drugs that ↑ [warfarin], liver dz, HF, bleeding risk ⇒ start ≤5mg"]

[Handwritten notes, bottom left: "sub 2C9 1A2 2C19 3A4"]

Warfarin – Pharmacokinetic Drug Interactions

- Warfarin is a substrate of CYP 2C9 (major), 1A2 (minor), 2C19 (minor) and 3A4 (minor) and an inhibitor of 2C9 (weak) and 2C19 (weak). Avoid use with tamoxifen.

- 2C9 inducers – including aprepitant, bosentan, carbamazepine, phenobarbital, phenytoin, primidone, rifampin (large ↓ INR), licorice and St. John's Wort – may ↓ INR.

- 2C9 inhibitors – including amiodarone, azole antifungals (e.g., fluconazole, ketoconazole, voriconazole), capecitabine, etravirine, fluvastatin, fluvoxamine, macrolide antibiotics, metronidazole, tigecycline, TMP/SMX and zafirlukast – can ↑ INR. See Drug Interactions chapter. *[Handwritten: ↓ warfarin dose, monitor]*

- Antibiotics: Penicillins, including amoxicillin, some cephalosporins, fluoroquinolones, macrolides, TMP/SMX and tetracyclines can enhance the anticoagulant effect of warfarin – monitor INR.

- Check for 1A2, 2C19 and 3A4 interactions; these occur, but usually have less of an effect on INR.

- When starting amiodarone, ↓ the dose of warfarin by 30-50%.

Mg salicylate (Doan's®) is don't use w/warfarin
acetaminophen safer

Warfarin – Pharmacodynamic Drug Interactions

- The most common pharmacodynamic interactions are with NSAIDs, antiplatelet agents, other anticoagulants, SSRIs and SNRIs. These interactions ↑ bleeding risk, but the INR may be in the usual range or slightly elevated.

- Drugs that ↑ clotting risk (including estrogen and SERMs) should be discontinued.

Herbal/Natural Product Drug Interactions

- Ginkgo biloba ↑ bleeding risk with no effect on the INR. Other natural products that can pose an ↑ bleeding risk include bromelain, danshen (can ↑ INR), dong quai (can ↑ INR), vitamin E, evening primrose oil, echinacea, high doses of fish oils, garlic, glucosamine (can ↑ INR), goldenseal, grapefruit (can ↑ INR), policosanol, willow bark and wintergreen oil (can ↑ INR). There are other herbal products that can increase the bleeding risk with warfarin.

- Alfalfa, American ginseng, green tea and coenzyme Q-10 can ↓ the effectiveness of warfarin.

- Any additions of vitamin K will ↓ the INR. Check any nutritional products for vitamin K content. Stay consistent with the amount of vitamin K consumed through the diet (see foods high in vitamin K in following table).

Warfarin Pharmacogenomics

The presence of variant alleles, such as CYP 2C9*2 and CYP 2C9*3, and polymorphisms in the VKORC1 gene can ↑ the risk of bleeding from warfarin. Patients with these polymorphisms may require lower doses of warfarin therapy. Genetic testing is not routinely recommended at this time. See Pharmacogenomics chapter.

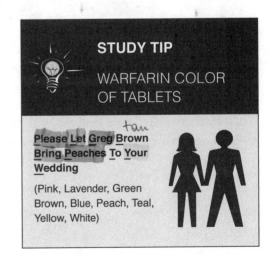

STUDY TIP

WARFARIN COLOR OF TABLETS

tan

Please Let Greg Brown Bring Peaches To Your Wedding

(Pink, Lavender, Green Brown, Blue, Peach, Teal, Yellow, White)

Warfarin Use – Key Points from CHEST 2012 Guidelines

- In healthy outpatients, the initial starting dose of warfarin should be 10 mg daily for the first 2 days, then adjust per INR values.

- For patients with stable therapeutic INRs presenting with a single subtherapeutic INR value, routinely bridging with heparin is not recommended.

- Routine pharmacogenomic testing is not recommended at this time.

- For patients with consistently stable INRs on warfarin therapy, INR testing can be done up to every 12 weeks rather than every 4 weeks.

- For patients with previously stable therapeutic INRs who present with a single out-of-range INR of ≤ 0.5 below or above the therapeutic range, continue current dose and obtain another INR within 1-2 weeks.

- Routine use of vitamin K supplementation is not recommended in patients taking warfarin.

- Start warfarin therapy on the same day as the parenteral anticoagulant (e.g., enoxaparin) and continue both anticoagulants for a minimum of 5 days and until the INR is 2 or above for at least 24 hours. Once the INR is therapeutic for 24 hours, the parenteral anticoagulant can be discontinued.

- Warfarin is highly protein bound, therefore caution is advised with other highly protein bound drugs that may displace warfarin such as phenytoin, valproic acid, furosemide, bumetanide, spironolactone, metolazone, doxycycline, glipizide, glyburide, ibuprofen, naproxen, and diphenhydramine.

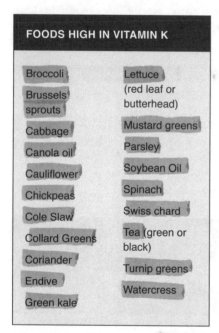

FOODS HIGH IN VITAMIN K

Broccoli	Lettuce (red leaf or butterhead)
Brussels sprouts	Mustard greens
Cabbage	Parsley
Canola oil	Soybean Oil
Cauliflower	Spinach
Chickpeas	Swiss chard
Cole Slaw	Tea (green or black)
Collard Greens	Turnip greens
Coriander	Watercress
Endive	
Green kale	

Use of Vitamin K for High (Supratherapeutic) INRs

Variable INRs are a norm of clinical practice. Elevated INRs can scare the clinician due to increased risk of bleeding. It is important to know how to treat patients with high INR values. Vitamin K is used for reversal (to ↓ INR quickly) by itself or with other agents described later in this section. Bleeding, at any INR, will warrant more serious intervention.

Oral formulations of vitamin K (generally at doses of 2.5-5 mg) are preferred in patients without significant or major bleeding. Vitamin K given subcutaneous (SC) produces a slow onset and a variable response; therefore, SC injections should be avoided. The intramuscular route should also be avoided due to the risk of hematoma formation. Intravenous administration should be given only when the patient is experiencing serious bleeding. IV injection is reported to cause anaphylaxis in 3 of out 100,000 patients: infuse slowly.

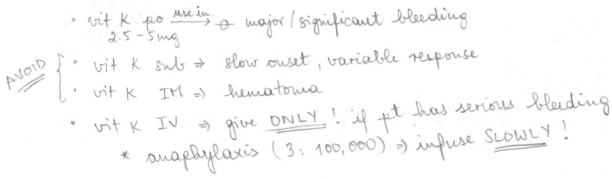

- vit K po $\xrightarrow{\text{use in}}$ major/significant bleeding
  2.5-5mg
AVOID {
- vit K sub ⇒ slow onset, variable response
- vit K IM ⇒ hematoma
- vit K IV ⇒ give ONLY! if pt has serious bleeding
  * anaphylaxis (3:100,000) ⇒ infuse SLOWLY!

Use of Vitamin K for Overanticoagulation

SYMPTOMS/INR VALUE	WHAT TO DO
INR above therapeutic range but < 4.5	Reduce or skip warfarin dose. Monitor INR. Resume warfarin when INR therapeutic. Dose reduction may not be needed if only slightly above therapeutic range.
For patients with a supratherapeutic INR of 4.5-10 without bleeding	Routine use of vitamin K is NOT recommended if no evidence of bleeding. Hold 1-2 doses of warfarin. Monitor INR. Resume warfarin at lower dose when INR therapeutic. Vitamin K can be used if urgent surgery needed (≤ 5 mg, with additional 1-2 mg in 24 hours if needed) or bleeding risk is high (1-2.5 mg).
For patients with INR > 10 without bleeding	Hold warfarin. Give oral vitamin K 2.5-5 mg even if not bleeding. Monitor INR. Resume warfarin at a lower dose when INR is therapeutic.
For patients with major bleeding from warfarin	Hold warfarin therapy. Give vitamin K 5-10 mg by slow IV injection and four-factor prothrombin complex concentrate (PCC). PCC suggested over fresh frozen plasma (FFP) due to risks of allergic reactions, infection transmission, longer preparation time, slower onset and higher volume.

Anticoagulant Antidotes

Protamine combines with strongly acidic heparin to form a stable salt complex neutralizing the anticoagulant activity of both drugs. Phytonadione provides an essential vitamin for liver synthesis of clotting factors (II, VII, IX, X). *Kcentra* is a newer product available as a single-use vial containing coagulation Factors II, VII, IX and X, and antithrombotic proteins C and S as a lyophilized concentrate. It is indicated for the urgent reversal of warfarin.

ANTIDOTE*	DOSING	SAFETY/SIDE EFFECTS/MONITORING

For heparin/LMWH reversal

| Protamine 10 mg/mL (5 mL, 25 mL) | 1 mg protamine will reverse ~ 100 units of heparin – reverse the amount of heparin given in the last 2-2.5 hours; max dose: 50 mg

Enoxaparin given within last 8 hours: 1 mg protamine will neutralize 1 mg of enoxaparin

Enoxaparin given > 8 hours ago: give 0.5 mg protamine per 1 mg of enoxaparin given

Give 1 mg protamine for each 100 anti-Xa units of dalteparin | **BOXED WARNING**
Hypotension, cardiovascular collapse, non-cardiogenic pulmonary edema, pulmonary vasoconstriction, and pulmonary hypertension may occur.

SIDE EFFECTS
Hypotension, bradycardia, flushing, anaphylaxis

MONITORING
aPTT, anti-Xa levels, cardiac monitoring required (ECG, BP, HR)

NOTES
For IV use only.
Rapid IV infusion causes hypotension. Administer slow IV push (50 mg over 10 minutes). Inject without further dilution over 1-3 minutes. |

Handwritten notes:

max 50 mg !!

- rapid infusion → ↓↓ bp
- slow IV push (50mg over 10min)
- inj w/o further dilution over 1-3 min

protamine
1 mg = ~ 100 units heparin (given last 2-2.5 hrs)
1 mg = 1 mg enoxaparin (8 hrs)
0.5 mg = 1 mg " (>8 hrs)
1 mg = 100 antiXa units dalteparin

Anticoagulant Antidotes Continued

ANTIDOTE*	DOSING	SAFETY/SIDE EFFECTS/MONITORING

For warfarin reversal

ANTIDOTE*	DOSING	SAFETY/SIDE EFFECTS/MONITORING
Vitamin K or Phytonadione *(Mephyton)* 5 mg tablets 1 mg/0.5 mL, 10 mg/mL inj.	1-10 mg PO/IV If given IV, infuse slowly; rate of infusion should (not) exceed 1 mg/min	**BOXED WARNING** Severe reactions resembling hypersensitivity reactions (e.g., anaphylaxis) have occurred rarely during or immediately after IV administration (even with proper dilution and rate of administration); some patients had no previous exposure to phytonadione. **SIDE EFFECTS** Anaphylaxis **NOTES** To ↓ risk of anaphylactoid reaction upon IV administration, dilute dose in a minimum of 50 mL of compatible solution and administer using an infusion pump over at least 20 minutes Requires light protection during administration SC route not recommended due to variable absorption IM route not recommended due to risk of hematoma Discontinue orlistat and mineral oil during vitamin K administration (decreases vitamin K absorption).
Four Factor Prothrombin Complex Concentrate (Human) *(Kcentra)* Factors II, VII, IX, X, Protein C, Protein S	Based on patient's INR and body weight – given IV Do not let drug back-up into line; will clot. Refrigerate. Reach room temp prior to administration. Protect from light.	**BOXED WARNING** Arterial and venous thromboembolic complications have been reported **CONTRAINDICATIONS** Disseminated intravascular coagulation and known heparin-induced thrombocytopenia (contains heparin) **WARNINGS** Made from human blood and may carry risk of transmitting infectious agents (e.g., viruses) **SIDE EFFECTS** Headache, nausea, vomiting, arthralgia, hypotension and thrombotic events **NOTES** Do (not) repeat dose Administer vitamin K concurrently
Three Factor Prothrombin Complex Concentrates (Human) *(Bebulin, Profilnine)* (Off) label	Weight-based dosing given IV slowly Given with Fresh Frozen Plasma (FFP) or Factor VIIa	**WARNING** *Bebulin* and *Profilnine* contain Factors II, IX and X but low or nonthera-peutic levels of factor VII and should not be confused with Prothrombin Complex Concentrate (Human) [(Factors II, VII, IX, X), Protein C, Protein S] *(Kcentra)* which contains therapeutic levels of factor VII. **SIDE EFFECTS** Chills, fever, flushing, nausea, headache, risk of thrombosis **NOTES** Due to ADRs may need to slow infusion and give antihistamine Administer vitamin K concurrently
Factor VIIa Recombinant *(NovoSeven RT)* Off label	10-20 mcg/kg IV bolus over 5 minutes	**BOXED WARNING** Serious thrombotic events are associated with the use of factor VIIa outside labeled indications.

*There are no available antidotes for dabigatran, rivaroxaban, or apixaban; however, drug-specific antidotes for each drug have been developed and are in clinical trials – FDA-approval may become available in 2015.

(handwritten margin notes: "light protect during admin", "light protect", "2, 7, 9, 10 protein C, S", "2, 9, 10 & 7 !!")

bridging = stop warfarin, use anticoag doses of UFH/LMWH

Perioperative Management of Patients on Warfarin

- Stop warfarin therapy approximately 5 days before major surgery. In patients with a mechanical heart valve, AFib, or VTE at high risk for thromboembolism, bridging therapy with LMWH or UFH is recommended (bridging means stopping the warfarin and using anticoagulant doses of the LMWH or UFH). Discontinue therapeutic-dose SC LMWH 24 hours before surgery (stop the UFH IV therapy 4-6 hours before surgery). Patients at low risk for thromboembolism do not require bridging – just stop the warfarin and restart after surgery when hemostasis is achieved (see below).

- If INR is still elevated 1-2 days before surgery, give low-dose vitamin K (1-2 mg).

- If reversal of warfarin is needed in a patient requiring an urgent surgical procedure, give low-dose (2.5-5 mg) IV or oral vitamin K.

- Resume warfarin therapy 12-24 hours after the surgery, when there is adequate hemostasis.

- In patients receiving bridge therapy with SC LMWH undergoing high-bleeding risk surgery, resume therapeutic dose of LMWH therapy 48-72 hours after surgery, when there is adequate hemostasis. If low bleeding risk, may resume therapeutic dose LMWH therapy 24 hours after surgery.

  pts @ ↑ risk for VTE, bridge w/ THERAPEUTIC dose! of Lovenox®

- Continue warfarin or aspirin in patients undergoing minor dental, dermatologic, or cataract surgery.

- Antiplatelet therapies (such as P2Y$_{12}$ inhibitors) may need to be stopped 5-10 days prior to major surgery. The risks/benefit of stopping therapy must be evaluated on a case-by-case basis.

Anticoagulation for Patients with Atrial Fibrillation

x 4 weeks after cardioversion

Anticoagulation for patients with AFib who are going to undergo cardioversion:

- For patients with AFib of > 48 hours or unknown duration, anticoagulation (if warfarin, target INR 2-3) is recommended for at least 3 weeks prior to and 4 weeks after cardioversion (regardless of method – electrical or pharmacologic) when normal sinus rhythm is restored.

- For patients with AFib ≤ 48 hours duration undergoing elective cardioversion, start full therapeutic anticoagulation at presentation, do cardioversion, and continue full anticoagulation for at least 4 weeks while patient is in normal sinus rhythm.

- For patients staying in AFib, chronic anticoagulation therapy may be needed for stroke prevention. Treatment depends on the number of risk factors present. See following tables.

Anticoagulation For Patients With AFib or AFlutter

This section refers only to non-valvular AFib and AFlutter anticoagulation. Valvular patients can have mechanical heart valves; these patients have the highest risk for VTE. Valvular patients with mechanical heart valves are treated with warfarin and the treatment is non-controversial.

The majority of patients with these two common arrhythmias (AFib/AFlutter) do not have heart valve involvement; they have one of these common rhythm disturbances, usually due to years of high blood pressure or coronary artery disease.

The latest 2012 CHEST guidelines use the $CHADS_2$ scoring system to estimate risk of stroke in AFib/AFlutter and to guide anticoagulation therapy. They do not include the newer anticoagulants rivaroxaban and apixiban. After the 2012 CHEST guideline was released, a newer guideline by the ACC/AHA/HRS group was released that does include the two newer drugs and uses the CHA_2DS_2-VASc scoring system. This means there are two current guidelines for the same condition – but this is not difficult: first, focus on the simpler CHEST guideline boxes (below), and then focus on the differences in the newer guideline (the 2nd set of boxes).

To use the $CHADS_2$ scoring system, first <u>count the risk factors</u> in the box on the <u>left</u>. Second, use the box on the <u>right</u> to <u>pick</u> the <u>correct anticoagulant</u>.

The higher the value the more intensive anticoagulation that is required to reduce the chance that the patient will have a stroke.

$CHADS_2$ SCORING SYSTEM
Add up the total number of risk factors for a given patient.
C – CHF...1
H – HTN...1
A – Age ≥ 75 years 1
D – Diabetes..............................1
S_2 – prior Stroke/TIA 2

RISK CATEGORY	RECOMMENDED THERAPY
$CHADS_2$ score = 0	No therapy. For patients wanting anticoagulant therapy, ASA 75-325 mg daily should be used over oral anticoagulation or combination therapy with ASA and clopidrogrel.
$CHADS_2$ score = 1	Oral anticoagulation* rather than ASA 75 mg-325 mg daily or combination therapy with ASA and clopidogrel. For patients unable to take oral anticoagulants, ASA and clopidogrel should be used.
$CHADS_2$ score ≥ 2	Oral anticoagulation*. For patients unable to take oral anticoagulants, ASA and clopidogrel should be used.

*Oral anticoagulation favors dabigatran 150 mg BID rather than adjusted-dose warfarin therapy (target INR 2-3).

Anticoagulation for Patients with Nonvalvular Atrial Fibrillation/Atrial Flutter (Per the ACC/AHA/HRS AFib Guideline)

The boxes below are the CHA_2DS_2-VASc scoring boxes. Notice that there are more risk factors than in the first table – the additions are the three on the bottom called "VASc" (Vascular disease, Age and Sex category). Notice that the newer agents rivaroxaban and apixiban are included as treatment options if the score is 2 or higher. Anticoagulation for patients with AFib who are undergoing cardioversion is the same as the CHEST guidelines.

CHA₂DS₂-VASc SCORING SYSTEM

Add up the total number of risk factors for a given patient.

C – CHF.................................... 1

H – HTN.................................... 1

A – Age ≥ 75 years .... ②

D – Diabetes.............................. 1

S₂ – prior Stroke/TIA 2

V – Vascular Disease 1
(prior MI, PAD, aortic plaque)

A – Age 65-74 years 1

S – Sex category, female.................. 1

RISK CATEGORY	RECOMMENDED THERAPY
CHA₂DS₂-VASc Score = 0	No anticoagulation recommended.
CHA₂DS₂-VASc Scoring = 1	No anticoagulation or oral anticoagulation or ASA may be considered.
CHA₂DS₂-VASc Scoring ≥ 2	Oral anticoagulation is recommended. Options include warfarin, dabigatran, rivaroxaban and apixaban.

For patients who are unable to maintain a therapeutic INR on warfarin, a direct thrombin inhibitor or factor Xa inhibitor is recommended.

Important – Patients with valvular AFib (those with mechanical heart valves) should only be treated with warfarin (with the INR goals given in the warfarin section of this chapter).

Patient Counseling: For All Anticoagulants

- This medication can interact with many other drugs. Check with your healthcare provider before taking any other medication, including over the counter medications, vitamins, and herbal products.
- This medication can cause you to bruise and/or bleed more easily. Report any unusual bleeding, bruising, or rashes to your healthcare provider.
- Tell physicians and dentists that you are using this medication before any surgery is performed.
- Call your healthcare provider right away if you fall or injure yourself, especially if you hit your head. Alcoholic drinks should be avoided.
- Do not start, stop, or change any medicine without talking with your healthcare provider.
- This medication is very important for your health, but it can cause serious and life-threatening bleeding problems.
- Call your healthcare provider right away if you develop any of these symptoms:
  - ❏ Unexpected pain, swelling, or discomfort
  - ❏ Headaches, dizziness, or weakness
  - ❏ Unusual bruising that develops without known cause
  - ❏ Frequent nose bleeds
  - ❏ Unusual bleeding gums ⇒ *metallic taste in mouth*
  - ❏ Bleeding from cuts that take longer than normal to stop
  - ❏ Menstrual bleeding or vaginal bleeding that is much heavier than normal
  - ❏ Pink or brown urine
  - ❏ Red or black stools that look like tar
  - ❏ Coughing up blood or blood clots
  - ❏ Vomiting blood or material that looks like coffee grounds

Enoxaparin

- Wash and dry hands.
- Sit or lie in a comfortable position so you can see your abdomen. Choose an area on the right or left side of your abdomen, at least 2 inches from the belly button.
- Clean the injection site with an alcohol swab and allow the site to dry.
- Remove the needle cap by pulling it straight off the syringe and discard it in a sharps collector. Do not twist the cap off as this can bend the needle.
- Hold the syringe like a pencil in your writing hand.
- Do not expel the air bubble in the syringe prior to injection unless your healthcare provider has advised you to do so.
- With your other hand, pinch an inch of the cleansed area to make a fold in the skin. Insert the full length of the needle straight down – at a 90 degree angle – into fold of skin.
- Press the plunger with your thumb until the syringe is empty.
- Pull the needle straight out at the same angle that it was inserted, and release the skin fold.
- Point the needle down and away from yourself and others, and push down on the plunger to activate the safety shield.
- Do not rub the site of injection as this can lead to bruising. Place the used syringe in the sharps collector.

Dabigatran

- Do not stop taking dabigatran without talking to your prescriber. Stopping dabigatran increases your risk of having a stroke.
- Take with a full glass of water and swallow the capsules whole. Do not break, chew, or empty the pellets from the capsule. It is fine to take with or without food.
- Common side effects of dabigatran include indigestion, upset stomach or stomach burning and/or pain.
- Only open 1 bottle of dabigatran at a time. Finish your opened bottle of dabigatran before opening a new bottle. After opening a bottle of dabigatran, use within 4 months.
- Keep dabigatran in the original bottle or blister package to keep it dry and protect the capsules from moisture. Do not put dabigatran in pill boxes or pill organizers.
- Tightly close your bottle of dabigatran right after you take your dose.
- If you miss a dose of dabigatran, take it as soon as you remember. If your next dose is less than 6 hours away, skip the missed dose. Do not take two doses of dabigatran at the same time.
- Dabigatran is not for patients with artificial heart valves.

Rivaroxaban

- Rivaroxaban is not for patients with artificial heart valves.
- If you take rivaroxaban for atrial fibrillation: Take rivaroxaban once daily with your evening meal.
  - ❑ If you miss a dose of rivaroxaban, take it as soon as you remember on the same day. Take your next dose at your regularly scheduled time.
- If you take rivaroxaban for blood clots in the veins of your legs or lungs: Take rivaroxaban once or twice daily as prescribed with food at the same time each day.
  - ❑ If you miss a dose of rivaroxaban and take rivaroxaban twice daily: Take rivaroxaban as soon as you remember on the same day. You may take 2 doses at the same time to make up for the missed dose. Take your next dose at your regularly scheduled time.

Xarelto®

❑ If you miss a dose of rivaroxaban and take rivaroxaban <u>once daily</u>: Take rivaroxaban as soon as you remember on the same day. Take your next dose at your regularly scheduled time.

■ If you take rivaroxaban for hip or knee replacement surgery: Take rivaroxaban once daily with or without food.

❑ Take rivaroxaban once daily with or without food.

❑ If you miss a dose of rivaroxaban, take it as soon as you remember on the same day. Take your next dose at your regularly scheduled time.

Warfarin

■ Take warfarin at the same time every day as prescribed by your doctor. You can take warfarin either with food or on an empty stomach.

■ Warfarin lowers the chance of blood clots forming in your body.

■ If you miss a dose, take the dose as soon as possible on the same day. Do not take a double dose the next day to make up for a missed dose.

■ You will need to have your blood tested frequently to monitor your response to this medication. This test is called an INR. Your dose may be adjusted to keep you INR in a target range.

■ Do not make changes in your diet, such as eating large amounts of green, leafy vegetables. Be consistent with the amount of leafy green vegetables and other foods rich in vitamin K.

■ Avoid drinking alcohol.

■ Other side effects besides bleeding include purple toe syndrome that can cause your toes to become painful and purple in color. Also, death of skin tissue can occur. Report any unusual changes or pain immediately to your healthcare provider.

° continue to monitor for signs/sx of bleeding 1 week after d/c warfarin

PRACTICE CASE

AM is a 57 y/o female who has been admitted to the hospital with shortness of breath, difficulty breathing, chest pain, coughing and sweating. She states she saw blood in a tissue that she coughed into while coming to the hospital. Her past medical history includes hypertension, neuropathic pain in her feet and atrial fibrillation. She is recovering from a bad fall two days ago but reports "no broken bones, just bruises." She states that she is having difficulty taking care of her grandson who she watches during the day because she is "too tired."

Medications:
Aspirin 325 mg one EC tablet daily
Cordarone 200 mg one daily
Lyrica 75 mg one capsule BID
Chlorthalidone 25 mg one daily
Effexor XR 150 mg one daily

Labs: Ca (mg/dL) = 8.3 (8.5 - 10.5)
Cl (mEq/L) = 98 (95 - 103)
Mg (mEq/L) = 1.3 (1.3 - 2.1)
K (mEq/L) = 4.2 (3.5-5)
PO_4 (mg/dL) = 3.9 (2.3 - 4.7)
Na (mEq/L) = 142 (135 - 145)
HCO_3 (mEq/L) = 22 (24 - 30)
BUN (mg/dL) = 41 (7 - 20)
SCr (mg/dL) = 1.5 (0.6 - 1.3)

AST (U/L) = 27 (0-33)
ALT (U/L) = 23 (0-45)

INR = 1.1 (0.00-1.2)
PTT (seconds) = 27.4 (24.8-35.6)

BP: 152/96 Temp: 98.4°F. Computerized tomography and ultrasound are ordered. Acute PE and DVT are confirmed. The patient will be started on a heparin drip.

Adult Heparin Drip Protocol

PTT	Rebolus or Hold	Rate Adjustment	Recheck PTT
≤ 60	Bolus: 80units/kg	↑ 4 units/kg/hr	6hrs
61-78	Bolus: 40units/kg	↑ 2 units/kg/hr	6hrs
GOAL 79-118	**NONE**	**NONE**	**In AM**
119-135	NONE	↓ 2 units/kg/hr	6hrs
≥ 136	HOLD 60 minutes	↓ 3 units/kg/hr	6hrs

[handwritten: wt = 80 kg, CrCl = 55]

QUESTIONS

[handwritten: wt not given]

1. The medical team asks the clinical pharmacist to dose the heparin for AM. Using the protocol provided, what should the correct bolus and infusion rate of heparin be for AM?

    a. 10,000 units bolus, followed by 2,300 units/hr infusion

    b. 14,000 units bolus, followed by 3,500 units/hr infusion

    c. 7,000 units bolus, followed by 1,400 units/hr infusion

    → d. 6,400 units bolus, followed by 1,440 units/hr infusion

    e. None of the above

2. The bolus and infusion are given. After 6 hours, the aPTT comes back at 66 sec. Per the protocol, what is the correct dose adjustment for heparin?

    a. Give a 6,400 unit bolus now and increase the infusion rate to 1,900 units/hr

    b. Give a 3,200 unit bolus now and increase the infusion rate to 1,600 units/hr

    c. Make no change to the dose

    d. Do not give a bolus and reduce the infusion rate to 1,500 units/hr

    e. None of the above

3. The pulmonary embolism was confirmed. It is AM's third day in the hospital, and the medical team would like to discharge her. She starts bridge therapy and receives 5 mg of warfarin at bedside. Which of the statements is true regarding warfarin? (Select **ALL** that apply.)

    a. Warfarin is a direct thrombin inhibitor that helps to prevent clot formation.

    b. Warfarin has a high risk of bleeding. Careful monitoring is advised.

    c. Warfarin should be taken with a low fat meal and never double up on the dose.

    d. Warfarin is a racemic mixture and the R-isomer is more potent than the S-isomer.

    e. Warfarin should overlap the heparin therapy until she is at a therapeutic INR for 24 at least hours.

4. In addition to warfarin, what other medication will AM need for bridge therapy until her INR is therapeutic? Select the appropriate agent, route of administration, and dose for AM's treatment of PE.

    a. Lovenox 30 mg SC daily *[handwritten:] prophylaxis]*

    b. Lovenox 30 mg SC Q12H

    c. Lovenox 80 mg SC Q12H *[handwritten: 1 mg/kg q 12 hrs]*

    d. Lovenox 80 mg SC daily

    e. Lovenox 180 mg SC daily

5. AM will need to be counseled on subcutaneous administration of enoxaparin. List the steps in order that the patient should take to administer the drug.

    [handwritten: 3] a. Place injection in the abdomen at least 2″ from the navel.

    [handwritten: 4] b. Insert full length of the needle at a 90 degree angle.

    [handwritten: 5] c. Place the used syringe in a sharps container.

    [handwritten: 1] d. Wash hands thoroughly.

    [handwritten: 2] e. The patient should clean the injection site with alcohol.

6. AM should be careful not to take other products that can increase the bleeding risk while on warfarin. Which of the following would not increase her risk of bleeding? (Select **ALL** that apply.)

    a. Calcium with Vitamin D

    b. Large amounts of garlic

    c. Dong quai

    d. Fidaxomicin

    e. Ginkgo biloba

Questions 7-10 do not relate to the case.

7. Which of the following medications can significantly interact with warfarin? (Select **ALL** that apply.)

    a. Amiodarone

    b. Morphine

    c. Rifampin

    d. Levetiracetam

    e. Fluconazole

8. A patient comes to the hospital with a DVT. He has developed HIT with thrombosis in the past. Which of the following agents is considered first-line treatment in this patient?

    a. Arixtra
    b. Argatroban
    c. Xarelto
    d. Fragmin
    e. Desirudin

9. Which of the following is a possible side effect of heparin? (Select **ALL** that apply.)

    a. Xerostomia
    b. Thrombocytopenia
    c. Osteoporosis
    d. Hyperkalemia
    e. Bleeding

10. Which of the following parameters need to be monitored during heparin therapy?

    a. Hematocrit, hemoglobin, platelets, AST, and ALT
    b. Hematocrit, hemoglobin, platelets, and aPTT
    c. Hematocrit, hemogloblin, platelets, and PT
    d. CBC and Chem 7 panel
    e. Chem 7 panel and aPTT

Answers

1-d, 2-b, 3-b,e, 4-c, 5-d,e,a,b,c, 6-a,d, 7-a,c,e, 8-b, 9-b,c,d,e, 10-b

Pirzmetal's
· UA: new onset, ↑ (frequency, intensity or duration) or @ rest
· stable (SIHD): predictable chest pain 2° to exertion/stress
    * due to atherosclerosis

CHRONIC STABLE ANGINA

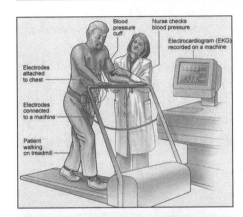

Blood pressure cuff
Nurse checks blood pressure
Electrocardiogram (EKG) recorded on a machine
Electrodes attached to chest
Electrodes connected to a machine
Patient walking on treadmill

GUIDELINES

Fihn SD, Blankenship JC, Alexander KP, et al. 2014 ACC/AHA/AATS/PCNA/SCAI/STS Focused Update of the Guideline for the Diagnosis and Management of Patients With Stable Ischemic Heart Disease. *Journal of the American College of Cardiology.* 2014; doi:10.1016/j.jacc.2014.07.017.

2012 ACCF/AHA/ACP/AATS/PCNA/SCAI/STS Guideline for the Diagnosis and Management of Patients with Stable Ischemic Heart Disease. *Circulation.* 2012;126(25):e354-471.

We gratefully acknowledge the assistance of Kim Jones, PharmD, BCPS, Assistant Dean of Student Services and Associate Professor of Pharmacy Practice, Union University, in preparing this chapter.

BACKGROUND

Angina is chest pain, pressure, tightness or discomfort. The chest pain is described as "squeezing," "grip-like," "heavy," or "suffocating," and typically does not vary with position or respiration. The patient presenting with angina is categorized as having stable angina or unstable angina (UA). UA is a medical emergency where the pain is increasing (in frequency, intensity or duration) or occurring at rest. Stable chronic angina, also known as stable ischemic heart disease (SIHD), is associated with predictable chest pain often brought on by exertion or emotional stress and relieved within minutes by rest or with nitroglycerin. Stable angina is due to plaque build up within the inner walls of the coronary arteries (atherosclerosis), causing narrowing of the arteries and reduced blood flow to the heart. The reduced blood flow causes ischemia (lack of oxygen) to the heart which causes the chest pain.

Angina can also be present in patients with normal coronary arteries, where symptoms are caused by vasospasm in the arteries. This type of angina is uncommon and is called Prinzmetal's (variant or vasospastic) angina.

Some patients (women, elderly and those with diabetes) may not develop the classic symptoms of angina and may not recognize the onset of cardiac symptoms and their need for medical attention. The ischemia can be silent, unnoticeable by the patient.

NON-DRUG TREATMENT

Multiple risk factors for heart disease, vascular disease and stroke are typically present in patients with SIHD, including hypertension, smoking, dyslipidemia, diabetes, obesity and physical inactivity. Patients should be encouraged to follow a heart healthy dietary pattern (saturated fats < 7% of total calories and *trans* fat < 1% of total calories, intake of fresh fruits and vegetables, low-fat dairy products, etc.) Encourage patients to stop smoking and avoid secondhand smoke, maintain a BMI of 18.5 – 24.9 kg/m^2, and maintain a waist circumference < 35 inches in females and < 40 inches in males. Encourage physical activity, 30 - 60 minutes of moderate-intensity aerobic activity, at least 5 days and preferably 7 days per week, supplemented by an increase in daily lifestyle activities (e.g., walking breaks at work, gardening) to improve cardiopulmonary fitness. Medically supervised programs such as cardiac rehabilitation, and physician-directed, home-based programs are recommended for at-risk patients at first diagnosis. Please note these recommendations are different from the obesity guideline recommendations (see Weight Loss chapter for more information).

TYPES OF ANGINA
Stable Angina
Decreased myocardial O$_2$ supply due to reduced blood flow from narrowed arteries by atherosclerotic plaque
Symptoms have been occurring for weeks but without worsening
Prinzmetal's Angina
Decreased myocardial O$_2$ supply due to vasospasm of the artery
Silent Ischemia
Transient myocardial ischemia without symptoms of angina
Unstable Angina
Severe, crushing chest pain unrelieved by rest; acute medical care is needed

DRUG TREATMENT

The treatment goals for chronic angina are to reduce the risk of an acute coronary syndrome (unstable angina/myocardial infarction) and provide relief from the anginal pain. An antiplatelet agent and an antianginal regimen are used together for this purpose. Aspirin is the recommended antiplatelet agent; clopidogrel *(Plavix)* is used in patients with an allergy or other contraindication to aspirin or in combination in high-risk patients with SIHD. Beta blockers are first line therapy for angina treatment. Calcium channel blockers or long-acting nitrates should be utilized when beta blockers are contraindicated or when additional symptomatic relief is needed. Ranolazine can also be utilized as a substitute or in addition to beta blocker therapy. Nitroglycerin as a sublingual tablet or translingual spray, is recommended for immediate relief of angina. Stable chronic angina is one of the atherosclerotic cardiovascular diseases (ASCVD), as defined by the ACC/AHA lipid guideline. Patients ≤ 75 years should be placed on high-intensity statin therapy. For patients > 75 years, moderate-intensity statin therapy is recommended. Patients should be aggressively managed if they have hypertension, heart failure and diabetes with the guideline-driven therapies for each of these conditions. A pneumococcal polysaccharide *(Pneumovax)* and an annual influenza vaccine is recommended. The acronym below summarizes the non-pharmacologic and pharmacologic approach to chronic angina:

DIAGNOSTIC PROCEDURES
History and physical
CBC, CK-MB, troponins (T or I), aPTT, PT/INR, lipid panel, glucose
ECG (at rest and during chest pain)
Exercise tolerance test/stress imaging
Cardiac catheterization/angiography

A – Antiplatelet and antianginal drugs

B – Blood pressure and beta blockers

C – Cholesterol (statins) and cigarettes (cessation)

D – Diet and diabetes

E – Exercise and education

ANTIPLATELET AGENTS ↓ MI risk (progression to ACS)

Aspirin binds irreversibly to cyclooxygenase-1 and 2 (COX-1 and 2) enzymes which results in ↓ prostaglandin (PG) and ↓ thromboxane A_2 (TxA_2) production; TxA_2 is a potent vasoconstrictor and facilitates platelet aggregation. Aspirin has anti-platelet, antipyretic, analgesic and anti-inflammatory properties. Clopidogrel inhibits $P2Y_{12}$ ADP-mediated platelet activation and aggregation.

DRUG	DOSING	SAFETY/SIDE EFFECTS/MONITORING
Aspirin (Bayer, Ascriptin, Bufferin, Ecotrin, others) See Pain chapter for more information on aspirin *irreversible*	75-162 mg daily	**CONTRAINDICATIONS** NSAID or salicylate allergy; patients with the syndrome of asthma, rhinitis, and nasal polyps; children < 16 years old with viral infection (due to Reye's syndrome risk) **SIDE EFFECTS** Dyspepsia, heartburn, GI upset, GI bleed/ulceration, bleeding, renal impairment, tinnitus (in toxicity) **MONITORING** Bleeding, bruising **NOTES** Shown to ↓ incidence of MI, CV events, and death; used in all acute and chronic ischemic heart disease patients indefinitely Enteric coated aspirin must be chewed if patient is having ACS

Handwritten notes:

antianginal + antiPLT

β-blocker (w/o ISA)
± CCB
± nitrate
± ranolazine

ASA – DOC
(or Plavix® if ASA contraindicated)
* high-risk pts (e.g. post-stent)
⇒ ASA + Plavix®

+ statin + other comorbidities mgt

+ sub/translingual NTG

+ Pneumovax
+ flu vaccine

Antiplatelet Agents Continued

DRUG	DOSING	SAFETY/SIDE EFFECTS/MONITORING
Clopidogrel *(Plavix)* *PRODRUG*	75 mg daily	**BOXED WARNING** Effectiveness depends on the activation to an active thiol metabolite mainly by CYP 2C19. Poor metabolizers exhibit higher cardiovascular events than patients with normal CYP 2C19 function. Tests to check CYP 2C19 genotype can be used as an aid in determining a therapeutic strategy. Consider alternative treatment strategies in patients identified as 2C19 poor metabolizers. The CYP 2C19*1 allele corresponds to fully functional metabolism while the CYP 2C19*2 and *3 alleles have reduced function. **CONTRAINDICATIONS** Active pathological bleed (e.g., PUD, ICH) **WARNINGS** CYP 2C19 inhibitors: Avoid concomitant use of omeprazole or esomeprazole. *tx: plasmapheresis* → Thrombotic thrombocytopenic purpura (TTP) has been reported; have patients report fever, weakness, extreme skin paleness, purple skin patches, yellowing of the skin or eyes, or neurological changes. *renal dysfxn, hemolytic anemia* **SIDE EFFECTS** Bleeding, bruising, rash, pruritus **MONITORING** Symptoms of bleeding; Hgb/Hct as necessary **NOTES** Do not start in patients likely to undergo CABG surgery and discontinue 5 days prior to any major surgery. Used in patients with a contraindication to aspirin or in addition to aspirin in certain high-risk patients with SIHD.

Aspirin Drug Interactions

- Most drug interactions are due to additive effects with other agents that can ↑ bleeding risk (e.g., anticoagulants, other antiplatelet drugs, ginkgo and other natural products, dextran, NSAIDs, SSRIs, SNRIs, thrombolytics and others). See Drug Interactions chapter for more information on drugs that can increase bleeding risk.

- NSAIDs (like aspirin) can ↑ the level of lithium (avoid concurrent use) and methotrexate.

- Caution with use of aspirin and other ototoxic agents (see Drug Interactions chapter).

Clopidogrel Drug Interactions

- Most drug interactions are due to additive effects with other agents that can ↑ bleeding risk (e.g., anticoagulants, other antiplatelet drugs, ginkgo and other natural products, dextran, NSAIDs, SSRIs, SNRIs, thrombolytics and others). See Drug Interactions chapter for more information on drugs that can increase bleeding risk.

- Clopidogrel is a prodrug metabolized mainly by CYP 2C19. Avoid concomitant use with strong or moderate 2C19 inhibitors (cimetidine, fluconazole, ketoconazole, voriconazole, fluoxetine, fluvoxamine and others). Avoid concomitant use with omeprazole and esomeprazole as these agents may reduce the effectiveness of clopidogrel due to 2C19 inhibition.

ANTI-ANGINAL THERAPY

DRUG	MECHANISM	CLINICAL NOTES
Beta Blockers Used 1st line See Hypertension chapter for a complete review of these agents	Reduce myocardial oxygen demand by ↓ HR (negative chronotropic effect), ↓ contractility (negative inotropic effect) and ↓ LV wall tension with long term use	Start low, go slow; titrate to resting HR of 55-60 BPM; avoid abrupt withdrawal. Do not use a beta blocker with intrinsic sympathomimetic activity (ISA). More effective than nitrates and CCBs in silent ischemia; avoid use in Prinzmetal's angina; effective as monotherapy or in combination with CCBs, nitrates, and/or ranolazine.
Calcium Channel Blockers Preferred agent for Prinzmetal's (variant) angina See Hypertension chapter for a complete review of these agents	Produces vasodilation, ↓ SVR and ↓ BP and improves myocardial oxygen supply; ↓ oxygen demand by ↓ contractility	Used when beta blockers are contraindicated or as add on therapy. Slow-release or long-acting dihydropyridine and nondihydropyridine CCBs are effective; avoid short-acting CCBs (e.g., nifedipine IR).
Nitrates	Forms free radical nitric oxide which ↑ cGMP, producing vasodilation of veins more than arteries, ↓ myocardial oxygen demand by ↓ preload; improves collateral blood flow	**SL tablets or spray** Recommended for all patients for fast relief of angina. Call 911 if chest pain does not go away after the first SL tab or first spray. **Long-acting nitrates** Long-acting nitrates are used as add-on therapy with beta-blockers and/or CCBs. Long-acting nitrates require a nitrate-free interval to prevent tolerance. See Nitroglycerin Formulations Table on next page.
Ranolazine (Ranexa)	Selectively inhibits the late phase Na+ current; ↓ intracellular Ca²⁺; may ↓ myocardial oxygen demand 500 mg BID (max 1,000 mg BID)	**CONTRAINDICATIONS** Hepatic cirrhosis, concurrent use of strong 3A4 inhibitors and inducers **WARNING** Can cause QT prolongation Acute renal failure has been observed in some patients with CrCl < 30 mL/min **SIDE EFFECTS** Dizziness, constipation, headache, nausea **MONITORING** ECG, K+, renal function **NOTES** Has little to no clinical effects on HR or BP Do not crush, break, or chew

Handwritten margin notes:
- do NOT use in Prinzmetal's
- for SIHD (next to "Used 1st line")
- muscles need Ca++ to contract (spas)
- Ø effect on bp or HR
- not 1st line (monotx), can be start in combo w/ β-blocker

NITROGLYCERIN FORMULATIONS

NITROGLYCERIN (NTG) FORMULATIONS	SAFETY/SIDE EFFECTS/MONITORING
Nitroglycerin SL tablet *(Nitrostat)* 0.3, 0.4, 0.6 mg	**CONTRAINDICATIONS** Hypersensitivity to organic nitrates, concurrent use with PDE-5 inhibitors; increased intracranial pressure; severe anemia **SIDE EFFECTS** Headache, dizziness, lightheadedness, flushing, hypotension, tachyphylaxis (↓ effectiveness/tolerance), syncope **MONITORING** BP (continuously if receiving IV), HR, chest pain **NOTES** Counsel patients to dose the medication so they have a 10-12 hour nitrate-free period to ↓ tolerance (some products require more than 12 hours of a nitrate-free interval).
Nitroglycerin translingual spray 0.4 mg/spray *(NitroMist, Nitrolingual Pump Spray)* *— shake, inhale spray*	
Nitroglycerin IV *glass bottles or nonPVC bags/tubes*	**Nitroglycerin SL tablets** Keep in the original amber glass bottle **Nitroglycerin IV** Prepare in glass bottles or polyolefin bags (non-PVC) due to sorption of the drug in PVC. Use administration sets intended for nitroglycerin (non-PVC as well). Use with infusion pump.
Nitroglycerin ointment 2% *dosed in inches* *BID (6 hrs apart)*	
Nitroglycerin transdermal patch *(Nitro-Dur, Minitran)* 0.1, 0.2, 0.3, 0.4, 0.6, 0.8 mg/hr *chest preferred* *any area on body EXCEPT extremities below elbow/knee*	**Nitroglycerin patch** On for 12-14 hours, off for 10-12 hours; rotate sites. Dispose of safely, away from children and pets. **Nitroglycerin ointment 2%** Dosed BID, 6 hours apart with 10-12 hour nitrate-free interval.
Isosorbide mononitrate IR/ER tablet/capsule *(Monoket)* IR: 10 mg, 20 mg *BID (7+ hrs apart)* ER: 30 mg, 60 mg, 120 mg *QAM*	**Isosorbide mononitrate** IR: BID at least 7 hours apart (e.g., 8 AM and 3 PM) ER: QAM
Isosorbide dinitrate IR/ER *(Isordil Titradose, Dilatrate-SR)* – preferred for systolic HF IR: 5 mg, 10 mg, 20 mg, 30 mg, 40 mg ER: 40 mg *BID-TID* ↳ *QAM* *or div BID* *8AM, 12PM, 4PM* *(18 hr NTG-free)* *(14 hr NTG-free)*	**Isosorbide dinitrate** IR is dosed BID-TID. If TID, give at 8 A.M., 12 P.M. and 4 P.M. for a 14 hour nitrate-free interval (or similar). SR/ER is daily in the morning or divided BID for an 18 hour nitrate-free interval.

Nitrate Drug Interactions

- Avoid concurrent use with PDE-5 inhibitors; use caution with other antihypertensive medications and alcohol as these can potentiate the hypotensive effect and cause a significant drop in blood pressure.

Ranolazine Drug Interactions

- Ranolazine is a substrate of 3A4 (major), 2D6 (minor) and P-gp and an inhibitor of 3A4 (weak), 2D6 (weak) and P-gp. Do not use with strong 3A4 inhibitors or CYP 3A4 inducers. Limit the dose to 500 mg BID in patients taking moderate CYP 3A4 inhibitors. Limit simvastatin to 20 mg/day if used concurrently.

Patient Counseling

Nitroglycerin Sublingual Tablet and Translingual Spray

- Nitroglycerin sublingual tablet should not be chewed, crushed or swallowed. Take one tablet at the first sign of chest pain. This medication may also be taken prophylactically 5 - 10 minutes before activities that bring on chest pain. The tablet should be placed under the tongue or in the area between the inside of the cheek and the gums/teeth.

- Take the medicine while sitting or lying down to avoid dizziness, lightheadedness or fainting which may be associated with use. Do not eat, drink, or smoke for at least 5 – 10 minutes after use of the product or while experiencing chest pain.

- Call 911 immediately if chest pain/angina persists after one dose of sublingual NTG. Continue to take 2 additional doses (up to 3 doses total) at 5 minute intervals while waiting for the ambulance to arrive.

- If NTG products are stored and handled properly, tablets should be stable until the manufacturer provided expiration date.

- If the tablets start to get powdery, get a new bottle.

- You may feel a slight burning or tingling sensation when taken sublingually. This sensation is not a sign of how well the medication is working. Do not use more medication just because you do not feel a burning or tingling sensation.

- Nitroglycerin SL tablets should be kept in the original amber glass bottle, at room temperature, and must be tightly capped after each use to prevent loss of potency. Shake out 1 tablet only, do not let the other tablets get wet.

- For the *Nitrolingual Pump Spray*: The pump must be sprayed 5 times into the air to prime the pump before use. If not used within 6 weeks, prime the pump with 1 spray before use. Do not shake. Press the button firmly with the forefinger to release the spray onto or under the tongue. Close your mouth after the spray. Do not inhale the spray and try not to swallow too quickly afterwards. Do not eat or drink or rinse the mouth for 5 – 10 minutes after the dose. You can use 1 spray every 5 minutes as needed for chest pain but no more than 3 sprays in 15 minutes.

- If you recently used a PDE-5 inhibitor like sildenafil *(Viagra, Revatio)*, tadalafil *(Cialis, Adcirca)*, vardenafil *(Levitra, Staxyn)*, or avanafil *(Stendra)*, avoid using nitroglycerin and inform your healthcare provider of PDE-5 inhibitor use immediately.

Nitroglycerin Patches

→ b/c if placed on elbows/knees in pt w/ atherosclerosis → ↓ perfusion to extremities

- Remove the patch from its pouch and remove the protective clear liner. Select any area of skin on the body EXCEPT the extremities below the knee or elbow. The chest is the preferred site.

- Apply the patch to a clean, dry, and hairless area. Hair in the area may be clipped, but not shaved. Avoid areas with cuts or irritation. Do not apply the patch immediately after bathing or showering. Wait until your skin is completely dry. However, you may bathe, shower, and swim while wearing the patch.

- Press the patch firmly in place with the palm of your hand. Wash your hands after applying the patch.

- Wear 1 patch a day for 12 to 14 hours.

- For the medicine to work well, there must be a 10 – 12 hour "patch free" interval between patches (where the patch is left off).

- To reduce skin irritation, apply each new patch to a different area of skin. After removing the old patch, fold it in half with the sticky sides together, and discard out of the reach of children and pets.

- This drug should not be used with the following medications: sildenafil *(Viagra, Revatio)*, tadalafil *(Cialis, Adcirca)*, vardenafil *(Levitra, Staxyn)* or avanafil *(Stendra)*. A dangerous drop in blood pressure could occur.

may/may not feel tingle

very sensitive to light & moisture

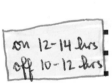

on 12-14 hrs
off 10-12 hrs

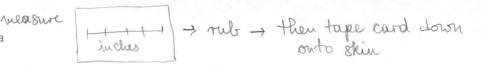

measure

inches → rub → then tape card down onto skin

Nitroglycerin Ointment

- Measure desired dosage of ointment with the dose measuring applicator supplied with the tube. Place the applicator on a flat surface, printed side down. Squeeze the necessary amount of ointment from the tube onto the applicator, and place the applicator (ointment side down) on the desired area of the skin.

- Spread the ointment using the dose measuring applicator lightly onto the chest (or other area of skin if preferred). Do not rub into the skin.

- Tape the applicator into place.

- This medication can stain clothing. Care should be taken to completely cover the dose measuring applicator.

Isosorbide Mononitrate

- Take this medication by mouth, once or twice daily or as directed by your healthcare provider. Take the first dose of the day when you wake up, then take the second dose 7 hours later. It is important to take the drug at the same times each day. Do not change the dosing times unless directed by your healthcare provider.

- Side effects can include headache (can be severe), dizziness, lightheadedness, redness, mild warmth, or nausea. The redness and mild warmth is called flushing which will go away when your body adjusts to the medicine. Headache is often a sign that this medication is working. Your healthcare provider may recommend treating headaches with the over-the-counter pain reliever acetaminophen. The headache should become less bothersome as your body gets used to the medicine. If the headaches continue or become severe, tell your healthcare provider promptly.

- This drug may make you dizzy. Do not drive, use machinery, or do any activity that requires alertness until you are sure you can perform such activities safely. Limit alcoholic beverages.

- To reduce the risk of dizziness and lightheadedness, get up slowly when rising from a sitting or lying position. Hold onto the side of the bed or chair to avoid falling.

- This drug should not be used with the following medications: sildenafil *(Viagra, Revatio)*, tadalafil *(Cialis, Adcirca)*, vardenafil *(Levitra, Staxyn)* or avanafil *(Stendra)*. A dangerous drop in blood pressure could occur.

Ranolazine

- Ranolazine is used to decrease the number of times you may get chest pain.

- Ranolazine works differently than other drugs for angina, so it can be used with your other angina medications (beta blockers, nitrates and calcium channel blockers).

- Take this medication by mouth twice daily with or without food or as directed by your healthcare provider. Swallow the tablet whole. Do not crush or chew the tablets.

- Use this medication regularly in order to get the most benefit from it. Take it at the same times each day. It should not be used to treat chest pain when it occurs. Use other medications (sublingual nitroglycerin) to relieve an angina attack as directed by your healthcare provider.

- Inform your healthcare provider if your condition does not improve or if it worsens (if the chest pain happens more often).

- Dizziness, headache, lightheadedness, nausea, and constipation may occur. If any of these effects persist or worsen, notify your healthcare provider or pharmacist promptly.

- Ranolazine may cause a condition that affects the heart rhythm (QT prolongation). This heart rhythm can infrequently result in serious fast/irregular heartbeat and other symptoms (such as severe dizziness, fainting) that require immediate medical attention. The risk may be increased if you are taking other drugs that may affect the heart rhythm. Check with your healthcare provider or pharmacist before using any herbal or over the counter medications.

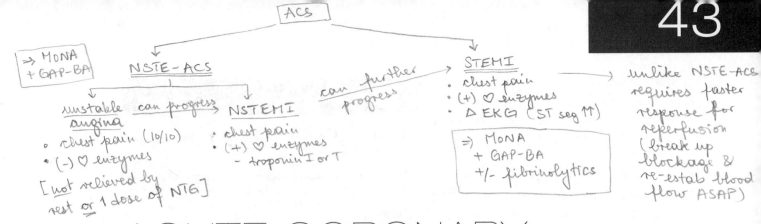

ACS

→ MONA + GAP-BA

NSTE-ACS

can progress → NSTEMI

can further progress →

STEMI
- chest pain
- (+) ♡ enzymes
- Δ EKG (ST seg ↑↑)

⟹ unlike NSTE-ACS requires faster response for reperfusion (break up blockage & re-estab blood flow ASAP)

unstable angina
- chest pain (10/10)
- (-) ♡ enzymes
[not relieved by rest or 1 dose of NTG]

NSTEMI
- chest pain
- (+) ♡ enzymes
  - troponin I or T

⟹ MONA + GAP-BA +/- fibrinolytics

ACUTE CORONARY SYNDROMES (ACS)

SCD = sudden cardiac death

atherosclerosis
⟹ plaque rupture
⟹ PLT aggregation

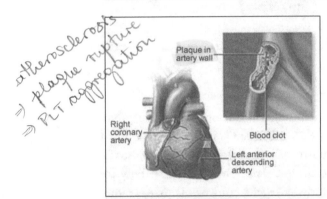

Plaque in artery wall

Right coronary artery

Blood clot

Left anterior descending artery

We gratefully acknowledge the assistance of Doug Humber, PharmD, Associate Clinical Professor, University of California San Diego Skaggs School of Pharmacy and Pharmaceutical Sciences, in preparing this chapter.

O_2 supply ≠ O_2 demand

BACKGROUND

Acute Coronary Syndrome (ACS) is a set of clinical conditions brought on by sudden, reduced blood flow causing an imbalance between myocardial oxygen supply and demand. This results from plaque buildup in the coronary arteries (coronary atherosclerosis). These plaques are made up of fatty deposits and cause the arteries to narrow, making blood flow more difficult. The surface of the plaque can rupture, leading to clot formation and the acute reduction in blood flow, causing ischemia. This ischemia leads to myocyte necrosis and subsequent release of biochemical markers into the bloodstream, mainly cardiac troponins I and T. The measurement of these enzymes is routine when establishing the diagnosis of acute myocardial infarction. The cardiac troponins T and I (TnT and TnI) are the most sensitive and specific biomarkers for ACS. The troponins are detectable in the blood within 2-12 hours (depending on the assay) after myocardial necrosis and can remain detectable for up to 5 – 14 days. Creatine kinase myocardial isoenzyme (CK-MB) and myoglobin are less sensitive markers than troponins, but may still be monitored in clinical practice.

↳ guidelines discourage routine monitoring of CK-MB, myoglobin

Acute coronary syndrome encompasses the clinical conditions of non-ST segment elevation acute coronary syndromes (NSTE-ACS) and ST segment elevation myocardial infarction (STEMI). NSTE-ACS describes both unstable angina (UA) and non-ST-segment elevation myo-

GUIDELINES

2014 AHA/ACC Guideline for the Management of Patients with Non-ST-Elevation Acute Coronary Syndromes. *Journal of the American College of Cardiology*. 2014; doi:10.1016/j.jacc.2014.09.017.

2013 ACCF/AHA Guideline for Management of ST-Elevation Myocardial Infarction: A Report of the American College of Cardiology Foundation/American Heart Association Task Force on Practice Guidelines. *Circulation*. 2013; 127:e362-e425.

cardial infarction (NSTEMI) since patients are indistinguishable upon presentation and the term emphasizes the continuum between UA and NSTEMI.

ACS is a medical emergency. When patients experience ACS symptoms, 911 should be called immediately. Emergency medical personnel should immediately perform a 12-lead ECG at the site of first medical contact. Patients who are having an acute MI (STEMI and NSTEMI) should be urgently transported to a hospital with percutaneous coronary intervention (PCI) capability. Coronary heart disease is the leading cause of death in the United States.

RISK FACTORS
Age (men > 45 years of age, women > 55 years of age or had early hysterectomy)
Family history of coronary event before 55 years of age (men) or 65 years of age (women)
Smoking
Hypertension
Dyslipidemia
Diabetes
Chronic angina
Known coronary artery disease
Sedentary lifestyle; lack of exercise

Signs and Symptoms of ACS

may go away & come back

The classic symptoms of ACS include chest pain ("pain" encompasses not only pain, but also symptoms of discomfort, pressure and squeezing) lasting ≥ 10 minutes, severe dyspnea, diaphoresis, syncope/presyncope, and/or palpitations. The pain may radiate to the arms, back, neck, jaw or epigastric area. However, female, elderly, and diabetic patients are less likely to present with classic symptoms. Precipitating factors include exercise, cold weather, extreme emotions, stress and sexual intercourse.

anxiety
↑↑ RR
sweating

Diagnosis

A 12-lead ECG should be performed and evaluated within 10 minutes upon the patient's arrival to the emergency department (ED). If not diagnostic, but the patient remains symptomatic, ECGs should be performed every 15-30 minutes to detect ischemic changes. Cardiac troponin I or T levels should be obtained at presentation and 3 – 6 hours after symptom onset in all patients with ACS symptoms. Additional troponin levels may be obtained afterwards. B-type natriuretic peptide (BNP) level may be obtained for prognostic information.

- UA: chest pain with negative cardiac enzymes; and no or transient ischemic ECG changes (ST-segment depression or prominent T-wave inversion).

- NSTEMI: chest pain with positive cardiac enzymes (↑ troponin I or T levels) and no or transient ischemic ECG changes (ST-segment depression or prominent T-wave inversion).

- STEMI: chest pain with positive cardiac enzymes and positive ST segment elevation in at least 2 contiguous leads of ≥ 0.2 mV (2 mm) in men or ≥ 0.15 mV (1.5 mm) in women in leads V2-V3 and/or ≥ 0.1 mV (1 mm) in other contiguous leads or a new left bundle branch block (LBBB).

DRUG TREATMENT

Acute treatment is aimed at providing immediate relief of ischemia and the prevention of MI and death. Treatment includes the use of antianginal, antiplatelet and anticoagulant therapy. A combination of morphine, oxygen, nitroglycerin and aspirin are given upon presentation (acronym MONA). Other mainstay therapies include P2Y$_{12}$ inhibitors and an anticoagulant such as heparin, low-molecular weight heparin or bivalirudin. Additionally a GP IIb/IIIa antagonist (eptifibatide, tirofiban or abciximab) may be given in select patients. All patients without contraindications should receive a beta blocker within 24 hours of presentation; ACE inhibitors and aldosterone antagonists should be used in select patients (see below). For patients presenting with STEMI, a fibrinolytic may be administered if the patient is not at a PCI-capable hospital or is not able to receive PCI within 2 hours (120 minutes) from presentation to the hospital.

When patients arrive at the hospital, the medical team decides on a treatment strategy for the patient depending on the diagnosis and symptom severity. Patients may be treated with medications alone (referred to as medical management) or with PCI (referred to as early invasive strategy). Patients may also go directly for urgent coronary artery bypass surgery (CABG) if there is significant multi-vessel disease.

Treatment of Non-ST-Segment Elevation Acute Coronary Syndrome (NSTE-ACS)

Treatment acronym is MONA + GAP-BA (see chart below).

Summary of Drugs Used Acutely for ACS

DRUG	MOA	CLINICAL COMMENTS
MONA (acronym)	*@ home / ambulance till get to hospital*	
Morphine	Produces arterial and venous dilation; leading to a ↓ in myocardial O$_2$ demand; pain relief	Morphine sulfate (2 to 5 mg IV repeated at 5- to 30-minute intervals PRN) may be used in patients with ongoing chest discomfort despite nitroglycerin (NTG) therapy. Side effects: hypotension, bradycardia, N/V, sedation, and respiratory depression. Avoid use in bradycardia, right ventricular infarct, confusion, and hypotension. Antidote: naloxone (Narcan). More information in the Pain chapter.
Oxygen	*nasal cannula*	Supplemental oxygen should be administered to patients with arterial oxygen saturation < 90% (SaO$_2$ < 90%), or who are in respiratory distress.
Nitrates	Dilates coronary arteries and improves collateral blood flow; ↓ cardiac oxygen demand by ↓ preload	Sublingual NTG (0.3-0.4 mg) every 5 minutes for up to 3 doses should be taken for immediate relief of ischemic pain. If chest pain/discomfort is not improved or worsening 5 minutes after the first dose, call 911. Administer IV NTG (start at 10 mcg/min, titrate to desired BP effect) for persistent ischemic pain, hypertension or heart failure. Do not use NTG if patient's SBP < 90 mmHg, HR < 50 BPM or experiencing a right ventricular infarction. NTG or other nitrates should not be administered to patients receiving PDE-5 inhibitors for erectile dysfunction within 12 hrs of avanafil, 24 hrs of sildenafil/vardenafil, or 48 hrs of tadalafil use. More information on nitrates in the Chronic Stable Angina chapter.
Aspirin	Inhibits platelet aggregation by inhibiting production of thromboxane A$_2$ (TxA$_2$) via COX-1 and COX-2 inhibition	Non-enteric-coated, chewable aspirin (162-325 mg) should be given to all patients immediately if no contraindications are present. Maintenance dose of aspirin 81-162 mg daily should be continued indefinitely. If intolerant to aspirin, use a P2Y$_{12}$ inhibitor. Give loading dose, followed by the maintenance dose (discussed later in this chapter).

Handwritten margin notes:

→ ↓ preload vasodilation + pain relief → ↓ anxiety

* counsel pt to sit down when taking NTG 1) ↓ bp 2) so pt does not pace (walk back/forth from anxiety) → ↓ O$_2$ demand

or spray (on/under tongue)

1 dose → 911 → 2 more doses

if chest pain still there, start NTG drip in hosp till pt is pain free

↳ if enteric coated, must chew for immediate onset (counsel pt to chew ASA whether EC or not; no harm if not & they chew)

* ASA inhibits PLT aggregation, stops thrombus formation stabilizes plaque, ↓ mortality in STEMI

731

Summary of Drugs Used Acutely for ACS Continued

DRUG	MOA	CLINICAL COMMENTS

GAP-BA (acronym) @ emergency dept (ED)

(handwritten left margin: glycoprotein inhibitors (GPIs))

Glycoprotein (GP) IIb/IIIa receptor antagonists	Blocks fibrinogen binding to the GPIIb/IIIa receptors on platelets, preventing platelet aggregation	Can be used in medical management or for patients going for a percutaneous coronary intervention (PCI +/- stent). Agents include abciximab, eptifibatide, or tirofiban. Abciximab should only be given to patients in whom PCI is planned. Of note: these agents are not used for all patients undergoing PCI; if used, they are given concurrently with heparin.
Anticoagulants	Inhibits clotting factors and can reduce infarct size	Used to prevent further clotting. Agents include heparin, LMWHs (enoxaparin, dalteparin), fondaparinux and bivalirudin. More information in Anticoagulation chapter.
P2Y$_{12}$ inhibitors	Inhibits P2Y$_{12}$ receptor on platelets	Ticagrelor (slightly preferred) or clopidogrel can be given for all patients (medical management as well as PCI). Prasugrel should only be given if the patient is going for PCI. Administer the loading dose followed by a maintenance dose. Do not give these agents if patient is going for urgent CABG surgery.
Beta Blockers	↓ O$_2$ demand by ↓ BP, HR, and contractility; ↓ ischemia, reinfarction, and arrhythmias and ↑ long-term survival	An oral low dose beta-1 selective blocker should be started within the first 24 hours in patients who do not have any of the following: 1) signs of HF, 2) evidence of a low-output state 3) ↑ risk for cardiogenic shock, 4) other contraindications to beta blockade (PR interval > 0.24 sec., 2nd or 3rd degree heart block without a pacemaker, active asthma or reactive airway disease). If patient has concomitant HF and is stable, choose 1 of the 3 beta blockers used in HF (bisoprolol, metoprolol succinate or carvedilol – see HF chapter). IV beta blocker therapy may be reasonable especially if ongoing ischemia or hypertension is present. Oral long-acting nondihydropyridine calcium channel blockers (verapamil or diltiazem) are reasonable to use in patients with recurrent ischemia without contraindications after beta blockers and nitrates have been fully used. See Hypertension chapter for more information.
ACE Inhibitors	Inhibits Angiotensin Converting Enzyme and blocks the production of Angiotensin II; prevents cardiac remodeling; ↓ preload and afterload	An oral ACE inhibitor should be started within the first 24 hours and continued indefinitely in all patients with left ventricular ejection fraction (LVEF) < 40%, those with HTN, DM, or stable CKD unless contraindicated (use ARB if patient is ACE inhibitor intolerant). ACE inhibitors may be reasonable in all patients with other cardiac or vascular disease. Do not use an IV ACE inhibitor within the first 24 hours due to the risk of hypotension. See Hypertension chapter for more information.

(handwritten margin notes: "more commonly given in cath lab than ED"; P2Y$_{12}$ "given only if pt candidate for PCI (not for CABG)"; Beta Blockers "UA/NSTEMI"; "may give IV in STEMI to quickly ↓ ♡ demand"; left bracket "to prevent ♡ remodeling")

Medications to Avoid in the Acute Setting

- NSAIDs (except for aspirin), whether nonselective or COX-2-selective agents, should not be administered during hospitalization due to ↑ risk of mortality, reinfarction, hypertension, cardiac rupture, renal insufficiency and heart failure associated with their use.

- Immediate-release nifedipine should not be used due to ↑ risk of mortality.

- IV fibrinolytic therapy should not be administered unless patient has ST-segment elevation MI or a new left bundle branch block (which is a STEMI equivalent).

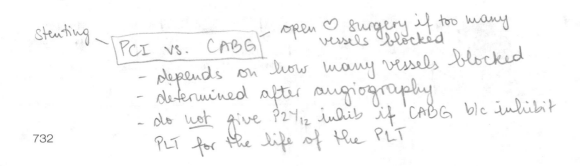

(handwritten: Stenting — PCI VS. CABG — open ♡ surgery if too many vessels blocked; - depends on how many vessels blocked; - determined after angiography; - do not give P2Y$_{12}$ inhib if CABG b/c inhibit PLT for the life of the PLT)

IV

Glycoprotein IIb/IIIa Receptor Antagonists

Blocks the platelet glycoprotein IIb/IIIa receptor, which is the binding site for fibrinogen, von Willebrand factor, and other ligands. Inhibition of binding at this final common receptor blocks platelet aggregation and prevents thrombosis. Eptifibatide and tirofiban have reversible blockade and abciximab has irreversible blockade.

DRUG	DOSING	SAFETY/SIDE EFFECTS/MONITORING
Abciximab *(ReoPro)*	LD: 0.25 mg/kg IV bolus MD: 0.125 mcg/kg/min (max 10 mcg/min) IV infusion for 12 hrs (PCI, STEMI with PCI) or 18-24 hrs (UA/NSTEMI unresponsive to conventional medical therapy with planned PCI within 24 hrs). Abciximab is not recommended for NSTE-ACS without PCI.	**CONTRAINDICATIONS** Thrombocytopenia (platelets < 100,000/mm³) History of bleeding diathesis (predisposition) Recent (within 6 weeks) GI or GU bleeding of clinical significance (abciximab) Active internal bleeding Recent (within 4-6 weeks) major surgery or trauma (4 weeks for tirofiban/eptifibatide and 6 weeks for abciximab) ↑ prothrombin time History of stroke within 2 years (abciximab); History of stroke within 30 days or any history of hemorrhagic stroke (eptifibatide/tirofiban) Severe uncontrolled HTN Hypersensitivity to murine proteins (abciximab) Dependency on renal dialysis (eptifibatide)
Eptifibatide *(Integrilin)*	LD:180 mcg/kg IV bolus (max 22.6 mg), repeat bolus in 10 mins if undergoing PCI MD: 2 mcg/kg/min (max 15 mg/hour) IV infusion started after the first bolus. Continue for 18-24 hours after PCI or for 12-72 hours if PCI was not performed. Reduce maintenance infusion to 1 mcg/kg/min in patients with CrCl < 50 mL/min (max 7.5 mg/hour)	**SIDE EFFECTS** Bleeding, thrombocytopenia (esp. abciximab), hypotension **MONITORING** Hgb, Hct, platelets, signs and symptoms of bleeding, SCr **NOTES** Do not shake vials upon reconstitution Must filter abciximab with administration
Tirofiban *(Aggrastat)*	NSTE-ACS dose: LD: 25 mcg/kg IV bolus over 3 min MD: 0.15 mcg/kg/min IV infusion for up to 18 hours Reduce infusion dose to 0.075 mcg/kg/min in patients with CrCl ≤ 60 mL/min	Platelet function returns in 24-48 hours after discontinuing abciximab, 2-4 hours after stopping eptifibatide and 4-8 hours after stopping tirofiban

P2Y$_{12}$ Inhibitors

Binds the adenosine diphosphate (ADP) P2Y$_{12}$ receptor on the platelet surface which prevents ADP-mediated activation of the GPIIb/IIIa receptor complex, thereby reducing platelet aggregation. Clopidogrel and prasugrel are prodrugs and have irreversible binding to the receptor. Ticagrelor is not a prodrug and has reversible binding to the receptor.

DRUG	DOSING	SAFETY/SIDE EFFECTS/MONITORING
Clopidogrel *(Plavix)*	LD: 300-600 mg (600 mg for PCI) MD: 75 mg PO daily If patient received fibrinolytic therapy for STEMI and is > 75 years of age, omit the loading dose and start 75 mg daily	**BOXED WARNING** Effectiveness depends on the activation to an active thiol metabolite mainly by CYP 2C19. Poor metabolizers exhibit higher cardiovascular events than patients with normal CYP 2C19 function. Tests to check CYP 2C19 genotype can be used to guide therapeutic strategy. Consider alternative treatment strategies in patients identified as 2C19 poor metabolizers. The CYP 2C19*1 allele corresponds to fully functional metabolism while the CYP 2C19*2 and *3 alleles have reduced function. **CONTRAINDICATIONS** Active pathological bleed (e.g., PUD, ICH) **WARNINGS** Avoid concurrent use of CYP2C19 inhibitors such as omeprazole or esomeprazole. Thrombotic thrombocytopenic purpura (TTP) has been reported; have patients report fever, weakness, extreme skin paleness, purple skin patches, yellowing of the skin or eyes, or neurological changes. **SIDE EFFECTS** Bleeding, bruising, rash, pruritus **MONITORING** Symptoms of bleeding; Hgb/Hct as necessary **NOTES** Do not start in patients likely to undergo CABG surgery and discontinue 5 days prior to any major surgery. MedGuide required
Prasugrel *(Effient)* Indicated for the reduction of thrombotic events in patients with ACS who are to be managed with PCI	LD: 60 mg PO (no later than 1 hour after PCI) MD: 10 mg PO daily (5 mg daily if patient weighs < 60 kg) Once PCI is planned, give the dose promptly and no later than 1 hour after the PCI. Keep in original container.	**BOXED WARNING (3)** Can cause significant or fatal bleeding In patients ≥ 75 years, prasugrel is generally not recommended due to ↑ risk of fatal and intracranial bleeding and uncertain benefit, except in high risk patients (DM and prior MI). Do not start in patients likely to undergo urgent CABG surgery; discontinue 7 days prior to any major surgery. **CONTRAINDICATIONS** Active pathological bleed; patients with a history of TIA or stroke **WARNINGS** Thrombotic thrombocytopenic purpura (TTP) has been reported **SIDE EFFECTS** Bleeding (more than clopidogrel) **NOTES** MedGuide required

Handwritten margin notes: 2C19 · PRODRUG irreversible · ≠ active patho bleed · PRODRUG irreversible · causes more bleeding than Plavix · ≠ active patho bleed · ≠ hx of stroke / TIA

P2Y₁₂ Inhibitors Continued

DRUG	DOSING	SAFETY/SIDE EFFECTS/MONITORING
Ticagrelor (*Brilinta*) Indicated for reduction of thrombotic events in patients with ACS	LD: 180 mg MD: 90 mg PO BID	**BOXED WARNINGS (2)** Can cause significant, sometimes fatal, bleeding Maintenance doses of aspirin above 100 mg reduce the effectiveness of ticagrelor and should be avoided. After any initial aspirin dose, maintenance aspirin dose should not exceed 100 mg daily. **CONTRAINDICATIONS** Active pathological bleed, history of ICH, severe hepatic impairment **SIDE EFFECTS** Bleeding, dyspnea (> 10%); ↑ SCr, bradyarrhythmias **NOTES** Do not start in patients likely to undergo CABG surgery and discontinue 5 days prior to any major surgery. MedGuide required

Handwritten notes:
3A4
avoid simvastatin lovastatin > 40 mg
monitor digoxin w/ initiation & dose Δ

Drug Interactions

- With all P2Y₁₂ inhibitors: Avoid use, if possible, with other agents that ↑ bleeding risk, including other antiplatelets (although P2Y₁₂ inhibitors are used with aspirin), NSAIDs, anticoagulants, SSRIs, SNRIs, thrombolytics and others. See Drug Interactions chapter for drugs that can ↑ bleeding risk. If a patient experiences bleeding while on a P2Y₁₂ inhibitor, manage bleeding without discontinuing the P2Y₁₂ inhibitor, if possible. Stopping the P2Y₁₂ inhibitor (particularly within the first few months after ACS) ↑ the risk of subsequent cardiovascular events.

- Clopidogrel is a prodrug metabolized mainly by CYP 2C19. Avoid concomitant use with strong or moderate 2C19 inhibitors (cimetidine, fluconazole, ketoconazole, voriconazole, fluoxetine, fluvoxamine and others). Avoid concomitant use with omeprazole and esomeprazole as these agents may reduce the effectiveness of clopidogrel due to 2C19 inhibition.

- Ticagrelor is a 3A4 (major) and P-gp substrate – avoid use with strong 3A4 inhibitors and inducers. See Drug Interactions chapter for more information. Avoid simvastatin and lovastatin doses greater than 40 mg/day. Monitor digoxin levels with initiation of or any change in ticagrelor dose.

Treatment of ST Segment Elevation Myocardial Infarction (STEMI)

MONA + GAP-BA + PCI or fibrinolytic therapy (PCI is preferred if facilities are available).

Handwritten note: ↳ pts do better on stents than by receiving fibrinolytics

Fibrinolytics   *"Clot busters"*

These agents cause fibrinolysis by binding to fibrin in a thrombus (clot) and converting entrapped plasminogen to plasmin. Once a STEMI is confirmed on 12-lead ECG performed by emergency medical services (EMS), a treatment course of PCI or fibrinolytic therapy must be determined. PCI is preferred if it can be performed within 90 minutes (optimal door-to-balloon time) or within 120 minutes of first medical contact. If PCI is not possible within 120

Handwritten note: PCI preferred over fibrinolytics
* if pt cannot get PCI or transferred to a facility that does PCI within 2 hrs of arriving at ED, give fibrinolytics

minutes of first medical contact, fibrinolytic therapy is recommended and should be given within 30 minutes of hospital arrival (door-to-needle time). In the absence of contraindications and when PCI is not available, fibrinolytic therapy is reasonable in STEMI patients who are still very symptomatic within 12-24 hours of symptom onset.

DRUG	SAFETY/SIDE EFFECTS/MONITORING
Alteplase *(t-PA, rt-PA, Activase)*	**CONTRAINDICATIONS** **Absolute** Active bleeding or bleeding diathesis Any prior intracranial hemorrhage Recent intracranial or intraspinal surgery or trauma (last 3 months) Intracranial neoplasm, arteriovenous malformation, or aneurysm Aortic dissection *tear in aortic wall, blood flow forces layers apart* Severe uncontrolled hypertension (unresponsive to emergency therapy) Ischemic stroke within past 3 months, except acute ischemic stroke within 4.5 hrs **Relative** Pregnancy Active peptic ulcer Current use of anticoagulants **SIDE EFFECTS** Bleeding, hypotension, intracranial hemorrhage, fever **MONITORING** Hgb, Hct, signs and symptoms of bleeding **NOTES** Door-to-needle time should be < 30 minutes (for fibrinolytics)
Tenecteplase *(TNKase)*	
Reteplase (r-PA) *(Retevase)*	

Long-Term Medical Management in Patients S/P MI (Secondary Prevention)

TREATMENT	CONSIDERATIONS
Aspirin *max 100 mg ASA if used w/ ticagrelor*	Use (81 mg – 325 mg daily) indefinitely unless there is a contraindication; 81 mg is the preferred maintenance dose, per the guidelines. The recommended maintenance dose of aspirin to be used with ticagrelor is 81 mg daily.
P2Y$_{12}$ inhibitor *1 yr*	Clopidogrel 75 mg daily, prasugrel 10 mg daily (or 5 mg daily if weight < 60 kg), ticagrelor 90 mg BID for 1 year in all patients. Continuation beyond 12 months may be considered in patients following drug eluting stent placement.
Nitroglycerin	SL tabs or spray PRN chest pain. Verbal or written instructions for its use should be reviewed with the patient.
Beta blocker *3 yrs*	Given for 3 years in the absence of HF or HTN, per ACC/AHA secondary prevention guidelines. Dose titrated to a resting HR of 50-60 BPM. Patient should take indefinitely if HF is present or needed as additional therapy for HTN.
ACE inhibitor *∞*	Indefinitiely if patient has LVEF < 40%, HTN, CKD, or diabetes. May be considered for patients with other cardiac and vascular diseases.

Long-Term Medical Management in Patients S/P MI (Secondary Prevention) Continued

TREATMENT	CONSIDERATIONS
Aldosterone Antagonist	Indefinitely for patients with LVEF ≤ 40% and either symptomatic HF or DM who are receiving target doses of an ACE inhibitor and beta blocker without significant renal impairment (SCr > 2.5 mg/dL in men, SCr > 2 mg/dL in women) or hyperkalemia (K⁺ > 5 mEq/L). *or CrCl < 30*
Statin	Patients ≤ 75 years of age, use high-intensity statin therapy
blc ACS is ASCVD	Patients > 75 years of age, use moderate-intensity statin therapy (see Dyslipidemia chapter)

Other Considerations for Patients S/P MI

use APAP, tramadol, ↓ dose warc, or NPX ∅ COX₂ sel.!!

- Pain relief – Patients with chronic musculoskeletal pain should use acetaminophen, nonacetylated salicylates, tramadol or small doses of narcotics before considering the use of NSAIDs. If these options are insufficient, it is reasonable to use nonselective NSAIDs such as naproxen (lowest CV risk). COX-2 selective agents have high CV risk and should be avoided.

- Warfarin use – if patients need to take warfarin (AFib patients, etc.) along with aspirin and P2Y$_{12}$ inhibitor, it may be reasonable to lower the INR goal to 2 - 2.5. Use this triple combination for the shortest time possible to limit the risk of bleeding. Proton pump inhibitors should be prescribed in any patient with a history of GI bleeding while taking triple antithrombotic therapy.

WHAT MEDICATIONS TO STOP/CONTINUE WHEN PATIENT GOES FOR CABG SURGERY

Continue:
Aspirin

UFH

Discontinue:
Clopidogrel and ticagrelor 5 days before elective CABG; prasugrel 7 days before elective CABG

Eptifibatide/tirofiban 2-4 hours before CABG; 12 hours before CABG for abciximab

Enoxaparin 12-24 hours before CABG and dose with UFH

Fondaparinux 24 hours before CABG and dose with UFH

Bivalirudin 3 hours before CABG and dose with UFH

- Lifestyle counseling – should include smoking cessation, managing chronic conditions (such as HTN, DM), encouraging physical exercise and a healthy diet. All patients should be referred to a comprehensive cardiovascular rehabilitation program.

PROTEASE-ACTIVATED RECEPTOR-1 (PAR-1) ANTAGONIST

Vorapaxar is a reversible antagonist of the protease-activated receptor-1 (PAR-1) expressed on platelets, but its long half-life makes it effectively irreversible. As an anti-platelet agent, it decreases platelet aggregation and clot formation, thereby decreasing the risk of heart attacks and strokes. Vorapaxar is indicated in patients with a history of myocardial infarction (MI) or with peripheral arterial disease (PAD) to reduce thrombotic cardiovascular events (CV death, MI, stroke and urgent coronary revascularization). This agent was used in addition to ASA and/or clopidogrel in clinical trials. Vorapaxar has not yet been incorporated into clinical guidelines.

DRUG	DOSING	SAFETY/SIDE EFFECTS/MONITORING
Vorapaxar (Zontivity)	One tablet (2.08 mg) PO daily	**BOXED WARNING** Use is contraindicated in patients with history of stroke, TIA, or ICH; or active pathological bleeding. Vorapaxar increases the risk of bleeding, including ICH and fatal bleeding. **WARNING** Do not use in severe liver impairment **SIDE EFFECTS** Bleeding, anemia **NOTES** Pregnancy Category B No antidote MedGuide required

(handwritten margin notes:)
indications: ↓ thrombotic CV events in
1) hx of MI
2) PAD

* 2.08 mg ≙ 2.5mg vorapax sulfate

Vorapaxar Drug Interactions

- Vorapaxar is a substrate of 3A4 and inhibitor of P-gp. Avoid concomitant use with strong inhibitors of CYP3A4 (e.g., ketoconazole, itraconazole, posaconazole, clarithromycin, nefazodone, ritonavir, saquinavir, nelfinavir, indinavir, boceprevir, telaprevir, telithromycin and conivaptan) and with strong inducers of CYP3A4 (e.g., rifampin, carbamazepine, St. John's Wort and phenytoin).

Patient Counseling for Clopidogrel

- Take this medication once daily. Clopidogrel can be taken with or without food.

- Clopidogrel helps prevent platelets from sticking together and forming a clot that can block an artery.

- It is important to take this medication every day. Do not stop taking clopidogrel without talking to your healthcare provider who prescribed it. Stopping this medication can put you at risk of developing a clot which can be life-threatening.

- If you miss a dose, take as soon as you remember. If it is almost time for your next dose, skip the missed dose. Take the next dose at your regular scheduled time. Do not take 2 doses at the same time unless instructed by your healthcare provider.

- You may bleed and bruise more easily, even from a minor scrape. It may take longer for you to stop bleeding.

- Call your healthcare provider at once if you have black or bloody stools, or if you cough up blood or vomit that looks like coffee grounds. These could be signs of bleeding in your digestive tract.

- One rare but serious side effect is thrombotic thrombocytopenic purpura (TTP). Seek prompt medical attention if you experience any of these symptoms that cannot otherwise be explained: fever, weakness, extreme skin paleness, purplish spots or skin patches (called purpura), yellowing of the skin or eyes (jaundice), or mental status changes.

- Avoid drinking alcohol while taking clopidogrel. Alcohol may increase your risk of bleeding in your stomach or intestines.

- If you need to have any type of surgery or dental work, tell the surgeon or dentist ahead of time that you are using clopidogrel. You may need to stop using the medicine for at least 5 days before having major surgery, to prevent excessive bleeding.

- While you are taking clopidogrel, do not take aspirin, other NSAIDs (non-steroidal anti-inflammatory drugs) or acid-reducing medications without consulting your healthcare provider.

PULMONARY ARTERIAL HYPERTENSION (PAH) & PULMONARY FIBROSIS (PF)

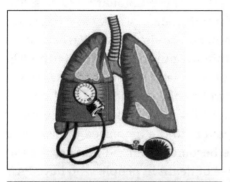

We gratefully acknowledge the assistance of Heather R. Bream-Rouwenhorst, PharmD, BCPS, Clinical Assistant Professor, University of Iowa College of Pharmacy, in preparing this chapter.

BACKGROUND

Pulmonary Arterial Hypertension (PAH) is characterized by continuous high blood pressure in the pulmonary arteries. The average blood pressure in a normal pulmonary artery (called pulmonary artery pressure) is about 14 mmHg when a person is resting. A mean pulmonary artery pressure (mPAP) greater than 25 mmHg in the setting of normal fluid status defines PAH. Other hemodynamic parameters are affected as well.

CLASSIFICATION

Pulmonary hypertension (PH) may occur with various disease states. The World Health Organization (WHO) classifies it into five groups.

Group 1 is PAH, which may arise from genetic inheritance, connective tissue disease, advanced liver disease, and HIV among others. Some patients have no identifiable cause of the disease; this is primary, or idiopathic, PAH (versus secondary, which has a known cause). Less commonly, medications can be the causative factor, including the chronic use of cocaine and methamphetamine. Recently, dasatinib *(Sprycel)* has been linked to causing PAH. Selective serotonin reuptake inhibitor (SSRI) use during pregnancy increases risk of persistent

GUIDELINE

ACCF/AHA 2009 Expert Consensus Document on Pulmonary Hypertension. J Am Coll Cardiol. 2009;53:1573-1619.

CLINICAL CLASSIFICATION OF PULMONARY HYPERTENSION

1. Pulmonary arterial hypertension (PAH)

Includes idiopathic PAH, heritable, drug and toxin induced, PAH associated with connective tissue diseases, HIV infection, portal hypertension, and persistent pulmonary hypertension of a newborn

2. Pulmonary hypertension owing to left heart disease

3. Pulmonary hypertension owing to lung diseases and/or hypoxia

4. Chronic thromboembolic pulmonary hypertension (CTEPH)

5. Pulmonary hypertension with unclear multifactorial mechanisms

pulmonary hypertension of the newborn (PPHN). <u>PH treatments discussed in this chapter have only been approved for the treatment of PAH with the exception of riociguat *(Adempas)*.</u>

Treatment of the other PH groups is aimed at the underlying causes. Group 2 is pulmonary venous hypertension, which arises from left-sided heart disease. Group 3 is PH from hypoxia or chronic lung disease, such as chronic obstructive pulmonary disease or interstitial lung disease. Group 4 is chronic thromboembolic PH (CTEPH), which occurs in a minority of PE survivors. Warfarin anticoagulation to an INR goal of 2-3 is recommended given the history of a clot, and for patients who are not thrombectomy candidates, riociguat *(Adempas)* is an approved treatment. Group 5 is PH due to causes that do not fit in the above categorization (e.g., sarcoidosis).

The pathology of PAH stems from an imbalance of vasoconstrictor and vasodilator substances and an imbalance of proliferation and apoptosis in the pulmonary arteries. The vasoconstrictor substances such as endothelin-1 and thromboxane A_2 (TxA_2) are increased in PAH, whereas the vasodilators (e.g., prostacyclins, others) are decreased. Vasoconstriction results in reduced blood flow and high pressure within the pulmonary vasculature. The walls of the pulmonary arteries thicken as the amount of muscle increases and scar tissue can form on the artery walls (vasoproliferation). As the walls thicken and scar, the arteries become increasingly narrower. These changes make it hard for the right ventricle to pump blood through the pulmonary arteries and into the lungs due to the increased pressure. As a result of the heart working harder, the right ventricle becomes enlarged and right heart failure can result. Heart failure is the most common cause of death in people who have PAH.

The biochemical changes mentioned above ($\uparrow TxA_2$, $\downarrow$ prostacyclin), along with other altered pathways, lead to a pro-thrombotic state, and anticoagulation is suggested to prevent blood clots from forming. <u>Warfarin, titrated to an INR of 1.5 – 2.5, is recommended in PAH.</u>

Symptoms of PAH include fatigue, dyspnea, chest pain, syncope, edema, tachycardia and/or Raynaud's phenomenon. In Raynaud's, the reduced blood supply causes discoloration and coldness in the fingers, toes, and occasionally other areas.

There is no cure for PAH, but in the last decade, the knowledge of PAH has increased significantly and many more treatment options have become available. Without treatment, life expectancy is three years. In some cases, a lung or heart-lung transplant may be an option, at least for younger patients.

NON-DRUG TREATMENT

Patients with PAH should follow a sodium restricted diet (< 2.4 grams/day) and manage volume status, especially if they have right ventricular failure. Routine immunizations against influenza and pneumococcal pneumonia are advised. Exposure to high altitudes may contribute to hypoxic pulmonary vasoconstriction and may not be tolerated by patients. Oxygen is used to maintain oxygen saturation above 90%.

PAH Treatment Algorithm

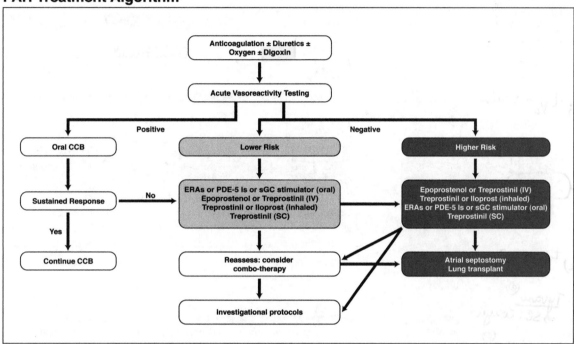

DRUG TREATMENT

Approximately 10 percent of patients respond to and are candidates for calcium channel blocker therapy, although only half have a sustained response. The calcium channel blockers used most frequently are long-acting nifedipine, diltiazem, and amlodipine. The use of verapamil is not recommended due to its more pronounced negative inotropic effects relative to diltiazem. Digoxin is sometimes used in patients with right heart failure and a low cardiac output and in patients with atrial arrhythmias.

[handwritten: nifedipine (Adalat®)]

[handwritten: do not use]

For most cases, drug therapy will reduce symptoms. Parenteral prostacyclin therapy appears to prolong life. Medications include prostacyclin analogues which cause vasodilation. These drugs may be given by continuous IV infusion, infusion under the skin, inhalation, or as oral therapy. Endothelin receptor antagonists block endothelin, a vasoconstrictor. Phosphodiesterase-5 inhibitors (the same drugs used for erectile dysfunction – but with different brand names and doses) and a soluble guanylate cyclase (sGC) stimulator relax the blood vessels in the lungs. Some patients may benefit from combination therapy.

Prostacyclin Analogues (or Prostanoids)

Prostacyclin analogues act as potent vasodilators (on both pulmonary and systemic vascular beds). They are also inhibitors of platelet aggregation. Prostacyclin synthase is reduced in PAH resulting in inadequate production of prostacyclin I_2, which normally stimulates cAMP, a vasodilator with antiproliferative effects, in pulmonary artery smooth muscle cells. Drugs which ↓ prostaglandins (NSAIDs) should be avoided in patients with PAH.

DRUG	DOSING	SAFETY/SIDE EFFECTS/MONITORING
Epoprostenol (Flolan, Veletri) AKA prostacyclin and PGI₂ *[handwritten: chill & pump on ice packs for cooling; light protect]* *[handwritten: t½ ~ 5 min]*	Start at 2 ng/kg/min and ↑ by 1 ng/kg/min in at least 15 minute increments. Normal dose is 25-40 ng/kg/min (may be up to 200 ng/kg/min titrated over months to years) via continuous IV infusion	**CONTRAINDICATIONS** Use of oral treprostinil in Child-Pugh class C hepatic impairment **WARNINGS** *[handwritten: Orenitram®]* Alcohol should be avoided with oral treprostinil due to accelerated absorption. Oral treprostinil's shell does not dissolve and may lodge in diverticuli. **SIDE EFFECTS** During Dose Titration – vasodilation (hypotension, headache, flushing; dose-limiting; if this happens, ↓ dose of the drug), nausea, vomiting, diarrhea, anxiety, chest pain/palpitations, tachycardia, edema, and jaw claudication – *[handwritten: cramping due to artery obstruction]* With Chronic Use – anxiety, flu-like symptoms, jaw pain, thrombocytopenia, neuropathy in addition to those seen during dose titration Treprostinil (inhaled) and iloprost: cough (in addition to above side effects) Treprostinil (oral): side effects as above with more pronounced gastrointestinal adverse effects
Treprostinil (Remodulin is SC/IV, Tyvaso is inhaled, Orenitram is oral) *[handwritten: very painful (may need analgesic) t½ ~ 4 hrs]* *[handwritten: Tyvaso® → SE: cough]* *[handwritten: Orenitram® → SE: more pronounced N/V/D]*	*Remodulin:* start at 1.25 ng/kg/min and ↑ by 1.25 ng/kg/min at weekly intervals for the first month and 2.5 ng/kg/min increments thereafter up to 40-160 ng/kg/min via continuous SC or IV infusion Inhalation form (*Tyvaso*) is given 4 times/day Oral, ER tablets (*Orenitram*): start at 0.25 mg BID with food and ↑ by 0.25-0.5 mg BID every 3-4 days up to ~ 20 mg BID as tolerated	**NOTES** Avoid interruptions in therapy. Immediate access to back up pump, infusion sets and medication is essential – particularly for epoprostenol – to prevent treatment interruptions (epoprostenol half-life ~ 5 minutes vs. treprostinil half-life ~ 4 hours). Avoid large, sudden reductions or increases in dose. *Flolan:* pump needs to be on ice packs for proper cooling. Requires light protection during administration. *Veletri:* thermostable (no need for ice packs). *Remodulin:* SC very painful (85% of patients), may need analgesic to tolerate. Also thermostable – no ice packs needed. The parenteral agents are considered the most potent of all PAH medications. Patients must be instructed on central catheter maintenance to ↓ infections and to avoid interruption of therapy – both which can be fatal.
Iloprost (Ventavis)	2.5-5 mcg/inhalation given 6-9 times/day	

Prostacyclin Analogue Drug Interactions

- Can ↑ the effects of antihypertensive and antiplatelet agents. *[handwritten: potent vasodilators + inhibit PLT aggregation]*

- Treprostinil levels are ↑ by the cytochrome P450 2C8 inhibitor gemfibrozil and ↓ by 2C8 inducers such as rifampin.

preg X
SE: anemia
(↓Hgb)

Endothelin Receptor Antagonists (ERAs)

These agents block endothelin receptors on pulmonary artery smooth muscle cells. Endothelin is a vasoconstrictor with cellular proliferative effects.

DRUG	DOSING	SAFETY/SIDE EFFECTS/MONITORING
Bosentan (Tracleer)	< 40 kg: 62.5 mg BID ≥ 40 kg: 62.5 mg BID (for 4 wks) then 125 mg BID	**BOXED WARNINGS (2)** Hepatotoxicity Use in pregnancy is contraindicated (Pregnancy Category X) Because of the risks of hepatic impairment and possible teratogenic effects, bosentan is only available through the *Tracleer* Access Program (T.A.P.). Prescribers and pharmacists must be certified and enroll patients in T.A.P. **CONTRAINDICATIONS** Pregnancy; concurrent use of cyclosporine or glyburide **WARNINGS** Avoid use in moderate-to-severe hepatic impairment **SIDE EFFECTS** Headache, ↓ Hgb (usually in first 6 weeks of therapy), ↑ LFTs (dose related), upper respiratory tract infections, edema (all > 10%) Spermatogenesis inhibition (25%) leading to male infertility (with bosentan only) **MONITORING** Monitor LFTs and bilirubin at baseline and every month thereafter. Monitor hemoglobin and hematocrit at baseline and at 1 month and 3 months, then every 3 months thereafter. **NOTES** Women of childbearing potential must have a negative pregnancy test prior to initiation of therapy and monthly thereafter (prior to shipment of the monthly refill). Barrier techniques of contraception are recommended. MedGuide required.

Endothelin Receptor Antagonists (ERAs) Continued

DRUG	DOSING	SAFETY/SIDE EFFECTS/MONITORING
Ambrisentan (Letairis)	5-10 mg daily	**BOXED WARNING** Use in pregnancy is contraindicated (Pregnancy Category X) Because of the risk of possible teratogenic effects, ambrisentan is only available through the *Letairis* Education and Access Program (LEAP) restricted distribution program. Prescribers and pharmacists must be certified and enroll patients in LEAP. **CONTRAINDICATIONS** Pregnancy, idiopathic pulmonary fibrosis **SIDE EFFECTS** Peripheral edema, headache, ↓ Hgb, flushing, palpitations, and nasal congestion **MONITORING** Monitor hemoglobin and hematocrit at baseline and at 1 month, then periodically thereafter. **NOTES** Women of childbearing potential must have a negative pregnancy test prior to initiation of therapy and monthly thereafter (prior to shipment of the monthly refill). Monitoring of LFTs was removed from the package insert on March 4, 2011 (FDA). MedGuide required.
Macitentan (Opsumit)	10 mg daily	**BOXED WARNING** Use in pregnancy is contraindicated (Pregnancy Category X) Because of the risk of possible teratogenic effects, macitentan is only available through the *Opsumit* restricted distribution program. Prescribers and pharmacists must be certified and enroll patients in the *Opsumit* REMS program. **CONTRAINDICATIONS** Pregnancy **SIDE EFFECTS** ↓ Hgb, headache, pharyngitis, bronchitis (all > 10%) **MONITORING** Monitor hemoglobin, hematocrit, and LFTs at baseline and repeat as clinically indicated. **NOTES** Women of childbearing potential must have a negative pregnancy test prior to initiation of therapy and monthly thereafter (prior to shipment of the monthly refill). MedGuide required.

Handwritten note: → LFT monitoring (no hepatotox BBW)

Endothelin Receptor Antagonist Drug Interactions

- Avoid use with St. John's wort or grapefruit juice.

- Bosentan is a substrate of 3A4 (major) and 2C9 (minor) and an inducer of 3A4 (weak/moderate) and 2C9 (weak/moderate); monitor for drug interactions. Levels of bosentan may ↑ with 2C8/9 and 3A4 inhibitors. Bosentan can ↓ the effectiveness of hormonal birth control. Avoid concurrent use of cyclosporine or glyburide.

- Ambrisentan is a substrate of 3A4 (major), 2C19 (minor), P-glycoprotein and other pathways. The dose should not exceed 5 mg/d when given concomitantly with cyclosporine.

- Macitentan is a substrate of 3A4 (major) and 2C19 (minor). Strong 3A4 inhibitors and inducers should be avoided with macitentan.

Phosphodiesterase-5 Inhibitors (PDE-5 Inhibitors)

These agents inhibit phosphodiesterase 5 (PDE-5) in smooth muscle cells of the pulmonary vasculature. PDE-5 is responsible for the degradation of cyclic guanosine monophosphate (cGMP); ↑ cGMP concentrations lead to pulmonary vasculature relaxation and vasodilation.

DRUG	DOSING	SAFETY/SIDE EFFECTS/MONITORING
Sildenafil *(Revatio)*	IV: 2.5 or 10 mg TID Oral: 5 or 20 mg TID, taken 4-6 hours apart	**CONTRAINDICATIONS** Concurrent use of nitrates. Avoid using sildenafil for PAH in patients taking PI-based (ritonavir) HAART regimens. **WARNINGS** Color discrimination impairment (dose related) Hearing loss, can be sudden, with our without tinnitus Vision loss, rare but may be due to nonarteritic anterior ischemic optic neuropathy (NAION)
Tadalafil *(Adcirca)*	40 mg daily (two 20 mg tabs) 20 mg daily if mild to moderate renal/hepatic impairment; avoid when CrCl < 30 mL/min	Priapism – seek emergency medical care if erection lasts > 4 hours **SIDE EFFECTS** Dizziness, sudden drop in blood pressure, headache, flushing, dyspepsia, back pain, and epistaxis **NOTES** Avoid use in severe hepatic impairment

PDE-5 Inhibitor Drug Interactions

- Do not give with PDE-5 inhibitors used for erectile dysfunction. Avoid concurrent use of nitrates, itraconazole, and ketoconazole. Avoid grapefruit juice.

- Concurrent use of nitrate medications [any nitroglycerin-containing drug including *Nitrolingual, Nitrostat*, isosorbide dinitrate/hydralazine *(BiDil)*, among others], increases the potential for excessively low blood pressure. Taking nitrates is an absolute contraindication to the use of these medicines. These include the illicit drugs such as amyl nitrate and butyl nitrate ("poppers").

- If a patient has taken a PDE-5 inhibitor and then develops angina, nitroglycerin should not be used until after 24 hours has elapsed for sildenafil and 48 hours has elapsed for tadalafil. (Sometimes nitrates are used in an acute emergency, despite this warning, with careful monitoring.)

- Caution with PDE-5 inhibitors and concurrent alpha blocker therapy: PDE-5 inhibitors can ↑ the hypotensive effect of an alpha blocker. When tadalafil is used for treatment of BPH, concurrent alpha 1-blockers are not recommended.

- These are 3A4 substrates; caution with the use of 3A4 inhibitors and inducers.

CTEPH = Chronic Thromboembolic Pulmonary HTN

preg X

Soluble Guanylate Cyclase (sGC) Stimulator

Increasing conversion of GTP to cGMP leads to ↑ relaxation and antiproliferative effects in the pulmonary artery smooth muscle cells. Riociguat is approved for use in both PAH and CTEPH.

DRUG	DOSING	SAFETY/SIDE EFFECTS/MONITORING
Riociguat *(Adempas)*	0.5-1 mg TID, increasing by 0.5 mg TID every 2 weeks to target 2.5 mg TID	**BOXED WARNING** Use in pregnancy is contraindicated (Pregnancy Category X) Because of the risk of possible teratogenic effects, riociguat is only available through the *Adempas* restricted distribution program. Prescribers and pharmacists must be certified and enroll patients in the *Adempas* REMS program. **CONTRAINDICATIONS** Pregnancy; concomitant use of PDE-5 inhibitors or nitrates **SIDE EFFECTS** Headache, dyspepsia, dizziness, hypotension, nausea, vomiting, and diarrhea (all > 10%). Bleeding appears to be more common with riociguat than placebo. **NOTES** MedGuide required.

sCG Stimulator Drug Interactions

- Smoking ↑ riociguat clearance; the dose may need to be ↓ with smoking cessation.

- Separate from antacids by > 1 hour.

- Strong enzyme inhibitors (e.g., ketoconazole, ritonavir) may warrant a lower starting dose.

new section:

PULMONARY FIBROSIS

Pulmonary fibrosis (PF) is scarred and damaged lung tissue. The common presentation is exertional dyspnea with a nonproductive cough. As the condition worsen, breathing becomes more labored. There are a variety of causes of PF: toxin exposure (including asbestos, silica and many others), medical conditions, drugs (see box) or due to a multitude of factors. Often the contributing factor is not identified and the PF is called idiopathic pulmonary fibrosis (IPF). Two drugs were approved over the past year for IPF; these are presented below. If the condition is drug-induced, the offending drug should be discontinued. In addition to the two new drugs below, several of the drugs approved for pulmonary arterial hypertension are used off-label for PF.

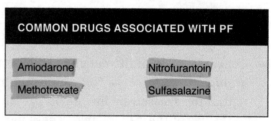

COMMON DRUGS ASSOCIATED WITH PF	
Amiodarone	Nitrofurantoin
Methotrexate	Sulfasalazine

DRUG	DOSING	SAFETY/SIDE EFFECTS/MONITORING
Pirfenidone *(Esbriet)* Mechanism fully unknown. May ↓ production of fibrosis-associated proteins & cytokines and fibroblast proliferation, may ↓ formation of collagen; anti-inflammatory properties	Days 1-7: 267 mg (1 cap) TID, Days 8-14: 534 mg (2 caps) TID, Days 15+: 801 mg (3 caps) TID (max 2,403 mg/day). Take with food, at same time of day.	**WARNINGS** Photosensitivity reactions, ↑ LFTs **SIDE EFFECTS** Nausea, diarrhea, rash, fatigue, dyspepsia, photosensitivity reaction
Nintedanib *(Ofev)* Tyrosine kinase inhibitor, blocks intracellular signaling and prevents proliferation, migration, and transformation of fibroblasts	150 mg Q12H (max 300 mg/d) Take with food, swallow whole with a full glass of water.	**WARNINGS** May ↑ bleeding, cause thromboembolic events (MI), ↑ LFTs **SIDE EFFECTS** N/V/D, abdominal pain, ↑ LFTs, ↓ appetite **NOTES** Pregnancy Category D. Avoid becoming pregnant during therapy and at least 3 months after use. Do not crush or chew. Use appropriate precautions when handling/disposing, drug is hazardous.

(handwritten in left margin, Arabic: عقار بتاع ; below: Nintendo)

(handwritten notes below table):

- $\dfrac{60,000 \text{ ng}}{\text{ml}} = \dfrac{x \text{ ng}}{76.8 \text{ ml}} \Rightarrow x = 4608000 \text{ ng/day} = 3200 \text{ ng/min} = 40 \text{ ng/kg/min}$

- $\dfrac{4.5 \times 10^6 \text{ ng}}{100 \text{ ml}} = \dfrac{x \text{ ng}}{74 \text{ ml}}$

  $3,330,000 \text{ ng/day}$

  $1 \text{ day} = 24 \text{ hrs} \cdot 60 \text{ min}$

  2312.5 ng/min

  ↳ : $\dfrac{210}{2.2} = 24.23 \dfrac{\text{ng}}{\text{kg min}}$

  ng 10^{-9}
  µg 10^{-6}
  mg 10^{-3}

- $\dfrac{96 \text{ ng}}{\text{kg min}} \cdot 60 \text{ kg} = 5760 \dfrac{\text{ng}}{\text{min}}$

  ↓ : 10^6

  $0.00576 \dfrac{\text{mg}}{\text{min}}$

  ↓ · 60

  $0.3456 \dfrac{\text{mg}}{\text{hr}}$

  $10 \text{ mg} = 1 \text{ ml}$
  $0.3456 \text{ mg} = ?$ $0.03456 \dfrac{\text{ml}}{\text{hr}}$

45

ASTHMA

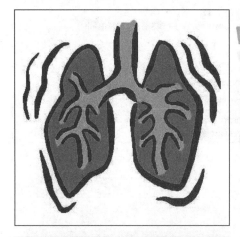

GUIDELINES

Expert Panel Report 3. Guidelines for the Diagnosis and Management of Asthma. National Heart, Lung and Blood Institute, August 2007. http://www.nhlbi.nih.gov/guidelines/asthma (accessed 2014 Oct. 17).

The Global Strategy for Asthma Management and Prevention, Global Initiative for Asthma (GINA) 2012. http://www.ginasthma.org/(accessed 2014 Oct. 17).

BACKGROUND

Asthma is characterized by a predisposition to chronic inflammation of the lungs in which the airways (bronchi) are reversibly narrowed. Asthma affects 8% of the population in the United States. During asthma attacks (exacerbations of asthma), the smooth muscle cells in the bronchi constrict, airways become inflamed and swollen, and breathing becomes difficult.

The National Heart, Lung and Blood Institute defines asthma as a common chronic disorder of the airways characterized by variable and recurring symptoms, airflow obstruction, bronchial hyperresponsiveness (bronchospasm), and underlying inflammation. Asthma is a chronic inflammatory disorder of the airways in which many cells and cellular elements play a role, in particular, mast cells, eosinophils, neutrophils, T lymphocytes, macrophages, and epithelial cells. This inflammation causes recurrent episodes of the classic signs and symptoms of asthma such as: wheezing, breathlessness, chest tightness, and coughing; particularly at night or early in the morning. These episodes are generally associated with variable airflow obstruction that is often reversible spontaneously or with treatment. Airway remodeling such as fibrosis and increased goblet (mucus-producing) cells can occur.

COMMON TRIGGERS OF ASTHMA

TRIGGERS	EXAMPLES
Allergens	Airborne pollens (grass, trees, weeds), house-dust mites, animal dander (cats, dogs, horses, rabbits, rats, mice), cockroaches, fungal spores
Drugs	Aspirin, NSAIDs, sulfites, beta-blockers (non-selective)
Environmental	Cold air, fog, ozone, sulfur dioxide, nitrogen dioxide, tobacco smoke, wood smoke
Exercise	Cold air or humid, hot air
Occupational	Bakers (flour dust), farmers (hay mold), spice and enzyme workers; painters (arabic gum), chemical workers (azo dyes, toluene diisocyanates, polyvinyl chloride); plastics, rubber, and wood workers (formaldehyde, dimethyethanolamine)
Respiratory Infections	Respiratory syncytial virus (RSV), rhinovirus, influenza, parainfluenza, *Mycoplasma pneumonia, Chlamydia*

DRUG TREATMENT

Drugs used to treat asthma are classified as controllers (maintenance) or relievers (rescue). All patients with asthma (Steps 1-6) need a "rescue" inhaler for acute asthma symptoms. Controllers are taken on a chronic, daily basis to keep asthma under control, primarily by reducing inflammation. Relievers are used as-needed to quickly reverse bronchoconstriction, or preventively for exercise-induced bronchospasm (EIB). Asthma drugs come in oral, inhaled and injectable formulations. Inhaled forms deliver drugs directly into the lungs, have reduced toxicity, and are the preferred delivery vehicle. Inhaled steroids (glucocorticosteroids) are the most effective and the recommended first-line maintenance medication. Short-acting beta-2 agonists (primarily albuterol) are the drugs of choice for acute bronchospasm, and for prevention of EIB, in both adults, children and during pregnancy. Increased use of a short-acting beta-2 agonist indicates worsening asthma control, and a need to reassess treatment. The primary treatment is to increase the inhaled steroid dose. Steroids can be given by injection in acute cases, and oral steroids are used for severely uncontrolled asthma, but the use of steroids in other formulations than inhaled is limited by the risk of adverse effects. Theophylline can be helpful in some cases, but has significant adverse effects and drug interactions. Cold air, pollutants and other "triggers" can worsen asthma control. Patients should attempt to identify what triggers their exacerbations and reduce trigger exposure. Adults aged 19-64 years old with asthma should receive the pneumococcal polysaccharide vaccine (PPSV23 or *Pneumovax)*. An annual flu vaccine should be given to those with asthma.

"RESCUERS" – THESE AGENTS ARE COMMONLY USED IN ASTHMA EXACERBATIONS	"CONTROLLERS" – OR LONG-TERM, MAINTENANCE THERAPY
Short-acting beta-2 agonists (SABA)	Inhaled steroids
Systemic steroids (inj. or oral)	Long-acting beta-2 agonists (taken with steroids)
Anticholinergics	Leukotriene Modifying Agents
	Theophylline
	Omalizumab *(Xolair)*

Classifying Asthma Severity & Initiating Treatment In Youths ≥ 12 Years Of Age and Adults

Components of Severity		Classification of Asthma Severity ≥12 years of age			
				Persistent	
		Intermittent	Mild	Moderate	Severe
Impairment Normal FEV₁/FVC: 8–19 yr 85% 20–39 yr 80% 40–59 yr 75% 60–80 yr 70%	Symptoms	≤2 days/week	>2 days/week but not daily	Daily	Throughout the day
	Nighttime awakenings	≤2x/month	3–4x/month	>1x/week but not nightly	Often 7x/week
	Short-acting beta₂-agonist use for symptom control (not prevention of EIB)	≤2 days/week	>2 days/week but not daily, and not more than 1x on any day	Daily	Several times per day
	Interference with normal activity	None	Minor limitation	Some limitation	Extremely limited
	Lung function	• Normal FEV₁ between exacerbations • FEV₁ >80% predicted • FEV₁/FVC normal	• FEV₁ >80% predicted • FEV₁/FVC normal	• FEV₁ >60% but <80% predicted • FEV₁/FVC reduced 5%	• FEV₁ <60% predicted • FEV₁/FVC reduced >5%
Risk	Exacerbations requiring oral systemic corticosteroids	0–1/year (see note)	≥2/year (see note)		
		Consider severity and interval since last exacerbation. Frequency and severity may fluctuate over time for patients in any severity category. Relative annual risk of exacerbations may be related to FEV₁			
Recommended Step for Initiating Treatment (See figure 4–5 for treatment steps.)		Step 1	Step 2	Step 3	Step 4 or 5 and consider short course of oral systemic corticosteroids
		In 2–6 weeks, evaluate level of asthma control that is achieved and adjust therapy accordingly.			

Key: FEV₁, forced expiratory volume in 1 second; FVC, forced vital capacity; ICU, intensive care unit

Notes:

- The stepwise approach is meant to assist, not replace, the clinical decisionmaking required to meet individual patient needs.

- Level of severity is determined by assessment of both impairment and risk. Assess impairment domain by patient's/caregiver's recall of previous 2–4 weeks and spirometry. Assign severity to the most severe category in which any feature occurs.

- At present, there are inadequate data to correspond frequencies of exacerbations with different levels of asthma severity. In general, more frequent and intense exacerbations (e.g., requiring urgent, unscheduled care, hospitalization, or ICU admission) indicate greater underlying disease severity. For treatment purposes, patients who had ≥2 exacerbations requiring oral systemic corticosteroids in the past year may be considered the same as patients who have persistent asthma, even in the absence of impairment levels consistent with persistent asthma.

Stepwise Approach For Managing Asthma In Youths ≥ 12 Years Of Age and Adults

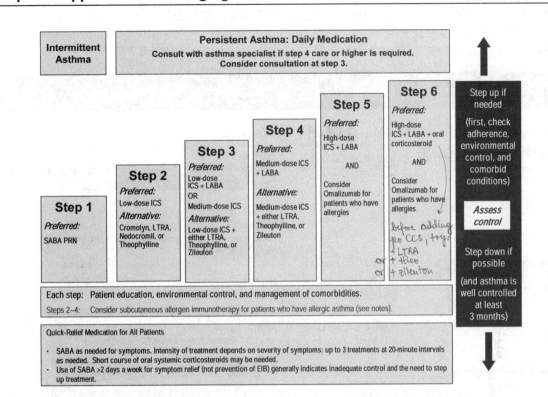

Key: Alphabetical order is used when more than one treatment option is listed within either preferred or alternative therapy. EIB, exercise-induced bronchospasm; ICS, inhaled corticosteroid; LABA, long-acting inhaled beta₂-agonist; LTRA, leukotriene receptor antagonist; SABA, inhaled short-acting beta₂-agonist

Notes:

- The stepwise approach is meant to assist, not replace, the clinical decisionmaking required to meet individual patient needs.
- If alternative treatment is used and response is inadequate, discontinue it and use the preferred treatment before stepping up.
- Zileuton is a less desirable alternative due to limited studies as adjunctive therapy and the need to monitor liver function. Theophylline requires monitoring of serum concentration levels.
- In step 6, before oral systemic corticosteroids are introduced, a trial of high-dose ICS + LABA + either LTRA, theophylline, or zileuton may be considered, although this approach has not been studied in clinical trials.
- Step 1, 2, and 3 preferred therapies are based on Evidence A; step 3 alternative therapy is based on Evidence A for LTRA, Evidence B for theophylline, and Evidence D for zileuton. Step 4 preferred therapy is based on Evidence B, and alternative therapy is based on Evidence B for LTRA and theophylline and Evidence D for zileuton. Step 5 preferred therapy is based on Evidence B. Step 6 preferred therapy is based on (EPR—2 1997) and Evidence B for omalizumab.
- Immunotherapy for steps 2–4 is based on Evidence B for house-dust mites, animal danders, and pollens; evidence is weak or lacking for molds and cockroaches. Evidence is strongest for immunotherapy with single allergens. The role of allergy in asthma is greater in children than in adults.
- Clinicians who administer immunotherapy or omalizumab should be prepared and equipped to identify and treat anaphylaxis that may occur.

Beta-2 Agonists

These agents bind to beta-2 receptors, causing relaxation of bronchial smooth muscle and leading to bronchodilation. Inhalation is the preferred route of administration. Inhaled devices come as metered-dose inhalers (MDI) or dry powder inhalers (DPI).

DRUG	DOSING	SAFETY/SIDE EFFECTS/MONITORING
Short-Acting Beta-2 Agonists (SABAs) *DOC for EIB*		
Racepinephrine *(Asthmanefrin EZ Breathe Atomizer)* OTC *racemic mixture*	Should not be used; not beta-2 selective	**SIDE EFFECTS** Tremor, shakiness, lightheadedness, cough, palpitations, hypokalemia, tachycardia, hyperglycemia **MONITORING** Number of days of use of SABA, symptom frequency, peak flow, pulmonary function tests, BP, HR, blood glucose, and K+ *↑BG ↓K+* **NOTES** Pregnancy Category C With MDIs, shake well before use. Prime prior to first use (3-4 sprays into the air away from face) and again if inhaler has not been used for > 2 weeks.
Albuterol *(Ventolin HFA, Proventil HFA, ProAir HFA, VoSpire ER)* *aerosol, po tab/ solution/ syrup*	MDI: 1-2 inhalations Q4-6H PRN Nebulizer: 1.25-5 mg Q4-8H PRN Tablet: 2-4 mg Q4-6H PO PRN	Prefer a beta-2 selective agent via inhaled route. These are rescue medications used PRN in asthma.
Levalbuterol *(Xopenex, Xopenex HFA)* *R-isomer systemic SE (tachy, h/a, nervousness) occur @ same rate as albuterol pirbuterol (Maxair®)*	MDI: 1-2 inhalations Q4-6H PRN Nebulizer: 0.63-1.25 mg Q6-8H PRN	If using SABA > 2 days/week, then need to ↑ maintenance therapy. Short acting beta-2 agonists are the drugs of choice for exercise-induced bronchospasm (EIB). Levalbuterol contains R-isomer of albuterol. Most albuterol inhalers contain 200 inhalations/canister.
Long-Acting Beta-2 Agonists (LABAs) *• ICS dose Δ • LABA dose stays same*		
Salmeterol *(Serevent Diskus)* **+ fluticasone** *(Advair Diskus, Advair HFA)* ***Advair Diskus*** – 100, 250, 500 mcg fluticasone + 50 mcg salmeterol/inh (ages ≥ 4 years) ***Advair HFA*** – 45, 115, 230 mcg fluticasone + 21 mcg salmeterol/ inh (ages ≥ 12 years)	*Diskus* DPI: 1 inhalation BID MDI: 2 inhalations BID	**BOXED WARNING** ↑ risk of asthma-related deaths. Monotherapy with LABA is contraindicated in the treatment of asthma; should only be used in asthma patients as adjunctive therapy in patients who are currently receiving but are not adequately controlled on a long-term asthma control medication (an inhaled corticosteroid). Once asthma control is achieved and maintained, assess the patient at regular intervals and step down therapy (discontinue LABA) if possible without loss of asthma control
Formoterol *(Foradil Aerolizer)* **+ budesonide *(Symbicort)*** ***Symbicort*** – 80, 160 mcg budesonide + 4.5 mcg formoterol/inh (ages ≥ 12 years) *+ mometasone (Dulera®) (≥ 12 y/o)*	DPI: 1 capsule (12 mcg) via *Aerolizer* BID MDI: 2 inhalations BID	**CONTRAINDICATIONS:** Monotherapy in treatment of asthma, treatment of status asthmaticus or other acute episides of asthma or COPD Similar side effects and monitoring as SABAs **NOTES** Pregnancy Category C ***Foradil*** Refrigerate capsules in the pharmacy, patient can keep at room temp. for 4 months

form. can cause palpitations

★ for both form/salm — Diskus: 1 inh BID MDI: 2 inh BID

Corticosteroids

Corticosteroids inhibit the inflammatory response, depressing migration of polymorphonu-clear (PMN) leukocytes and fibroblasts, and reversing capillary permeability and lysosomal stabilization at the cellular level.

Inhaled Corticosteroids

DRUG	DOSING	SAFETY/SIDE EFFECTS/MONITORING
Beclomethasone HFA *(QVAR)* – solution, do not need to shake	Low dose: 80-240 mcg/day Medium dose: > 240-480 mcg/day High dose: > 480 mcg/day	**CONTRAINDICATIONS** Primary treatment of status asthmaticus or acute episodes of asthma or COPD (not for relief of acute bronchospasm)
Budesonide *(Pulmicort Flexhaler, Pulmicort Respules)* **+ formoterol** *(Symbicort)*	Low dose: 180-600 mcg/day Medium dose: > 600-1,200 mcg/day High dose: > 1,200 mcg/day *Pulmicort Respules* – suspension for nebulization (ages 1-8 years) *jet nebulizer only*	**SIDE EFFECTS (INHALED)** Dysphonia (difficulty speaking), oral candidiasis (thrush), cough, hoarseness, URTI's, hyperglycemia, ↑ risk of fractures and pneumonia (with high dose, long-term use), growth retardation (in children with high doses) **MONITORING** Use of SABA, symptom frequency, peak flow, growth (children/adolescents) and signs/symptoms of HPA axis suppression/adrenal insufficiency, signs/symptoms of oral candidiasis, bone mineral density
Ciclesonide *(Alvesco)* – do not need to shake	Low dose: 80-160 mcg/day Medium dose: > 160-320 mcg/day High dose: > 320 mcg/day	**NOTES** To prevent oral candidiasis, rinse mouth and throat with warm water and spit out or use a spacer device if using a MDI
Flunisolide HFA *(Aerospan HFA)* – has built-in spacer	Low dose: 320 mcg/day Medium dose: > 320-640 mcg/day High dose: > 640 mcg/day	Inhaled steroids are first-line for long term control for all ages with persistent asthma *QVAR* and *Alvesco* are MDIs that do not need to be shaken before use Only use *Pulmicort Respules* with a jet nebulizer machine that is connected to an air compressor. Do not use an ultrasonic nebulizer. Pregnancy Category C/B (budesonide)
Fluticasone *(Flovent HFA,* Flovent Diskus, Arnuity Ellipta)* **+ salmeterol** *(Advair Diskus, Advair HFA)* *Flonase® for allergic rhinitis*	**For MDI:** Low dose: 88-264 mcg/day Medium dose: 264-440 mcg/day High dose: > 440 mcg/day **For *Diskus*:** Low dose: 100-300 mcg/day Medium dose: > 300-500 mcg/day High dose: > 500 mcg/day	To ↓ fracture risk, recommend: smoking cessation, exercise, using lowest, effective steroid dose, Ca²⁺ and vitamin D supplementation with prescription therapies if needed and obtaining regular bone density screening.
Mometasone *(Asmanex Twisthaler, Asmanex HFA)* **+ formoterol** *(Dulera)* *Dulera* – 100, 200 mcg mometasone + 5 mcg formoterol/inh (ages ≥ 12 years)	Low dose: 200 mcg/day Medium dose: 400 mcg/day High dose: > 400 mcg/day	*Nasonex® for allergic rhinitis*

Oral Corticosteroids

The two types of steroids are glu-cocorticoids, produced by the body as a reaction to stress or given ex-ogenously, and mineralocorticoids (fludrocortisone), which regulates sodium and water balance. Miner-alocorticoids are used to raise so-dium levels and to replace some of the function of aldosterone in Addi-son's disease.

Steroids (glucocorticoids) are used clinically primarily to reduce in-flammation, which can require high doses. In some cases, a few high doses are given and then stopped, such as with a methylprednisolone injection. In other cases, the ini-tial dose is started high and then sequentially tapered down to con-tinue to control the inflammation or to prevent a rebound attack. These tapered dosing regimens often come prepackaged such as prednisone, methylprednisolone *(Medrol Dosepak)* and dexametha-sone *(Dexpak)*.

The above tapered dosing regimens are different than what is typi-cally referred to as a steroid taper, which is used to wean patients off therapy by a steady reduction in dose for patients using steroids for longer than 14 days. Some package inserts state to taper if used lon-ger than 10-14 days. This taper is needed due to suppression of the hypothalamic-pituitary-adrenal (HPA) axis and is designed to give the patient's body time to increase its own endogenous cortisol pro-duction, which would have de-creased during the extended peri-od of systemic steroid use.

LONG-TERM SIDE EFFECTS OF SYSTEMIC STEROIDS

Cushing Syndrome
A condition due to excess endogenous cortisol from the pituitary gland or exogenous steroid therapy.

- Central redistribution of fat (fat deposits in the abdo-men)
- Moon facies (fat deposits in the face)
- Buffalo hump (fat deposits between the shoulders)
- Impaired wound healing
- Dermal thinning/bruising

Other Side Effects
Psychiatric disturbances (mood swings, delirium, psychoses)

Sodium and water retention/hypertension

Hypokalemia   ↓K⁺

Hyperglycemia/diabetes

Increased appetite/weight gain

Immunosuppression

Glaucoma/cataracts

Growth retardation

Amenorrhea

Osteoporosis/fractures

Hirsutism (in women)

Acne

Insomnia/nervousness

GI bleeding/esophagitis/ulcers (do not use with NSAIDs due to ↑ risk)

ORAL STEROIDS – DOSE EQUIVALENTS

Short-acting
Cortisone – 25 mg
Hydrocortisone – 20 mg

Intermediate-acting
Methylprednisolone/
Triamcinolone – 4 mg   4mg
Prednisone/
Prednisolone – 5 mg   5mg

Long-acting
Betamethasone – 0.6 mg
Dexamethasone – 0.75 mg

Mineralcorticoids
Fludrocortisone – no anti-inflammatory effect; used for mineralcorticoid proper-ties (primarily to ↑ Na⁺ and consequently fluid volume) in Addison's disease and other salt-wasting conditions

Florinef®

Oral Corticosteroids

DRUG	DOSING	SAFETY/SIDE EFFECTS/MONITORING
Cortisone *(handwritten: PRODRUG for cortisol)*	Dosing varies by disease severity and patient response Used as pulse therapy for acute exacerbations; used for maintenance therapy in very severe disease (Step 6) at doses of 5-60 mg daily or every other day	**CONTRAINDICATIONS** Live vaccines and most serious systemic infections **SIDE EFFECTS** Short-term side effects (used < 1 month): ↑ appetite/ weight gain, fluid retention, emotional instability (euphoria, mood swings, irritability), insomnia, indigestion, bitter taste. Higher doses ↑ in BP and ↑ blood glucose. Long-term side effects are listed in chart on previous page. **MONITORING** BP, weight, appetite, mood, symptoms of asthma, peak flow, growth (children/adolescents), mineral bone density, glucose, electrolytes, presence of infection, IOP if > 6 weeks therapy **NOTES** Cortisone is a prodrug for cortisol. Prednisone is a prodrug for prednisolone. Prednisolone is used most commonly in children (comes in many formulations). Steroids should be given between 7-8 AM to mimic the body's diurnal release of cortisol. Systemic steroids have a rapid onset of action and are used as "pulse" therapy – for up to 15 days after an asthma attack If taking longer than 10-14 days, must taper slowly due to suppression of the hypothalamic-pituitary-adrenal axis
Hydrocortisone *(Solu-CORTEF* – inj., *Cortef* – tablet, inj.)		
MethylPREDNISolone *(Medrol* – tablet *Medrol Dosepak* – tablet *Solu-MEDROL* – inj. *A-Methapred* – inj. *Depo-Medrol* – inj.)		
PredniSONE *(PredniSONE Intensol* – solution *Rayos* – delayed release tablet) *(handwritten: PRODRUG of prednisolone)*		
PrednisoLONE *(Millipred* – tablet, ODT, solution *Orapred* – tablet, ODT, solution *Pediapred* – solution *Veripred* – solution *Prelone* – syrup *Flo-Pred* – suspension) *(handwritten margin: commonly used in children)*		Tapering dose packs available for treating the acute, massive inflammation where the patient needs high doses up front and smaller doses later on to control the inflammation. Asthma exacerbations are generally treated with steroids for 3-10 days.
Triamcinolone *(Aristospan* – inj. *Kenalog* – inj. *Trivaris* inj.)		

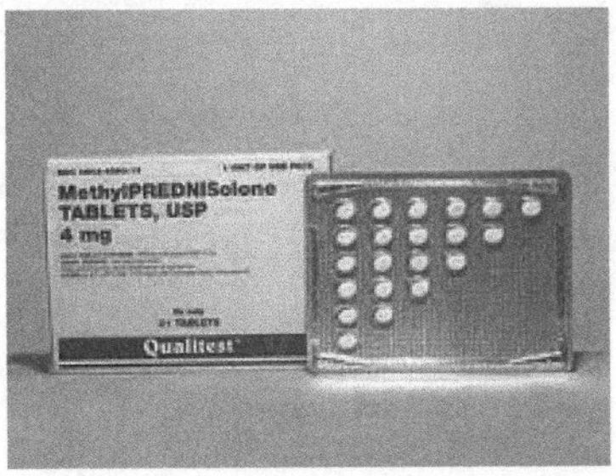

Relative antiinflammatory potency: betamethasone/dexamethasone > methylprednisolone/triamcinolone > prednisone/prednisolone > hydrocortisone > cortisone

Fludrocortisone has the highest mineralcorticoid potency causing Na$^+$ and H$_2$O retention – indicated for Addison's disease; not for inflammation

(handwritten notes at bottom:)

relative antiinflammatory potency/ dose equivalents

most potent
1. betamethasone 0.6 mg
   dexamethasone 0.75 mg
2. methylpred } 4 mg
   triamcinolone
3. prednisone } 5 mg
   prednisolone
least potent
4. hydrocortisone 20 mg
5. cortisone 25 mg

montelukast granules ⇒ take w/in 15 min of mixing
OR cold { 1. directly in mouth
room temp { 2. dissolved in 1 tsp baby formula/breast milk
3. dissolved in 1 spoonful of • applesauce • ice cream
• mashed carrots • rice

Leukotriene Modifying Agents

Zafirlukast and montelukast are leukotriene receptor antagonists (LTRAs) of leukotriene D4 (LTD4 – both drugs) and E4 (LTE4 – just zafirlukast). Zileuton is a 5-lipoxygenase inhibitor which inhibits leukotriene formation. All agents help ↓ airway edema, constriction and inflammation.

• LTD4 receptor antag ↑
• indicated in children

+ LTE4 inhib
≠ hepatic

5-lipoxy-genase inhibitor ⇒ inhibits LT formation

≠ active liver dz
OR LFT ≥ 3x normal

DRUG	DOSING	SAFETY/SIDE EFFECTS/MONITORING
Zafirlukast (*Accolate*)	20 mg BID Age 5-11 years: 10 mg BID Taken 1 hr before or 2 hrs after meals (empty stomach)	**CONTRAINDICATIONS** Hepatic impairment – zafirlukast Active liver disease or LFTs ≥ 3 x ULN – zileuton **WARNINGS** Neuropsychiatric events; monitor for signs of aggressive behavior, hostility, agitation, depression, suicidal thinking (vivid dreams, disorientation/confusion) Systemic eosinophilia, sometimes presenting with clinical features of vasculitis consistent with Churg-Strauss syndrome (rare)
Montelukast (*Singulair*)	10 mg daily in the evening Age 6-14 years: 5 mg daily in the evening Age 1-5 years: 4 mg daily in the evening	**SIDE EFFECTS** Headache, dizziness, abdominal pain, ↑LFTs, URTIs, pharyngitis, sinusitis
Zileuton (*Zyflo, Zyflo CR*)	*Zyflo*: 600 mg QID *Zyflo CR*: 1,200 mg BID within 1 hour of morning and evening meals Age < 12 years: not recommended	**MONITORING** Zileuton – need to monitor LFTs every month for first 3 months, every 2-3 months for the rest of the first year of therapy; use of SABAs **NOTES** Pregnancy Category B/C (zileuton) Zafirlukast: keep in the original container

Leukotriene Modifying Agents Drug Interactions

- Zafirlukast: substrate of 2C9 (major); inhibitor of 1A2 (weak), 2C9 (moderate), 2C19 (weak), 2D6 (weak), 2C8 (weak) and 3A4 (weak) – may ↑ levels of carvedilol, pimozide, theophylline, warfarin and 2C9 substrates. Levels of zafirlukast may be ↓ by erythromycin, theophylline, and food (↓ bioavailability by 40%) – take 1 hour before or 2 hours after meals

- Montelukast: substrate of 3A4 (major) and 2C9 (major); inhibitor of 2C8/9 (weak)

- Zileuton: substrate of 1A2 (minor), 2C9 (minor), 3A4 (minor); inhibitor of 1A2 (weak) – may ↑ levels of pimozide, propranolol, theophylline, and warfarin

Theophylline

Blocks phosphodiesterase causing ↑ cyclic adenosine monophosphate (cAMP) which promotes release of epinephrine from adrenal medulla cells. This results in bronchodilation, diuresis, CNS and cardiac stimulation and gastric acid secretion. Theophylline may help as add-on therapy in some patients, but it is not most effective and drug interactions and adverse effects limit its use.

* HF ↑ [theo] ⇒ ↓ dose needed

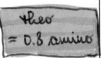

theo
≈ 0.8 amino

DRUG	DOSING	SAFETY/SIDE EFFECTS/MONITORING
Theophylline Immediate Release *(Elixophyllin)* Extended Release *(Theo-24, Theochron)* active metabolites are caffeine and 3-methylxanthine	300-600 mg daily Therapeutic range: 5-15 mcg/mL (measure peak level after 3 days of oral dosing, at steady state)	**WARNINGS** Caution in patients with cardiovascular disease, hyperthyroidism, PUD and seizure disorder since use may exacerbate these conditions **SIDE EFFECTS** Nausea, loose stools, headache, tachycardia, insomnia, tremor, and nervousness Signs of toxicity – persistent and repetitive vomiting, ventricular tachycardias, seizures **MONITORING** Theophylline levels, use of SABA, HR, respiratory rate, CNS effects **NOTES** **** Dosing is based on IBW. **** If no theophyilline given within past 24 hrs, LD = 5 mg/kg If theophylline given within past 24 hrs, LD = (Cp-Co)(Vd) where Vd = 0.5 L/kg; Cp = desired theophylline concentration; Co = initial theophylline concentration If using IV aminophylline, then multiply by 0.8 (aminophylline contains 80% theophylline) Pregnancy Category C

ALWAYS dose based on IBW

• no theo w/in past 24 hrs ⇒ LD = 5 mg/kg

• theo given w/in past 24 hrs ⇒ LD = Vd (Cp - Co)
  * Vd = 0.5 L/kg
  * Cp = desired [theo]
  * Co = initial [theo]

Theophylline Drug Interactions

Theophylline is a substrate of 1A2 (major) and 3A4 (major), 2C9 (minor) and 2D6 (minor) and an inhibitor of 1A2 (weak). It has first order kinetics, followed by zero order kinetics. A small increase in dose can result in a large increase in the theophylline concentration.

- Drugs that may ↑ theophylline levels due to 1A2 inhibition: ciprofloxacin, fluvoxamine, propranolol, zafirlukast, zileuton and possibly others

- Drugs that may ↑ theophylline levels due to 3A4 inhibition: clarithromycin, conivaptan, erythromycin and possibly others

- Drugs that may ↑ theophylline levels due to other mechanisms: alcohol, allopurinol antithyroid agents, disulfiram, estrogen containing oral contraceptives, methotrexate, pentoxifylline, propafenone, verapamil and possibly others. Also conditions such as acute pulmonary edema, CHF, cirrhosis or liver disease, cor-pulmonale, fever, hypothyroidism or shock can ↓ clearance.

?? marijuana 3A4 inhib

- Drugs that may ↓ theophylline levels: carbamazepine, fosphenytoin, phenobarbital, phenytoin, primidone, rifampin, ritonavir, tobacco/marijuana smoking, St. John's wort, thyroid hormones (levothyroxine), high-protein diet and charbroiled meats. Conditions such as hyperthyroidism and cystic fibrosis can ↑ clearance.

- Theophylline will ↓ lithium (theophylline ↑ renal excretion of lithium) and will ↓ zafirlukast

Anticholinergics

Mainly used with other medications in the emergency department for bronchodilation in acute attacks. See COPD chapter for more information on these drugs.

Omalizumab *(Xolair)*

IgG monoclonal antibody that inhibits IgE binding to the IgE receptor on mast cells and basophils. Omalizumab is indicated for moderate to severe persistent, allergic asthma in patients with a positive skin test to perennial aeroallergen and inadequately controlled symptoms on inhaled steroids (Step 5 or 6 per guidelines).

DRUG	DOSING	SAFETY/SIDE EFFECTS/MONITORING
Omalizumab *(Xolair)*	Dose and frequency based on pretreatment total IgE serum levels and body weight – given SC every 2 or 4 weeks Drug should always be given in the doctor's office	**BOXED WARNING** Anaphylaxis, including delayed-onset, can occur. Anaphylaxis has occurred after the first dose but also has occurred beyond 1 year after beginning treatment. Closely observe patients for an appropriate period of time after administration and be prepared to manage anaphylaxis that can be life-threatening. **WARNING** Slightly ↑ risk of serious cardiovascular and cerebrovascular adverse events Malignancies have been observed in clinical studies **SIDE EFFECTS** Injection site reactions, arthralgias, pain, dizziness, fatigue, leg pain, arm pain, pruritus, dermatitis, bone fracture **MONITORING** Baseline IgE, FEV$_1$, peak flow, signs of infection **NOTES** Pregnancy Category B Doses > 150 mg should be divided over more than one injection site

handwritten notes in left margin:
* 8mb Q
  q2-4 wks
* age 12+
* dosed based on
  1. baseline IgE
  and 2. actual body wt

SPECIAL POPULATIONS

Exercise-Induced Bronchospasm (EIB)

- Pretreatment before exercise with SABAs, LABAs or montelukast is recommended. SABAs are the drugs of choice generally.

- SABAs can be taken 5 – 15 minutes before exercise and have a duration of 2 – 3 hours.

- If longer duration of symptom control is needed, LABAs can be used. These agents need to be taken 15 minutes (formoterol) or 30 minutes (salmeterol) prior to exercise. If already using a LABA for asthma maintenance, then do not use additional doses for exercise-induced bronchospasm. Remember LABAs should not be used as monotherapy in patients with persistent asthma.

- Montelukast must be taken 2 hours prior to exercise and it lasts up to 24 hours. However, it only works in 50% of patients. Daily administration to prevent exercise-induced bronchoconstriction has not been evaluated. Patients receiving montelukast for asthma or another indication should not take an additional dose to prevent exercise-induced bronchoconstriction.

Pregnancy

- Albuterol is the preferred short-acting beta-2 agonist.

- Budesonide is the preferred inhaled corticosteroid due to more studies in pregnancy.

- Monitor asthma as it may get worse. It is safer to be treated with asthma medications than to have poorly controlled asthma to ensure oxygen supply to the fetus.

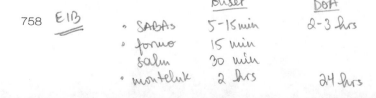

handwritten notes:
EIB

	onset	DOA
SABAs	5-15 min	2-3 hrs
formo	15 min	
salm	30 min	
monteluk	2 hrs	24 hrs

Sample Asthma Action Plan (Adult)

ENGLISH

My Asthma Action Plan

Patient Name:_____

Medical Record #:_____

Physician's Name:_____ DOB:_____

Physician's Phone #:_____ Completed by:_____ Date:_____

Long-Term-Control Medicines	How Much To Take	How Often	Other Instructions
		_____ times per day EVERY DAY!	
		_____ times per day EVERY DAY!	
		_____ times per day EVERY DAY!	
		_____ times per day EVERY DAY!	

Quick-Relief Medicines	How Much To Take	How Often	Other Instructions
		Take ONLY as needed	NOTE: If this medicine is needed frequently, call physician to consider increasing long-term-control medications.

Special instructions when I feel ● good, ○ not good, and ● awful.

GREEN ZONE

I feel *good.*
(My peak flow is in the GREEN zone.)

My Personal Best Peak Flow

PREVENT asthma symptoms everyday:

☐ Take my long-term-control medicines (above) every day.

☐ Before exercise, take _____ puffs of _____

☐ Avoid things that make my asthma worse like:

YELLOW ZONE

I do *not* feel *good.*
(My peak flow is in the YELLOW zone.)

My symptoms may include one or more of the following:
- Wheeze
- Tight chest
- Cough
- Shortness of breath
- Waking up at night with asthma symptoms
- Decreased ability to do usual activities
- _____

80% Personal Best

CAUTION. I should continue taking my long-term-control asthma medicines every day AND:

☐ Take _____

If I still do not feel good, or my peak flow is not back in the *Green Zone* within 1 hour, then I should:

☐ Increase _____

☐ Add _____

☐ Call _____

RED ZONE

I feel *awful.*
(My peak flow is in the RED zone.)

Warning signs may include one or more of the following:
- It's getting harder and harder to breathe
- Unable to sleep or do usual activities because of trouble breathing

50% Personal Best

Liters/Min.

Peak Flow Meter

MEDICAL ALERT! Get help!

☐ Take _____ until I get help immediately.

☐ Take _____

☐ Call _____

Danger! Get help immediately! Call 9-1-1 if you have trouble walking or talking due to shortness of breath or lips or fingernails are gray or blue.

PEAK FLOW METERS

Introduction

Peak flow meters are devices that measure a patient's peak expiratory flow rate (PEFR) – the greatest velocity attained during a forced expiration starting from fully inflated lungs. The patient's best PEFR is known as a Personal Best (PB) and is determined by spirometry, taking into account the patient's height, gender, and age. The PEFR and PB is effort-dependent. Peak flow meters are beneficial in patients with frequent asthma exacerbations. These devices can identify exacerbations early (even before the patient is symptomatic), allowing the patient to initiate treatment sooner. A treatment action plan, is developed by the health care provider so the patient can avoid hospitalizations due to an exacerbation (see previous page).

Technique

- Use the peak flow meter every morning upon awakening and before the use of any asthma medications. Proper technique and best effort are essential. Less than best effort can lead to false 'exacerbation' and unnecessary medication treatment.

- Move the indicator to bottom of numbered scale. Stand up straight. Exhale comfortably.

- Inhale as deeply as possible. Place lips firmly around mouthpiece, creating a tight seal.

- Blow out as hard and as fast as possible. Write down the PEFR.

- Repeat steps two more times, allowing enough rest in between. Record the highest value.

Zones

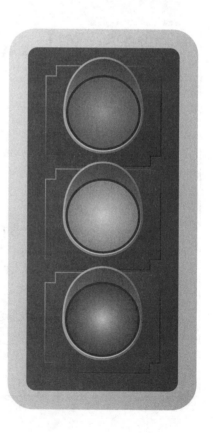

Green zone (80-100% of personal best)

- Indicates "all clear" – good control

- Patients are instructed to follow routine maintenance plan

Yellow zone (50-80% of personal best)

- Indicates "caution" – worsening lung function

- Patient-specific intervention required (action plan) – usually an increase in beta-2 agonist use and the addition or increase in other medications

Red zone (< 50% of personal best)

- Indicates "medical alert" and patient needs to seek medical attention – action plan includes using SABA, possibly steroids and going to the emergency department

Peak Flow Meter Care

- Always use the same brand of peak flow meter.

- Peak flow meters should be cleaned at least once a week; if patient has an infection, they should clean more frequently. Wash peak flow meters in warm water with mild soap. Rinse gently but thoroughly. Do not use brushes to clean inside the peak flow meters. Do not place peak flow meters in boiling water. Allow to air dry before taking next reading.

SPACERS

- Some spacer devices and chambers greatly enhance the coordination necessary to administer inhaled medication from a MDI.

- Spacer devices help prevent thrush from inhaled corticosteroids and can reduce cough associated with some inhalers.

- Clean at least once a week in warm, soapy water.

- Spacer devices are not to be shared.

DEVICES

Nebulizers

A nebulizer is a device that turns liquid medication into a fine mist. This fine mist can be inhaled through a face mask or mouthpiece and into the lungs. Nebulizers use natural breathing, making medication delivery easy for infants, children and the elderly. There are two types of nebulizers, jet nebulizers and ultrasound nebulizers. Check the medication information to see which nebulizer device is indicated. Please see online video course for a demonstration of the nebulizer devices and accessory parts that are required for appropriate use.

Nebulizers are covered by CMS' Durable Medical Equipment (DME) under the medical insurance component (Part B). See the Drug Formulations & DME chapter.

Metered-Dose Inhalers (MDIs)

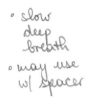

◦ slow deep breath
◦ may use w/ spacer

- A metered-dose inhaler is a handheld device that delivers a specific amount of medication in aerosol form. MDIs consist of a pressurized canister inside a plastic case, with a mouthpiece attached. MDIs use a chemical propellant (HFA) to push medication out of the inhaler. MDIs require a slow and deep breathe in from the device. All MDIs need to be shaken since they are suspensions except *QVAR* and *Alvesco*. They can be used with spacer devices.

Dry Powder Inhaler (DPIs)

◦ quick forceful breath
◦ ∅ spacer

- DPIs are devices that contain the drug in a dry powder. They do not contain propellants; therefore, they require a quick and forceful breathe in during use. Once the medication has been loaded (after "clicking" in place - see directions on the next few pages), the device needs to remain flat so the medication does not spill inside the device. These devices cannot be used with spacers (since they do not fit the back of the spacer - please see online video course for complete demonstration of all devices).

PATIENT COUNSELING

Metered Dose Inhalers

Shake x 5 sec (except QVAR, Alvesco®)
hold breath x 10 sec

Ventolin, ProAir, Proventil, Symbicort, QVAR, Flovent HFA, Alvesco, others

STEP 1	STEP 2	STEP 3
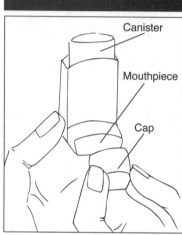	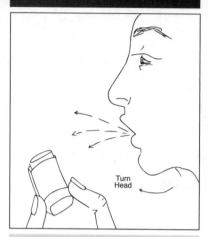	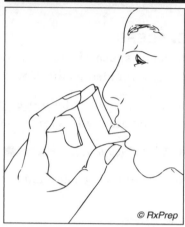

© RxPrep

Make sure the canister is fully inserted into the actuator (if it comes separately). Always use the actuator that came with the canister. Shake the inhaler well for 5 seconds immediately before each spray (except for *QVAR* or *Alvesco* which do not need to be shaken). Remove cap from the mouthpiece and check mouthpiece for foreign objects prior to use.

Breathe out fully through your mouth expelling as much air from your lungs as possible. Holding the inhaler upright (as shown in the picture), place the mouthpiece into your mouth and close your lips around it.

While breathing in slowly and deeply through your mouth, press the top of the canister all the way down with your index finger. Right after the spray comes out, take your finger off the canister. After you have inhaled all the way, take the inhaler out of your mouth and close your mouth. Hold your breath as long as possible, up to 10 seconds, then breathe normally. If another inhalation is needed, wait 1 minute and repeat Steps 1-3. Place cap back on the mouthpiece after use.

TO PRIME

prime x 3-4
again >14d

Albuterol
Spray 3-4 times (shaking between sprays) away from the face. Prime again if >14 days from last use.

prime x 4
again >7d

Flovent HFA
Spray 4 times (shaking between sprays) away from the face. Prime again if > 7 days from last use with just 1 spray.

prime x 2
again >7d

Symbicort
Spray 2 times (shaking between sprays) away from the face. Prime again if > 7 days from last use.

TO CLEAN

Albuterol
Rinse mouthpiece under warm running water (but not the metal canister) for 30 seconds to prevent medication buildup and blockage. Shake to remove excess water and let air dry. Clean weekly.

Flovent HFA
Use a clean cotton swab dampened with water to clean the small circular opening where the medicine sprays out. Gently twist the swab in a circular motion to remove the medicine buildup. Do not take the canister out of the plastic actuator. Wipe the inside of the mouthpiece with a damp tissue. Let air dry overnight.

Symbicort
Wipe the inside and outside of the mouthpiece opening with a clean, dry cloth. Do not put into water.

Dry Powder Inhalers

Advair Diskus

hold breath x 10sec

STEP 1	STEP 2	STEP 3	STEP 4	STEP 5

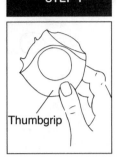 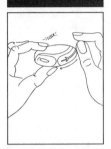 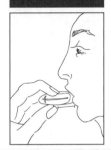 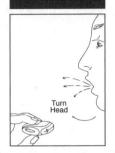 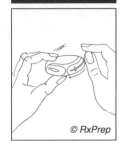

Thumbgrip

Turn Head

© RxPrep

Hold the *Diskus* in your left hand and put the thumb of your right hand in the thumb grip. Push the thumb grip away from you as far as it will go until the mouthpiece appears and the *Diskus* snaps into position.	Hold the *Diskus* in a level, flat position with the mouthpiece towards you. Slide the lever away from the mouthpiece until it clicks.	Before using, breathe out fully while holding the *Diskus* away from your mouth. Do not tilt the *Diskus*.	Put the mouthpiece to your lips. Breathe in quickly and deeply through the inhaler. Do not breathe in through your nose. Remove the *Diskus* from your mouth and hold your breath for 10 seconds, or as long as comfortable. Then, breathe out slowly.	Close the *Diskus* inhaler by putting your thumb in the thumb grip and slide as far back towards you as it will go, until the *Diskus* clicks shut. Rinse your mouth with water and spit out the water to prevent thrush.

TO CLEAN

Do not wash the *Diskus* and store in a dry place.

Pulmicort Flexhaler

STEP 1	STEP 2	STEP 3
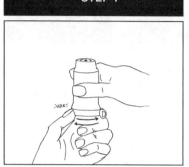	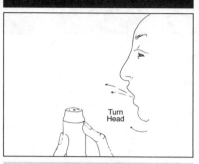	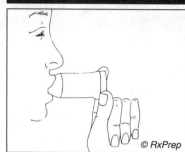

© RxPrep

Twist off the white cover. Holding the middle of the inhaler with one hand, twist the brown base fully in one direction as far as it will go with the other hand. Twist it fully back again in the other direction as far as it will go. You will hear a "click" during one of the twisting movements. The dose is now loaded. Do not shake the inhaler after it is loaded. (Of note, only one dose is loaded at a time, no matter how often you twist the brown base, but the dose counter will continue to advance).

Turn your head away from the inhaler and breathe out fully.

Place the mouthpiece in your mouth and close your lips around the mouthpiece. Breathe in deeply and forcefully through the inhaler. Remove the inhaler from your mouth and breathe out. Replace the white cover on the inhaler and twist shut. Rinse your mouth with water and spit water out to prevent thrush.

TO PRIME

Twist off the white cover. Holding the inhaler upright, twist the brown base fully in one direction as far as it will go and the fully back. You will hear a click during one of the twisting motions. Repeat twisting motion again (back and forth). The inhaler is now primed and ready to load your first dose. This inhaler does not need to be primed again (even after long periods of no use).

TO CLEAN

Wipe the mouthpiece with a dry tissue weekly. Do not use water or immerse it in water.

Foradil Aerolizer

STEP 1	STEP 2	STEP 3	STEP 4	STEP 5
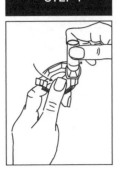	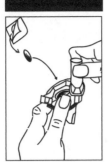	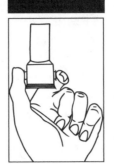	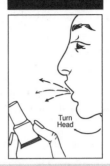	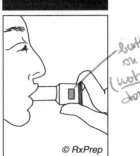

buttons on sides (not up/down)

Turn Head

© RxPrep

| Do not remove a *Foradil* capsule from the blister card until time to take the dose. Pull off the *Aerolizer* inhaler cover. Hold the base of the *Aerolizer* firmly and twist the mouthpiece in the direction of the arrow to open. | Place the capsule in the capsule-chamber in the base of the *Aerolizer*. Twist the mouthpiece back to the closed position. | Hold with mouthpiece upright and press both buttons at the same time on the base of the *Aerolizer*. Only press the buttons once. You should hear the capsule being pierced. | Exhale fully away from the device. | Tilt head back slightly. Place mouthpiece in mouth with the buttons on the side (not facing up and down) and close your lips around the mouthpiece. Breathe in quickly and deeply through the inhaler. (You should hear a whirring noise. If not, open the inhaler and loosen the capsule so it can spin freely). Hold your breath as long as you can, then breathe out. Open the *Aerolizer* and make sure capsule is empty, then discard. Close inhaler and replace the cover. |

TO CLEAN

Never wash the *Aerolizer*; keep it dry. Always use the new *Aerolizer* that comes with your refill. Always use the *Aerolizer* in a level position.

Patient Counseling for *Singulair*

- For adults and children 12 months of age and older with asthma:
- Take this medication once a day in the evening. You may take this medication with food or without food.
- Take every day for as long as your healthcare provider prescribes it, even if you have no asthma symptoms.
- If your asthma symptoms get worse, or if you need to increase the use of your rescue inhaler for asthma attacks, call your healthcare provider right away.
- Do not take this medication for the immediate relief of an asthma attack. If you have an asthma attack, you should follow the instructions your healthcare provider gave you for treating asthma attacks. Always have your rescue inhaler with you.
- The most common side effects with this medication include: stomach pain, upper respiratory infections, headache, flu and sinus infection.

- Rarely, this medication has been associated with behavior and mood changes such as aggressive behavior, hostility, anxiousness, depression and/or suicidal thoughts and actions. Please report any of the symptoms to your healthcare provider immediately.

For patients 6 years of age and older for the prevention of exercise-induced asthma:

- Take this medication at least 2 hours before exercise.
- Always have your rescue inhaler with you for asthma attacks.
- If you are taking *Singulair* daily for chronic asthma or allergies, do not take another dose to prevent exercise-induced asthma. Talk to your healthcare provider about your treatment of exercise-induced asthma.
- Do not take an additional dose of *Singulair* within 24 hours of a previous dose.
- *Singulair* 4-mg oral granules can be given:
  - directly in the mouth;
  - dissolved in 1 teaspoonful (5 mL) of cold or room temperature baby formula or breast milk;
  - mixed with 1 spoonful of one of the following soft foods at cold or room temperature:
    - applesauce, mashed carrots, rice, or ice cream. Give the child all of the mixture right away (within 15 minutes).
- Important: Never store any oral granules mixed with food, baby formula, or breast milk for use at a later time. Throw away any unused portion. Do not mix *Singulair* oral granules with any liquid drink other than baby formula or breast milk.

Suspension age 1-8

Patient Counseling for *Pulmicort Respules*

- Take one ampule out of the sealed aluminum envelope, recording the date you opened the envelope.
- Place any unused ampules back into the envelope and store upright, protected from light, at room temperature. Keep in mind, any remaining ampules should be used within two weeks.
- Gently swirl the ampule using a circular motion, making sure to not squeeze the ampule and keeping it in an upright position.
- Twist off the top of the ampule and squeeze all the liquid into the nebulizer and use right away. If using a face mask, make sure it fi ts snugly.
- Turn the compressor on and continue treatment until the mist stops, generally within 5 to 10 minutes.
- Rinse mouth with water after each dose, and wash face after treatment if a face mask was used.

- Suspension → JET nebulizer only!!
- age 1-8
- use ampules w/in 2 weeks of opening aluminum envelope
- full dose takes ~ 5-10 min (mist will stop when full dose admin)

PRACTICE CASE

Patient Profile

Patient Name Terri Price
Address 108 Morning Road
Age 22
Sex Female
Race White
Height 5'3"
Weight 130 lbs
Allergies NKDA

DIAGNOSES

Asthma - Step 3   GERD
Anemia

MEDICATIONS

Date	No.	Prescriber	Drug and Strength	Quantity	Sig	Refills
7/14	35421	May	*Maxair*	#1	1-2 puffs Q4-6H PRN	6
7/14	35422	May	*Flovent Diskus* 100 mcg/inh	#1	2 inh BID	6
7/14	35423	May	*Singulair* 10 mg	#30	1 PO daily	6
7/14	35424	May	*Aciphex* 20 mg	#30	1 PO daily	6
7/14	35425	May	*Advil* 200 mg		TID PRN headaches	
7/14	35426	May	Ferrous sulfate 325 mg		1 PO daily	

LAB/DIAGNOSTIC TESTS

Test	Reference Value	Results 4/1/12	7/4/14
Glu	65-99 mg/dL		
Na	135-146 mEq/L	135	137
K	3.5-5.3 mEq/L	4.2	4.7
Cl	98-110 mEq/L	102	105
CO_2	21-33 mmHg	26	26
BUN	7-25 mg/dL	10	12
Creatinine	0.6-1.2 mg/dL	0.6	0.7
Calcium	8.6-10.2 mg/dL		9.8
WBC	4-11 cells/mm3		10.2
RBC	3.8-5.1 mL/mm3		4.6

10/29/14 Here for refills on all her asthma medications. Using *Maxair* 4 x/week. Last refilled *Maxair* 18 days ago. Last refilled *Flovent, Singulair* and *Aciphex* 27 days ago. Requests recommendation for sleep agent. Also buying OTC ferrous sulfate, aspirin, *Dexatrim*, Sucrets lozenges and *Maalox*. Per discussion, she is a college student who lives at home with her parents.

Questions

1. TP seems to be exhibiting signs of uncontrolled asthma. Which of the following would be the best recommendation for better control?

   a. Take *Maxair* on a scheduled basis.
   b. Change the *Flovent Diskus* to 3 inhalations BID. *Δ baseline meds*
   c. Take *Singulair* 10 mg BID.
   d. Go to the emergency room as she is having an acute asthma attack.
   e. Elevate the head of the bed by 30 degrees when she sleeps.

2. TP states that she doesn't understand why her asthma is worsening. Which of the following could be a trigger for her symptoms?

   a. Living in the same place for many years
   b. NSAID use
   c. Ferrous sulfate use
   d. *Aciphex* use
   e. She could be sleeping on her stomach more

3. TP asks you if the *Sucrets* lozenges will help the sore throat. She was told by her doctor that she has signs of thrush. Which of the following recommendations would you give that would help prevent this from happening in the future? (Select **ALL** that apply.)

   a. Take the *Sucrets* lozenges because they will help with her sore throat and cure thrush.
   b. Recommend that she switch to *Symbicort* instead of *Flovent*.
   c. Recommend that she rinse her mouth after her *Flovent Diskus*, if not already doing so.
   d. Tell her to save her money; *Sucrets* will not work for treating thrush.
   e. Tell her to purchase a spacer device for the *Flovent Diskus*. *spacer ≠ Diskus*

   spacers prevent thrush from ICS & cough

4. TP comes back to your pharmacy with a prescription for *Foradil*. Which of the following statements is correct?

   a. The patient can store the medication at room temperature. *x 4 mo*
   b. This medication needs to be taken with 8 oz of water.

   c. This medication is not recommended in Step 3 asthma.
   d. This medication is taken once daily.
   e. This medication will interact with *Aciphex*.

5. Which of the following side effects is most likely to occur when using *Foradil* therapy?

   a. Neuropsychiatric behavior *LT modifiers*
   b. Palpitations
   c. Stomach upset
   d. Enuresis
   e. Depression

6. TP comes to you 2 days after a severe asthma exacerbation. She is currently taking dexamethasone 3 mg PO daily. Convert her to an equivalent dose of prednisone. Choose the correct dose of prednisone:

   a. 20 mg
   b. 12 mg
   c. 3.75 mg
   d. 2 mg
   e. 0.75 mg

   $$\frac{dex}{pred} \quad \frac{0.75mg}{5mg} = \frac{3 mg}{x\ mg}$$

   $$\Rightarrow x = 20mg$$

7. TP is placed on theophylline therapy for treatment of her asthma. Which of the following can decrease theophylline levels? (Select **ALL** that apply.)

   a. Ciprofloxacin
   b. Carbamazepine
   c. Erythromycin
   d. Cirrhosis
   e. High protein diet *& charbroiled foods*

Questions 8-11 do not relate to the above case.

8. Omalizumab has a black box warning for:

   a. Increased risk of MI
   b. Stevens-Johnson syndrome
   c. Thrombocytopenia
   d. GI ulcers
   e. Anaphylaxis

9. A patient with asthma has been prescribed *Advair Diskus*. Which of the following statements is correct?

    salmeterol + fluticasone

   a. *Advair Diskus* contains fluticasone, a long-acting beta$_2$ agonist.

   b. *Advair Diskus* contains flunisolide, an inhaled corticosteroid.

   c. *Advair Diskus* is usually dosed 2 inhalations once daily.   MDI   1 inhalation BID

   d. *Advair Diskus* treats both airway constriction and inflammation.

   e. *Advair Diskus* contains formoterol, an anticholinergic agent.   LABA

   * formoterol
     + mometasone (Dulera®)
     + budesonide (Symbicort®)

10. Carla is a 10 year old girl with asthma. The physician wants to give her montelukast, but is not sure of the correct dose. Choose the correct dose of montelukast for a 10-year old child:

   1-5 y/o ⇒ 4 mg
   6-14 y/o ⇒ 5 mg

   a. A 5 mg chewable tablet taken BID

   b. A 5 mg chewable tablet taken once daily

   c. A 10 mg chewable tablet taken once daily

   d. A 10 mg chewable tablet taken BID

   e. A 4 mg packet of granules mixed with milk   → mix w/any liquids other than baby formula/breast milk

11. The therapeutic range for theophylline is:

   a. 10-20 mcg/mL

   b. 5-10 mcg/mL   ALWAYS dosed based on IBW

   c. 5-15 mg/mL

   d. 8-12 mg/mL

   e. 5-15 mcg/mL

Answers

1-b, 2-b, 3-c,d, 4-a, 5-b, 6-a, 7-b,e, 8-e, 9-d, 10-b, 11-e

1. betameth   0.6 mg
   dexameth   0.75 mg

2. methylpred } 4 mg
   triamcinol }

3. prednisone   } 5 mg
   prednisolone }

4. hydrocort   20 mg

5. cortisone   25 mg

46

CHRONIC OBSTRUCTIVE PULMONARY DISEASE (COPD)

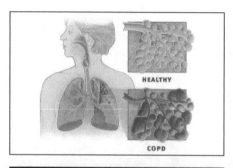

GUIDELINE

Global Strategy for the Diagnosis, Management and Prevention of COPD, Global Initiative for Chronic Obstructive Lung Disease (GOLD) 2013 update. http://www.goldcopd.org/uploads/users/files/GOLD_Report_2013_Feb20.pdf (accessed 2014 Oct. 10).

BACKGROUND

Chronic obstructive pulmonary disease (COPD) is a common preventable and somewhat treatable disease characterized by persistent airflow limitation that is usually progressive and associated with an enhanced chronic inflammatory response in the airways to noxious particles or gases. In contrast to asthma, the limitation of airflow is not fully reversible and generally worsens over time. COPD is the 4th leading cause of death in the world and the incidence is increasing, primarily due to tobacco use and secondhand smoke.

COPD is caused by inhalation of cigarette smoke and other noxious particles or gas (such as from biomass fuels) which triggers an abnormal inflammatory response in the lungs. This chronic inflammatory response can lead to lung tissue destruction (resulting in emphysema), and alter normal repair and defense mechanisms (resulting in small airway narrowing and fibrosis). These changes lead to air trapping and worsening airflow limitation, and to the breathlessness and other classic symptoms of COPD.

A clinical diagnosis of COPD should be considered in any patient who has dyspnea (shortness of breath, which is chronic and progressive), chronic cough or sputum production, and a history of exposure to risk factors for the disease, especially cigarette smoke. Spirometry (testing to measure lung function) is required to make the diagnosis; the presence of a post-bronchodilator $FEV_1/FVC < 0.70$ confirms the presence of persistent airflow limitation and thus of COPD. Smoking cessation is the only management strategy proven to slow progression of disease. Other important management strategies include vaccinations, pulmonary rehabilitation programs, and drug therapy (often using inhalers). Some patients go on to require long-term oxygen therapy, either given in the hospital for acute exacerbations, or used chronically outpatient with the use of portable oxygen systems. In rare cases, lung transplantation is needed.

RISK FACTORS

The major risk factors for developing COPD include <u>smoking or smoke exposure</u>, alpha-1 antitrypsin deficiency, occupational dusts and chemicals (chemical agents and fumes), and indoor and outdoor air pollution.

ASSESSMENT OF COPD

The goals of COPD assessment are to determine the severity of disease, its impact on the patient's health status and the risk of future events (exacerbations, hospital admissions, death) in order to guide therapy. Assess the following aspects of the disease separately:

- Symptoms

- Degree of airflow limitation (using spirometry)

- Risk of exacerbations

- Comorbidities

Symptoms

Symptoms can be assessed using validated questionnaires such as the COPD Assessment Test (CAT) or the Modified British Medical Research Council (mMRC) breathlessness scale.

Degree of Airflow Limitation

Degree of airflow limitation is assessed using spirometry. Please see table below for classification of severity.

Classification of Severity of Airflow Limitation in COPD (Based on Post-Bronchodilator FEV_1)

CLASSIFICATION	SEVERITY	AIRFLOW
In patients with $FEV_1/FVC < 0.70$		
GOLD 1	Mild	$FEV_1 \geq 80\%$ predicted
GOLD 2	Moderate	$50\% \leq FEV_1 < 80\%$ predicted
GOLD 3	Severe	$30\% \leq FEV_1 < 50\%$ predicted
GOLD 4	Very Severe	$FEV_1 < 30\%$ predicted

Risk of Exacerbations

An exacerbation of COPD is defined as an acute event characterized by a worsening of the patient's respiratory symptoms that is beyond normal day-to-day variations and leads to a change in medication. The best predictor of having frequent exacerbations (2 or more per year) is a history of previous treated events. The risk of exacerbations will also increase as airflow limitation worsens.

Comorbidities

Comorbid conditions such as cardiovascular diseases, osteoporosis, depression and anxiety, skeletal muscle dysfunction, metabolic syndrome, and lung cancer may influence mortality and hospitalizations, and should be monitored routinely and treated appropriately.

The combined assessment of COPD takes into account the symptoms, airflow limitation and exacerbation risk of the patient (see table below).

Combined Assessment of COPD

When assessing risk, choose the <u>highest risk</u> according to GOLD grade or exacerbation history.

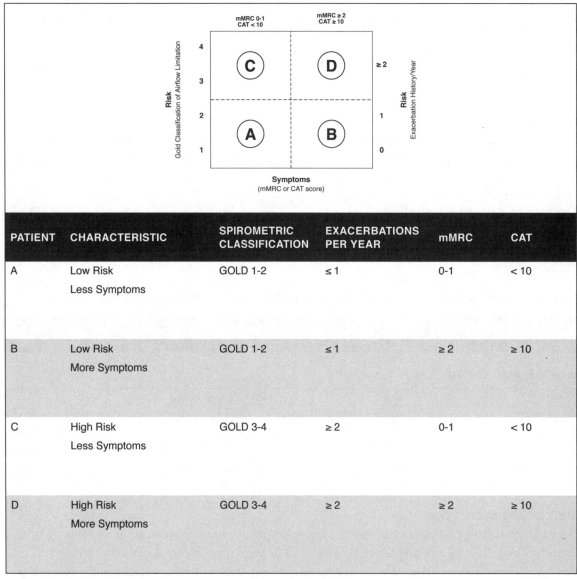

PATIENT	CHARACTERISTIC	SPIROMETRIC CLASSIFICATION	EXACERBATIONS PER YEAR	mMRC	CAT
A	Low Risk Less Symptoms	GOLD 1-2	≤ 1	0-1	< 10
B	Low Risk More Symptoms	GOLD 1-2	≤ 1	≥ 2	≥ 10
C	High Risk Less Symptoms	GOLD 3-4	≥ 2	0-1	< 10
D	High Risk More Symptoms	GOLD 3-4	≥ 2	≥ 2	≥ 10

CAT: COPD Assessment Test, mMRC: Modified British Medical Research Council

Pharmacologic Therapy for Stable COPD*

PATIENT GROUP	RECOMMENDED FIRST CHOICE	ALTERNATIVE CHOICE	OTHER POSSIBLE TREATMENTS**
A	SA anticholinergic PRN or SABA PRN	LA anticholinergic or LABA or SABA and SA anticholinergic	Theophylline
B	LA anticholinergic or LABA	LA anticholinergic and LABA	SABA and/or SA anticholinergic Theophylline
C	ICS + LABA or LA anticholinergic	LA anticholinergic and LABA or LA anticholinergic and PDE-4 inhibitor or LABA and PDE-4 inhibitor	SABA and/or SA anticholinergic Theophylline
D	ICS + LABA and/or LA anticholinergic	ICS + LABA and LA anticholinergic or ICS + LABA and PDE-4 inhibitor or LA anticholinergic and LABA or LA anticholinergic and PDE-4 inhibitor	Carbocysteine SABA and/or SA anticholinergic Theophylline

* Medications in each box are mentioned in alphabetical order and therefore not necessarily in order of preference

** Medications in this column can be used alone or in combination with other options in the First and Alternative Choice columns

SA: short-acting, LA: long-acting, SABA: short-acting beta-2 agonist, LABA: long-acting beta-2 agonist, ICS: inhaled corticosteroid, PDE-4: phosphodiesterase-4, PRN: when necessary

DRUG TREATMENT

No medication used in COPD has been shown to modify the long-term decline in lung function that is the hallmark of COPD. Therefore, pharmacotherapy is used to decrease symptoms and/or complications. Carbocysteine is a mucolytic that has shown a small benefit in patients with viscous sputum. Bronchodilators (beta-2 agonists, anticholinergics) are used as-needed or on a regular basis, depending on symptom severity. If used on a regular basis, long-acting inhaled bronchodilators are more effective and more convenient than treatment with short-acting inhaled bronchodilators. Combining bronchodilators of different pharmacologic classes may improve efficacy and decrease the risk of side effects compared to increasing the dose of a single agent. Long-term monotherapy with oral or inhaled corticosteroids is not recommended in COPD. PDE-4 inhibitors reduce inflammation by inhibiting the breakdown of intracellular cyclic AMP and should always be used in combination with at least one long-acting bronchodilator. Treatment with theophylline is not recommended unless other long-term treatment bronchodilators are unavailable or unaffordable.

<u>Influenza</u> (annually) and <u>pneumococcal</u> (PPSV23, *Pneumovax)* (x 1, repeat when 65 years or older, and if received vaccine more than 5 years ago) should be given to patients with COPD, unless contraindications exist. Vaccines are used to prevent infections and reduce the risk of acute exacerbations.

If patients have severe hereditary alpha-1 antitrypsin deficiency, they may be placed on an alpha-1 proteinase inhibitor *(Prolastin, Aralast, or Zemaira)* for chronic augmentation therapy. These agents are very expensive, given as weekly IV infusions and are associated with many side effects, including anaphylaxis.

For treatment of acute COPD exacerbations, see the Infectious Diseases chapter. Outside of antibiotics, an inhaled anticholinergic bronchodilator plus oral steroids (tapered over 2 weeks) are effective treatments. The use of azithromycin 250 mg/day reduces the risk of acute exacerbations due to its anti-inflammatory and immunomodulatory properties; however, treatment is not recommended because of an unfavorable balance between benefits and side effects (e.g., decreased hearing).

PHARMACOLOGIC AGENTS

DRUG	DOSING	SAFETY/SIDE EFFECTS/MONITORING

Anticholinergics – block the action of acetylcholine and ↓ cyclic guanosine monophosphate (cGMP) at parasympathetic sites in bronchial smooth muscle causing bronchodilation.

DRUG	DOSING	SAFETY/SIDE EFFECTS/MONITORING
Short-acting anticholinergics		**WARNINGS** Use with caution in patients with myasthenia gravis, narrow-angle glaucoma, urinary retention, benign prostatic hyperplasia, or bladder neck obstruction
Ipratropium bromide *(Atrovent HFA)*	*Atrovent* MDI: 2 inhalations QID	
	Nebulizer: 0.5 mg TID-QID	**SIDE EFFECTS** <u>Dry mouth</u> (much more common with tiotropium), upper respiratory tract infections, nasopharyngitis, sinusitis, cough and bitter taste
+ albuterol *(Combivent Respimat*, DuoNeb)	*Combivent Respimat* MDI: 1 inhalation QID Nebulizer: 0.5/2.5 mg (3 mL) QID	
		MONITORING Signs and symptoms at each visit, smoking status, COPD questionnaires, annual spirometry
Long-acting anticholinergics		
Aclidinium *(Tudorza Pressair)*	DPI: 1 inhalation BID	**NOTES** <u>Avoid spraying in the eyes</u> <u>Do NOT swallow capsules of tiotropium</u> *Combivent Respimat* – Discard 3 months from when cartridge is inserted into device.
Tiotropium *(Spiriva HandiHaler)*	DPI: 1 capsule (18 mcg) inhaled daily via the *HandiHaler* device (requires 2 puffs)	*Tudorza* – Discard product 45 days after opening pouch, when device locks out, or when dose indicator displays "0", whichever comes first.
Umeclidinium *(Incruse Ellipta)*	DPI: 1 inhalation (62.5 mg) daily	

Pharmacologic Agents Continued

DRUG	DOSING	SAFETY/SIDE EFFECTS/MONITORING

Beta-2 agonists – bind to beta-2 receptors causing relaxation of bronchial smooth muscle, resulting in bronchodilation – inhaled route is the preferred route of administration. For short-acting beta-2 agonists, see Asthma chapter.

DRUG	DOSING	SAFETY/SIDE EFFECTS/MONITORING
Long-acting Beta-2-agonists		**BOXED WARNING** Long-acting beta-2 agonists (LABAs) increase the risk of asthma-related deaths and should only be used in asthma patients who are currently receiving but are not adequately controlled on a long-term asthma control medication (inhaled corticosteroid)
Salmeterol *(Serevent Diskus)*	DPI: 1 inhalation BID	
+ fluticasone *(Advair Diskus)* ***Advair Diskus:*** 100, 250, 500 mcg fluticasone + 50 mcg salmeterol/inh	DPI: 1 inhalation BID	**CONTRAINDICATIONS** Status asthmaticus, acute episodes of asthma or COPD, monotherapy in treatment of asthma
Formoterol *(Foradil Aerolizer, Perforomist* – nebulizer*)* **+ budesonide** *(Symbicort)* ***Symbicort:*** 80, 160 mcg budesonide + 4.5 mcg formeterol/inh	DPI: 12 mcg capsule via *Aerolizer* BID Nebulizer: 20 mcg BID *Symbicort* MDI: 2 inhalations BID	**SIDE EFFECTS** Tachycardia, tremor, shakiness, lightheadedness, cough, palpitations, hypokalemia and hyperglycemia **MONITORING** Signs and symptoms at each visit, smoking status, COPD questionnaires, annual spirometry
Arformoterol *(Brovana)*	Nebulizer: 15 mcg BID	**NOTES** Bronchodilators are used on a PRN or scheduled basis to reduce symptoms. Long-acting inhaled bronchodilators are more effective and convenient. Combination therapy with inhaled steroids can ↑ the risk of pneumonia, however, the combination showed a ↓ in exacerbations and improvement in lung function when compared to the individual components. Arformoterol contains R-isomer of formoterol.
Indacaterol *(Arcapta Neohaler)*	DPI: 75 mcg capsule via *Neohaler* device daily	Do NOT swallow capsules of indacaterol or formoterol. All steroid-containing inhalers – rinse mouth with water after use and spit. *Advair* – discard device 1 month after removal from pouch.
Vilanterol/fluticasone *(Breo Ellipta)* 25 mcg vilanterol + 100 mcg fluticasone/inh	DPI: 1 inhalation daily	*Symbicort* – discard inhaler after the labeled number of inhalations have been used or within 3 months after removal from foil pouch. *Serevent Diskus/Breo Ellipta* – discard device 6 weeks after removal from the foil tray or when the dose counter reads "0" (whichever comes first).
Olodaterol *(Striverdi Respimat)*	MDI: 2 inhalations daily	*Striverdi Respimat* - discard device 3 months from the date when the cartridge is inserted into the inhaler or when the inhaler locks (which indicates no doses are left).

Pharmacologic Agents Continued

DRUG	DOSING	SAFETY/SIDE EFFECTS/MONITORING

Phosphodiesterase 4 inhibitor – PDE-4 inhibitor that ↑ cAMP levels, leading to a reduction in lung inflammation.

Roflumilast *(Daliresp)*	Tablet: 500 mcg PO daily	**CONTRAINDICATIONS** Moderate to severe liver impairment **SIDE EFFECTS** Diarrhea, weight loss, nausea, ↓ appetite, insomnia, depression and psychiatric events including suicidality **MONITORING** Signs and symptoms at each visit, LFTs, smoking status, COPD questionnaires, spirometry yearly **NOTES** Use only in severe COPD due to modest benefit

See asthma section for details on theophylline and inhaled corticosteroids

Drug Interactions with Roflumilast

Roflumilast is a substrate of 3A4 (major) and 1A2 (minor). Use with strong enzyme inducers (carbamazepine, phenobarbital, phenytoin, rifampin) is not recommended. Use with 3A4 inhibitors or dual 3A4 and 1A2 inhibitors (erythromycin, ketoconazole, fluvoxamine, cimetidine) will ↑ roflumilast levels.

PATIENT COUNSELING

Metered Dose Inhalers

Atrovent HFA

STEP 1	STEP 2	STEP 3

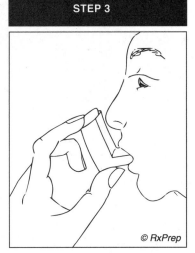

© RxPrep

Insert the metal canister into the actuator. The *Atrovent HFA* plastic actuator should only be used with the *Atrovent HFA* canister. Remove the protective dust cap from the mouthpiece and check mouthpiece for foreign objects prior to use.

Breathe out deeply through your mouth. Holding the inhaler upright (as shown in the picture), place the mouthpiece into your mouth and close your lips around it. Keep your eyes closed so that no medicine will be sprayed into your eyes.

While breathing in slowly and deeply through your mouth, press the top of the canister all the way down with your index finger. Hold your breath as long as possible, up to 10 seconds, then breathe normally. If another inhalation is needed, wait at least 15 seconds and repeat Steps 1-3. Place cap back on the mouthpiece after use.

TO PRIME
Spray 2 times away from the face. Prime again if > 3 days from last use.

TO CLEAN
Rinse mouthpiece under warm running water (but not the metal canister) for 30 seconds to prevent medication buildup and blockage. Shake to remove excess water and let air dry. Clean at least weekly.

Combivent Respimat

STEP 1	STEP 2	STEP 3
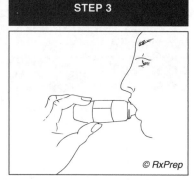 © RxPrep		

STEP 1: Hold the inhaler upright with the orange cap closed to avoid accidentally releasing a dose. Turn the clear base in the direction of the white arrows on the label until it clicks (half a turn).

STEP 2: Flip the orange cap until it snaps fully open. Turn head away from the inhaler and breath out slowly and fully.

STEP 3: Close lips around the end of the mouthpiece without covering the air vents. While taking a slow, deep breath through your mouth, press the dose release button and continue to breathe in slowly. Hold your breath for 10 seconds or as long as comfortable. Close the orange cap when finished.

Tips

ASSEMBLE DEVICE FOR FIRST TIME USE

With the orange cap closed, press the safety catch while pulling off the clear base. Do not touch the piercing element located inside the bottom of the clear base. Write the discard by date on the label of the inhaler (which is 3 months from the date the cartridge is inserted). Remove the cartridge from packet and place narrow end into the inhaler. The base of the cartridge will not sit flush with the inhaler; about 1/8 of an inch will stick out when the cartridge is correctly inserted.

PRIMING

Hold the inhaler upright with the orange cap closed, to avoid accidentally releasing a dose. Turn the clear base in the direction of the white arrows on the label until it clicks (half a turn). Flip the orange cap until it snaps fully open. Point the inhaler toward the ground away from your face. Press the dose release button. Close orange cap. Repeat these steps over again until a spray is visible. Once the spray is visible, repeat the steps 3 more times to make sure inhaler is prepared for use. If inhaler is not used for > 3 days, spray 1 puff toward the ground to prepare the inhaler. If inhaler has not been used for > 21 days, follow priming for initial use instructions.

CLEANING

Clean the mouthpiece, including the metal part inside the mouthpiece, with a damp cloth or tissue weekly.

Dry Powder Inhalers

Spiriva HandiHaler

STEP 1	STEP 2	STEP 3	STEP 4	STEP 5
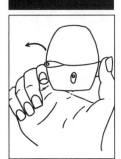	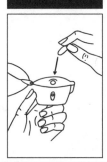	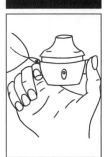	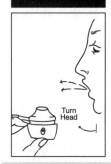	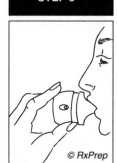
Open the Handi-Haler device by pressing on the green button and lifting the cap upwards. Open the mouthpiece by pulling up and away from the base.	Insert the *SPIRIVA* capsule in the chamber and close the mouthpiece firmly against the gray base until you hear a click.	Press the green piercing button once until it is flat (flush) against the base, then release. Do not shake the device.	Turn head away from the inhaler and breathe out fully.	Raise your *Handihaler* to your mouth in a horizontal position and close your lips around the mouthpiece. Breathe in deeply and fully. You should hear or feel the *SPIRIVA* capsule vibrate (rattle). Remove inhaler from your mouth and hold your breath for a few seconds. Breathe normally. Breathe out again and breathe in deeply and fully through the inhaler (you must inhale twice from each capsule). Discard capsule after 2 inhalations. Close the lid of the device.

© RxPrep

Tips

CLEANING

Clean inhaler as needed. Rinse inhaler with warm water, pressing the green button a few times so the chamber and piercing needle are under the running water. Make sure any powder build up is removed. Air dry. It takes 24 hours to air dry the *Handihaler* device after it is cleaned.

Turdorza

STEP 1	STEP 2	STEP 3	STEP 4

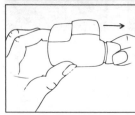 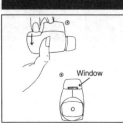 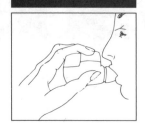 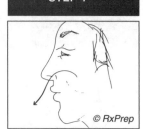

Remove the protective cap by lightly squeezing the arrows marked on each side of the cap and pulling outwards. Check the mouthpiece for foreign objects.	A. Before putting into mouth, press the back (green) button all the way down and release. B. Check the control window to make sure the dose is ready for inhalation; the window will change from red to green. Breathe out completely, away from the inhaler.	Put your lips tightly around the mouthpiece. Breathe in quickly and deeply through your mouth. Breathe in until you hear a "click" sound and keep breathing in to get the full dose. Note. Do not hold down the back (green) button while breathing in.	Remove the inhaler from your mouth and hold your breath for as long as is comfortable. Then breathe out slowly through your nose. Place the protective cap on the inhaler. Note. Check that the control window has turned to red which indicates the full dose has been inhaled correctly.

Tips

CLEANING

You do not need to clean your inhaler. If you wish to clean it, wipe the outside of the mouthpiece with a dry tissue or paper towel. Do not use water.

Breo Ellipta

STEP 1	STEP 2	STEP 3

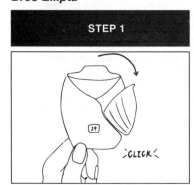 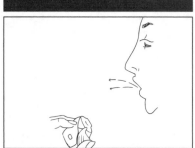 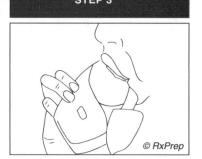

Open the cover of the inhaler by sliding the cover down to expose the mouthpiece. You should hear a "click." The counter will count down by 1 number, indicating that the inhaler is ready to use.	While holding the inhaler away from your mouth, breathe out fully. Do not breathe out into the mouthpiece.	Put the mouthpiece between your lips, and close your lips firmly around it. Take one long, steady, deep breath in through your mouth. Do not block the air vent with your fingers. Remove inhaler from mouth and hold your breath for 3-4 seconds, or as long as comfortable. Breathe out slowly and gently. Close the inhaler. Rinse your mouth.

Tips

CLEANING

You can clean the mouthpiece if needed, using a dry tissue, before you close the cover. Routine cleaning is not required.

Arcapta Neohaler

STEP 1	STEP 2	STEP 3	STEP 4
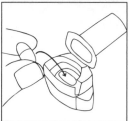	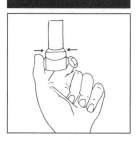		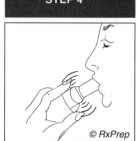
Pull off cap.	Hold the base of the inhaler firmly and tilt the mouthpiece to open the inhaler. Place the capsule into the capsule chamber. Close the inhaler fully, until you hear a "click" sound.	Hold the inhaler upright. Press both buttons fully one time. You should hear a "click" as the capsule is being pierced. Release the buttons fully. The inhaler is now ready to be used. Before using, breathe out fully, away from the inhaler.	Place the mouthpiece in your mouth and close your lips around the mouthpiece. Hold the inhaler with the buttons to the side (not up and down). Breathe in rapidly and deeply (you should hear a whirring sound when breathing in). Hold your breathe as long as comfortable and remove inhaler from mouth. Then, breath out. The capsule should be empty of all powder. If it is not, inhale again. Remove capsule and replace the cap.

© RxPrep

Tips

CLEANING

Cleaning the device is not necessary, however, if desired, a clean, dry, lint-free cloth or a clean, dry soft brush may be used to wipe the inhaler between uses.

47

SMOKING CESSATION

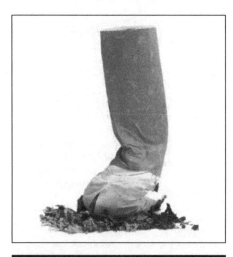

GUIDELINES/REFERENCES

Agency for Healthcare Research and Quality. Treating tobacco use and dependence: 2008 update. http://www.ahrq.gov/professionals/clinicians-providers/guidelines-recommendations/tobacco/clinicians/update/index.html (accessed 2014 Nov 17).

FDA Drug Safety Communication: Safety review update of Chantix (varenicline) and risk of neuropsychiatric adverse events, Available at: http://www.fda.gov/Drugs/DrugSafety/ucm276737.htm (accessed 2014 Nov 17).

The American College of Obstetricians and Gynecologists – Committee Opinion: Smoking Cessation During Pregnancy. Number 471, November 2010 (Reaffirmed 2013).

BACKGROUND

Tobacco dependence is a chronic disease that often requires repeated intervention and multiple attempts to quit. Effective treatments exist that can significantly increase rates of long-term abstinence. It is essential that clinicians and healthcare delivery systems consistently identify and document tobacco use status and treat every tobacco user seen in a healthcare setting.

Counseling and medication are more effective when used together than either modality used alone. Two counseling components that are especially effective are practical counseling (problem-solving/skills training) and social support delivered as part of treatment. There is a strong correlation between counseling intensity and quitting success (counseling sessions should be > 10 minutes in length and number of sessions should be ≥ 4).

Smoking accounts for more than 435,000 deaths per year in the U.S. It is a known cause of multiple cancers, heart disease, stroke, complications of pregnancy, COPD, and many other diseases. Still, roughly 20% of adult Americans smoke representing ~45 million current adult smokers.

Numerous effective medications (5 nicotine and 2 non-nicotine) are available for treating tobacco dependence and clinicians should encourage their use by all patients attempting to quit smoking except when medically contraindicated. Use a combination of two nicotine products (use extreme caution if any underlying cardiovascular condition due to additive side effects) or combination with bupropion, if a single agent is not enough (e.g., patch + gum or nasal spray or inhaler or bupropion SR + patch). Bupropion plus a nicotine product is sometimes used initially; however, there is less evidence of benefit with this combination versus using two nicotine agents. There is benefit (and increased side effects) with the use of bupropion and two nicotine products. <u>Do not use varenicline with nicotine products due to increased side effects</u>.

Recently, electronic cigarettes (e-cigarettes) have gained popularity as an alternative to traditional cigarettes and as a potential smoking cessation aid. E-cigarettes use an electronic delivery system to aerosolize nicotine without the traditional carcinogenic toxins present in cigarettes. They reduce the user's desire to smoke traditional cigarettes and thus, are sometimes recommended to help smoking cessation. The FDA has not approved the use of any e-cigarettes thus far, citing potential safety concerns (e.g., potential for toxic ingestion in children, rising use in adolescents).

THE "5 A'S" MODEL FOR TREATING TOBACCO USE AND DEPENDENCE

Ask about tobacco use
Identify and document tobacco use status for every patient at every visit.

Advise to quit
In a clear, strong, and personalized manner, urge every tobacco user to quit.

Assess
For current tobacco user, is the tobacco user willing to make a quit attempt at this time?

For the ex-tobacco user, how recently did you quit and are there any challenges to remaining abstinent?

Assist
For the patient willing to make a quit attempt, offer medication and provide or refer for counseling or additional behavioral treatment to help the patient quit.

For patients unwilling to quit at this time, provide motivational interventions designed to increase future quit attempts.

For the recent quitter and any with remaining challenges, provide relapse prevention.

Arrange
All those receiving the previous A's should receive follow up.

Smoking causes an induction of some isoforms of the CYP450 system. Therefore, <u>smokers who quit can experience side effects from supratherapeutic drug levels of caffeine, estrogens (oral), theophylline, fluvoxamine, olanzapine and clozapine</u>. High levels of clozapine have increased risk for agranulocytosis. Ensure that smokers get <u>required vaccines</u>, including pneumococcal *(Pneumovax 23)* and an annual (fall) influenza vaccine. If no local programs are available smokers can get free assistance by calling the U.S. national quitline network at 1-800-QUIT-NOW (1-800-784-8669). The help line has services available in multiple languages.

Smoking in Pregnancy

Smoking in pregnancy can cause adverse outcomes for the child, including spontaneous abortion, low birth weight and sudden infant death. If women smoke 5 or less cigarettes daily (occasional, "nervous" type smokers), they should be encouraged to quit with behavioral support. If they smoke more than 5 cigarettes daily, more intensive therapy along with bupropion (Pregnancy Category C) may be used, although evidence to support its use in pregnant patients is lacking. Nicotine products may also be considered; however, the efficacy is not as high as it is in non-pregnant patients. All nicotine products are Pregnancy Category D, except the gum and lozenge are Pregnancy Category C.

Vaccinations in Smokers

Smokers 19-64 years old should receive the pneumococcal polysaccharide vaccine (PPSV23, Pneumovax). If 65 and older and it has been more than 5 years since your last vaccination, a 2nd dose is needed. Everyone should receive the influenza vaccine in the fall, including people who smoke. The ACIP has no recommendation on vaccine use with e-cigarettes. See Immunizations chapter for further discussion.

Nicotine Replacement Therapy (NRT)

DRUG	DOSING	SAFETY/SIDE EFFECTS/MONITORING
Nicotine polacrilex gum (Nicorette, Nicorette Starter Kit, Nicorelief, Thrive) OTC	If < 25 cigs/day, use 2 mg gum If ≥ 25 cigs/day, use 4 mg gum 1 gum Q1-2H x 6 wks, then 1 gum Q2-4H x 3 wks, then 1 gum Q4-8H hrs x 3 wks; max 24 pieces/day Use up to 12 weeks	**CONTRAINDICATIONS** Recent MI (within 2 weeks), life-threating arrhythmia, severe or worsening angina, pregnancy **SIDE EFFECTS** Headache, dizziness, nervousness, insomnia, dyspepsia (all products)
Nicotine Inhaler (Nicotrol Inhaler) Rx	6-16 cartridges daily; taper frequency of use over 6-12 weeks Use up to 6 months	Local irritation in the mouth and throat, coughing, rhinitis (inhaler) Nasal irritation, transient changes in taste and smell (nasal spray) Application site reaction, local erythema (patch) **NOTES** Nicotine patch has highest adherence rate; however, may need additional product for acute cravings
Nicotine nasal spray (Nicotrol NS) Rx	1 dose = 2 sprays (1 spray in each nostril), give 1-2 doses per hour, ↑ PRN for symptom relief; max: 5 doses/hr or 40 doses/day Use 3-6 months	Patients must show identification for proof of age prior to purchase of nicotine products since the FDA prohibits sale of nicotine products to individuals younger than 18 years of age (REMS).
Nicotine patch (NicoDerm CQ, Habitrol) OTC	7 mg/day, 14 mg/day, 21 mg/day; apply upon waking on quit date If > 10 cigs/day, use 21 mg x 6 wk, then 14 mg x 2 wk, then 7 mg x 2 wk If ≤ 10 cigs/day, use 14 mg x 6 wk, then 7 mg x 2 wk	Gum has been shown to reduce or delay weight gain – review gum counseling at end of this section. Inhaler has a hand to mouth use; mimics smoking action, providing a coping mechanism Nasal spray has the fastest delivery system; useful for rapid relief of withdrawal; highest dependence potential among NRTs. Avoid in severe reactive airway disease
Nicotine Lozenge (Nicorette, Nicorette Mini) OTC	1st cigarette smoked > 30 min after waking up: use 2 mg lozenge 1st cigarette smoked ≤ 30 min of waking up: use 4 mg lozenge Do not exceed 20 lozenges/day Minimum of 9 lozenges/day 1 lozenge Q1-2H x 6 wks, then 1 lozenge Q2-4H x 3 wks, then 1 lozenge Q4-8H x 3 wks.	Patch is typically worn for 24 hours; however, can remove at bedtime to avoid insomnia Pregnancy Category C (gum, lozenge)/D (all others)

Oral Prescription Agents

Bupropion blocks neural re-uptake of dopamine and/or norepinephrine and blocks nicotinic acetylcholinergic receptors. Varenicline is a partial neuronal α4-β2 nicotinic receptor agonist. It also stimulates dopamine activity, resulting in reduced withdrawal symptoms, including cravings.

DRUG	DOSING	SAFETY/SIDE EFFECTS/MONITORING
BuPROPion SR *(Zyban, Buproban)*	150 mg QAM for 3 days, then 150 mg BID. Start 1 week before quit date If no significant progress by week 7, consider discontinuation.	**BOXED WARNINGS (2)** Serious neuropsychiatric events, including depression, suicidal thoughts and suicide have been reported in patients taking bupropion; not approved for use in children; not approved for bipolar; ↑ risk of suicidal thinking and behavior in young adults (18-24 years) with depression or other psychiatric disorders **CONTRAINDICATIONS** Seizure disorder; history of anorexia/bulimia; patients undergoing abrupt discontinuation of ethanol or sedatives, including benzodiazepines; use of MAO inhibitors or MAO inhibitors intended to treat psychiatric disorders (concurrently or within 14 days of discontinuing either bupropion or the MAO inhibitor); initiation of bupropion in a patient receiving linezolid or intravenous methylene blue; patients receiving other dosage forms of bupropion **WARNINGS** Use with caution in patients with underlying psychiatric disorders and while driving or operating machinery, traffic accidents have occurred. Avoid use in pilots, air traffic controllers, commercial truckers, bus drivers. **SIDE EFFECTS** Dry mouth, insomnia, headache/migraine, weight loss, nausea/vomiting, constipation, and tremors/seizures (dose-related), possible blood pressure changes (more hypertension than hypotension – monitor) No effects on 5HT and therefore no sexual dysfunction **NOTES** Can be used in combination with NRT Delays weight gain, can be used with CVD risk Do not exceed 450 mg/day due to seizure risk Pregnancy Category C (but used in pregnancy) MedGuide required

Oral Prescription Agents Continued

DRUG	DOSING	SAFETY/SIDE EFFECTS/MONITORING
Varenicline *(Chantix)*	Start one week before the quit date Days 1-3: 0.5 mg daily Days 4-7: 0.5 mg BID Days 8 (quit date) and beyond: 1 mg BID	**BOXED WARNING** Serious neuropsychiatric events including depression, suicidal ideation, suicide attempt and completed suicide have been reported in patients taking varenicline. Stop taking this medication if patients become hostile, agitated, depressed, or have changes in behavior or thinking that are not typical for the patient. **WARNINGS** Angioedema, hypersensitivity rxns, seizures, ↑ intoxicating effect of alcohol, and serious skin reactions have occurred. Use with caution in patients with underlying psychiatric disorders and while driving or operating machinery, traffic accidents have occurred. Avoid use in pilots, air traffic controllers, commercial truckers, bus drivers. **SIDE EFFECTS** Nausea (~30% and dose dependent), insomnia, abnormal dreams, headache, constipation, flatulence, vomiting **NOTES** To reduce nausea, can use lower dosage and/or take with food and a full glass of water. To reduce insomnia, take 2nd dose at dinner rather than bedtime. CrCl < 30 mL/min: dose 0.5 mg daily If patient has cardiovascular disease they can use if stable but need to stop smoking as varenicline may exacerbate CVD, but at this point it is thought that risk may be worth the benefit. Pregnancy Category C MedGuide required

Nicotine Replacement Counseling

Counseling with the Nicotine Gum

- Gum should be chewed slowly until a "peppery" or "flavored" taste emerges, then "parked" between cheek and gum to facilitate nicotine absorption through the oral mucosa. Gum should be slowly and intermittently chewed and parked for about 30 minutes or until the taste or tingle goes away.

- Acidic beverages (e.g., coffee, juices, soft drinks) interfere with the buccal absorption of nicotine, so eating and drinking anything except water should be avoided for 15 minutes before or during chewing.

- Patients often do not use enough gum to obtain optimal clinical effects. Instruct to use at least 1 piece Q1-2 hours.

Counseling with Inhaler

- Frequent, continuous puffing for 20 minutes is advised with each cartridge. Once a cartridge is opened, it is only good for one day. Peak effect is achieved within 15 minutes. After your dose is established, it is generally maintained for 3 months and then gradually tapered during the following 3 months. Clean mouthpiece with soap and water regularly. Delivery of nicotine from the inhaler declines significantly below 40°F. In cold weather, the inhaler and cartridge should be kept in an inside pocket or other warm area.

ADDITIONAL RESOURCES FOR YOU AND YOUR PATIENTS ON SMOKING CESSATION

http://www.surgeongeneral.gov/initiatives/tobacco/index.html

http://www.cdc.gov/tobacco/campaign/tips/

http://smokefree.gov

http://www.cancer.org/healthy/stayawayfromtobacco/guidetoquittingsmoking/index

http://www.heart.org/HEARTORG/GettingHealthy/QuitSmoking/Quit-Smoking_UCM_001085_SubHomePage.jsp

- Acidic beverages (e.g., coffee, juices, soft drinks) interfere with the buccal absorption of nicotine, so eating and drinking anything except water should be avoided for 15 minutes before or during the use of the nicotine inhaler.

Counseling with the Lozenge

- The lozenge should be allowed to <u>dissolve in the mouth</u> rather than chewing or swallowing it. It could take 20-30 minutes to completely dissolve.

- <u>Acidic beverages (e.g., coffee, juices, soft drinks) interfere with the buccal absorption of nicotine</u>, so eating and drinking anything <u>except water</u> should be avoided for 15 minutes before or during use of the nicotine lozenge.

- Patients often do not use enough PRN nicotine replacement medications to obtain optimal clinical effects. <u>Generally, patients should use 1 lozenge every 1-2 hours</u> during the first 6 weeks of treatment, using a minimum of 9 lozenges/day, then decrease over time.

Counseling with Nasal Spray

- Patients should not sniff, swallow, or inhale through the nose while administering doses, as this increases irritating effects. The spray is best delivered with the <u>head tilted slightly back</u>.

Counseling with the Nicotine Patch

- At the start of each day, place the patch on a relatively hairless location, typically between the neck and waist, rotating the site to reduce local skin irritation.

- Patches should be applied <u>as soon as the patient wakes on the quit day</u>. With patients who experience <u>sleep disruption, have the patient remove the 24-hour patch prior to bedtime, or use the 16 hour patch</u>.

- Up to 50% of patients using the nicotine patch will experience a <u>local skin reaction</u>. Skin reactions usually are mild and self-limiting, but occasionally worsen over the course of therapy. Local treatment with hydrocortisone cream (1%) or triamcinolone cream (0.5%) and rotating patch sites may lessen the reaction. Fewer than 5% of patients discontinue patch treatment due to skin reactions.

Bupropion Counseling

- <u>It takes about 1 week for the medication to start working. For your best chance of quitting, you should not stop smoking until you have been taking this medicine for 1 week. Set a date to stop smoking during the second week of starting this medication.</u>

- The most common side effects are dry mouth and trouble sleeping. These side effects are generally mild and often disappear after a few weeks.

- Some people have severe allergic reactions to bupropion. Stop taking and call your healthcare provider right away if you get a rash, itching, hives, fever, swollen lymph glands, painful sores in your mouth or around your eyes, swelling of your lips or tongue, chest pain, or have trouble breathing. These could be signs of a serious allergic reaction.

- <u>Do not take if have a seizure disorder, are taking other forms of bupropion, or have taken an MAO inhibitor within the last 14 days or had an eating disorder</u>.

- Do not chew, cut, or crush the tablets. If you do, the medicine will be released into your body too quickly. If this happens you may be more likely to get side effects including seizures. Tablets must be swallowed whole. <u>Do not exceed 450 mg daily</u>, or 150 mg at each dose if using the IR formulation, due to seizure risk.

- Take the doses at least 8 hours apart.

- <u>If you, your family, or caregiver notice agitation, hostility, depression or changes in behavior or thinking</u> that are not typical for you, or you develop any of the following symptoms, stop taking the medication and call your healthcare provider right away:

- ❏ thoughts about suicide or dying, or attempts to commit suicide
- ❏ new or worse depression, anxiety or panic attacks
- ❏ feeling very agitated or restless
- ❏ acting aggressive, being angry, or violent
- ❏ acting on dangerous impulses
- ❏ an extreme increase in activity and talking (mania)
- ❏ abnormal thoughts or sensations
- ❏ seeing or hearing things that are not there (hallucinations)
- ❏ feeling people are against you (paranoia)
- ❏ feeling confused
- ❏ other unusual changes in behavior or mood
- If you are able to quit smoking with this medicine, your healthcare provider may keep you on it for several months so you don't go back to smoking.

Varenicline Counseling

- Choose a quit date to stop smoking.
- Start taking the medication 1 week (7 days) before the quit date. This allows the medication to build up in the body. You may continue to smoke during this time. Try to stop smoking on the quit date. If it doesn't happen, try again. Some people need to take the medication for a few weeks to work best.
- Take the medication after eating and with a full glass (8 ounces) of water.
- Most people will take this medicine for up to 12 weeks. If you do not quit smoking by 12 weeks, another 12 weeks of therapy may be helpful to stay cigarette-free.
- Symptoms of nicotine withdrawal include the urge to smoke, depressed mood, trouble sleeping, irritability, frustration, anger, feeling anxious, difficulty concentrating, restlessness, decreased heart rate, and increased appetite or weight gain.
- Before taking this medication, tell your healthcare provider if you have ever had depression or other mental health problems.
- If you, your family, or caregiver notice agitation, hostility, depression or changes in behavior or thinking that are not typical for you, or you develop any of the following symptoms, stop taking the medication and call your healthcare provider right away:
  - ❏ thoughts about suicide or dying, or attempts to commit suicide
  - ❏ new or worse depression, anxiety or panic attacks
  - ❏ feeling very agitated or restless
  - ❏ acting aggressive, being angry, or violent
  - ❏ acting on dangerous impulses
  - ❏ an extreme increase in activity and talking (mania)
  - ❏ abnormal thoughts or sensations
  - ❏ seeing or hearing things that are not there (hallucinations)
  - ❏ feeling people are against you (paranoia)
  - ❏ feeling confused
  - ❏ other unusual changes in behavior or mood
- Some people can have allergic reactions to this medication. Some of these allergic reactions can be life-threatening and include: swelling of the face, mouth, and throat that can cause trouble breathing. If these symptoms occur, stop taking the medication and get medical attention right away.

- Some people can have <u>serious skin reactions</u> while taking this medication. These can include rash, swelling, redness, and peeling of the skin. Some of these reactions can become life-threatening. If a rash with peeling skin or blisters in your mouth occurs, stop taking the medication and get medical attention right away.

- Tell your pharmacist about all your other medicines including prescription and nonprescription medicines, vitamins and herbal supplements.

- <u>Use caution driving or operating machinery</u> until you know how this medication may affect you. Some people may become sleepy, dizzy, or have trouble concentrating, that can make it hard to drive or perform other activities safely.

48

ALLERGIC RHINITIS, COUGH & COLD

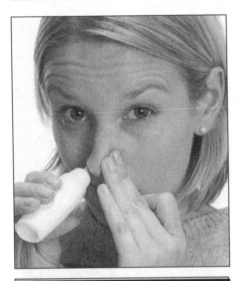

We gratefully acknowledge the assistance of Renu F. Singh, PharmD, BCACP, CDE, Associate Clinical Professor, University of California San Diego Skaggs School of Pharmacy and Pharmaceutical Sciences, in preparing this chapter.

ALLERGIC RHINITIS

Background

Allergic Rhinitis is inflammation of the nasal airways and is very common, affecting up to 20% – 40% of the population. It is classified as intermittent (infrequent or seasonal) or persistent (chronic or perennial), and symptoms can be mild, moderate or severe. It represents an opportunity for pharmacists to help patients select self care over the counter products, and to use prescription medication correctly. Allergic rhinitis is a major reason for decreased work productivity, or lost work or school days each year. Symptoms include sneezing, itchy nose, eyes or throat, watery eyes, rhinorrhea, nasal congestion, and postnasal drip. It can also result in fatigue, sleep disturbance and reduced cognitive ability. Untreated allergic rhinitis can lead to sinusitis, otitis media (in children) and asthma exacerbation in susceptible people. Unlike the common cold or the flu, onset of symptoms occurs quickly (within minutes) after allergen exposure.

REFERENCES

Joint Task Force on Practice Parameters: American Academy of Allergy, Asthma & Immunology; the American College of Allergy, Asthma and Immunology; and the Joint Council of Allergy, Asthma and Immunology. The diagnosis and Management of Rhinitis: An Updated Practice Parameter. J Allergy Clin Immunol. 2008; 122:S1-84.

Krinsky DL, Berardi RR, Ferreri SP, eds. Handbook of Nonprescription Drugs. 17th ed. Washington DC: APhA; 2012:179-204.

NON-DRUG TREATMENT

Environmental control is required to minimize allergic symptoms and involves <u>avoiding exposure to known or suspected allergens</u>, if possible. An IgE-mediated skin or blood allergy test by an allergy or pulmonary specialist can help determine patient-specific allergens. Ventilation systems with high-efficiency particulate air (HEPA) filters can help with some allergens (pollen, mold), however, these systems are expensive and ineffective for some patients. Vacuuming carpets, drapes, and upholstery with a HEPA vacuum cleaner weekly or more often will reduce household allergens. Removing carpets, upholstered furniture, encasing mattresses, pillows and boxsprings in allergen-impermeable covers, and washing bedding and soft toys in hot water weekly reduces dust mite allergens. Patients with air pollutants as triggers should be aware of the air quality index (AQI) and plan outdoor activities accordingly. Patients with pollen as a trigger should monitor pollen counts and plan accordingly. Staying indoors, closing windows in the house or car and using air-conditioning can help reduce exposure. However, keeping an environment that is "too clean" reduces exposure to microbes and helminths and may not be ideal: children need exposure to various "germs" to build a healthy immune system.

Nasal Irrigation and Wetting Agents

Nasal wetting agents (saline, propylene and polyethylene glycol sprays) or nasal irrigation with warm saline (isotonic or hypertonic) may reduce symptoms. Nasal irrigation rinses out allergens and mucus, increases ciliary function and reduces swelling. Saline solutions are either isotonic (0.9%) or hypertonic (2 - 3.5%). A popular product, the "neti pot", looks like a small genie lamp or teapot. It is used to hold salt water (saline solution) that is poured into one nostril and drained out of the other nostril. Nasal irrigation is safe for children and pregnant women. Instruct to use <u>boiled, bottled or distilled</u> water (not tap). The most common side effects are nasal burning, stinging, pain or irritation, which are increased with higher concentrations of saline. Pots and rinse bottles should be washed with hot soapy water after every use and should never be shared with others. Nasal gels with petrolatum *(Allergen Block)* can be applied around the nostrils to physically block pollens and allergens from entering the nose.

DRUG TREATMENT

Selecting appropriate pharmacologic management depends on the illness's severity and symptoms. <u>Intranasal corticosteroids are first-line for chronic, moderate-to-severe rhinitis. Milder, intermittent symptoms can be treated with oral antihistamines</u>. Decongestants are used for congestion (if present) and come in nasal and oral formulations. Agents for itchy eyes can be found in the Glaucoma, Ophthalmics & Otics chapter. A variety of other agents can be modestly useful.

Intranasal Corticosteroids

Intranasal corticosteroids work by decreasing inflammation. They are the <u>most effective medication class</u> in controlling symptoms of chronic allergic rhinitis and are considered <u>first-line treatment for moderate-severe rhinitis.</u> They are especially effective in reducing the nasal symptoms of allergic rhinitis (sneezing, itching, rhinorrhea, congestion). Take note that steroids used to treat chronic allergic rhinitis have <u>different brand names</u> and delivery vehicles in those used to treat asthma. For example, fluticasone for nasal allergy relief is *Flonase* (nase for nose) and for asthma is *Flovent*.

DRUG	DOSING	SAFETY/SIDE EFFECTS/MONITORING
Beclomethasone *(Beconase AQ, Qnasl)*	Adult: 1-2 sprays per nostril BID *(Beconase AQ)*; 2 sprays per nostril daily *(Qnasl)* Age 6-11 yrs.: 1-2 sprays per nostril BID *(Beconase AQ)*	**WARNINGS** Adrenal suppression can occur when used in high doses for prolonged periods Delayed wound healing, avoid use if recent nasal septal ulcers, nasal surgery, or nasal trauma until healing has occurred.
Budesonide *(Rhinocort Aqua)*	Adult: 1 spray per nostril daily Age ≥ 6 yrs.: use adult dose	Pediatrics: can ↓ growth velocity in pediatric patients (~1 centimeter/yr and is dose and duration related). To minimize, use lowest effective dose. Monitor growth. Prolonged use can ↑ the risk of secondary infection or limit response to vaccines. Avoid exposure to chickenpox. Caution in patients with untreated fungal, viral, or bacterial infections.
Ciclesonide *(Omnaris, Zetonna)*	Adult: 2 sprays per nostril daily *(Omnaris)*; 1 spray per nostril daily *(Zetonna)* Age ≥ 6 yrs.: use adult dose	Caution in patients with cataracts and/or glaucoma; ↑ intraocular pressure, open-angle glaucoma, and cataracts have occurred with prolonged use. Consider routine eye exams in chronic users.
Flunisolide	Adult: 2 sprays per nostril BID or TID Age 6-14 yrs.: 1 spray per nostril TID or 2 sprays per nostril BID	**SIDE EFFECTS** Headache, dry nose, epistaxis (nose bleeds), unpleasant taste, localized infection **NOTES** Can take up to one week to get full relief.
Fluticasone *(Flonase, Veramyst)* + azelastine *(Dymista)*	Adult: 1-2 sprays per nostril daily or BID *(Flonase)*; 1-2 sprays per nostril daily *(Veramyst)* Age ≥ 4 yrs.: 1-2 sprays per nostril daily *(Flonase)* Age ≥ 2 yrs.: 1-2 sprays per nostril daily *(Veramyst)* *Dymista:* Adult: 1 spray per nostril BID	Budesonide is Pregnancy Category B and is the preferred inhaled steroid in pregnancy. If using regularly for several months, recommend periodic nasal exams to evaluate for nasal septal perforation or ulcers. Advise patients to discontinue if they come into contact with a person who has chickenpox, measles or TB, if they develop symptoms of an infection, have a change in vision, or experience frequent nose bleeds.
Mometasone *(Nasonex)*	Adult: 2 sprays per nostril daily Age 2-11 yrs.: 1 spray per nostril daily	
Triamcinolone *(Nasacort AQ,* **Nasacort Allergy 24HR OTC)**	Adult: 1-2 sprays per nostril daily Age ≥ 6 yrs.: use adult dose Age 2-5 yrs.: 1 spray per nostril daily	

Oral Antihistamines

Oral antihistamines are considered <u>first-line agents for patients with mild-moderate disease. They are effective in reducing symptoms of itching, sneezing, and rhinorrhea, but have little effect on nasal congestion.</u> Antihistamines work by blocking histamine at the histamine-1 (H1) receptor site. The <u>second-generation agents are generally preferred</u> since they cause less sedation and cognitive impairment. Antihistamines can help if symptoms of allergic conjunctivitis (itchy, red eyes) are present. See Glaucoma, Ophthalmics & Otics chapter.

DRUG	DOSING	SAFETY/SIDE EFFECTS/MONITORING

Select First Generation Oral Antihistamines

DRUG	DOSING	SAFETY/SIDE EFFECTS/MONITORING
Clemastine *(Tavist, Dayhist Allergy 12 HR Relief)* Tablet, syrup	Adult: 1.34-2.68 mg PO Q8-12H (max 8.04 mg/day) Age 6-12 yrs.: 0.67-1.34 mg PO BID (max 4.02 mg/day) Age < 6 yrs.: 0.335-0.67 mg/day divided 2-3 doses (max 1.34 mg/day)	**CONTRAINDICATIONS** Carbinoxamine: Do not use in children < 2 years, lactation, avoid use of MAO inhibitors. Clemastine: narrow-angle glaucoma. Diphenhydramine: neonates or premature infants, lactation Chlorpheniramine: narrow-angle glaucoma, bladder neck obstruction, BPH, acute asthmatic attacks, stenosing peptic ulcer, pyloroduodenal obstruction, premature and term newborns
DiphenhydrAMINE HCl *(**Benadryl**, many others)* Capsule, tablet, chewable, elixir, strip, syrup, suspension, injection, cream, gel, solution, stick	Adult: <u>25-50 mg PO Q4-6H</u> (max 300 mg/day) Age 6-11 yrs.: 12.5-25 mg PO Q4-6H (max 150 mg/day) Age < 6 yrs.: <u>do not use</u> for self care	**WARNINGS** Due to strong anticholinergic effects, avoid use in elderly (Beers criteria), caution with cardiovascular disease, prostate enlargement, glaucoma, asthma, pyloroduodenal obstruction, thyroid disease. Caution for excessive sedation. In 2008 the FDA advised that OTC cough and cold preparations, including first generation antihistamines (chlorpheniramine, diphenhydramine, brompheniramine and clemastine) should not be used in children < 2 years due to the risk of potentially serious and life threatening side effects.
Carbinoxamine *(Arbinoxa Karbinal ER)* Capsule, tablet, solution	**IR** Adult: 4-8 mg PO Q6-8H 6-11 yrs.: 2-4 mg PO Q6-8H 2-5 yrs.: 1-2 mg PO Q6-8H **ER** Adult: 6-16 mg PO Q12H 6-11 yrs.: 6-12 mg PO Q12H 4-5 yrs.: 3-8 mg PO Q12H 2-3 yrs.: 3-4 mg PO Q12H	**SIDE EFFECTS** <u>Somnolence</u>, cognitive impairment, strong anticholinergic effects (dry mouth, blurred vision, urinary retention, constipation), and seizures/arrhythmias in higher doses **NOTES** First generation antihistamines should not be taken in lactating women; second generation agents, such as loratadine or fexofenadine, are preferred. All first generation antihistamines are Pregnancy Category B except carbinoxamine, which is Pregnancy Category C.
Chlorpheniramine *(Chlor-Trimeton, Chlorphen, Ed ChlorPed,* others)* Tablet, liquid, suspension, syrup	**IR** Adult: 4 mg PO Q4-6H (max 24 mg/day) 6-11 yrs.: 2 mg PO Q4-6H (max 12 mg/day) 2-5 yrs.: 1 mg PO Q4-6H (max 6 mg/day) **ER** Adult: 12 mg PO Q12H (max 24 mg/day) no pediatric dosing	

Oral Antihistamines Continued

DRUG	DOSING	SAFETY/SIDE EFFECTS/MONITORING

Second Generation Oral Antihistamines

DRUG	DOSING	SAFETY/SIDE EFFECTS/MONITORING
Cetirizine *(ZyrTEC, ZyrTEC D*, others)* Capsule, tablet, solution, syrup, chewable, ODT	Adult: 5-10 mg PO daily ≥ 6 yrs.: use adult dose 2-5 yrs.: 2.5-5 mg PO daily	**CONTRAINDICATIONS** Levocertirizine: end-stage renal disease, hemodialysis, infants and children 6 months to 11 years of age with renal impairment **WARNINGS** CNS depression: can cause sedation when used with other sedating drugs **SIDE EFFECTS** Somnolence can still be seen occasionally with the 2nd generation agents (more with cetirizine and levocetirizine) **NOTES** Fexofenadine: take with water (not juice due to ↓ absorption). Avoid concurrent administration with aluminum or magnesium-containing products.
Levocetirizine *(Xyzal)* Tablet, solution	Adult: 5 mg PO QHS 6-11 yrs.: 2.5 mg PO QHS 6 mos-5 yrs.: 1.25 mg PO QHS	
Fexofenadine *(Allegra, Allegra D 12H, Allegra D 24H, Children's Allegra ODT, Mucinex Allergy)* Tablet, suspension, ODT	Adult: 60 mg PO BID or 180 mg daily 2-11 yrs.: 30 mg PO BID	
Loratadine *(Claritin, Claritin-D 24 hour, Claritin RediTabs, Alavert)* Tablet, capsule, chewable, solution, syrup, ODT	Adult: 10 mg PO daily or 5 mg PO BID *(RediTabs)* Age ≥ 6 yrs.: use adult dose 2-5 yrs.: 5 mg PO daily	
Desloratadine *(Clarinex, Clarinex D, Clarinex RediTabs)* Tablet, syrup, ODT	Adult: 5 mg PO daily 6-11 yrs.: 2.5 mg PO daily 12 mos-5 yrs.: 1.25 mg PO daily 6-11 mos.: 1 mg PO daily	

Intranasal Antihistamines

DRUG	DOSING	SAFETY/SIDE EFFECTS/MONITORING
Azelastine *(Astelin, Astepro)* + fluticasone *(Dymista)*	Adult: 1-2 sprays per nostril BID 6-11 yrs.: 1 spray per nostril BID	**SIDE EFFECTS** Bitter taste, headache, somnolence, nasal irritation, minor nosebleed, sinus pain **NOTES** Helps with nasal congestion as well.
Olopatadine *(Patanase)*	Adult: 2 sprays per nostril BID 6-11 yrs.: 1 spray per nostril BID	

Decongestants

These agents are effective in reducing sinus and nasal congestion. Decongestants are <u>alpha-adrenergic agonists</u> (sympathomimetics) that work by causing vasoconstriction. If <u>a product contains a D after the name (such as *Mucinex D* or *Robitussin D*), it usually contains a decongestant (phenylephrine or pseudoephedrine).</u>

DRUG	DOSING	SAFETY/SIDE EFFECTS/MONITORING
Systemic (oral)		
Phenylephrine HCl *(Sudafed PE*, others)* Tablet, liquid, solution, injection	Adult: 10 mg PO Q4H PRN (max 60 mg/day) 6-11 yrs.: 5 mg PO Q4H PRN (max 30 mg/day) 4-5 yrs.: 2.5 mg PO Q4H PRN (max 15 mg/day)	**CONTRAINDICATIONS** Do not use within 14 days of MAOIs. **WARNINGS** Avoid in children < 2 years Use with caution in patients with CV disease and uncontrolled hypertension (can ↑ BP), hyperthyroidism (can worsen), diabetes (can ↑ blood glucose), bowel obstruction, glaucoma (can ↑ IOP), BPH (can cause urinary retention), and in the elderly
Pseudoephedrine *(Sudafed, Nexafed, Zephrex-D*, others)* Tablet, liquid, syrup	Adult: 60 mg PO Q4-6H PRN, or 120 mg PO ER Q12H, or 240 mg PO ER daily (max 240 mg/day) 6-12 yrs.: 30 mg PO Q4-6H PRN (max 120 mg/day) 4-5 yrs.: 15 mg PO Q4-6H PRN (max 60 mg/day)	**SIDE EFFECTS** Cardiovascular stimulation (tachycardia, palpitations, ↑ BP), CNS stimulation (anxiety, tremors, insomnia, nervousness, restlessness), dizziness, headache, anorexia **NOTES** Pregnancy Category C Phenylephrine has low bioavailability (~38%); pseudoephedrine is more effective Onset of 30-60 minutes
Topicals (Intranasal)		
Naphazoline 0.05% *(Privine)*	Adult: 1-2 sprays per nostril Q6H PRN	**CONTRAINDICATIONS** Phenylephrine: hypertension, ventricular tachycardia **WARNINGS** Do not use with MAOIs, or if have closed angle glaucoma
Oxymetazoline 0.05% *(Afrin*, Neo-Synephrine Nighttime 12-Hour)*	Adult: 2-3 sprays per nostril Q12H PRN ≥ 6 yrs.: use adult dose	
Phenylephrine 0.125%, 0.25%, 0.5%, 1% *(Neo-Synephrine 4-Hour)*	Adult: 2-3 sprays of 0.25% to 1% per nostril Q4H PRN 6-12 yrs.: 2-3 sprays of 0.25% per nostril Q4H PRN 2-5 yrs.: 1 spray of 0.125% per nostril Q2-4H PRN	**SIDE EFFECTS** Stinging, burning, sneezing, dryness (vehicle-related), trauma from the tip of the device, rhinitis medicamentosa (rebound congestion if used longer than 3 days) **NOTES** Effective with a fast onset of 5-10 minutes
Tetrahydrozoline 0.05%, 0.1% *(Tyzine)* – Rx	Adult: 3-4 sprays of 0.1% per nostril Q3-4H PRN or 2-4 drops per nostril Q3-4H PRN > 6 yrs.: use adult dose 2-6 yrs.: 2-3 drops of 0.05% per nostril Q4-6H PRN	<u>Limit use to ≤ 3 days to prevent rebound congestion</u>

Additional Allergy Agents

Intranasal cromolyn *(Nasalcrom)*

Cromolyn is a mast cell stablizer used for treatment and prophylaxis. It must be started at the onset of allergy season and used regularly (not PRN), every 6-8 hours, to be effective. Symptoms start to improve in 4-7 days but can take as long as 2-4 weeks of continued use to see maximal effect. Although generally not as effective as other agents, it is used in children and pregnancy due to its safety profile.

Intranasal ipratropium bromide

(Atrovent Nasal Spray)

This agent is effective for ↓ rhinorrhea by causing nasal dryness (not effective for other nasal symptoms).

Oral antileukotrienes

(Montelukast – *Singulair*)

Montelukast has similar efficacy to anti-histamines or pseudoephedrine. The dose of montelukast is 10 mg PO daily (15 years and up), 5 mg chewable tablet PO daily (ages 6-14 years), 4 mg chewable tablet PO daily (ages 2-5 years), or one packet of 4 mg oral granules PO daily (ages 6 months-5 years). See Asthma chapter for more information.

COMBAT METHAMPHETAMINE EPIDEMIC ACT 2005

Pseudoephedrine (PSE) is located behind pharmacy counters as part of the "Combat Meth Act" (CMEA), under the Patriot Act, to crack down on the methamphetamine epidemic. Meth causes unpredictable and often violent behavior. The waste created in the production is very toxic and is usually dumped illegally. The act applies to any non-prescription product containing pseudoephedrine, phenylpropanolamine and ephedrine, all of which can be converted rather easily into methamphetamine.

To sell these products (primarily PSE, the others are not easily available), they must be kept behind the counter or in a locked cabinet. They often are, but do not need to be, located in the pharmacy. Stores must keep a logbook of sales (exception is the single dose package that contains a maximum of 60 mg – this is 2 of the 30 mg tablets.) For any sale above this amount, customer must show photo ID issued by the state (e.g., license, ID card, expired or unexpired US passport, unexpired foreign passport).

Customers record their name, date and time of sale, and sign the logbook. Store staff must verify the name matches the photo ID and that the date and time are correct. Record the address. Some stores can swipe the drivers license to get the name and address recorded. The store staff must record what the person received. The maximum dose allowed for purchase is 3.6 grams or 120 of the 30 mg tablets, and 9 grams (300 tablets) in a 30-day period. Keep logbook for at least 2 years. The logbook has to be kept secured and readily available upon request by board inspectors or law enforcement. The logbook cannot be shared with the public.

Many states now have their own restrictions in addition to the federal restriction, such as age restrictions, prescription required or stricter limits.

Sublingual Immunotherapy

In 2014 the FDA approved 3 new sublingual treatments for allergic rhinitis due to specific types of grass pollen. They are alternatives to allergy shots, which must be given in a physician office. The first dose must be given in the doctor's office with all 3 of these agents, but subsequent doses can be taken at home. The patient must be monitored for at least 30 minutes for signs of allergic reactions (boxed warning) and the patient should be prescribed autoinjectable epinephrine.

- *Oralair* contains 5 different grass pollen extracts. Place 1 SL tablet under the tongue daily; initiate treatment 4 months before and during grass pollen season.

- *Grastek* contains Timothy grass pollen extract. Place 1 SL tablet under the tongue daily; initiate treatment 3 months before and during grass pollen season.

- *Ragwitek* contains ragweed pollen extract. Place 1 SL tablet under the tongue daily; initiate treatment 3 months before and during pollen season.

COUGH AND COLD AGENTS

Background

The common cold, is a viral infection of the upper respiratory tract, caused by over 200 viruses including rhinoviruses, coronaviruses, influenza, and transmitted primarily by mucus secretions via patient's hands or by the air from coughing or sneezing. Coughing or sneezing into the elbow or into a tissue is preferable over coughing into a hand, which can then touch surfaces and spread illness. Frequent hand cleansing with soap or soap substitutes (e.g., hand sanitizers) should be encouraged. Refer to the Medication Safety chapter for correct hand washing technique. Refer to the Infectious Diseases chapter for a table that compares viral and bacteria infections.

Natural Products used for Colds

Zinc, in various formulations including lozenges, is used for cold prevention and treatment. There is little efficacy data for cold prevention, but zinc lozenges may decrease cold duration if used correctly (taken every 2 hrs hours while awake, starting within 48 hours of symptom onset). For this purpose zinc supplements are rated as "possibly effective" by the Natural Medicines Database. Zinc lozenges can cause mouth irritation, a metallic taste and nausea. Do not use for more than 5-7 days as long term use can cause copper deficiency. Do not recommend zinc nasal swabs or sprays due to the risk of loss of smell. Vitamin C supplements are commonly used, with no efficacy for cold prevention. Some data has shown a decrease in the duration of the cold by 1-1.5 days at dose of 1-3 gm/day. There may also be a dose-dependent response; doses of at least 2 grams/day appears to work better than 1 gram/day. Vitamin C is rated as "possibly effective" for cold treatment by the Natural Medicines Database. However, the high doses of vitamin C recommended for cold treatment (1-3 gm/day) may cause diarrhea. Echinacea is also rated as "possibly effective" for cold treatment. With any of these products it is important to use the correct dose from a reputable manufacturer. *Airborne* is a popular product that contains a variety of ingredients, including vitamins C, vitamin E, zinc and echinacea. It is costly and has no proven benefit in the combinations provided.

Expectorants

Expectorants are used for a productive cough to ↓ phlegm viscosity in the lower respiratory tract and ↑ secretions in the upper respiratory tract to help move phlegm upwards and out.

DRUG	ADULT DOSING	SAFETY/SIDE EFFECTS/MONITORING
GuaiFENesin *(Mucinex)* Tablet, packet, solution, syrup	200-400 mg Q4H PRN, or 600-1,200 mg XR Q12H (max 2.4 g/day)	**WARNINGS** Some formulations may contain phenylalanine. **SIDE EFFECTS** Nausea (dose-related), vomiting, dizziness, headache **NOTES** Not for OTC use in children < 2 years of age

Cough Suppressants

Cough suppressants are used for dry, unproductive cough, or to suppress productive cough at night to allow for restful sleep. Dextromethorphan (DM) and codeine have high affinity to several regions of the brain, including the medullary cough center, suppressing the cough reflex. DM also acts as a serotonin reuptake inhibitor. DM is a drug of abuse as it acts as a NMDA-receptor blocker in high doses leading to euphoric and hallucinogenic properties similar to PCP. In 2012, California became the first state to ban the sale of DM to minors < 18 years of age. A few other states have followed, some with more stringent requirements. Benzonatate suppresses cough by topical anesthetic action on the respiratory stretch receptors.

DRUG	ADULT DOSING	SAFETY/SIDE EFFECTS/MONITORING
Dextromethorphan *(Delsym)* <u>Most commonly used</u>	10-20 mg Q4H PRN, or 30 mg Q6-8H PRN, or 60 mg XR Q12H PRN (max 120 mg/day)	**CONTRAINDICATIONS** All dextromethophan-containing products should not be used within 14 days of MAOI use. **SIDE EFFECTS** Serotonin syndrome if co-administered with other serotonergic drugs **NOTES** If the product name has DM at the end, such as *Robitussin DM*, it contains dextromethorphan.
Codeine C-II	7.5-120 mg daily or divided	**BOXED WARNING** Respiratory depression and death have occurred in children who received codeine following tonsillectomy and/or adenoidectomy and had evidence of being ultra-rapid metabolizers of codeine due to a CYP2D6 polymorphism, avoid. **CONTRAINDICATIONS** Paralytic ileus, children who have undergone tonsillectomy and/or adenoidectomy **SIDE EFFECTS** CNS depression, constipation, hypotension
Benzonatate *(Tessalon Perles, Zonatuss)*	100-200 mg TID PRN (max 600 mg/day)	**WARNINGS** Accidental ingestion and fatal overdose has been reported in children < 10 years of age, avoid. **SIDE EFFECTS** Somnolence, confusion, hallucinations
Diphenhydramine *(Benadryl)*	25 mg Q4H PRN (max 150 mg/day)	See First Generation Oral Antihistamine table

Decongestants

Systemic and nasal decongestants are used to relieve congestion and rhinorrhea. These agents are discussed in the previous section.

Analgesics/Antipyretics

Analgesics and antipyretics such as acetaminophen and ibuprofen are used to relieve sore throat, body malaise, and/or fever. See Pain chapter for more information.

Select Cough and Cold Products

DRUG	ADULT DOSING
Dextromethorphan/promethazine	15 mg/6.25 mg per 5 mL; 5 mL Q4-6H PRN (max 30 mL/day)
Brompheniramine/pseudoephedrine/ dextromethorphan *(Bromfed DM)*	2 mg/30 mg/10 mg per 5 mL; 10 mL Q4H PRN (max 60 mL/day)
Promethazine/phenylephrine/codeine (Promethazine VC/Codeine) C-V	6.25 mg/5 mg/10 mg per 5 mL; 5 mL Q4-6H PRN (max 30 mL/day)
GuaiFENesin/codeine *(Robafen AC, Virtussin AC)* C-V	100 mg/10 mg per 5 mL; 10 mL PO Q4H PRN (max 60 mL/day)
GuaiFENesin/codeine/pseudoephedrine *(Cheratussin DAC, Mytussin DAC)* C-V	100 mg/10 mg/30 mg per 5 mL; 10 mL Q4H PRN (max 40 mL/day)
Chlorpheniramine/hydrocodone *(TussiCaps, Tussionex, Vituz)* C-II	8 mg/10 mg ER per 5 mL; 5 mL Q12H PRN (max 10 mL/day)

Cough and Cold Products in Children

In 2008, the FDA warned that OTC cough and cold products should not be used in children under age 2 years old due to safety concerns (under 6 years old per the American Academy of Pediatrics). Later that same year, many manufactures voluntarily re-labeled these cough and cold products to state: "do not use in children under 4 years of age." These cough and cold products include any product containing decongestants and the antihistamines diphenhydramine, brompheniramine or chlorpheniramine. Do not use promethazine in any form in children less than 2 years old. The FDA advises against the use of promethazine with codeine cough syrups in children ≤ 6 years of age, due to the risk of respiratory depression, cardiac arrest and neurological problems.

If a young child has a cold, it is safe and useful to recommend proper hydration, nasal bulbs for gentle suctioning, saline drops/sprays (*Ocean* and generics), vaporizers/humidifiers, and ibuprofen and acetaminophen, if needed for fever or pain. Do not use aspirin in children due to the risk of Reye's syndrome. OTC cough and cold medications have not been shown to work in young children and can be dangerous. Over the past year there have been rare cases of severe skin reactions in patients using acetaminophen and NSAIDs. Symptoms of the common cold usually resolve in a few days (up to 2 weeks). If the child is a small infant, seems seriously ill, or if symptoms worsen or do not go away, the child should be seen by a pediatrician.

Non-pharmacological treatments should be initiated first. A cool mist humidifier helps nasal passages shrink and allow easier breathing. Avoid using warm mist humidifiers as they can cause nasal passages to swell (making breathing more difficult) and can cause burns if spilled. Wash humidifiers daily when in use. Saline nose drops or sprays keep nasal passages moist and reduces congestion. Nasal suctioning with a bulb syringe, either with or without saline nose drops, works especially well for infants less than a year old. Older children often resist its use.

Acetaminophen or ibuprofen can be used to reduce fever, aches and pains. If a parent purchases OTC infant drops for ibuprofen (let pediatrician recommend if under age 2), remind them to use the calibrated dropper or oral syringe that <u>came with the bottle</u> and do not mix and match dosing devices or overdose can occur. Advise against using kitchen teaspoons to measure out medication since these come in different sizes.

- Acetaminophen infants' or children's liquid suspensions (<u>both 160 mg/5 mL</u>): <u>10-15 mg/ kg/dose</u> Q4-6H PRN, max 5 doses/24H.

- Ibuprofen infants' drops (<u>50 mg/1.25 mL</u>) or children's liquid suspensions (<u>100 mg/5 mL</u>): <u>5-10 mg/kg/dose</u> Q6-8H PRN. Max daily dose 40 mg/kg/day for both formulations.

Some doctors recommend alternating ibuprofen with acetaminophen at each dosing interval to avoid acetaminophen toxicity or ibuprofen-induced GI discomfort.

Menthol and camphor used topically, such as in *Vick's VapoRub*, do not work well and should not be used in children less than 2 years. Menthol can result in aspiration and cardiac and CNS toxicity if ingested. Camphor is generally considered safe but lacks sufficient data. *Vick's BabyRub* contains petrolatum, eucalyptus oil, lavendar oil, rosemary oil and aloe extract and is also considered relatively safe but lacks sufficient efficacy data.

Patient Counseling for *Flonase* (Fluticasone Nasal Inhaler) and *Nasacort 24 HR OTC* (Triamcinolone Nasal Spray)

Before using

- Shake the bottle gently and then remove the dust cover/cap.
- It is necessary to prime the pump into the air the first time it is used, or when you have not used

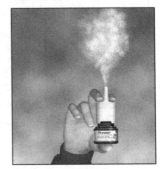

it for awhile (7 days for *Flonase*, 14 days for *Nasacort*). To prime the pump, hold the bottle with the nasal applicator pointing away from you and with your forefinger and middle finger on either side of the nasal applicator and your thumb underneath the bottle. When you prime the pump for the first time, press down and release the pump a few times (6 times for *Flonase*, as many times as it takes until a fine mist appears for *Nasacort*). The pump is now ready for use. If the pump is not used for awhile (7 days for *Flonase*, 14 days for *Nasacort*) prime until a fine spray appears.

Using the spray

- Blow your nose to clear your nostrils.
- Close one nostril. Tilt your head forward slightly and, keeping the bottle upright, carefully insert the nasal applicator into the other nostril.

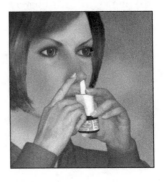

- Start to breathe in through your nose, and while breathing in, press firmly and quickly down once on the applicator to release the spray. To get a full actuation, use your forefinger and middle finger to spray while supporting the base of the bottle with your thumb. Avoid spraying in eyes. Breathe gently inwards through the nostril.
- Breathe out through your mouth.

- If a second spray is needed in that nostril, repeat the above 3 steps. Repeat the above 3 steps in the other nostril.

- Wipe the nasal applicator with a clean tissue and replace with dust cover.

- Do not use the bottle for more than the labeled number of sprays even though the bottle is not completely empty.

- Do not blow your nose right after using the nasal spray. Clean the nasal applicator tip regularly (at least once a week for *Flonase*, after every use for *Nasacort)* by gently pulling it off and rinsing it under warm water. Let it air dry before replacing back onto bottle.

49

CYSTIC FIBROSIS (CF)

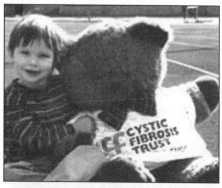

We gratefully acknowledge the assistance of Paul Beringer, PharmD, Associate Professor of Clinical Pharmacy and Clinical Medicine, University of Southern California, in preparing this chapter.

BACKGROUND

Cystic fibrosis (CF) is an autosomal recessive genetic disorder that leads to abnormal transport of chloride, bicarbonate, and sodium ions across the epithelium, leading to thick, viscous secretions. The thick mucus mostly affects the lungs, pancreas, liver and intestine, primarily causing difficulty breathing and lung infections as well as digestive complications. The name cystic fibrosis refers to the characteristic scarring (fibrosis) and cyst formation that occurs within the pancreas.

CF is caused by a mutation in the gene for the protein cystic fibrosis transmembrane conductance regulator (CFTR). This protein is required to regulate the components of sweat, digestive juices, and mucus. CFTR regulates the movement of chloride, bicarbonate, and sodium ions across epithelial membranes and mutations can lead to a chronic cycle of lung infection, inflammation, and obstruction which results in a progressive loss of pulmonary function and eventual respiratory failure. CFTR dysfunction also leads to pancreatic insufficiency, infertility, biliary cirrhosis as well as a range of other defects.

GUIDELINES

Cystic Fibrosis Pulmonary Guidelines: Chronic Medications for Maintenance of Lung Health. *Am J Respir Crit Care Med.* 2013; 187:680–689.

Cystic Fibrosis Pulmonary Guidelines: Treatment of Pulmonary Exacerbations. *Am J Respir Crit Care Med.* 2009; 180:802–808.

CLINICAL PRESENTATION

The classic symptoms of CF are salty tasting skin, poor growth and poor weight gain despite adequate food intake, thick and sticky mucus production, frequent lung infections, coughing and shortness of breath. Digital clubbing is often present. Digestive symptoms include steatorrhea, malnutrition due to poor absorption of nutrients, including fat-soluble vitamins, and a failure to thrive if not treated.

PHARMACOLOGIC TREATMENT

An early diagnosis of CF and a comprehensive treatment plan can improve both survival and quality of life. Specialty clinics for cystic fibrosis are helpful and are found in many communities. Many drugs are used in the treatment of CF (see below for specifics). If the patient is taking several medications, the recommended order is as follows: bronchodilator, hypertonic saline, dornase alfa, chest physiotherapy, then inhaled antibiotics.

Treatment for Lung Problems

- Inhaled bronchodilators to help open the airways.

- Hypertonic saline *(HyperSal)* for hydrating the airway mucus secretions and facilitating mucociliary clearance.

- DNAse enzyme to breakdown extracellular DNA from accumulated neutrophils. DNAse therapy is designed to thin mucus and facilitate mucociliary clearance.

- Inhaled antibiotics for prevention and treatment of lung and sinus infections.

- Oral azithromycin to reduce airway inflammation and disrupt *P. aeruginosa* biofilm formation.

- Transplantation, in patients with end-stage lung disease.

Treatment for Intestinal and Nutritional Problems

- A high-fat and calorically-dense diet to help with nutrition.

- Pancreatic enzyme replacement to optimize growth and nutritional status and promote healthy bowels.

- Proton pump inhibitors to prevent degradation of pancreatic enzymes in the stomach and for treatment of GERD.

- Vitamin supplements, especially the fat-soluble vitamins A, D, E, and K.

- Insulin for treatment of CF-related diabetes mellitus.

Controlling Infections in the Lungs

Intermittent Infection

- Impaired mucociliary clearance predisposes patients with CF to lung infections. The most common organisms early in the disease are _Staphylococcus aureus_ and _Haemophilus influenzae_ followed by _P. aeruginosa_ in adolescents and adults. Acute pulmonary exacerbations characterized by an increase in cough, sputum production with a change in sputum color (greenish), shortness of breath, a rapid decline in FEV1, loss of appetite and weight are a frequent complication of CF. Treatment often includes an extended course of antibiotics (2-4 weeks), modalities to increase airway clearance and nutritional therapies.

- If the patient has a _P. aeruginosa_ infection, 2 drugs given IV are recommended to provide potential synergy and prevent resistance. These include aminoglycosides, beta lactams, quinolones, and others that cover _P. aeruginosa_. See Infectious Diseases chapter for a complete discussion on treatment of _P. aeruginosa_. Doses tend to be larger than normal due to the need to obtain a therapeutic concentration in lung tissue and the reduced susceptibility of the bacteria chronically colonizing the airways of these patients.

- Lung infections occur intermittently at first, but eventually become chronic. In particular, chronic lung infections with _P. aeruginosa_ are associated with more rapid decline in pulmonary function. Inhaled antibiotics may be used to eradicate _P. aeruginosa_ from the lungs. See agents below. If patient is using a bronchodilator and/or mucolytic, make sure these are given prior to the antibiotic inhalation.

Chronic Infection

Inhaled antibiotics are recommended for patients with chronic _P. aeruginosa_ lung infections to reduce the bacterial burden. Treatment is associated with an improvement in lung function and a reduction in the frequency of acute pulmonary exacerbations. The frequency of acute pulmonary exacerbations is strongly associated with lung function decline and shortened survival in CF.

DRUG	DOSE/INDICATION	SAFETY/SIDE EFFECTS/MONITORING

Antibiotics, Inhaled

DRUG	DOSE/INDICATION	SAFETY/SIDE EFFECTS/MONITORING
Tobramycin Inhalation Solution (TOBI, Bethkis) _TOBI:_ 300 mg/5mL single use ampule _Bethkis:_ 300 mg/4mL single use ampule	300 mg via nebulizer Q12H x 28 days, followed by 28 days off cycle Indicated in CF patients ≥ 6 years who are colonized with _P. aeruginosa_ to reduce infection/hospitalization	**SIDE EFFECTS** Ototoxicity, tinnitus, voice alteration, dizziness, bronchospasm **NOTES** Little systemic absorption _TOBI:_ Use with _PARI LC Plus_ reusable nebulizer and _DeVilbiss Pulmo-Aide_ air compressor _Bethkis:_ Use with _PARI LC Plus_ nebulizer and _Vios_ air compressor Doses should be taken at least 6 hours apart Recommended to store in refrigerator; can be kept at room temperature up to 28 days In foil to protect from light Not for use if FEV1 < 40% or > 80% predicted, or if colonized with _Burkholderia cepacia._

Chronic Infection Continued

DRUG	DOSE/INDICATION	SAFETY/SIDE EFFECTS/MONITORING
Tobramycin Inhalation Powder *(TOBI Podhaler)* 28 mg capsules in blister card	112 mg (4 x 28 mg caps) via podhaler Q12H x 28 days, followed by 28 days off cycle. Indicated in CF patients ≥ 6 years who are colonized with *P. aeruginosa* to reduce infection/hospitalization	**SIDE EFFECTS** Similar to above **NOTES** Little systemic absorption Use with *Podhaler* Doses should be taken at least <u>6 hours apart</u> <u>Store capsules at room temperature in a dry place</u> Not for use if FEV1 < 25% or > 80% predicted, or if colonized with *Burkholderia cepacia*.
Aztreonam Lysine Inhalation Solution *(Cayston)* 75 mg vial	75 mg TID x 28 days, followed by 28 days off cycle Indicated in CF patients ≥ 7 years with *P. aeruginosa* in the lungs	**SIDE EFFECTS** <u>Allergic reactions (may be severe), bronchospasm, fever, wheezing, cough, chest discomfort</u> **NOTES** Doses should be taken at least <u>4 hours apart</u> Use with *Altera* nebulizer system Need to <u>reconstitute</u> with 1 mL of <u>sterile diluent (provided)</u>; <u>give immediately</u> Recommend to <u>refrigerate</u>; can be kept at <u>room temperature</u> up to <u>28 days</u> <u>Protect from light</u>

Antibiotic, Oral

Azithromycin *(Zithromax)*	< 40 kg: 250 mg 3 times/week > 40 kg: 500 mg 3 times/week Used to decrease inflammation and reduce exacerbations; not an FDA-indicated use.	**SIDE EFFECTS** In CF patients: Tinnitus, nausea, risk of QT prolongation **NOTES** Do not use as monotherapy in individuals with nontuberculous mycobacteria lung infections

Select Patient Instructions on Using *TOBI Podhaler*

- *TOBI* should be taken using the <u>*Podhaler* device</u>.

- Do not swallow the capsules.

- Use a new *Podhaler* device every 7 days.

- Each dose of 4 *TOBI Podhaler* capsules should be taken as close to 12 hours but <u>no less</u> than 6 hours apart.

- Make sure to finish the whole dose of *TOBI*. Do not leave any medication in the capsules.

- *TOBI* comes in 4 weekly packs containing 7 blister cards of 8 capsules each (4 for each morning and evening) and 2 *Podhaler* devices. <u>Store capsules at room temperature in a dry place</u>.

- Only remove 1 capsule at a time immediately before administration.

Agents to Promote Mucus Clearance

DRUG	DOSING	SAFETY/SIDE EFFECTS/MONITORING
Albuterol (*AccuNeb, Proventil HFA*, others)	2-4 times daily	Well-tolerated if taken correctly; refer to Asthma chapter for complete information
Hypertonic saline (*HyperSal*) 4 mL unit dose vials	4 mL via a nebulizer 2-4 times daily	Hypertonic saline is a high-alert drug, especially with IV administration. For CF therapy, hypertonic saline is supplied as small ampules that are delivered via a nebulizer.
Dornase alfa (*Pulmozyme*) 2.5 mg single use ampule	2.5 mg daily with recommended nebulizer and compressor system	**CONTRAINDICATIONS** Hypersensitivity to Chinese Hamster Ovary (CHO) products **SIDE EFFECTS** Chest pain, fever, rash, rhinitis, laryngitis, voice alteration, throat irritation **NOTES** Store the ampules in the refrigerator (do not expose to room temperature ≥ 24 hours) Do not mix with any other drug in the nebulizer Protect from light

ADEQUATE NUTRITION

Dietary measures must ensure adequate nutrition and include high calorie, high protein, and high fat diets with liberal use of salt to encourage normal weight and growth. The needs are high due to the extra work involved with breathing and a hyper-metabolic state associated with bronchial infection. Due to poor fat absorption, patients use 1-2 multivitamins daily (with A, D, E and K), and some require additional doses.

Pancreatic Enzyme Products (PEPs)

The thick mucus obstructs pancreatic enzyme flow, resulting in a paucity of these enzymes reaching the gastrointestinal tract. Frequently, greasy, foul-smelling stools are manifestations of pancreatic insufficiency. Most CF patients need to supplement their diet with appropriate amounts of pancreatic enzyme supplements.

Pancrelipase is a natural product harvested from porcine pancreatic glands which contains a combination of lipase, amylase, and protease. PEPs are formulated to dissolve in the more basic pH of the duodenum so they can act locally to break down fat, starches and protein. The dose is individualized for each patient and is based on the lipase component. Once enzyme therapy is started, the dose is adjusted every 3-4 days until stools are normalized. Do not use doses > 6,000 units/kg/meal of lipase due to colonic stricture risk.

Enzymes are given prior to meals and snacks: full doses are given before meals and 50% of the mealtime dose is given with snacks. Meals with high fat content require higher doses. Counsel patients not to chew or crush the capsules. If a patient cannot swallow them whole, the microsphere-contents can be sprinkled on soft food with a low pH that does not require chewing (such as applesauce, gelatin, baby food). Do not mix with milk-based foods, such as yogurt or pudding since these have a higher pH. There is also a powder formulation. Take the entire dose at the beginning of each meal or snack along with a generous amount of liquid. Retention in the mouth before swallowing may cause mucosal irritation and stomatitis.

Do not substitute pancreatic enzyme products. This is an FDA recommendation. They do not require refrigeration. If infants spit them out, immediately follow with liquid until swallowed.

DRUG	DOSING	SAFETY/SIDE EFFECTS/MONITORING
Pancrelipase (Creon, Lip-Prot-Amyl, Pancreaze, Pertzye, Ultresa, Viokace, Zenpep)	**Initial** Age < 4 years: Lipase 1,000 units/kg/meal Age ≥ 4 years: Lipase 500 units/kg/meal **Max (all ages)** Lipase ≤ 2,500 units/kg/meal or ≤ 10,000 units/kg/day. Doses > 6,000 units/kg/meal are associated with colonic stricture. Take before or with food, avoid foods with high pH such as dairy. Use 1/2 meal-time dose with snacks. Keep in original container; protect from moisture.	**WARNING** Caution for risk of (rare) fibrosing colonopathy: Symptoms include severe abdominal pain, bloating, difficulty passing stools, nausea, vomiting, diarrhea. Risk higher with doses > 10,000 lipase units/kg/day. **SIDE EFFECTS** Mucosal irritation, abdominal pain, nausea, headache, neck pain **MONITORING** Abdominal symptoms, nutritional intake, weight, height (children), stool, fecal fat **NOTES** MedGuide required. *Viokace* is the only formulation not enteric coated and needs to be given with PPI. All formulations are porcine derived and are not interchangeable. Do not crush or chew contents of capsules. Delayed-release capsules with enteric coated microspheres or microtablets may be opened and sprinkled on soft, acidic foods (pH ≤ 4.5). MedGuide required

Pancreatic Enzyme Counseling (Children)

- This medication comes with an extra patient fact sheet called a Medication Guide. Read it carefully. The Medication Guide discusses a rare, but serious allergic reaction that can happen with some people.

- This medication is taken at the beginning of a meal or snack. At snacks give half the meal-time dose.

- Have your child swallow whole. Do not let your child chew or crush or hold in the mouth or the medicine will cause the mouth to become sore.

- If it is difficult to swallow the capsules, the contents can be sprinkled on a spoonful of soft food such as applesauce, pureed bananas, or pears. Once the contents are sprinkled on the food it needs to be used right away. Do not let your child chew it, just swallow.

- Do not mix with dairy products such as milk or yogurt.

- Have your child drink lots of non-caffeinated liquids every day.

- It is important to follow the diet plan you received for your child to get adequate nutrition and to keep as healthy as possible.

- Common side effects can include stomach pain, nausea, headache, and neck pain.

- If you forget to give the medicine before the meal give it as soon you remember, but if it is close to time for the next dose, skip it and go back to the usual schedule.

Cystic Fibrosis Transmembrane Conductance Regulator (CFTR) Potentiator

Ivacaftor is approved for the treatment of CF in patients ≥ 6 years of age who have one of the following mutations in the cystic fibrosis transmembrane conductance regulator (CFTR) gene: G551D, G1244E, G1349D, G178R, G551S, S1251N, S1255P, S549N, or S549R. Ivacaftor works by increasing the time CFTR channels remain open, augmenting chloride transport activity.

DRUG	DOSING/INDICATIONS	SAFETY/SIDE EFFECTS/MONITORING
Ivacaftor (Kalydeco)	150 mg PO Q12H with high fat containing food With CYP3A4 moderate inhibitors or moderate-severe hepatic impairment: 150 mg daily With CYP3A4 strong inhibitors: 150 mg twice weekly	**SIDE EFFECTS** Headache, URTIs, nasal congestion, oropharyngeal pain, abdominal pain, rash **MONITORING** LFTs (baseline, every 3 months for 1 year, then annually), CF mutation test, FEV_1

PRACTICE CASE

GA is a 6 y/o white female with cystic fibrosis. Her parents brought her to the pediatric clinic today because of a 2-day history of mild cough and increased sputum production. Her pulmonary function tests are at her baseline.

Allergies: NKDA

Medications:
Multivitamin daily
ZenPep 20,000 units TID with meals
Albuterol nebulization solution 2.5 mg BID

Vitals:
BP: 101/69 mmHg   HR: 112 BPM   RR: 20 BPM   Temp: 98.6°F

Labs: Na (mEq/L) = 142 (135 - 145)
K (mEq/L) = 3.5 (3.5 - 5)
Cl (mEq/L) = 97 (95 - 103)
HCO_3 (mEq/L) = 27 (24 - 30)
BUN (mg/dL) = 13 (7 - 20)
SCr (mg/dL) = 1.1 (0.6 - 1.3)
Glucose (mg/dL) = 129 (100 - 125)
Ca (mg/dL) = 10.1 (8.5 - 10.5)
Mg (mEq/L) = 2.0 (1.3 - 2.1)
PO_4 (mg/dL) = 4.2 (2.3 - 4.7)
Hgb (g/dL) = 13.3 (13.5 - 18 male, 12 - 16 female)
Hct (%) = 42 (38 - 50 male, 36 - 46 female)
Plt (cells/mm^3) = 315 (150 - 450 x 10^3)
PMNs (%) = 90 (45 - 73)
Bands (%) = 7 (3 - 5)
Eosinophils (%) = 2 (0 - 5)
Basophils (%) = 0 (0 - 1)
Lymphocytes (%) = 37 (20 - 40)
Monocytes (%) = 3 (2 - 8)

Tests: Sputum culture: *Staphylococcus aureus*

Questions

1. Which one of the following is the best pharmacologic intervention for management of GA's airway disease at this time?

    a. Tobramycin via *Podhaler* 112 mg twice daily for 28 days

    b. Aztreonam 75 mg via *Altera nebulizer* three times daily for 28 days

    c. Dornase alfa 2.5 mg once daily via nebulizer

    d. Increase albuterol to four times daily

    e. Decrease albuterol to once daily

2. GA returns to clinic 2 weeks later and her parents report that her symptoms are not improved. Her pulmonary function tests are reduced by 10%. Based on the above culture only, which of the following represents the best pharmacologic intervention at the present time?

    a. Cephalexin 500 mg 4 times/day

    b. Tobramycin via *Podhaler* 112 mg twice daily for 28 days

    c. Dornase alfa 2.5 mg once daily via nebulizer

    d. Aztreonam 75 mg via *Altera* nebulizer three times daily for 28 days

    e. Imipenem 500 mg IV Q 6 hours

3. Which of the following is a correct patient counseling recommendation for pancreatic enzyme replacement therapy?

    a. If the patient has difficulty swallowing the capsules the microspheres can be crushed and sprinkled over food.

    b. The enzymes should be taken with meals.

    c. The enzyme products are equivalent and can be interchanged, depending on formulary requirements.

    d. *Viokace* should be administered with an acidic liquid such as orange juice.

    e. Pancreatic enzymes should not be taken if the meal contains little or no fat content.

Questions 4-7 do not apply to the above case.

4. Which of the following are potential adverse effects associated with *TOBI* therapy? (Select **ALL** that apply.)

    a. Voice alteration

    b. Bronchospasm

    c. Ototoxicity

    d. Tinnitus

    e. Pulmonary infiltrates

5. Which of the following is an appropriate counseling recommendation for *TOBI Podhaler* therapy?

    a. Store capsules in the freezer at all times.

    b. Capsules should be taken orally on an empty stomach.

    c. Take twice daily; doses may be taken 4 hours apart.

    d. Remove only 1 capsule at a time immediately before administration.

    e. Instruct the patient to thoroughly chew (or crush) the tablets.

6. Which of the following therapies are used in promoting mucus clearance in patients with cystic fibrosis?

    a. Pseudoephedrine

    b. Hypertonic saline

    c. Tiotroprium

    d. Inhaled aztreonam

    e. Inhaled tobramycin

7. Which of the following are correct statements regarding dosing considerations for ivacaftor? (Select **ALL** that apply).

    a. The brand name is *Kaleidoscope XR*.

    b. Ivacaftor should be administered with a high fat containing meal.

    c. Dosage adjustment is necessary when co-administered with CYP3A4 inhibitors.

    d. Ivacaftor is nephrotoxic and is contraindicated in severe renal insufficiency.

    e. The normal dose is 150 mg by mouth every 12 hours.

Answers

1-c, 2-a, 3-b, 4-a,b,c,d, 5-d, 6-b, 7-b,c,e

50

ONCOLOGY I: OVERVIEW, PREVENTION, SCREENING & SIDE EFFECT MANAGEMENT

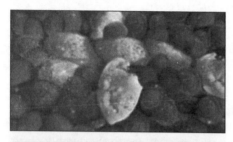

We gratefully acknowledge the assistance of Muoi Gi, PharmD, BCPS, BCOP, Oncology Pharmacy Residency Director, VA San Diego Healthcare System and D. Raymond Weber, PharmD, BSPharm, BCOP, BCPS, RPh, Associate Professor, University of Maryland Eastern Shore School of Pharmacy and Health Professions (rweberpharmd@umes.edu) and Amine Ale-Ali, PharmD, BCOP, Hematology-Oncology Pharmacist UCSD Moores Cancer Center, in preparing this chapter.

GUIDELINES

National Comprehensive Cancer Network (NCCN) website (www.nccn.org – by cancer type) and through the American Society of Clinical Oncology (ASCO) website (www.asco.org).

WARNING SIGNS

The American Cancer Society lists seven warning signs of cancer in an adult. Any of these warning signs should warrant referral to a physician:

Change in bowel or bladder habits

A sore that does not heal

Unusual bleeding or discharge

Thickening or lump in breast or elsewhere

Indigestion or difficulty swallowing

Obvious change in wart or mole

Nagging cough or hoarseness

BACKGROUND

Cancer is a group of diseases characterized by uncontrolled growth and spread of abnormal cells. If the spread is not controlled, it can result in death. Cancer is caused by both external factors (such as chemicals, radiation, bacteria and viruses) and internal factors (heredity, hormones, immune disorders, and genetic mutations). Age is certainly a factor. Sunlight exposure, tobacco use, excessive alcohol intake, obesity, poor diet and low physical activity level increases the risk for certain types of cancer.

CLASSIFICATION

Malignancies are classified based on the tissue type as epithelial, connective, lymphoid or nerve. A sample of tissue (biopsy) should be taken for diagnosis along with X-rays, CT scans, MRIs and other diagnostic tools to evaluate the cancer's stage. Lab work is required for blood chemistries and tumor markers.

CANCER SCREENING RECOMMENDATIONS

Cancer Screening Guidelines (Average Risk)

CANCER	ACS GUIDELINES	NCCN GUIDELINES	USPSTF
Breast	Age: 20-39 (CBE every 3 years) Age: ≥ 40 (CBE + mammography yearly)	Age: 25-39 (CBE every 1-3 years) Age: ≥ 40 (CBE + mammography yearly)	Age: 40s (start discussion) Age: 50-74 (mammography every 2 years)
Cervical	Age: 21-29 (Pap smear only every 3 years) Age: 30-65 [Pap only every 3 years or Pap + HPV testing (preferred) every 5 years]	Same as ACS guidelines	Same as ACS guidelines
Colon	Age: ≥ 50 [(annual FOBT or FIT or stool DNA every 3 years; and 1 of the following: every 5 years sigmoidoscopy, contrast enema, CT scan, or colonoscopy (every 10 years)]	Age: ≥ 50 (Colonoscopy every 10 years, or sigmoidoscopy every 5 years ± interval stool-based testing at year 3, or annual FOBT or FIT)	Age: 50-75 (annual FOBT, sigmoidoscopy every 5 years with FOBT every 3 years, or colonoscopy every 10 years)
Prostate	Age: 50s (start discussion) (if screened: PSA with or without DRE)	Age: 45-49 (if DRE normal, PSA > 1 ng/mL, repeat test Q1-2 years, if DRE normal, PSA ≤1 ng/mL, repeat test at age 50) Age: ≥ 50 (if DRE normal, PSA < 3 ng/mL, repeat test Q1-2 years)	Recommend against screening for prostate cancer
Lung (High Risk)	Age: 55-74 (in fairly good health) with ≥ 30 pack year smoking Hx and are either still smoking or have quit for < 15 years (low dose CT scan)	Age: 55-74 with ≥ 30 pack year smoking Hx and quit for < 15 years (low dose CT scan) Age: ≥ 50 with ≥ 20 pack year smoking Hx and 1 additional risk factor other than 2nd hand smoke (low dose CT scan)	Age: 55-80 with ≥ 30 pack year smoking Hx and are either still smoking or have quit for < 15 years (annual low dose CT scan)

ACS: American Cancer Society; CBE: Clinical Breast Exam; DRE: Digital Rectal Exam; FIT: Fecal Immunochemical Test; FOBT: Fecal Occult Blood Test; HPV: Human Papilloma Virus; NCCN: National Comprehensive Cancer Network; PSA: Prostate-Specific Antigen; USPSTF; United States Preventive Services Task Force

Everyone should be encouraged to maintain a healthy lifestyle to reduce cancer risk:

- Avoid tobacco (enroll in smoking cessation program if needed).

- Maintain a healthy weight.

- Exercise regularly.

- Eat healthy with plenty of fruits and vegetables.

- Limit alcohol intake.

- Protect skin from harmful UV rays.

- Assess cancer risk, family history, and individual history.

- Have regular check-ups and cancer screening tests.

TREATMENT OVERVIEW

Cancer can be treated with surgery, radiation, chemotherapy, hormone therapy, biological therapy, targeted therapy, immunotherapy and/or vaccines. Treatment decisions are based on the cancer type and stage and patient characteristics such as tumor markers. For most cancers (including breast, lung, prostate and colon cancer), the stage is classified by the size of the tumor and whether it has spread. Goals of treatment depend on prognosis. The plan may attempt to achieve remission (with curative intent) or be palliative (to reduce tumor size and symptoms). Most cancers will not relapse if a patient remains cancer-free for 5 years. These patients may be "cured" but are really considered cancer-free survivors. Response to treatment is classified as complete (no evidence of disease for at least 1 month) or partial (≥ ↓ in tumor size). Stable disease means < 25% decrease or increase in tumor size, and progression is ≥ 25% tumor growth or tumor growth in a new site.

Often, the primary treatment modality is surgery if the cancer is resectable. Neoadjuvant therapy (e.g., radiation or chemotherapy) may be used prior to surgery to shrink the tumor initially. Adjuvant therapy (may include radiation and/or chemotherapy) is given after surgery in an attempt to eradicate residual disease and ↓ recurrence.

Sometimes, surgery is not an option for initial treatment and the treatment regimen begins with chemotherapy. This is called primary induction chemotherapy.

Chemotherapeutic regimens are usually designed for synergism. Drugs with different mechanisms of action that complement each other are chosen. Synergy will not work unless each drug is active on the tumor independently. Most drugs work on rapidly dividing DNA since they work by damaging the replication cycle. They may work on different phases of the cell cycle or are phase non-specific (discussed in the next chapter). The success or failure of previous treatments is an important consideration in recurrent disease.

Chemotherapeutic regimens can be highly toxic, therefore managing adverse events is part of the treatment plan. The majority of adverse effects are due to damaging effects on non-cancerous, rapidly dividing cells in the GI tract, hair follicles and bone marrow (blood cells). Thus, nausea and vomiting, alopecia, and myelosuppression are common side effects of most chemotherapy. Due to these severe side effects, the patient's quality of life must be assessed with rating systems such as the Karnofsky and the ECOG (Eastern Cooperative Oncology Group) toxicity and performance status scales. Many patient factors can affect treatment choice such as: age, co-morbidities and/or previous treatments. A patient's quality of life may lead the clinician and family to choose palliative measures (to reduce the symptoms) over a more aggressive treatment plan with side effects that could be intolerable to the patient.

Danger During Pregnancy & Breastfeeding

Chemotherapy should be avoided during pregnancy and breastfeeding, although some patients treated while pregnant have delivered healthy babies. Counsel both male and female patients to avoid conceiving during treatment and to consider using barrier methods to avoid contact with body fluids. Some of the medications can cause long-term sterility.

SUMMARY OF TOXICITIES

For studying purposes, it is best to group drugs based on similar side effects. These side effects are discussed here and the drug/drug classes are discussed in more detail in the next chapter.

- Myelosuppression: (↓ in bone marrow activity leading to ↓ RBCs, WBCs and platelets) caused by most oncology drugs, therefore complete blood cell count with differential must be routinely monitored. The few that do not cause this side effect include: asparaginase, bleomycin, vincristine and most of the monoclonal antibodies (mAbs).

- Neuropathy: associated with platinum agents, proteosome inhibitors, taxanes and vinca alkaloids.

- Cardiotoxicity: caused by chest radiation and drugs such as anthracyclines, tyrosine kinase inhibitors (such as imatinib, nilotinib, and dasatinib), and breast cancer drugs (trastuzumab and lapatinib). These drugs require monitoring via ECG, ECHO or MUGA. Arsenic trioxide requires ECG and electrolyte (Mg^{2+}, K^+) monitoring at baseline and weekly while on treatment to assess for QT prolongation.

- Pulmonary toxicity: associated with require pulmonary function tests if a high-risk agent, including alkylators (busulfan, carmustine, and lomustine), bleomycin and methotrexate. Monitor pulmonary function tests.

- Nephrotoxicity/Bladder toxicity: nephrotoxicity is caused by bevacizumab, methotrexate, and platinum agents (cisplatin and carboplatin). Amifostine (Ethyol) may be used to reduce the risk of cisplatin-induced renal toxicity. Cyclophosphamide and ifosfamide cause bladder toxicity. Mesna (Mesnex) is always given with ifosfamide to prevent hemorrhagic cystitis and with high-doses of cyclophosphamide. Hydration is used to flush the drug out and prevent bladder and/or renal toxicity. Monitor the BUN, SCr, urinalysis, and urine output.

- Acneiform rash: caused by cetuximab, erlotinib, panitumumab, sorafenib, sunitinib. These are all agents that inhibit EGFR.

- Mucositis: inflammation of the GI tract and can develop into painful, burning ulcers. High risk agents include 5-fluorouracil, capecitabine, irinotecan, and methotrexate.

- Hand-foot syndrome: occurs with many oral chemotherapy agents, including capecitabine, pazopanib, sorafenib, sunitinib and vemurafenib, and the IV agents, 5-fluorouracil, liposomal doxorubicin and cytarabine.

(Doxil®)
and liposomal daunorubicin (DaunoXome®)
* liposomal formulations cause hand & foot syndrome,
   not so much non-liposomal formulations

- **Hepatotoxicity**: caused by antiandrogens, the folate and pyrimidine analog antimetabolites (including methotrexate), aromatase inhibitors, busulfan, ixabepilone, SERMs, taxanes, some tyrosine kinase inhibitors and the vinca alkaloids. Monitor liver enzymes and symptoms.

- **Clotting risk**: occurs with the SERMs, bevacizumab (anti-VEGF agents) and some immunomodulators (thalidomide, lenalidamide, pomalidomide). Monitor for DVT/PE.

- **Alopecia**: thinning or complete loss of hair. Most notably the taxanes and anthracyclines cause hair loss in nearly 100% of patients including loss of the eyebrows, eyelashes and pubic hair. Other agents that cause alopecia include carboplatin, cyclophosphamide, etoposide, ifosfamide and the vinca alkaloids.

- **Extravasation**: leakage of drug from the vein into the extravascular space. Vesicants are drugs known to cause tissue necrosis with extravasation, which can require surgical debridement and skin grafting. Each oncology agent should have an extravasation protocol which needs to be followed. Minimally, stop the infusion, elevate the limb, use cold compresses (except with the vinca alkaloids and etoposide, use warm compresses – as cold worsens tissue ulceration). Tissue damage from extravasation can occur with these agents: anthracyclines, ixabepilone, mitomycin, mechlorethamine, teniposide and the vinca alkaloids. Common antidotes used for extravasation include:

  - Dimethyl sulfoxide (DMSO) or dexrazoxane *(Totect)* for the anthracyclines.
  - Hyaluronidase for the vinca alkaloids. *[handwritten: also for extravasation from nafcillin]*
  - Sodium thiosulfate for mechlorethamine.

MANAGEMENT OF SIDE EFFECTS

Chemotherapeutic agents are toxic to the tumor and to the rest of the patient. Many pharmacists are directly involved with cancer treatment and assist patients with the complications of chemotherapy. All pharmacists should be able to assist with the related therapies while specialists are required to help manage the chemotherapeutic regimens.

This section discusses the treatment of myelosuppression (primarily anemia, neutropenia and thrombocytopenia), nausea/vomiting, mucositis, hand-foot syndrome and hypercalcemia of malignancy. Weight loss/gain is a separate chapter, and the drugs used for tumor lysis syndrome are discussed in the Gout chapter.

[handwritten: dexrazoxane (Totec®, Zinecard®)
• FDA - ① ♡ myopathy 2° to doxorubicin
② cytotoxic inj site extravasation]

Myelosuppression Overview

Myelosuppression (↓ in bone marrow activity resulting in fewer RBCs, WBCs and platelets) is a complication of most chemotherapeutic agents. Neutrophils and platelets are often affected since these cells have short lifespans and rapid turnover. If WBCs decrease, the immune system will become depressed and the patient will have trouble fighting an infection. If RBCs decrease, the patient becomes anemic, experiencing weakness and fatigue. If platelets decrease, there is an increased risk of severe bleeding.

The lowest point that WBCs and platelets reach (the nadir) occurs about 7-14 days after chemotherapy, although some agents have a delayed effect. RBC nadir is much later due to their long life span (~120 days). WBCs and platelets generally recover 3-4 weeks post treatment. The next dose of chemotherapy is given after the cells have returned to a safe level. Medications may be necessary to help restore blood cell counts. Severe cases may require a transfusion (providing the deficient cell line directly, such as giving packed RBCs for severe anemia). All agents used for myelosuppression discussed here are usually given by subcutaneous injection, either by the patient, caregiver or medical provider.

Anemia

In the past, anemia was routinely treated with an erythropoiesis-stimulating agent (ESA). However, most anemias are not life-threatening and there is now awareness that ESAs can shorten survival and ↑ tumor progression in some cancers. This has resulted in much less frequent use of ESAs. To make sure that patients are aware of the risks, MedGuides are dispensed at the initiation of therapy. For cancer, the use of ESAs must fulfill the requirements of the ESA APPRISE Oncology Program. This is a REMS (Risk Evaluation and Mitigation Strategies) program to make sure healthcare providers are trained and patients receive proper counseling on the risks and benefits of therapy. ESAs are associated with this and other boxed warnings and are not commonly used in oncology.

Hemoglobin (Hgb) levels are used to assess anemia. Anemia may recover on its own, be treated with a RBC transfusion, or rarely, with an ESA. Normal Hgb levels are 12-16 g/dL for females and 13.5-18 g/dL for males (hematocrit is 36-46% females; 38-50% males). Serum ferritin, transferrin saturation (TSAT) and total iron-binding capacity (TIBC) may be ordered to assess iron storage and transport since the ESAs will not work well to correct the anemia if iron levels are inadequate. Levels of folate and vitamin B12 may need to be evaluated, especially if there is a poor response to the ESA.

normal Hgb		Hct
♀	12-16 g/dl	36-46%
♂	13.5-18 g/dl	38-50%

Erythropoiesis-Stimulating Agents (ESAs)

Hgb must be <10 g/dl to use

DRUG	DOSING	SAFETY/SIDE EFFECTS/MONITORING
Epoetin alfa **(Epogen, Procrit)**	150 units/kg SC 3x/week or 40,000 units SC weekly Initiate ESA when Hgb < 10 g/dL and when at least 2 additional months of chemo planned.	**BOXED WARNINGS** ESAs ↑ risk of death, MI, stroke, VTE, thrombosis of vascular access, and tumor progression or recurrence. **CANCER** ESAs ↓ overall survival and/or ↑ risk of tumor progression or recurrence in clinical studies of patients with breast, head and neck, nonsmall cell lung, lymphoid, and cervical cancers. Prescribers and hospitals must enroll in and comply with the ESA APPRISE Oncology Program to prescribe and/or dispense these agents to cancer patients. Use ESAs only for anemia due to myelosuppressive chemotherapy. ESAs are not indicated when the anticipated outcome is cure. Use the lowest effective dose to avoid RBC transfusions.
Darbepoetin **(Aranesp)**	2.25 mcg/kg weekly or 500 mcg SC every 3 weeks Initiate ESA when Hgb < 10 g/dL and when at least 2 additional months of chemo planned.	Discontinue following completion of a chemotherapy course. **CONTRAINDICATIONS** Uncontrolled hypertension; pure red cell aplasia (PRCA) that begins after treatment; multidose vials containing benzyl alcohol contraindicated in neonates, infants, pregnancy and lactation. **SIDE EFFECTS** Hypertension, fever, headache, arthralgia/bone pain, pruritus/rash, nausea, cough, injection site pain, thrombosis, edema, chills, dizziness **MONITORING** Hgb, Hct, transferrin saturation, serum ferritin, BP **NOTES** Store in refrigerator. Protect vials from light. The doses of ESAs for chemo-induced anemia are much higher than the doses used for anemia due to chronic renal disease. If Hgb increases > 1 g/dL in any 2-week period, ↓ dose by 25% for epoetin alfa and ↓ dose by 40% for darbepoetin alfa. MedGuide required

if Hgb ↑ by > 1 g/dl in 2 wks ⇒ ↓ dose by 25%

if Hgb ↑ by > 1 g/dl in 2 wks ⇒ ↓ dose by 40%

Neutropenia

A low neutrophil count ↑ infection risk and makes it difficult for the human body to fight an infection. The more neutropenic the patient is, the higher the risk of infection.

Neutropenia Definition (American Society of Clinical Oncology)

CATEGORY	ANC
Neutropenia	< 1,000 mmol/L
Severe Neutropenia	< 500 mmol/L
Profound Neutropenia	< 100 mmol/L

Know how to calculate the ANC; this is reviewed in the Calculations chapter.

The colony stimulating factors (CSFs) are called "myeloid growth factors." Myeloid refers to the granulocyte precursor cell, which differentiates into neutrophils, eosinophils, and basophils. These agents are expensive and have not been shown to improve overall survival outcomes. They do shorten the time that a patient is at risk for infection due to neutropenia and reduce mortality from infections when given prophylactically in patients at high risk for febrile neutropenia. Consequently, their use is usually limited to conditions outlined in an institution's protocol which define criteria for use. There are three types: GM-CSF (sargramostim), G-CSF (filgrastim) and pegylated G-CSF (pegfilgrastim). GM-CSF is limited to use in stem cell transplantation. Both forms of G-CSF are indicated in febrile neutropenia.

The NCCN recommends all patients with > 20% chance of developing chemotherapy-induced febrile neutropenia to receive myeloid growth factors. The use of growth factors in intermediate-risk patients is more controversial.

DRUG	DOSING	SAFETY/SIDE EFFECTS/MONITORING
Sargramostim (Leukine) GM-CSF Limited to use in stem cell transplantation	250 mcg/m²/day given IV/SC daily; treat through post-nadir recovery	**SIDE EFFECTS** Filgrastim/pegfilgrastim/tbo-filgrastim: bone pain, fever, generalized rash, injection site reaction Sargramostim: fever, bone pain, arthralgias, myalgias, rash, dyspnea, peripheral edema, pericardial effusion, cardiovascular edema, HTN, chest pain
Filgrastim (Neupogen) G-CSF	5-10 mcg/kg/day given IV/SC daily (round to the nearest 300 mcg or 480 mcg vial size); treat through post-nadir recovery	**MONITORING** CBC with differential, pulmonary function, weight, vital signs
Pegfilgrastim (Neulasta) Pegylated G-CSF Long acting: relatively equivalent to 14 daily doses of filgrastim	1 prefilled syringe (6 mg) SC once per chemo cycle	**NOTES** Store in refrigerator. Protect vials from light. Administer first dose 24-72 hours after chemo. Patients should report any signs of enlarged spleen (pain in left upper abdomen or respiratory distress syndrome). Must document when pegfilgrastim was given; it should not be given within 14 days before or 24 hours after chemo. All others should not be given before or within 24 hours after chemo.
Tbo-filgrastim (Granix) G-CSF	5 mcg/kg/day given SC daily (round to nearest 300 mcg or 480 mcg pre-filled syringe); treat through post-nadir recovery	

Handwritten notes: "for febrile neutropenia" (pointing to Filgrastim/Pegfilgrastim); "DON'T GIVE W/IN 14 DAYS BEFORE OR 24 HRS AFTER CHEMO"

Thrombocytopenia

Handwritten note: oprelvekin (Neumega®) to ↑ PLTs

Low platelets (thrombocytes) can result in spontaneous, uncontrolled bleeding. The normal range for platelets is 150,000-450,000/mm³. Chemotherapy dose may be reduced or placed on hold until the platelet count recovers. Platelet transfusions are generally indicated when the count falls below 10,000/mm³ (or 20,000/mm³ if active bleed is present).

Chemotherapy-Induced Nausea and Vomiting (CINV)

Nausea and vomiting are common with chemotherapy. Patient factors which ↑ risk of nausea and vomiting include: female gender, < 50 years of age, dehydration, history of motion sickness, and history of nausea and vomiting with prior regimens. For chemotherapy-induced nausea and vomiting (CINV), administer anti-emetics at least 30 minutes prior to chemotherapy and provide take-home anti-emetic medication (such as ondansetron, prochlorperazine, or metoclopramide) for breakthrough nausea and vomiting.

Emetic Risk Potential of IV Antineoplastic Agents (per NCCN guidelines)

HIGH EMETIC RISK	MODERATE EMETIC RISK	LOW EMETIC RISK	MINIMAL EMETIC RISK
> 90% frequency of emesis	30%-90% frequency of emesis	10%-30% frequency of emesis	< 10% frequency of emesis
AC combination (doxorubicin or epirubicin with cyclophosphamide)	Aldesleukin > 12-15 million units/m²	Aldesleukin ≤ 12 million units/m²	Majority of the monoclonal antibodies (bevacizumab, cetuximab, ipilimumab, panitumumab, pertuzumab, rituximab, trastuzumab)
Cisplatin	Arsenic trioxide	Cabazitaxel	
Cyclophosphamide > 1,500 mg/m²	Bendamustine	Carfilzomib	Bleomycin
Doxorubicin ≥ 60 mg/m²	Carboplatin	Docetaxel	Bortezomib
Dacarbazine	Cyclophosphamide ≤ 1,500 mg/m²	5-FU	Vinca alkaloids
Epirubicin > 90 mg/m²	Daunorubicin	Gemcitabine	
Ifosfamide ≥ 2 g/m² per dose	Doxorubicin < 60 mg/m²	Paclitaxel	
	Epirubicin ≤ 90 mg/m²	Pemetrexed	
	Idarubicin	Etoposide	
	Ifosfamide < 2 g/m² per dose	Ixabepilone	
	Interferon alfa ≥ 10 million units/m²	Mitoxantrone	
	Irinotecan	Topotecan	
	Oxaliplatin		

Emetic Risk Potential of Oral Antineoplastic Agents (per NCCN guidelines)

MODERATE TO HIGH RISK	MINIMAL TO LOW RISK
Cyclophosphamide ≥ 100 mg/m²/day	Capecitabine
Crizotinib	Mercaptopurine
Etoposide	Methotrexate
Lomustine (single day)	Temozolomide ≤ 75 mg/m²/day
Procarbazine	Majority of the TKIs (dasatinib, erlotinib, imatinib, nilotinib, sunitinib, sorafenib)
Temozolomide > 75 mg/m²/day	Immunomodulators (lenalidomide, pomalidomide, thalidomide)
Vismodegib	

Anti-Emetic Regimens for Acute/Delayed Nausea & Vomiting

High Emetic Risk Chemotherapy

steroid + 5HT₃ antag + olanzapine or NK 1 antag

High emetic risk is managed by a 3-drug combination based on either a neurokinin 1 receptor antagonist or olanzapine. Both regimens include a steroid and a 5HT$_3$ antagonist.

NEUROKININ 1 RECEPTOR ANTAGONIST CONTAINING REGIMEN

DRUG	DAY 1	DAY 2	DAY 3	DAY 4
Neuokinin 1 receptor antagonist and	Aprepitant 125 mg PO or	80 mg PO	80 mg PO	–
	Fosaprepitant 150 mg IV*	–	–	–
Dexamethasone and	12 mg PO/IV (with aprepitant) or	8 mg PO	8 mg PO	8 mg PO
	12 mg PO/IV (with fosaprepitant)*	8 mg PO*	8 mg PO BID*	8 mg PO BID*
Ondansetron or	16-24 mg PO or	–	–	–
	8-16 mg IV			
Granisetron or	2 mg PO or	–	–	–
	0.01 mg/kg IV (max 1 mg) or			
	3.1 mg patch (applied 24-48 hrs before chemo)			
Dolasetron† or	100 mg PO	–	–	–
Palonosetron	0.25 mg IV (preferred)	–	–	–

± Lorazepam 0.5-2 mg PO/IV/SL Q4-6H on days 1-4

± H$_2$RA or proton pump inhibitor

* Fosaprepitant 150 mg IV once on Day 1 lasts up to 72 hours post chemotherapy, thus neuokinin 1 receptor antagonist regimen is not needed on days 2-4.

† Dolasetron IV is contraindicated in CINV due to incidence of QT prolongation

Note: Use this regimen for patients receiving combination of an anthracycline and cyclophosphamide and select patients receiving other chemotherapies of moderate emetic risk (e.g., carboplatin, cisplatin, doxorubicin, epirubicin, ifosfamide, irinotecan or methotrexate).

OLANZAPINE-CONTAINING REGIMEN

DRUG	DAY 1	DAY 2	DAY 3	DAY 4
Olanzapine and	10 mg PO	10 mg PO	10 mg PO	10 mg PO
Dexamethasone and	20 mg IV	–	–	–
Palonosetron	0.25 mg IV	–	–	–

± Lorazepam 0.5-2 mg PO/IV/SL Q4-6H on days 1-4

± H$_2$RA or proton pump inhibitor

Moderate Emetic Risk Chemotherapy

→ steroid + 5HT₃ antag ± NK 1 antag
alternative: olanzapine regimen

Moderate emetic risk is managed by a 2-drug combination of a steroid and 5-HT$_3$ antagonist, with or without a neurokinin 1 antagonist (for select patients, where appropriate). As an alternative, an olanzapine-containing regimen could be used as well.

Low Emetic Risk Chemotherapy

[handwritten annotation: 1 drug]

[handwritten annotation: 5HT₃ antag OR steroid OR prochlorperazine OR metoclopramide]

Low emetic risk is managed by a 1-drug regimen of either a 5-HT₃ antagonist, dexamethasone, prochlorperazine or metoclopramide.

Delayed emesis (defined as vomiting ocurring > 24 hours after chemotherapy) can be prevented with dexamethasone, aprepitant or palonosetron, alone or in combination depending on the risk and severity (note that palonosetron is the only 5-HT₃ receptor antagonist with proven efficacy in delayed CINV). At any point, an adjunct such as lorazepam (Ativan) may be added for anxiety/amnestic response or a H₂RA or PPI if upper GI symptoms similar to GERD are present.

Prochlorperazine or a similar phenothiazine-like agent, antihistamines (diphenhydramine or others), or metoclopramide (Reglan) are sometimes used, however each has safety concerns. Phenothiazines and metoclopramide are dopamine-blocking agents and could cause or worsen movement disorders. Both classes are sedating and can cause cognitive dysfunction. Metoclopramide requires a reduced dose with renal dysfunction. When overdosed, the side effect profile is worsened. Centrally-acting antihistamines such as diphenhydramine can cause central and peripheral anticholinergic side effects, which may be intolerable in elderly patients (refer to discussion in the Overactive Bladder chapter).

Dronabinol (Marinol) and nabilone (Cesamet) can be used as second line agents. These are synthetic analogs of delta-9-tetrahydrocannabinol, a naturally occurring component of Cannabis sativa (marijuana). The DEA classifies Cannabis, (marijuana, used in the plant form) as a schedule I drug, however it can be purchased for medical and nonmedical use in some states, and in some jurisdictions can be purchased for medical use only.

[handwritten notes:]

delayed emesis = vomiting > 24 hrs after chemo
↳ prevent w/ [dexamethasone / aprepitant / palonosetron — only 5HT₃ antag w/ proven efficacy in delayed CINV]
  alone or combo

* may + lorazepam (for anxiety/amnestic response)
  OR   H₂ blocker or PPI (for GERD-like sx)

• DA blockers ⟵ prochlorperazine / antihistamines (Benadryl®, etc.) / metoclopramide (Reglan®) } may also use but safety concerns
  ⟹ movement d/o
• sedating
• cogn. dysfxn

2nd line
dronabinol (Marinol®) } synthetic analogs
nabilone (Cesamet®) } of marijuana

Antiemetic Agents

DRUG	DOSING	SAFETY/SIDE EFFECTS/MONITORING

5-HT₃ receptor antagonists work by blocking serotonin, both peripherally on vagal nerve terminals and centrally in the chemoreceptor trigger zone.

DRUG	DOSING	SAFETY/SIDE EFFECTS/MONITORING
Ondansetron (Zofran, Zuplenz film) Tablet, injection, solution, ODT, film	High risk: 8-16 mg IV or 16-24 mg PO on day 1 of chemo Moderate risk: 8-16 mg IV or 16-24 mg PO on day 1 of chemo, 8-16 mg IV/PO on days 2 and 3 Low risk: 16-24 mg PO daily Breakthrough nausea: 16 mg IV/PO daily PRN Single max IV dose is 16 mg; max PO dose is 24 mg	**CONTRAINDICATIONS** Concomitant use of apomorphine (Apokyn) with ondansetron; do not use dolasetron IV for acute CINV (due to QT prolongation). **WARNINGS** Dose-dependent ↑ in QT interval (torsade de pointes) - more common with IV Serotonin syndrome when used in combination with other serotonergic agents **SIDE EFFECTS** Headache, fatigue, dizziness, constipation **NOTES** Pregnancy Category B
Granisetron (Sancuso transdermal patch) Tablet, injection, solution, patch *Sancuso patch* 3.1 mg/24 hr	High, moderate, and low risk and breakthrough: 2 mg PO or 0.01 mg/kg (max 1 mg) IV on day 1 of chemo for high risk, 1-2 mg all days of chemo for moderate risk; PRN for breakthrough *Sancuso patch* - apply to upper arm 24-48 hrs before day 1 of chemo, leave on at least 24 hrs after last chemo session Can be worn up to 7 days	*Sancuso patch*: may be preferred in patients with mucositis, dysphagia or if expected to need up to 5 days of nausea prevention. Avoid sunlight near patch site. IV and oral 5-HT₃ antagonists are equally efficacious. If a patient failed one 5-HT₃ antagonist, try switching to another 5-HT₃ antagonist. Give 30 minutes prior to chemo (except patch). Palonosetron is preferred in the guidelines for high and moderate emetic risk.
Dolasetron (Anzemet)	High, moderate, and low risk and breakthrough: 100 mg PO once on day 1 of chemo for high risk and on all days of chemo for moderate/low risk; PRN for breakthrough	
Palonosetron (Aloxi) + netupitant (Akynzeo)	High and moderate risk: 0.25 mg IV once on day 1 of chemo One capsule 1 hour prior to chemotherapy	

Phenothiazines work by blocking dopamine receptors in the CNS, including the chemoreceptor trigger zone (among other mechanisms).

DRUG	DOSING	SAFETY/SIDE EFFECTS/MONITORING
Prochlorperazine (Compro)	10 mg IV/PO Q6H PRN May give 25 mg suppository PR Q12H PRN	**BOXED WARNING** Prochlorperazine: ↑ mortality in elderly patients with dementia-related psychosis. Promethazine: Do not use in children < 2 years old due to risk of respiratory depression. Do not give via intra-arterial or SC administration. Intravenous route can cause serious tissue injury if extravasation occurs.
Promethazine (Phenergan, Phenadoz, Promethegan)	12.5-25 mg PO/IV/PR Q4-6H PRN	**SIDE EFFECTS** Sedation, lethargy, hypotension, neuroleptic malignant syndrome (NMS), QT prolongation, acute EPS (common in children – antidote is diphenhydramine or benztropine), can lower seizure threshold, strong anticholinergic side effects.

Handwritten annotations:

avoid apomorphine w/ other 5HT₃ antag as well (Q #5 p.852)

≠ apomorphine (Apokyn®)

Kytril®

IV ≠ acute CINV (QT prolong)

preferred in high & mod emetic risk (guidelines)

↑ mortality in elderly (dementia-related psychosis)

⊖ subQ → gangrene!

⊖ children < 2 y/o - resp. depression intra-arterial or subQ

* IV → extravasation

dantrolene to cool pt?

↳ Cogentin®

Antiemetic Agents Continued

DRUG	DOSING	SAFETY/SIDE EFFECTS/MONITORING

Corticosteroid's mechanism of action of antiemetic activity is unknown.

| Dexamethasone (*Decadron*) | High risk: 12 mg PO/IV on day 1 of chemo, then 8 mg PO daily days 2-4 (with aprepitant) or 8 mg PO day 2, then 8 mg PO BID days 3 and 4 (with fosaprepitant)

Moderate risk: 12 mg PO/IV on day 1 of chemo, then 8 mg PO/IV days 2-3

Low risk and breakthrough: 12 mg PO/IV on day(s) of chemo or PRN for breakthrough | **CONTRAINDICATIONS**
Systemic fungal infections, cerebral malaria

SIDE EFFECTS
Short-term side effects include ↑ appetite/weight gain, fluid retention, emotional instability (euphoria, mood swings, irritability, acute psychosis), insomnia, GI upset. Higher doses can cause ↑ in BP and blood glucose (especially in patients with diabetes). |

Cannabinoids may work by activating cannabinoid receptors within the central nervous system and/or by inhibiting the vomiting control mechanism in the medulla oblongata.

| Dronabinol (*Marinol*)
Refrigerate capsules
C-III | 5-10 mg PO Q3H or Q6H | **SIDE EFFECTS**
Somnolence, euphoria, ↑ appetite, orthostatic hypotension |
| Nabilone (*Cesamet*)
No refrigeration needed
C-II | 1-2 mg PO BID, continue for up to 48H after last of chemo dose | |

Substance P/Neurokinin-1 receptor antagonists inhibit the substance P/neurokinin 1 receptor, therefore augmenting the antiemetic activity of 5HT$_3$ receptor antagonists and corticosteroids to inhibit acute and delayed phases of chemotherapy-induced emesis.

| Aprepitant (*Emend*) | PO: 125 mg given 1 hour before chemo, then 80 mg daily x 2 days or | **SIDE EFFECTS**
Dizziness, fatigue, constipation, weakness, hiccups |
| Fosaprepitant (*Emend for injection*) – prodrug of aprepitant IV
PRODRUG | IV: 150 mg given 30 minutes before chemo as single dose only (lasts up to 72 hours) | **NOTES**
Aprepitant ↑ the concentration of corticosteroids |

Mucositis

Inflammation of the GI tract can cause pain, ulceration and considerable suffering. There are some agents used to prevent and treat mucositis, such as "Magic Mouthwash" and chlorhexidine rinse, but only palifermin (*Kepivance*) is FDA approved for mucositis due to high dose chemo prior to stem cell transplant. Patients at risk for mucositis should be counseled to use saline rinses several times daily. Use of agents containing viscous lidocaine are effective in numbing the affected area locally. Patients can swish and spit the suspension.

Hand-Foot Syndrome

Hand-foot syndrome (also known as palmar-plantar erythrodysesthesia) can occur following the chemotherapy drugs listed previously. Small amounts of drug leak out of the capillaries and into the palms of the hands and the soles of the feet. Exposure of the hands and feet to heat as well as friction increases the amount of drug in the capillaries. This leakage results in redness, swelling, tenderness, pain, blisters and possibly peeling of the palms and soles. Dose reductions or delays in treatment are recommended if symptoms do not improve. Pyridoxine (vitamin B6) is no longer recommended as prophylaxis or treatment as it was found to be no better than placebo.

Prevention is very important in trying to reduce the development of hand-foot syndrome (see box).

Cooling procedures provide temporary relief of pain and tenderness. Using cold compresses like ice packs or frozen vegetables may reduce the severity of the pain (alternate cold packs on and off for 15-20 minutes at a time). Emollients such as petrolatum, *Udderly Smooth Cream* and *Bag Balm* provide excellent moisturizing for hands and feet; lotions do not provide adequate protection. Corticosteroids and pain medications may be used to help alleviate inflammation and pain.

HAND-FOOT SYNDROME PREVENTION

Limit daily activities to reduce friction and heat exposure to hands and feet for 1 week after IV medication (e.g., 5-Fluorouracil) or during the duration of oral exposure (e.g., capecitabine).

Avoid long exposure to hot water (washing dishes, showers). Take short showers in tepid water.

Avoid use of dishwashing gloves as the rubber will hold in the heat.

Avoid increased pressure on soles of feet (no jogging, aerobics, power walking, jumping).

Avoid increased pressure on palms of hands (do not use garden tools, screwdrivers, knives for chopping or performing other tasks that require squeezing hand(s) on a hard surface).

HYPERCALCEMIA OF MALIGNANCY

Prior to the therapeutic use of bisphosphonates in metastatic bone cancer, hypercalcemia occurred in ~25% of cancer patients and was the most common metabolic complication of breast cancer. It also occurs commonly with lung cancer and multiple myeloma. The bone destruction that results in hypercalcemia causes significant symptoms for the patient, including nausea, vomiting, fatigue, dehydration and mental status changes. Bone pain can be significant, and the complication carries a high risk of long-term skeletal damage (fractures, spinal cord compression, etc.) which is why bisphosphonates or denosumab *(Xgeva)* are used early in metastatic disease to prevent skeletal-related events. Denosumab blocks the interaction between RANKL and RANK (a receptor located on osteoclast surfaces), preventing osteoclast formation and leading to ↓ bone resorption. Denosumab, used in the prevention of skeletal-related events, is also indicated for osteoporosis under the brand name *Prolia*. Do not confuse *Xgeva* (120 mg SC monthly) with *Prolia* (60 mg SC every 6 months), see Osteoporosis chapter for further information.

Zoledronic also comes as two brand names for different indications, *Reclast* (5 mg/year) is used for osteoporosis while *Zometa* (4 mg/month) is used in oncology. Bisphosphonates require renal adjustment whereas denosumab, a monoclonal antibody, does not. All of these have a risk of osteonecrosis of the jaw (ONJ) which require discontinuation of therapy. Treatment for hypercalcemia of malignancy is summarized in the following table.

Hypercalcemia of Malignancy Treatment

TREATMENT	MOA	ONSET	DURATION	DEGREE OF HYPERCALCEMIA*
Hydration with normal saline and loop diuretics	↑ renal calcium excretion	Minutes to hours	Only during length of infusion	Mild Moderate Severe
Calcitonin	Inhibits bone resorption, ↑ renal calcium excretion	4-6 hours	48 hours max (risk of tachyphylaxis)	Moderate Severe
IV Bisphosphonates zoledronic acid (Zometa) 4 mg pamidronate (Aredia) 30-90 mg	Inhibits bone resorption by stopping osteoclast function	24-72 hours	2-4 weeks	Mild Moderate Severe

for osteoporosis Reclast© 5mg/yr *gmo*

Mild: corrected calcium < 12 mg/dL, Moderate: corrected calcium 12-14 mg/dL, Severe: corrected calcium > 14 mg/dL

Safe Handling of Hazardous Agents

Chemotherapy agents are hazardous drugs that are considered carcinogenic, mutagenic, and teratogenic. To limit exposure to these agents, pharmacies should have written procedures for handling these drugs safely. The United States Pharmacopeia (USP) chapter 800 regulates the preparation and handling of hazardous drugs and should be used by centers that prepare chemotherapy. Refer to the Medication Safety chapter for further information.

Routes of exposure include inhalation, ingestion, dermal contact, and accidental injections. The most common type of accidental exposure is inhalation of the aerosolized drug. A class II biologic safety cabinet should be used at all times in addition to chemo-gowns and chemo-block gloves (preferably double gloving). The gowns should be made of lint-free, low-permeability fabric with a solid front, long sleeves, and tight-fitting elastic cuffs. Negative-pressure techniques should be employed during drug preparation. Chemotherapy spill kits should be readily available and located in areas of the institution in which chemotherapy is handled. Cytotoxic waste should be disposed of properly, IV bags should be labeled "Chemotherapeutic: Dispose of Properly" or similar, and patients should be informed of proper methods of disposing of potentially contaminated body waste (such as flushing the toilet twice).

Timing of Vaccinations

Vaccination during chemotherapy should be avoided because the antibody response is suboptimal. When chemotherapy is being planned, vaccination should precede the initiation of chemotherapy by ≥ 2 weeks. The administration of live vaccines to immunocompromised patients must be avoided.

give vaccines 2+ weeks before chemo initiation

ONCOLOGY II: COMMON CANCER TYPES & TREATMENT

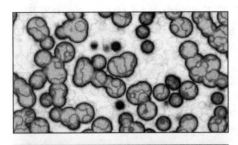

We gratefully acknowledge the assistance of Muoi Gi, PharmD, BCPS, BCOP, Oncology Pharmacy Residency Director at the VA San Diego Healthcare System, D. Raymond Weber, PharmD, BSPharm, BCOP, BCPS, RPh, University of Maryland Eastern Shore, School of Pharmacy and Health Professions (rweberpharmd@umes.edu) and Amine Ale-Ali, PharmD, BCOP, Hematology-Oncology Pharmacist UCSD Moores Cancer Center, in preparing this chapter.

GUIDELINES

National Comprehensive Cancer Network (NCCN). www.nccn.org (accessed 2014 November 10)

American Society of Clinical Oncology (ASCO). www.asco.org (accessed 2014 November 10)

CHEMOTHERAPY REGIMENS AND DOSING

In the preceeding section an overview of cancer treatment and management of major side effects were discussed. Cancer treatment depends on multiple factors, including cancer type, extent of disease and patient factors. When chemotherapy is used, the regimens are usually in combinations chosen for efficacy, synergy and ability to target cells with different resistance mechanisms and different stages of replication. There are many regimens such as the ABVD regimen used for Hodgkin's lymphoma [Adriamycin (doxorubicin), Bleomycin, Vinblastine, Dacarbazine] and the FOLFOX regimen used for colorectal cancer [FOLinic acid (leucovorin), Fluorouracil, OXaliplatin].

Regimens are usually administered in cycles involving one or more drugs, given once, or multiple times, such as over several consecutive days, followed by days or weeks without treatment. The break in treatment will give the patient, including the patient's cell lines, time to recover.

Body Surface Area (BSA) Calculations

Chemotherapy may be dosed using flat or fixed dosing, patient's weight (mg/kg), or patient's body surface area (BSA). There are four BSA formulas: 1. DuBois and DuBois, 2. Mosteller, 3.

Haycock, and 4. Gehan and George. These formulas may produce slightly different BSAs and, consequently, a different drug dosage. The one most commonly used in adult oncology practice is the DuBois and DuBois formula. Oncology pharmacists will use a plug-in calculator to get the result as the formula is complex. This is followed by the Mosteller formula, which is also used in adults. The weight that is commonly used for calculating the dose in oncology is the actual weight; sometimes the adjusted weight is used if the patient is overweight or treatment intent is palliative. Use the actual weight unless instructed otherwise by the oncologist or the exam. In practice, note the weight used since the weight changes the dose.

Dubois and Dubois Equation

$$\text{BSA (m}^2) = 0.007184 \times \text{Height(cm)}^{0.725} \times \text{Weight(kg)}^{0.425} \quad \times 250 \times 2$$

(handwritten: 162.56 above Height; 61.36 above Weight)

Example

A patient has a weight of 175 pounds and height of 6'1". Calculate the patient's BSA using the DuBois and DuBois formula. Round to the nearest hundredth.

Convert weight in pounds to kilograms by dividing by 2.2: 175/2.2 = 79.5 kg
Convert height in inches to centimeters by multiplying by 2.54: 73" x 2.54 = 185.4 cm

$$\text{BSA (m}^2) = 0.007184 \times \text{Height(cm)}^{0.725} \times \text{Weight(kg)}^{0.425}$$

$$\text{BSA (m}^2) = 0.007184 \times (185.4)^{0.725} \times (79.5)^{0.425}$$

$$\text{BSA (m}^2) = 2.03 \text{ m}^2$$

Mosteller Equation

$$\text{BSA (m}^2) = \sqrt{\frac{\text{Ht (cm)} \times \text{Wt (kg)}}{3{,}600}}$$

Examples

A patient has a weight of 175 pounds and height of 6'1". Calculate the patient's BSA using the Mosteller formula. Round to the nearest hundredth.

Convert weight in pounds to kilograms by dividing by 2.2: 175/2.2 = 79.5 kg
Convert height in inches to centimeters by multiplying by 2.54: 73" x 2.54 = 185.4 cm

$$\text{BSA (m}^2) = \sqrt{\frac{185.4 \text{ cm} \times 79.5 \text{ kg}}{3{,}600}} = 2.02 \text{ m}^2$$

A patient with a BSA of 2.02 m² is going to receive paclitaxel for lung cancer at a dose of 175 mg/m². Calculate the dose of paclitaxel that this patient will receive.

$$175 \text{ mg/m}^2 \times 2.02 \text{ m}^2 = 354 \text{ mg}$$

A patient with a BSA of 2.02 m² is going to receive paclitaxel for lung cancer at a dose of 175 mg/m². Paclitaxel is available as a 6 mg/mL solution. If the patient's dose is 354 mg, how many milliliters will be needed for the dose?

$$354 \text{ mg} \ \times \ \frac{1 \text{ mL}}{6 \text{ mg}} \ = \ 59 \text{ mL}$$

CHEMOTHERAPEUTIC AGENTS

Chemotherapeutic regimens are designed to complement each other (with different mechanisms of action, toxicities and cell cycle specificity). It is important to note where in the cell cycle the drugs work in order to target tumor cells which will be at different stages in the cycle.

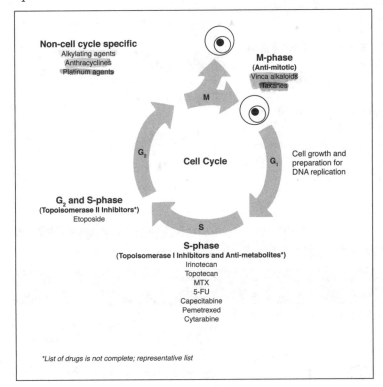

PHASES OF THE CELL CYCLE

M
Mitosis – cell divides into 2 daughter cells

G₀
Resting phase post mitosis – no cell division occurs

G₁
Post-mitotic phase – where enzymes and proteins are synthesized

S
DNA synthesis and duplication occurs

G₂
Pre-mitotic phase – RNA and topoisomerase I and II are produced to prepare for cell division

In the following sections, the drugs are listed in alphabetical order for general adult oncology practice. Specific areas of oncology (pediatrics, urology, transplantation) would place a higher level of importance on less common agents and there are also regional differences in which agents may be considered more important.

The initial groups of chemotherapy agents that follow are commonly used in a multitude of cancers and share similar toxicities. These are followed by more targeted agents accompanied by brief descriptions of some of the more common cancers they treat. This review focuses on the medications and does not go into detail on the actual cancers or treatment regimens which are generally protocol based.

Alkylators

Non-cell cycle specific: Cross-links DNA, preventing cell replication.

DRUG	UNIQUE CONCERNS	SAFETY/SIDE EFFECTS/MONITORING
Cyclophosphamide (Cytoxan) Ifosfamide (Ifex) Altretamine (Hexalen) Bendamustine (Treanda) Busulfan (Myleran) Carmustine (BiCNU, Gliadel wafer for brain cancer) Chlorambucil (Leukeran) – requires refrigeration Dacarbazine (DTIC) Lomustine (CeeNU) Mechlorethamine (Mustargen) Melphalan (Alkeran) – tablets require refrigeration Procarbazine (Matulane) Streptozocin (Zanosar) Temozolomide (Temodar) Thiotepa (Thioplex)	Bladder toxicity with high-dose cyclophosphamide and all doses of ifosfamide – give mesna (Mesnex) to protect against hemorrhagic cystitis and ensure adequate hydration. Temozolomide crosses the blood brain barrier and is used primarily in brain cancers such as glioblastoma multiforme. Best taken on an empty stomach or QHS to ↓ nausea. Prophylaxis against Pneumocystis pneumonia is important while on temozolomide + radiation. Lomustine PO is dosed QHS with an antiemetic. Procarbazine is a MAO inhibitor, avoid interacting drugs/foods. Carmustine: use non-PVC bag and tubing due to leaching of DEHP. Dacarbazine requires light protection during administration. Decomposed drug turns pink.	**BOXED WARNINGS** Hemorrhagic cystitis (ifosfamide, cyclophosphamide), severe bone marrow suppression, secondary malignancy **CONTRAINDICATIONS** Severe bone marrow suppression, bladder or urinary obstruction **SIDE EFFECTS** Myelosuppression, nausea/vomiting, alopecia Pulmonary toxicity (busulfan, carmustine, lomustine) Neurologic toxicity such as seizures, encephalopathy (chlorambucil, ifosfamide, temozolamide, thiotepa) Skin pigmentation changes (busulfan, carmustine) Dacarbazine is highly emetogenic and can cause flu-like symptoms Impairs fertility

Anthracyclines

Non-cell cycle specific: Work by several mechanisms, including intercalation into DNA, inhibiting topoisomerase II, and creating oxygen-free radicals that damage cells.

DRUG	UNIQUE CONCERNS	SAFETY/SIDE EFFECTS/MONITORING
DOXOrubicin (Adriamycin) DOXOrubicin liposomal (Doxil) EPIrubicin (Ellence) IDArubicin (Idamycin) DAUNOrubicin (Cerubidine) DAUNOrubicin liposomal (DaunoXome) MitoXANtrone (Novantrone) Valrubicin (Valstar) intravesicular bladder irrigation only	Very effective but limited use due to cardiac toxicity and N/V. Vesicants: High risk of severe tissue damage with extravasation, antidote is dexrazoxane (Totect) or dimethyl sulfoxide. Do not use both. Serial monitoring of cardiac output is necessary at baseline and with anthracycline doses exceeding: 250 mg/m² doxorubicin; 320 mg/m² daunorubicin. The liposomal products have higher incidence of hand-foot syndrome and allergic reactions. Do not exceed max lifetime doxorubicin dose of 450-550 mg/m² (450 mg/m² with mediastinal radiation) due to cardiotoxicity. The cardioprotective agent dexrazoxane (Zinecard) should be considered when cumulative doxorubicin dose > 300 mg/m². Mitoxantrone is an anthracenedione similar to anthracyclines in toxicity and turns body fluids blue rather than red as with the other anthraclines. Requires light protection during administration.	**BOXED WARNINGS** Irreversible myocardial toxicity may occur as total dosage approaches cumulative max dose Secondary malignancy (AML or MDS) Severe myelosuppression in patients with impaired hepatic function Potent vesicant – avoid extravasation. Conventional and liposomal formulations are not bioequivalent, do not substitute **CONTRAINDICATIONS** HF, MI or arrhythmias; pre-existing bone marrow suppression (ANC < 1,500), previous therapy with high cumulative dose of anthracyclines, severe liver impairment **SIDE EFFECTS** Myelosuppression, alopecia, N/V, mucositis, injection site extravasation, radiation recall, hepatitis, red urine and body secretions (blue with mitoxantrone)

Anthracycline and Mitoxantrone Maximum Lifetime Doses

(handwritten left margin:) ♡ monitor
> 250 mg/m²
> 320 mg/m²

DRUG	LIFETIME DOSE
Doxorubicin *Adriamycin®*	450-550 mg/m², 450 mg/m² with chest radiation *(handwritten:)* → mediastinal
Daunorubicin *Cerubidine®*	400-550 mg/m²
Epirubicin *Ellence®*	800-900 mg/m²
Idarubicin *Idamycin®*	120-150 mg/m²
Mitoxantrone *Novantrone®*	140 mg/m²

Platinum-Based Compounds

Non-cell cycle specific: Cross-links DNA, leading to apoptosis (programmed cell death)

DRUG	UNIQUE CONCERNS	SAFETY/SIDE EFFECTS/MONITORING
CISplatin *(Platinol)*	Nephrotoxicity is managed with vigorous hydration and sometimes mannitol, electrolyte wasting requires magnesium and potassium supplementation. Amifostine *(Ethyol)* may also be used prophylactically for renal protection. Recommend audiograms prior to each cycle to screen for ototoxicity. Manage acute and delayed N/V with 3 drug combination antiemetic regimen.	**BOXED WARNINGS** **Cisplatin** Anaphylactic-like reactions, cumulative renal toxicity, ototoxicity, caution against cisplatin overdose (doses > 100 mg/m² Q 3-4 weeks are rarely used and should be verified) **Carboplatin** Anaphylactic-like reactions, myelosuppression, nausea and vomiting **Oxaliplatin** Anaphylactic-like reactions **CONTRAINDICATIONS** **Cisplatin** Pre-existing renal impairment, myelosuppression, hearing impairment **Carboplatin** Myelosuppression, bleeding **SIDE EFFECTS** Myelosuppression, neuropathy (cumulative, dose-dependent), hypersensitivity reactions (including anaphylaxis); may respond to pretreatment with steroids and antihistamines.
CARBOplatin *(Paraplatin-AQ)* *(handwritten:)* target AUC = 1-7 1-2 → radio-sensitizer 4-6 ⇒ in combo 7 ⇒ as single agent	Calvert Formula: Total Carboplatin Dose (mg) = (Target AUC) x (GFR + 25). Target AUC ranges from 1 to 7 with 1-2 as a radiosensitizer (makes cancer cells sensitive to radiation therapy); 4-6 in combination therapy and 7 as a single agent. Commonly used max GFR for calculating carboplatin dose is 125 mL/min.	
Oxaliplatin *(Eloxatin)*	Anaphylaxis, pancreatitis, pulmonary toxicity, hepatotoxicity. Neuropathy exacerbated by exposure to cold	

Folate Antimetabolites
Cell cycle specific, S-phase: Prevent DNA synthesis.

DRUG	UNIQUE CONCERNS	SAFETY/SIDE EFFECTS/MONITORING
Methotrexate *(Trexall, Rheumatrex)* Lower doses used in RA and psoriasis	High-dose regimens are needed to penetrate the blood-brain barrier and overcomes relative resistance in malignancies such as osteosarcoma. High-doses also require leucovorin or levoleucovorin rescue to ↓ toxicity. Leucovorin is the active form of folic acid, which bypasses the enzyme block of dihydrofolate reductase by methotrexate. Avoid renal transport inhibitors that can ↓ elimination, resulting in MTX toxicity: aspirin, beta lactams, probenecid and NSAIDs. Maintain proper hydration. Alkalinize urine with IV sodium bicarbonate to ↓ toxicity.	**BOXED WARNINGS (MANY)** Pregnancy, hepatotoxicity, ascites diarrhea, SJS/TEN, infection, renal impairment, tumor lysis syndrome, stomatitis, pulmonary disease, lymphoma, preserved formulation not for intrathecal administration or high-dose therapy, radiation therapy (if is used as a radiation sensitizer, it may cause more soft tissue or bone necrosis), myelosuppression, death **SIDE EFFECTS** Myelosuppression, mucositis, hepatic and renal toxicity (renal is dose-related), pulmonary toxicity (rare), hand-foot syndrome, tumor lysis syndrome
PEMEtrexed *(Alimta)*	To ↓ side effects (hematologic, mucositis, diarrhea, dermatologic): give folic acid supplements (1 mg PO daily), vitamin B12 (cyanocobalamin) and dexamethasone.	**SIDE EFFECTS** Renal toxicity, bone marrow suppression, dermatologic toxicity, mucositis, N/V/D
PRALAtrexate *(Folotyn)*	Similar to above, use vitamin B12 and folate to ↓ toxicity.	**SIDE EFFECTS** Myelosuppression, mucositis, anemia, renal toxicity, hepatic toxicity, tumor lysis syndrome, fetal harm

Pyrimidine Analog Antimetabolites
Cell cycle specific, S-phase: Inhibits pyrimidine synthesis.

DRUG	UNIQUE CONCERNS	SAFETY/SIDE EFFECTS/MONITORING
Capecitabine *(Xeloda)* Prodrug of 5-fluorouracil Given PO as 2 divided doses taken 12 hours apart, take within 30 minutes after a meal	Pharmacogenomic testing for dihydropyrimidine dehydrogenase (DPD) – deficiency ↑ risk of severe toxicity. Capecitabine can ↑ INR up to 91% due to CYP 2C9 inhibition – dose adjust based on severity of interaction.	**BOXED WARNING** ↑ INR during and up to 1 month after discontinuation; reduce warfarin dose, monitor carefully; fatal bleeding can occur **CONTRAINDICATIONS** Dihydropyrimidine dehydrogenase (DPD) deficiency, severe renal impairment (CrCl < 30 mL/min) **SIDE EFFECTS** Hand-foot syndrome (more than 5-fluorouracil), diarrhea, mucositis, gastritis, N/V, dermatitis, cardiotoxicity, edema, myelosuppression
Cytarabine conventional, (AKA ara-C) Cytarabine liposomal *(DepoCyt)*: for intrathecal administration	Cytarabine syndrome includes fever, weakness, fatigue, skin rash, reddened eyes, bone, muscle, joint and/or chest pain – treat with corticosteroids.	**BOXED WARNING** Bone marrow suppression (conventional formulation) **CONTRAINDICATIONS** Active meningeal infection (*DepoCyt* only) **SIDE EFFECTS** Mucositis, myelosuppression, hepatotoxicity, pulmonary toxicity, encephalopathy, severe N/V and peripheral neuropathy at high doses, hand-foot syndrome

Pyrimidine Analog Antimetabolites Continued

DRUG	UNIQUE CONCERNS	SAFETY/SIDE EFFECTS/MONITORING
Fluorouracil, 5-FU *(Adrucil)* *Efudex*, *Carac* and *Fluoroplex* are topical formulations used for actinic keratosis. *Efudex* is also used for superficial basal cell carcinoma.	Pharmacogenomic testing for dihydropyrimidine dehydrogenase (DPD) – deficiency ↑ risk of severe toxicity. Given with leucovorin to ↑ efficacy of 5-FU	**CONTRAINDICATIONS** Bone marrow suppression, infection, malnutrition **SIDE EFFECTS** Myelosuppression, mucositis, dermatitis, diarrhea, cardiotoxicity, hand-foot syndrome (with continuous infusions), photosensitivity
Gemcitabine *(Gemzar)*	Flu-like syndrome during first 24 hours: use acetaminophen. Prolonged infusion time may ↑ toxicities, use infusion rates per protocol.	**SIDE EFFECTS** Myelosuppression, hepatotoxicity, arthralgia, rash, fatigue, headache, N/V/D, stomatitis, radiation recall, peripheral edema, dyspnea

Taxanes

(handwritten note in left margin: ≠ neutropenia)

(handwritten note at top: GIVE TAXANES BEFORE CIS/CARBOPLATIN!)

M-phase specific: Inhibit microtubule function and angiogenesis (dysfunctional microtubule bundling). Elimination of taxanes is reduced when given immediately after administration of cisplatin or carboplatin. Give taxanes first.

(handwritten note in left margin: use non-PVC IV bag & tubing w/ ALL taxanes)

DRUG	UNIQUE CONCERNS	SAFETY/SIDE EFFECTS/MONITORING
PACLitaxel *(Taxol)* Paclitaxel albumin-bound *(Abraxane)* has less hypersensitivity reactions	Anaphylaxis, hypersensitivity reaction (78%) due to polyoxyethylated castor oil solvent system, can be severe in 2-4% of patients. Pre-treat with dexamethasone, diphenhydramine and H₂RA (not needed with *Abraxane*). For all taxanes, use non-PVC IV bag and tubing due to leaching of DEHP (except *Abraxane*). Do not extravasate. Will ↑ INR if on warfarin; monitor closely.	**CONTRAINDICATIONS** Neutropenia **SIDE EFFECTS** Myelosuppression, peripheral neuropathy, anaphylactoid reaction, alopecia (can be entire body), fever, skin reaction, cardiotoxicity, hepatotoxicity, myalgia/arthralgia, N/V, radiation recall
DOCEtaxel *(Taxotere)*	Hypersensitivity (40-50%) due to polysorbate 80 solvent system. Cardio-pulmonary side effects (41-70%) include fluid retention, pericardial effusion, pleural effusion and edema. Pre-treat with dexamethasone to ↓ fluid retention. For all taxanes, use non-PVC IV bag and tubing due to leaching of DEHP.	**BOXED WARNINGS (5)** Neutropenia, edema, hepatic disease, hypersensitivity, ↑ mortality **CONTRAINDICATIONS** Neutropenia **SIDE EFFECTS** Myelosuppression, fluid retention, peripheral neuropathy, anaphylactoid reaction, cutaneous reactions, N/V/D, mucositis, myalgias, arthralgias, fatigue, alopecia

Taxanes Continued

DRUG	UNIQUE CONCERNS	SAFETY/SIDE EFFECTS/MONITORING
Cabazitaxel *(Jevtana)*	Hypersensitivity reaction (40-50%) due to polysorbate 80 solvent system. Pre-treat with antihistamines and corticosteroids. For all taxanes, use non-PVC IV bag and tubing due to leaching of DEHP.	**BOXED WARNING** Neutropenia, hypersensitivity **CONTRAINDICATIONS** Neutropenia, hypersensitivity **SIDE EFFECTS** Myelosuppression, peripheral neuropathy, anaphylactoid reaction, N/V/D, peripheral edema, fatigue, alopecia, myalgias, arthralgias

Vinca Alkaloids

M-phase specific: Inhibit microtubule function (destabilizers).

DRUG	UNIQUE CONCERNS	SAFETY/SIDE EFFECTS/MONITORING
VinCRIStine (Vincasar) Max single dose: 2 mg Vincristine liposomal (Marqibo) **VinBLASTine (Velban)** **VinORELbine (Navelbine)**	These agents are vesicants. Best to administer with a central line. Avoid extravasation as tissue damage may occur. Use warm compress and hyaluronidase if extravasation occurs. IV only, accidental intrathecal administration is fatal. Vincristine is NOT myelosuppressive, vinblastine and vinorelbine are myelosuppressive.	**BOXED WARNINGS** Extravasation, intrathecal administration (fatal), vincristine conventional injection and liposomal injection are not interchangeable **SIDE EFFECTS** Cumulative (dose-dependent) peripheral neuropathy (paresthesias, gastroparesis, constipation, paralytic ileus, ↑ risk of falls), alopecia, rash, SIADH, tumor lysis syndrome, ↑ LFTs, myelosuppression (vinblastine and vinorelbine only)

Handwritten margin notes: "NOT myelo-suppressive", "not interchange-able", "myelo-suppressive ↑"

Topoisomerase I Inhibitors

S-phase specific: Block the coiling and uncoiling of the DNA helix. Topoisomerase I facilitates single strand breaks followed by religation (putting the DNA strands back together).

DRUG	UNIQUE CONCERNS	SAFETY/SIDE EFFECTS/MONITORING
Irinotecan *(Camptosar)*	Acute diarrhea is a cholinergic symptom, treat with atropine. Delayed diarrhea is treated with loperamide (up to 24 mg daily). Pharmacogenomic testing: Those who are homozygous for the UGT1A1*28 allele are at an ↑ risk for neutropenia, dose adjust as needed.	**BOXED WARNINGS (2)** Bone marrow suppression, diarrhea **SIDE EFFECTS** Diarrhea, myelosuppression, mucositis, acute cholinergic syndrome (rhinitis, hypersalivation, sweating, etc), N/V, asthenia, fever, pain, headache, chills, pulmonary reactions (dyspnea, cough), ↑ LFTs, alopecia
Topotecan *(Hycamtin)*	Used typically as a second line agent for cervical, ovarian or small cell lung cancer.	**BOXED WARNING** Bone marrow suppression **SIDE EFFECTS** Myelosuppression, N/V/D, alopecia, dyspnea, flu-like symptoms, infertility

Topoisomerase II Inhibitors

G2-phase specific: Block the coiling and uncoiling of the DNA helix by facilitating single strand breaks followed by religation.

DRUG	UNIQUE CONCERNS	SAFETY/SIDE EFFECTS/MONITORING
Etoposide *(VePesid)* *VePesid* capsules require refrigeration Teniposide *(Vumon)*	IV administration can cause hypotension due to rapid infusion rate, infuse slowly over at least 30-60 minutes. Precipitation may occur, to ↓ risk: use a large volume infusion for etoposide concentrations > 0.4 mg/mL, administer all teniposide concentrations within 4 hours of preparation. Use non-PVC IV bag and tubing due to leaching of DEHP. Irritant: use hyaluronidase and warm compresses to treat extravasation. Etoposide IV:PO ratio is 1:2, round to nearest 50 mg capsule. If total dose is > 400 mg, administer BID.	**BOXED WARNING** Bone marrow suppression **SIDE EFFECTS** Myelosuppression, hypotension, bronchospasm, anaphylactoid reaction, neuropathy, hepatotoxicity, alopecia, N/V, mucositis, secondary malignancies

(handwritten margin note: non-PVC bag & tubing)

Epothilone

M-phase specific: Microtubule stabilizer enhancing polymerization of tubules halting cell division; mechanism similar to taxanes.

DRUG	UNIQUE CONCERNS	SAFETY/SIDE EFFECTS/MONITORING
Ixabepilone *(Ixempra)*	Similar mechanism to taxanes but retains efficacy in taxane-resistant breast cancer. Hypersensitivity due to *Cremophor EL* (polyoxyethylated castor oil solvent), requires pre-treatment with antihistamines +/- steroids. Use 0.2 – 1.2 micron filter. Use non-PVC IV bag and tubing due to leaching of DEHP.	**BOXED WARNING** Hepatic disease **CONTRAINDICATIONS** Hypersensitivity to castor oil, neutropenia, thrombocytopenia, hepatic disease **SIDE EFFECTS** Myelosuppression, neuropathy, hypersensitivity reaction (flushing, rash, dyspnea, bronchospasm), fatigue, asthenia, mucositis, N/V/D, alopecia, hand-foot syndrome

(handwritten margin note: non-PVC bag & tubing)

Miscellaneous Agents

DRUG	UNIQUE CONCERNS	SAFETY/SIDE EFFECTS/MONITORING
Tretinoin, AKA **All-trans Retinoic Acid**, *ATRA* ↓ proliferation and ↑ differentiation of APL cells First line therapy for acute promyelocytic leukemia (APL)	Retinoids (vitamin A analogues) Pregnancy Category D Retinoic Acid-Acute Promyelocytic Leukemia (RA-APL) differentiation syndrome: fever, dyspnea, weight gain, edema, pulmonary infiltrates, pericardial or pleural effusions – treat with dexamethasone.	**BOXED WARNINGS (3)** RA-APL differentiation syndrome, leukocytosis, pregnancy **CONTRAINDICATIONS** Hypersensitivity to paraben or retinoid **SIDE EFFECTS** Leukocytosis, RA-APL differentiation syndrome, QT prolongation, N/V/D, skin/mucous membrane dryness, hyperlipidemia, GI bleeding

Miscellaneous Agents Continued

DRUG	UNIQUE CONCERNS	SAFETY/SIDE EFFECTS/MONITORING
Arsenic trioxide *(Trisenox)* ↑ apoptosis of APL cells and damages fusion protein PML-RAR alpha Second line therapy for acute promyelocytic leukemia (APL)	QT prolongation: monitor ECG, avoid concurrent QT prolonging agents, keep Mg^{2+}, Ca^{2+}, and K^+ within normal range. APL Differentiation Syndrome (see above). If acute vasomotor reactions (lightheadedness, dizziness, or hypotension) occur, prolong infusion.	**BOXED WARNINGS (5)** RA-APL differentiation syndrome, ECG abnormalities (AV block, QT prolongation), ECG and electrolyte monitoring **SIDE EFFECTS** Leukocytosis, APL differentiation syndrome, QT prolongation, N/V/D, GI bleeding, stomatitis, electrolyte imbalance, acute vasomotor reactions (lightheadedness, dizziness, or hypotension), fatigue, edema, headache, insomnia, anxiety, infection
L-Asparaginase *(Elspar)* – derived from *Escherichia coli* Asparaginase (Erwinaze) – derived from Erwinia chrysanthemi Pegaspargase *(Oncaspar)* – modified form of L-asparaginase conjugated with polyethylene glycol	Deprives leukemia cells of asparagine which is an essential amino acid in leukemia. *Erwinaze* is FDA approved for patients who develop allergic reactions to the *E. coli* derived asparaginase. The pegylated form allows for every 2 week dosing and ↓ incidence of allergic reactions. Monitor fibrinogen.	**CONTRAINDICATIONS** Hypersensitivity to *E. coli* or L-asparaginase; bleeding or pancreatitis with prior asparaginase treatment **SIDE EFFECTS** Hypersensitivity reactions, pancreatitis, hyperglycemia, hepatotoxicity, CNS toxicity (lethargy, somnolence), N/V, encephalopathy, prolonged prothrombin time (PT/INR) and thrombin time (TT)
Bleomycin Intercalating agent blocking topoisomerase II	Due to risk of anaphylactoid reaction, a test dose may be given to lymphoma patients. May pre-medicate with acetaminophen to ↓ incidence of fever or chills. ↑ risk of pulmonary fibrosis when given with G-CSF (filgrastim). Recommended not using G-CSF on days of bleomycin administration. Not myelosuppressive. Maximum lifetime dose of 400 units due to pulmonary toxicity risk.	**BOXED WARNINGS (2)** Pulmonary fibrosis, anaphylaxis **SIDE EFFECTS** Hypersensitivity reaction, pulmonary reactions (10%) – such as pneumonitis, which may progress to pulmonary fibrosis, mucositis, hyperpigmentation, fever, chills, N/V (mild)
Mitomycin *(Mutamycin)* Derived from *Streptomyces caespitosus* Free radical formation and alkylator	Vesicant, do not extravasate. Antidote is dimethyl sulfoxide (DMSO) and cool compresses. Mitomycin IV solutions are a hazy blue or purple color.	**BOXED WARNINGS (2)** Bone marrow suppression (thrombocytopenia, leukopenia), hemolytic-uremic syndrome **CONTRAINDICATIONS** Thrombocytopenia, coagulopathy, bleeding **SIDE EFFECTS** Leukopenia, thrombocytopenia, N/V, fatigue, alopecia, mucous membrane toxicity, cystitis or dysuria (from intravesical administration into bladder)

Monoclonal Antibodies Nomenclature

PREFIX	TARGET			SOURCE				STEM
	Substem	Meaning	Example	Substem	Meaning	% Human	Example	
variable	*ci*	circulatory system	beva*ci*zumab	*o*	m*o*use	0	Tositum*o*mab	-mab
	li	immune system	ipi*li*mumab	*xi*	*Chi*meric*	~34	Cetu*xi*mab	
	so	bone	den*os*umab	*zu*	Humani*z*ed*	~90-95	Bevaci*zu*mab	
	tu	tumor	per*tu*zumab	*u*	h*u*man	100	Panitum*u*mab	

Chimeric/humanized are designated as human and animal source

"AMA (USAN) Monoclonal antibodies". United States Adopted Names. 2007-08-07.

"The use of stems in the selection of International Nonproprietary Names (INN) for pharmaceutical substances" (PDF). World Health Organization. 2009. pp. 107–109, 168–169.

COMMON MABs	TARGET
Bevacizumab *(Avastin)*	Binds to VEGF-A
Cetuximab *(Erbitux)*	Binds to EGFR
Trastuzumab *(Herceptin)*	Binds to HER2/neu
Rituximab *(Rituxan)*	Binds to CD20
Ipilimumab *(Yervoy)*	Binds to Cytotoxic T-lymphocyte antigen-4 (CTL4) receptor

Monoclonal Antibodies

Over-expression targeted: Inhibit growth factors that are promoting cancer cell growth.

DRUG	UNIQUE CONCERNS	SAFETY/SIDE EFFECTS/MONITORING
Bevacizumab *(Avastin)* Binds to VEGF-A Angiogenesis inhibitor: Limits tumor's blood supply.	Impairs wound healing: stop at least 28 days before elective surgery and may restart bevacizumab 28 days after surgery. Monitor blood pressure and urinalysis prior to each dose. Used with other agents in numerous types of cancer but a high cost for modest benefit.	**BOXED WARNINGS (3)** Bleeding, GI perforation, wound dehiscence **SIDE EFFECTS** Bleeding, hypertension, HF, thrombosis (including DVT, PE and stroke), GI perforation, wound dehiscence, nephrotic syndrome, proteinuria, exfoliative dermatitis

Monoclonal Antibodies Continued

DRUG	UNIQUE CONCERNS	SAFETY/SIDE EFFECTS/MONITORING
Trastuzumab *(Herceptin)* HER2/neu over-expression required for use Synergistic efficacy with some chemotherapeutics but avoid use with anthracyclines due to ↑ cardiotoxicity.	Pharmacogenomics: trastuzumab binds to and reverses effects of overactive HER2 receptors. HER2 gene is over-expressed in ~25% of early-stage breast tumors. Must be ≥ 2+ by immunohistochemical (IHC) testing to respond/use this drug. Obtain MUGA or ECHO at baseline and during treatment. Not interchangeable with ado-trastuzumab emtansine.	**BOXED WARNINGS** Heart failure, severe infusion-related reactions (including hypersensitivity, infusion reactions or pulmonary); may give acetaminophen, diphenhydramine, corticosteroids or meperidine for management. **SIDE EFFECTS** Cardiomyopathy (HF, ↓ LVEF), infusion reaction, weakness, pain, chills, fever, cough, pulmonary toxicity, N/V/D, rash, edema
Ado-Trastuzumab Emtansine *(Kadcyla)* HER2/neu over-expression required for use	*Kadcyla* is a conjugate of trastuzumab linked to DM-1, a highly potent anti-microtubule derivative of maytansine which provides targeted delivery. Pharmacogenomics: HER2 gene over-expression required for use Use 0.22 micron filter. Obtain MUGA or ECHO at baseline and during treatment. Do not confuse with conventional trastuzumab; not interchangeable.	**BOXED WARNINGS (4)** Heart failure, hepatotoxicity, embryo-fetal death and birth defects, ado-trastuzumab emtansine and conventional trastuzumab are not interchangeable **SIDE EFFECTS** Cardiac dysfunction, constipation, nausea, headache, thrombocytopenia, ↑ LFTs, myalgia, fatigue, N/V/D
Pertuzumab *(Perjeta)* HER2/neu over-expression required for use	Pharmacogenomics: HER2 gene over-expression. Obtain MUGA or ECHO at baseline and during treatment.	**BOXED WARNINGS (2)** Embryo-fetal death and birth defects; cardiac failure **SIDE EFFECTS** Cardiomyopathy (HF, ↓ LVEF), alopecia, rash, N/V/D, anemia, asthenia, fatigue, anaphylaxis, peripheral neuropathy
Cetuximab *(Erbitux)* EGFR positive expression correlates with better response rates. K-ras mutation indicates poor response; requires EGFR postive and K-ras wildtype.	Pharmacogenomics: Must test for EGFR and K-ras mutations before treatment. Premedicate with diphenhydramine for at least the first dose. Presence of rash correlates with high survival rate.	**BOXED WARNINGS (2)** Severe infusion reactions, cardiopulmonary arrest. $\downarrow Mg^{++}, Ca^{++}$ **SIDE EFFECTS** Acne-like rash onset in 1st few weeks of treatment, severe rash possible. N/V/D, fatigue, magnesium and calcium wasting
Panitumumab *(Vectibix)* Same EGFR and K-ras issues as cetuximab	Pharmacogenomics: Must test for EGFR and K-ras mutations before treatment. Presence of rash correlates with a higher survival rate.	**BOXED WARNING** Dermatologic toxicities $\downarrow Mg^{++}, Ca^{++}$ **SIDE EFFECTS** Acne-like rash onset in 2 weeks of treatment, severe rash possible. Infusion reactions (can be fatal); N/V/D, fatigue, magnesium and calcium wasting

Monoclonal Antibodies Continued

DRUG	UNIQUE CONCERNS	SAFETY/SIDE EFFECTS/MONITORING
RiTUXimab (Rituxan) Targets CD20 antigen on B lymphocytes, killing the cancer and releasing cytokines	Must be administered in hospital or clinic to monitor for infusion reactions which may occur within 30-120 minutes, and may include: urticaria, hypotension, angioedema, hypoxia, bronchospasm, acute respiratory distress syndrome, myocardial infarction, ventricular fibrillation, cardiogenic shock, anaphylaxis, and death. Administer diphenhydramine and acetaminophen prior to infusion.	**BOXED WARNINGS (4)** Severe infusion reactions, hepatitis B reactivation, fatal mucocutaneous reactions, progressive multifocal leukoencephalopathy (PML) from JC virus **SIDE EFFECTS** Infusion reaction Tumor lysis syndrome, rash, pruritus, toxic epidermal necrolysis. Myelosuppression with prolonged immune suppression ↑ risk of opportunistic infections and reactivation of hepatitis B

PROSTATE CANCER

1 out of 6 males may be diagnosed with prostate cancer in his lifetime. After surgery or radiation therapy has been considered, oral or injectable agents for prostate cancer are used. Typically, "castration sensitive" patients are started on Luteinizing Hormone-Releasing Hormone (LHRH) agonists for chronic suppression of testosterone. Antiandrogens are started 1-4 weeks prior (to help mitigate the tumor flare) to the LHRH agonists. Many clinicians will discontinue the anti-androgens a week or more after starting the LHRH agonists. PSA levels are checked routinely as a marker of treatment response. IV chemotherapy (with docetaxel/prednisone) or abiraterone (a more potent oral antiandrogen) are used in metastatic disease.

Antiandrogens: Androgen Receptor Antagonists

Blocks androgens at the receptor site, thus preventing testosterone stimulation of cell growth in prostate cancer.

DRUG	UNIQUE CONCERNS	SAFETY/SIDE EFFECTS/MONITORING
Bicalutamide (Casodex) 50 mg PO daily **Flutamide (Eulexin)** 250 mg PO Q8H SE: diarrhea **Nilutamide (Nilandron)** 300 mg PO daily x 30 days, then 150 mg PO daily SE: visual disturbances, night blindness	Used 1-4 weeks prior to starting LHRH agonists to mitigate tumor flare.	**SIDE EFFECTS** Hot flashes, edema, pain, asthenia, heart failure, hepatotoxicity, gynecomastia, N/V/D, visual disturbances (nilutamide only) **NOTES** Nilutamide causes night blindness Flutamide causes more diarrhea

Antiandrogen-Antiestrogen: LHRH (Luteinizing Hormone-Releasing Hormone) Agonists

Used for prostate cancer in males and for endometriosis, fibroids and breast cancer in females: initially ↑ production of androgens and estrogens, which can cause an initial tumor flare; followed by down regulation through a negative feedback loop which ↓ gonadotropin release, ↓ LH, and ↓ FSH, resulting in a chemical castration/oophorectomy.

DRUG	UNIQUE CONCERNS	SAFETY/SIDE EFFECTS/ MONITORING
Goserelin *(Zoladex)* **Leuprolide** *(Lupron, Eligard, Viadur)* # breastfeeding vaginal bleed Histrelin *(Vantas)* Triptorelin *(Trelstar)* Given SQ or IM monthly or less frequently (up to once/yr) depending on formulation and indication.	↓ bone density and ↑ risk for osteoporosis: consider calcium and vitamin D supplementation, weight bearing exercise and DEXA screening. Typically patients should start an anti-androgen at least 1 week prior to mitigate tumor flare.	**CONTRAINDICATIONS** Pregnancy, breastfeeding (leuprolide), vaginal bleeding (leuprolide) **SIDE EFFECTS** Hot flashes, bone pain, impotence, injection site pain/swelling, dyslipidemia, QT prolongation, gynecomastia (men), peripheral edema

Antiandrogen: Gonadotropin-Releasing Hormone (GRH) Antagonist

DRUG	UNIQUE CONCERNS	SAFETY/SIDE EFFECTS/MONITORING
Degarelix *(Firmagon)*	Similar efficacy/toxicity to LHRH agonists (above) but true blockade of GnRH so does not cause ↑ testosterone with tumor flare. No need for concomitant antiandrogens.	**CONTRAINDICATIONS** Pregnancy **SIDE EFFECTS** Same as LHRH agonists above plus QT prolongation

Antiandrogen: Pregnenolone Analog

A pregnenolone analog that irreversibly inhibits CYPC17, the rate limiting enzyme in androgen production in the testes, adrenal gland and prostate without causing adrenal insufficiency.

DRUG	UNIQUE CONCERNS	SAFETY/SIDE EFFECTS/MONITORING
Abiraterone acetate *(Zytiga)* 1,000 mg (4 x 250 mg tabs) PO daily on an empty stomach *more potent ⇒ used in metastatic dz*	Substrate of CYP 3A4 and inhibitor of CYP 2D6, requires caution with inhibitors/substrates. Taken in combination with prednisone	**CONTRAINDICATION** Pregnancy **SIDE EFFECTS** Mineralocorticoid elevation with fluid retention, hypertension, hypokalemia, hepatotoxicity, joint swelling, hot flashes, diarrhea, nocturia, osteoporosis (fractures)

Antiandrogen: Receptor-Signaling Pathway Inhibitor

Blocks the downstream transfer of information from the activated receptor. Used in patients with castration-resistant metastatic prostate cancer who failed docetaxel chemotherapy.

DRUG	UNIQUE CONCERNS	SAFETY/SIDE EFFECTS/MONITORING
Enzalutamide *(Xtandi)* 160 mg (4 x 40 mg caps) PO once daily	CYP 2C8 and 3A4 substrate; avoid use with inhibitors. If used concurrently with a strong CYP 2C8 inhibitor, reduce dose to 80 mg daily. CYP 2C9, 3A4 and 2C19 inducer, caution with substrates.	**CONTRAINDICATION** Pregnancy **SIDE EFFECTS** Fatigue, insomnia, weakness, diarrhea, edema, pulmonary infections, dizziness, flushing, neutropenia, seizures (~1%).

Prostate Cancer Vaccine

Autologous cellular immunotherapy which stimulates an immune response targeting prostatic acid phosphatase (PAP), an antigen expressed in most prostate cancer cells.

DRUG	UNIQUE CONCERNS	SAFETY/SIDE EFFECTS/MONITORING
Sipuleucel-T *(Provenge)*	Infusion of CD 54+ antigen presenting cells obtained through leukapheresis. Patient's own WBCs are harvested and activated against PAP to target cancer prostate cells, and then patients own cells are re-infused.	**SIDE EFFECTS** Acute infusion reactions, nausea, vomiting, hypersensitivity, back pain, hypertension
	Requires premedication with acetaminophen and diphenhydramine due to acute flu-like infusion reactions.	

BREAST CANCER

1 out of 8 females may be diagnosed with breast cancer in her lifetime. Approximately 1% of all breast cancer patients are male. Risk factors include: family history, genetics (BRCA1 or BRCA2 mutations), early menarche or late menopause (which ↑ lifetime exposure to estrogen), late pregnancy (age > 30 years old), nulliparity (no pregnancy), smoking, obesity and lack of exercise. Typically, breast cancer patients will receive conventional chemotherapy for a limited number of cycles (in the adjuvant setting) or until disease progression (in the metastatic setting).

To prevent recurrence, hormonal therapy is recommended for the following patients:

1. ER/PR⁺ (pre-menopausal and peri-menopausal) female patients: tamoxifen for 5 years, after which they should receive additional therapy based on menopausal status. If pre-menopausal, continue tamoxifen for a total duration of 10 years. If post-menopausal, continue tamoxifen for a total duration of 10 years or an aromatase inhibitor (AI) for a total duration of up to 10 years.

2. ER/PR⁺ (post-menopausal) female patients: one of the following options should be used – tamoxifen for 10 years; an AI for 5 years; tamoxifen for 5 years then switching to an AI for up to 5 years; or tamoxifen for 2-3 years then switching to an AI for up to 5 years.

3. ER/PR⁻ patients: do not have benefit with hormonal agents.

4. ER/PR⁺ male patients: oral hormonal therapy (SERM agent for 5-10 years; tamoxifen is typically the first line agent).

In the metastatic setting, standard IV chemotherapy combinations may be used. However, in HER2/neu positive patients, the first line combination includes pertuzumab, trastuzumab and docetaxel. Second line therapies can also use other standard IV chemotherapy combinations. However, if oral therapy is preferred, lapatinib with capecitabine is a viable option.

Antiestrogens/SERMs

Selective Estrogen Receptor Modulators (SERMs) are estrogen antagonists in breast tissue, but act as estrogen agonists in some other tissues, including bone. These are used for breast cancer in hormone receptor+ tumors (estrogen/progesterone). Most SERMs are used in post-menopausal women, except tamoxifen, which is indicated for pre- and post- menopausal women and in men.

DRUG	UNIQUE CONCERNS	SAFETY/SIDE EFFECTS/MONITORING
Tamoxifen *(Soltamox)* 20 mg PO daily **Fulvestrant** *(Faslodex)* 500 mg IM days 1, 15, 29, then monthly **Raloxifene (Evista)** Used for osteoporosis in women at risk of breast cancer 60 mg PO daily **Toremifene (Fareston)**	Tamoxifen ↑ risk of endometrial cancers: others ↓ risk. Tamoxifen CYP 2D6 polymorphism *4/*5 may result in shorter disease free survival. Consider alternative therapy (aromatase inhibitor). Tamoxifen is a substrate of CYP 3A4, 2C9 and 2D6. Watch for drug-drug interactions (especially with agents used for hot flashes). Recommend venlafaxine for hot flashes (over fluoxetine and paroxetine) for patients on tamoxifen. Fulvestrant may cause osteoporosis, other SERMs ↑ bone density	**BOXED WARNINGS** Uterine malignancy (tamoxifen); ↑ risk of thromboembolic events such as DVT, PE, stroke (tamoxifen, raloxifene), QT prolongation (toremifene) **CONTRAINDICATIONS** Tamoxifen: DVT/PE, concomitant warfarin therapy Raloxifene: DVT/PE, pregnancy, breastfeeding Toremifene: QT prolongation, hypokalemia, hypomagnesemia **SIDE EFFECTS** DVT/PE, menopausal symptoms, hot flashes, flushing, N/V, edema, weight gain, hypertension, mood changes, amenorrhea, vaginal bleeding/discharge, skin changes, cataracts (tamoxifen) **NOTES** Pregnancy Category D (tamoxifen, fulvestrant, toremifene) Pregnancy Category X (raloxifene) MedGuide required for tamoxifen and raloxifene

Handwritten annotations:
- 1st line in ♀ → MedGuide (for thrombosis (DVT/PE, stroke))
- SE: cataracts
- preg X
- ‡ ↓K+, Mg++ QT prolong
- Evista® d/c (72 hrs) prior & during prolonged immobilization (bed rest, post-surgical recovery, etc.); avoid prolonged restriction of movement (VTE risk)

Aromatase Inhibitors

Blocks conversion to active estrogen/androgen/corticosteroid/mineralocorticoid to reduce cell growth in breast, prostate and/or adrenal cancer. These agents are approved for post-menopausal women and are not FDA-approved for men with breast cancer.

DRUG	UNIQUE CONCERNS	SAFETY/SIDE EFFECTS/MONITORING
Anastrozole (Arimidex) 1 mg PO daily **Letrozole (Femara)** 2.5 mg PO daily **Exemestane (Aromasin)** 25 mg PO daily **Mitotane (Lysodren)** non-selective	↓ bone density and ↑ risk for osteoporosis: consider calcium and vitamin D supplementation, weight bearing exercise, DEXA screening. ↑ cardiovascular disease risk compared to SERMs. Mitotane is a non-selective aromatase inhibitor requiring glucocorticoid and mineralocorticoid supplementation.	**CONTRAINDICATION** Pregnancy **SIDE EFFECTS** Arthralgia, edema, lethargy/fatigue, rash, menopausal symptoms/hot flashes, hepatotoxicity, nausea, vomiting, weakness, joint pain, bone pain, HTN, depression ↑ cholesterol

Tyrosine Kinase Inhibitor (TKI) Targeting HER-2 neu

HER-2 neu is a tyrosine kinase that regulates cell proliferation and survival in over-expressed cancers (~25% of breast cancer). Blocking this results in a halt to cancer cell growth and possibly apoptosis. All TKIs are substrates of CYP 3A4 and have many drug-drug interactions – some of which require dose modification.

DRUG	UNIQUE CONCERNS	SAFETY/SIDE EFFECTS/MONITORING
Lapatinib (Tykerb) 1,250-1,500 mg PO daily on empty stomach	Inhibits HER-2/neu (ErbB2) and EGFR (Erb1) tyrosine kinases. Used in metastatic breast cancer. Pharmacogenomics: HER2 gene over-expression.	**BOXED WARNING** Hepatotoxicity **SIDE EFFECTS** Myelosuppression, hand-foot syndrome, acneiform rash, N/V/D, fatigue, ↑ LFTs, interstitial lung disease hepatotoxicity, HF, ↓ LVEF and QT-prolongation

NON-SMALL CELL LUNG CANCER

Lung cancer is the most common cause of cancer-related death in men and women. The most important risk factor is smoking. About 80–90% of lung cancers are caused by long-term exposure to tobacco smoke. Nonsmokers account for 10–15% of lung cancer cases. Other risk factors include genetic factors, radon gas, asbestos, and second-hand smoke. Treatment options include surgery, radiation and chemotherapy. Non-small cell lung cancer (NSCLC) is sometimes treated with surgery. Small cell lung cancer (SCLC) usually responds better to chemotherapy and radiation.

Tyrosine Kinase Inhibitors (TKIs) Targeting EGFR

Epidermal growth factor receptors (1, 2, 3 and 4) control cell growth, angiogenesis, invasion, metastasis and resistance to apoptosis. Inhibition of EGFR results in a halt to cancer cell growth and possibly apoptosis (programmed cell death, in which the cells self-destruct). Pharmacogenomic testing for the EGFR mutation in the adenocarcinoma NSCLC subtype is required. An EGFR mutation predicts response.

DRUG	UNIQUE CONCERNS	SAFETY/SIDE EFFECTS/MONITORING
Erlotinib (Tarceva) 150 mg daily PO (1 hour before or 2 hours after meal)	Works best in EGFR positive mutation, adenocarcinoma histology, non-smokers, Asians, females Pharmacogenomics: Must test for EGFR mutation status. Must be positive to use. Dose reductions by 50 mg are based on toxicities.	**SIDE EFFECTS** Acneiform rash, diarrhea, hepatotoxicity, GI perforation, severe skin reactions, eye damage, nephrotoxicity, stomatitis, interstitial lung disease, cough, headache, fatigue, fever
Afatinib (Gilotrif) 40 mg PO daily on an empty stomach (1 hour before or 2 hours after meal)	Inhibits EGFR 1, 2, 4. Approved for patients with metastatic NSCLC with known EGFR exon 19 deletions or exon 21 substitution mutations detected by FDA-approved test (EGFR, RGQ, PCR, Kit). Pharmacogenomics: Must test for EGFR mutation status. Must be positive to use.	**SIDE EFFECTS** Acneiform rash, diarrhea, stomatitis, dry skin, paronychia, ↓ appetite, pruritus *nail dz (bacterial/fungal) of finger/toe nail*

Tyrosine Kinase Inhibitors (TKIs) Targeting Anaplastic Lymphoma Kinase (ALK)

In ALK-positive lung cancer (~1-7% of NSCLC), the ALK fusion protein is responsible for tumor growth. Inhibition of ALK causes stabilization or regression of tumors. ALK is prevalent in non-smokers or those with a history of light smoking and an adenocarcinoma subtype.

DRUG	UNIQUE CONCERNS	SAFETY/SIDE EFFECTS/MONITORING
Crizotinib (Xalkori) 250 mg PO BID	Pharmacogenomics: Must test for ALK mutation status. Must be positive. Primary target is ALK but also inhibits cMET (Mesenchymal Epithelial Transition Factor)	**SIDE EFFECTS** Edema, N/V/D, constipation, vision disturbances (visual impairment, flashes of light, blurred vision, floaters, double vision, sensitivity to light, visual field defects), interstitial pneumonitis
Ceritinib (Zykadia) 750 mg PO daily on an empty stomach (2 hour before or 2 hours after meal)	Pharmacogenomics: Must test for ALK mutation status. Must be positive. Primary target is ALK. Used as 2nd line agent.	**SIDE EFFECTS** Interstitial pneumonitis, hepatotoxicity, GI toxicity, QT prolongation, hyperglycemia, bradycardia

RENAL CELL CANCER (RCC)

RCC is the most common type of kidney cancer in adults (~80% of the cases). Risk factors include smoking, obesity and hypertension. Primary therapy is surgery (radical or partial nephrectomy) with curative intent. RCC is fairly resistant to radiation therapy and chemotherapy. Below is a list of commonly used targeted cancer therapies for RCC.

Tyrosine Kinase Inhibitors (TKIs) Targeting Multiple Kinases

DRUG	UNIQUE CONCERNS	SAFETY/SIDE EFFECTS/MONITORING
SUNitinib (Sutent) 50 mg PO daily for 4 weeks on and 2 weeks off Dosing varies depending on indication	Inhibits multiple tyrosine kinases: PDGF, VEGF-R 1/2, SCF-R, cKIT and others.	**BOXED WARNING** Hepatotoxicity **SIDE EFFECTS** Rash, hand-foot syndrome, N/V/D, mucositis/stomatitis, dyspepsia, anorexia, taste disturbance, skin discoloration, alopecia, neutropenia, anemia, thrombocytopenia, lymphopenia, hypertension, edema, HF, ↓ LVEF, QT prolongation, fatigue, electrolyte imbalance, ↑ LFTs, elevated lipase, hypothyroidism MedGuide required ↳ *like lapatinib (Tykerb®)*
PAZOPanib (Votrient) 800 mg PO daily on empty stomach (1 hour before or 2 hours after a meal), do not crush	Inhibits PDGF-R alpha and beta, VEGF-R 1/2/3, FGFR 1/3, cKit, and others.	**BOXED WARNING** Hepatotoxicity **SIDE EFFECTS** ↑ LFTs, hyperglycemia, hypothyroidism, electrolyte loss (phosphorus, Na+, Mg2+), fatigue, diarrhea, weight loss, hypertension, anorexia, headache, dysguesia, dyspnea, QT prolongation, thromboembolic events, hemorrhagic events, color changes in skin and hair MedGuide required

Tyrosine Kinase Inhibitors (TKIs) Targeting Multiple Kinases Continued

DRUG	UNIQUE CONCERNS	SAFETY/SIDE EFFECTS/MONITORING
SORAfenib *(NexAVAR)* 400 mg PO BID on an empty stomach (1 hour before or 2 hours after a meal)	Inhibits raf-mek pathway kinases (CRAF, BRAF), PDGF, EGFR, VEGF-R 2/3, SCF R, cKIT, FLT-3.	**CONTRAINDICATIONS** Combination with carboplatin and paclitaxel (squamous cell lung cancer) causing aplastic anemia **SIDE EFFECTS** Fatigue, hypertension, hand-foot syndrome, diarrhea, N/V, mucositis/stomatitis, dyspepsia, GI bleed, acneiform rash, alopecia, neutropenia, anemia, thrombocytopenia, lymphopenia, electrolyte imbalance, ↑ LFTs, ↑ lipase/amylase, impaired wound healing (dehiscence), interstitial pneumonitis, hair color changes *↳ like bevacizumab (Avastin®)*

Tyrosine Kinase Inhibitors (TKIs) Targeting VEGF

The VEGF family of protein kinases regulate angiogenesis which is blocked by these TKIs, thus reducing to the tumor's blood supply.

DRUG	UNIQUE CONCERNS	SAFETY/SIDE EFFECTS/MONITORING
Axitinib *(Inlyta)* 5 mg PO Q12H After 2 weeks, may increase to 7 mg PO Q12H, and further to 10 mg Q12H (if tolerated)	Inhibits: VEGF receptors 1, 2 and 3. CYP 3A4/5 substrate: caution with inhibitors.	**SIDE EFFECTS** Hypertension, hepatotoxicity, hand-foot syndrome, dysphonia, weight loss, anorexia, fatigue, asthenia, N/V/D, constipation, thromboembolic events, hemorrhagic events, hypothyroidism

Mammalian Target of Rapamycin (mTOR) Inhibitors

Inhibit downstream regulation of VEGF reducing cell growth, metabolism, proliferation and angiogenesis

DRUG	UNIQUE CONCERNS	SAFETY/SIDE EFFECTS/MONITORING
po Everolimus *(Afinitor)* 10 mg PO daily *Zortress* is indicated for transplantation and used in various doses	CYP 3A4 inhibitor/substrate	**BOXED WARNINGS** See Transplant chapter for *Zostress* **CONTRAINDICATIONS** Hypersensitivity to rapamycin derivatives **SIDE EFFECTS** Dyslipidemia, hyperglycemia, myelosuppression, rash, pruritus, hand-foot syndrome, stomatitis, fatigue, N/V/D, peripheral edema, interstitial lung disease, elevated creatinine with ↓ renal function, ↑ LFTs MedGuide required
IV Temsirolimus *(Torisel)* 25 mg IVPB over 30-60 minutes once weekly	CYP 3A4 inhibitor/substrate Pre-medicate with diphenhydramine Use non-PVC bag & tubing due to leaching of DEHP.	**CONTRAINDICATION** Hepatotoxicity **SIDE EFFECTS** Dyslipidemia, hyperglycemia, myelosuppression, interstitial lung disease, acute hypersensitivity reactions (polysorbate 80 solvent system), N/V/D, peripheral edema, pain, dyspnea, cough, fever, asthenia, rashes, acne

non-PVC bag & tubing

CHRONIC MYELOID LEUKEMIA (CML)

Chronic myelogenous (or myeloid) leukemia (CML) is a type of myeloproliferative disease of mature granulocytes (neutrophils, eosinophils and basophils) with a characteristic chromosomal translocation called the Philadelphia (Ph) chromosome (bcr-abl fusion gene). CML is primarily treated with oral tyrosine kinase inhibitors (TKIs), which have led to dramatically improved long term survival rates (mean 47 months to over 10 years) since the introduction of imatinib in 2001.

CHRONIC LYPHOMCYTIC LEUKEMIA (CLL)

Many of the BCR-ABL targeting TKIs used in CML are also used in treatment of CLL. Recent approvals include: ibrutinib *(Imbruvica)*, idelalisib *(Zydelig)*, ofatumumab *(Arzerra)* and obinutuzumab *(Gazyva)*.

Tyrosine Kinase Inhibitors (TKIs) Targeting BCR-ABL

A fusion gene is created when the ABL gene on chromosome 9 is translocated to the Breakpoint Cluster Region (BCR) gene on chromosome 22 resulting in cancer cell growth, replication and immortality. Blocking this results in a halt to cancer cell growth and likely apoptosis. Use of TKIs require pharmacogenomic testing for the presence of bcr-abl fusion gene.

DRUG	UNIQUE CONCERNS	SAFETY/SIDE EFFECTS/MONITORING
Imatinib *(Gleevec)* 400-600 mg PO daily with water and full meal Various doses used for other cancers	Indications: Philadelphia-chromosome positive (Ph+) chronic myelogenous leukemia (CML) or cKIT (CD117)-positive gastrointestinal stromal tumors (GIST).	**SIDE EFFECTS** Fluid retention, skin rash, diarrhea, edema, leukopenia, thrombocytopenia, N/V, HF, muscle spasms
Dasatinib *(Sprycel)* 100-180 mg PO daily Needs acid for absorption, avoid PPIs and H$_2$RAs	Maintains clinical activity in CML resistant to imatinib but more expensive as first line therapy. ~ 300 times more potent than imatinib. Also inhibits cKit, PDGFR, SCF, SRC tyrosine kinases.	**SIDE EFFECTS** Pleural effusions, fluid retention, edema, leukopenia, thrombocytopenia, N/V/D, skin rash, headache, musculoskeletal pain
Nilotinib *(Tasigna)* 300-400 mg PO BID on an empty stomach (1 hour before, 2 hours after meal)	Maintains clinical activity in CML resistant to imatinib but more expensive as first line therapy. Major CYP3A4 substrate, avoid strong CYP3A4 inhibitors	**BOXED WARNINGS** QT prolongation **CONTRAINDICATIONS** Hypomagnesemia, hypokalemia, QT prolongation **SIDE EFFECTS** QT prolongation, hypo- and hyperkalemia, hypomagnesemia, leukopenia, thrombocytopenia, N/V/D, fluid retention, edema, skin rashes, pruritus, alopecia
Bosutinib *(Bosulif)* 500-600 mg PO daily with food	Maintains clinical activity in CML in ~ 33% of imatinib resistant and ~ 27% of dasatinib or nilotinib resistant patients. CYP3A4 and P-gp substrate; avoid use with inhibitors.	**SIDE EFFECTS** Diarrhea, fluid retention (pleural effusions, pericardial effusion, pulmonary edema, and/or peripheral edema), anemia, rash, fever, fatigue, ↑ LFTs, nausea, vomiting, abdominal pain, thrombocytopenia, neutropenia

Tyrosine Kinase Inhibitors (TKIs) Targeting BCR-ABL Continued

DRUG	UNIQUE CONCERNS	SAFETY/SIDE EFFECTS/MONITORING
PONATinib *(Iclusig)* 45 mg PO daily	Maintains clinical activity in CML imatinib, dasatinib or nilotinib resistant patients, including T315I mutation. Distributed by exclusive specialty pharmacy due to brief FDA suspension from life threatening blood clots. Enrollment in *Iclusig* REMS program required.	**BOXED WARNINGS (3)** Vascular occlusions (thrombotic events, stroke, MI), heart failure and hepatotoxicity **SIDE EFFECTS** Hypertension, dry skin, abdominal pain, fluid retention (pleural effusions, pericardial effusion, pulmonary edema, and/or peripheral edema), anemia, thrombocytopenia, neutropenia, rash, fever, fatigue, ↑ LFTs, N/V/D **NOTES** MedGuide required

EARLY SIGNS OF MELANOMA (ABCDE)

- Asymmetry

- Borders (irregular)

- Color (variegated – with different colors)

- Diameter (greater than 6 mm, or 0.24 in, about the size of a pencil eraser)

- Evolving over time

However, these classifications do not, apply to the most dangerous form of melanoma, nodular melanoma, which has its own classifications:

- Elevated above the skin surface

- Firm to the touch

- Growing

MELANOMA

Melanoma is usually caused by damage from UV light from the sun or tanning beds. Early signs of melanoma are summarized by the mnemonic "ABCDE" (see box). If melanoma is found early, surgery has a high cure rate (> 80%). For melanomas that return or spread, symptoms can be non-specific and include loss of appetite, nausea, vomiting and fatigue. Treatments include surgery, radiation, chemotherapy or immunotherapy. Stage IV (metastatic) melanoma can spread to the brain, bone, liver, abdomen or distant lymph nodes.

Tyrosine Kinase Inhibitors (TKIs) Targeting BRAF: BRAF Protein Kinase Mutation

DRUG	UNIQUE CONCERNS	SAFETY/SIDE EFFECTS/MONITORING
Vemurafenib *(Zelboraf)* 960 mg PO BID	Pharmacogenetic testing required. Use only in BRAF positive melanoma with the V600E mutation (~50% of patients). Inhibitor of CYP 1A2, 2D6, P-gp; substrate of CYP 3A4, P-gp; inducer of 3A4	**WARNINGS** Not recommended in BRAF wild types as vemurafenib paradoxically activates the MAPK pathway promoting tumor growth. **SIDE EFFECTS** Dermatologic disorders (rashes, photosensitivity, alopecia, pruritus, SJS/TEN), QT prolongation, N/V/D, constipation, anorexia, weight loss, dysgeusia, arthralgia, arrhythmia, headache, uveitis, fatigue, asthenia, ↑ LFTs, squamous cell and basal cell carcinomas
Dabrafenib *(Tafinlar)* 150 mg PO BID on an empty stomach (1 hour before or 2 hours after food)	For metastatic melanoma patients with BRAF V600E or V600K mutation. Less skin toxicities compared with vemurafenib.	**WARNINGS** Not recommended in BRAF wild types **SIDE EFFECTS** Pyrexia, hyperglycemia, hypophosphatemia, alopecia, hand-foot syndrome, headache, arthralgia, squamous cell and basal cell carcinomas

Inhibitor of Mitogen-Activated Extracellular Signal Kinase 1 and 2 (MEK1 and MEK2)

DRUG	UNIQUE CONCERNS	SAFETY/SIDE EFFECTS/MONITORING
Trametinib (*Mekinist*) 2 mg PO daily on an empty stomach (1 hour before or 2 hours after food)	For metastatic melanoma patients with BRAF V600E or V600K mutations.	**WARNINGS** Not recommended in BRAF wild types **SIDE EFFECTS** Hand foot syndrome, ↑ LFTs, diarrhea, anemia, lymphedema, stomatitis, bleeding, cardiomyopathy, hypertension, rhabdomyolysis, infection, skin rashes, interstitial lung disease (can be fatal)

Immunotherapy

Blocks the Cytotoxic T-lymphocyte antigen-4 (CTL4) receptor, which effectively takes the brake off T-cell activation. Activated T-cells then can recognize melanoma cells for removal but at a risk of autoimmune activity

DRUG	UNIQUE SIDE EFFECTS/NOTES	SAFETY/SIDE EFFECTS/MONITORING
Ipilimumab (*Yervoy*)	Primarily autoimmune system unchecked *Yervoy* REMS program MedGuide required	**BOXED WARNING** Fatal immune-mediated reactions (enterocolitis, hepatitis, dermatitis, neuropathy) – discontinue drug and start high doses of steroids. **SIDE EFFECTS** Dermatologic (rash, pruritus), gastrointestinal (N/V/D, colitis, esophagitis, gastritis, jejunitis, ulcers), endocrine (hypophysitis, hypothyroidism, hypoadrenalism, hyponatremia, pancreatitis), neuropathies, hepatitis, uveitis, and nephritis

↳ inflammation of eye middle layer (handwritten)

Human Programmed Death Receptor-1 (PD-1) Blocking Antibody

Blocks the programmed cell death protein 1 (PD-1) receptor pathway mediated inhibition of the immune response, reversing T-cell suppression and inducing antitumor responses

DRUG	UNIQUE CONCERNS	SAFETY/SIDE EFFECTS/MONITORING
Pembrolizumab (*Keytruda*)	Indication: unresectable or metastatic melanoma and disease progression following ipilimumab and, if BRAF V600 mutation positive, a BRAF inhibitor	**SIDE EFFECTS** Immune-mediated reactions (pneumonitis, colitis, hepatitis, nephritis, hyper- and hypothyroidism), renal failure, pruritus, rash, arthralgia, N/V/D MedGuide required

MULTIPLE MYELOMA

In multiple myeloma, abnormal plasma cells accumulate in the bone marrow. A mnemonic used to remember the common tetrad of multiple myeloma is CRAB: C = Calcium (elevated), R = Renal failure, A = Anemia, B = Bone lesions. Most cases of myeloma have high levels of paraprotein (also known as M protein) – an abnormal antibody that can cause renal failure.

Myeloma is generally incurable but highly treatable. With conventional treatment, median survival is 3–4 years, which may be extended to 5–7 years or longer with advanced treatments. Remission can be induced with steroids, chemotherapy, proteasome inhibitors, immunomodulators, and stem cell transplant.

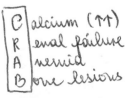

C alcium (↑↑)
R enal failure
A nemia
B one lesions (handwritten)

Immunomodulators *♀ must have (-) hCG and use 2 forms of birth control*

The immunomodulatory drugs are thalidomide or thalidomide-derivatives; the primary toxicity is severe birth defects (Pregnancy Category X) and patients must not become pregnant while using these drugs. All three have strict REMS programs designed to prevent pregnancy. They block angiogenesis and kill abnormal cells in the bone marrow while stimulating the bone marrow to produce normal healthy cells.

BBW:
here

BEs
↑↑ Ca++ ←

SE: confusion,
somnolence,
neuropathy

DRUG	UNIQUE CONCERNS	SAFETY/SIDE EFFECTS/MONITORING
Lenalidomide (Revlimid) 25 mg PO daily for 21 days and 7 days off	Pregnancy Category X Severe birth defects. Only available under restricted distribution program: patient, prescriber and pharmacist must be registered with *Revlimid* REMS program, *Pomalyst* REMS program and/or *Thalomid* REMS program if using drug.	**BOXED WARNINGS** Fetal risk/pregnancy, thrombosis (DVT/PE), hematologic toxicity (lenalidomide) **CONTRAINDICATIONS** Pregnancy
Pomalidomide (Pomalyst) 4 mg PO daily for 21 days and 7 days off For relapsed multiple myeloma after at least 2 prior therapies (including lenalidomide and bortezomib)	Consider prophylactic anticoagulation due to ↑ VTE risk, seek medical care if signs and symptoms of DVT/PE develop: shortness of breath, chest pain, or arm or leg swelling.	**SIDE EFFECTS** Neutropenia, thrombocytopenia, constipation, N/V/D, fatigue, fever, cough, pruritus, rash, arthralgias, back pain, peripheral edema, DVT/PE. Neuropathy, confusion, somnolence (thalidomide)
Thalidomide (Thalomid) 100-400 mg PO daily with water and at least 1 hour after a meal		Hypercalcemia (pomalidomide)

Proteasome Inhibitors

Proteasomes are large protein complexes responsible for degrading intracellular proteins, enzymes and transcription factors. This maintains protein homeostasis upon which cancer cells are highly dependent. The 26S proteasome inhibitors block this pathway, inhibiting cell cycle progression and inducing apoptosis.

DRUG	UNIQUE CONCERNS	SAFETY/SIDE EFFECTS/MONITORING
Bortezomib (Velcade) Very active drug for multiple myeloma (typically part of first line regimen) SC administration has less neuropathy than IV administration 1.3 mg/m² SC/IV or 1.5mg/m² IV	Substrate/Inhibitor of CYP1A2, 2C9, 2C19, 2D6, 3A4 Give acyclovir to prevent zoster reactivation.	**CONTRAINDICATIONS** Hypersensitivity to boron or mannitol, intrathecal administration (fatal) **SIDE EFFECTS** Peripheral neuropathy, psychiatric disturbances, insomnia, weakness, paresthesias, arthralgias/myalgias, cardiotoxicity, pulmonary toxicity, hypotension, thrombocytopenia, neutropenia, N/V/D, tumor lysis syndrome
Carfilzomib (Kyprolis) Cycle 1: 20 mg/m² daily for 2 days for 3 consecutive weeks followed by 1 week off. Cycle 2 and on: 27 mg/m² daily for 2 days for 3 consecutive weeks followed by 1 week off. Cycles repeated monthly. IVPB For relapsed multiple myeloma after at least 2 prior therapies	More specific for the 26S-proteasome so maintains activity in some patients refractory to bortezomib. Premedicate with dexamethasone and fluids. ↑ alkaline phosphatase correlates with ↑ efficacy.	**SIDE EFFECTS** Peripheral neuropathy (but less than bortezomib), fatigue, pulmonary toxicity, acute renal failure, tumor lysis syndrome, hepatic toxicity, anemia, thrombocytopenia, N/V/D, pyrexia, cardiotoxicity

Administration and Safe Handling of Oral Chemotherapeutic Agents

GENERIC (BRAND)	PREGNANCY CATEGORY	ADMINISTRATION	SPECIAL HANDLING
Imatinib (Gleevac)	D	Take with food or within 1 hour after a meal	Thalidomide, pomalidomide, and lenalidomide: female patients of reproductive potential must have negative pregnancy tests and use 2 forms of birth control. REMS drugs and only available through a specialty pharmacy.
Thalidomide (Thalomid)	X		
Capecitabine (Xeloda)	D		
Nilotinib (Tasigna)	D	Take on an empty stomach (1 hour before or 2 hours after food, pomalidomide is taken 2 hours before or 2 hours after food)	
Erlotinib (Tarceva)	D		
Sorafenib (Nexavar)	D		
Pazopanib (Votrient)	D		
Temozolomide (Temodar)	D		
Abiraterone (Zytiga)	X		
Pomalidomide (Pomalyst)	X		
Dasatinib (Sprycel)	D	Take without regards to food	
Sunitinib (Sutent)	D		
Tamoxifen (Soltamox)	D		
Anastrozole (Arimidex)	X		
Bicalutamide (Casodex)	X		
Lenalidomide (Revlimid)	X		

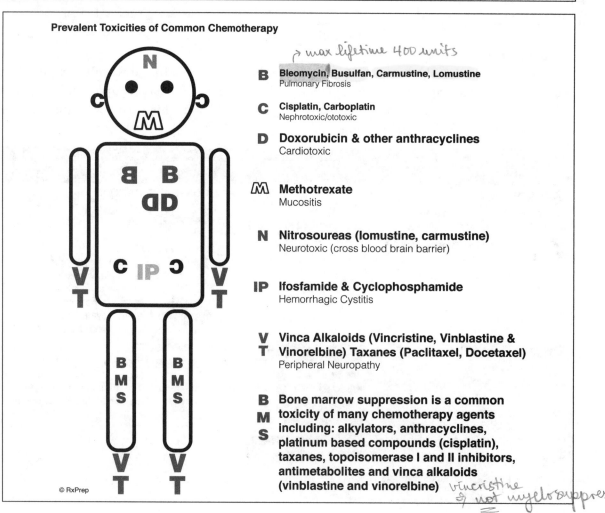

Prevalent Toxicities of Common Chemotherapy

→ max lifetime 400 units

B **Bleomycin, Busulfan, Carmustine, Lomustine**
Pulmonary Fibrosis

C **Cisplatin, Carboplatin**
Nephrotoxic/ototoxic

D **Doxorubicin & other anthracyclines**
Cardiotoxic

M **Methotrexate**
Mucositis

N **Nitrosoureas (lomustine, carmustine)**
Neurotoxic (cross blood brain barrier)

IP **Ifosfamide & Cyclophosphamide**
Hemorrhagic Cystitis

V **Vinca Alkaloids (Vincristine, Vinblastine &**
T **Vinorelbine) Taxanes (Paclitaxel, Docetaxel)**
Peripheral Neuropathy

B **Bone marrow suppression is a common**
M **toxicity of many chemotherapy agents**
S **including: alkylators, anthracyclines,**
platinum based compounds (cisplatin),
taxanes, topoisomerase I and II inhibitors,
antimetabolites and vinca alkaloids
(vinblastine and vinorelbine) vincristine
→ not myelosuppressive

© RxPrep

Patient Counseling Examples

Selective Estrogen Receptor Modulators (Using Tamoxifen as an Example)

- This medication can be used to reduce your chance of getting breast cancer, reduce the spread of breast cancer or be used to cure breast cancer.

- Swallow the tablet whole daily, with water or another non-alcoholic liquid. You can take it with or without food.

- If you forget a dose, take it when you remember, then take the next dose as usual. If it is almost time for your next dose or you remember at your next dose, do not take extra tablets to make up the missed dose.

- Do not become pregnant while taking this medication or for 2 months after you stop. This medication can stop hormonal birth control methods from working correctly (birth control pills, patches, injections, rings and implants). Therefore, while taking this medication, another method of contraception should be used, such as condoms, diaphragms with spermicide, or IUDs.

- If you become pregnant, stop taking this medication right away and call your healthcare provider.

- Be sure to have regular gynecology check-ups, breast exams and mammograms. Your healthcare provider will tell you how often. These will check for signs of breast cancer and cancer of the endometrium (lining of the uterus).

- This medication can cause some serious, but rare, side effects such as endometrial cancer, stroke, or a blood clot. This medication can also increase the risk of getting cataracts.

- The most common side effects include hot flashes, hypertension, peripheral edema, mood changes, depression, skin changes, and vaginal discharge.

- You should call your healthcare provider right away if you develop:

  - vaginal bleeding or bloody discharge that could be a rusty or brown color, change in your monthly bleeding, such as in the amount or timing of bleeding or increased clotting, or pain or pressure in your pelvis (below your belly button).

  - sudden chest pain, shortness of breath, coughing up blood, pain, tenderness, or swelling in one or both of your legs. *[handwritten: DVT/ PE]*

  - sudden weakness, tingling, or numbness (in your face, arm or leg, especially on one side of your body), sudden confusion, trouble speaking or sudden trouble seeing in one or both eyes, sudden trouble walking, dizziness, loss of balance or coordination, or sudden severe headache with no known cause. *[handwritten: stroke]*

  - signs of liver problems like lack of appetite and yellowing of your skin or whites of your eyes.

- For *Evista* – discontinue at least <u>72 hours</u> prior to and during prolonged immobilization (e.g., post-surgical recovery, prolonged bed rest), and avoid prolonged restrictions of movement during travel because of the increased risk of thromboembolic event (blood clots).

Aromatase Inhibitors

- This medication is used to treat breast cancer in women who have <u>finished menopause</u>. This medication does not work in women who have not finished menopause. It can be taken with or without food.

- If you miss a dose, take it as soon as you remember. If it is almost time for your next dose, skip the missed dose. Take your next regularly scheduled dose. Do not take two doses at the same time.

- Common side effects include hot flashes, weakness, <u>joint pain</u>, bone pain, <u>osteoporosis</u>, mood changes, high blood pressure, depression, and rash.

- This medication can cause rare, but serious, adverse effects such as heart disease, increased cholesterol, skin reactions, allergic reactions, and liver problems.

- Call your healthcare provider right away if you develop:
  - chest pain, shortness of breath.
  - any skin lesions, ulcers, or blisters.
  - swelling of the face, lips, tongue, or throat, trouble swallowing, or trouble breathing.
  - a general feeling of not being well with yellowing of the skin or whites of the eyes or pain on the right side of your abdomen.
- Tell your healthcare provider about all the medicines you take, including prescription and non-prescription medicines, vitamins, and herbal supplements. This medication should not be taken with tamoxifen or any medicines containing estrogen regardless of formulation (pills, patches, creams, rings, or suppositories).

Leuprolide

- This medication is used to treat your prostrate cancer and will lower sex hormones (testosterone and estrogen) produced by the body.
- Some patients experience worsening of their prostate cancer upon starting the LHRH agonist due to "tumor flare". To minimize this side effect, an anti-androgen (such as bicalutamide) is started at least 1 week prior to your injection.
- Common side effects include hot flashes and impotence.
- During the first few weeks of treatment you may experience increased bone pain and increased difficulty in urinating.
- If you have a change in strength on one side of your body that is greater than the other side, trouble speaking or thinking, change in balance, or blurred eyesight you will need to see a healthcare provider right away.

Ondansetron

- Take this medicine by mouth with a glass of water. It may be taken as needed or at scheduled times. Follow the directions on your prescription label. Do not take your medicine more often than directed.
- Do not take this medicine if you are taking apomorphine.
- Common side effects of this medication include headache, constipation, fatigue and dizziness.
- If you are prescribed the oral disintegrating tablets (Zofran ODT): Do not attempt to push the tablets through foil backing. With dry hands, peel back the foil of 1 blister and remove the tablet. Place tablet on the tongue; it will dissolve in seconds. Once dissolved, you may swallow with saliva. Administration with liquid is not necessary. Wash hands after administration.
- If you are prescribed the oral soluble film (Zuplenz): with dry hands, fold the pouch along the dotted line to expose the tear notch. While still folded, tear the pouch carefully along the edge and remove the oral soluble film just prior to dosing. Place the film on the tongue, it will dissolve in a few seconds. Allow each film to dissolve completely before taking the next film if more than one is needed to reach the desired dose (i.e., 16 mg given as two 8 mg films).
- The maximum oral dose of ondansetron is 24 mg/day.

PRACTICE CASE

TO is a 53 y/o Indian male diagnosed with non-Hodgkin's lymphoma. His past medical history is significant for mild heart failure (NYHA Class I). He is to receive 6 cycles of "CHOP" chemotherapy.

Allergies: NKDA

Chemotherapy Regimen:
Cyclophosphamide 750 mg/m² IV on Day 1
Doxorubicin 50 mg/m² IV on Day 1
Vincristine 1.4 mg/m² IV on Day 1
Prednisone 100 mg PO on Days 1-5 given first

Vitals:
Height: 5'10" Weight: 200 pounds
BP: 145/97 mmHg HR: 79 BPM RR: 15 BPM Temp: 98.5°F Pain: 0/10

Labs:
Na (mEq/L) = 136 (135 - 145)
K (mEq/L) = 3.7 (3.5 - 5)
Cl (mEq/L) = 98 (95 - 103)
HCO_3 (mEq/L) = 26 (24 - 30)
BUN (mg/dL) = 15 (7 - 20)
SCr (mg/dL) = 1.1 (0.6 - 1.3)
Glucose (mg/dL) = 106 (100 - 125)
Ca (mg/dL) = 9.1 (8.5 - 10.5)
Mg (mEq/L) = 1.5 (1.3 - 2.1)
PO_4 (mg/dL) = 2.9 (2.3 - 4.7)
AST (IU/L) = 20 (8 - 48)
ALT (IU/L) = 12 (7 - 55)
Albumin (g/dL) = 3.4 (3.5 - 5)
T Bili (mg/dL) = 0.8 (0.1 - 1.2)

Start chemotherapy today. Monitor for acute toxicities from chemotherapy regimen and begin any supportive care as needed.

Questions

Questions 1-5 refer to the above case.

1. The pharmacist must first calculate the patient's BSA and will use the Dubois and Dubois equation: BSA (m²) = 0.007184 x [weight (kg)$^{0.425}$] x [height (cm)$^{0.725}$]. The patient's BSA is:

   a. 1.15 m²
   b. 1.03 m²
   c. 2.09 m²
   d. 2.18 m²
   e. 3.15 m²

2. What is the correct milligram dose of doxorubicin that the patient should receive on Day 1?

   a. 104.5 mg
   b. 510 mg
   c. 949.5 mg
   d. 948.5 mg
   e. 300 mg

(handwritten) $\frac{50mg}{m^2} \cdot 2.09 m^2 = 104.5 mg$

(handwritten) $BSA = 0.007184 \times \left(\frac{200}{2.2}\right)^{0.425} \times (177.8)^{0.725} = 2.089$

3. The physician wants to know if there are any medications that can reduce the likelihood of cardiotoxicity with doxorubicin therapy. Which of the following would you suggest?

   dexrazoxane

   a. Totect — *for extravasation*
   b. Zinecard — *for cardioprotection*
   c. Lasix
   d. Epogen
   e. Mesna

4. What is the dose limiting toxicity of vincristine?

   a. Neuropathy
   b. Nephrotoxicity
   c. Hypersensitivity reaction
   d. Ototoxicity
   e. Pulmonary toxicity

Questions 5-13 do not relate to the above case.

5. A patient is using apomorphine *(Apokyn)* injections for advanced Parkinson disease. The patient has been suffering from nausea. Which of the following antiemetics should be avoided with apomorphine?

   a. Lorazepam
   b. Metoclopramide
   c. Prochlorperazine
   d. Granisetron *↳ ≠ w/ ondansetron*
   e. All of the above

6. A patient will begin raloxifene therapy. Choose the correct counseling points: (Select **ALL** that apply.)

   a. This drug can increase your risk of breast cancer.
   b. Avoid long periods of immobility, such as during long airplane flights – get up and move when you can.
   c. This medication can cause weakened bones and fractures. *used for osteoporosis*
   d. This medication should only be used by men.
   e. This drug should be taken once daily.

7. Which of the following medications should be taken with food? (Select **ALL** that apply.)

   a. Gleevec
   b. Xeloda
   c. Nexavar
   d. Votrient
   e. Zytiga

8. An antidote for toxicity from high-dose methotrexate is:

   a. Folic acid
   b. Leucovorin
   c. Vitamin B12
   d. Cholestyramine
   e. Vitamin D

9. A pharmacist received a prescription for *Gleevec*. An appropriate generic interchange is:

   a. Aprepitant
   b. Imatinib
   c. Temozolomide
   d. Anastrozole
   e. Capecitabine

10. A pharmacist received a prescription for *Arimidex*. An appropriate generic interchange is:

    a. Aprepitant
    b. Anastrozole
    c. Exemestane
    d. Letrozole
    e. Tamoxifen

11. A patient is receiving dronabinol for nausea. Appropriate counseling points should include: *Marinol®*

    a. The capsules should be kept in the refrigerator.
    b. Your appetite may increase.
    c. This medication cannot be shared with others.
    d. A and B only.
    e. A, B and C.

12. A patient has chemotherapy-induced anemia. She states she is weak. The pharmacist has access to her labs and finds that the current hemoglobin level is (11) g/dL. Ferritin, serum iron, TIBC, folate and vitamin B12 are all at acceptable levels. Her oncologist has prescribed *Procrit*. The patient has brought the *Procrit* prescription to the pharmacy. Choose the correct statement:

a. The prescription can be filled after the pharmacist confirms that the patient is registered with the ESA APPRISE program.

b. The generic name of *Procrit* is darbepoetin.

c. The patient should be aware that they may experience euphoria and increased appetite.

d. The prescription should not be filled; the pharmacist should contact the prescriber.

e. A and B only.

13. A patient with end stage breast cancer has been experiencing fatigue and dehydration. She has a corrected calcium of 11.5 mg/dL. What is most appropriate for treating her hypercalcemia?

8.5 - 10.5

a. Instruct patient to drink 8 glasses of water

b. IV hydration, loop diuretic, and zoledronic acid

c. Calcitonin

d. Vitamin D

e. No treatment is necessary since her calcium is within the normal range

Answers

1-c, 2-a, 3-b, 4-a, 5-d, 6-b,e, 7-a,b, 8-b, 9-b, 10-b, 11-e, 12-d, 13-b

anemia normal MCV = 80-100

microcytic
⇒ MCV ≤ 80 mm³
• small cell size
• Fe deficiency

macrocytic
= megaloblastic
⇒ MCV > 100 mm³
• folate deficiency
• vit B₁₂ deficiency
Schilling's test [↳ pernicious anemia
= ↓ intrinsic factor
⇒ ↓ vit B₁₂ absorption

normocytic
⇒ MCV = 80-100 mm³
• acute blood loss (surgery/trauma)
• hemolysis
• bone marrow failure (aplastic anemia)
• anemia of chronic dz (e.g. CKD)

ANEMIA = ↓ Hct or Hgb

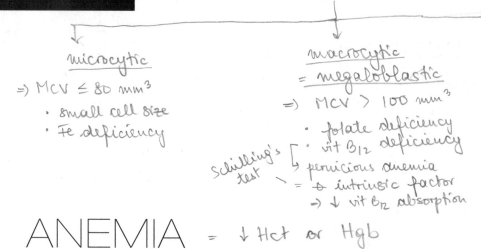

Normal amount of red blood cells   Anemic amount of red blood cells

GUIDELINES/REFERENCES

Kidney Disease: Improving Global Outcomes (KDIGO) Anemia Work Group. KDIGO Clinical Practice Guideline for Anemia in Chronic Kidney Disease. Kidney International. Suppl 2012; 2:279-335.

FDA Drug Safety Communication: Modified dosing recommendations to improve the safe use of erythropoiesis-stimulating agents in chronic kidney disease. www.fda.gov/Drugs/Drug-Safety/ucm259639.htm (accessed 2014 November 3).

National Institute of Health Dietary Supplement Fact Sheet: Iron. http://ods.od.nih.gov/factsheets/Iron-HealthProfessional/(accessed 2014 November 3).

Note: Iron requirements for infants, per the American Pediatric Association, are in the Natural Products and Vitamins chapter.

BACKGROUND

Anemia is the most common blood disorder and affects approximately 3.5 million Americans. It is characterized by a decrease in hematocrit (Hct) or hemoglobin (Hgb) concentration below the normal range for age and gender. Red blood cells (RBCs), known as erythrocytes, are the most common type of blood cell whereas Hgb is an iron-rich protein in RBCs that carries oxygen from the lungs to the tissues. Reticulocytes are immature RBCs which circulate in the blood for 1-2 days before maturing into an erythrocyte. Normally, RBCs have a lifespan of about 120 days after which they are removed from circulation by macrophages, mainly in the spleen. A decrease in Hgb or RBC volume results in decreased oxygen carrying capacity of the blood. The main cause of anemia can be classified as impaired RBC production, increased RBC destruction (hemolysis), and blood loss. Anemia can be a sign of many medical disorders, including chronic renal disease and malignancy. Therefore, rapid diagnosis of the cause is essential.

↓ Hgb or RBC volume = ↓ O₂ carrying capacity

SYMPTOMS OF ANEMIA

Most patients with mild or early stage anemia are asymtomatic. If anemia becomes severe and prolonged, the lack of oxygen in the blood can lead to classic symptoms including fatigue, malaise, weakness, shortness of breath, exercise intolerance, headache, dizziness, anorexia, and/or pallor. More severe symptoms, usually due to acute blood loss, may include chest pain, angina, fainting, palpitations, and tachycardia. Glossitis (an inflamed, sore tongue), koilonychias

Sx from ↓ O₂
1) fatigue/malaise/weakness
2) SOB
3) exercise intolerance
4) h/a
5) dizziness
6) anorexia
7) pallor
dry skin/thin hair

& restless leg syndrome (RLS)

(thin, concave, spoon-shaped nails), or pica (craving and eating non-foods such as chalk or clay) may develop in iron deficiency anemia.

A decreased oxygen supply can cause ischemic damage to many organs. Chronic anemia is most notable in causing heart damage, the heart will try to compensate for low oxygen levels by pumping faster (tachycardia) and by increasing the mass of the ventricular wall, which can eventually lead to heart failure.

TYPES OF ANEMIA

The most common way to classify anemia is by the mean corpuscular volume (MCV) or the average volume of RBCs. While the symptoms may be similar for both macrocytic and microcytic anemia, the MCV will differ. The MCV is small, < 80 mm^3, in microcytic anemia due to a small cell size and can be due to iron deficiency. The MCV is large, > 100 mm^3, in macrocytic (megaloblastic) anemia and can be due to folate or vitamin B12 deficiency. An anemia presenting with a normal MCV, 80 - 100 mm^3, is called normocytic anemia. This type of anemia can result from acute blood loss (surgery or trauma), hemolysis, bone marrow failure (aplastic anemia), or anemia of chronic disease. Certain genetic conditions cause dysfunctional RBCs resulting in anemia, such as sickle cell anemia. Please refer to the Sickle Cell Disease chapter for more information.

TEST	NORMAL ADULT RANGE
Red Blood Cell Count (RBCs)	Males: 4.5-5.5 x 10^6 cells/μL Females: 4.1-4.9 x 10^6 cells/μL
Hemoglobin (Hgb)	Males: 13.5-18 g/dL Females: 12-16 g/dL
Hematocrit (Hct)	Males: 38-50% Females: 36-46%
Mean Corpuscular Volume (MCV)	80-100 mm^3
Mean Corpuscular Hemoglobin Concentration (MCHC)	31-37 g/dL
Reticulocyte Count	0.5-2.5% of RBCs
Total Iron-Binding Capacity (TIBC)	250-400 mcg/dL
Serum Iron	65-150 mcg/dL
Serum Ferritin	11-300 ng/mL
Transferrin Saturation (TSAT)	Males: 15-50% Females: 12-45%
Serum Folate	5-25 mcg/L

MICROCYTIC ANEMIA

Iron deficiency is the most common nutritional deficiency in the United States. It can result from inadequate dietary intake (e.g., vegetarian diet, malnutrition, dementia, psychiatric illnesses), ↑ iron loss (e.g., acute/chronic hemorrhage, blood donation), ↓ iron absorption (e.g., antacid therapy or high gastric pH, celiac disease, partial gastrectomy), or ↑ iron requirements (e.g., pregnancy and lactation). Dietary iron is available in two forms: heme iron (found in meat) and non-heme iron (found in plant and dairy foods). Absorption of heme iron is minimally affected by dietary factors and is much more absorbable than non-heme iron. The bioavailability of non-heme iron requires gastric acid and varies greatly depending on the concentration of enhancers (e.g., meat, ascorbate) and inhibitors (tannins found in tea, calcium, phytates found in legumes, and whole grain) in the diet. Vegetarians may or may not require iron supplementation; even if the intake is adequate, the absorption can be decreased by concurrent foods. Microcytic anemia is diagnosed by a low hemoglobin and a low mean corpuscular volume (MCV) ≤ 80 mm^3. Other abnormal laboratory findings include $\downarrow$ ferritin level (most sensitive marker), $\downarrow$ serum iron and $\downarrow$ TSAT, and $\uparrow$ TIBC. Iron deficiency anemia is generally treated with oral ferrous sulfate and takes 3-6 months to adequately replete iron stores.

QUANTITATIVE LABORATORY FINDINGS	TEST
Low	RBC, Hct, Hgb, MCV (< 80 mm^3), ferritin, serum iron, TSAT, MCHC, reticulocyte count
High	RDW, TIBC

At-Risk Patients

@ 4-6 mo old until they start eating Fe-rich food
even breast-fed babies require Fe suppl 1 mg/kg/day

Pregnant women, pre-term and low birth weight infants, older infants and toddlers, teenage girls, women with heavy menstrual periods, and renal failure patients are at an increased risk for iron deficiency. Gastrointestinal diseases, including Crohn's, celiac disease and weight loss surgery, can reduce absorption and require replacement therapy. Total dietary iron intake in vegetarian diets may meet recommended levels; however, that iron is less available (non-heme iron) for absorption than in diets that include meat (heme-containing iron). As stated above, vegetarians may need iron replacement.

Women taking hormonal contraception experience less bleeding during menstrual periods, and therefore have a lower risk of developing iron deficiency. A pharmacist may occasionally dispense hormonal contraception to a female to reduce anemia, this is usually in younger females since young women tend to have heavier blood loss.

The CDC recommends routine low-dose iron supplementation (30 mg/day) for all pregnant women, beginning at the first prenatal visit. Usually the low iron dose is provided in the prenatal vitamin. When a low hemoglobin or hematocrit is confirmed by testing, larger doses of iron are required.

TREATMENT OF IRON DEFICIENCY ANEMIA

Oral Iron Therapy

- Oral iron therapy (ferrous sulfate) can adequately treat patients with iron-deficiency anemia, except for patients on hemodialysis (discussed in parenteral iron therapy section).

- Ferrous iron (Fe^{2+}) is absorbed more readily than the ferric (Fe^{3+}) form.

ferrous > ferric absorption
(Fe^{2+})   (Fe^{3+})

may start seeing initial ↑ Fe @ ~ 3 wks

- An increase in Hgb level by (1)g/dL should occur every (2-3) weeks on iron therapy. Treatment should continue for (3-6) months after the anemia is resolved to allow for iron stores to return to normal and to prevent relapse.

- Sustained-release formulations or enteric coated formulations of iron are not recommended as initial therapy because they reduce the amount of iron that is present for absorption in the duodenum.

- Absorption of iron is enhanced in an acidic gastric environment. Administering iron with ascorbic acid (vitamin C 200 mg) may enhance absorption to a minimal extent.

food ↓ Fe absorp
- Food will decrease the absorption of iron. It is best to take iron at least 1 hour before meals. However, many patients must take iron with food because they experience GI upset (nausea) when iron is administered on an empty stomach.

Oral Iron Therapy

→ Fer-In-Sol® ⇒ Fe-only drops for infants
Poly-Vi-Sol® ⇒ Fe + vit D infant drops

elemental

DRUG	DOSING	SAFETY/SIDE EFFECTS/MONITORING	
Ferrous sulfate (*Ferro-Bob, FerrouSul, Fer-In-Sol, Poly-Vi-Sol Wlth Iron, Flinstones MVI With Iron*) *20%*	325 mg PO daily to TID (65 mg elemental iron) Most commonly prescribed and is the least expensive	**Iron Salt**	**Elemental Iron**
		Ferrous gluconate	12%
		Ferrous sulfate	20%
		Ferrous sulfate, exsiccated	30%
Ferrous fumarate (*Ferretts, Hemocyte*) *33%*	324 mg PO daily to TID (other doses available) (106 mg elemental iron)	Ferrous fumarate	33%
		Carbonyl iron	100%
		Polysaccharide iron complex	100%
Ferrous gluconate (*Fergon*) *12%*	324 mg PO daily to TID (other doses available) (38 mg elemental iron)	**CONTRAINDICATIONS** Hemochromatosis, hemolytic anemia **WARNING** Accidental overdose of iron-containing products is a leading cause of fatal poisoning in children under 6. Keep iron out of reach of children. In case of accidental overdose, go to ED or call poison control center immediately.	
Ferrous sulfate, dried (exsiccated) **Controlled Release** (*Slow Fe, Feosol*) CR *31%*	160 mg PO daily to TID (other doses available) (50 mg elemental iron)	**SIDE EFFECTS** Nausea, stomach upset, constipation (dose related), dark and tarry stools	
Carbonyl iron (*Feosol with Carbonyl Iron, Ferracap, Ferralet 90*) *100%*	varies	**MONITORING** Hgb, serum iron, TIBC, reticulocyte count, transferrin **NOTES** Enteric coated and delayed-release products are not recommended due to ↓ iron absorption since it passes the duodenum (site of maximal absorption) and is released into the ileum of the small intestine. Although fiber is first line treatment for constipation, a stool softener such as docusate is often recommended for iron-induced constipation. Although carbonyl iron has the highest amount of iron (100% elemental iron), it does not have any advantage over other formulations. Some patients may tolerate it better.	

→ advantage over other formulations (better tolerated)

Oral Iron Drug Interactions

- Antacids and agents that raise pH (H_2RAs, PPIs) will ↓ iron absorption by ↑ pH. Thus, patients should take iron 2 hours prior to, or 4 hours after antacids.

- Antibiotics, primarily tetracycline (less of a concern with doxycycline and minocycline) and quinolones, can decrease iron absorption through chelation. Take iron 1-2 hours before or 4 hours after tetracycline; 2 hours before or 6 hours after ciprofloxacin; 2 hours before or 2 hours after levofloxacin; 4 hours before or 8 hours after moxifloxacin.

p. 350
cipro 2/6
levo 2/2
moxi 4/8

- Iron should be taken 60 minutes after oral ibandronate or 30 minutes after alendronate/risedronate. (Actonel®, Atelvia®) ⌐Boniva®   ⌐Fosamax®

- Iron can interact and ↓ the levels of the following medications: levodopa, methyldopa, levothyroxine, cefdinir and mycophenolate. Separate the doses by 2-4 hours.

- High dose vitamin C (~200 mg) will ↑ acidity, and thus ↑ the absorption of iron; little benefit with low doses.

- Food ↓ absorption as much as 50%; advise patients to take on an empty stomach. If unable to tolerate, take with a small amount of food. If taken with food, it will take longer to correct the anemia.

Iron Toxicity

Accidental iron poisoning is the leading cause of poisoning deaths among young children. As little as 5 tablets in a small child can lead to overdose. The child can initially appear asymptomatic or have already developed severe nausea, vomiting, gastrointestinal bleeding (most often vomiting blood), and diarrhea. If a parent suspects their child ingested iron pills or liquid, they should be directed to the nearest emergency room immediately – whether symptomatic or not. Left untreated, iron overdose will damage most organs, including the brain, and can be fatal. The antidote for iron overdose is deferoxamine. This is different from deferiprone (*Ferriprox*), which is for transfusional iron overload unresponsive to chelation therapy.

Desferal®

Parenteral Iron Therapy

Parenteral iron therapy is as effective but can be more dangerous and is much more expensive than oral therapy. The following clinical situations can warrant IV administration:

causes loss of 6-7 mg on day of dialysis

- Hemodialysis (most common use of IV iron) – the National Kidney Foundation (NKF) guidelines state that to achieve and maintain a hemoglobin level of 11-12 g/dL (and hematocrit of 33-36%), most hemodialysis patients will require IV iron on a regular basis.

- Unable to tolerate oral iron or losing iron too fast for oral replacement.

- Intestinal malabsorption, such as Crohn's disease.

- Patients donating large amounts of blood for autoinfusion.

all stable in NS

Intravenous (Parenteral) Iron Supplementation

DRUG	SAFETY/SIDE EFFECTS/MONITORING
Iron Dextran (INFeD, Dexferrum)	**Boxed Warning (Iron Dextran only)** *→ monitor x 15-20 min* Risk of anaphylactic reactions. A test dose should be given to all patients prior to first therapeutic dose. Fatal reactions have occurred even in patients who tolerated the test dose. History of drug allergy and/or concomitant use of ACE inhibitor may ↑ risk.
Sodium Ferric Gluconate (Ferrlecit)	
	SIDE EFFECTS Hypotension, chest tightness, peripheral edema, risk of anaphylaxis with all agents (especially with iron dextran, which requires a test dose)
Iron Sucrose (Venofer)	
Ferumoxytol (Feraheme) *NS or D5W*	**MONITORING** Hgb, serum ferritin, serum iron, transferrin saturation, TIBC, vital signs, electrolytes, anaphylaxis
	NOTES Give by slow IV injection to ↓ risk of hypotension
Ferric carboxymaltose (Injectafer)	All agents are stable in NS; maximum of 100 mL of NS for *Ferrlecit* and *Venofer*. *Feraheme* is stable in NS or D5W.

BBW: anaphylaxis → test dose

max 100 ml NS

MACROCYTIC ANEMIA

Macrocytic anemia is caused by either a vitamin B12 or folate deficiency or both. If macrocytic anemia continues long-term, the patient is at risk for serious neurological consequences including cognitive dysfunction (dementia) and peripheral nerve damage. Pernicious anemia is a type of macrocytic anemia that results in low vitamin B12 levels due to lack of intrinsic factor, which is required for adequate vitamin B12 absorption in the small intestine. Since gut absorption of vitamin B12 is impaired in those who lack intrinsic factor, pernicious anemia requires lifelong vitamin B12 replacement therapy. The Schilling test can diagnose vitamin B12 deficiency due to lack of intrinsic factor.

Alcoholism, Crohn's disease, and celiac disease are other causes of macrocytic anemia. Macrocytic anemia is diagnosed by a low hemoglobin and a high mean corpuscular volume (MCV > 100 mm^3). Vitamin B12 and/or serum folate levels will be low.

QUANTITATIVE LABORATORY FINDINGS	TEST
Low	Hct, Hbg, RBC, reticulocyte count, serum folate and/or serum vitamin B12
Normal	MCHC
High	MCV (> 100 mm^3), RDW, serum homocysteine
	Serum methylmalonate in vitamin B12 deficiency

Treatment of Macrocytic Anemia

Vitamin B12 deficiency is generally treated initially with vitamin B12 injections (since injections bypass absorption barriers) and followed with oral supplements. Vitamin B12 injections are preferred for anyone with a severe deficiency or neurological symptoms.

DRUG	DOSING	SAFETY/SIDE EFFECTS/MONITORING
Cyanocobalamin, vitamin B12 *(Physicians EZ Use B-12* inj, *Nasocobal* nasal spray, oral generics)	IM or deep SC: 100-1,000 mcg daily/weekly/monthly (various dosing regimens depending on severity of deficiency) Oral/Sublingual: 1,000-2,000 mcg/day for mild-moderate deficiencies Intranasal *(Nascobal)*: 500 mcg in one nostril once weekly	**CONTRAINDICATIONS** Cobalt allergy **SIDE EFFECTS** Pain with injection, rash **MONITORING** Hgb, Hct, vitamin B12, folate, iron, reticulocyte count **NOTES** Do not use sustained-release B12 supplements as the absorption is not adequate.
Folic Acid, folate *(FA-8)* 0.4, 0.8 mg tab (OTC) 1 mg tab (Rx)	0.4-1 mg daily	**SIDE EFFECTS** Bronchospasm, flushing, rash, pruritus, malaise **MONITORING** Hgb, Hct, folate, vitamin B12, iron

folic acid = vit B9

Drug Interactions

Vitamin B12

- Chloramphenicol, colchicine, ethanol and long-term treatment with metformin may ↓ B12 absorption.

Folic Acid

- Folic acid decreases the efficacy of raltitrexed; avoid concurrent use. *→ antimetabolite (like MTX)*
- Folic acid may ↓ the serum concentration of primidone, phenobarbital, phenytoin and fosphenytoin. Monitor therapy. *fos/PHT → SE: folate deficiency ⇒ supplementation*
- Green tea and sulfasalazine may ↓ the serum concentration of folic acid. Monitor therapy.

NORMOCYTIC ANEMIA

Anemia Of Chronic Kidney Disease

Chronic kidney disease (CKD) causes anemia due to a deficiency in erythropoietin (EPO), a hormone produced by the kidneys. Erythropoietin stimulates the bone marrow to produce RBCs in response to falling levels of oxygen in the tissues. To a lesser degree, this type of anemia is also attributed to a shortened red cell survival and reduced responsiveness to the hormone. Before treating this type of anemia, iron levels are important to assess. If the iron stores are low, ESAs will be ineffective. Iron therapy and ESAs are the mainstay of anemia treatment in patients with CKD. The majority of patients who receive iron by injection are on hemodialysis since hemodialysis results 6-7 mg of iron loss per day of dialysis and is further compounded by physiologic and venipuncture losses.

For CKD, ESAs should be used at the lowest effective dose to reduce the need for blood transfusions. Start when Hgb is < 10 g/dL and reduce or stop therapy when the Hgb is near 11 g/dL. Transferring *(trn)* saturation should be at least 20%, and ferritin levels should be at least 100

TSAT

ESA
start
① Hgb < 10
② TSAT 20+ %
③ ferritin 100+ ng/ml

↓/d/c
Hgb ~ 11

ng/mL prior to starting ESA therapy. Levels of folate and vitamin B12 may also be assessed, especially if there is a poor response to ESA.

[Handwritten margin notes: "if Hgb ↑ > ① g/dl over ② wks → ↓ dose of ESA by 25%) (CKD)"]

[Handwritten top notes: "↓ need for blood transfusions", "start when Hgb < 10", "ineffective if Fe is low!"]

Erythropoiesis-Stimulating Agents (ESAs)

DRUG	DOSING	SAFETY/SIDE EFFECTS/MONITORING
Epoetin alfa (Epogen, Procrit) IV, SC	**Chronic Kidney Disease** 50-100 units/kg 3x/week, then individualize maintenance dose. Initiate when Hgb < 10 g/dL. Reduce or interrupt dose when Hgb approaches or exceeds 11 g/dL for CKD on HD, or > 10 g/dL for CKD not on HD. **Cancer** 150 units/kg 3x/week or 40,000 units weekly. Initiate when Hgb < 10 g/dL and when at least 2 additional months of chemotherapy planned. If Hgb increases > 1 g/dL in any 2-week period, interrupt or ↓ dose by 25% for CKD and cancer patients.	**BOXED WARNINGS** ESAs ↑ risk of death, MI, stroke, VTE, thrombosis of vascular access, and tumor progression or recurrence. **Chronic Kidney Disease** ESAs ↑ risk of death, serious cardiovascular events, and stroke when administered to target a Hgb level > 11 g/dL. No trial has identified a Hgb target level, ESA dose, or dosing strategy to minimize these risks. Use the lowest effective dose to avoid RBC transfusions. **Cancer** ESAs ↓ overall survival and/or ↑ risk of tumor progression or recurrence in clinical studies of patients with breast, head and neck, non-small cell lung, lymphoid, and cervical cancers. Prescribers and hospitals must enroll in and comply with the ESA APPRISE Oncology Program to prescribe and/or dispense these agents to cancer patients. Use ESAs only for anemia due to myelosuppressive chemotherapy. ESAs are not indicated when the anticipated outcome is cure. Use the lowest effective dose to avoid RBC transfusions. Discontinue following completion of a chemotherapy course.
Darbepoetin (Aranesp) IV, SC	**Chronic Kidney Disease on HD** 0.45 mcg/kg weekly or 0.75 mcg/kg every 2 weeks. **Chronic Kidney Disease Not on HD** 0.45 mcg/kg every 4 weeks. Initiate when Hgb < 10 g/dL. Reduce or interrupt dose when Hgb approaches or exceeds 11 g/dL for CKD on HD, or > 10 g/dL for CKD not on HD. **Cancer** 2.25 mcg/kg weekly or 500 mcg every 3 weeks. Initiate when Hgb < 10 g/dL and when at least 2 additional months of chemotherapy planned. If Hgb increases > 1 g/dL in any 2-week period, ↓ dose by 25% for CKD patients, 40% for cancer patients.	**Perisurgery** Due to ↑ risk of DVT, DVT prophylaxis is recommended. **CONTRAINDICATIONS** Uncontrolled HTN; pure red cell aplasia (PRCA) that begins after treatment; multidose vials containing benzyl alcohol contraindicated in neonates, infants, pregnancy and lactation. **SIDE EFFECTS** Hypertension, fever, headache, arthralgia/bone pain, pruritus/rash, nausea, cough, injection site pain, thrombosis, edema, chills, dizziness *[handwritten: Seizures]* **MONITORING** Hgb, Hct, transferrin saturation, serum ferritin, BP **NOTES** IV route is recommended for patients on hemodialysis. Do not ↑ the dose more frequently than once every 4 weeks. Store in refrigerator. Protect vials from light. MedGuide required.

[Handwritten margin notes: "keep Hgb rate of ↑ ~ to ↓", "less frequent dosing but does NOT normalize Hgb any quicker"]

Aplastic Anemia

Aplastic anemia occurs when the bone marrow fails to make enough RBCs, WBCs and platelets. It can be caused by drugs, infectious disease, autoimmune disorders, or hereditary conditions, but in many cases the cause is unknown. Patients become at risk for life-threatening infections or bleeding. Treatment may include immunosuppressants, blood transfusions or

*[Handwritten bottom notes: "aplastic anemia tx: ① immunosuppressants ② blood transfusions ③ stem cell transplant * eltrombopag (Promacta®) ↑ PLT - initial 50 mg po qd"]*

a stem cell transplant. Eltrombopag *(Promacta)*, a thrombopoietin nonpeptide agonist which increases platelet counts, was recently approved for treatment of severe aplastic anemia. The initial dose is 50 mg PO daily.

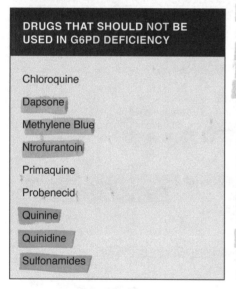

SELECT DRUGS THAT CAN CAUSE A POSITIVE COOMBS TEST

Cephalosporins

Isoniazid

Levodopa

Methyldopa

Nitrofurantoin

Penicillins

Quinidine

Quinine

Rifampin

Sulfonamides

DRUGS THAT SHOULD NOT BE USED IN G6PD DEFICIENCY

Chloroquine

Dapsone

Methylene Blue

Ntrofurantoin

Primaquine

Probenecid

Quinine

Quinidine

Sulfonamides

Hemolytic Anemia

Hemolytic anemia is a type of anemia where RBCs are destroyed and removed from the bloodstream before their normal lifespan of 120 days. This type of anemia can be acquired (e.g., drug induced) or inherited (e.g., sickle cell anemia, G6PD deficiency). Acquired hemolytic anemia, such as drug induced, occurs when the medication binds to the RBCs surface and cause antibodies to develop against the RBC proteins. This autoimmune reaction can persist for several weeks despite the medication being discontinued. The direct Coombs test is used to detect antibodies that are stuck to the surface of red blood cells. Medications that can causes a positive Coombs test are listed to the left.

Glucose-6-phosphate dehydrogenase (G6PD) is an X-linked inherited disorder that most commonly affects persons of African, Asian, Mediterranean, or Middle Eastern descent. G6PD deficiency is the result of a deficient enzyme produced from RBCs or a nonfunctional enzyme. Without sufficient levels of the enzyme to protect the RBCs, the RBCs become damaged or destroyed via hemolysis 24 to 72 hours after exposure to oxidative stress such as infections, certain foods (e.g., fava beans), severe stress, and certain drugs (see box to the left). When hemolysis is severe, patients present with weakness, tachycardia, jaundice, and hematuria, but these symptoms are self-limiting with resolution after 8 to 14 days. Most individuals do not need treatment but should be instructed on what foods and medications to avoid that cause oxidant stress.

Oral Iron Patient Counseling

- This medication will work faster if taken on an empty stomach. If taking it on an empty stomach is too nauseating, it can be taken with food, but this will mean that it will take more time to correct the anemia.
- Limit consumption of tannins, calcium, polyphenols, and phytates (found in legumes and whole grains), as these can decrease iron absorption.
- This medication needs to be taken for at least a few months for your anemia symptoms to improve, do not stop until directed by your healthcare provider.
- Iron can cause your stool to become dark. This is expected.

- If you develop constipation, ask your pharmacist for a recommendation for a stool softener (such as docusate) and a fiber product (such as psyllium).

ESA Patient Counseling

- This drug can increase your risk of life-threatening heart or circulation problems, including heart attack or stroke. This risk will increase the longer you use this drug. Seek emergency medical help if you have symptoms of blood clots, such as: crushing chest pain, or a sudden numbing pain spreading to the arm or shoulder, sudden trouble thinking/seeing/walking, or feeling short of breath, even with mild exertion.

- This drug may increase risk of disease progression or recurrence for breast cancer, non-small cell lung cancer, head and neck cancer, cervical cancer, or lymphoid cancer. Talk with your healthcare provider about your individual risk.

- This drug may cause other serious side effects such as high blood pressure, seizures, or serious allergic reactions (causing rash, shortness of breath, wheezing, fainting, sweating, facial swelling). If you experience any of these, stop using the drug and contact your healthcare provider right away.

- Less serious side effects may include dizziness, mild headache, fever, sore throat, body aches, nausea, vomiting, diarrhea, or pain or tenderness where you injected the medication. Do not shake the medication vial (bottle). Vigorous shaking will ruin the medicine. Do not draw up the drug dose into a syringe until you are ready to give yourself an injection. Do not use the medication if it has changed colors or has any particles in it. Use each disposable needle only once. Throw away used needles in a puncture-proof container (ask your pharmacist where you can get one and how to dispose of it). Keep this container out of the reach of children and pets.

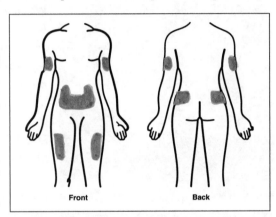

- Do not inject into an area that is tender, red, bruised, hard, or has scars or stretch marks. Recommended sites for injection are the outer area of the upper arms, the abdomen (except for 2 inches around the navel), the front of the middle thighs, and the upper outer area of the buttocks. See shaded areas for injection above.

- Store this drug in the refrigerator and do not allow it to freeze.

- Your healthcare provider may occasionally change your dose to make sure you get the best results from this medication.

- To be sure this medication is helping your body produce red blood cells, your blood will need to be tested on a regular basis. You may also need to check your blood pressure during treatment. Do not miss any scheduled appointments.

do NOT inject into deltoid → muscle
⇒ ESAs are subQ, not IM!

53

SICKLE CELL DISEASE

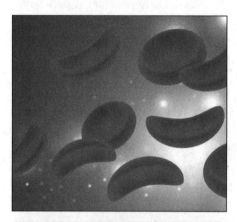

We gratefully acknowledge the assistance of Kimberly B. Tallian, PharmD, BCPP, FASHP, FCCP, FCSHP, Assistant Dean and Chair for Clinical and Administrative Sciences, Professor at Keck Graduate Institute, School of Pharmacy, Claremont Colleges, in preparing this chapter.

BACKGROUND

Sickle cell disease (SCD) is a group of disorders that affects the hemoglobin in red blood cells (RBCs). The hemoglobin molecule has an alpha chain and a beta chain. Patients with SCD have a single base substitution on chromosome 11 in the DNA sequence of the gene encoding the beta chain. Sickle cell hemoglobin is designated HbS, and normal hemoglobin is designated HbA. This causes the hemoglobin to be misshapen, which makes the RBCs rigid with a concave "sickle" shape. The irregularly shaped RBCs are unable to transport oxygen effectively and get stuck in smaller blood vessels. When the tissue is deprived of oxygen-rich blood it is ischemic, and painful. An acute episode of ischemic pain is called a sickle cell crisis or vaso-occlusive crisis (VOC) and is the hallmark of sickle cell disease. These are severe painful episodes that usually begin at night, are most common in the lower back, legs, hips, abdomen and chest, and last from 3 to 14 days. If the pain is in the chest it is called acute chest syndrome (ACS), which is very painful and can be life-threatening. ACS is the leading cause of illness in SCD and is the most common condition at the time of death. Other common conditions with SCD include:

Infections: 35% of infants with SCD die from infections most commonly due to *Streptococcus pneumoniae* and *Haemophilus influenza*. Infections are also common in children and young adults, with a higher prevalence of *Chlamydia* and *Mycoplasma pneumonia* infections. Patients with SCD should seek medical attention whenever temperature > 101.3°F occurs.

Pulmonary hypertension: 30% of patients with SCD have pulmonary hypertension, which leads to *cor pulmonale,* (increase in size in the right side of the heart), which can lead to heart failure.

Stroke: is a common killer in SCD, primarily due to blockages of coronary blood vessels. Multiple aneurysms are common. Patients with SCD should be screened for HTN and treated according to guidelines.

Anemia: sickle cell anemia (SCA) is caused when sickled cells collect in the spleen. Chronic hemolytic anemia develops due to the shortened lifespan of the RBCs; the bone marrow is not able to replace the damaged RBCs as quickly as they are destroyed. The chronic anemia is a major contributor to overall poor health and heart failure.

Kidneys: are chronically infected, urination problems are common, including uncontrolled urination during sleep, and there is high-risk for renal medullary carcinoma. Treatment with an ACE inhibitor should be started for proteinuria or microalbinuria in adults

Priapism: occurs in over 30% of male patients and must be treated.

Liver enlargement: is present in over half of SCD patients and acute liver damage is common during hospitalization. In previous years there was a high risk of hepatitis infections from chronic transfusions; this risk has decreased in recent years due to screening procedures.

Gallstones: are common, which are asymptomatic or painful.

Spleen: the spleen becomes nonfunctional due to recurrent episodes of oxygen deprivation. Spleen injury increases the risk for serious infections. Acute splenic sequestration crisis (sudden spleen enlargement) occurs when the spleen suddenly becomes enlarged from trapped blood.

Pregnancy/Contraception: Pregnancies in women with SCD have a high risk of miscarriage, premature birth and low birth weight. Men and women with SCD should consider their plans for having children. Due to the ↑ risk of stroke in SCD, progestin-only contraceptives, levonorgestrel IUDs, and barrier methods of contraception are recommended.

Other concerns: excessive production of blood cells causes the bones to grow abnormally, resulting in long legs and long arms. Sickled cells that block oxygen to bone cause severe bone pain, and sickled cells in the small capillaries cause painful hand-foot syndrome (described in the Oncology I chapter). Eye problems can develop.

Children with severe sickle cell disease have been cured with bone marrow transplant after undergoing a regimen in which their own marrow was completely destroyed with chemotherapy first, followed by the healthy donor marrow replacement. This regimen is considered too toxic for adults who have accumulated organ damage. Some adults have been successfully treated in recent years with a partial bone marrow transplant in combination with immune-suppressants.

DRUG TREATMENT

The primary drug classes used in SCD are immunizations and antibiotics (primarily penicillin) to reduce infection risk, analgesics to control pain, folic acid to help control anemia, hydroxyurea to reduce the frequency of pain episodes and acute chest syndrome, and iron chelation therapy.

- infen - PCN, immunizations
- pain - analgesics
- anemia - folic acid
- ↓ pain episodes frequency / ACS - hydroxyurea

\+ Fe chelation

Blood transfusions are often essential for treating SCD. Transfusions protect against many of the life-threatening complications by providing healthy red blood cells. These are given either chronically or for acute episodes of ACS, stroke and anemia. The goal hemoglobin level is no higher than 10 g/dL post-infusion. Transfusions carry risk, including iron overload. Chelation therapy and drugs used for iron overload are discussed in the last section.

Immunizations and Antibiotics

The major cause of death for children with SCD under 5 years of age is infection. Due to the repetitive sickling and infarctions, the spleen becomes fibrotic and eventually shrinks in size. Bacteria proliferates and causes increased risk of infection, including septicemia with encapsulated bacteria (S. pneumonia, H. influenza, Salmonella spp.)

Children under the age of 2 years are at highest risk for invasive pneumococcal disease and should receive the pneumococcal conjugate vaccine. SCD children older than 2 years, with either surgical splenectomy or functional asplenia, should receive the pneumococcal poly-saccharide vaccine and the meningococcal conjugate vaccine. Prophylactic penicillin has been shown to dramatically reduce the mortality associated with invasive pneumococcal infection in young children and should be initiated at age 2 months and continued minimally until age 5 years. If invasive pneumococcal infection develops despite antibiotic prophy-laxis, indefinite antibiotic prophylaxis should be used.

AGE	VACCINATIONS*
< 2 years	13-valent pneumococcal conjugate vaccine (Prevnar 13) H. influenza vaccine
≥ 2 years	23-valent pneumococcal polysaccharide vaccine (Pneumovax) x 2 Administer at ≥ 2 years (at least 2 months apart from Prevnar 13) and at 5 years Meningococcal conjugate vaccine x 2, given between 2-6 years and 5-9 years

* In addition to normal childhood vaccine schedule (see Immunizations chapter)

PNEUMOCOCCAL PROPHYLAXIS	DRUGS AND DOSE
Penicillin	Penicillin V Potassium 125 mg PO BID for age < 3 years and 250 mg BID for age ≥ 3-5 years or Benzathine penicillin 600,000 million units IM Q 4 weeks in nonadherent patients from 6 months to 6 years
Penicillin Allergy	Erythromycin 10 mg/kg PO BID

handwritten: p.411 also used for tx of syphilis, pen G

(see Infectious Disease chapter for further information on the antibiotics)

Pain Management and VOC *= vasoocclusive crisis*

Mild to moderate pain can often be managed at home with rest, fluids, application of warm compresses applied to affected areas, and the use of NSAIDs or acetaminophen. For severe pain and VOC, opioids are recommended. There is no test or lab to definitively diagnose VOC. Pain management must be guided by the patient's self-reported pain severity. Outpatient an-algesic use should be reviewed and treatment initiated within 30 minutes of triage. Many

handwritten: septicemia in children < 5 y/o

handwritten: ① Strep. pneumo ② H. influen ③ Salmonella

patients will require patient-controlled analgesia (PCA) for severe pain. Blood transfusion is (not) recommended in (un)complicated VOC.

Anemia Management

Folic acid is recommended in children with SCD with chronic hemolytic anemia at a dose of 0.1 mg/day up to age 1 year, 0.3 mg/day from 1-4 years, and 0.4-1 mg/day from 4 years through adolescence.

might need to give w/ vit B₁₂ inj if pernicious anemia (⊖ intrinsic factor)

SICKLE CELL PAIN MANAGEMENT PRINCIPLES

Appoint one healthcare provider to write prescriptions for long-term opioids

Believe the patient's pain

Patient should be seen every 2-3 months

Encourage fluids, fiber, stool softeners, and stimulant laxatives PRN

Use a partnership agreement and individualized treatment plan (patient rights and responsibilities, including random drug testing)

Hydroxyurea to Stimulate HbF Production

Fetal hemoglobin, or HbF, is the form of hemoglobin present in the fetus and young infants. Fetal hemoglobin blocks the sickling action of red blood cells, which is why infants with SCD do not develop symptoms until HbF levels have dropped. Hydroxyurea reduces the severity of sickle cell disease by stimulating production of HbF, by blocking the enzyme ribonucleotide reductase. This reduces the frequency of acute pain crises and episodes of ACS. Hydroxyurea is indicated for adults with ≥ 3 moderate-severe pain crises in 1 year or patients with severe ACS, anemia, or disability. May use in children > 9 months regardless of disease severity.

age > 9 months

DRUG	DOSE	SAFETY/SIDE EFFECTS/MONITORING
Hydroxyurea (Droxia, Hydrea)	Initiate: 15 mg/kg PO daily (round to nearest capsule), max 35 mg/kg/day (divide higher doses)	**BOXED WARNING** Serious and life-threatening adverse events may occur. Should be administered under the supervision of a physician experienced in the treatment of SCD (or in cancer chemotherapy). **CONTRAINDICATIONS** Significant myelosuppression: WBC < 2,500/mm³ or platelet count < 100,000/mm³ or severe anemia **SIDE EFFECTS** Leukopenia, anemia, thrombocytopenia, anorexia, nausea, diarrhea, constipation, hyperpigmentation, scaling, headache, dizziness, rash, skin and nail atrophy **MONITORING** HgF levels, CBC with differential; monitor for toxicity every 2 weeks; if toxicity, withhold until bone marrow recovers, then restart with dose reduction. If no toxicity, then can increase dose to maximum tolerated. **NOTES** Pregnancy Category D Wear gloves when handling and wash hands before and after contact

• monitor for toxicity (q 2 wks)
• if toxicity, hold until bone marrow recovers
  * then restart @ ↓ dose
• if no toxicity, ↑ dose to max tolerated

Hydroxyurea Drug Interactions

- Hydroxyurea can increase the effects of clozapine, didanosine, natalizumab, pimecrolimus, stavudine, tacrolimus (topical), tofacitinib, and live vaccines. Concomitant use should be avoided. Concurrent treatment with antiretrovirals (including didanosine and stavudine), is higher risk for potentially fatal pancreatitis, hepatotoxicity, hepatic failure, and severe peripheral neuropathy.

Hydroxyurea Patient Counseling

- For males and females of reproductive age: this medicine can harm an unborn baby and is not recommended during pregnancy. Discuss reliable birth control and family planning with your healthcare provider.

- Hydroxyurea can lower your body's ability to fight infection and make you more prone to bleeding or becoming ill.

- Call your healthcare provider immediately if you experience fever, chills, sores in the mouth, easy bruising/bleeding, purple or red point spots under the skin, pale skin, rash, shortness of breath, rapid heart rate, painful or difficulty urinating, and/or confusion.

- Wear disposable gloves when handling to reduce risk of exposure. Wash hands before and after handling. If you accidentally spill any of the contents, immediately wipe up with a damp cloth and throw cloth away in a sealed plastic bag.

Chelation to Reduce Iron Overload from Transfusions

Chronic RBC transfusions cause iron overload, which damages the liver, heart and other organs. Chelation therapy is used to remove excess iron stores in the body. Historically, deferoxamine, the antidote for iron toxicity, has been used but requires a pump for about 12 hours/day and has significant toxicities. Many patients will choose not to use it. Deferasirox (*Exjade*) is taken once daily by mouth, mixed with liquid. It is easier to take with less toxicity. Deferasirox is indicated for the treatment of chronically elevated levels of iron in the blood caused by repeated blood transfusions (transfusional hemosiderosis) in patients 2 years of age and older. It is also used for iron overload from chronic transfusions in patients with beta-thallassemia, a blood disorder causing decreased hemoglobin production.

DRUG	DOSING	SAFETY/SIDE EFFECTS/MONITORING
Deferoxamine *(Desferal)* Injection	Start at 20 mg/kg/day SC, max 2,000 mg/day. Infuse over 8-24 hours via pump. After 1 month add: ascorbic acid 50-200 mg/d	**CONTRAINDICATIONS** Severe renal disease **SIDE EFFECTS** Ototoxicity, visual impairment, arthralgia, headache, acute respiratory distress syndrome (dyspnea, cyanosis, and/or interstitial infiltrates), agranulocytosis, growth failure, hypersensitivity reactions (e.g., urticaria, angioedema), injection-site reactions (erythema, pruritus), hypotension **MONITORING** Serum iron, ferritin, total iron-binding capacity, CBC with differential, SCr, LFTs, chemistry panel, growth and body weight (baseline and every 3 months in children), audiometry and ophthalmologic exams (if used long-term) **NOTES** Pregnancy Category C

Chelation Drugs Continued

FDA
2+ y/o
transfusional
hemosiderosis

DRUG	DOSING	SAFETY/SIDE EFFECTS/MONITORING
Deferasirox (Exjade)	Start at 20 mg/kg PO daily (round to nearest tablet), max 40 mg/kg/day Must be taken on an empty stomach at least 30 minutes before eating, mixed into orange juice, apple juice or water. Instruct patients using the Drop-Stir-Drink counseling method (refer to counseling section).	**BOXED WARNINGS (3)** Gastrointestinal hemorrhage (including fatalities) may occur; monitor. Hepatic injury and failure (including fatalities) may occur. Acute renal failure (including fatalities and cases requiring dialysis) may occur; monitor carefully. **CONTRAINDICATIONS** CrCl < 40 mL/min or SCr > two-fold the age-appropriate upper limit of normal, platelet counts < 50,000/mm³, advanced malignancies **SIDE EFFECTS** Headache, rash, abdominal pain, nausea, arthralgia, visual impairment, hepatic dysfunction, kidney impairment **MONITORING** LFTs, bilirubin, SCr/CrCl, ferritin, iron, CBC **NOTES** Pregnancy Category C May cause reddish discoloration of urine

comes a tablet
MUST! be dissolved in liquid

Deferasirox Drug Interactions

- Deferasirox is a substrate of UGT1A1 as well as an inhibitor of CYP450 1A2, 2C8, and an inducer of 3A4 and can be affected by many drugs; check prior to dispensing.

- Avoid concomitant use of aluminum hydroxide, bile acid sequestrants (e.g., cholestyramine), and potent UGT inducers (e.g., rifampin, phenobarbital, phenytoin) as they may reduce the efficacy of chelation therapy.

Deferasirox Patient Counseling

- Administer tablets by making an oral suspension in water, juice or in apple sauce. Do not chew or swallow tablet whole. Take on an empty stomach at least 30 minutes before eating. Use this method:
  - DROP the *Exjade* tablet(s) into a glass of orange juice, apple juice, or water. You can also use the *Exjade* mixer each day when taking your *Exjade*. Make sure that you use the amount of liquid directed by your healthcare provider.
  - STIR the liquid and *Exjade* tablet(s) until you have an even mixture. The consistency of the mixture may be thick.
  - DRINK all of the *Exjade* mixture. Add more juice or water to mix anything that's left over. And then drink that.
- Avoid aluminum containing or milk products as they can bind the chelation therapy and reduce its effectiveness. Avoid carbonated drinks due to foaming. Seek immediate medical attention if you experience any of these signs of an allergic reaction, including difficulty breathing, hives, and/or swelling of your face, lips, tongue, or throat.

p. 858   deferiprone (Ferriprox®)
=> for transfusional Fe overload unresponsive to chelation

* alcoholics @ risk for Wernicke's encephalopathy
=> supplement vit B₁ (thiamine)
* scurvy
=> vit C

54

DEPRESSION

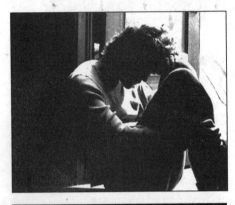

GUIDELINES

Institute for Clinical Systems Improvement (ICSI). Major depression in adults in primary care. Bloomington (MN): Institute for Clinical Systems Improvement (ICSI); September 2013.

Diagnostic and Statistical Manual of Mental Disorders (DSM-5).

Addtl guidelines included with the video files (RxPrep Online).

BACKGROUND

Major Depressive Disorder (MDD, or referred to here as "depression") is one of the most common health conditions in the world. The statistics are sobering. In any given year, approximately 15 million U.S. citizens will experience an episode of MDD. Although approximately half of these people seek help for this condition, only 20 percent – 10 percent of the total population with MDD – receive adequate treatment, and just 30 percent of those who receive adequate treatment reach the treatment goal of remission. People with depression suffer greatly with persistent feelings of hopelessness, dejection, constant worry, poor concentration, a lack of energy, an inability to sleep and, sometimes, suicidal tendencies.

Healthcare providers should remember that depression is usually a chronic illness that requires long-term treatment, much like diabetes or high blood pressure. Although some people experience only one episode, the majority have recurrent episodes. A significant treatment problem is patients who discontinue their medication, or, continue medication despite an inadequate response. This is discussed under "Treatment-Resistant Depression." Due to high rates of inadequate response, pharmacists should attempt to ensure adequate treatment trials: 6-8 weeks, at a therapeutic dose (the VA/DoD guideline recommends an 8-12 week trial).

CAUSES OF DEPRESSION

Depression's causes are poorly understood, but involve some combination of genetic, biologic and environmental factors. Pharmacists are most concerned with biological factors, since these are treated with medications. Serotonin (5HT) may be the most important neurotransmitter (NT) involved with feelings of well being. Other NTs include acetylcholine (ACh) and catecholamines [including dopamine (DA), norepinephrine (NE), and epinephrine (EPI)]. Recent research has focused on complex or completely novel pathways that may be involved in depression. Since it is not possible at this time to measure brain chemical imbalances, treatment for mood disorders, including depression, depends on a competent assessment and trial. If a drug does not work, after a suitable trial of at least 6 – 8 weeks, a combination or different set of NTs can be targeted (see treatment resistance section). Patient history is critical in treating any mental illness; what worked in the past, or did not work, should help guide current and future therapy. Pharmacists should always counsel patients, family and caregivers that mood may worsen; this is essential, since the majority of antidepressants are prescribed by primary care providers, and patient follow-up (after the prescription has been written) rarely occurs. The patient needs instructions on how to respond to worsened mood. This is critical for adolescents and young adults in particular.

DEPRESSION DIAGNOSIS

DSM-5 criteria includes presence of at least 5 of the following symptoms (even if they are in response to a significant loss like bereavement or financial ruin) during the same two week period (must include symptom 1 or 2):

1. Depressed mood
2. Marked diminished interest/pleasure
3. Significant weight loss or weight gain
4. Insomnia or hypersomnia
5. Psychomotor agitation or retardation
6. Fatigue or loss of energy
7. Feelings of worthlessness
8. Diminished ability to concentrate
9. Recurrent suicidal ideation

CONCURRENT BIPOLAR OR ANXIETY DISORDERS

It is necessary to rule-out bipolar disorder prior to initiating antidepressant therapy in order to treat the patient properly and avoid rapid-cycling (cycling rapidly from one phase to the other). This is why screening forms for MDD now include questions designed to identify mania symptoms such as "There are times when I get into moods where I feel very speeded up or irritable." Benzodiazepines (BZDs) are often used adjunctively in depression with concurrent anxiety, although in many cases the BZD is the only "treatment" and the depression itself is left untreated. BZDs can cause and/or mask depression and put the patient at risk for physiological dependence and withdrawal symptoms when the dose is wearing off (tachycardia, anxiety, amongst others). Prescribers should also select BZDs carefully and monitor closely if patients have co-occurring substance use disorders.

LAG EFFECT AND SUICIDE PREVENTION

Patients should be told that the medicine must be used daily, and will take time to work. It is important to inform the patient that physical symptoms such as low energy improve within a few weeks but psychological symptoms, such as low mood, may take a month or longer. If a patient reports suicidal ideation, refer to the ED or elsewhere for help. If someone has a plan to commit suicide, it is more likely that the threat is real.

DRUG TREATMENT

The guidelines state that because the effectiveness of the different antidepressant classes is generally comparable, the initial choice of an agent should be based on the side effect profile,

MEDICATIONS THAT CAN CAUSE OR WORSEN DEPRESSION

Beta-blockers
(particularly propranolol)

Clonidine

Corticosteroids

Cyclosporine

Ethanol

Isotretinoin

Indomethacin

Interferons   *Pegasys® for hep C*

common SE: depression (20%)

Methadone, and possibly other chronic opioid use that can lower testosterone or estrogen levels

Oral contraceptives, anabolic steroids (medication-specific, patient specific)

Methyldopa

Methylphenidate/Other ADHD Stimulants/Atomoxetine: Monitor mood

Procainamide

Reserpine

Statins (patient specific, some cases)

Varenicline

Antidepressants require monitoring for worsening mood, especially among younger people

---

In addition to the medications listed, medical conditions such as stroke, Parkinson disease, dementia, multiple sclerosis, thyroid disorders (particularly hypothyroidism), low vitamin D levels (possible link), metabolic conditions (e.g., hypercalcemia), malignancy, OAB and infectious diseases can be contributory.

safety concerns and the patient-specific symptoms. For most patients an SSRI, SNRI or (with specific concurrent conditions or considerations) mirtazapine or bupropion is preferred.

Due to safety concerns (the risk of drug-drug and drug-food interactions) the use of the oral nonselective monoamine oxidase inhibitors (MAO Is) such as phenelzine, tranylcypromine and isocarboxazid is restricted to patients unresponsive to other treatments. Serotonin syndrome can occur with administration of one or more serotonergic medications (and higher doses increase risk) but is most severe when an MAO I is administered with another serotonergic medication.

All drug therapy trials should preferably be given with competent, concurrent psychotherapy, although this is not typically done. If a drug is being discontinued it should be tapered off over several weeks. In some instances a drug with a longer half-life (e.g., fluoxetine) can be used to minimize withdrawal symptoms. Withdrawal symptoms (anxiety, agitation, insomnia, dizziness, flu-like symptoms) can be quite distressing to the patient. Paroxetine and some other agents carry a high risk of withdrawal symptoms and must be tapered upon discontinuation.   *due to short t½*

→ *+ nightmares, confusion, depressed mood, weakness, nausea*

Treatment-Resistant Depression

Prescribers should supervise a trial of 6-8 weeks at an adequate (therapeutic) dose before concluding that it is not working well. Only about half of patients respond to the prescribed antidepressant and just about one-third will reach remission (the elimination of depressive symptoms). The goal of therapy is remission. An incomplete response can necessitate any of the following:

- A dosage increase.

- A combination of antidepressants (which may or may not be appropriate).

- Augmentation with buspirone *(BuSpar)* or a low dose of an atypical antipsychotic. Agents approved as augmentation therapy with antidepressants are aripiprazole *(Abilify)*, olanzapine + fluoxetine *(Symbyax)* and quetiapine ext-rel *(Seroquel XR)*.

- Other guideline recommendations (as there are several, with various recommendations) include augmentation with lithium, thyroid hormone, and in some cases, electroconvulsive therapy (ECT).

- In 2012, good trial results were reported with the use of ketamine, which suggests alternative mechanisms may be targeted for improved treatment response.

Antidepressant Use in Pregnancy, Postpartum Depression

Untreated maternal depression, especially in the late second or early third trimesters, is associated with increased rates of adverse outcomes (e.g., premature birth, low birth weight, fetal growth restriction, postnatal complications). Depression in pregnant women often goes unrecognized and untreated in part because of safety concerns. All drugs carry risk, and the risk/benefit must be considered individually.

If a woman is on antidepressants and wishes to become pregnant, it may be possible to taper the drug if the depression is mild and she has been symptom-free for the previous six months. In more severe cases, medications may need to be continued, or started. The ACOG guidelines for mild depression in pregnancy recommend psychotherapy first, followed by drug treatment if-needed. SSRIs are often used initially and are pregnancy category C, except for paroxetine, which is D, due to potential cardiac effects. Paroxetine is the most difficult SSRI to discontinue, and requires a slow titration [tapering] if stopped. The new formulation of paroxetine, *Brisdelle*, is pregnancy category X. Although SSRIs have historically been preferred, in December of 2011 the FDA issued a warning regarding SSRI use during pregnancy and the potential risk of persistent pulmonary hypertension of the newborn (PPHN). Tricyclics, also pregnancy category C, are the second group most commonly used.

Postpartum depression is common but often unrecognized and undertreated, with adverse outcomes for the mother, baby, and family. Breast-feeding is helpful for most women for physical and emotional symptoms, and is considered beneficial for the baby. Drug safety in breastfeeding, therefore, is essential. SSRIs or tricyclics are generally preferred (with the exception of doxepin, per the ACOG recommendations).

NATURAL PRODUCTS

St. John's wort or SAMe (S-adenosyl-L- methionine) may be helpful. Both are classified as "likely effective" for treating depression in the *Natural Medicines Database*, but there is less evidence of efficacy than with standard treatments. Both agents cannot be used with other serotonergic agents. St. John's wort is a broad-spectrum CYP 450 enzyme inducer and has many significant drug interactions. It is a photosensitizer and is serotonergic; use caution with other 5HT drugs. L-methylfolate *(Deplin)* is a medical food product being used for depression.

medications w/ 5HT properties
- meperidine (Demerol®)
- lithium
- tramadol (Ultram®)
- St. John's wort

* Chantix® works on DA, not 5-HT

all SSRIs preg C
* except paroxetine => D [Brisdelle® => X]

SSRIs: Selective Serotonin Reuptake Inhibitors

DRUG	DOSING	SAFETY/SIDE EFFECTS/MONITORING
FLUoxetine ***(PROzac,*** *Sarafem, PROzac Weekly)* + OLANZapine *(Symbyax)* – taken QHS, for resistant depression q AM stimulating ⊁ thioridazine (Mellaril®)	10-60 mg/day (titrate to 60 mg/d for bulimia) 90 mg weekly 20 mg/5 mL liquid Premenstrual dysphoric disorder (PMDD): *Sarafem* 20 mg every day of menstrual cycle or 20 mg daily starting 14 days prior to menstruation through 1st full day of bleeding	**BOXED WARNING** Antidepressants increase the risk of suicidal thinking and behavior in children, adolescents, and young adults (18-24 years of age) with major depressive disorder (MDD) and other psychiatric disorders; consider risk prior to prescribing. **CONTRAINDICATIONS** Concurrent use with MAO Is, linezolid, IV methylene blue (MAOI properties), or pimozide; concurrent use with thioridazine (fluoextine, paroxetine); concurrent use with alosetrom, ramelteon, or tizanidine (fluvoxamine); concurrent use with disulfiram (sertraline); pregnancy *(Brisdelle)*
PARoxetine ***(Paxil,*** *Pexeva, Paxil CR, Brisdelle)* Preg Cat D *Briselle:* Preg Cat X ⊁ thioridazine	IR: 10–60 mg/day CR: 12.5–75 mg/day 10 mg/5mL Each 10 mg IR = 12.5 mg CR	**SIDE EFFECTS** Sexual side effects: include ↓ libido, ejaculation difficulties, anorgasmia (ability to have erection unaffected) Somnolence, insomnia, nausea, xerostomia, diaphoresis (dose-related), weakness, tremor, dizziness, headache (but may help for migraines if taken continuously)
FluvoxaMINE *(Luvox, Luvox CR)* FDA for OCD ONLY! ⊁ alosetron, ramelteon, tizanidine	100-300 mg/day Fluvoxamine has more drug interactions	Fluoxetine can cause activation; take dose in AM, others AM (usually) or PM, if sedating SIADH, hyponatremia (elderly at higher risk) Restless leg syndrome (see if this began when treatment was started) ↑ bleeding risk with concurrent use of anticoagulants, antiplatelets, NSAIDs, gingko, thrombolytics ↑ fall risk; use extreme caution in frail patients, osteopenia/ osteoporosis, use of CNS depressants
Sertraline ***(Zoloft)*** ⊁ disulfiram SSRI of choice in ♡ pts	50-200 mg/day 20 mg/mL liquid Premenstrual dysphoric disorder (PMDD): 50-150 mg every day of menstrual cycle or 50-150 mg daily starting 14 days prior to menstruation through 1st full day of bleeding	**NOTES** All approved for depression and a variety of anxiety disorders except fluvoxamine which is only approved for OCD. Note FDA warning regarding QT risk and citalopram at > 40 mg/day or > 20 mg/day if 60+ years, if liver disease, with 2C19 poor metabolizers or on 2C19 inhibitors. Similar, but lower risk for escitalopram at > 20 mg/day; do not exceed 10 mg/day in elderly. Bottom line: if cardiac risk is present, best to avoid citalopram. Sertraline is often the top choice for an SSRI in cardiac patients.
Citalopram (CeleXA) 2C19 do not exceed 20mg/d • 60+ y/o • liver dz • poor 2C19 metab or • on 2C19 inhib	20-40 mg/day 2011 FDA warning not to use > 40 mg/day due to QT risk; Max 20 mg/day in poor CYP2C19 metabolizers or concurrent use of CYP2C19 inhibitors	In 2011, the FDA issued a warning regarding SSRI use during pregnancy and the potential risk of persistent pulmonary hypertension of the newborn (PPHN). SSRIs are pregnancy category C, except paroxetine, which is considered more dangerous, and is D/X *(Briselle)*. Citalopram/escitalopram not approved for use in children.
Escitalopram ***(Lexapro*** **– S-enantiomer of citalopram)**	10 mg/day (can ↑ 20 mg/d) 1 mg/mL liquid Do not exceed > 20 mg/day due to QT risk; Max 10 mg/day in CYP 2C19 poor metabolizers. or elderly	To switch to fluoxetine 90 mg/weekly from fluoxetine daily, start 7 days after last daily dose.

↓ Na

PMDD: Sarafem®, Zoloft®, Yaz®
* only condition for which antidepressants are not always taken continuously

SSRI and Combined Mechanism

DRUG	DOSING	SAFETY/SIDE EFFECTS/MONITORING

SSRI and 5-HT$_{1A}$ Partial Agonist

DRUG	DOSING	SAFETY/SIDE EFFECTS/MONITORING
Vilazodone (*Viibryd*) Dosing to the right is in the patient starter kit.	Start at 10 mg x 7 days, then 20 mg x 7 days, then 40 mg <u>all with food</u>	**BOXED WARNING** Antidepressants increase the risk of suicidal thinking and behavior in children, adolescents, and young adults (18-24 years of age) with major depressive disorder (MDD) and other psychiatric disorders; consider risk prior to prescribing. **CONTRAINDICATIONS** Potentially lethal drug interaction with MAO Is; see wash-out information. Do not initiate in patients being treated with linezolid or methylene blue IV. **SIDE EFFECTS** Diarrhea, nausea/vomiting, insomnia, ↓ libido (less sexual SEs compared to SSRIs and SNRIs) **NOTES** ↑ bleeding risk with concurrent use of anticoagulants, anti-platelets, NSAIDs, gingko, thrombolytics. Pregnancy Category C

Handwritten note: 10 mg x 7 days / then 20 mg x 7 days / then 40 mg } w/ FOOD!

SSRI, 5-HT Receptor Antagonist, 5-HT$_{1A}$ Agonist

DRUG	DOSING	SAFETY/SIDE EFFECTS/MONITORING
Vortioxetine (*Brintellix*)	10 mg/d, can ↑ 20 mg/day, with or without food (5 mg/d if higher doses not tolerated)	**BOXED WARNING** Antidepressants increase the risk of suicidal thinking and behavior in children, adolescents, and young adults (18-24 years of age) with major depressive disorder (MDD) and other psychiatric disorders; consider risk prior to prescribing. **CONTRAINDICATIONS** Potentially lethal drug interaction with MAO Is; see washout information. Do not initiate in patients being treated with linezolid or methylene blue IV. **SIDE EFFECTS** Nausea, constipation, vomiting ↑ bleeding risk with concurrent use of anticoagulants, antiplatelets, NSAIDs, gingko, thrombolytics **NOTES** Pregnancy Category C

Handwritten note at bottom: ✱ STOP 5-HT PSYCHIATRIC DRUGS AT LEAST [2 WEEKS] PRIOR TO METHYLENE BLUE OR LINEZOLID TX!! (stop fluoxetine 5 weeks prior tx)

SSRI Drug Interactions

- MAO Is and hypertensive crisis: allow 2 weeks either going to an MAO I or from an MAO I to an SSRI except fluoxetine which requires a 5 week wash-out period if going from fluoxetine to a MAO I (due to the long half-life of fluoxetine of at least 7 days).

- Fluoxetine: 2D6, 2C19 inhibitor. Fluvoxamine: 1A2, 2D6, 2C9, 2C19, 3A4 inhibitor. Paroxetine: 2D6 inhibitor. Note all three are 2D6 inhibitors and some other psych drugs are 2D6 substrates. Psych drugs are sometimes used in combination.

- Tamoxifen's effectiveness decreases with fluoxetine, paroxetine and sertraline (and duloxetine and bupropion).

- ↑ bleeding risk with concurrent use of anticoagulants, antiplatelets, NSAIDs, gingko, thrombolytics.

  fluvoxamine + methadone ⇒ ↑↑ [methadone]
  ↓
  pro-arrhythmic @ higher [ ]s

- Do not use with thioridazine or pimozide.

- Do not use with cimetidine.

- Do not initiate in patients receiving linezolid or methylene blue IV.

- Caution with drugs that cause orthostasis or CNS depressants due to risk of falls.

- FDA warning regarding QT risk and citalopram at > 40 mg/day or > 20 mg if 60+ years, if liver disease, with 2C19 poor metabolizers and on 2C19 inhibitors. Similar, but lower risk for escitalopram at > 20 mg/day; do not exceed 10 mg/day in elderly. Bottom line: if cardiac risk is present, avoid citalopram. Sertraline is often the top choice for an SSRI in cardiac patients.

SSRI Counseling

- Dispense MedGuide and instruct patient to read it. Especially in adolescents and young adults; counsel on risk of suicide – particularly during therapy initiation.

- Fluoxetine is taken in the morning; the others morning or at bedtime.

- To reduce your risk of side effects, your healthcare provider may direct you to start taking this drug at a low dose and gradually increase your dose.

- Take this medication exactly as prescribed. To help you remember, use it at the same time each day. Antidepressants do not work if they are taken as-needed.

- It is important to continue taking this medication even if you feel well. Do not stop taking this medication without consulting your healthcare provider. Some conditions may become worse when the drug is suddenly stopped. Your dose may need to be gradually decreased.

- It may take 1 to 2 weeks to feel a benefit from this drug and 6-8 weeks to feel the full effect on your mood. Tell the healthcare provider if your condition persists or worsens. You can try a medication in a different class. One will work or it may take different tries to find the right medicine that will help you feel better.

- Some patients, but not all, have sexual difficulties when using this medicine. If this happens, talk with the healthcare provider. They can change you to a medicine that does not cause these problems.

- Sertraline oral concentrate must be diluted before use. Immediately before administration, use the dropper provided to measure the required amount of concentrate; mix with 4 ounces (1/2 cup) of water, ginger ale, lemon/lime soda, lemonade, or orange juice only. Do not use with disulfiram.

Handwritten annotations:
ALL ↑ bp ‼
SE: ↑ HR (pulse)
↓ Na+

SNRIs – Serotonin and Norepinephrine Reuptake Inhibitors

DRUG	DOSING	SAFETY/SIDE EFFECTS/MONITORING
Venlafaxine (Effexor, Effexor XR) Depression, GAD, Panic Disorder, Social Anxiety Disorder	150-375 mg/day Can start low with 37.5 or 75 mg Different generics; check orange book	**BOXED WARNING** Antidepressants increase the risk of suicidal thinking and behavior in children, adolescents, and young adults (18-24 years of age) with major depressive disorder (MDD) and other psychiatric disorders; consider risk prior to prescribing.
DULoxetine (Cymbalta) Depression, Peripheral Neuropathy (Pain), Fibromyalgia, GAD, Chronic Musculoskeletal Pain	40-60 mg/day (daily, or 20-30 BID); max dose 120 mg/day; doses > 60 mg/day not more effective Duloxetine is a good choice if the patient has both pain and depression	**CONTRAINDICATIONS** Potentially lethal DI: SNRIs and MAO Is – see wash out information. Do not initiate in a patient receiving linezolid or intravenous methylene blue. **SIDE EFFECTS** Similar to SSRIs (due to serotonin reuptake) and side effects due to ↑ NE uptake: ↑ pulse, dilated pupils (possibly leading to an episode of narrow angle glaucoma), dry mouth, excessive sweating and constipation
Desvenlafaxine (Pristiq) Depression	50 mg/day, can ↑ 100 mg/day	SNRIs can affect urethral resistance. Caution is advised when using SNRIs in patients prone to obstructive urinary disorders. All have warning for ↑ BP, but risk is greatest with venlafaxine when dosed > 150 mg/day; yet all have risk especially at higher doses. ↑ BP may respond to dose reduction, use of antihypertensive or change in therapy.
Levomilnacipran (Fetzima) Depression	40-120 mg/day Start at 20 mg/day x 2 days Do not open, chew or crush capsules; take whole. Do not take with alcohol.	↑ bleeding risk with concurrent use of anticoagulants, antiplatelets, NSAIDs, gingko, thrombolytics. **NOTES** The SNRI dose is ↓ in renal impairment. Do not use levomilnacipran or duloxetine with CrCl < 30 mL/min.

Handwritten annotations (left margin):
↑ bp @ > 150mg/d
* 5-14 day washout before MAOIs
* CrCl < 30
ghost shell → dose titration needed
⊘ EtOH

SNRI Drug Interactions

- MAO Is and hypertensive crisis: 5-14 day (duloxetine) or 7 day (venlafaxine, desvenlafaxine, levomilnacipran) wash out if going from SNRI to MAO I, 14 day wash out if going from MAO I to SNRI.

- Duloxetine is a moderate 2D6 inhibitor.

- Tamoxifen's effectiveness decreases with duloxetine.

- Do not initiate in patients receiving linezolid or methylene blue IV.

- ↑ bleeding risk with concurrent use of anticoagulants, antiplatelets, NSAIDs, gingko, thrombolytics.

- If on antihypertensive medications, use caution and monitor (can ↑ BP), especially at higher doses.

SNRI Counseling

- Dispense MedGuide and instruct patient to read it. Especially in adolescents and young adults: counsel on risk of suicide – particularly during therapy initiation.

- This medication may cause nausea and stomach upset (if venlafaxine IR can try change to XR).

- You may experience increased sweating; if so, discuss with your healthcare provider. You should check your blood pressure regularly to make sure it stays in a safe range.

- Desvenlafaxine: When you take this medicine, you may see something in your stool that looks like a tablet. This is the empty shell from the tablet after the medicine has been absorbed by your body.

- Levomilnacipran: Take capsules whole. Do not open, chew or crush the capsules. Do not take with alcohol; this could cause the medicine to be released too quickly.

- To reduce your risk of side effects, your healthcare provider may direct you to start taking this drug at a low dose and gradually increase your dose.

- Do not crush or chew extended-release formulations.

- Take this medication exactly as directed. To help you remember, use it at the same time each day. Antidepressants do not work if they are taken as-needed.

- It is important to continue taking this medication even if you feel well. Do not stop taking this medication without consulting your healthcare provider. Some conditions may become worse when the drug is suddenly stopped. Your dose may need to be gradually decreased.

- It may take 1 to 2 weeks to feel a benefit from this drug and 6-8 weeks to feel the full effect on your mood. Tell the healthcare provider if your condition persists or worsens. You can try a medication in a different class. One will work it may take different tries to find the right medicine that will help you feel better.

- Some patients, but not all, have sexual difficulties when using this medicine. If this happens, talk with the healthcare provider. They can change you to a medicine that does not cause these problems.

TRICYCLICS

NE and 5HT reuptake inhibitors (primarily, and block ACh and histamine receptors which contributes to the SE profile).

DRUG	DOSING	SAFETY/SIDE EFFECTS/MONITORING
TERTIARY AMINES **Amitriptyline** (Elavil – brand N/A) **Doxepin** – Zonalon cream is for pruritus, Silenor is for insomnia ClomiPRAMINE (Anafranil) Imipramine (Tofranil, Tofranil PM – this is different salt, not interchangeable) Trimipramine (Surmontil) **SECONDARY AMINES** Amoxapine Desipramine (Norpramine) Maprotiline Nortriptyline (Pamelor) Protriptyline (Vivactil) (Secondary amines are relatively selective for NE – tertiary amines may be slightly more effective but have worse SE profile)	**AMITRIPTYLINE** Depression: 100-150 mg BID Neuropathic pain/migraine prophylaxis: 10-50 mg QHS **NORTRIPTYLINE** Depression: 25 mg TID-QID **DOXEPIN** Depression: 100-300 mg daily	**BOXED WARNING** Antidepressants ↑ the risk of suicidal thinking and behavior in children, adolescents, and young adults (18-24 years of age) with major depressive disorder (MDD) and other psychiatric disorders; consider risk prior to prescribing. **CONTRAINDICATIONS** Concurrent use with MAO Is, linezolid, IV methylene blue; myocardial infarction, glaucoma (doxepin), urinary retention (doxepin) **SIDE EFFECTS** **Cardiotoxicity** QT-prolongation with overdose – can be used for suicide-counsel carefully; obtain baseline ECG if cardiac risk factors or age > 50 years old Orthostasis, tachycardia **Anticholinergic** Dry mouth, blurred vision, urinary retention, constipation (taper off to avoid cholinergic rebound) Vivid dreams Weight gain (varies by agent and patient), sedation, sweating Myoclonus (muscle twitching-may be symptoms of drug toxicity) **NOTES** ↑ fall risk – especially in elderly due to combination of orthostasis and sedation Tertiary amines more likely to cause sedation and weight gain

(handwritten margin notes:) more sedation & wt gain; + glaucoma; + urinary retention

Tricyclic Drug Interactions

- MAO Is and hypertensive crisis: 2 week wash-out if going to or from a MAO I.

- Additive QT prolongation risk; see Drug Interaction chapter for other high-risk QT drugs to attempt to avoid additive risk.

- Metabolized by 2D6 (up to 10% of Caucasians are slow metabolizers); check for DIs

Tricyclic Counseling

- Dispense MedGuide and instruct patient to read it. Especially in adolescents and young adults: counsel on risk of suicide – particularly during therapy initiation. TCAs are dangerous if the patient wishes to kill themselves; a month's supply can be deadly. Counseling is critical.

- This drug can cause constipation. You may need to use a stool softener or laxative if this becomes a problem.

- This drug may cause dry/blurry vision. You may need to use an eye drop lubricant.

- This drug may make it more difficult to urinate.

- This drug may cause dry mouth. This can contribute to dental decay (cavities) and difficulty chewing food. It is important to use proper dental hygiene when taking any medication that causes dry mouth, including brushing and flossing. Sugar free lozenges may be helpful.

- This drug may cause changes in your blood pressure. Use caution when changing from lying down or sitting to a standing position. Hold onto the bed or rail until you are steady.

- If you experience anxiety, or insomnia (sometimes with vivid dreams), these usually go away. If they do not, contact your healthcare provider.

- Take this medication exactly as prescribed. To help you remember, use it at the same time each day. Antidepressants do not work if they are taken as-needed.

- It is important to continue taking this medication even if you feel well. Do not stop taking this medication without consulting your healthcare provider. Some conditions may become worse when the drug is suddenly stopped. Your dose may need to be gradually decreased.

- It may take 1 to 2 weeks to feel a benefit from this drug and 6-8 weeks to feel the full effect on your mood. Tell the healthcare provider if your condition persists or worsens. You can try a medication in a different class. It may take several tries to find the right medicine that will help you feel better.

MAO Is: Monoamine Oxidase Inhibitors

Inhibit the enzyme monoamine oxidase, which breaks down catecholamines, including 5-HT, NE, EPI, DA. If these NTs ↑ dramatically, hypertensive crisis, and death can result.

DRUG	DOSING	SAFETY/SIDE EFFECTS/MONITORING/
Isocarboxazid (*Marplan*)	20 mg/day, divided, max 60 mg/day	**BOXED WARNING** Antidepressants increase the risk of suicidal thinking and behavior in children, adolescents, and young adults (18-24 years of age) with major depressive disorder (MDD) and other psychiatric disorders; consider risk prior to prescribing.
Phenelzine (*Nardil*)	15 mg TID, max 60-90 mg/day	**CONTRAINDICATIONS** Cardiovascular disease, cerebrovascular defect, history of headache, history of hepatic disease, pheochromocytoma. Concurrent use of sympathomimetics and related compounds, CNS depressants, dextromethorphan, ethanol, meperidine, bupropion, or buspirone.
Tranylcypromine (*Parnate*)	30 mg/day in divided doses, max 60 mg/day	**WARNINGS** Not commonly used but watch for drug-drug and drug-food interactions – if missed could be fatal. Hypertensive crisis (VERY high blood pressure) can occur when taken with TCAs, SSRIs, SNRIs, many other drugs and tyramine-rich foods (see interactions below). **SIDE EFFECTS** Anticholinergic effects (taper upon discontinuation to avoid cholinergic rebound) Orthostasis Sedation (except tranylcypromine causes stimulation) Sexual dysfunction, weight gain, headache, insomnia
Selegiline transdermal patch (*EMSAM*) MAO I B Selective Inhibitor Selegiline as *Eldepryl* and *Zelapar* (ODT) are oral drugs for Parkinson disease.	Start at 6 mg patch/day, can ↑ to 9 or 12 mg/day	**CONTRAINDICATIONS** Discontinue at least 10 days prior to elective surgery requiring general anesthesia, do not use with local anesthesia containing sympathomimetic vasoconstrictors, foods high in tyramine, supplements containing tyrosine, phenylalanine, tryptophan, or caffeine. No dietary issues with 6 mg patch. **SIDE EFFECTS** Constipation, gas, dry mouth, loss of appetite, sexual problems

Handwritten note alongside Tranylcypromine row: ⊖ sedation (stimulating)

MAO I Drug Interactions

- MAO Is and hypertensive crisis: allow 2 week wash-out if going to or from a MAO I and an SSRI, SNRI or TCA antidepressant (exception: if going from fluoxetine back to MAO I need to wait 5 weeks).

Handwritten note: ≠ stimulants

- MAO Is <u>cannot</u> be used with many other drugs or the drugs will not be broken down and hypertensive crisis, serotonin syndrome or psychosis may result. The interaction could be fatal. These include any drugs with effects on the concentrations of epinephrine, norepinephrine, serotonin or dopamine. This includes bupropion, carbamazepine, oxcarbazepine, ephedrine and analogs (pseudoephedrine, etc), buspirone, levodopa, linezolid, lithium, meperidine, SSRIs, SNRIs, TCAs, tramadol, methadone, mirtazapine, dextromethorphan, cyclobenzaprine (and other skeletal muscle relaxants), OTC diet pills/herbal weight loss products and St. John's wort.

- Patients taking MAO Is must avoid tyramine-rich foods, including aged cheese, pickled herring, yeast extract, air-dried meats, sauerkraut, soy sauce, fava beans and some red wines and beers (tap beer and any beer that has not been pasteurized – canned and bottled beers contain little or no tyramine). Foods can become high in tyramine when they have been aged, fermented, pickled or smoked.

MAO I Inhibitor Counseling

- Dispense MedGuide and instruct patient to read it. Especially in adolescents and young adults: counsel on risk of suicide – particularly during therapy initiation.

- Warn patients regarding the need to avoid interacting foods and drugs. See list in above drug interaction section. Stay away from tyramine-rich containing foods.

- Seek immediate medical care if you experience any of these symptoms: sudden severe headache, nausea, stiff neck, vomiting, a fast or slow heartbeat or a change in the way your heart beats (palpitations), tight chest pain, a lot of sweating, confusion, dilated pupils, and sensitivity to light.

- Use this medication regularly in order to get the most benefit from it. Take this medication exactly as prescribed. To help you remember, use it at the same time each day. Antidepressants do not work if they are taken as-needed.

- It is important to continue taking this medication even if you feel well. Do not stop taking this medication without consulting your healthcare provider. Some conditions may become worse when the drug is suddenly stopped. Your dose may need to be gradually decreased.

- It may take 1 to 2 weeks to feel a benefit from this drug and 6-8 weeks to feel the full effect on your mood. Tell the healthcare provider if your condition persists or worsens. You can try a medication in a different class. One will work – it may take different tries to find the right medicine that will help you feel better.

- *EMSAM* Patch Application: Change once daily. Pick a time of day you can remember. Apply to either upper chest or back (below the neck and above the waist), upper thigh, or to the outer surface of the upper arm. Rotate site and do not use same site 2 days in a row. Wash hands with soap after applying patch. Do not expose to heat. The wash-out period counseling above includes the patch.

Dopamine (DA) and Norepinephrine (NE) Reuptake Inhibitor

DRUG	DOSING	SAFETY/SIDE EFFECTS/MONITORING
BuPROPion *(Aplenzin, Wellbutrin SR, Wellbutrin XL, Wellbutrin, Forfivo XL)* *Buproban, Zyban* – for smoking cessation *Wellbutrin XL* is approved for Seasonal Affective Disorder (SAD) – start in early fall, titrate to 300 mg/day, if desired can discontinue in late spring by cutting to 150 mg daily x 2 weeks	300-450 mg daily *Wellbutrin IR* is TID *Wellbutrin SR* is BID (to 200 mg BID) *Wellbutrin XL* is daily Hydrobromide salt *(Aplenzin)*: Initial: 174 mg once daily in the morning; may increase as early as day 4 of dosing to 348 mg once daily (target dose); maximum dose: 522 mg daily. In patients receiving 348 mg once daily, taper dose down to 174 mg once daily prior to discontinuing. Do not exceed 450 mg/day due to seizure risk	**BOXED WARNING** Antidepressants increase the risk of suicidal thinking and behavior in children, adolescents, and young adults (18-24 years of age) with major depressive disorder (MDD) and other psychiatric disorders; consider risk prior to prescribing. **CONTRAINDICATIONS** Seizure disorder; history of anorexia/bulimia, abrupt discontinuation of ethanol or sedatives; concurrent use with MAO Is, linezolid, IV methylene blue, or other forms of bupropion **SIDE EFFECTS** Dry mouth, insomnia, headache/migraine, nausea/vomiting, constipation, and tremors/seizures (dose-related), possible blood pressure changes (more hypertension than hypotension – monitor), weight loss No effects on 5HT and therefore no sexual dysfunction; may be used if issues with other antidepressants

Handwritten notes:
- for SAD, start @ 150mg qd then ↑ to 300mg qd
- if condition warrants, may continue ∞

IR – TID
SR – BID
XL – QD

↓ seizure threshold

or 150mg/dose (IR)

DRUG	DOSING	SAFETY/SIDE EFFECTS/MONITORING
Mirtazapine *(Remeron, Remeron SolTab)* Used commonly in oncology and skilled nursing since it helps with sleep at night (dosed QHS) & increases appetite (good for weight gain in frail elderly)	Tetracyclic antidepressant, central presynaptic alpha$_2$–adrenergic blocker, which increases NE and 5HT. It also blocks 5-HT$_2$ and 5-HT$_3$ receptors, H1 receptors and is a moderate peripheral alpha1-adrenergic and muscarinic blocker. 15-45 mg QHS	**BOXED WARNING** Antidepressants increase the risk of suicidal thinking and behavior in children, adolescents, and young adults (18-24 years of age) with major depressive disorder (MDD) and other psychiatric disorders; consider risk prior to prescribing. **WARNINGS** Anticholinergic effects, QT prolongation, blood dyscrasias, CNS depression **SIDE EFFECTS** Sedation and ↑ appetite, weight gain, dry mouth, dizziness Agranulocytosis (rare)

ODT

Handwritten notes:
- tetracyclic antidepressant
- central presynaptic α$_2$ blocker ⇒ ↑ NE, 5-HT
- 5-HT$_2$, 5-HT$_3$, H$_1$ receptors blocker
- α$_1$, muscarinic blocker

DRUG	DOSING	SAFETY/SIDE EFFECTS/MONITORING
TraZODone *(Oleptro)* Rarely used as an antidepressant due to sedation. Used primarily off-label for sleep (dosed 50-100 mg QHS)	100-300 mg BID TraZODone ER *(Oleptro)* may be less sedating and is dosed 150-375 mg QHS	**BOXED WARNING** Antidepressants increase the risk of suicidal thinking and behavior in children, adolescents, and young adults (18-24 years of age) with major depressive disorder (MDD) and other psychiatric disorders; consider risk prior to prescribing. **CONTRAINDICATIONS** Concurrent use with MAO Is, linezolid, or IV methylene blue **SIDE EFFECTS** Sedation Orthostasis (risk in elderly for falls) Sexual dysfunction and risk of priapism (medical emergency – requires immediate medical attention if painful erection longer than 4 hrs)
Nefazodone	150-600 mg BID	**BOXED WARNINGS (2)** Antidepressants increase the risk of suicidal thinking and behavior in children, adolescents, and young adults (18-24 years of age) with major depressive disorder (MDD) and other psychiatric disorders; consider risk prior to prescribing, hepatotoxicity. **CONTRAINDICATIONS** Hepatic disease, concurrent use with MAO Is, carbamazepine, cisapride, pimozide, or triazolam **SIDE EFFECTS** Similar to trazodone, but less sedating **NOTES** Rarely used due to hepatotoxicity; monitor LFTs, counsel on symptoms of liver damage

Handwritten annotations:
- Desyrel® – IR
- Oleptro® – ER
- @ ER, penis will be drained + vasoconstrictor admin

Bupropion Drug Interactions

- Do not use with *Buproban* or *Zyban* for smoking cessation; same drug.

- Do not use in patients with seizure history; drug ↓ seizure threshold. Do not exceed 450 mg daily in anyone.

Key Counseling Points For Above Agents

- Dispense MedGuide and instruct patient to read it. Especially in adolescents and young adults: counsel on risk of suicide – particularly during therapy initiation.
- Counsel on lag time, need to take daily as with other agents.
- Bupropion: Include not to exceed 450 mg daily, or 150 mg at each dose if using immediate-release formulations due to seizure risk.
- Mirtazapine: Counsel to take at night, drug is sedating, and should increase appetite.

FOR TREATMENT RESISTANCE DEPRESSION ONLY

Rule-out bipolar disorder, check if antidepressant is at optimal dose, sometimes use combination standard antidepressants, or augment with various options. The antipsychotics below are approved for treatment-resistant depression.

All antipsychotics require MedGuides with this Warning:

Medicines like this one can raise the risk of death in elderly people who have lost touch with reality (psychosis) due to confusion and memory loss (dementia). This medicine is not approved for the treatment of patients with dementia-related psychosis.

And because it is being used to augment AD therapy:

Antidepressants have increased the risk of suicidal thoughts and actions in some children, teenagers, and young adults. See Schizophrenia/Psychosis chapter for more detail on the antipsychotics.

DRUG	DOSING	SAFETY/SIDE EFFECTS/MONITORING
ARIPiprazole (Abilify, Abilify Discmelt)	Start 2-5 mg/day (QAM), can ↑ to 15 mg	**BOXED WARNINGS (2)** Antidepressants increase the risk of suicidal thinking and behavior in children, adolescents, and young adults (18-24 years of age) with major depressive disorder (MDD) and other psychiatric disorders; consider risk prior to prescribing. Elderly patients with dementia-related psychosis treated with antipsychotic drugs are at ↑ risk of death. **WARNINGS** Risk of Neuroleptic Malignant Syndrome Risk of Tardive Dyskinesia (TD) Risk of leukopenia, neutropenia, agranulocytosis
OLANZapine/fluoxetine (Symbyax)	Usually started at 6 mg/25 mg capsule QHS (fluoxetine is activating, but olanzapine is more sedating), can ↑ cautiously.	**CONTRAINDICATIONS** *Symbyax:* Do not use with pimozide, thioridazine & caution with other QT prolongating drugs/conditions **SIDE EFFECTS** Each of these drugs can cause metabolic issues, including dyslipidemia, weight gain, diabetes (less with aripiprazole) All can cause orthostasis/dizziness **Abilify** Anxiety, insomnia, constipation
QUEtiapine extended release (SEROquel, SEROquel XR)	Start 50 mg QHS, ↑ nightly to 150-300 mg QHS	**Olanzapine** Sedation Weight gain, ↑ lipids, ↑ glucose, EPS, QT prolongation (lower risk) **Quetiapine** Sedation, orthostasis Weight gain, ↑ lipids, ↑ glucose Little risk EPS

PRACTICE CASE

SA is a 57 y/o male who appears thin and anxious. He is married with two children. His wife brought him to the clinic today due to constant worry, anxiety, and feelings of worthlessness. When he was in college, he had several bouts of depression and was successfully treated with doxepin at that time. He stopped taking the medication when he graduated and moved to California, because he felt the sunshine made him feel better. His wife reports that this is the third or fourth time in the past few years that her husband has felt so low that she became concerned he might harm himself. She reports that he stays up all night with constant worry and probably has not had a good night's sleep in months.

Per clinic records, SA was seen 2 months ago and started on *Celexa* 40 mg daily and lorazepam 1 mg 1-3 times daily as needed. SA has been using these medications, and states that they "help a little, but not much". He is taking the lorazepam 1 mg TID each day. He does not smoke, drink alcohol, or use illicit drugs.

Allergies: shellfish, contrast dye, latex

Medications:
Inderal LA 120 mg daily
Celexa 40 mg daily
Lorazepam 1 mg 1-3 times daily PRN
Fosinopril 20 mg daily

Vitals:
Height: 5'10" Weight: 155 lbs
BP: 158/102 mmHg HR: 80 BPM RR: 16 BPM Temp: 98.2°F Pain: 1/10

Labs: Na (mEq/L) = 140 (135 - 145)
K (mEq/L) = 4.1 (3.5 - 5)
Cl (mEq/L) = 99 (95 - 103)
HCO_3 (mEq/L) = 26 (24 - 30)
BUN (mg/dL) = 12 (7 - 20)
SCr (mg/dL) = 0.7 (0.6 - 1.3)
Glucose (mg/dL) = 100 (100 - 125)
Ca (mg/dL) = 10.1 (8.5 - 10.5)
Mg (mEq/L) = 2.0 (1.3 - 2.1)
PO_4 (mg/dL) = 4.1 (2.3 - 4.7)

AST (IU/L) = 27 (8 - 48)
ALT (IU/L) = 39 (7 - 55)
Albumin (g/dL) = 3.7 (3.5 - 5)

Patient reports minimal improvement of depression with current prescriptions.

Questions

1. SA has depression that has not responded to an adequate trial of fluoxetine or citalopram. Which of the following options represents the best alternative?

   a. Sertraline
   b. Venlafaxine
   c. Fluvoxamine
   d. Escitalopram
   e. Mirtazapine

2. If SA was started on *Effexor XR* (he won't be), which of the following parameters should be carefully monitored in this patient? (Select **ALL** that apply.)

   a. Blood pressure
   b. Thyroid parameters
   c. White blood cell count
   d. Metabolic acidosis
   e. Symptoms of depression

3. A pharmacist counseling a patient on the use of any antidepressant should include the following counseling points:

   a. Your energy level may pick up before your mood starts to feels better.
   b. Your mood should improve; this usually takes about a month.
   c. If this medicine does not work, the doctor will try a different agent, which may work better.
   d. This medication needs to be taken every day; it does not work if it is taken occasionally.
   e. All of the above.

4. What is the mechanism of action of venlafaxine?

   a. Selective serotonin reuptake inhibitor
   b. Serotonin and dopamine reuptake inhibitor
   c. Serotonin and norepinephrine reuptake inhibitor
   d. Norepinephrine and dopamine reuptake inhibitor
   e. Norepinephrine and acetylcholine reuptake inhibitor

5. The doctor takes a thorough medication history and decides that it would be worthwhile to try doxepin, since the patient had a good history of use with this agent. Which of the following statements is correct? (Select **ALL** that apply.)

   a. Doxepin is a monoamine oxidase inhibitor.
   b. Doxepin can cause excess salivation and has significant food interactions.
   c. He should be carefully evaluated for suicide risk.
   d. The brand name is *Sular*.
   e. The brand name is *Silenor*.

Questions 6-7 do not apply to the case.

6. A patient has been started on bupropion for depression. His other medications include *Lopid*, *Pravachol* and *Zyban*. Which of the following statement is correct?

   a. Bupropion will raise his triglycerides.
   b. Bupropion will raise his HDL cholesterol.
   c. Bupropion will lower his HDL cholesterol.
   d. Bupropion should not be used in this patient.
   e. *Lopid* is an inducer and will decrease the level of bupropion.

7. A patient has been started on bupropion 200 mg TID for depression. His medical conditions include partial seizures and obsessive compulsive disorder. His medications include fluvoxamine and phenytoin. Which of the following statements is correct? (Select **ALL** that apply.)

   a. Bupropion will induce the metabolism of phenytoin.
   b. The bupropion dose is too high.
   c. Bupropion should not be used in this patient.
   d. One of the brand formulation used for depression is called *Contrave*.
   e. Patients with sexual dysfunction should avoid the use of this drug.

Answers

1-e, 2-a,e, 3-e, 4-c, 5-c,e, 6-d, 7-b,c

SCHIZOPHRENIA/ PSYCHOSIS

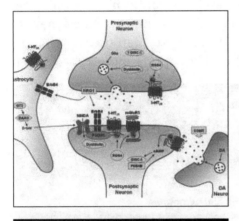

We gratefully acknowledge the assistance of Robin Wackernah, PharmD, BCPP, Regis University School of Pharmacy, Rueckert-Hartman College for Health Professions, in preparing this chapter.

GUIDELINES

Diagnostic and Statistical Manual of Mental Disorders. Fifth Edition (DSM-5).

American Psychiatric Association Guideline Watch (September 2009): Practice Guideline for the Treatment of Patients with Schizophrenia. http://psychiatryonline.org/pdfaccess.ashx?ResourceID=243181&PDFSource=6 (accessed 2014 Sept 30).

BACKGROUND

Schizophrenia is a chronic, severe and disabling thought disorder. The cause is multifactorial and includes altered brain structure and chemistry, primarily involving dopamine and glutamine. The patient's genes (inherited susceptibility) and environmental factors are important in the disease development. Patients suffer from hallucinations, delusions (false beliefs), disorganized thinking and behavior. They can withdraw from the world around them and enter a world of psychosis, where they struggle differentiating reality from altered perceptions. Schizophrenia ranges from relatively mild to severe. Some people may be able to function adequately in daily life, while others need specialized, intensive care. Treatment adherence is important and often difficult to obtain, primarily due to the patient's inability to recognize their illness. This is regrettable to the patient's family and to themselves since the patient with schizophrenia typically lives a life of torment where they may not be able to care for themselves. This condition has one of the highest suicide rates.

The onset of symptoms usually begins in young adulthood. A diagnosis is not based on lab tests, but on the patient's behavior, which should include negative and positive signs and symptoms (described on the following page). Schizophrenia occurs in ~1% in all societies regardless of class, color, religion, culture or national origin. The Diagnostic and Statistical Manual of Mental Disorders, 5th Edition (DSM-5) is the current tool used to diagnose schizophrenia and other psychiatric disorders.

CAUSES OF SCHIZOPHRENIA

Schizophrenia is a thought disorder that manifests in the brain. Genetics, environment, stressors and some illicit drugs can be contributing factors. Abnormalities in the role of neurotransmitters is central. There is increased dopamine in the mesolimbic pathway. Antipsychotics primarily block dopamine receptors, although newer agents that block serotonin and additional receptors have benefit. The older "dopaminergic model" is being supplemented with a more recent understanding of the role of the glutamatergic N-methyl-D aspartate (NMDA) receptor and its role in the pathogenesis of schizophrenia.

Antipsychotics target the positive symptoms, but the lack of motivation, cognitive and functional impairment remain challenges for many patients and often take longer to respond to antipsychotic treatment, if at all. Researchers hope that a better understanding of glutamate receptors will improve functional levels. A problem with current therapy is that the drugs that target dopamine hyperactivity also target dopamine involved in focus and the ability to pay attention; dopamine and glutamine modulate each other. Glutamine synaptic dysfunction is a large area of current research. It is hoped that as the pathways are better understood, along with drug development, a "fine tuning" of therapy will improve treatment.

DSM 5 DIAGNOSTIC CRITERIA FOR SCHIZOPHRENIA

Patients must have 2 or more of the following symptoms
(delusions, hallucinations or disorganized speech must be present)

Negative signs and symptoms	Positive signs and symptoms
Loss of interest in everyday activities	Hallucinations; hearing voices (auditory hallucinations are common), visual hallucinations
Lack of emotion	
Inability to plan or carry out activities	Delusions; beliefs the patient has, but are without a basis in reality
Poor hygiene	Disorganized thinking/behavior, incoherent speech, often on unrelated topics, purposeless behavior, or difficulty speaking and organizing thoughts, such as stopping in mid-sentence or jumbling together meaningless words
Social withdrawal	
Loss of motivation (avolition)	
Poverty (lack) of speech (alogia)	Difficulty paying attention

NATURAL PRODUCTS

Fish oils are being used for psychosis, as well as other psychiatric disorders including ADHD and depression. The evidence is preliminary, but promising. Considering the debilitating nature of schizophrenia, natural products are not used in lieu of antipsychotic medications in patients that require them. Do not recommend cod liver oil due to risk of vitamin A toxicity. Keep in mind that natural products have dose-response relationships; check the Natural Medicines Database for dosing recommendations that appear to have benefit from clinical trials.

DRUG THERAPY

Second-generation antipsychotic agents (SGAs) are commonly used <u>first-line</u> due to a lower risk of extrapyramidal side effects (EPS), however, they are not first-line in all patients and some respond better to a first-generation antipsychotic agent (FGA).

In assessing treatment resistance or evaluating the best option for a partial response, it is important to evaluate whether the patient has had an <u>adequate trial</u> (at least 4-6 weeks) of an antipsychotic, including whether the dose is adequate and whether the patient has been <u>taking the medication</u> as prescribed. <u>A previous positive or negative history</u> with antipsychotics should be used <u>to guide therapy</u>.

Clozapine has superior efficacy, but has multiple black box warnings and is particularly known for <u>agranulocytosis</u>, seizures and myocarditis – in addition to having high metabolic risk. <u>A clozapine trial should be considered for a patient who has had no or poor response to two trials of antipsychotic medication</u> (at least one should be a SGA) or for a patient with significant ADRs.

<u>High-potency FGAs</u> such as haloperidol are associated with a <u>high risk of EPS effects, a moderate risk of sedation</u> and a lower risk of orthostatic hypotension, tachycardia, and anticholinergic effects compared to low-potency FGAs. In contrast, <u>low-potency FGAs</u> are associated with a <u>lower risk of EPS, a high degree of sedation, a high risk of orthostatic hypotension, tachycardia, and a high risk of anticholinergic effects</u>. Although other side effects also vary with the specific medication, in general, the first-generation antipsychotic medications are associated with a moderate risk of weight gain, a low risk of metabolic effects, and a risk of sexual side effects. <u>With certain agents (thioridazine particularly), QT risk is significant</u>.

Other possible side effects of FGAs include seizures, temperature dysregulation, allergic reactions, and dermatological, hepatic, ophthalmological, and hematological effects.

<u>With the commonly used SGAs, weight gain, lipid and glucose abnormalities (metabolic side effects) are common with clozapine, olanzapine, and quetiapine. Risperidone and paliperidone have a moderate risk of metabolic side effects</u>. Aripiprazole, ziprasidone, lurasidone and asenapine have lower metabolic risk. The American Diabetes Association (ADA) screening and monitoring recommendations when initiating antipsychotics state that patients should first be screened for <u>overweight and obesity, dyslipidemia and hyperglycemia, hypertension, and personal or family history</u> of risk. While being treated, the patient should be <u>monitored</u> for treatment-emergent changes in weight, waist circumference, plasma lipid and

MEDICATIONS/ILLICIT DRUGS THAT CAN CAUSE PSYCHOTIC SYMPTOMS
Amphetamines
Bath salts (synthetic cathinones)
Methamphetamine, ice, crack
Cannabis
Cocaine, esp. "crack" cocaine
Dextromethorphan (DM)
Phencyclidine (PCP), MDPV (bath salts)
Lysergic acid diethylamide (LSD) and other hallucinogenics
Anticholinergics (centrally-acting, high doses)
Dopamine or dopamine agonists used for Parkinson disease (Requip, Mirapex, Sinemet, etc.)
Interferons
Steroids (typically with lack of sleep – ICU psychosis)
Stimulants (especially if already at risk), including ADHD drugs

glucose levels, and acute symptoms of diabetes (e.g., polyuria, polydipsia). <u>QT prolongation</u> with SGAs can be present and <u>ziprasidone</u> has the <u>highest</u> risk.

FORMULATIONS

<u>Long-Acting Injections:</u> Haloperidol is an older agent and comes in various formulations, including an IM injection for acute use, a long-acting decanoate, tablets and a solution. Long-acting injectables, including *Haldol* decanoate (every 4 weeks), *Risperdal Consta* (every 2 weeks), *Invega Sustenna* (every 4 weeks), *Abilify Maintena* (every 4 weeks), and a few others provide the benefit of increased adherence, or compliance, with the medication. They are also used in acute care settings prior to the release of patients to the street (such as with homelessness).

<u>Orally Disintegrating Tablets (ODTs):</u> These are used to help solve the problem of "cheeking" where the patient holds the medication in their cheek and then spits it in the toilet. With ODTs the tablet dissolves rapidly in the mouth, without the need for water. Several of the SGAs come as ODTs (clozapine, olanzapine, risperidone, aripiprazole and asenapine).

<u>Acute IM Injections:</u> Intramuscular (IM) injections provide "stat" relief to help calm down an acutely agitated, psychotic patient for their own safety and the safety of others. They are often mixed with other drugs, such as benzodiazepines for anxiolytic and sedative effects and anticholinergics to reduce EPS risk. In contrast, oral absorption could take up to an hour to calm the patient down. The patient will be sedated and hopefully sleep through the acute symptoms. Olanzapine and benzodiazepines should not be given together (IM) due to orthostasis risk.

CHOOSING A SGA BASED ON THE SIDE EFFECT PROFILE

Clinicians choose among the various SGAs based on the formulary availability and the following considerations:

- If a patient has <u>cardiovascular risk</u> do not choose an agent that has a high risk of QT prolongation/arrhythmia (ziprasidone-greatest risk). Although this is a review of SGAs, keep in mind that phenothiazines (a class of FGAs) in general, and thioridazine in particular, are high QT-risk. The other SGAs are moderate or lower risk.

- If a patient is <u>overweight, has little physical activity or has metabolic issues</u> (elevated blood glucose and/or lipids) avoid agents that have significant metabolic risk (most notably olanzapine and quetiapine). Aripiprazole, ziprasidone, asenapine and lurasidone have the least risk of metabolic side effects and weight gain. Clozapine has high metabolic risk but is used in refractive cases and might be required. Olanzapine has the highest risk of metabolic issues (but does not have a high risk of QT prolongation).

- High <u>prolactin levels</u> cause galactorrhea, or milk production without pregnancy, sexual dysfunction, gynecomastia (painful, swollen breast tissue) and irregular or missed periods. After several years this can contribute to osteoporosis. This is a concern with <u>risperidone</u> and <u>paliperidone</u>, especially with higher doses.

- If the patient has a history of tardive dyskinesia (TD), or any type of movement disorder, avoid risperidone, paliperidone and lurasidone. Quetiapine has low risk of movement disorders and is the recommended agent for psychosis in a patient with Parkinson disease. Clozapine has very low risk but is not used lightly.

- Adherence Issues: see formulation section above. In addition, an agent that comes as once-daily dosing (versus BID or TID) would be preferred.

Boxed Warning

Antipsychotics (APs) increase the risk of mortality in elderly patients with dementia-related psychosis, primarily due to an increased risk of stroke and infection. Note that APs are not particularly helpful to treat dementia-related anger/outbursts, but they are used and pharmacists are required to counsel on this risk. See the counseling section for wording suggestion. Additional drug-specific warnings are listed separately with the drugs.

Neuroleptic Malignant Syndrome (NMS)

Antipsychotics used to be called neuroleptics. NMS is rare but is highly lethal. It occurs most commonly with the FGAs and is due to D_2 blockade. NMS occurs less commonly with SGAs and with other dopamine blocking agents including metoclopramide (*Reglan*). The majority of cases occur within two weeks of starting therapy or immediately following high doses of injectables given alongside multiple oral doses. Occasionally, patients develop NMS even after years of antipsychotic use. NMS is a medical emergency as the intense muscle contractions can lead to acute renal injury (due to rhabdomyolysis from the destruction of muscle tissue), suffocation and death.

Signs Include

- Hyperthermia (high fever, with profuse sweating)

- Extreme muscle rigidity (called "lead pipe" rigidity)

- Mental status changes

- Other signs can include tachycardia and tachypnea and blood pressure changes

Laboratory results

- ↑ creatine phosphokinase and ↑ white blood cells

Treatment

STOP the antipsychotic.

- Provide supportive care: cardiorespiratory and hemodynamic support, body temperature modulation and control of electrolyte balance.

- Cool them down: cooling bed, antipyretics, cooled IV fluids.

- Muscle relaxation with benzodiazepines or dantrolene (*Ryanodex*), a muscle relaxant, is sometimes used, and some cases may require a dopamine antagonist such as bromocriptine.

First-Generation Antipsychotics (FGAs) block D$_2$ receptors. Minimal 5HT$_{2A}$ receptor blockade.

DRUG	DOSING	SAFETY/SIDE EFFECTS/MONITORING
Low Potency		**BOXED WARNING (ALL APs)** Elderly patients with dementia-related psychosis treated with antipsychotics are at an increased risk of death compared to placebo. Most deaths appeared to be either cardiovascular (e.g., heart failure, sudden death) or infectious in nature. This drug is not approved for the treatment of dementia-related psychosis.
ChlorproMAZINE	300-1,000 mg/day, divided	
Thioridazine BOXED WARNING: QT prolongation	300-800 mg/day, divided	**SIDE EFFECTS** All are sedating and all cause EPS, however the lower-potency agents have ↑ somnolence and ↓ incidence EPS (e.g., chlorpromazine), and the higher-potency agents have ↓ sedation (but still sedating) with ↑ EPS (e.g., haloperidol).
Mid-potency		Dystonias, which are prolonged contraction of muscles (including painful muscle spasms) can occur during initiation. There is higher risk with younger males. Consider use of centrally-acting anticholinergic (diphenhydramine, benztropine) for prophylaxis during therapy initiation. May be life-threatening if airway is compromised.
Loxapine (*Loxitane, Adasuve* inhalation powder for acute agitation)	30-100 mg/day, divided	Akathisia, which is restlessness with anxiety and an inability to remain still. May be treated with anticholinergics, benzodiazepines or propranolol.
Perphenazine	16-64 mg/day, divided	Parkinsonism, which looks similar to Parkinson's disease, with tremors, abnormal gait, bradykinesia, etc. Treat with anticholinergics or propranolol if tremor is the main symptom.
High Potency		Tardive dyskinesias (TD), which are abnormal facial movements, primarily in the tongue or mouth. The risk is higher in elderly females. If TD occurs the drug should be stopped as soon as possible and replaced with a SGA with low EPS risk (quetiapine, clozapine). TD can be irreversible.
FluPHENAZine Available in **2-wk decanoate**	5-20 mg/day, divided	Dyskinesias, which are abnormal movements, are possible however this is more of an issue with the Parkinson drugs. Seizures (phenothiazines, butyrophenones) Cardiovascular Effects: orthostasis, tachycardia, QT prolongation; IV haloperidol has high risk.
Haloperidol (*Haldol*), see formulations to right Class: butyrophenone (and DA-blocker) Haloperidol is also used for tics and vocal outbursts due to Tourette syndrome	Oral (tablet, solution): start 0.5-2 mg BID-TID, up to 100 mg/day IV: usually 5-10 mg Decanoate (monthly): IM only, for conversion from PO, use 10-20x the oral dose	Sexual dysfunction *Adasuve*: dysgeusia (bad, bitter, or metallic taste in mouth), sedation, bronchospasm risk, REMS drug
Trifluoperazine	15-50 mg/day, divided	
Thiothixene (*Navane*)	15-60 mg/day, divided	

Second-Generation Antipsychotics (SGAs) block D$_2$ and 5HT$_{2A}$ receptors. Aripiprazole is unique; it also acts as a D$_2$ and 5HT$_{1A}$ partial agonist.

DRUG	DOSING	SAFETY/SIDE EFFECTS/MONITORING
CloZAPine *(Clozaril, FazaClo ODT, Versacloz* suspension) Only if failed to respond to treatment with 2 standard AP treatments, or had significant ADRs	300-900 mg/day, divided (start at 12.5 mg and titrate, also titrate off since abrupt discontinuation can cause seizures) Clozapine has ↓ risk EPS/TD	**BOXED WARNINGS, CLOZAPINE-SPECIFIC (4)** Significant risk of potentially life-threatening agranulocytosis. Tachycardia, orthostatic hypotension, syncope, and cardiac arrest; risk is highest during the initial titration period especially with rapid dose increases. Titrate slowly. Myocarditis and cardiomyopathy; discontinue if suspect. Seizures, dose-correlated; start at no higher than 12.5 mg once or twice daily, titrate slowly, using divided doses. Use with caution in patients at seizure risk: seizure history, head trauma, alcoholism, or concurrent therapy with medications which lower seizure threshold. **SIDE EFFECTS** Orthostasis, syncope, weight gain, ↑ lipids, ↑ glucose, somnolence, dizziness, insomnia, GI upset, sialorrhea (hypersalivation), QT prolongation Risk of agranulocytosis, seizures, myocarditis **MONITORING** REMS: Patient must register with *Clozaril* Registry. Only pharmacies using Registry can fill this drug: To start: WBC must be ≥ 3,500/mm^3 and ANC must be ≥ 2,000/mm^3. Check WBC and ANC weekly x 6 months, then every 2 weeks x 6 months, then monthly. Monitor for metabolic effects; see counseling section. **NOTES** Smoking reduces drug levels.
OLANZapine *(ZyPREXA, Zydis ODT, Relprevv* injection)	10-20 mg QHS IM Injection (acute agitation) *Relprevv* inj suspension lasts 2-4 weeks, restricted use, REMS drug	**BOXED WARNING, OLANZAPINE-SPECIFIC** Sedation (including coma) and delirium (including agitation, anxiety, confusion, disorientation) have been observed following use of *Zyprexa Relprevv.* (3-hr monitoring post-injection) **SIDE EFFECTS** Somnolence Weight gain, ↑ lipids, ↑ glucose EPS, QT prolongation (lower risk) **MONITORING** For metabolic effects; see counseling section **NOTES** Smoking reduces drug levels.

Second-Generation (SGA) Antipsychotics Continued

DRUG	DOSING	SAFETY/SIDE EFFECTS/MONITORING
RisperiDONE (RisperDAL, RisperDAL M-TAB ODT), see injection to right Also approved for irritability associated with autism	4-16 mg/day, divided *Risperdal Consta*, 2 week injection, 25-50 mg	**SIDE EFFECTS** Somnolence EPS, especially at higher doses ↑ prolactin – sexual dysfunction, galactorrhea, irregular/missed periods Orthostasis Weight gain, ↑ lipids, ↑ glucose QT prolongation **MONITORING** For metabolic effects; see counseling section **NOTES** > 6 mg ↑ prolactin and ↑ EPS
QUEtiapine (SEROquel, SEROquel XR)	400-800 mg/day, divided BID or XR QHS	**SIDE EFFECTS** Somnolence, orthostasis Weight gain, ↑ lipids, ↑ glucose Little risk EPS – often used for psychosis in Parkinson's disease, QT prolongation (lower risk) **MONITORING** For metabolic effects; see counseling section **NOTES** Take XR at night, without food or with a light meal (≤ 300 calories).
Ziprasidone (Geodon), *Geodon* injection	40-160 mg/day, divided BID Acute injection: *Geodon IM* 10-20 mg	**CONTRAINDICATIONS** QT prolongation; contraindicated with QT risk **SIDE EFFECTS** Somnolence, respiratory tract infection (some have insomnia), headache, dizziness, nausea **NOTES** Take with food.
ARIPiprazole (Abilify, Abilify Discmelt ODT, *Maintena* injection) Also approved for irritability associated with autism	10-30 mg Q AM IM Injection, for acute agitation, *Abilify Maintena* is monthly injection	**SIDE EFFECTS** Akathisia, anxiety, insomnia Constipation Less weight gain, some degree QT prolongation
Paliperidone (Invega, *Invega Sustenna* is long-acting injection) Similar SEs to parent compound risperidone	3-12 mg/day (3 mg if CrCl < 50 mL/min; not rec. CrCl < 10 mL/min) Active metabolite of risperidone; OROS delivery, enables once daily dosing *Invega Sustenna*, IM injection, give monthly	**SIDE EFFECTS** ↑ prolactin – sexual dysfunction, galactorrhea, irregular/missed periods EPS, especially at higher doses Tachycardia, headache, sedation, anxiety QT prolongation; avoid use with QT risk Weight gain, ↑ lipids, ↑ glucose **MONITORING** For metabolic effects; see counseling section

Second-Generation (SGA) Antipsychotics Continued

DRUG	DOSING	SAFETY/SIDE EFFECTS/MONITORING
Iloperidone *(Fanapt)*	12-24 mg/day, divided	**SIDE EFFECTS** Dizziness, somnolence, orthostasis, tachycardia QT prolongation; avoid use with QT risk Titrate slowly due to orthostasis/dizziness
Asenapine *(Saphris)*	10-20 mg/day, divided, taken SL No food/drink for 10 min after dose	**SIDE EFFECTS** Somnolence, tongue/mouth numbness EPS (5% more than placebo), QT prolongation; avoid use with QT risk
Lurasidone *(Latuda)*	40-160 mg/day, divided	**SIDE EFFECTS** Somnolence, EPS, dystonias, nausea, agitation, akathisia Nearly weight, lipid and blood glucose neutral **NOTES** Take with food ≥ 350 kcal

Antipsychotic Drug Interactions

- Smoking can reduce plasma levels of olanzapine and clozapine, patients who smoke may require higher doses.

- All antipsychotics can prolong the QT interval – note that some are considered higher risk than others. The higher risk QT SGAs are noted. Thioridazine is a high risk FGA QT prolongating drug (boxed warning).

- High plasma levels of risperidone and paliperidone can ↑ prolactin and cause EPS. Caution when using risperidone concomitantly with CYP 2D6 inhibitors, including paroxetine and fluoxetine.

- With clozapine: avoid concurrent drugs that lower the seizure threshhold. Some of the APs have CYP450 drug interactions which could require dosing adjustments. Monitoring is also required for an increased risk of respiratory depression and hypotension when administered with benzodiazepines.

ALL ANTIPSYCHOTIC COUNSELING

- Dispense Med Guide and instruct patient to read it. In addition to individual warnings, several of the agents have anti-depressive properties and these include a warning for suicidality, particularly among adolescents.

- This medication can decrease hallucinations and improve your concentration. It helps you to think more clearly and feel positively about yourself, feel less nervous, and take a more active part in everyday life.

- There may be a slightly increased risk of serious, possibly fatal, side effects when this medication is used in older adults with dementia. This medication is not approved for the treatment of dementia-related behavior problems. Discuss the risks and benefits of this medication, as well as other effective and possibly safer treatments for dementia-related behavior problems, with your healthcare provider. The pharmacist should review symptoms of stroke with family/caregivers.

- Contact your healthcare provider right away if you experience uncontrollable movements of the mouth, tongue, cheeks, jaw, arms, or legs.

- Contact your healthcare provider immediately and seek immediate medical attention if you experience fever, sweating, severe muscle stiffness (rigidity) and confusion.

- Use caution when driving, operating machinery, or performing other hazardous activities. This drug may cause dizziness, confusion and sedation.

- Dizziness may be more likely to occur when you rise from a sitting or lying position. Rise slowly to prevent dizziness and a possible fall.

- To reduce the dizziness and lightheadedness that may occur when you first start to take this drug, you will be starting with a low dose, which will be slowly increased. You may be started with the immediate-release (IR) form of this drug, and then switched to the sustained-release form or an injectable form taken less often once you are taking a regular dose.

- Avoid consuming alcohol during treatment with this drug. Alcohol may increase sleepiness and dizziness and interfere with the drug's ability to work properly.

- Tell your healthcare provider if your condition persists or worsens.

Clozapine

- This medication can cause a serious immune system problem called agranulocytosis (low white blood cells). To make sure you have enough white blood cells, you will need to have a blood test before you begin taking clozapine and then have your blood tested regularly during your treatment.

- Clozapine can also cause seizures, especially with higher doses, or if it is increased too quickly when starting therapy. Let your healthcare provider know if you have ever had seizures. While taking this medication, avoid activities during which a sudden loss of consciousness could be dangerous (e.g., driving, operating machinery, swimming).

- This medication may rarely cause an inflammation of the heart muscle (myocarditis). Seek immediate medical attention if you have weakness, difficult/rapid breathing, chest pain, or swelling of the ankles/legs. The risk is highest during the first month of treatment.

Olanzapine, Clozapine, Risperidone, Paliperidone and Quetiapine

- This drug has a risk of weight gain, elevated cholesterol, blood pressure and blood glucose (hyperglycemia). These must be monitored, and treated if they occur. Talk to your healthcare provider if you experience any signs of hyperglycemia including excessive thirst, frequent urination, excessive hunger, or weakness.

- Your healthcare provider will order blood tests during treatment to monitor progress and side effects.

Different Types of Oral Formulations

- *Asenapine*: Place the sublingual tablet under the tongue and allow it to dissolve completely. The tablet will dissolve in saliva within seconds. Do not eat or drink for 10 minutes after taking this medication. The tongue will feel numb afterwards.

- *FazaClo, Abilify Discmelt, Risperdal M-Tab, Zyprexa Zydis*: Immediately upon opening the foil blister, using dry hands, remove tablet and place in mouth. Do not push the tablet through the foil because it may crumble. Tablet disintegration occurs rapidly so it can be easily swallowed with or without liquid. Use liquid only if you need it.

- Most ODTs contain phenylalanine. Do not dispense ODTs to patients with phenylketonuria (PKU).

- *Risperdal* oral solution can be administered directly from the calibrated pipette, or mixed with water, coffee, orange juice, and low-fat milk; it is not compatible with cola or tea.

- *Latuda* is taken with food, at least 350 kcal. *Geodon* is taken with food.

- Quetiapine immediate-release tablet may be taken without regard to meals. The extended-release tablet *(Seroquel XR)* should be taken without food or with a light meal (up to 300 kcal).

- Olanzapine is usually taken once daily at night (QHS), since it is long-acting and sedating.

PRACTICE CASE

Ruby is a 24 year-old college student. Her parents have attempted to help Ruby over the past year. Her academic performance deteriorated and she began to look unkempt. About a month ago, her Mom was sure she saw Ruby mumbling to herself. Ruby began to call her mother "evil" and told her mother that she was destroying her life. Later, Ruby accused her mother of trying to feed her poisoned food. Ruby has dropped her old high-school friendships, except for one girl who her mother feels is more troubled than Ruby. When the mother went to talk to one of Ruby's instructors, they found out that Ruby had accused the teacher of changing what Ruby had written on an exam, and that the teacher had seen Ruby mumbling to herself in class. The teacher also complained that Ruby lacks attention in class, and reported that her work is sloppy and disorganized. The teacher had assumed there was difficulty at home, since Ruby told her that her mother is dying from cancer. This report from Ruby was not truthful.

The crisis in the family came to a head recently when Ruby stole a bottle of vodka from the local convenience store and was caught. Fortunately, the store manager knew the family and declined to press charges. However, later that night Ruby took some unknown medication and attempted to drown herself in the bathtub. She was taken by ambulance to the hospital.

The psychiatric team, after a brief visit with Ruby and a history taken from her family, gave Ruby a tentative diagnosis of schizophrenia. She received an injection of haloperidol and lorazepam, and is sleeping soundly. The psychiatric resident has come to the family to discuss treatment options.

No current medications; no known medical history. Height 5'5", weight 125 lbs.

Questions

1. The physician gave the patient an injection of haloperidol. This medication comes in the following formulations. (Select **ALL** that apply.)

   a. Oral tablets
   b. IM injection
   c. Long-lasting (monthly) decanoate
   d. Oral solution
   e. Orally disintegrating tablet (ODT)

2. If Ruby is continued on haloperidol, she will be at risk for these side effects. (Select **ALL** that apply.)

   a. Painful dystonic reactions (including painful neck and back muscle contractions)
   b. Tardive dyskinesias, or abnormal facial movements
   c. Gynecomastia
   d. Agranulocytosis
   e. QT prolongation and possible arrhythmia risk

3. If Ruby were to experience neuroleptic malignant syndrome while receiving haloperidol, what therapies would likely be administered in this emergency situation? (Select **ALL** that apply.)

   a. Switch to fluphenazine
   b. Cooled IV fluids, ice beds
   c. Heating blankets
   d. Muscle relaxants
   e. Airway support

Questions 4-10 do not apply to the case.

4. Choose the potential adverse reaction from haloperidol which can be <u>irreversible</u> (and, if it occurs, the medicine should be stopped right away):

   a. Dystonic reaction
   b. Tardive dyskinesia
   c. Akathisia
   d. Dizziness
   e. Orthostatic hypotension

5. A patient is started on olanzapine for psychotic symptoms. This agent puts the patient at high risk for the following side effects: (Select **ALL** that apply.)

    a. Weight loss

    b. Elevated blood glucose

    c. Increased risk lymphoma or other malignancies

    d. Elevated cholesterol

    e. Elevated creatine phosphokinase

6. A patient has been prescribed *Risperdal Consta*. Choose the correct statement:

    a. The medication lasts four weeks.

    b. The medication is given by slow IV infusion.

    c. *Risperdal Consta* is an orally-dissolving formulation for use with dysphagia.

    d. There remains a risk of EPS with this formulation.

    e. The benefit with the *Consta* formulation is little or no risk of elevated prolactin levels.

7. A patient has schizophrenia, with constant auditory hallucinations which have instructed the patient to harm himself and others. He has failed olanzapine and chlorpromazine. His other medications include sertraline for anxiety. His WBC ranges from 2.3-3.4 cells/mm³. He also has a low platelet count of 120. Which of the following statements is correct?

    a. He should begin clozapine therapy.

    b. Clozapine therapy is contraindicated due to his WBC count.

    c. Clozapine therapy is contraindicated due to his platelet count.

    d. Clozapine therapy is not indicated since he has not tried haloperidol.

    e. He should begin treatment with *Zyprexa*.

8. A patient with psychotic symptoms takes the following medications for chronic conditions: metoprolol, warfarin, amiodarone, lisinopril and insulin. His physician wishes to begin an antipsychotic. Which of the following agents represents the best option for this patient?

    a. Thioridazine

    b. Haloperidol

    c. Ziprasidone

    d. Risperidone

    e. Aripiprazole

9. A patient is using olanzapine in the morning. He takes 10 mg daily. He is tired all the time, but has trouble sleeping at night. Which option is best?

    a. Add temazepam at bedtime.

    b. Add zolpidem at bedtime.

    c. Move the olanzapine to bedtime.

    d. Add modafinil in the morning.

    e. Add mirtazapine at bedtime.

10. A physician wrote a prescription for *Fanapt*. Which medication should be dispensed?

    a. Asenapine

    b. Olanzapine

    c. Aripiprazole

    d. Iloperidone

    e. Thioridazine

Answers

1-a,b,c,d, 2-a,b,e, 3-b,d,e, 4-b, 5-b,d, 6-d, 7-b, 8-e, 9-c, 10-d,

BIPOLAR DISORDER

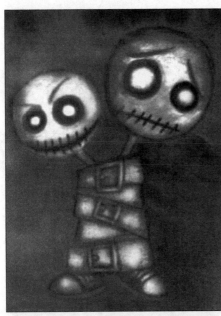

We gratefully acknowledge the assistance of Robin Wackernah, PharmD, BCPP, Regis University, School of Pharmacy, in preparing this chapter.

BACKGROUND

Bipolar disorder is a mood disorder where moods can fluctuate from depression to elevated moods referred to as "mania." Each mood episode represents a drastic change from a person's usual mood and behavior. Bipolar disorder is currently broken up into bipolar I disorder and bipolar II disorder and a milder form called "cyclothymic disorder" where the criteria for depression or mania are not fully met. The Diagnostic and Statistical Manual of Mental Disorders, Fifth Edition (DSM-5) is the current tool used to diagnose bipolar disorder and other psychiatric disorders.

Bipolar I disorder is the most severe version of the disorder. The classic diagnostic symptom is mania, but patients may also experience bouts of depression. Mania is characterized as an elevated mood where patients have a lot of energy, may feel euphoric, "on top of the world," and/or irritable. The symptoms of mania in bipolar I disorder can be so severe that they can require psychiatric hospitalization, impair social or occupational functioning or have features of psychosis such as hearing voices or delusions (false beliefs).

Bipolar II disorder has the same symptoms of bipolar I disorder, however the symptoms are described as "hypomania" because they are less severe than in pure mania.

GUIDELINES

Diagnostic and Statistical Manual of Mental Disorders, Fifth Edition (DSM-5).

WFSBP: Update 2012 on the long-term treatment of bipolar disorder. The World Journal of Biological Psychiatry, 2013; 14: 154–219.

APA, Treatment of Patients with Bipolar Disorder. http://psychiatryonline.org/content.aspx?bookid=28&sectionid=1669577 (accessed Oct 5 2014).

VA/DOD, Management of Bipolar Disorder in Adults, 2010. http://www.healthquality.va.gov/bipolar/bd_305_full.pdf (accessed Oct 5 2014).

Hypomania by definition will not affect social or occupational functioning, patients do not require hospitalization for mania, and do not have psychosis.

The estimated prevalence of bipolar I disorder ranges from 0.4 – 1.6%. Bipolar II disorder is less common in the general population, but is more common in women. Bipolar disorder can lead to problems with relationships, employment, disrupt lives, lead to suicide and/or a variety of risky behaviors.

Diagnostic Criteria

In addition to the elevated or irritable mood, the DSM-5 diagnostic criteria for mania include 3 or more of the following symptoms. Note that 4 symptoms are required if the mood is only irritable:

- Inflated self-esteem or grandiosity (having an exaggerated belief in one's importance or talents)

- Decreased need for sleep

- More talkative than usual

- Flight of ideas (jumping from one topic to the next) or racing thoughts (the mind switches between thoughts very quickly)

- Distractibility

- Increase in goal-directed activity (either social, at work or at school)

- Excessive involvement in pleasurable activities that have a high potential for painful consequences (e.g., buying sprees, sexual indiscretions, gambling)

DRUG TREATMENT

Mood stabilizers (lithium, valproate, lamotrigine, carbamazepine), and the second-generation antipsychotics (SGAs) are first-line for treating mania and maintaining a stable mood (preventing the patient's mood from swinging into mania or depression). The definition of a mood stabilizer is a medication that can treat either mania or depression without inducing either. Antidepressants are not considered mood stabilizers. Do not start an antidepressant unless there is a mood stabilizer in the patient's regimen. Otherwise, there is risk of inducing mania. MedGuides are required with all antidepressants (primarily due to suicide risk) and with all antipsychotics (primarily due to increased risk of death in elderly patients with dementia-related psychosis).

First generation antipsychotics (FGAs), such as haloperidol, have been used in the past for bipolar mania but have fallen out of favor due to the increased risk of extrapyramidal side effects (EPS). Patients with bipolar disorder are more susceptible to EPS and antipsychotic agents should be used with caution in this population, particularly the FGAs.

While some of the FGAs have been associated with causing depression, the SGAs do not induce depressive episodes, and some of them have antidepressant effects. The most current guidelines recommend either a mood stabilizer, a SGA, or a combination of a mood stabilizer and SGA. If psychotic features are present, it makes sense to begin with a SGA. In deciding which SGA to use, clinicians should consider the primary treatment goal: treating mania, treating depression or for maintenance, and the side effect profile.

Lamotrigine is used in bipolar depression and for maintenance, however it is not beneficial in mania due to the slow titration that is required to reach a target dose. Lithium is used in mania, depression and maintenance. Lithium is still commonly used today and is often paired with a SGA in severe cases. Valproate and carbamazepine (as *Equetro*) are both approved for bipolar mania. Refer to the Epilepsy/Seizures chapter for information on these agents; and, there is a summary table further in this chapter.

MOOD STABILIZERS & PREGNANCY

Valproate, carbamazepine and lithium are pregnancy category D for treatment of bipolar and have known fetal risk. The benefit must outweigh the risk. Lamotrigine (pregnancy category C) is often considered the safer option, relative to the other agents. During pregnancy if the risk is not well quantified an attempt should be made to avoid unnecessary drugs during the first trimester when organogenesis takes place. The SGAs that are approved for bipolar disorder are pregnancy category C. Lurasidone is pregnancy category B.

- Lithium exposure in pregnancy is associated with an increase in congenital cardiac malformations.

- Valproate exposure in pregnancy is associated with increased risk of fetal anomalies, including neural tube defects, fetal valproate syndrome, and long term adverse cognitive effects. It should be avoided in pregnancy, if possible, especially during the first trimester.

- Carbamazepine exposure in pregnancy is associated with fetal carbamazepine syndrome. It should be avoided in pregnancy, if possible, especially during the first trimester. Carbamazepine is a third-line agent for treating bipolar but is occasionally used and a formulation was approved recently that is indicated for bipolar *(Equetro)*.

- If an antidepressant is used, paroxetine should be avoided. It is rated as pregnancy category D due to the risk of cardiac defects, particularly in the 1st trimester. Other SSRIs and SNRIs should be considered to have some degree of risk as well.

Bipolar Mania or Illicit Drug Use?

A toxicology screen should be taken first (prior to start of treatment, and as-needed) to rule-out mania due to illicit drug use.

ANTIEPILEPTIC DRUGS (AEDs) USED IN BIPOLAR DISORDER

See Epilepsy/Seizure chapter for a full discussion including drug interactions and patient counseling.

DRUG	DOSING	SAFETY/SIDE EFFECTS/MONITORING
LamoTRIgine (*LaMICtal* [tabs/chewables], *LaMICtal ODT*) Various formulations, including chewables, ODT	Dosing requires slow titration (↑ every other week) due to risk of rash. Dose depends on inhibitors (lower doses) and inducers (higher doses): Usual dose: 25 mg Q daily, max 200 mg/day If using valproic acid, start at 25 mg every other day, max 100 mg Q daily If using carbamazepine, phenytoin, phenobarbital or primidone (and not on valproic acid), start at 50 mg Q daily, max 400 mg/day Divided BID; XR is daily	**BOXED WARNING** Serious skin reactions, including SJS/TEN **WARNINGS** Risk of aseptic meningitis, blood dyscrasias (aplastic anemia, agranulocytosis) **SIDE EFFECTS CAN ↓ ADHERENCE** Somnolence, dizziness, rash (non-serious, 7%), vision changes/diplopia, nausea, insomnia
Valproate/Valproic acid (*Depakene, Stavzor, Depacon*) Supplementation with calcium and vitamin D recommended	Start at 25 mg/kg/day, max 60 mg/kg/day Therapeutic Range 50-125 mcg/mL	**BOXED WARNINGS (4)** Hepatic Failure Teratogenicity Pancreatitis Mitochondrial disease ↑ risk acute liver failure **CONTRAINDICATIONS** Hepatic disease, urea cycle disorders, prophylaxis of migraine in pregnancy, known mitochondrial disorders **WARNINGS** Hyperammonemia, hypothermia **SIDE EFFECTS CAN ↓ ADHERENCE** Nausea, alopecia, (treat with a multivitamin containing selenium and zinc), weight gain, tremor Dose-related: thrombocytopenia, diplopia, blurred vision **NOTES** Pregnancy Category D/X (for migraine prophylaxis)
CarBAMazepine (*Equetro*) – for bipolar Potent CYP450 inducer and autoinducer – ↓ level of many other drugs and of itself Supplementation with calcium and vitamin D recommended	Start at 200 mg BID, max 1600 mg/day Therapeutic Range 4-12 mcg/mL	**BOXED WARNINGS (2)** Serious skin reactions, including SJS/TEN; if Asian descent, test for HLA-B*1502 allele prior to use Blood cell abnormalities, incl. risk agranulocytosis **WARNINGS** SIADH, others **SIDE EFFECTS CAN ↓ ADHERENCE** Dizziness, somnolence, headache, nausea, ataxia, rash

Lithium

Lithium has various proposed mechanisms, including influencing the reuptake of serotonin and/or norepinephrine and inhibiting postsynaptic D_2 receptor supersensitivity.

DRUG	DOSING	SAFETY/SIDE EFFECTS/MONITORING
Lithium *(Lithobid)*	Start at 150-900 mg/day, divided, max 900-2,400 mg/day, with the extended-release given BID **Therapeutic Range** 0.6-1.2 mEq/L (trough level) Acute mania may need up to 1.5 mEq initially Titrate slowly to help patient tolerate SEs Take with food (post-meal) if nausea, or try split dosing If tremor, thirst, confusion, or nocturia, try QHS dosing	Cannot use with renal impairment: lithium is 100% renally cleared – and if not eliminated, toxicity will result **SIDE EFFECTS** GI upset (take with food in the stomach, can change to ER forms) Cognitive effects, cogwheel rigidity, fine hand tremor, weight gain Polyuria/polydipsia, hypothyroidism – must monitor, serotonergic; avoid co-admin with other serotonergic agents Cardiac abnormalities (inverted T waves) Edema, worsening of psoriasis **TOXICITY** > 1.5 mEq/L (coarse hand tremor, vomiting, persistent diarrhea, confusion, ataxia) > 3 mEq/L (CNS depression, arrhythmia, seizures, irreversible brain damage, coma) **MONITORING** BMP (renal function), thyroid function (TSH, FT4), ECG in patients over 40 Pregnancy Category D

Lithium Drug Interactions

- These will ↑ lithium: ↓ salt intake, NSAIDs, ACE Is, ARBs, thiazide diuretics; aspirin and sulindac are safer NSAID options.

- These will ↓ lithium: ↑ salt intake, caffeine, and theophylline.

- These will ↑ risk 5HT-syndrome if given with lithium: SSRIs, SNRIs, triptans, linezolid and other serotonergic drugs.

- ↑ neurotoxicity risk (ataxia, tremors, nausea) with lithium in combination with these drugs: verapamil, diltiazem, phenytoin and carbamazepine.

Lithium Counseling

- Call your healthcare provider if you experience severe nausea, vomiting, worsened diarrhea, slurred speech, extreme drowsiness, weakness, and noticeable (worsened) tremor. These symptoms may indicate that the lithium level is too high in your blood.

- Do not crush, chew, or break any extended-release forms of lithium (*Lithobid*). The drug is specially formulated to release slowly in the body.

- Lithium can cause you to feel confused or "dizzy," especially when the dose is started or increased. Use caution when driving or performing other hazardous activities until you know how you feel taking this medication.

- Lithium is FDA pregnancy category D. This means that lithium is known to be harmful to an unborn baby. Do not take lithium without first talking to your healthcare provider if you are pregnant or are planning a pregnancy. Lithium can pass into breast milk. Discuss with your healthcare provider if you are breastfeeding.

- Maintain adequate fluid intake by drinking 8 to 12 glasses of water or other fluids (do not count any caffeinated sodas, coffee or tea) every day while taking lithium. Vigorous exercise, prolonged exposure to heat or sun, excessive sweating, diarrhea, or vomiting can cause dehydration and increased side effects from lithium. Call your doctor if you lose a significant amount of body fluid as a result of sweating, diarrhea, or vomiting.

- Do not change the amount of salt you consume. There is a lot of salt in many fast foods, luncheon meats, "TV dinners" and canned goods.

- You will need to have your blood checked occasionally during treatment.

- Do not stop taking this medication, even if you are feeling better.

SECOND-GENERATION ANTIPSYCHOTICS USED IN BIPOLAR DISORDER

The 2010 VA guidelines list other second generation antipsychotics as treatment options. These are the agents with FDA approval. For a more complete review of the SGAs, including mechanism, drug interactions and counseling, refer to the Schizophrenia and Psychosis chapter.

DRUG	DOSING	SAFETY/SIDE EFFECTS/MONITORING
Aripiprazole (Abilify, Abilify Discmelt, Abilify Maintena) Approved for manic & mixed symptoms, maintenance, +/- lithium or valproate	PO: 15-30 mg QAM IM: 400 mg monthly	**COMMON SIDE EFFECTS** These drugs can cause metabolic issues, including dyslipidemia, weight gain, diabetes Risk of Neuroleptic Malignant Syndrome Risk of Tardive Dyskinesia (TD) Risk of leukopenia, neutropenia, agranulocytosis All can cause orthostasis/dizziness **SPECIFIC SIDE EFFECTS** **Aripiprazole** Akathisia (esp in younger patients), restlessness, insomnia, constipation, fatigue, blurred vision
OLANZapine/FLUoxetine (Symbyax) Approved for bipolar depression, 2nd line option due to metabolic effects from olanzapine	Usually started at 6 mg/25 mg capsule QHS (fluoxetine is activating, but olanzapine is more sedating), can ↑ cautiously. CI with pimozide, thioridazine, & caution with other QT prolonging drugs/conditions	
OLANZapine (ZyPREXA, Zydis ODT, Relprevv Inj.) Approved for manic or mixed episodes +/- lithium or valproate, or for monotherapy maintenance	5-20 mg/day, generally QHS	**Olanzapine** Cognitive dysfunction, dry mouth, fatigue, sedation, ↑ appetite/weight, peripheral edema, tremor, blurred vision. ↓ CVD risk than other listed APs, some QT risk with the IM injection.
QUEtiapine extended release (SEROquel, SEROquel XR) Approved for mania/maintenance with lithium or divalproex, and for bipolar depression	Bipolar mania/maintenance: 400-800 mg QHS Bipolar depression: 300 mg QHS	**Quetiapine** QT risk, sedation, dry mouth, constipation, dizziness, ↑ appetite/weight
RisperiDONE (RisperDAL, RisperDAL Consta, RisperDAL M-TAB) Approved alone or with lithium or valproate for acute mania or mixed episodes	Start at 2-3 mg/d, can ↑ to 6 mg In children start 0.5 mg/d Tablets, oral solution, M-tabs (ODT)	**Risperidone** Sedation, ↑ appetite, fatigue, insomnia, Parkinsonism, akathisia, nausea, some QT risk, EPS **Ziprasidone** QT risk (greatest), sedation or insomnia, EPS, dizziness, akathisia, abnormal vision, asthenia, nausea
Ziprasidone (Geodon) Approved with lithium or valproate for maintenance, or alone for manic/mixed episodes	Start at 40 mg BID, can ↑ to 80 mg BID Take with food	**Asenapine** Numbs mouth, sedation, dizziness, weight gain (less than risperidone and olanzapine). Some QT risk.
Asenapine (Saphris) Approved for acute manic or mixed episodes, +/- lithium or valproate	5-20 mg Sublingual (SL) only: must dissolve under tongue, & no food/drink for 10 min after taking	**ADA Screening/Monitoring Recommendations** Patients being started on APs should first be screened for overweight and obesity, dyslipidemia and hyperglycemia, hypertension, and personal or family history of risk. While being treated, the patient should be monitored for treatment-emergent changes in weight, waist circumference, plasma lipid and glucose levels, and acute symptoms of diabetes (e.g., polyuria, polydipsia).
Lurasidone (Latuda) Approved for bipolar depression, +/- lithium or valproate	20-120 mg/day Dose titration NOT required Take with food	

PRACTICE CASE

MH is a 65 y/o white female brought to the clinic today by her sister. She has a long history of bipolar I that has been reasonably controlled on lithium therapy for many years. MH lives with her sister, who takes good care of her medical and social needs. Occasionally, her sister reports, MH gets "back to her old thing" and becomes convinced that she is on a mission to "change the world." MH can never explain what is involved with this mission. Her sister states that MH has always had a fine hand tremor, but today her hand is visibly shaking. She is nauseous and vomited the little she ate this morning. Her speech is slurred and confused. She appears to have difficulty walking into the examination room. She also has a cold with nasal congestion. Additional past medical history includes hypertension.

Allergies: NKDA

Medications:
Lithobid 450 mg BID
Lopressor 50 mg BID
Oscal 500 mg BID with meals
B-complex tablet daily

Vitals:
BP: 129/80 mmHg   HR: 75 BPM   RR: 15 BPM   Temp: 38.1°C   Pain: 2/10

Labs:

Previous Labs (10/1/2013)
Na (mEq/L) = 136 (135 - 145)
K (mEq/L) = 3.9 (3.5 - 5)
Cl (mEq/L) = 104 (95 - 103)
HCO3 (mEq/L) = 24 (24 - 30)
BUN (mg/dL) = 14 (7 - 20)
SCr (mg/dL) = 0.7 (0.6 - 1.3)
Glucose (mg/dL) = 120 (100 - 125)
WBC (cells/mm3) = 8.2 (4 - 11 x 103)
Hgb (g/dL) = 12.4
(13.5 - 18 male, 12 - 16 female)
Hct (%) = 39.2 (38 - 50 male, 36 - 46 female)
Plt (cells/mm3) = 201 (150 - 450 x 103)
Lithium (mEq/L) = 0.9 (0.6 - 1.2)

Today (11/1/2014)
Na (mEq/L) = 140 (135 - 145)
K (mEq/L) = 4.6 (3.5 - 5)
Cl (mEq/L) = 101 (95 - 103)
HCO3 (mEq/L) = 25 (24 - 30)
BUN (mg/dL) = 28 (7 - 20)
SCr (mg/dL) = 1.7 (0.6 - 1.3)
Glucose (mg/dL) = 108 (100 - 125)
WBC (cells/mm3) = 5.6 (4 - 11 x 103)
Hgb (g/dL) = 14.3
(13.5 - 18 male, 12 - 16 female)
Hct (%) = 42.1 (38 - 50 male, 36 - 46 female)
Plt (cells/mm3) = 250 (150 - 450 x 103)
Lithium (mEq/L) = 1.8 (0.6 - 1.2)

Sept 9th: Increased lithium level and increased BUN/SCr compared to visit last year. Diovan added to control BP.

Questions

1. The following factors are likely contributing to the current symptoms of GI distress, coarse hand tremor, ataxia and confusion: (Select **ALL** that apply.)

   a. The use of a calcium supplement
   b. The patient's decline in renal function
   c. Lithium level of 1.8 mEq/L
   d. The use of a vitamin supplement (B-complex)
   e. The patient's ethnicity

2. Margie is using *Lithobid*. Describe *Lithobid* clearance:

   a. 100% renal clearance; no hepatic metabolism.
   b. 50% metabolized by 3A4, 50% excreted unchanged in the urine.
   c. 75% metabolized by 2D6, 25% excreted unchanged in the urine.
   d. 100% metabolized by 2C9, 100% metabolites cleared renally.
   e. Metabolized by 2C19, metabolites cleared renally.

3. Select the correct statement regarding the medication added to the patient's regimen on September 9th:

   a. It will increase the risk of bradycardia.
   b. It will increase her blood pressure.
   c. It will contribute to rapid-cycling.
   d. It will increase appetite and could contribute to weight gain.
   e. It will increase lithium levels.

Questions 4-7 are NOT based on the above case.

4. A patient has a history of two myocardial infarctions. He has bipolar II which is moderately controlled with lithium monotherapy. He has been using lithium for many years. His physician wishes to use an antipsychotic as augmentation therapy. Which of the following antipsychotics can cause QT prolongation? (Select **ALL** that apply.)

   a. *Seroquel*
   b. *Risperdal*
   c. *Geodon*
   d. *Mellaril*
   e. *Haldol*

5. Patient counseling for lithium should include the following points (Select **ALL** that apply.):

   a. Lithium could become unsafe if taken with over-the-counter ibuprofen or naproxen.
   b. You may notice that your hands develop a fine (light) tremor.
   c. If the tremor becomes worse and you feel nauseated, contact the doctor at once.
   d. A safe level for this drug is 0.6-1.2 mg/L
   e. You must keep the salt level in your diet around the same amount each day.

6. A patient is using valproate therapy. Boxed warnings for this medication include: (Select **ALL** that apply.)

   a. Neuroleptic Malignant Syndrome
   b. Mitochondrial disease
   c. Hepatotoxicity
   d. Pancreatitis
   e. Teratogenicity

7. A patient has been diagnosed with bipolar II. Which of the following statement/s concerning bipolar II are correct?

   a. The mania symptoms are generally worse in bipolar II than in bipolar I.
   b. The depressive symptoms are generally worse in bipolar II than in bipolar I.
   c. Bipolar II is much less common than bipolar I.
   d. Bipolar II is much more common in men.
   e. In bipolar I, mania and psychosis can require hospitalization.

Answers

1-b,c, 2-a, 3-e, 4-a,b,c,d,e, 5-a,b,c,e, 6-b,c,d,e, 7-e

PARKINSON DISEASE

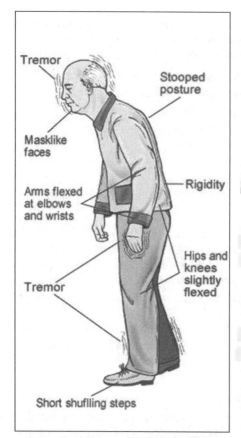

Tremor
Stooped posture
Masklike faces
Arms flexed at elbows and wrists
Rigidity
Hips and knees slightly flexed
Tremor
Short shufling steps

GUIDELINE

Diagnosis and prognosis of new onset Parkinson disease (an evidence-based review): Report of the Quality Standards Subcommittee of the American Academy of Neurology. *Neurology.* 2006 Apr 11;66(7):968-75.

We gratefully acknowledge the assistance of George De-Maagd, PharmD, BCPS, Associate Dean of Academic Administration, Professor of Pharmacy, Union University School of Pharmacy, in preparing this chapter.

BACKGROUND

Parkinson disease (PD) is a brain disorder. It occurs when neurons in a part of the brain called the substantia nigra die or become impaired. The cause of neuronal death is not well understood, but is multi-factorial. Normally, these cells produce dopamine. Dopamine allows smooth, coordinated function of the body's muscles and movement. When ~80% of the dopamine-producing cells are damaged, the motor symptoms of the disease appear. Non-motor symptoms can precede motor symptoms and may appear much earlier. These include loss of sense of smell (anosmia), constipation, sleep difficulties, low mood and orthostasis. While this disease usually develops after the age of 65, 15% of those diagnosed are under 50. Initially (in what is called Stage I) the disease appears as tremor on one-side (unilateral) and eventually spreads bilaterally. Bradykinesia (slow movement) refers to a reduction in spontaneous movement, which can give the appearance of abnormal stiffness and a decrease in facial expression. This causes difficulty with everyday functions, such as buttoning clothes and cutting food. Walking appears as shuffling steps. Speech is also affected. Rigidity causes stiffness and difficulty with movement. "Cogwheel rigidity" is a ratchet-like movement of arms. Postural instability, another cardinal feature of this condition, is a tendency

PRIMARY SIGNS/SYMPTOMS

TRAP:

Tremor – seen during resting, usually worsened by anxiety

Rigidity – arms, legs, trunk and face (mask-like face)

Akinesia/bradykinesia – lack of movement or slow initiation of movement

Postural instability – poor balance, which may lead to frequent falls

Other Signs of Parkinson Disease
Small, cramped handwriting (micrographia)

Shuffling walk, bent (over) posture

Stiff "masked" facial expression, reduced eye blinking

Muffled speech, drooling, dysphagia

Depression, anxiety (psychosis in advanced disease)

Constipation, incontinence

---

to be unstable when standing upright, and is due to a decline in reflexes. Some patients will sway backwards, which causes falls. Eventually, even with high doses of the two most effective classes of drugs (carbidopa/levodopa and the dopamine agonists), the "off" periods will increase – this is among the most frustrating and challenging aspects of disease management. An off episode is a period of time with muscle stiffness, slow movements, and difficulty starting movements. Eventually, the patient will be unable to walk and have difficulty feeding themselves or swallowing foods. Amantadine can be useful to help with dyskinesias in later stage disease due to it's antagonism of the NMDA receptor. Apomorphine treats later stage severe freezing episodes, but it requires subcutaneous (SC) administration, has difficult side effects, and provides increased movement for just about an hour. Patients with Parkinson disease have high incidence of depression. The agents with the highest efficacy for treatment in these patients are the tricyclic antidepressants, and the secondary amines (such as desipramine and nortriptyline) are preferred due to less side effects than the tertiary amines. The majority of PD patients, however, use SSRIs since many clinicians are familiar with this class and think that they are better tolerated. Psychosis can present with advanced disease. Although the SSRIs are commonly used, they may contribute to tremor or increase the risk of serotonin syndrome in Parkinson disease patients who are taking MAO-B inhibitors. Quetiapine is the preferred antipsychotic, due to a low risk of [OR iloperidone (Fanapt®)] movement disorders, but will require monitoring due to metabolic complications, including increased blood glucose and cholesterol. The benefit of helping the psychosis is contradictory. Clozapine also has low risk of aggravating movement disorders and has been studied for this purpose, but the use is limited by the risk of severe complications and the requirement of frequent monitoring.

Drug-induced Parkinson Disease

Certain drugs can cause Parkinsonism due to their antagonism of dopamine receptors. These include phenothiazines (prochlorperazine, others), first generation antipsychotics (including haloperidol) the second-generation antipsychotics risperidone *(Risperdal)*, at higher doses, [> 6 mg/day] and the newer agent paliperidone *(Invega)*, and the dopamine-blocking agent metoclopramide *(Reglan)*. Metoclopramide is mostly likely to produce Parkinsonism when it is overdosed, especially in elderly patients who require a dose reduction with renal dysfunction. CNS effects (sedation, dizziness) from this drug are another reason to avoid use in the elderly, if possible. Disorders with these drugs are always dose-dependent; higher doses (especially in elderly patients) are highest risk. Keep in mind that with PD patients drugs that cause tremor (lithium, etc.) will aggravate the pre-existing condition.

FL BLUE   877 352 2583   benefits
      ?
                 877 504 2583   appeal

DRUG TREATMENT

Medications can help improve movement, and may be used for related issues, such as psychosis and constipation. Levodopa, which is in the commonly used agent carbidopa-levodopa (Sinemet), is the most effective agent and is sometimes better tolerated for initial treatment in the elderly than the dopamine agonists. Initial treatment of tremor in younger patients may be treated with an anticholinergic. The considerable side effects of the anticholinergics prohibit use in elderly patients. Amantadine is sometimes used for initial treatment of tremor, usually in younger patients. A monoamine oxidase inhibitor may also be used for a mild benefit as initial treatment. The dopamine agonists are often given as the initial option in younger patients (< 65 years). As the disease progresses treatment will be directed at both reducing off periods and limiting dyskinesias, using multiple combinations and adjunctive therapies to manage the progressive nature of the disease. In 2014 a new drug was approved for orthostatic hypotension, which (primarily) affects patients with Parkinson's, although other conditions can present with this complication and in some cases it is idiopathic. The drug is called droxipoda (Northera). It is reviewed at the end of the PD drugs in this chapter.

Dopamine Replacement Agents & Agonists

DRUG	DOSING	SAFETY/SIDE EFFECTS/MONITORING
Carbidopa/Levodopa MOA: Levodopa is a precursor of dopamine. Carbidopa inhibits dopa decarboxylase, preventing peripheral metabolism of levodopa		
Carbidopa/Levodopa (Sinemet, Sinemet CR) *Parcopa RapiTab* rapidly dissolves on the tongue without water. Levodopa and carbidopa are available separately. If switching from levodopa IR to levodopa-carbidopa CR, dosage should be substituted at an amount that provides ~10% more of levodopa/day.	Usual starting dose 25/100 TID IR: 10/100, 25/100, 25/250 mg tab CR: 25/100, 50/200 *Parcopa* comes in 10/100, 25/100 mg, 25/250 ODT SR tab can be cut into half – do not crush or chew 70-100 mg of carbidopa is required to to inhibit the peripheral conversion (dopa decarboxylase) and to ↓ nausea Titrate cautiously due to orthostasis/dizziness risk; these are often titrated quickly (such as every few days) to help with movement.	**CONTRAINDICATIONS** Non-selective MAOIs within last 14 days, narrow angle glaucoma **SIDE EFFECTS** Nausea, dizziness, orthostasis, vomiting, dry mouth, Dyskinesias (abnormal movements), dystonias (occasional, painful) ~1/3 of patients develop confusion, hallucinations, or psychosis (with disease progression; not initially) Can cause brown, black or dark urine, saliva or sweat, and discolor clothing, positive Coombs test **NOTES** Possibility of unusual sexual urges, priapism Response fluctuations and dyskinesias after long-term use Separate from iron, possibly separate from protein (see counseling) May slightly increase uric acid

Handwritten annotations:

↓ nausea from levodopa by inhib peripheral conversion

min dose of carbi required for effectiveness; ↑↑ dose of carbi → nausea

per day

↑ UA

} after long-term use

elderly
** Sinemet Ⓡ **
- most effective
- better tolerated than DA agonists

younger
- DA agonists ⇒ <65 y/o
- antiACh ⇒ initial tremor
- amantadine

→ pts may be on Sinemet Ⓡ IR to get them going in AM (be able to eat breakfast, etc.) and Sinemet Ⓡ CR dosed TID to cover rest of day.

→ faster onset than CR

Dopamine Replacement Agents & Agonists Continued

DRUG	DOSING	SAFETY/SIDE EFFECTS/MONITORING

COMT-INHIBITOR: Used only with levodopa to ↑ levodopa duration of action. Inhibits the enzyme COMT to prevent peripheral and central conversion of levodopa

DRUG	DOSING	SAFETY/SIDE EFFECTS/MONITORING
Entacapone *(Comtan)* Levodopa/carbidopa + entacapone *(Stalevo)* Tolcapone *(Tasmar)* – not used much due to hepatotoxicity	200 mg with each dose of carbidopa/levodopa (max 1,600 mg/day) *Stalevo* 12.5/50/200 mg 18.75/75/200 mg 25/100/200 mg 31.25/125/200 mg 37.5/150/200 mg 50/200/200 mg	**SIDE EFFECTS** Similar to levodopa, due to extending levodopa duration of action: Nausea, dyskinesias Dizziness, orthostasis, hypotension Urine discoloration, diarrhea **NOTES** ↓ in levodopa dose of 10-30% is usually necessary when adding on COMT inhibitor

DA-AGONISTS – Act Similar to dopamine at the dopamine receptor   *TITRATE WEEKLY! ⇒ DIZZINESS / ORTHOSTASIS*

DRUG	DOSING	SAFETY/SIDE EFFECTS/MONITORING
Pramipexole *(Mirapex, Mirapex ER)* Both dopamine agonists approved in IR formulations (not long-acting) for restless leg syndrome (dosed QHS) *IR* *★ CrCl<50 ⇒ ↓ dose*	Start 0.125 mg TID, titrate 5-7 d to 0.5–1.5 mg TID ER: Start 0.375 mg daily, can ↑ ~5-7 d to max dose of 4.5 mg/d A slow dose titration (no more than weekly) is required due to orthostasis, dizziness, sleepiness	**SIDE EFFECTS** Drowsiness, including sudden daytime sleep attacks Nausea, dizziness, orthostasis, vomiting, dry mouth, peripheral edema, constipation Hallucinations, dyskinesias, impulse control disorders **NOTES** Renal ↓ pramipexole dose if CrCl < 50 mL/min
Ropinirole *(Requip, Requip XL)* Restless leg syndrome, see above *IR* *1A2*	Start 0.25 mg TID, titrate weekly to 4-8 mg TID, max 24 mg/d XL: Start 2 mg daily, can ~1-2 weeks to max dose of 24 mg/d	Ropinirole: CYP 450 1A2 substrate; caution with 1A2 inhibitors due to increased drug levels. Bromocriptine *(Parlodel)* – no longer used for PD due to serious pulmonary complications; used as *Cycloset* for type 2 diabetes. *P.472*
Rotigotine *(Neupro)* Patch formulation Like the other dopamine agonists, approved for both PD and restless leg syndrome RLS: 1 mg/24 hours, can increase by 1 mg weekly *Press in place x 30 sec ↳ like Transderm Scop®*	Patch: 1, 2, 3, 4, 6 or 8 mg/24 hours *↑ sweating remove before MRI/cardioversion*	**SIDE EFFECTS** Peripheral edema, drowsiness, headache, fatigue, orthostasis, sleep disturbance (trouble initiating/maintaining sleep), hallucinations, application site (skin) reactions, hyperhidrosis, nausea, dyskinesias, arthralgias. **NOTES** Apply once daily, same time each day Do not apply to same site for at least 14 days *14 days like rivastigmine (Exelon®)* Do not apply heat source over patch Remove patch in MRI, avoid if sensitivity/allergy to sulfites

Dopamine Replacement Agents & Agonists Continued

DRUG	DOSING	SAFETY/SIDE EFFECTS/MONITORING

DA-agonist injection for advanced disease; a "rescue" movement agent; FOR "OFF" PERIODS

Apomorphine *(Apokyn)* Lasts 45-90 minutes For hypomobility in advanced disease – SC injection restores temporary movement Used by patients for "off" periods; can be injected up to 5x/day. Taken in addition to other PD medications.	SC injection Start at 0.2 mL (this is 2 mg, but do not write in mg) and can increase to a maximum recommended dose of 0.6 mL (6 mg). CAUTION, this drug is dosed in milliliters, not milligrams.	**CONTRAINDICATIONS** Do not use with 5HT$_3$-antagonists (ondansetron, others), due to severe hypotension and loss of consciousness **SIDE EFFECTS** *dizziness, orthostasis* Severe nausea and vomiting, hypotension; monitor BP Supine and standing blood pressure should be checked pre-dose and at 20, 40, and 60 minutes post dose Trimethobenzamide *(Tigan)* 300 mg PO TID or a similar antiemetic should be started 3 days prior to the initial dose of apomorphine and continued at least during the first two months of therapy. This is used to manage the severe nausea and vomiting due to apomorphine use. Yawning, dyskinesias, somnolence, dizziness, QT-prolongation

Handwritten margin note: ↑ 5HT$_3$ outing (→) ↑↑↑ bp, loss of consciousness)

Carbidopa/Levodopa *(Sinemet)* Drug Interactions

- Contraindicated with non-selective MAO inhibitors (2 week separation).

- Do not use with dopamine blockers – which will worsen Parkinson disease symptoms (see front section) – this includes phenothiazines, metoclopramide, etc.

- Iron can ↓ absorption.

- Protein-rich foods can ↓ absorption.

Carbidopa/Levodopa *(Sinemet)* Counseling

- Do not stop taking this medicine suddenly. It may take several weeks before you feel the full effects of this medicine. Stopping suddenly could make your condition much worse.

- Do not crush or chew any controlled-release forms of carbidopa and levodopa *(Sinemet CR)*. They are specially formulated to release slowly into your system. If necessary, the tablets can be split in half where they are scored, then swallowed without crushing or chewing.

- Use caution when driving, operating machinery, or performing other hazardous activities. Carbidopa and levodopa may cause dizziness or drowsiness. If you experience dizziness or drowsiness, avoid these activities.

- Call your doctor right away if you have uncontrollable movements of the mouth, tongue, cheeks, jaw, arms, or legs. Contact your doctor if you experience fever or if your body feels very hot.

- Do not take carbidopa and levodopa if you are taking or have taken a monoamine oxidase inhibitor (MAOI) such as isocarboxazid *(Marplan)*, phenelzine *(Nardil)*, or tranylcypromine *(Parnate)* in the past 14 days.

- You may have unusual sexual urges – if this develops, discuss with your doctor.

- This drug may cause the urine to become darker, even dark brown, and can stain clothing.

- Iron can decrease the amount of medicine that gets into your body; if you take iron pills they should be taken at a different time.

- Foods high in protein may reduce the amount of drug that gets into your body (however, protein intake is important and usually not reduced).

- For males, in the very unlikely event you have a painful or prolonged erection (lasting more than 4 hours), stop using this drug and seek immediate medical attention or permanent problems could result.

- The *Parcopa RapiTab* disintegrating tablet contains phenylalanine. If you have phenylketonuria, you should not use this medicine.

Ropinirole & Pramipexole *(Requip & Mirapex)* Counseling

- This medicine can be taken with or without food. Taking it with food is helpful if the medicine causes nausea.

- Nausea and sleepiness are the most common side effects. If your ankles get swollen, let the doctor know.

- This medicine may cause you to fall asleep while you are doing daily activities such as driving, talking with other people, watching TV, or eating. If you experience increased drowsiness or dizziness, or episodes of falling asleep while performing daily activities, do not drive or participate in potentially dangerous activities and contact your doctor.

- This drug can cause dizziness, which may be more likely to occur when you rise from a sitting or lying position. Rise slowly and use caution to prevent a fall.

- Alcohol, sleeping pills, antihistamines, antidepressants, pain medicine and other medicines that cause drowsiness can make the drowsiness worse, which could be dangerous. Do not use alcohol.

- Hallucinations may occur, and may be more common in elderly patients. Please tell your doctor if you experience thoughts which seem like they are paranoid, or excessive worry, or hearing voices. There is medicine that may help, or the dose may need to be changed.

- It is likely that the doctor will increase the dose slowly, over time. This is normal since the dose has to start low due to dizziness and sleepiness.

Rotigotine *(Neupro)* Patch Counseling

- Side effects from the patch can include ankle swelling, headache, fatigue, nausea, changes in blood pressure, difficulty getting a good night's sleep, and unusual thoughts. If any of these occur and are troublesome, discuss with your doctor.

- This medicine can cause you to become very sleepy. Do not drive a car or operate dangerous machinery until you are sure this can be done safely.

- If you have any unusual body movements, please contact your doctor.

- You may find that you sweat more than usual. It is important to drink enough fluids and avoid direct sunlight.

- The patch contains aluminum, which can burn your skin if you have certain medical procedures. The patch must be removed prior to magnetic resonance imaging (MRI) or "cardioversion."

- The patch can irritate the skin. It is important to rotate the patch site.

- Do not expose the patch to heat sources, such as heating pads.

- To apply the patch:
  - Choose the time of day that works best for you so it is easiest to remember.
  - Wear the patch for 24 hours. Remove before applying the next patch.
  - Do not apply to hairy skin, or skin that has cuts. Do not use moisturizer before applying the patch or it will not stick well.
  - After peeling off one side of the backing, apply to dry skin on the stomach, thigh, hip, side of the body, shoulder or upper arm. PRESS in place for 30 seconds. *like Transderm Scop®*
  - Do not cut the patch. If the patch falls off, you can reapply with bandage tape.
  - The patch can irritate the skin. Report to the doctor if you get a rash, swelling or itching that persists. Rotate the place where you place the patch. Wait at least 14 days before applying in the same location.

Apomorphine (Apokyn) Counseling

- Do not take with any of these drugs: ondansetron, dolasetron, granisetron, palonosetron, and alosetron or any drug of the 5HT₃ antagonist class or group if using apomorphine.

- This drug causes severe nausea, and vomiting. A drug called trimethobenzamide (Tigan), started before using this medicine and during treatment, will help reduce nausea.

- Other possible side effects include yawning, a runny nose, and swelling of your hands, arms, legs, and feet.

- Do not drink alcohol or take any medicines that make you sleepy while you are using this medicine.

- Do not drive a car, operate machinery, or do anything that might put you or others at risk of getting hurt until you know how the medicine affects you.

- This medicine can cause dizziness or fainting. Do not change your body position too fast. Get up slowly from sitting or lying.

- Choose an injection site on your stomach area, upper arm, or upper leg. Change your injection site each time the medicine is used. This will lower your chances of having a skin reaction at the site where you inject.

- This medicine is given by subcutaneous (SC) injection. Never inject into a vein.

Additional Parkinson Disease Medications

DRUG	DOSING	SAFETY/SIDE EFFECTS/MONITORING
Amantadine: blocks dopamine reuptake into presynaptic neurons, increases dopamine release from presynaptic fibers; Used for mild disease, or for dyskinesias in advanced disease *for early sx (tremor-predominant dz)*		
Amantadine (Symmetrel)	100 mg BID-TID ↓ dose in renal impairment	**SIDE EFFECTS** Dizziness (lightheadedness) and insomnia, abnormal dreams, hallucinations Toxic delirium (with renal impairment, ↓ dose) Cutaneous reaction called *livedo reticularis* (reddish skin mottling – requires drug discontinuation)

also approved for tx/ prevention of influenza A

NMDA receptor antagonist

DRUG	DOSING	SAFETY/SIDE EFFECTS/MONITORING
Selective MAO-B Inhibitors: used as adjunctive therapy with levodopa or as monotherapy (rasagiline has this indication)		
Selegiline (Eldepryl) Emsam – patch for depression May need to reduce levodopa dose when beginning therapy w/selective MAO-B Inhibitor--watch for side effects	5 mg BID, with breakfast & lunch Selegiline can be activating; do not dose at bedtime. If dosed twice, take 2nd dose at mid-day. Selegiline only has benefit when used with levodopa	**CONTRAINDICATIONS** *Flexeril®* Concomitant use of cyclobenzaprine, dextromethorphan, methadone, propoxyphene, St John's wort, or tramadol; concomitant use of meperidine or an MAO inhibitor. **SIDE EFFECTS** Due to DA-excess, similar to levodopa Rasagiline, when taken as monotherapy, can cause headache, joint pain and indigestion. If taken with levodopa, any of the side effects from dopamine excess are possible.
Selegiline (Zelapar ODT)	1.25-2.5 mg daily	**NOTES** Selegiline is metabolized by several CYP450 enzymes to amphetamine metabolites. *Zelapar* ODT has greater liver bypass, with ↓ formation of amphetamine metabolites. Rasagiline is metabolized by CYP1A2 and has no amphetamine metabolites.
Rasagiline (Azilect)	0.5-1 mg daily Can be used as initial monotherapy or adjunctive with levodopa.	

amphetamine metabolites

↓ amph metab

∅ amph. metab

RASAGILINE !! *→ coma/ death*

* tyramine

* selegiline – MAO-B selective @ ↓ doses BUT nonselective @ ↑ doses

Additional Parkinson Disease Medications Continued

DRUG	DOSING	SAFETY/SIDE EFFECTS/MONITORING

Centrally-Acting Anticholinergics: used primarily for tremor in younger patients

Benztropine *(Cogentin)*	0.5-2 mg TID (start QHS)	Used primarily for tremor; avoid use in elderly
Trihexyphenidyl	1-5 mg TID (start 1 mg QHS)	**SIDE EFFECTS** Dry mouth, constipation, urinary retention, blurred vision Drowsiness, confusion, tachycardia, high incidence peripheral and central anticholinergic side effects

[handwritten: 2 indications: ① adjunct for PD ② EPS prevention]

Alpha/Beta Agonist: used for neurogenic orthostatic hypotension

Droxidopa *(Northera)* *[handwritten: α/β agonist]*	Start at 100 mg TID, can titrate Q 24-48 hour to max 1800 mg/day Take with or without food, with last dose at least 3 hours prior to bedtime (to avoid supine hypertension during sleep)	**BOXED WARNING** Supine hypertension: monitor supine BP prior to and during treatment and more frequently when titrating. To reduce risk, elevate the head of the bed and measure BP in this position. If supine hypertension cannot be managed by elevation of the head of the bed, reduce or discontinue droxidopa **SIDE EFFECTS** Syncope, falls, headache, UTI **NOTES** Take capsule whole; do not open. Sound-alike drug name (levodopa, carbidopa, *Droxia*).

MAO-B Inhibitor Drug Interactions

- Rasagiline is risky in combination with drugs (above) and tyramine-rich foods, while selegiline has interactions with mostly drugs – this is dose dependent, keep doses at MAO-B selective levels or drugs become non-selective and the risk is higher.

- 5HT Interactions: Do not use with meperidine (can be fatal), tramadol, methadone, propoxyphene, dextromethorphan, St. John's wort, mirtazapine, cyclobenzaprine, other agents with 5HT risk. *[handwritten: ↳ ↑NE (α₂ blockade)]*

- Tyramine Interactions: Low risk, but possible, of hypertensive crisis if used with tyramine rich foods – see Drug Interactions and Depression chapters.

PRACTICE CASE

Patient Profile

Patient Name Benjamin Chen
Address 6401 Wisteria Drive
Age 70
Sex Male
Race Asian
Height 5'11"
Weight 185 lbs
Allergies none

DIAGNOSES

Sleepiness
Diziness

MEDICATIONS

Date	No.	Prescriber	Drug and Strength	Quantity	Sig
8/30	76525	Hayes	Carbidopa/Levodopa 25/250 mg	#30	TID
8/30	76526	Hayes	Ropinirole 1 mg	#30	TID (not using, per patient)
8/30	67527	Hayes	Ramipril 10 mg daily	#30	one capsule BID
8/30	76528	Hayes	Amlodipine 10 mg	#30	daily
8/30	76549	Hayes	Multivitamin	#30	daily

(handwritten note near Carbidopa/Levodopa: "need 70-100 mg per day")

LAB/DIAGNOSTIC TESTS

Test	Reference Value	Results 9/15
Ca (mg/dL)	8.5 - 10.5	8.8
Cl (mEq/L)	95 - 103	99
Mg (mEq/L)	1.3 - 2.1	1.4
K (mEq/L)	3.5-5	4.1
P04 (mg/dL)	2.3 - 4.7	4.2
Na (mEq/L)	135 - 145	140
HC03 (mEq/L)	24 - 30	27
BUN (mg/dL)	7 - 20	16
SCr (mg/dL)	0.6 - 1.3	0.9
WBC (mm3)	4,000 - 11,000	5.3
RBC (106/-L)	4.5 - 5.5 male, 4 - 4.9 female	4.8
Hgb (g/dL)	13.5 - 18 male, 12 - 16 female	12.2
Hct (%)	38 - 50 male, 36 - 46 female	36
MCV (mm3)	80 - 96	82
MCHC (g/dL)	31 - 37	33
RDW (%)	11.5 - 14.5	12.1
BP		108/64
Temp		98.6oF
HR		84 BPM

01/11/2015 (today): Patient here for a follow-up due to worsening clinical state. Sinemet use x 3 years, he states it "worked fine" but is now "nearly useless." States he is choking swallowing his food and cannot move well.

Questions

1. Choose the correct statement concerning the patient's carbidopa/levodopa therapy:

   a. The dose of carbidopa is too low.

   b. The dose of carbidopa is too high.

   c. The medication may make his urine turn brown.

   d. The medication will worsen his hypertension.

   e. The medication can cause severe rash.

2. When Benjamin started ropinirole, he found he could not tolerate the medicine due to excessive sleepiness. Choose the correct statement:

   a. The starting dose of ropinirole was too high.

   b. Pramipexole would be less sedating.

   c. The brand name of ropinirole is *Mirapex*.

   d. He should have been started on benztropine instead. *antiACh → younger*

   e. He should have been counseled to increase his caffeine intake during therapy initiation.

3. Choose the correct titration schedule for ropinirole or pramipexole:

   a. Wait at least 2 days before increasing the dose.

   b. Wait at least one week before increasing the dose.

   c. Wait at least two weeks before increasing the dose.

   d. Wait at least three weeks before increasing the dose.

   e. Wait at least four weeks before increasing the dose.

4. Benjamin is using levodopa therapy. He is taking carbidopa concurrently, in the combination medicine *Sinemet*. Choose the correct statements concerning Sinemet. (Select **ALL** that apply.)

   a. Carbidopa inhibits decarboxylase and prevents the breakdown of levodopa outside the CNS.

   b. The dose of carbidopa should stay between 30-50 mg. *70 - 100 mg*

   c. Using carbidopa with levodopa will decrease nausea.

   d. A typical starting dose of *Sinemet* is 25/250 mg TID.

   e. *Sinemet* is preferred for initial treatment in younger patients with tremor as the only presenting symptom.

5. Which of the following is a common side effect from ropinirole therapy?

   a. Brown urine

   b. Extreme hunger

   c. Somnolence

   d. Loss of consciousness

   e. Hyperglycemia

Questions 6-11 do not apply to the case.

6. A patient has been started on selegiline therapy. What is the mechanism of action of selegiline?

   a. Selective inhibitor of monoamine oxidase A

   b. Selective inhibitor of monoamine oxidase B

   c. Dopamine reuptake inhibitor

   d. Dopamine agonist

   e. Anticholinergic

7. Which of the following medications will require a dose reduction with renal impairment?

   a. Rasagiline

   b. Pramipexole *Mirapex®*

   c. Benztropine

   d. Levodopa

   e. *Stalevo*

8. Choose the drug which can be safely administered to a patient receiving *Azilect* therapy:

   a. Tramadol

   b. Meperidine

   c. Dextromethorphan

   d. Methadone

   e. Polyethylene glycol

9.   Which of the following side effects can be expected with the use of *Cogentin?*

   a. Dyskinetic movements
   b. Unusual sexual urges
   c. Confusion
   d. Tremor
   e. Insomnia, difficulty sleeping

10.   A patient is having a difficult time swallowing pills. Which of the following medications would be the best option for this type of patient?

   a. Comtan
   b. Cogentin
   c. Azilect
   d. Zelapar ODT
   e. Symmetrel

11.   Which of the following medications can worsen or cause Parkinson-like symptoms? (Select **ALL** that apply.)

   a. Metoclopramide, especially in a patient with renal insufficiency
   b. Risperdal, especially when dosed high (> 6 mg daily)
   c. Clozapine
   d. Symmetrel
   e. Haloperidol

Answers

1-c, 2-a, 3-b, 4-a,c, 5-c, 6-b, 7-b, 8-e, 9-c, 10-d, 11-a,b,e

ALZHEIMER'S DISEASE

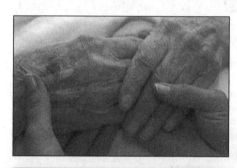

We gratefully acknowledge the assistance of George DeMaagd, PharmD, BCPS, Associate Dean of Academic Administration, Professor of Pharmacy, Union University School of Pharmacy, in preparing this chapter.

BACKGROUND

Dementia is a group of symptoms affecting intellectual and social abilities severely enough to interfere with daily functioning. There are several types of dementia and Alzheimer's disease is the most common type and the type with well-defined treatment. Unfortunately, the treatments provide modest benefit.

Diagnosis

Initial screening should attempt to rule out causes of memory impairment which could be reversible, such as vitamin B12 deficiency, depression and infection. In some patients, analgesics and benzodiazepines can cause memory loss. Mild memory loss could be age-related. Exams used to identify or screen for dementia include the Folstein Mini-Mental State Exam (MMSE, score <24 indicates memory disorder), DSM V criteria, National Institute of Neurological and Communicative Disorders and Stroke and the Alzheimer's Disease and Related Diseases Association (NINCDS-ARDA) criteria. The prescriber uses various tests to diagnose dementia. Studies continue to evaluate markers and tests that may help identify the disease at earlier stages. A definitive diagnosis of the actual cause and type of the dementia cannot be made unless an autopsy is conducted post-mortem. If the diagnosis is a dementia that will progressively worsen over time, such as Alzheimer's disease, early diagnosis gives a person time to plan for the future while he or she can still participate in making decisions.

GUIDELINES

American Geriatrics Society. Guide to the management of psychotic disorders and neuropsychiatric symptoms of dementia in older adults. April 2011. http://dementia.americangeriatrics.org/AGSGeriPsychConsult.pdf (accessed 17 Oct 2014).

Qaseem, A, Snow, V, Cross JT Jr et al. Current pharmacologic treatment of dementia: a clinical practice guideline from the American College of Physicians and the American Academy of Family Physicians. Ann Intern Med. 2008;148(5):370-8.

NATURAL PRODUCTS USED FOR DEMENTIA

Vitamin E is sometimes tried for dementia, but doses (> 150 IU) carry risk. *Ginkgo biloba* is commonly used for memory; a well-designed, 8-year study completed in 2008 did not find benefit for prevention of dementia with the use of ginkgo, but many patients still use it, and in some earlier studies the use of ginkgo provided modest benefit – for both dementia and in slowing age-related memory decline. At this point, the benefit is not well-defined. *Ginkgo* can increase bleeding risk. But remember, there is not much available to treat this disease and the patient and family may want "something" to help. Huperzine A (derived from chinese club moss) is being used for dementia with promising efficacy. The adverse effects are similar to acetylcholinesterase inhibitors, and are mostly gastrointestinal, such as nausea. Other natural products such as A-phosphatidylserine and acetyl-L-carnitine may be helpful. Recent data suggests older adults with low serum vitamin D levels have an increased risk of developing Alzheimer's disease. If vitamin D is low, it should be supplemented.

NON-DRUG TREATMENT

In all age groups, physical activity enhances the growth and survival of brain cells. Studies have shown increased brain volume in regions important for memory, learning, concentration and planning in individuals with higher levels of physical activity. The vascular health of the blood vessels in the brain is vital for cognitive function. Healthy blood glucose, blood pressure and cholesterol values will reduce the risk of systemic atherosclerosis and preserve brain function. To help stave off cognitive deterioration in older adults, games and "thinking" activities can provide benefit in slowing decline.

DRUG TREATMENT

Acetylcholinesterase inhibitors, such as donepezil, are the mainstay of therapy. These are used alone, or with memantine for more advanced disease. At best, one in twelve patients has improvement with these medications. However, for a family, this may mean that the patient who responds can feed themselves for a little while longer, or use the bathroom independently for several more months. Many others do not have noticeable improvement and likely experience side effects (nausea, diarrhea, dizziness). A key clinical pearl with the acetylcho-

---

SYMPTOMS

Memory loss

Difficulty communicating

Inability to learn or remember new information

Difficulty with planning and organizing

Poor coordination & motor functions

Personality changes

Inappropriate behavior

Paranoia, agitation, hallucinations

Pathophysiology
Neuritic plaques & tangles in brain tissue; neuron signaling is interrupted

Alteration of neurotransmitters (e.g., decreased acetylcholine)

DRUGS THAT CAN WORSEN DEMENTIA

Peripheral anticholinergics (including incontinence & IBS drugs)

Central anticholinergics (benztropine, etc.)

Antihistamines & antiemetics

Antipsychotics

Barbiturates

Benzodiazepines

Skeletal muscle relaxants

Other CNS depressants

linesterase inhibitors is that although patients may not improve clinically, they may have a slower clinical progression versus if they were not on therapy.

A higher dose of donepezil *(Aricept)* was released in 2010 for advanced disease, however the benefit is very mild (2-point improvement on a 100-point cognition scale). The motivation for the release of this product was the availability of generic donepezil. If a prescriber writes for the higher dose the patient will need to purchase the brand medication. With acetylcholinesterase inhibitors the patient should be monitored for both improvement and side effects; if no improvement or intolerable side effects the drug may be discontinued – this may also be advisable if the dementia has advanced to the point where it lacks clinical benefit. However, it may not be acceptable to the family and in some patients there will be noticeable deterioration when the medicine is discontinued. The timing of the dose should be considered: if nausea is present, evening administration can be helpful. Donepezil is administered QHS for this reason. If insomnia is a concern, the dose can be moved to the morning.

It has become more common to add memantine *(Namenda)* to an acetylcholinesterase inhibitor. It is approved for use alone or with donepezil.

Antidepressants (e.g., sertraline, citalopram, escitalopram) can be used to treat related depression and anxiety. Antipsychotics can be used to treat delusion/anger, but they increase the risk of death in elderly patients (see Boxed Warning in the Schizophrenia chapter) and provide little benefit.

ANTICHOLINERGICS & MEMORY IMPAIRMENT RISK

Anticholinergics are used to treat incontinence (e.g., oxybutinin), allergies or insomnia (e.g., diphenhydramine), dystonic reactions (e.g., benztropine, diphenhydramine), and a few other conditions. A drug with strong central anticholinergic effects (e.g., benztropine) can cause acute cognitive impairment and, occasionally, confusion and hallucinations. The effect depends on patient's baseline cognitive function, the sensitivity to the medication, the clearance, and the number of drugs and dosing used. In elderly patients, anticholinergics are commonly avoided due to these risks except for the use of anticholinergics used for overactive bladder (OAB). Incontinence is distressing to the patient, to the family, and can lead to nursing home placement; it is not a minor concern. It is difficult to treat adequately – and the cost of disposable diapers is beyond the reach of many families. If an OAB is added to a patient with baseline memory impairment, the following issues should be considered: does the patient have functional versus urge incontinence? Can scheduled toileting and pelvic floor muscle exercises help? Can the dose of the OAB drug be reduced? If used, the effectiveness should be evaluated and if no improvement in OAB symptoms at 6 weeks the drug should be discontinued.

benztropine (Cogentin®)

DRUGS TO TREAT ALZHEIMER'S DISEASE

DRUG	DOSING	SAFETY/SIDE EFFECTS/MONITORING
Acetylcholinesterase Inhibitors – Inhibits centrally-active acetylcholinesterase, the enzyme responsible for hydrolysis (breakdown) of acetylcholine, which results in ↑ ACh		
Donepezil (Aricept, Aricept ODT) Used alone or with memantine in more severe disease *Aricept 23 mg* used for advanced disease – minimal additional benefit	5-10 mg QHS for mild to moderate disease 23 mg QHS, for advanced disease, if stable on lower dose 1st x 3 mos Do not crush or chew	FOR MILD-MODERATE DISEASE (& IN COMBO FOR MODERATE-SEVERE AD) **SIDE EFFECTS** GI side effects (nausea, vomiting, loose stools) Donepezil given QHS to help tolerate nausea Bradycardia, fainting, insomnia, tremors, weight loss
Rivastigmine (Exelon, Exelon Patch)	1.5-6 mg BID 4.6, 9.5, 13.3 mg/24 hr patch < 6 mg PO daily = 4.6 mg patch 6-12 mg PO daily = 9.5 mg Can ↑ to 13.3 mg patch If 9.5 mg tolerated x 4 weeks	**NOTES** Other oral formulations are BID or daily if long-acting Rivastigmine and galantamine IR is with food (breakfast and dinner), galantamine ER with breakfast. Galantamine solution can be mixed with liquid and taken within 4 hours.
Galantamine (Razadyne, Razadyne ER)	IR: 4-12 mg BID 4mg/mL solution ER: start at 8 mg daily x 4 weeks, then ↑ to 16-24 mg	Recommend *Exelon* patch or *Aricept ODT* to decrease GI side effects – if the cost difference is acceptable *Exelon* patch: titrate Q 4 weeks, apply first patch the day after last oral dose *Razadyne* solution: can mix in 100 mL of non-alcohol liquid
Memantine – blocks NMDA (N-methyl-D-aspartate), which inhibits glutamate from binding to NMDA receptors & ↓ abnormal activation		
Memantine (Namenda, Namenda XR) Approved for use alone or in combination with donepezil (Aricept) for moderate to severe AD XR caps can be opened and sprinkled on applesauce	5-10 mg BID (start at 5 mg Q daily) XR: 7, 14 or 28 mg daily (start at 7 mg daily and titrate not faster than weekly) Can switch 10 mg BID to 28 mg daily; start daily; begin XR the next day (not same day) Oral Solution 2 mg/mL (10 mg = 5 mL)	FOR MODERATE-SEVERE DISEASE **SIDE EFFECTS** Dizziness, constipation, headache Rare SEs: flu-like symptoms, arthralgia, UTIs, urinary retention, small risk seizures, hypertension **NOTES** Mostly excreted unchanged in urine; do not exceed 5 mg BID or 14 mg XR daily if CrCl < 30 mL/min

Acetylcholinesterase Drug Interactions

- Use caution with concurrent use of drugs that can lower heart rate (beta blockers, diltiazem, verapamil, digoxin, etc.) and with drugs that cause dizziness (antipsychotics, antihypertensives, alpha blockers, skeletal muscle relaxants, hypnotics, opioids, etc.) due to the risk of dizziness and falls.

- Drugs that have anticholinergic effects can reduce efficacy (see previous table for drugs that can worsen symptoms). Discontinue incontinence drugs if there is no benefit.

Acetylcholinesterase Counseling

- These medicines can cause nausea and stomach upset. If this remains a problem, talk to your doctor about changing to the longer-acting formulations, or the *Exelon* patch, which has the least nausea. Taking the medicine with food should help.

- The dose of this medication may be increased, but is started low due to the risk of dizziness, falls, and nausea. Use caution when moving from a sitting to a standing position. Try not to use with other drugs that can lower your heart rate and make you feel dizzy. Try not to use alcohol when using this medicine.

- Please tell the pharmacist about all medicine you purchase over-the-counter since some of these can worsen memory problems.

- Please make sure the pharmacist knows about all prescription drugs you are using. Some of them can worsen memory problems.

- Donepezil is started at 5 mg, at bedtime. It is taken at night to help with nausea. If you experience sleep problems (insomnia), you can take it in the morning. If you have trouble swallowing the medicine, there is a formulation that dissolves in your mouth that can be used instead. Your doctor may increase the dose to 10 mg after about 4 weeks. In a small number of people even higher doses (to 23 mg daily) may be helpful.

- Rivastigmine is started at 1.5 mg twice daily, with food. Taking this medicine with food should help reduce nausea. Your doctor may increase the dose after about 4 weeks. The maximum dose is 6 mg, taken twice daily.

- Galantamine is started at 4 mg twice daily, with or without food. Your doctor may increase the dose after ~ 4 weeks. The maximum dose is 12 mg, taken twice daily.

Handwritten margin notes: 5mg qhs, max 10mg (23mg) qhs; 1.5mg BID w/ food, max 6mg BID; 4mg BID w/ food, max 12mg BID

Exelon patch application instructions

- Apply a new patch each day to the upper or lower back, upper arm, or chest; rotate applications site. Do not use the same site within 14 days. Do not apply to an area of the skin that is hairy, oily, irritated, broken, scarred, or calloused.

- Do not apply to an area where cream, lotion, or powder has recently been applied. Do not place the patch under tight clothing.

- Do not remove the patch from the sealed pouch until you are ready to apply it.

- Remove the protective liner from one side of the patch.

- Place the sticky side of the patch on the application site, then remove the second side of the protective liner.

- Press the patch down firmly until the edges stick well.

- After 24 hours, remove the used patch.

- Do not touch the sticky side. Fold the patch in half with the sticky sides together.

Handwritten margin notes: 14 days like rotigotine (Neupro); may leave patch on during MRI

Memantine Counseling (Caregivers)

- Take this medication by mouth, with or without food. When you first start taking this medication, you will usually take it once daily. Your dose will be gradually increased to avoid risk of side effects. Once your dose increases to more than 5 mg daily, take this medication twice daily (5 mg twice daily, and then it usually increases to 10 mg twice daily).

- If you are taking memantine oral liquid, read the instruction sheet that comes with the bottle. Follow the directions exactly. Use the oral syringe that comes with the product to measure out your dose. Swallow the medication directly from the syringe. Do not mix it with water or other liquids. Rinse the syringe with water after each use.

Handwritten: 469 648 5131 Sandra Parkland HR

- You may experience dizziness; use caution when moving from a sitting to a standing position. Try not to use with other drugs that can make you feel dizzy. Try not to use alcohol when using this medicine.

- If you become constipated from this medicine, please ask your pharmacist, who can recommend an over-the-counter stool softener (if the stool is hard) or a different type of laxative that is taken at bedtime. The laxatives come in chewable or liquid formulations.

Memantine Extended Release *(Namenda XR)*

Same as above except:

- If you have trouble swallowing can open capsule and sprinkle on applesauce (do not divide dose) but do not crush or chew the capsule.

- Start at 7 mg daily. Titrate weekly (as tolerated) to 28 mg daily.

ATTENTION DEFICIT HYPERACTIVITY DISORDER (ADHD)

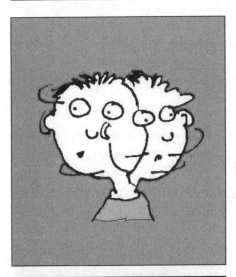

We gratefully acknowledge the assistance of Robin Wackernah, PharmD, BCPP, Regis University School of Pharmacy, Rueckert-Hartman College for Health Professions, in preparing this chapter.

BACKGROUND

The core symptoms of ADHD are <u>inattention, hyperactivity, and impulsivity</u>. People with ADHD often have difficulty focusing, are easily distracted, have trouble staying still, and frequently are unable to control impulsive behavior. Primary symptoms vary; some patients are more inattentive, and others are more impulsive.

The primary treatments for ADHD are <u>stimulant</u> medications, primarily methylphenidate formulations *(Concerta, Ritalin,* others) and lisdexamfetamine *(Vyvanse).* Stimulants raise dopamine and norepinephrine levels. In ADHD it is thought that there may be defects or alterations in the dopamine pathways, that regulate reward anticipation and emotional self regulation in the brains of persons with ADHD. Providing medications is challenging since, like other psychiatric conditions, ADHD is marked by a wide variation in treatment response and dosing range. The range in treatment response and dosing has led research into the hypothesis that genetic factors may underlie such differences. Due to the positive response from using methylphenidate, the primary focus of research is on the catecholamine system (dopamine is catalyzed to the two other primary catecholamines, epinephrine and norepinephrine.)

GUIDELINES

Diagnostic and Statistical Manual of Mental Disorders, Fifth Edition (DSM-5).

Dobie C, Donald WB, Hanson M, et al. Institute for Clinical Systems Improvement's Diagnosis and Management of Attention Deficit Hyperactivity Disorder in Primary Care for School-Age Children and Adolescents. https://www.icsi.org/_asset/60nzr5/ADHD-Interactive0312.pdf (accessed 05 Oct 2014).

ADHD: Clinical Practice Guideline for the Diagnosis, Evaluation, and Treatment of Attention-Deficit/Hyperactivity Disorder in Children and Adolescents. *Pediatric Peds.* 2011; 2011-2654.

Keep in mind that a focus on genetics alone is a mechanistic view; it is likely that <u>stressors</u> alter the brains pattern of catecholamine use in some patients, which leads to ADHD symptoms. In the popular book *Scattered* (Gabor Maté, MD), the author focuses on altering the environment to help control symptoms. Environment, as well as genetics, is a determinant in brain chemistry and alterations in the environment can change the chemistry. However, some require medications even with strong social support.

ADHD can cause an emotional response from those who feel stimulant drugs are over-used. Parents who rely on the drugs to help their children do better in school, and adults who use ADHD medications may be negatively viewed. As pharmacists, we should do our best to remain nonjudgmental and make sure that when medications are prescribed, they are used safely. <u>Stimulants are C-II</u>, which means the prescriptions can only be prescribed for one month at a time, which makes it convenient to check blood pressure and heart rate (and weight and height, periodically, in children). Many prescribers issue three months of prescriptions at a time, which are post-dated. Stimulants are a common drug of abuse and have a high street value; these should be dispensed with caution, and counseling must include instructions <u>not to share with others and to store in a safe place</u>. Occasionally the "ADHD" stimulants are used for other conditions, including narcolepsy and shift work sleep disorder; this condition is discussed in the Sleep Disorders chapter.

About 10% of school-aged children are using ADHD medications, with boys outnumbering girls. The guidelines have age-specific treatment recommendations for children ages 4-18 years. ADHD should be considered a chronic illness; up to 80% of children will continue to exhibit symptoms into adolescence and up to 65% of children will still exhibit symptoms into adulthood. Inattention and impulsivity often remain as the patient ages, and hyperactivity can be decreased.

DSM-5 DIAGNOSTIC CRITERIA

People with ADHD show a persistent pattern of inattention and/or hyperactivity-impulsivity that interferes with functioning or development. The DSM-5 requirements for an ADHD diagnosis:

<u>Inattention</u>: Six or more symptoms of inattention for children up to age 16, or five or more for ages 17 to adults; symptoms of inattention have been present for at least 6 months, and they are inappropriate for the developmental level:

- Fails to pay attention, has trouble holding attention, does not pay attention when someone is talking, does not follow through on instructions, fails to finish schoolwork, has difficulty organizing tasks, avoids or dislikes tasks which require mental effort, loses things, is easily distracted, and is forgetful.

<u>Hyperactivity and Impulsivity</u>: Six or more symptoms of hyperactivity-impulsivity for children up to age 16, or five or more for ages 17 to adults; symptoms of hyperactivity-impulsivity have been present for at least 6 months to an extent that is disruptive and inappropriate for the person's developmental level:

- Often fidgets or squirms, leaves seat unexpectedly, runs about when not appropriate, unable to play quietly, is "on the go" as if "driven by a motor", talks excessively, blurts out answers, has trouble waiting his/her turn, and interrupts or intrudes on others.

In addition, the following conditions must be met:

- Several inattentive or hyperactive-impulsive symptoms were present before age 12 years, symptoms must have been present in 2 or more settings (at home, school, at work, with friends or relatives), symptoms interfere with functioning, and symptoms are not caused by another psychiatric disorder.

NATURAL PRODUCTS

Fish oils are a natural product increasingly used for a variety of psychiatric conditions, including ADHD. Fish oil supplements (which provide omega-3 fatty acids) with or without evening primrose oil (which provides omega-6 fatty acids) may be helpful in some patients. Fish oils are rated as "possibly effective" to improve cognitive function and behavior in children with ADHD by the *Natural Medicines Database*. Check the dose prior to making a recommendation. The combo product used in the study that showed benefit used 6 capsules daily. Other products are occasionally used for ADHD, including SAMe, St. John's wort and ginkgo. If St. John's wort is used, check for drug interactions since this herbal induces CYP 450 enzymes and will lower the concentration of the majority of other drugs. It is serotonergic, and has phototoxicity risk.

DRUG TREATMENT

First-line drug therapy for ADHD are stimulants. When stimulants do not work well enough (after trials of 2-3 agents), atomoxetine (Strattera), a non-stimulant medication, can be tried next, or will be used first-line by prescribers who are concerned about the possibility of abuse by the patient or family.

The stimulant agent methylphenidate, which is available in various formulations, is tried first, or lisdexamfetamine (*Vyvanse*), the pro-drug of dextroamphetamine. Longer-acting formulations are preferred for children who would otherwise need dosing at school (which would require a nurse's office visit) and to help maintain more steady symptom control. Other stimulant classes can be tried.

Guanfacine (approved in the extended-release (ER) formulation *Intuniv*), and clonidine (in the ER formulation *Kapvay*) are used most often as adjunctive treatments. For example, it is common to see *Concerta* with *Intuniv*, or *Vyvanse* with *Kapvay*, or vice versa. The guanfacine or clonidine formulation is being added-on to the stimulant after the stimulant was tried and additional benefit was needed. *Intuniv* or *Kapvay* can also be used to help with sleep in the evening as they are sedating. They are also used alone. Diphenhydramine is used to help with sleep at night, however it is important to monitor for a paradoxical reaction in some children (e.g., hyperactive). Another option to help with sleep is immediate-release clonidine, taken at bedtime.

Family therapy/psychotherapy may be required for an improved prognosis. The drugs described in this section are used off-label to help with some of the symptoms of autism.

Stimulants for narcolepsy: modafinil (Provigil®) & MedGuide armodafinil (Nuvigil®) for severe rash; CIV; also for sleep apnea, shift work d/o

STIMULANTS FOR ADHD

CNS stimulants that block the reuptake of norepinephrine [NE] and dopamine [DA].

DRUG	DOSING	SAFETY/SIDE EFFECTS/MONITORING
Methylphenidate		
Methylphenidate IR (Ritalin, Methylin chewable, oral susp)	20-30 mg BID-TID, 30 min before meals	**BOXED WARNINGS**
All of the stimulants (including modafinil and armodafinil) and atomoxetine require a MedGuide. Clonidine ER (Kapvay) and guanfacine ER (Intuniv) do not.	All C-II Methylphenidate approved for 6+ yrs	Potential for drug dependency; use caution if a history of ethanol or drug abuse. Avoid abrupt discontinuation in patients who have been taking drug for prolonged period. *Adderall:* Misuse may cause sudden death and serious cardiovascular adverse events.
Methylphenidate long-acting (Ritalin LA) ½ IR, ½ SR in one capsule	10-40 mg LA caps OPEN	**CONTRAINDICATIONS** Marked anxiety, tension, and agitation, glaucoma, MAO inhibitor use within the past 14 days, family history or diagnosis of Tourette's syndrome or tics. *Metadate CD* and *Metadate ER* only: Severe hypertension, heart failure, arrhythmia, hyperthyroidism, recent MI or angina; concomitant use of halogenated anesthetics. *Ritalin* and *Ritalin SR* only: Pheochromocytoma.
Methylphenidate sustained release (Ritalin SR)	20 mg SR tabs	**SIDE EFFECTS** Nausea, loss of appetite, insomnia, dizziness, headache, lightheadedness, irritability, blurry vision, difficulty with visual accomodation, dry mouth ↑BP ~2-4 mmHg, ↑HR ~3-8 BPM, monitor and avoid use with known cardiac issues/defects
Methylphenidate ER (Methylin ER, Metadate ER, Quillivant XR – ER oral suspension; reconstitute at pharmacy)	10-20 mg ER tabs	Exacerbation of mixed/mania episodes if bipolar disorder, use caution with any pre-existing psychiatric condition, including depression, aggressive behavior, hostility Peripheral vasculopathy may worsen, including in Raynaud's Risk of seizures (caution with seizure history), priapism
Methylphenidate IR – ER (Concerta) OROS system (GI) Somewhat harder to abuse (harder to crush)	18, 27, 36, 54 mg ER tabs QAM, with or without food, swallow whole	**MONITORING** Consider ECG prior to treatment, monitor BP and HR during treatment (all). Monitor height and weight (children). Conduct cardiac evaluation if chest pain, unexplained syncope, or other cardiac symptoms develop.
Methylphenidate IR – ER (Metadate CD) Beads that dissolve at different rates	10-60 mg ER caps OPEN	Monitor CNS activity in all patients; signs of peripheral vasculopathy (e.g., digital changes), signs of misuse, abuse, or addiction.
Methylphenidate transdermal patch (Daytrana)	1.1 mg/hr (10 mg/9 hr)-3.3 mg/hr (30 mg/9 hr)	**NOTES** *Focalin XR, Ritalin LA, Metadate CD* and *Adderall XR* can be taken whole or the capsules sprinkled on applesauce (if not warm and used right away, do not chew). *Concerta* OROS delivery The capsule's outer coat dissolves fast to give immediate action, and the rest is released slowly. *Concerta, Metadate CD* and *Ritalin LA* are all QAM (IRs and some others are divided), and *Daytrana* patch is QAM, applied to alternate hip 2 hours before desired effect (or as soon as the child awakens so it starts to deliver prior to school). Remove after 9 hours (at night, so the patient can sleep). If overdosed, symptoms (anxiety, tachycardia) can be ↓ with a benzodiazepine. Titrate dose up (to ↓ nausea, headache, anxiety) and down (to ↓ any withdrawal symptoms).

Handwritten annotations:

stimulants used for narcolepsy require MedGuide for risk of severe rash

qAM (×3, next to Concerta, Metadate CD, Daytrana)

titrate!!

Mrs. Brickler!

* apply to alternate hip 2 hrs before desired effect
* remove after 9 hrs + observation

may need antiHTN ⇒ β-blockers (DOC)

w/ injection, may experience seizures, psychosis ⇒ may require tx

* Ritalin/SR ≠ pheochromocytoma
* Metadate CD/ER ≠ severe HTN, HF, arrhythmia, angina, recent MI, hyperthyroidism, concurrent use of halogenated anesthetics

Stimulants for ADHD Continued

DRUG	DOSING	SAFETY/SIDE EFFECTS/MONITORING

Dexmethylphenidate

Dexmethylphenidate IR *(Focalin)*	2.5-10 mg tabs BID, 4+ hrs apart, with or without food	see Methylphenidate
Dexmethylphenidate ER *(Focalin XR)*	5-20 mg caps OPEN 30 mg max/d children 6 years + 40 mg max/d adults	

Dextroamphetamine and amphetamine *(handwritten: all given qAM; IR may also be dosed BID)*

Dextroamphetamine/ Amphetamine IR *(Adderall)*	5-30 mg scored tabs Given QAM or BID without regard to meals. First dose on awakening, additional dose 4-6 h later.	see Methylphenidate **NOTES** Although FDA approved, American Academy of Pediatrics (2011) does not recommend use of dextroamphetamine in children ≤ 5 years due to insufficient evidence Patients should avoid use of acidic foods, juice or vitamin C as amphetamine levels may decrease when taken together
Dextroamphetamine/ Amphetamine ER *(Adderall XR)*	5-30 mg ER caps OPEN QAM, with or without food	
Dextroamphetamine IR *(Dexedrine, Zenzedi, ProCentra)*	5-10 mg tabs QAM or BID, with or without food.	
Dextroamphetamine SR and IR *(Dexedrine Spansules, ProCentra – solution)*	5, 10, 15 mg SR caps QAM, with or without food.	

Lisdexamfetamine (prodrug of dextroamphetamine)

Lisdexamfetamine *(Vyvanse)*	20, 30, 40, 50, 60, 70 mg caps Can mix capsule contents with water, yogurt or orange juice. Take right away. QAM, with or without food	see Methylphenidate *(handwritten: converted via 1st pass hepatic & intestinal metab)* **NOTES** Lisdexamfetamine is a prodrug composed of l-lysine (amino acid) bonded to dextroamphetamine (d-amphetamine). It is hydrolyzed in the blood to active d-amphetamine. If injected or snorted the fast effect would be muted. The design is to ↓ the abuse potential.

Handwritten left margin notes:
- *BBW misuse → sudden death, CV events*
- *qAM*
- *PRODRUG*
- *yogurt water orange juice*
- *put more water in same glass, drink again to get full dose*

Stimulant Drug Interactions

- 14-Day wash out period after MAO I use.

Patient Counseling for Stimulants

- Dispense MedGuide and instruct parents/patient to read it. Stimulants should not be used in patients with heart problems or serious psychiatric conditions. Report at once if the child has chest pain, shortness of breath, or fainting. Report at once if the child is seeing or hearing things that are not real, believing things that are not real, or are paranoid.

- The healthcare provider should check the child's blood pressure, heart rate, height and weight.

- Some children get nausea or headache when the dose is increased or can act "wired." This is why the dose is increased slowly at the beginning.

- This is a controlled medication and has potential to be abused. Do not share this medicine with anyone else and store in a safe place.

- Your child may not have much of an appetite. Children seem to be less hungry during the middle of the day, but they are often hungry by dinnertime as the medication wears off. Your child should eat a healthy breakfast. Pack healthy snacks for school, such as nuts, cheese and fruit.

- Certain food colorings and preservatives that are common in "junk" foods and candies can worsen hyperactive behavior in some children. If these foods affect your child, you can limit them.

- If the child has trouble sleeping, the formulation may be changed. Or, the prescriber may recommend OTC diphenhydramine or prescription clonidine to take before bedtime.

- Less commonly, a few children develop sudden, repetitive movements or sounds called tics. Changing the medication dosage may make tics go away. Some children also may appear to have a personality change, such as appearing "flat" or without emotion. Talk with your child's healthcare provider if you see any of these side effects.

- If your child develops an erection lasting longer than 4 hours he will need to get immediate medical help to prevent long-term problems with the penis.

- If using a capsule formulation that can be mixed with applesauce *(Focalin XR, Ritalin LA, Metadate CD* and *Adderall XR)* and your child has difficulty swallowing the capsules, they can be sprinkled on a small amount of applesauce (if not warm and used right away). Do not chew the applesauce; just swallow. A small amount only so it is not chewed.

- If the child is using the medicine *Vyvanse*, the capsule contents can be mixed in water, yogurt or orange juice. Take right away. It must be taken right after putting into the water.

- *Daytrana* Patch Instructions

- Each morning put a new patch on the hip and alternate the side each day (left hip odd days, right hip even days). Do not apply where the waist of the pants could rub it off. Apply 2 hours before effect is needed.

- Hold patch on skin for 30 seconds and smooth down edges. It should stay on during swimming or bathing. Remove the patch after 9 hours so your child can sleep well at night.

- Wash your hands immediately after applying the patch. Patches should not be reapplied with bandages, tape, or other household adhesives. Do not use hair dryers, heating pads, electric blankets, or other heat sources directly on the patch. If you have to replace a patch that has fallen off, the total wear-time for the first and second patch should not be more than a total of 9 hours in 1 day. Do not reapply the same patch that fell off.

- When peeling off to discard, fold in half, put down the toilet or lidded trash can.

Quillivant XR Suspension Instructions

- The bottle must contain liquid. Return to the pharmacist if it is powder.

- First, shake the bottle for at least 10 seconds. Use the dosing dispenser to measure the milliliters (mL) dose.

- Insert the tip of the dispenser into the upright bottle and push the plunger all the way down. Turn the bottle upside down and remove the correct amount; measure to the white end of the plunger.

- Use the dosing dispenser to slowly squirt the medication into the child's mouth. Cap tightly and rinse the dispenser with tap water or in a dishwasher.

- The medicine can be stored at room temperature for up to 4 months.

NON-STIMULANTS FOR ADHD – 2ND LINE AGENTS – NOT CONTROLLED

DRUG	DOSING	SAFETY/SIDE EFFECTS/MONITORING

Selective Norepinephrine Reuptake Inhibitor

[handwritten margin note: selective NRI]

[handwritten margin note: 2D6]

Atomoxetine (*Strattera*)	40-100 mg/day, max 80 mg/day with CYP 2D6 inhibitors or if poor 2D6 metabolizer Take daily, or can divide BID	**BOXED WARNING** Risk of suicidal ideation; monitor for suicidal thinking or behavior, worsening, or unusual behavior. **CONTRAINDICATIONS** Glaucoma, pheochromocytoma, MAO I use within past 14 days. **WARNINGS** Aggressive behavior, treatment-emergent psychotic or manic symptoms, orthostasis and syncope, priapism. Rare, but severe hepatotoxicity (most within 120 days of start of treatment). Risk of serious cardiovascular events; avoid use if known problems; conduct cardiac evaluation if needed. Use with caution if BP elevated. **SIDE EFFECTS** Headache, insomnia, somnolence, dry mouth, nausea, abdominal pain, ↓ appetite, nausea, hyperhidrosis, fatigue, dizziness, hot flashes, dysmenorrhea, ↓ libido, menstrual changes Orthostasis; use caution in patients at risk. Psychiatric effects, including hallucinations and mania, discontinue if symptoms. Urinary retention in patients with history or with outlet obstruction. Priapism (more common than with methylphenidate). **NOTES** Do not open capsule – irritant Evaluate for CVD risk (HR, BP, consider ECG) prior to initiation. Primarily a CYP450 2D6 substrate; 2D6 inducers or inhibitors may necessitate a change in atomoxetine dose.

[handwritten margin note: ⊖ open capsule (irritant) hepatotox]

Central Alpha2A Adrenergic Receptor Agonist

These agents stimulate alpha-2 adrenergic receptors in the brain. Both are (old) hypertension drugs and are more recently used in longer-acting formulations for ADHD.

GuanFACINE ER (*Intuniv*) For patients using stimulants for additional benefit, or alone *Tenex* – for hypertension	1-4 mg, max 4 mg/day Start at 1 mg daily Do not take with high-fat meal (↑ absorption) With CYP 3A4 inducers, max dose 8 mg/day With CYP 3A4 inhibitors, max dose 2 mg/day	**SIDE EFFECTS** Somnolence, dizziness, headache, fatigue, hypotension, nausea, constipation, abdominal pain, skin rash (rare, discontinue if occurs), bradycardia **NOTES** All cardiovascular effects (bradycardia, hypotension, orthostasis, syncope) are dose-dependent; titrate carefully. Sedation can cause risk with physical and mental activities. Cases of skin rash with exfoliation; discontinue if rash develops. Do not interchange with other guanfacine formulations. Do not crush.

Non-Stimulants for ADHD – 2nd Line Agents – Not Controlled Continued

DRUG	DOSING	SAFETY/SIDE EFFECTS/MONITORING
CloNIDine ER *(Kapvay)* For patients using stimulants for additional benefit, or alone *Catapres* – for hypertension	0.1-0.4 mg/day Start at 0.1 mg at bedtime, ↑ 0.1 mg/day Q 7 days until desired response Dose BID, if uneven give higher dose QHS Start 0.1 mg QHS, titrate weekly, using BID dosing	**SIDE EFFECTS** Headache, somnolence, abdominal pain, upper resp tract infections **NOTES** Rebound hypertension (with sweating/anxiety/tremors), if stopped abruptly – taper off by ↓ 0.1 mg Q 3-7 days. ER formulation has ↓ SEs. Do not crush.

Atomoxetine Drug Interactions

- Decrease dose if on strong CYP 2D6 inhibitors (e.g., paroxetine, fluoxetine, bupropion, quinidine) or if 2D6 poor metabolizer, up to max 80 mg/day.

- 14-Day wash out period after MAO I use.

Patient Counseling for Atomoxetine

- Dispense MedGuide and instruct parents/patient to read it. The MedGuide includes a warning for risk of suicidal ideation in children and risk of liver injury.

- Common side effects can include headache, insomnia, somnolence, dry mouth, nausea, stomach pain, lessened appetite, nausea, sweating, dizziness and fatigue. Girls and women can get hot flashes, dysmenorrhea, ↓ sexual interest or menstrual changes.

- You may have suicidal thoughts or behavior while taking atomoxetine. Watch for symptoms of depression, unusual behavior, or thoughts of hurting yourself. Your healthcare provider may need to check you at regular visits while you are taking this medication.

- The capsule cannot be opened. Do not use an open or broken capsule. If the medicine from inside the capsule gets into your eyes, rinse thoroughly with water and call your healthcare provider.

- Atomoxetine can cause side effects that may impair your thinking or reactions. Be careful if you drive or do anything that requires you to be awake and alert.

- Monitor for symptoms of liver damage: weakness, abdominal pain, yellowed skin, light colored stool or darkened urine.

Clonidine and Guanfacine Drug Interactions

- Both clonidine and guanfacine are sedating; use caution with other CNS depressants.

- Both clonidine and guanfacine lower blood pressure; use caution with other anti-hypertensives.

- Both clonidine and guanfacine come as other formulations; do not use concurrently.

- Guanfacine is a CYP 3A4 substrate; see dosing in table for use with inducers or inhibitors.

ANXIETY DISORDERS

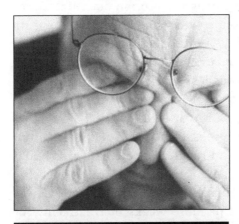

We gratefully acknowledge the assistance of Robin Wackernah, PharmD, BCPP, Regis University School of Pharmacy, Rueckert-Hartman College for Health Professions, in preparing this chapter.

BACKGROUND

Anxiety exists to protect us from harm. For example, if an aggressive dog or bear comes along, fear (a symptom of anxiety) is important to avoid getting attacked and can help us escape from the situation. Normal, occasional anxiety can occur in the general population when faced with challenging issues at work, home or school. The symptoms of <u>occasional</u> anxiety (fear, worry) should dissipate once the issue is gone. Any physical symptoms (tachycardia, palpitations, shortness of breath, stomach upset, chest pain or other pain, insomnia and fatigue) should also resolve.

GUIDELINES

Diagnostic and Statistical Manual of Mental Disorders, Fifth Edition (DSM-5)

Baldwin DS, Waldman S, Allgulander C. "Evidence-based pharmacological treatment of generalized anxiety disorder (DSM-IV-TR)." *Int J Neuropsychopharmacol.* 2011 Jun;14(5):697-710.

When a person has an anxiety <u>disorder</u>, the symptoms are <u>continuous and severe</u> and cause great distress. The disorder can interfere with the ability to do well at school or work, and can harm relationships. The major types of anxiety disorders are generalized anxiety disorder (GAD), panic disorder (PD) and social anxiety disorder (SAD). Disorders that have symptoms of anxiety include obsessive compulsive disorder (OCD) and posttraumatic stress disorder (PTSD). Although OCD and PTSD have symptoms of anxiety, the Diagnostic and Statistical Manual of Mental Disorders, Fifth Edition (DSM-5) classifies these disorders differently. OCD has its own category called "obsessive-compulsive and related disorders" and PTSD is categorized under "trauma-and stressor- related disorders."

Lifestyle changes can improve symptoms. Increasing physical activity, talk therapy (with friends or a trained therapist), helping others, community involvement) yoga, meditation,

ANTIDEPRESSANTS WITH ANXIETY INDICATION

Escitalopram – GAD

Fluoxetine – OCD, PD

Fluvoxamine – OCD

Paroxetine – GAD, OCD, SAD, PD, PTSD

Sertraline – OCD, PD, PTSD

Duloxetine – GAD

Venlafaxine – GAD, PD

Doxepin – Anxiety

Clomipramine – OCD

COMMON MEDICATIONS THAT CAN WORSEN ANXIETY

Theophylline

Levothyroxine

Acetazolamide

Albuterol (if used incorrectly-swallowed)

Aripiprazole, haloperidol

Caffeine, in high doses

Stimulants

Decongestants (pseudoephedrine and nasally inhaled agents)

Steroids

Bupropion

Fluoxetine, paroxetine

Illicit drugs, including cocaine, LSD, methamphetamine, others

and other methods can broaden the patient's outlook and reduce stress. Currently, financial stress and uncertainty about the future is causing considerable stress and anxiety in many people.

The primary agents used to treat anxiety disorders are selective serotonin reuptake inhibitors (SSRIs) and Serotonin norepinephrine reuptake inhibitors (SNRIs). Although only some of the antidepressants (ADs) have specific indications (see chart), these agents are often chosen based on the healthcare provider's familiarity and/or the side effect profile. For example, although fluvoxamine was the first SSRI indicated for OCD, it is rarely used due to its drug interaction potential. Other SSRIs should be used instead. SSRI and SNRI agents are initiated at half the initial dose used for depression and are slowly titrated to minimize stimulatory adverse events, such as anxiousness and jitteriness that is common during the first couple of weeks of treatment. Clinicians may overlap SSRIs or SNRIs with a benzodiazepine (BZD) for 2-4 weeks to help alleviate the initial stimulatory effects and regulate sleep. Patients should be advised that immediate relief is not to be expected when initiating AD treatment. Noticeable improvement may be seen after 4 or more weeks of treatment. For specifics on the antidepressants see the Depression chapter.

Buspirone *(BuSpar)* is a second-line option for GAD (only FDA approved indication). It is an alternative for patients who do not respond to antidepressants, are at risk for BZD abuse or added as adjunctive therapy. It has a delayed onset of 2-4 weeks, shorter than SSRIs but longer than BZDs.

Hydroxyzine *(Vistaril)* is FDA approved for anxiety and is considered second-line. It is occasionally used for short-term anxiety in lieu of BZDs that have the potential for abuse. This is a sedating antihistamine and works by sedating the patient, rather than treating any underlying cause. It should not be used long-term. Review hydroxyzine in the Common Skin Conditions chapter. it is used more commonly for pruritus.

Pregabalin *(Lyrica)* is not FDA approved for anxiety but is useful if a patient has anxiety with neuropathic pain. Pregabalin has immediate anxiolytic effects similar to BZDs. It is scheduled C-V due to its euphoric properties, which can have a calming effect.

Propranolol *(Inderal,* others) is used to reduce symptoms of stage fright or performance anxiety (e.g., tremor, tachycardia). It is dosed at 10-40 mg 1 hour prior to an event such as a public speech. Use caution with this approach due to CNS effects (e.g., confusion, dizziness). This is a non-selective beta blocker and is not used with asthma or COPD.

NATURAL PRODUCTS USED FOR ANXIETY

Natural products used for anxiety include valerian, lemon balm, glutamine, passion flower and hops (both as teas), chamomile tea, theanine and skullcap. Kava is used as a relaxant but can damage the liver and should not be recommended. Valerian may rarely be hepatotoxic (or some valerian products may have been contaminated with liver toxins); this is unclear at present. Passionflower is rated as "possibly effective" by the Natural Medicines Database. For most of the other agents evidence of efficacy is scant or poor but individual patients may get benefit from the various agents.

DRUG TREATMENT

Benzodiazepine (BZD) Treatment for Anxiety

BZDs are often used for anxiety. They provide fast relief for acute symptoms, and relaxation is felt within 30 minutes – 2 hours. Situations in which BZDs are appropriate include short-term situations where anxiety is acute and can cause extreme stress, prevent proper sleep, and disrupt life. These symptoms can be the result of a recent death of a loved one, an earthquake, a motor vehicle accident, or other stressful situations. In such cases, they are used less than 1-2 weeks and then discontinued. BZDs can cover-up these symptoms, but do not treat the causes of anxiety, and, in most cases, should not be used long-term.

When BZDs are used in the elderly, they pose significant risks for confusion, dizziness and falls – the risk increases with concurrent use of other CNS depressants. The BEERS Criteria for BZD use in the elderly: May be potentially inappropriate for use in geriatric patients (Quality of evidence – high; Strength of recommendation – strong). Additionally, elderly patients may have a "paradoxidal" reaction to BZDs and present with insomnia, agitation and excitement.

BZDs all have the same mechanism of action (potentiation of GABA). They are differentiated by onset of action and duration of activity.

Benzodiazepines

Potentiate GABA, an inhibitory neurotransmitter, causing CNS depression and providing anxiolytic, anticonvulsant, sedative and/or muscle relaxant properties.

DRUG	DOSING	SAFETY/SIDE EFFECTS/MONITORING
LORazepam (Ativan) Available: Tablet, solution, injection *LORazepam Intensol* is solution (sol for solution) LORazepam injection--used commonly for agitation, sedation	1-3 mg PO BID-TID All C-IV All given PRN or scheduled, depending on condition	**CONTRAINDICATIONS** Myasthenia gravis, severe respiratory insufficiency, severe hepatic insufficiency, sleep apnea syndrome, acute narrow-angle glaucoma, not for use in infants < 6 months of age (oral) **WARNINGS** Anterograde amnesia (after drug is taken some events may not be stored as memories), CNS depression, extravasation with IV administration (vesicant), paradoxical reactions (discontinue if hyperactive/aggressive behavior), potential for abuse, safety risks in elderly (risk of impaired cognition, delirium falls/fractures, development of tolerance, withdrawal following abrupt discontinuation or large decrease in dose; taper off slowly.
ALPRAZolam (Xanax, Xanax XR, Niravam ODT) Tablet *Alprazolam Intensol* (solution), ODT	0.25-0.5 mg PO TID	Potential for abuse Physiological dependence and tolerance develop with chronic use
ChlordiazePOXIDE (*Librium*) Capsule	5-25 mg TID-QID	**SIDE EFFECTS** Somnolence, dizziness, weakness, ataxia, lightheadedness, and with chronic use: tolerance, withdrawal symptoms if stopped
ClonazePAM (KlonoPIN) Tablet, ODT	0.25-0.5 mg PO BID-TID	**NOTES** L-O-T (lorazepam, oxazepam, and temazepam): these are considered less potentially harmful for elderly or with liver impairment since they are metabolized to inactive compounds (glucuronides).
Clorazepate (*Tranxene, Gen-Xene*) Tablet	0.75-15 mg BID-QID	Diazepam: Lipophilic, fast onset, long half-life, high abuse potential. Alprazolam: Fast onset, often abused due to quick action. To avoid withdrawal symptoms (anxiety, shakiness, insomnia, tachycardia, muscle pain) taper off slowly.
Diazepam (Valium) Tablet, injection, *Diazepam Intensol* (solution) *Diastat* – rectal, for acute seizure control	2-10 mg PO BID-QID	Alcohol withdrawal: chlordiazepoxide, diazepam (fastest onset, comes as injection), lorazepam (has injection) or oxazepam (preferred BZD if liver disease). Pregnancy Category D; possible risk of cleft lip and/or palate or "floppy baby syndrome" if used during pregnancy. For lactation, if a benzodiazepine is required, use short-acting agents such as alprazolam or lorazepam.
Oxazepam (*Serax*) Capsule	10-30 mg PO TID-QID	Overdose causes respiratory depression. BZD antidote is flumazenil.

Benzodiazepine Drug Interactions

- Additive effects with sedating drugs, including most pain medicines, muscle relaxants, antihistamines, antipsychotics, anticonvulsants, the antidepressant mirtazapine (*Remeron*), trazodone, alcohol, among others.

- Alprazolam is contraindicated with potent CYP 3A4 inhibitors.

- Diazepam, clonazepam, chlordiazepoxide: ↑ levels with CYP 3A4 inhibitors; caution/lower doses if used in combination.

- Caution if used with clozapine due to ↑ risk of delirium and sedation.

Benzodiazepine Counseling

- Common side effects include drowsiness, dizziness, unsteadiness on your feet, slow reactions, lightheadedness and difficulty remembering what happened after you had taken the medicine. If any of these persist or worsen, contact your healthcare provider promptly.

- If you have been using the medication regularly on a daily basis it cannot be stopped suddenly. To stop using it the dose will have to be decreased slowly or you will experience withdrawal, which is uncomfortable and can be dangerous.

- This medication can cause drug-seeking behavior (addiction/habit forming). Do not increase your dose, take it more frequently or use it for a longer time than prescribed. Keep the bottle in a safe place to prevent others from taking it.

- When used for an extended time, this medication may not work as well and may require different dosing. This is called "tolerance." Talk with your healthcare provider if this medication stops working well. Do not increase the amount or take it more frequently than prescribed.

- Do not take with other medications that can make you sleepy, unless directed by your healthcare provider. Other sedating medications could cause a great deal of sedation and confusion if taken together with this medications. Do not use alcohol with this medications.

- Do not drive a car or do anything that could be dangerous after taking this medication. Car accidents are twice as likely because will not be alert enough to drive and will not be able to respond quickly.

- Taking this drug during pregnancy can cause harm to the baby. This medication is not recommended during breastfeeding.

Buspirone

5-HT1 and 5-HT$_2$ agonist. Only approved for GAD. <u>Not controlled, no abuse or physiological dependence potential</u>.

DRUG	DOSING	SAFETY/SIDE EFFECTS/MONITORING
BusPIRone Available: Tablet	Start 7.5 mg PO BID Can increase by 5 mg/day Q 2-3 days until 30 mg/day, if needed. Max: 60 mg/day	2-4 weeks for optimal effect No potential for abuse, tolerance or physiological dependence <u>Nausea, dizziness, headache</u>, lightheadedness, excitement Avoid use if severe kidney or liver dysfunction When switching from a benzodiazepine to buspirone, the benzodiazepine should be tapered slowly **NOTES** Pregnancy category B

Buspirone Drug Interactions

- Do not use with MAO Inhibitors.

- ↓ dose with erythromycin, diltiazem, itraconazole, verapamil; consider dose reduction with any 3A4 inhibitor.

- 3A4 inducers, including rifampin, may require an increase in the buspirone dose.

- Grapefruit increases the buspirone level; avoid consuming large amounts of grapefruit.

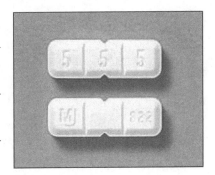

Buspirone Counseling

- Buspirone comes in a *Dividose* tablet designed to make dose adjustments easy. Each tablet is scored and can be broken accurately on the score lines into thirds. It snaps into pieces with finger pressure.

- Take this medication by mouth, usually 2 or 3 times a day or as directed by your healthcare provider. You may take this medication with or without food, but it is important to choose one way and always take it the same way so that the amount of drug absorbed will always stay the same. This medication does not have immediate effects but takes 2 to 4 weeks to see its full benefit.

- Do not take with other medicines that can make you sleepy, unless directed by your healthcare provider. Other sedating medications can have additive effects when this medicine is taken together.

- Do not use alcohol with this medicine.

- Common side effects include dizziness, nausea, or headache. If any of these persist or worsen, contact your healthcare provider or pharmacist promptly.

- Grapefruit will increase the amount of buspirone in your bloodstream.

- Dosage is based on your medical condition and response to therapy. Use this medication regularly in order to get the most benefit from it. To help you remember, use it at the same times each day. When this medication is started, symptoms of anxiety (e.g., restlessness) may sometimes get worse before they improve. It may take up to a month or more to get the full effect of this medication.

- This medication is not recommended during breastfeeding.

SLEEP DISORDERS: INSOMNIA, RESTLESS LEGS SYNDROME (RLS) & NARCOLEPSY

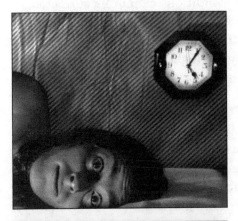

GUIDELINES

American Academy of Sleep Medicine: Practice Parameters for the Treatment of Narcolepsy and other Hypersomnias of Central Origin. *Sleep*. 2006; 29:11:1705-1711.

American Academy of Sleep Medicine: Practice Parameters for the Treatment of Insomnia. *Sleep*. 2007; 30:2:1415-1419.

Cappuccio FP, D'Elia L, Strazzullo P, Miller MA. Sleep duration and all-cause mortality: a systematic review and meta-analysis of prospective studies. *Sleep*. 2010; 33:585-92.

BACKGROUND

There are several types of common sleep disorders. This chapter discusses the primary types for which common prescription drug treatments are available: insomnia, restless leg syndrome and narcolepsy. A lack of restful sleep contributes to poor health and is linked to development of a number of chronic conditions, including cardiovascular disease and depression. Patients who are using chronic OTC sleep agents should be referred to a healthcare provider. The other sleep condition in the "top 4" is sleep apnea, which is treated by non-drug measures.

Insomnia

Insomnia is when a person wants to sleep but cannot. This is the most common sleep condition and occurs either when trying to get sleep (sleep initiation), with reduced duration (sleep is normally 7-9 hours) or is due to a poor sleep quality. A problem with either sleep initiation, duration or quality will contribute to daytime impairment with fatigue, somnolence, poor memory and concentration and, if long-term, chronic health conditions.

Primary treatments for insomnia include cognitive therapy and drug treatment. Cognitive therapy is preferred and includes changes to sleep hygiene (these are called "lifestyle" changes and are in the following box) that can reduce the need for drugs entirely. If a retired elderly person has a daily routine that includes watching television and napping for much of the day they may be able to eliminate night-time sleep problems by reducing the naps and taking a brisk walk earlier in the day. In some cases avoidance of caffeine later in the day is the answer. There is concern about increased mortality with the use of hypnotics--even with occasional use. The hypnotics are

DRUGS LIKELY TO CONTRIBUTE TO INSOMNIA

Bupropion

Stimulants (methylphenidate, etc.)

OTC appetite suppressants

Decongestants (pseudoephedrine, etc.)

MAO-B Inhibitors, if taken late in the day

Fluoxetine, if taken late in the day

Caffeine

Steroids

Alcohol (initially induces sleep, but prevents deeper stages of sleep and causes nocturia)

Any drug that causes urinary retention or nocturia, including antihistamines and diuretics taken later in the day.

SLEEP (INCLUDE WITH COUNSELING) HYGIENE METHODS TO IMPROVE SLEEP

Keep the bedroom dark, comfortable, and quiet

Keep a regular sleep schedule

Avoid daytime naps even after a poor night of sleep – or limit to 30 minutes

Reserve bedroom for only sleep and sex

Turn the face of clock aside to minimize anxiety about falling asleep

If unable to sleep, get up and do something to take your mind off sleeping

Establish a pre-bedtime ritual to condition your body for sleep

Relax before bedtime with soft music, mild stretching, yoga, or pleasurable reading

Avoid exercising right before bedtime

Do not eat heavy meals before bedtime

Do not take any caffeine in the afternoon

over-prescribed. Other cognitive therapy that can be helpful includes biofeedback where the patient is educated to monitor heart rate and muscle tension and record the daily patterns. They receive instruction on how to modify patterns to improve sleep.

Heart failure or any condition that causes shortness of breath can worsen sleep. Anxiety and depression cause insomnia; if the condition can be corrected with psychotherapy, a prescription agent, or both, a hypnotic may not be required. When sleep hygiene issues or medical conditions cannot be corrected, or when a problem causing the insomnia has not been identified, hypnotics may be used to help provide a good night's rest.

Natural Products used for Insomnia

If insomnia is due to depression, taking St. John's wort may be helpful but this will interact with many prescription drugs. St. John's wort induces CYP 450, is a photosensitizer and is serotonergic. Chamomile tea taken in the evening helps many people feel calmer. Melatonin is useful for some patients. Valerian can be useful. There have been isolated reports of valerian causing liver toxicity; this risk is unclear at present. Check the Natural Medicines Database for doses and the current safety profile.

DRUG TREATMENT

The OTC first-generation antihistamines diphenhydramine and doxylamine are used for insomnia. Neither should be used chronically but can be helpful short-term for problems with sleep initiation and duration. Diphenydramine has better evidence of efficacy and is available in many formulations and in less-expensive store brands. In patients using prescription agents long-term the non-benzodiazepines are preferred over benzodiazepines due to a decreased risk of physical dependence and less daytime cognitive effects. The non-controlled prescription agents are not as effective in most patients but are useful in select cases. Most commonly non-benzodiazepines, such as zolpidem, are used chronically and are preferred over the benzodiazepines that are used as hypnotics. Although this is accurate keep in mind that, if possible, drugs used chronically for sleep are now discouraged. Suvorexant *(Belsomra)* is a new agent with a unique mechanism: it blocks the orexin neuropeptide signaling system, which is involved with promoting wakefulness. Non-24-Hour Sleep-Wake Disorder, or "Non-24" is a condition where patients have difficulty with obtaining restful sleep because their circadian rhythm is not synchronized with the 24-hour day-night cycle. This can be present in persons who are totally visually blind and non-blind. Tasimelteon *(Hetlioz)* is the first drug approved for this condition. It is a melatonin receptor agonist (similar to ramelteon).

DRUG	DOSING	SAFETY/SIDE EFFECTS/MONITORING
Non-benzodiazepines: Acts selectively at the benzodiazepine receptors to increase GABA		
Zolpidem *(Ambien, Ambien CR,* generic) C-IV *Zolpimist*-spray *Edluar SL* tabs *Intermezzo SL* – for night-time awakening	5-10 mg PO QHS *Ambien CR*: 6.25-12.5 mg PO QHS *Zolpimist* 5 mg/spray (1-2 sprays) QHS *Edluar* 5-10 mg PO QHS *Intermezzo SL* 3.5 mg males, 1.75 mg females, and if using CNS depressants (decrease dose of these as well, if possible)	**WARNINGS** ↑ risk mortality (interferes with breathing at night, causes accidents/falls, confusion, and may ↑ risk infection and cancer) Potential for abuse and dependence **SIDE EFFECTS** Somnolence Dizziness, ataxia Lightheadedness "pins and needles" feeling on skin May cause parasomnias (unusual actions while sleeping – of which the patient may not be aware) Withdrawal symptoms if used longer than 2 weeks **NOTES** ***Intermezzo SL*** Do not take unless planning to sleep 4+ more hours. Lifestyle changes should be the primary method to improve sleep, not drugs.
Zaleplon *(Sonata)* C-IV	5-10 mg PO QHS	
Eszopiclone *(Lunesta)* C-IV Not limited to short-term use (officially, although all 3 used long-term commonly)	1-3 mg PO QHS 1 mg if difficulty falling asleep, 2 mg if difficulty staying asleep, 3 mg if helpful for longer duration	Preferred over benzodiazepines for 1st line treatment of insomnia due to ↓ abuse, dependence and tolerance. Do not take with fatty food, a heavy meal or alcohol.

Insomnia Drugs Continued

DRUG	DOSING	SAFETY/SIDE EFFECTS/MONITORING

Orexin-receptor antagonist: The orexin neuropeptide signaling system promotes wakefulness.

DRUG	DOSING	SAFETY/SIDE EFFECTS/MONITORING
Suvorexant *(Belsomra)* C-IV	10 mg QHS if at least 7 hours sleep remaining, max 20 mg	**CONTRAINDICATIONS** Narcolepsy **WARNINGS** Abnormal thinking and behavioral changes, worsening of depression/suicidal ideation, sleep paralysis, hypnagogic/hypnopompic hallucinations, cataplexy-like symptoms **SIDE EFFECTS** Somnolence, headache, dizziness, abnormal dreams, cough, upper respiratory tract infection **NOTES** *Belsomra* may cause sleep-driving and other complex behaviors while not being fully awake. Use lower dose (5 mg) with moderate CYP 3A4 inhibitors; avoid use with strong CYP3A4 inhibitors.

Melatonin Receptor Agonists

DRUG	DOSING	SAFETY/SIDE EFFECTS/MONITORING
Ramelteon *(Rozerem)* For insomnia, not controlled Not limited to short-term use	8 mg PO QHS	**SIDE EFFECTS** <u>Somnolence</u>, dizziness **NOTES** Do not take with fatty food.
Tasimelteon *(Hetlioz)* For Non-24-Hour Sleep-Wake Disorder	20 mg PO QHS	**WARNINGS** Use is not recommended in patients with severe hepatic impairment, may have significant drug interactions; check prior to dispensing ↑<u>ALT</u>, URI **SIDE EFFECTS** <u>Headache, abnormal dreams</u>, ALT, URI **NOTES** Can take weeks to take effect. Take without food.

Tricyclic Antidepressant

DRUG	DOSING	SAFETY/SIDE EFFECTS/MONITORING
Doxepin extended-release *(Silenor)* Not controlled Generic doxepin, traZODone, mirtazapine used off-label for sleep Used for difficulty staying asleep (sleep maintenance)	6 mg PO QHS 3 mg if ≥ 65 years	**CONTRAINDICATIONS** Requires 2 week washout for MAO Is This is an antidepressant and requires MedGuide for unusual thoughts/suicide risk **SIDE EFFECTS** Somnolence, low incidence nausea and upper respiratory infections, possibility of anticholinergic SEs

Ambien, Sonata and *Lunesta* Drug Interactions

- Caution with the use of non-benzodiazepines with potent 3A4 inhibitors (e.g., ritonavir, indinavir, saquinavir, atazanavir, ketoconazole, itraconazole, erythromycin and clarithromycin).

- Additive effects with sedating drugs, including most pain medicines, muscle relaxants, antihistamines, the antidepressant mirtazapine *(Remeron)*, trazodone, alcohol and others.

Ambien, Sonata and *Lunesta* Counseling

- If using *Zolpimist*, spray directly into your mouth over your tongue (once for a 5 mg dose, twice for a 10 mg dose). Prime the bottle if 1st-time use. If using *Edluar* SL tablets, allow tablet to dissolve under tongue; do not swallow. For *Intermezzo*: this drug is not swallowed, it dissolves under the tongue. Do not take unless you are planning to sleep 4 or more hours.

- You should not eat a heavy/high-fat meal within 2 hours of taking this medication; this may prevent the medicine from working properly.

- Call your healthcare provider if the insomnia worsens or is not better within 7 to 10 days. This may mean that there is another condition causing your sleep problem.

- Common side effects include sleepiness, lightheadedness, dizziness, "pins and needles" feeling on your skin and difficulty with coordination.

- You may still feel drowsy the next day after taking this medicine.

- This drug may (rarely) cause abnormal thoughts and behavior. Symptoms include more outgoing or aggressive behavior than normal, confusion, agitation, hallucinations, worsening of depression, and suicidal thoughts or actions. Some people have found that they get out of bed while not being fully awake and do an activity that they do not know they are doing.

- You may have withdrawal symptoms when you stop taking this medicine, if you have been taking it for more than a couple of weeks. Withdrawal symptoms include unpleasant feelings, stomach and muscle cramps, vomiting, sweating and shakiness. You may also have more trouble sleeping the first few nights after the medicine is stopped. The problem usually goes away on its own after 1 or 2 nights.

- Do not take with other medicines that can make you sleepy, unless directed by your healthcare provider. Do not use alcohol with any sleep medicine.

- After taking this medicine, you should not be driving a car or using any dangerous machinery.

- This medicine is a federally controlled substance (C-IV) because it can be abused or lead to dependence. Keep the bottle in a safe place to prevent misuse and abuse.

BENZODIAZEPINES

Potentiate GABA, an inhibitory neurotransmitter, causing CNS depression. BEERS Criteria for use in elderly: May be potentially inappropriate for use in geriatric patients.

DRUG	DOSING	SAFETY/SIDE EFFECTS/MONITORING
LORazepam (Ativan) LORazepam Intensol is solution (sol for solution) Further information on the BZDs is in the Anxiety chapter. C-IV	0.5-2 mg PO QHS	See Anxiety chapter for a full discussion; these are important agents and cause risk of physical (physiological) dependence, abuse (addiction) and tolerance. L-O-T (lorazepam, oxazepam, and temazepam): these are considered less potentially harmful for elderly or those with liver impairment since they are
Temazepam (Restoril) C-IV	7.5-30 mg PO QHS	metabolized to inactive compounds (glucuronides); choose L-O-T if need BZD in elderly patient and for sleep. Lorazepam and Oxazepam are approved for sleep (not Temazepam).
Estazolam (Prosom) C-IV		Cannot use with potent 3A4 inhibitors
Quazepam (Doral) C-IV		Caution when use in elderly due to its long half-life: risk of falls, fractures
Flurazepam C-IV		Caution when use in elderly due to its long half-life: risk of falls, fractures
Triazolam (Halcion) C-IV		Associated with higher rebound insomnia and daytime anxiety; Tapering upon discontinuation. Contraindicated with efavirenz (Sustiva), delavirdine (Rescriptor), azole antifungals, and protease inhibitors & all 3A4 Inhibitors

Benzodiazepine Drug Interactions: refer to Anxiety chapter for complete counseling.

Additional Counseling when Used for Sleep

- This medication should be taken before bedtime. Take the medicine immediately prior to sleep. Do not do anything dangerous, such as driving a car, after taking the medicine. Do not mix with alcohol.

ANTIHISTAMINES

Compete with (block) histamine H1 receptors.

DRUG	DOSING	SAFETY/SIDE EFFECTS/MONITORING
Diphenhydramine (Benadryl, Sominex, Unisom, others, store brands)	25-50 mg PO QHS	SIDE EFFECTS Due to the side-effect profile, considered "DO NOT USE DRUGS IN ELDERLY" Possible anticholinergic side effects: Sedation; tolerance to sedative effects can develop after 10 days use.
Doxylamine (Aldex, Unisom Nighttime, store brands)	25 mg PO QHS	Confusion (can exaccerbate memory/cognition difficulty) Peripheral anticholinergic side effects: Dry mouth Urinary retention (will make it very difficult for males with BPH to urinate, can slow down/delay urination in females) Dry/blurry vision, risk increased IOP Constipation Best to avoid use in BPH (may worsen symptoms) and glaucoma (may elevate IOP)

Diphenhydramine *(Benadryl)* Counseling (for all indications – applies to other sedating antihistamines)

- Diphenhydramine is an antihistamine used to relieve symptoms of allergy, hay fever and the common cold. These symptoms include rash, itching, watery eyes, itchy eyes/nose/throat, cough, runny nose and sneezing. It is also used to prevent and treat nausea, vomiting and dizziness caused by motion sickness. Diphenhydramine can also be used to help you relax and fall asleep. It is occasionally used for involuntary movements and muscle stiffness from Parkinson's disease.

- When using this medicine, you will become sleepy. It can also make you feel confused and make it difficult to concentrate.

- Do not take with other medicines that can make you sleepy, unless directed by your doctor. Do not use alcohol with any sleep medicine.

- This medicine should not be used by patients with an enlarged prostate, or BPH, without getting approval. It will temporarily make urination more difficult.

- If you have glaucoma, discuss use with your eye doctor. It may raise your the pressure in your eyes.

- If you have problems with constipation, this medicine will worsen the constipation.

- This medicine can cause your eyes to become dry and your vision to become blurry. It can also cause dry mouth.

- This medicine can make it difficult to urinate (it will take longer for the urine to come out).

- Although this drug is meant to be sedating, some children will experience excitability instead.

- After taking this medicine, you should not drive a car or use any dangerous machinery.

- Take the tablet, capsule, or liquid form by mouth, with or without food. Diphenhydramine may be taken with food or milk if stomach upset occurs. If you are taking the suspension, shake the bottle well before each dose. Measure liquid forms of this medication with a dose-measuring spoon or device, not a regular teaspoon, to make sure you have the correct dose.

- The rapidly-dissolving tablet or strip should be allowed to dissolve on the tongue and then swallowed, with or without water. A second strip may be taken after the first strip has dissolved. The chewable tablets should be chewed thoroughly before being swallowed.

- To prevent motion sickness, take your dose 30 minutes before starting activity such as travel. To help you sleep, take your dose about 30 minutes before bedtime. If you continue to have difficulty sleeping for longer than 2 weeks, contact your doctor.

RESTLESS LEGS SYNDROME

Restless legs syndrome (RLS) is an urge to move the lower legs which is sometimes described as a "creeping" sensation. RLS is worse at night and is relieved with movement. RLS is thought to be due to a dysfunction with dopamine in the brain's basal ganglia circuits. The primary treatment is dopamine agonists (most commonly) and the anticonvulsant gabapentin.

Drug Treatment

Pramipexole *(Mirapex)* and ropinirole *(Requip)* are dopamine agonists primarily used in longer-acting formulations for Parkinson disease, or are taken TID. For RLS these are taken in the immediate-release (IR) formulations 1-3 hours before bedtime. Rotigotine *(Neupro)* is a dopamine agonist that comes in a patch formulation that is also used for Parkinson disease and RLS. For both conditions the patch is applied once daily. Parkinson patients usually start with the 2 mg patch and RLS treatment begins with the 1 mg patch. Patients must be told not to apply a heat source over the patch and to remove the patch if receiving an MRI procedure. This patch causes skin irritation; the same site cannot be used again <u>for 14 days</u>. The patch contains a sulfite (metabisulfite) and in sulfite-sensitive patients will cause an allergic reaction.

Dopamine agonists cause <u>orthostasis, somnolence</u>, and nausea that is dose-related. Even when used for RLS the dose is titrated upwards carefully (slowly). Patients should be monitored for <u>psychiatric</u> concerns (hallucinations, abnormal dreams) and movement disorders.

<u>Gabapentin</u> enacarbil <u>*(Horizant)*</u> is approved for postherpetic neuralgia (PHN) and RLS. With any indication gabapentin requires a <u>reduced</u> dose with renal impairment (CrCl < 60 mL/min) to avoid increased side effects (dizziness, somnolence, ataxia, peripheral edema, weight gain, diplopia, blurred vision, dry mouth). The tablet is taken with food and must be swallowed whole (it cannot be crushed or chewed). For RLS it is taken at ~5:00 PM daily. The IR formulation of gabapentin is used off-label as a less-expensive alternative. Refer to the Parkinson Disease chapter for additional information on the dopamine agonists, and the Epilepsy/Seizures chapter for additional information on gabapentin.

NARCOLEPSY

Narcolepsy is excessive daytime sleepiness with cataplexy (sudden loss of muscle tone) and sleep paralysis. Narcolepsy causes sudden daytime "sleep attacks" especially when the person is in a relaxed setting due to poor control of normal sleep-wake cycles. The sleep attacks last a few seconds to several minutes. Patients have difficulty managing with narcolepsy; they can fall asleep while at work, school, or in the middle of a conversation. And, the sleep quality at night is poor.

Drug Treatment

Narcolepsy is treated with stimulants, such as modafinil or armodafinil or with sodium oxybate, which is derived from the inhibitory neurotransmitter gamma aminobutyric acid (GABA). Several of the stimulants used primarily for ADHD have narcolepsy indications, including dextroamphetamine, dextroamphetamine/amphetamine *(Adderall)* and various methylphenidate formulations (*Metadate ER, Methylin, Ritalin* and *Ritalin SR)*. Patients may be using drugs approved for other indications: selegiline can be useful for daytime sleepiness, and tricyclic antidepressants or fluoxetine can be useful for cataplexy. These are drugs used to improve wakefulness in adult patients with excessive sleepiness associated with narcolepsy, obstructive sleep apnea/hypopnea syndrome, and shift work sleep disorder.

Stimulants for Wakefulness

DRUG	DOSING	SAFETY/SIDE EFFECTS/MONITORING
Modafinil *(Provigil)* C-IV	200 mg daily	**SIDE EFFECTS** Headache, dizziness, anxiety, agitation, nausea, diarrhea, insomnia, dry mouth, risk of severe rash. **WARNINGS** Avoid use with pre-existing cardiac conditions. Use with caution with hepatic impairment, renal impairment, psychiatric disorders and Tourette's. **NOTES** Both of these agents require a MedGuide due to risk of severe rash, which can be life-threatening.
Armodafanil *(Nuvigil)* R-isomer of modafinil; similar drug C-IV	150-250 mg daily	Similar side effects, similar drug to modafinil, including risk of severe rash – give MedGuide.

Note: Additional stimulants indicated for weight loss in weight loss/gain chapter, and the ADHD stimulants are sometimes used for these conditions.

Sodium oxybate is derived from GABA. Indicated for narcolepsy with cataplexy (sudden loss of muscle strength). Helps with sleep at night, generally used with daytime stimulants.

DRUG	DOSING	SAFETY/SIDE EFFECTS/MONITORING
Sodium oxybate *(Xyrem)* C-III (narcolepsy) C-I (abuse) REMS program: this is a "date rape" drug (sedative, called GHB) that requires strict measures to ensure it is going to narcolepsy with cataplexy patients only.	Start 2.25 g QHS and again 2.5-4 hours later after 1st dose; titrate to effect, dosing range ~6-9 g/night	**BOXED WARNINGS (3)** Respiratory depression (strong CNS depressant). Sodium oxybate is a salt form of hydroxybutyrate (GHB), a drug of abuse. Danger is increased when taken with other CNS depressants; coma and death can result. Restricted access through the REMS *Xyrem* Success Program. **SIDE EFFECTS** Dizziness, nausea, somnolence, enuresis (dose-related), daytime hangover effect **NOTES** Taken in ¼ cup water, usually in an empty pharmacy pill container. Patient should lie down immediately after taking and stay in bed. The second dose is taken 2.5-4 hours after the first. Will typically fall asleep within 5-15 minutes after taking 1st dose. Contains a high sodium content.

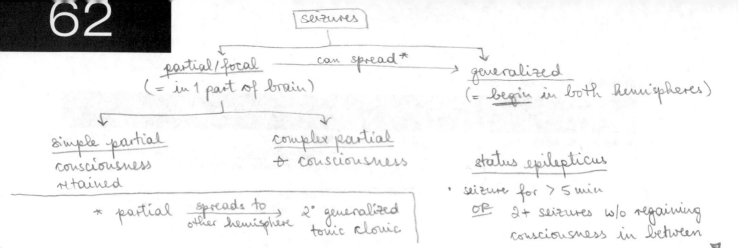

seizures

partial/focal ———— can spread* ————→ generalized
(= in 1 part of brain)   (= begin in both hemispheres)

simple partial   complex partial   status epilepticus
consciousness   ∅ consciousness   • seizure for > 5 min
retained   OR 2+ seizures w/o regaining
                                                     consciousness in between
* partial spreads to 2° generalized
  other hemisphere   tonic clonic   ⇒ MEDICAL EMERGENCY!

EPILEPSY/SEIZURES

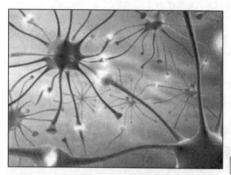

We gratefully acknowledge the assistance of Kimberly B. Tallian, PharmD, BCPP, FASHP, FCCP, FCSHP, Assistant Dean and Chair for Clinical and Administrative Sciences, Professor at Keck Graduate Institute, School of Pharmacy, Claremont Colleges, in preparing this chapter.

BACKGROUND

Epilepsy is a common neurological disorder, affecting up to 2.3 million Americans with approximately 150,000 new cases diagnosed in the United States each year. It is defined by unprovoked seizures or abnormal "electrical storms" in the brain. Unfortunately, many patients do not have complete seizure control, even with current medications. Seizures can damage and destroy neurons, which can cause cognitive deficits and be life-threatening.

Seizures are generally classified into two basic groups: partial and generalized. Partial seizures start in one part of the brain. If there is no loss of consciousness, the seizure is called simple partial. If there is a loss of consciousness, the seizure is termed complex partial. Partial seizures can spread to the other hemisphere of the brain, resulting in secondarily generalized tonic-clonic seizures. Generalized seizures, however, begin in both hemispheres of the brain and consciousness is impaired. Seizures that last longer than 5 minutes or 2 or more seizures between which the patient does not regain consciousness are called status epilepticus, which is a medical emergency.

GUIDELINES

Drugs for Epilepsy Treatment Guidelines, Medical Letter 2013;11(126):9-18.

Efficacy and tolerability of the new antiepileptic drugs I: Treatment of new onset epilepsy: Report of the Therapeutics and Technology Assessment Subcommittee and Quality Standards Subcommittee of the American Academy of Neurology and the American Epilepsy Society. *Neurology.* 2004;62:1252-1260.

Practice Parameter Update: Management Issues for Women with Epilepsy – Focus on Pregnancy (an Evidence-Based Review): Obstetrical Complications and Change in Seizure Frequency: Report of the Quality Standards Subcommittee and Therapeutics and Technology Assessment Subcommittee of the American Academy of Neurology and American Epilepsy Society. *Neurology.* 2009;73:133-141.

INTERNATIONAL CLASSIFICATION OF SEIZURES

SEIZURE TYPE	SYMPTOMS

Partial/Focal Seizures

Simple Partial Seizures (consciousness not impaired)	Motor (muscles contract/relax, eye movements, head turning)
	Autonomic (incontinence, nausea, sweating, tachycardia)
	Sensory (flashes of light, noises, dizziness, unpleasant odors/tastes)
	Psychic (detachment, time/memory distortions, unprovoked emotions)
Complex Partial Seizures (impaired consciousness)	Simple partial features (see above)
	Automatisms (repetitive behaviors that serve no purpose, such as lip smacking, fumbling, picking at something)

Generalized Seizures

Absence Seizures (formerly called petit mal)	Brief and abrupt staring spells lasting 10–30 seconds
Myoclonic Seizures	Brief, lightning-like jerk movements of entire body
Tonic-Clonic Seizures (formerly called grand mal)	Characterized by five phases: flexion, extension, tremor, clonic, and loss of consciousness
Tonic Seizures	Flexion and/or extension only (flexion ↓ angle, extension ↑ angle--the hand/arms/feet/legs open and close, or thrash)
Clonic Seizures	Rhythmic, repetitive, jerking muscle movements
Atonic Seizures	Loss of muscle tone and falls to the ground; known as "drop attacks"

RISKS ASSOCIATED WITH ANTIEPILEPTIC DRUGS

When anticonvulsants (or antiepileptic drugs, or AEDs) are used in women of reproductive age, it is important to consider teratogenicity and provide proper counseling. Carbamazepine, clonazepam, phenobarbital/primidone, phenytoin/fosphenytoin, topiramate and valproate are pregnancy category D – this means that there is known fetal risk, and the benefit must outweigh the risk. Health care providers should always consider that untreated or inadequately treated epilepsy during pregnancy ↑ the risk of complications in both the pregnant mother and her developing baby. Valproate is thought to have the highest risk of fetal harm. Valproate is pregnancy category X for migraine prophylaxis; otherwise, it is category D. There are much safer alternatives to treat migraine in pregnancy. Recently, the FDA issued a warning that valproate is associated with ↓ IQ scores in children following *in utero* exposure. All other AEDs are pregnancy category C. The metabolism of some of the AEDs increases during pregnancy (lamotrigine and others), resulting in breakthrough seizures. This can require a higher dose, which can ↑ risk to the baby. Managing epilepsy during pregnancy is complex.

The most common side effects with AEDs are CNS-related, including somnolence, fatigue, cognitive impairment and coordination abnormalities such as ataxia and dizziness since these drugs have to penetrate the CNS to work. Side effects such as mental confusion and sedation can make it difficult for children to do well in school and for adults to perform well at work or to drive safely.

There are many drug interactions with most of the antiepileptic drugs. Several of the AEDs are strong inducers and can ↓ the concentration of other drugs, including other AEDs the patient may be taking. AEDs that are strong inducers include carbamazepine, oxcarbazepine, fosphenytoin, phenytoin, phenobarbital, primidone, and topiramate (≥ 200 mg/d).

Individuals with epilepsy have ↑ fracture risk. Bone loss can occur as soon as two years after the start of AED therapy. Modifiable factors that affect bone density should be addressed (see Osteoporosis chapter). The mechanism of AED-induced bone loss is not completely understood. Hepatic enzyme inducers ↓ vitamin D levels by ↑ metabolism, which ↓ calcium absorption. All patients on enzyme-inducing AEDs should supplement with vitamin D and calcium.

All AEDs require a MedGuide due to the risk of suicidality. The MedGuide warning states: "Like other antiepileptic drugs, this medication may cause suicidal thoughts or actions in a very small number of people, about 1 in 500."

Seizure drugs are titrated upwards when initiated to ↓ side effects and ↓ toxicity risk. Never discontinue abruptly. This will cause or worsen seizures. Taper the medication off slowly. [over 2+ months] Often, the new drug is being titrated up while the old drug is being titrated off (to continue providing seizure control), unless the patient is discontinuing treatment entirely.

STATUS EPILEPTICUS

Status epilepticus (SE) is an acute continuous epileptic crisis lasting > 5 minutes or ≥ 2 discrete seizures between which there is incomplete recovery of consciousness.

- SE is a medical emergency.

- Treatment consists of using a rapid-acting benzodiazepine first (e.g., lorazepam), followed by AED therapy (loading dose followed by maintenance dose).

DRUGS/CONDITIONS THAT MAY LOWER THE SEIZURE THRESHOLD

Antipsychotics (e.g., clozapine, phenothiazines, butyrophenones)

Antivirals (e.g., amantadine, rimantadine, foscarnet, ganciclovir, valganciclovir, acyclovir IV)

Bupropion

Carbapenems (with higher doses/renal impairment – especially imipenem)

Cephalosporins

Fluoroquinolones

Lindane

Lithium and theophylline (in toxicity)

Mefloquine

metabolite: normeperidine

Meperidine (chronic dosing with poor renal function)

Metoclopramide *also induces PC (overdose, elderly, ↓ renal fxn)*

Natural products such as dendrobium, evening primrose oil, gingko, melatonin

Penicillins

Sleep deprivation, alcohol intoxication, menstruation, infection and fever (especially in children) can worsen seizure.

Tramadol

Status Epilepticus: First Line Treatment with Benzodiazepines

 DOC

- Lorazepam *(Ativan)* is the benzodiazepine of choice for treating status epilepticus due to the longer duration of action in the CNS which provides longer protection. Diazepam is highly lipophilic (quick onset) but rapidly redistributes into fat causing the CNS half-life to be shorter, with a shorter duration of effect.

- Lorazepam: 4 mg given slow IV (adults); max rate 2 mg/min – may repeat in 5-10 minutes if no response. May be given IM but IV preferred. If IV access is not established midazolam can be given IM.

- Diazepam: 5-10 mg given slow IV – may repeat every 5-10 min at a dose of ≤ 5 mg/minute; max dose: 30 mg.

- Diazepam rectal gel *(DIASTAT AcuDial)*: 2.5 – 20 mg PR (age and weight-based). May repeat once if necessary. It is important to check that the dose has been dialed correctly and locked for both syringes prior to dispensing.

- Follow initial benzodiazepine (BDZ) treatment with phenytoin (max rate 50 mg/minute) or fosphenytoin (max rate 150 mg PE/min).

- If the initial bolus did not control the seizure activity, the patient will be switched to an alternative AED or given a continuous infusion.

FIRST AID FOR SEIZURES

First aid for seizures involves responding in ways that can keep the person safe until the seizure stops by itself:

- Keep calm and reassure other people who may be nearby.

- Prevent injury by clearing the area around the person of anything hard or sharp.

- Ease the person to the floor and put something soft and flat, like a folded jacket, under the head. Turn the person gently onto one side. This will help keep the airway clear.

- Remove eyeglasses and loosen ties or anything around the neck that may make breathing difficult.

- Time the seizure with a watch. If the seizure continues for longer than five minutes without signs of slowing down or if the person has trouble breathing afterwards, appears to be injured, in pain, or has an unusual recovery, call 911.

- Do not hold people down or try to stop their movements.

- Contrary to popular belief, it is not true that people having a seizure can swallow their tongue. Do not put anything in the person's mouth. Efforts to hold the tongue down can injure the teeth or jaw.

- Do not attempt artificial respiration except in the unlikely event that a person does not start breathing again after the seizure has stopped.

- Stay with the person until the seizure ends naturally and the person is fully awake.

- Do not offer the person water or food until fully alert.

- Be friendly and reassuring as consciousness returns.

- Offer to call a taxi, friend or relative to help the person get home safely, particularly if the person seems confused or unable to get home without help.

DOC

lorazepam OR **diazepam** then **phenytoin**

lorazepam
- 4 mg slow IV (max rate 2 mg/min)
- repeat in 5-10 min if 0 response
- IV preferred over IM
  - if no IV access
    => midazolam IM

diazepam
- 5-10 mg slow IV
- repeat q 5-10 min @ ≤ 5 mg/min (max dose 30 mg)

* rectal gel (DIASTAT AcuDial®) 2.5-20 mg PR ⌐ age ⌐ wt
- may repeat x 1

phenytoin
max rate 50 mg/min
OR
fosphenytoin
max rate 150 mg PE/min

ANTIEPILEPTIC DRUGS (AEDs)

Treatment of Choice (Variable, Depends on Literature and Clinician Preference)

SEIZURE TYPE	1ST LINE TREATMENT
Partial, including secondarily generalized	Carbamazepine
	Lamotrigine
	Levetiracetam
	Oxcarbazepine
Primary Generalized Tonic-Clonic	Lamotrigine
	Levetiracetam
	Valproate
Absence	Ethosuximide
	Valproate
Atypical Absence, Myoclonic, Atonic	Ethosuximide
	Lamotrigine
	Levetiracetam
	Valproate

MEDICAL MARIJUANA AND EPILEPSY

Presently, it is unknown if marijuana is a safe and effective treatment for epilepsy, including the impact on cognitive function. Safety concerns coupled with a lack of evidence of efficacy in clinical trials does not support the use of marijuana for the treatment of seizures. Pharmacists should keep in mind that there are parents who have seen improved seizure control in their child; these are select cases. In such situations, consider the impact of drug induction, which may require dose adjustments of other medications.

COMMONLY USED/IMPORTANT ANTICONVULSANTS

Levetiracetam   *inhibits the "kindling effect" of seizures*

Mechanism of action is unknown; may inhibit voltage-dependent N-type calcium channels, facilitate GABA-ergic inhibitory transmission through displacement of negative modulators, reduce delayed rectifier potassium current and/or bind to synaptic proteins which modulate neurotransmitter release.

DRUG	DOSING	SAFETY/SIDE EFFECTS/MONITORING
LevETIRAcetam *(Keppra, Keppra XR)* Adjunctive therapy for several seizure types Tablet, solution, injection	Initial: 500 mg BID or 1,000 mg daily (XR) Maximum: 3,000 mg/d ↓ dose if CrCl ≤ 80 mL/min	**SIDE EFFECTS** Somnolence, dizziness, weakness, infection, behavior changes (aggression, irritability, etc.), vomiting, anorexia, asthenia *= weakness* **MONITORING** Mental status and seizure frequency **NOTES** Pregnancy Category C No significant drug interactions

Lamotrigine

Lamotrigine inhibits release of glutamate and aspartate (excitatory amino acids), and is also a fast sodium channel blocker and a t-type calcium channel blocker, thus stabilizing neuronal membranes.

DRUG	DOSING	SAFETY/SIDE EFFECTS/MONITORING
LamoTRIgine (LaMICtal [tabs/chewables], LaMICtal ODT Adjunctive therapy for partial seizures, or conversion to primary therapy from older drugs, bipolar Tablet, chewable, ODT	Week 1 and 2: 25 mg daily Week 3 and 4: 50 mg daily Week 5 and on: can ↑ by 50 mg daily every 1-2 weeks. Dosing is different if on enzyme inducers such as carbamazepine, phenytoin, phenobarbital or primidone. Also different dosing if on valproate (start with 25 mg every other day). Divide BID, unless using XR (daily)	**BOXED WARNING** Serious skin reactions, including SJS/TEN (rate of rash is greater in pediatrics than adults); ↑ risk with higher than recommended starting doses, rapid dose escalation, or co-administration of valproic acid which ↑ lamotrigine levels > 2-fold. To ↓ risk of rash, follow titration schedule– *Lamictal Starter Kit* and *Lamictal ODT Patient Titration Kits* provide the recommended titration schedule for the first 5 weeks. Titration schedule is based on whether patient is on valproate, inducer anticonvulsant, or no concomitant anticonvulsant. **WARNINGS** Risk of aseptic meningitis, blood dyscrasias. **SIDE EFFECTS** Nausea, vomiting, insomnia, somnolence, rash, headache, ataxia, impaired coordination, dizziness, diplopia, alopecia (treat with a multivitamin containing selenium and zinc), blurred vision. **NOTES** Pregnancy Category C Discontinue if any sign of hypersensitivity reaction or unspecified rash Comes in C-R (child-resistant) packaging. Starter kit packaging for those not taking interacting medications is orange; for those taking valproate is blue; for those taking inducers is green.

does not cause photosensitivity

Lamotrigine Drug Interactions

- Valproate ↑ lamotrigine concentrations more than 2-fold.

- Strong inducers (including carbamazepine, phenytoin phenobarbital and primidone) ↓ lamotrigine. There are higher titration schedules when using these drugs concurrently.

- Lamotrigine levels are ↓ with oral estrogen-containing contraceptives.

- Caution for additive CNS effects, including dizziness, somnolence, fatigue.

cause alopecia ⇒ tx w/ MVI w/ Se and Zn
lamotrigine
CBZ
valproate

FOA for migraine proph
1. topiramate
2. divalproex (Depakote®)

folate deficiency ⇒ anemia
(fos) phenytoin
phenobarb

Carbamazepine

Fast sodium channel blocker; structurally similar to tricyclic antidepressants (TCAs); stimulates release of antidiuretic hormone (ADH), promoting reabsorption of water. In addition to anticonvulsant effects, carbamazepine has anticholinergic, antineuralgic, antidiuretic, muscle relaxant, antimanic, antidepressive, and antiarrhythmic properties.

DRUG	DOSING	SAFETY/SIDE EFFECTS/MONITORING
CarBAMazepine *(TEGretol, TEGretol XR, Carbatrol, Epitol)* *Equetro* – for bipolar Indicated for many seizure types (except absence seizures) and indicated for trigeminal neuralgia Capsule, tablet, suspension	Initial: 200 mg BID or divided QID (suspension) Maximum: 1,600 mg/day (some patients may require more) **Therapeutic Range** 4-12 mcg/mL	**BOXED WARNINGS (2)** Serious skin reactions, including SJS and TEN: All Asians MUST be tested for HLA-B*1502 allele prior to initiation; if test positive for this allele, carbamazepine cannot be used (unless benefit clearly outweighs risk). Fatal blood cell abnormalities (including aplastic anemia and agranulocytosis). Monitor CBC, platelets, and differential prior to and during therapy; discontinue if significant bone marrow suppression occurs. **CONTRAINDICATIONS** Bone marrow suppression, hypersensitivity to TCAs, use of MAO inhibitors within past 14 days, concurrent use of nefazodone, concomitant use of delavirdine or other non-nucleoside reverse transcriptase inhibitors **WARNINGS** Risk of developing a hypersensitivity reaction may be ↑ in patients with the variant HLA-A*3101 allele. Hyponatremia (SIADH) Mild anticholinergic effects Cardiac conduction abnormalities Renal impairment Hypothyroidism can occur **SIDE EFFECTS** Dizziness, somnolence, headache, nausea, vomiting, ataxia, dry mouth, pruritus, photosensitivity, blurred vision, rash, vitamin D and calcium deficiency (bone loss), ↑ LFTs, alopecia (treat with a multivitamin containing selenium and zinc), risk SJS/DRESS. **MONITORING** CBC with differential, platelets, LFTs, signs of rash, ophthalmic exam, thyroid function tests, electrolytes (especially Na⁺), BUN, SCr, mental status, seizure frequency. Carbamazepine levels should be monitored within 3-5 days of initiation and again after 4 weeks due to autoinduction. **NOTES** Pregnancy Category D Potent CYP450 inducer and autoinducer – ↓ level of many other drugs and of itself Supplementation with calcium and vitamin D recommended

Handwritten annotations:

→ Rescriptor®

↓ Na⁺

↑ ADH ⇒ dilution ↓ [Na] — CBZ toxicity

CBZ or CBZ (fos) phenytoin

HLA-B* 1502 (must test Asians)
3101
↳ CBZ only

doxycycline

CBZ rash may be mild/ transitory or serious/ life-threatening

DRESS = drug rash w/ eosinophilia & systemic sx
1. doxycycline
2. CBZ
3. (fos) phenytoin
4. ethosuximide

Carbamazepine Drug Interactions

- Carbamazepine is a strong inducer of many enzymes (1A2, (2C19) 2C8/9, 3A4), P-glycoprotein (P-gp) and is an underlineautoinducer. It will ↓ the levels of many drugs, including hormonal contraceptives, other seizure medications, levothyroxine, warfarin and others. Use of an alternative, nonhormonal contraceptive is recommended.

- Carbamazepine is a major 3A4 substrate. 3A4 inhibitors will ↑ carbamazepine levels and 3A4 inducers will ↓ carbamazepine levels. Avoid use of nefazodone and non-nucleoside reverse transcriptase inhibitors.

- Caution for additive CNS effects, including dizziness, somnolence, fatigue.

Oxcarbazepine

Voltage-sensitive sodium channel blocker, inhibiting repetitive firing and reducing the propogation of synaptic impulse. Oxcarbazepine is a prodrug that converts to active 10-monohydroxy derivative (MHD).

DRUG	DOSING	SAFETY/SIDE EFFECTS/MONITORING
OXcarbazepine (Trileptal, Oxtellar XR) Partial seizures Tablet, suspension (Trileptal), extended-release tablet (Oxtellar XR) *PRODRUG → active 10-monohydroxy derivative (MHD)*	Initial: 300 mg BID (Trileptal); 600 mg daily (Oxtellar XR) Maximum: 2,400 mg/day Reduce dose in severe renal impairment (CrCl < 30 mL/min) start 300 mg daily Carbamazepine to oxcarbazepine dose conversion: 1.2 – 1.5x carbamazepine dose Extended release – take on empty stomach 1 hour before or 2 hours after meals	**WARNINGS** Hypersensitivity reactions to carbamazepine have 25-30% cross-sensitivity to oxcarbazepine ↑ risk for SJS/TEN, consider screening patients of Asian descent for HLA-B*1502 prior to initiating therapy. Hyponatremia – *more than w/ CBZ* Cardiac conduction abnormalities Hypothyroidism **SIDE EFFECTS** Somnolence, dizziness, headache, GI effects (nausea, vomiting, abdominal pain), diplopia, nystagmus, abnormal visual disturbances, ataxia, tremor, vitamin D and calcium deficiency (bone loss) **MONITORING** Serum Na⁺ levels especially during first 3 months of therapy (hyponatremia more common than with carbamazepine), thyroid function, CBC, mental status, seizure frequency **NOTES** Pregnancy Category C Supplementation with calcium and vitamin D recommended *Trileptal* oral suspension – once bottle is open use within 7 weeks.

Oxcarbazepine Drug Interactions

- Oxcarbazepine is a strong 3A4 inducer, but is not an auto-inducer.

- Oxcarbazepine is a strong 3A4/5 inducer. Oxcarbazepine can ↑ fosphenytoin, ↑ phenytoin, and ↓ hormonal contraceptive levels significantly. Use of an alternative, nonhormonal contraceptive is recommended.

- Caution for additive CNS effects, including dizziness, somnolence, fatigue.

Valproic Acid/Valproate

T-type calcium channel blocker and fast sodium channel blocker that ↑ gamma (γ)-aminobutyric activity (GABA), an inhibitory neurotransmitter. Valproic acid and divalproex dissociate to valproate in the GI tract.

DRUG	DOSING	SAFETY/SIDE EFFECTS/MONITORING
Valproate/Valproic acid (*Depakene, Stavzor, Depacon*) *Depakene* – capsule, syrup *Stavzor* – delayed-release capsule *Depacon* – IV **Divalproex** (*Depakote, Depakote ER, Depakote Sprinkle*) *Depakote* – delayed release tablet → ↓↓GI [handwritten: NOT bioequiv] *Depakote ER* – extended-release tablet 125-250mg BID [handwritten] *Depakote Sprinkle* – capsules can be opened and sprinkled on food Also used for bipolar and migraine prophylaxis Delayed-release divalproex ↓ GI upset	Initial: 10-15 mg/kg/day Maximum: 60 mg/kg/day **Therapeutic Range** 50-100 mcg/mL (some patients may need higher levels) Extended release tablets (*Depakote ER*) are not bioequivalent to delayed release tablets (*Depakote*). If the albumin is low (< 3.5 g/dL) the true valproate level will be higher than it appears – adjust with the same formula used for phenytoin.	**BOXED WARNINGS (4)** Hepatic Failure: Occurs rarely in adults (1:50,000) usually during first 6 months of therapy. Children (1:600) under the age of two years and patients with mitochondrial disorders are at higher risk. Monitor LFTs frequently during the first 6 months. Teratogenicity: Including neural tube defects (e.g., spina bifida) and ↓ IQ scores following *in utero* exposure. Pancreatitis: Can be fatal in children and adults. Mitochondrial Disease: ↑ risk of valproate-induced acute liver failure and death in patients with hereditary neurometabolic syndromes caused by DNA mutations in mitochondrial DNA polymerase gamma (POLG) gene. **CONTRAINDICATIONS** Significant hepatic disease, urea cycle disorders, prophylaxis of migraine in pregnancy, known mitochondrial disorders caused by mutations in mitochondrial DNA POLG or children < 2 years of age suspected of having a POLG-related disorder **WARNINGS** Hyperammonemia (treat with carnitine in symptomatic adults only), hypothermia [handwritten: ↑NH3] **SIDE EFFECTS** Nausea, vomiting, anorexia, abdominal pain, dizziness, somnolence, headache, tremor, alopecia (treat with a multivitamin containing selenium and zinc), weight gain, edema, polycystic ovary syndrome (PCOS), vitamin D and calcium deficiency (bone loss) Dose-related: thrombocytopenia, diplopia, blurred vision **MONITORING** * LFTs (at baseline and frequently during first 6 months), CBC with differential, platelets, serum drug concentrations, mental status changes, seizures **NOTES** Pregnancy Category D/X (for migraine prophylaxis) [handwritten: VA + pregnancy for migraine prophylaxis] Supplementation with calcium and vitamin D recommended

Valproic Acid/Valproate Drug Interactions

- Valproate is an inhibitor of 2C9 (weak) and can ↑ levels of lamotrigine [handwritten: 2-fold], phenobarbital, phenytoin, warfarin and zidovudine.

- Valproate is a substrate for several CYP450 enzymes; check for interactions.

- Use special caution with combination of valproate and lamotrigine due to risk of serious rash. Titrate slowly. Combination is synergistic.

- Combination with topiramate can lead to hyperammonemia ± encephalopathy. Salicylates displace valproate from albumin and ↑ levels.

- Carbapenems (imipenem, etc.) can ↓ the levels of valproic acid.

- Caution for additive CNS effects, including dizziness, somnolence, fatigue.

Phenytoin/Fosphenytoin

Fast sodium channel blockers that stabilize neuronal membranes and reduce seizures by increasing efflux or decreasing influx of Na+ ions.

DRUG	DOSING	SAFETY/SIDE EFFECTS/MONITORING
Phenytoin *(Dilantin, Dilantin Infatabs, Phenytek)* Capsule, chewable, suspension, injection Generalized tonic-clonic, complex partial; prevention of seizures following neurosurgery	Phenytoin: 15-20 mg/kg loading dose; up to 300-600 mg/d Fosphenytoin is dosed in phenytoin equivalents (PE): 1 mg PE = 1 mg phenytoin **Therapeutic Range** Total PHT: 10-20 mcg/mL Free PHT: 1-2.5 mcg/mL Exhibits saturable, or Michaelis-Menten, kinetics; a small change in dose can cause a large change in serum level If the albumin (alb) is low (< 3.5 g/dL), the true phenytoin level will be higher than it appears – adjust with formula below (if CrCl ≥ 10 mL/min) or measure a free phenytoin level. $$PHT\ correction = \frac{PHT\ measured}{(0.2 \times alb) + 0.1}$$ With CrCl < 10 mL/min and low albumin, use correction formula: $$PHT\ correction = \frac{PHT\ measured}{(0.1 \times alb) + 0.1}$$	**BOXED WARNINGS** Phenytoin IV administration should not exceed 50 mg/minute and fosphenytoin IV administration should not exceed 150 mg PE/minute; if faster hypotension and cardiac arrhythmias can occur. **WARNINGS** IV phenytoin is a vesicant; can cause venous irritation and "purple glove syndrome" (discoloration with edema and pain of distal limb); inject into a large vein slowly and follow with a saline flush. ↑ risk of SJS/TEN, Asian patients should be screened for HLA-B*1502 **SIDE EFFECTS** With IV route (may need to lower rate): Hypotension, bradycardia, arrhythmias, cardiovascular collapse Dose-related (toxicity): Ataxia, dizziness, somnolence, lethargy, nystagmus, slurred speech, confusion, blurred vision and diplopia Chronic: Skin thickening (children), gingival hyperplasia, hair growth, vitamin D and calcium deficiency (bone loss), connective tissue changes, coarsening of facial features, folate deficiency, hepatotoxicity Risk of SJS/DRESS
Fosphenytoin *(Cerebyx)* Prodrug of phenytoin (IV/IM) Injection		**MONITORING** LFTs, CBC with differential, serum trough concentration, mental status, seizure frequency. For IV, continuous cardiac monitoring (ECG, BP, HR). **NOTES** Pregnancy Category D Supplementation with folic acid, calcium and vitamin D recommended Strong CYP450 enzyme inducer Phenytoin IV is compatible with NS only, requires a filter and is stable for 4 hours; do not refrigerate as may cause precipitation (which may dissolve upon warming). Fosphenytoin can be mixed with NS or D5W and is refrigerated (stable for 48 hrs at room temperature; 30 days if refrigerated). IV:PO ratio is 1:1 Enteral feedings ↓ phenytoin absorption; hold feedings 1-2 hours prior and 1-2 hours after phenytoin administration

Handwritten annotations:

IV max 50 mg/min (faster ⇒ ↓↓↓ bp, ♡ arrhythmias)

extravasation phlebitis

IV vesicant!

IV mix w/ NS [ONLY] filter stable x 4 hrs ⊘ fridge

LUPUS

↓ macrocytic anemia

PRODRUG dosed in PE (phenytoin equiv.)

IV max 150 mg PE/min (faster ⇒ ↓↓↓ bp, ♡ arrhythmias)

mix w/ NS or D5W fridge (stable x 30 days) * room temp ⇒ stable x 48 hrs

* takes 15-30 min to be converted to phenytoin

* causes less ↓bp than phenytoin ⇒ can be pushed in faster

folate sources bread cereal Rx - supplement (1mg folic acid qd) * OR OTC ⇒ 800 µg

Phenytoin/Fosphenytoin Drug Interactions

- Phenytoin and fosphenytoin are strong inducers of several CYP450 enzymes, including 2C19, 2C8/9, 3A4 and P-gp. These 2 drugs can lower the concentration of many drugs including other anticonvulsants, contraceptives, warfarin, etc.

- Use of an alternative, non-hormonal contraceptive is recommended.

- Caution for additive CNS effects, including dizziness, somnolence, fatigue.

- These agents have high protein binding [fosphenytoin (95-99%)/phenytoin (90-95%)]; they can displace other highly-protein bound drugs. Other drugs can displace fosphenytoin/phenytoin, causing an ↑ in levels and potential toxicity.

Topiramate

Fast sodium channel blocker, enhances γ-aminobutyric activity, antagonizes the alpha-amino-3-hydroxy-5-methyl-4-isoxazolepropionic acid (AMPA)/kainate subtype of the glutamate receptors, and weakly inhibits carbonic anhydrase.

DRUG	DOSING	SAFETY/SIDE EFFECTS/MONITORING
Topiramate (*Topamax, Topiragen, Topamax Sprinkle*) Topiramate extended-release (*Qudexy XR, Trokendi XR*) Adjunctive therapy for partial seizure, primary generalized tonic-clonic seizure, or Lennox-Gastaut syndrome, or conversion to primary therapy from older drugs Capsule, extended-release capsule, tablet Also used for migraine prophylaxis *Topamax* Sprinkle Capsules: May be swallowed whole or opened to sprinkle the contents on a small amount (~1 teaspoon) of soft food (drug/food mixture should not be chewed; swallow immediately)	Week 1: 25 mg BID (IR) or 50 mg daily (XR) Week 2: 50 mg BID (IR) or 100 mg daily (XR) Week 3: 75 mg BID (IR) or 150 mg daily (XR) Week 4: 100 mg BID (IR) or 200 mg daily (XR) ↑ by 100 mg weekly until max dose or therapeutic effect Maximum: 400 mg/day ↓ dose by 50% if CrCl < 70 mL/min	**CONTRAINDICATIONS** *Trokendi XR* only – recent alcohol use (within 6 hours prior to and 6 hours after dose) **WARNINGS** Hyperchloremic nonanion gap metabolic acidosis due to inhibition of carbonic anhydrase and ↑ renal bicarbonate loss. Dose reduction or discontinuation (by tapering dose) should be considered in patients with persistent or severe metabolic acidosis. Oligohydrosis (reduced perspiration)/hyperthermia (mostly in children) – try to limit sun and hydrate Nephrolithiasis (kidney stones) – keep hydrated Acute myopia and secondary angle closure glaucoma Hyperammonemia – alone and with co-administration of valproate Visual problems (reversible) – consider discontinuation **SIDE EFFECTS** Somnolence, dizziness, difficulty with memory, difficulty with concentration/attention, cognitive problems, psychomotor slowing, paresthesias, weight loss, anorexia, mood changes, ↓ sodium bicarbonate concentrations, vitamin D and calcium deficiency (bone loss) **MONITORING** Hydration status, electrolytes (especially bicarbonate), SCr, BUN, mental status, seizure frequency **NOTES** Pregnancy Category D – use during pregnancy can cause cleft lip and/or palate in newborn Supplementation with calcium and vitamin D recommended

Handwritten margin notes: ≠ EtOH use w/in 6-hrs of dose; tingling in arms/legs

Topiramate Drug Interactions

- Topiramate is an inhibitor of (2C19) (weak) and inducer of 3A4 (weak/moderate).

- Topiramate may ↓ oral contraceptive effectiveness, especially with higher doses (≥ 200 mg/day). Use of an alternative, non-hormonal contraceptive is recommended.

- Caution for additive CNS effects, including dizziness, somnolence, fatigue.

Pregabalin/Gabapentin

These agents bind to the alpha-2-delta subunit of voltage-dependent calcium channels within the CNS, inhibiting excitatory neurotransmitter release.

DRUG	DOSING	SAFETY/SIDE EFFECTS/MONITORING
Pregabalin *(Lyrica)* Adjunctive therapy for adult patients with partial onset seizures Diabetic or spinal cord injury neuropathic pain, postherpetic neuralgia, fibromyalgia C-V Capsule, solution	Initial: 75 mg BID Maximum: 600 mg/day ↓ dose and/or extend the interval if CrCl < 60 mL/min	**WARNINGS** Angioedema and peripheral edema **SIDE EFFECTS** Dizziness, somnolence, peripheral edema, weight gain, ataxia, diplopia, blurred vision, dry mouth, mild euphoria ✳ ↳ CX **MONITORING** Edema/weight gain, mental status, seizure frequency **NOTES** Pregnancy Category C Often used for neuropathic pain treatment
Gabapentin *(Neurontin)* *Gralise* – postherpetic neuralgia *Horizant* – postherpetic neuralgia and restless leg syndrome Capsule, tablet, solution XR ~ w/ food	Initial: 300 mg TID Maximum: 3,600 mg/day ↓ dose and/or extend the interval if CrCl < 60 mL/min	**SIDE EFFECTS** Dizziness, somnolence, ataxia, peripheral edema, weight gain, diplopia, blurred vision, dry mouth **MONITORING** Edema/weight gain, mental status, seizure frequency **NOTES** Pregnancy Category C Used more often for off-labeled uses such as fibromyalgia, pain, headache, peripheral neuropathy, drug abuse, alcohol withdrawal Take extended-release formulation with food

Pregabalin/Gabapentin Drug Interactions

- No significant drug-drug interactions; renally eliminated. Use caution with pregabalin and glitazones concurrently due to risk of additive edema.

- Caution for additive CNS effects, including dizziness, somnolence, fatigue.

Phenobarbital/Primidone

These agents enhance gamma (γ)-aminobutyric acid (GABA)-mediated chloride influx; shift in Cl⁻ ions results in hyperpolarization (a less excitable state) and membrane stabilization.

DRUG	DOSING	SAFETY/SIDE EFFECTS/MONITORING
PHENobarbital C-IV Barbiturate Tablet, solution, elixir, injection Generalized tonic-clonic, status epilepticus, and partial seizures	Initial: 50-100 mg 2 or 3 times daily t½:~100 hrs **Therapeutic Range** 20-40 mcg/mL in adults 15-40 mcg/mL in children	**CONTRAINDICATIONS** Marked hepatic impairment, dyspnea or airway obstruction, SC administration **WARNINGS** *anxiety, tremor, weakness, dizziness, insomnia, orthostasis, seizures, delirium* Do not discontinue abruptly as seizures can result (applies to all anticonvulsants); withdrawal symptoms will ↑ seizure risk Paradoxical reactions, including hyperactive or aggressive behavior, particularly in acute pain and pediatric patients Hypotension especially when given IV Serious skin reactions, including SJS/TEN
Primidone *(Mysoline)* Prodrug of phenobarbital and phenylethylmalonamide (PEMA) – both are active metabolites Barbiturate Tablet Generalized tonic-clonic, pyschmotor, and focal seizures	Initial: 100-125 mg QHS Maximum: 2 g/day	**SIDE EFFECTS** Somnolence, cognitive impairment, dizziness/ataxia, physiological dependence, tolerance, hangover effect, depression, vitamin D and calcium deficiency (bone loss), respiratory depression, folate deficiency **MONITORING** LFTs, CBC with differential, mental status, serum drug concentration, seizure frequency **NOTES** Pregnancy Category D Supplementation with calcium and vitamin D recommended Strong CYP450 enzyme inducers

Phenobarbital/Primidone Drug Interactions

- Phenobarbital (primidone is the prodrug) is a strong inducer of most CYP enzymes, including 1A2, 2C8/9, 3A4 and P-gp. These two drugs will lower the levels of the many drugs metabolized by these enzymes.

- Use of an alternative, non-hormonal contraceptive is recommended.

- Caution for additive CNS effects, including dizziness, somnolence, fatigue.

digoxin
0.5-0.9 ng/ml (HF)
0.8 - 2 ng/ml (a fib)

tx ranges
CBZ = 4-12 µg/ml
valproate = 50 - 100 µg/ml
total PHT = 10 - 20 µg/ml
ethosux = 40 - 100 µg/ml
phenobarb = 20 - 40 µg/ml (adults)
15 - 40 µg/ml (children)

Ethosuximide

T-type calcium channel blocker that ↑ seizure threshold and suppresses paroxysmal spike-and-wave pattern in absence seizures.

DRUG	DOSING	SAFETY/SIDE EFFECTS/MONITORING
Ethosuximide *(Zarontin)* One of the drugs of choice for absence Capsule, solution	Initial: 500 mg daily Maximum: 1,500 mg/day Therapeutic range 40-100 mcg/mL	**WARNINGS** Rash, including SJS/TEN and drug rash with eosinophilia and systemic symptoms (DRESS) **SIDE EFFECTS** GI upset (weight loss, abdominal pain, nausea and vomiting), hiccups, dizziness, somnolence **MONITORING** LFTs, CBC with differential, platelets, signs of rash, serum drug concentrations, seizure frequency.

Ethosuximide Drug Interactions

- Ethosuximide is a major 3A4 substrate; look for 3A4 inducers and inhibitors.

- Valproic acid can ↑ ethosuximide levels.

- Caution for additive CNS effects, including dizziness, somnolence, fatigue.

Lacosamide

Slow sodium channel blocker, thereby stabilizing hyperexcitable neuronal membranes.

DRUG	DOSING	SAFETY/SIDE EFFECTS/MONITORING
Lacosamide *(Vimpat)* C-V Tablet, solution, injection Monotherapy or adjunctive therapy for partial-onset seizures ↑ PR	Initial: 50-100 mg BID Maximum: 400 mg/day Max dose is 300 mg if CrCl ≤ 30 mL/min	**WARNINGS** Lacosamide prolongs PR interval and ↑ risk of arrhythmias. Obtain an ECG prior to use and after titrated to steady state. Use with caution in patients with cardiac conduction problems and severe cardiac disease (MI, HF). **SIDE EFFECTS** Dizziness, headache, fatigue, ataxia, nausea, vomiting, diplopia, blurred vision, tremor, euphoria **MONITORING** ECG (baseline and at steady state), mental status, seizure frequency **NOTES** Pregnancy Category C

Lacosamide Drug Interactions

- No clinically significant drug interactions.

OTHER ANTICONVULSANTS

DRUG	MOA	SAFETY/SIDE EFFECTS/MONITORING
Benzodiazepines, including: CloBAZam (*Onfi*) Adjunctive with Lennox-Gastaut syndrome C-IV	Enhances GABA	**WARNINGS** Serious skin reactions, including SJS/TEN **NOTES** Causes physiological dependence, tolerance, drooling, pyrexia Inducer of 3A4 (weak/moderate) Supplementation with calcium and vitamin D recommended
Eslicarbazepine (*Aptiom*) Major active metabolite of oxcarbazepine Tablet	Fast Na+ channel blocker	**NOTES** Same warnings and side effects as oxcarbazepine including ↓ Na↑; monitor. Inducer of 3A4 (weak/moderate) Supplementation with calcium and vitamin D recommended
Ezogabine (*Potiga*) Refractory partial seizures C-V Tablet	Binds the KCNQ voltage-gated K+ channels, enhancing the M-current and suppressing seizure activity	**BOXED WARNING** Retinal abnormalities that can progress to vision loss in ~33% of patients after 4 years of treatment **WARNINGS** Skin discoloration (mostly blue) Urinary retention QT prolongation **NOTES** Requires eye exam at baseline and every 6 months Monitor QT interval Urine discoloration (orange, red, brown)
Felbamate (*Felbatol*) Refractory seizures Tablet, suspension	↑ GABA activity, NMDA receptor blocker	**BOXED WARNINGS (2)** Hepatic Failure and Aplastic Anemia **NOTES** Requires LFT and CBC monitoring Informed consent needs to be signed by patient and prescriber prior to dispensing
Perampanel (*Fycompa*) C-III Tablet	Alpha-amino-3-hydroxy-5-methyl-4-isoxazolepropionic acid (AMPA) glutamate receptor blocker	**BOXED WARNING** Risk of neuropsychiatric events (dose related), including irritability, aggression, anger, paranoia and others mostly in the first 6 weeks **NOTES** Inducer of 3A4 (weak/moderate) Supplementation with calcium and vitamin D recommended
Rufinamide (*Banzel*) Lennox-Gastaut syndrome only Tablet, suspension	Fast Na+ channel blocker	**CONTRAINDICATIONS** Familial short QT syndrome due to QT shortening (dose related) **NOTES** Take with food
TiaGABine (*Gabitril*) Tablet	Blocks GABA reuptake in the presynaptic neurons	**WARNINGS** Worsening of seizures/new onset seizures when used off-label for other indications, SJS/TEN **NOTES** Take with food

(handwritten annotations: "↑QT" next to Ezogabine; "↓QT" next to Rufinamide)

DRUG	MOA	SAFETY/SIDE EFFECTS/MONITORING
Vigabatrin (*Sabril*) Refractory complex partial seizures and infantile spasms Tablet, packet for solution	Irreversibly inhibits GABA transaminase, ↑ levels of GABA	**BOXED WARNING** Causes permanent vision loss (≥ 30% of patients) **MONITORING** Eye exam at baseline, every 3 months during therapy and every 3-6 months after discontinuation of therapy **NOTES** Only available through SHARE distribution program (Support, Help And Resources for Epilepsy)
Zonisamide (*Zonegran*) Capsule *topiramate's cousin* *⊖ ↑NH₃*	Fast Na⁺ channel blocker, T-type Ca²⁺ channel blocker and weak carbonic anhydrase inhibitor	**CONTRAINDICATIONS** Hypersensitivity to sulfonamides **WARNINGS** Same as topiramate but no hyperammonemia warning **SIDE EFFECTS** Side effects similar to topiramate, including oligohydrosis (primarily in children) and risk of nephrolithiasis; requires hydration, risk SJS/TEN **NOTES** Pregnancy Category C Supplementation with calcium and vitamin D recommended

Significant Toxicities

ADVERSE EFFECT	ASSOCIATED DRUGS	
Teratogenicity*	Carbamazepine Clonazepam Phenobarbital	Phenytoin Topiramate Valproic Acid
Hepatotoxicity	Carbamazepine Felbamate Phenobarbital/Primidone	Phenytoin Valproic Acid
Decreases efficacy of oral contraceptives	Carbamazepine Clobazam Oxcarbazepine Perampanel	Phenobarbital Phenytoin Primidone Topiramate (≥ 200 mg/day)
Fatal pancreatitis	Valproic Acid	
Aplastic anemia	Carbamazepine (and agranulocytosis)	Felbamate
Skin rash (Stevens-Johnson syndrome)	Carbamazepine Lamotrigine Oxcarbazepine Phenobarbital	Phenytoin/Fosphenytoin Tiagabine Zonisamide

Other Anticonvulsants Continued

ADVERSE EFFECT	ASSOCIATED DRUGS	
Oligohydrosis – inability to sweat, risk of heat stroke – highest risk in children	Topiramate	Zonisamide
Nephrolithiasis (kidney stones)	Topiramate	Zonisamide
Weight gain	Valproic Acid Gabapentin	Pregabalin
Weight loss	Felbamate Ethosuximide	Topiramate Zonisamide
Hyponatremia	Carbamazepine	Oxcarbazepine (more common)

*   *Patients should be encouraged to enroll in the North American Antiepileptic Drug (NAAED) Pregnancy Registry if they become pregnant. This registry is collecting information about the safety of antiepileptic drugs during pregnancy (aed-pregnancyregistry.org).*

Patient Counseling for All Anticonvulsants

- Like other seizure medications, this drug can cause suicidal thoughts or actions in a very small number of people (about 1 in 500). Call your healthcare provider right away if you experience thoughts about suicide or dying, new or worsening depression or anxiety, panic attacks, irritability or other unusual behavior. Dispense MedGuide and instruct patient/family to read it.

- Do not stop taking this medication without consulting your healthcare provider. Seizures may become worse when the drug is suddenly stopped. When stopping therapy, the dose needs to be gradually decreased.

- Seizure medications can impair judgment, thinking and coordination. You may experience dizziness and drowsiness, especially when starting therapy.

- Do not drive, operate heavy machinery, or do other dangerous activities until you know how this medication affects you.

- Pharmacist: all have additive sedative/dizziness/confusion side effects with CNS depressants, including alcohol, barbiturates, benzodiazepines, hypnotics, opioids and skeletal muscle relaxants. Avoid use of other sedating drugs, if possible. Counsel patients about additive risk.

- Avoid drugs that can lower the seizure threshold (see chart at the beginning of the chapter). Avoid St. John's Wort with all anticonvulsants.

- Use caution with different generic substitutions; try to stick to the same manufacturer. Small dosage variations can result in loss of seizure control.

Carbamazepine

- The most common side effects include sleepiness, dizziness, nausea, vomiting and problems with coordination. Take with food to decrease stomach upset.

- Carbamazepine can cause rare but very serious (possibly fatal) skin reactions. If you are of Asian descent, you must have a blood test prior to using this medicine to determine if you are at greater risk of developing a serious skin reaction. The serious skin reactions usually develop within the first few months of treatment. Seek immediate medical attention if you feel weak and feverish, develop a skin rash, hives, sores in your mouth, or blistering or peeling of the skin.

SJS 1st few months

CBZ rash may be mild/ transitory or serious/ life-threatening (SJS)

Significant Toxicities Continued

- Carbamazepine can cause rare but serious blood problems (aplastic anemia or agranulocytosis). You will need to have your blood checked to make sure this is not occurring. Contact your healthcare provider right away if you develop fever, sore throat, other infections, easy bruising or bleeding, red or purple spots on your body or severe weakness and tiredness.

- Carbamazepine is FDA pregnancy category D. This means that the drug is known to be harmful to an unborn baby. Do not take this drug without first talking to your doctor if you are pregnant or are planning a pregnancy.

- This medication can lower the amount of vitamin D and calcium in your body; it is recommended to supplement with calcium and vitamin D while taking this medication.

Lamotrigine

- Side effects of this medication include sleepiness, dizziness, rash, nausea, vomiting, insomnia, lack of coordination, headache, or blurred or double vision.

- This medication can cause a serious skin rash. These serious skin reactions are more likely to happen in the first 2 to 8 weeks of treatment (but it can happen in people who have taken the medication for any period of time). Call your healthcare provider right away if you develop a fever, skin rash, hives, swollen lymph glands, sores in the mouth or around your eyes or unusual bleeding or bruising.

- This medication can rarely cause aseptic meningitis, which is a serious inflammation of the protective membrane of the brain. Call your healthcare provider right away if you develop a stiff neck, headache, fever, abnormal sensitivity to light, muscle pains, chills and/or confusion.

- Swallow tablets whole.

- The ODT formulation should be placed on the tongue and moved around the mouth to rapidly disintegrate.

- Chewable tablets can be swallowed whole, chewed, or mixed in water or diluted fruit juice. If mixed, take the whole amount right away.

Levetiracetam

- Take levetiracetam with or without food.

- Swallow the tablets whole. Do not chew, break, or crush tablets. Ask your healthcare provider for levetiracetam oral solution if you cannot swallow tablets.

- If taking levetiracetam oral solution, be sure to use a medicine dropper or medicine cup to help you measure the correct amount of levetiracetam oral solution. Do not use a household teaspoon or tablespoon.

Oxcarbazepine

- This medication can cause low sodium concentrations in the blood. Symptoms of low blood sodium include nausea, tiredness or lack of energy, headache, more frequent or more severe seizures and confusion.

- Take oxcarbazepine with or without food. Take oxcarbazepine extended release (*Oxtellar XR*) on an empty stomach.

- Before taking oxcarbazepine oral suspension, shake the bottle for at least 10 seconds and use the oral dosing syringe to withdraw the amount of medicine needed. The dose may be taken directly from the oral syringe or may be mixed in a small glass of water immediately prior to swallowing. Rinse syringe with warm water after use and allow to dry thoroughly. Discard any unused portion after 7 weeks of first opening the bottle.

- This medication can lower the amount of vitamin D and calcium in your body; it is recommended to supplement with calcium and vitamin D while taking this medication.

Phenobarbital ↓ folic acid (like (fos) phenytoin) but don't supplement ??

- This is a federally controlled substance (C-IV) because it can cause abuse and dependence.
- This medication can slow your thinking and reflexes. Do not drive, operate heavy machinery, or do other dangerous activities until you know how this medication affects you.
- This medication can lower the amount of vitamin D and calcium in your body; it is recommended to supplement with calcium and vitamin D while taking this medication.

Phenytoin

- This medication can lower the amount of folic acid, vitamin D and calcium in your body; it is recommended to supplement with folic acid, calcium and vitamin D while taking this medication.
- Call your healthcare provider right away if you develop a skin rash, hives, fever, swollen lymph glands, sores in the mouth or unusual bleeding or bruising.
- This medicine can cause inflammation of your gums. Brush and floss regularly; do not miss dental cleanings or appointments.
- Phenytoin is FDA pregnancy category D. This means the drug is known to be harmful to an unborn baby. Do not take phenytoin without first talking to your doctor if you are pregnant or are planning a pregnancy.
- If using the suspension, shake the bottle well before each dose.
- Use this medication regularly in order to get the most benefit from it. It is important to take all doses on time to keep the amount of medicine in your body at a constant level.

Topiramate → paresthesia

- The most common side effects of this medication include sleepiness, dizziness, difficulty with memory, tingling of the arms and legs, weight loss and loss of appetite.
- This medication may cause eye problems. Please contact your healthcare provider right away if you experience a sudden decrease in vision with or without eye pain and redness. Rarely, this medicine can increase the pressure in the eye. This can lead to permanent loss of vision if not treated.
- Topiramate may cause decreased sweating and increased body temperature. Children in particular should be watched for signs of decreased sweating and fever especially in hot weather. Keep your child out of direct sunlight and heat and have the child drink plenty of water when going outside when it is hot.
- Topiramate can increase the level of acid in your blood (metabolic acidosis). Contact your healthcare provider right away if you feel tired, have a loss of appetite, feel changes in heartbeat, or have trouble thinking clearly.
- Topiramate Sprinkle Capsules may be swallowed whole or may be opened and sprinkled on a teaspoon of soft food. Drink fluids right after eating the food and medicine mixture to make sure it is all swallowed. Do not chew the food and medicine mixture. Do not store any medicine and food mixture for later use.
- Drink plenty of fluids during the day. This helps prevent kidney stones while taking this medication.
- This medication may affect how you think and can cause confusion, problems with concentration, attention, memory, or speech. It may also cause depression or mood problems, tiredness, and sleepiness.
- Topiramate is FDA pregnancy category D. This means the drug is known to be harmful to an unborn baby. An increased risk of oral clefts (cleft lip and/or palate) has been observed, particularly following first trimester exposure.
- This medication can lower the amount of vitamin D and calcium in your body; it is recommended to supplement with calcium and vitamin D while taking this medication.

Valproic Acid

- This medication can rarely cause liver failure. This is more likely to occur in the first 6 months of therapy. Call your healthcare provider right away if you develop severe fatigue, vomiting, loss of appetite, pain on the right side of your stomach, dark urine, light stools or yellowing of your skin or whites of your eyes.

- In rare cases, valproic acid has caused severe, sometimes fatal, cases of pancreatitis (inflammation of the pancreas). Call your healthcare provider right away if you have severe stomach pain that you may also feel in your back or have nausea or vomiting that does not go away. These symptoms may be early signs of pancreatitis.

- Do not crush, chew, or break the capsules. Swallow them whole.

- Measure the liquid form of valproic acid with a special dose-measuring spoon or cup, not a regular teaspoon or tablespoon. If you do not have a dose-measuring device, ask your pharmacist for one.

- Valproic acid is FDA pregnancy category D for treating seizures. This means the drug is known to be harmful to an unborn baby. Malformations of the face and head, heart, and nervous system have been reported. In addition, children born to mothers taking valproate products while pregnant may have impaired mental development. Do not take valproic acid without first talking to your healthcare provider if you are pregnant or could become pregnant.

- Take with food to help avoid stomach upset.

- You will need to have blood tests during treatment. It is important for your healthcare provider to know how much medication is in the blood and how well your liver is working.

- Common side effects with this medication include nausea, vomiting, sleepiness, weakness, increased appetite, weight gain, double or blurry vision and hair loss.

- This medication can lower the amount of vitamin D and calcium in your body; it is recommended to supplement with calcium and vitamin D while taking this medication.

PRACTICE CASE

LK is a 35 y/o white female s/p MVA. She suffered a closed head injury, two broken ribs and a concussion. She had one seizure in the emergency room. During her hospital stay, she was initially treated with fosphenytoin then continued on phenytoin. She has no past medical history and does not smoke or drink alcohol. Her medications, vitals, and labs on the day of discharge are as follows:

Allergies: PCN, sulfa, "quinolones" and latex

Discharge Medications:
Phenytoin 100 mg PO TID
Norco 5/325 mg 1-2 tabs Q6 hours PRN pain #10
Patient states that she will continue her home medications, which include:
Loestrin 1 tab PO daily
Fish oil softgels 2 with dinner for "cholesterol"
Valerian root 3 capsules at bedtime for "calm sleep"
B complex tablet daily with lunch

Vitals:
BP: 138/76 mmHg   HR: 85 BPM   RR: 14 BPM   Temp: 38°C   Pain: 4/10

Labs: Na (mEq/L) = 133 (135 - 145)
K (mEq/L) = 3.8 (3.5 - 5)
Cl (mEq/L) = 101 (95 - 103)
HCO_3 (mEq/L) = 26 (24 - 30)
BUN (mg/dL) = 10 (7 - 20)
SCr (mg/dL) = 0.7 (0.6 - 1.3)
Glucose (mg/dL) = 98 (100 - 125)
Ca (mg/dL) = 9.9 (8.5 - 10.5)
Mg (mEq/L) = 1.9 (1.3 - 2.1)
PO_4 (mg/dL) = 3.1 (2.3 - 4.7)
AST (IU/L) = 34 (8 - 48)
ALT (IU/L) = 42 (7 - 55)
Albumin (g/dL) = 4.2 (3.5 - 5)
Phenytoin (mcg/mL) = 11.7 (10 - 20)

Discharge patient with follow up in 1 week in the Internal Medicine clinic.

Questions

1. Lucinda is receiving phenytoin for her seizure control. What is one of the brand names for phenytoin?

    a. Trileptal
    b. Keppra
    c. Phenytek
    d. Stavzor
    e. Diastat _diazepam_ !

2. The medical resident asks the pharmacist to explain when a total phenytoin level needs to be adjusted for the albumin level. The pharmacist should give this response:

    a. The total phenytoin level will appear artificially low if the albumin is low – and should be adjusted.
    b. The total phenytoin level will appear artificially high if the albumin is low – and should be adjusted.
    c. The total phenytoin level will appear artificially low if the albumin is high – and should be adjusted.
    d. The total phenytoin level will appear artificially high if the albumin is high – and should be adjusted.
    e. Albumin levels have no effect on total phenytoin levels.

3. Lucinda will be counseled to recognize symptoms of acute phenytoin toxicity. Which of the following should be included? (Select **ALL** that apply.)

    a. Shakiness/walking unsteady
    b. Severe rash
    c. Double vision
    d. Nystagmus
    e. Osteomalacia

4. There is a serious drug interaction between Lucinda's birth control pills and phenytoin. Choose the correct counseling statement(s):

    a. Phenytoin will lower the amount of contraceptive medicine in her body.
    b. She will need to use a different type of contraceptive method.
    c. Phenytoin will increase the amount of contraceptive medicine in her body.
    d. A and B
    e. B and C

5. If Lucinda continues phenytoin long-term, which of the following medical condition(s) could result if she does not use proper supplementation? (Select **ALL** that apply.)

    a. Osteoporosis
    b. Vision loss
    c. Alopecia
    d. Arrhythmias
    e. Anemia

Questions 6-13 do not apply to the case.

6. A patient is going to receive phenytoin via infusion. Which of the following statements are correct? (Select **ALL** that apply.)

    a. Phenytoin has saturable kinetics.
    b. The maximum infusion rate is 100 mg/minute.
    c. The therapeutic level of total phenytoin is 10-20 mcg/mL.
    d. Phenytoin should be mixed in dextrose only. NS [for PHT = NS or D5W]
    e. The brand name of phenytoin is _Felbatol_.

7. A child has been receiving divalproex for seizure control. Unfortunately, the seizures are not well-controlled. The physician has ordered lamotrigine as adjunctive therapy, with a careful dose-titration. What is the reason that a slow titration is required when initiating lamotrigine?

    a. Risk of multi-organ hypersensitivity reaction
    b. Risk of cardiac myopathy
    c. Risk of fluid retention and heart failure
    d. Risk of severe, and potentially fatal, rash
    e. Risk of fulminant hepatic failure

8. What is the mechanism of action of phenobarbital?

    a. Enhances dopamine
    b. Enhances GABA
    c. Suppresses dopamine
    d. Suppresses GABA
    e. Fast sodium channel blocker

9. Which of the following drugs decrease sweating and can cause heat stroke in children, and requires counseling to parents to help children avoid the sun and keep hydrated? (Select **ALL** that apply.)

   a. Rufinamide
   b. Zonisamide
   c. Felbamate
   d. Topiramate
   e. Oxcarbazepine

10. Which of the following drugs can cause kidney stones and require counseling for adequate fluid intake?

    a. Topiramate
    b. Tiagabine
    c. Pregabalin
    d. Valproic Acid
    e. Carbamazepine

11. Which of the following drugs is a preferred agent for treating typical absence seizures?

    a. Ethosuximide
    b. Lamotrigine
    c. Felbamate
    d. Topiramate
    e. Ezogabine

12. You find a patient actively seizing and call 911. What steps should you take to ensure the patient is safe? (Select **ALL** that apply.)

    a. Turn the patient on their side
    b. Remove sharp or hard objects away from the patient seizing and support their head
    c. Insert a stick into the seizing patient's mouth to prevent them from swallowing their tongue
    d. Loosen the patient's clothes
    e. Time the seizure

13. Which of the following statements are true regarding status epilepticus? (Select **ALL** that apply.)

    a. It is a medical emergency.
    b. Lorazepam is preferred over other benzodiazepines since it has a longer duration of action in the CNS.
    c. Phenobarbital is preferred for patients still having seizure activity after the first-line agent is given.
    d. It is defined as sub-clinical seizure activity on an EEG.
    e. Phenytoin is the drug that should be used first-line to break status epilepticus.

Answers

1-c, 2-a, 3-a,c,d, 4-d, 5-a,e, 6-a,c, 7-d, 8-b, 9-b,d, 10-a, 11-a, 12-a,b,d,e, 13-a,b

Stroke vs. TIA
* TIA = "warning/mini stroke"
   ↳ stroke-like sx but no lasting damage
      (short duration of sx, ⊖ permanent brain injury)

STROKE

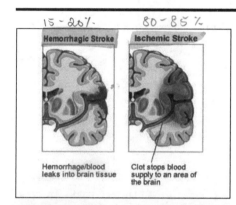

15-20%   80-85%

Hemorrhagic Stroke   Ischemic Stroke

Hemorrhage/blood leaks into brain tissue

Clot stops blood supply to an area of the brain

GUIDELINES

Guidelines for the Prevention of Stroke in Patients with Stroke and Transient Ischemic Attack. AHA/ASA. *Stroke* 2014; 45:2160-2236.

Guidelines for the Early Management of Patients with Acute Ischemic Stroke. AHA/ASA. *Stroke* 2013; 44:870-947.

Guidelines for the Management of Aneurysmal Subarachnoid Hemorrhage. AHA/ASA. *Stroke* 2012; 43:1711-1737.

Guidelines for the Management of Spontaneous Intracerebral Hemorrhage. AHA/ASA. *Stroke* 2010; 41:2108-2129.

BACKGROUND

A stroke, or cerebrovascular accident (CVA), occurs when blood flow to an area of the brain is interrupted by ischemia due to a clot (thrombus or emboli) or a ruptured blood vessel (hemorrhage). When a stroke occurs, brain cells in the immediate area are killed. When brain cells die, they release chemicals that set off a chain reaction that endanger brain cells in the larger, surrounding area of brain tissue called the penumbra. Without prompt medical treatment, this larger area of brain cells can also die. Acute ischemic stroke refers to a stroke caused by a thrombus or embolus and is more common than a hemorrhagic stroke. Intracerebral hemorrhage (ICH), subarachnoid hemorrhage (SAH) and subdural hematoma are all hemorrhagic strokes which indicate bleeding in the brain. Using agents that increase the risk of bleeding can be harmful (and fatal) in these cases.

When brain cells die, the abilities controlled by that area of the brain can be lost or impaired. Some people recover completely from less serious strokes, while others face chronic disability or loss of life. Stroke is the leading cause of disability and the 4th leading cause of death in the United States.

CLINICAL PRESENTATION & DIAGNOSIS

Signs and symptoms of a stroke can include the 5 "suddens":

- Sudden numbness or weakness of the face, arm or leg, especially on one side of the body (hemiplegia-paralysis on one side of the body, hemiparesis-weakness on one side of the body).

- Sudden confusion, trouble speaking or understanding

- Sudden trouble seeing in one or both eyes

- Sudden trouble walking, dizziness, loss of balance or co-ordination

- Sudden, severe headache with no known cause

Instruct the patient to call 9-1-1 immediately if any of these symptoms are present.

The evaluation of a stroke patient should be done expeditiously as time is brain. The clinical assessment (history, general exam, labs, and neurological exam) and stroke scales such as the National Institutes of Health Stroke Scale (NIHSS) assess severity of the stroke and provide prognostic information. Initial treatment includes supportive cardiac and respiratory care and quickly determining the nature of the lesion as ischemic or hemorrhagic via brain imaging. Brain imaging, either by computed tomography (CT) or, less commonly with magnetic resonance imaging (MRI), is essential to the diagnostic process and in selecting the appropriate treatment. Imaging should be interpreted within 45 minutes of the patient's arrival in the emergency department by a physician with expertise in reading these studies.

RISK FACTORS FOR STROKE
Hypertension – most common risk factor
Atrial Fibrillation
Gender (males > females)
Ethnicity (highest risk in African Americans)
Age ≥ 55 years
Atherosclerosis
Diabetes
Transient Ischemic Attack (TIA)
Prior history of stroke
Smoking
Dyslipidemia
Patent Foramen Ovale (PFO)
Sickle Cell Disease

ACT F.A.S.T. (TEST TO LOOK FOR SIGNS/SYMPTOMS OF STROKE)	
Face	Ask the person to smile. Does one side of the face droop or is it numb?
Arms	Ask the person to raise both arms. Does one arm drift downward?
Speech	Ask the person to repeat a simple sentence. Are the words slurred? Is the sentence repeated correctly?
Time	If the person shows any of these symptoms, even if the symptoms go away, call 9-1-1 immediately. Check the time so you know when the symptoms appeared. Brain cells are dying.

HEMORRHAGIC STROKE

Hemorrhagic strokes include intracerebral hemorrhage (ICH), subarachnoid hemorrhage (SAH) and subdural hematoma. Patients with hemorrhagic stroke should use intermittent pneumatic compression for the prevention of venous thromboembolism in addition to elastic stockings since anticoagulants should not be used while the patient is bleeding. Overall, treatment of a hemorrhagic stroke is largely supportive.

Drug Treatment of Intracerebral Hemorrhage

ICH has the highest mortality rate of all stroke subtypes. The progression of neurological deficits in many patients is frequently due to ongoing bleeding and enlargement of the he-

can cause herniated brainstem ⇒ death

matoma during the first few hours of the bleed. This can lead to an increase in ICP. Measures should be taken to lower the ICP such as elevating the head of the bed by 30 degrees and using mannitol. Patients with a severe coagulation factor deficiency or severe thrombocytopenia should receive appropriate factor replacement therapy or platelets, respectively. Prophylactic anticonvulsant medication should not be used.

Mannitol

Produces osmotic diuresis by increasing the osmotic pressure of glomerular filtrate, which inhibits tubular reabsorption of water and electrolytes and increases urinary output. Mannitol reduces ICP by withdrawing water from the brain parenchyma and excreting water in the urine.

DRUG	DOSING	SAFETY/SIDE EFFECTS/MONITORING
Mannitol (Osmitrol)	5%, 10%, 15%, 20%, 25% Mannitol 20% – 0.25-1 g/kg/dose IV every 6-8H: give over 20-30 minutes	**CONTRAINDICATIONS** Severe renal disease (anuria), severe dehydration, progressive heart failure, pulmonary congestion **WARNINGS** May accumulate in the brain (causing rebound increases in intracranial pressure) if circulating for long periods of time as with continuous infusion; intermittent boluses preferred. **SIDE EFFECTS** Fluid and electrolyte loss, dehydration, hyperosmolar-induced hyperkalemia, acidosis, ↑ osmolar gap **MONITORING** Renal function, daily fluid in's and out's, serum electrolytes, serum and urine osmolality, CPP, ICP, and BP *cerebral perfusion pressure* **NOTES** Vesicant Maintain serum osmolality < 300-320 mOsm/kg

Drug Treatment of Acute Subarachnoid Hemorrhage

Subarachnoid hemorrhage (SAH) is bleeding occurring in the space between the brain and the surrounding membrane (subarachnoid space). SAH usually results from rupture of a cerebral aneurysm or an arteriovenous malformation (AVM) or from traumatic brain injury. Surgical clipping, endovascular coiling or complete obliteration, when feasible, may be performed in patients with an aneurysm or AVM. SAH is associated with a high incidence of delayed cerebral ischemia 2 weeks following the stroke. Vasospasm is thought to be the cause of the delayed ischemia and can occur 4-21 days after the bleed. Oral nimodipine is used to prevent the vasospasm associated with delayed ischemia. The use of prophylactic anticonvulsants may be considered in the acute post hemorrhagic period to prevent seizures. The routine use of long-term anticonvulsants is not recommended, but may be considered for patients with known risk factors for delayed seizure disorder (e.g., prior seizure, intracerebral hematoma).

no drug tx for SAH
but prevent 2° stroke w/ po nimodipine

Nimodipine

Dihydropyridine calcium channel blocker shown to be more selective for cerebral arteries due to increased lipophilicity.

DRUG	DOSING	SAFETY/SIDE EFFECTS/MONITORING
NiMODipine *(Nymalize)* Capsule, solution	60 mg PO Q4H for 21 days Start therapy within 96 hours of the onset of subarachnoid hemorrhage Administer on an empty stomach, at least 1 hour before or 2 hours after meals	**BOXED WARNING** Nimodipine has inadvertently been administered IV when withdrawn from capsules into a syringe for subsequent nasogastric administration. Severe cardiovascular adverse events including death have occurred. *severe ↓↓ bp* **SIDE EFFECTS** Hypotension, bradycardia, headache, nausea **MONITORING** Cerebral perfusion pressure (CPP), ICP, BP, HR, neurological checks **NOTES** Label oral syringes "For oral use only". Pharmacy should draw up the medication to reduce medication errors.

Nimodipine Drug Interactions

- Nimodipine is a major 3A4 substrate; strong 3A4 inhibitors can increase the levels of nimodipine and strong 3A4 inducers can decrease the levels of nimodipine. Avoid concurrent use of grapefruit juice.

ISCHEMIC STROKE

Drug Treatment of Acute Ischemic Stroke

The goal of therapy is to maintain cerebral perfusion pressure (CPP) to the ischemic area, maintain normal ICP, control blood pressure and possibly remove the clot (e.g., *Merci Retrieval System* device, others) or dissolve the clot with alteplase *(Activase)* if within the safe time frame.

• nicardipine (Cardene®) } *favorable*
labetalol (Trandate®) } *data*
• ⊘ nitroprusside ⟹ ↑↑ ICP

Alteplase

Recombinant tissue plasminogen activator (rt-PA) causes fibrinolysis by binding to fibrin in a thrombus (clot) and converts entrapped plasminogen to plasmin.

dissolves fibrin

- only fibrinolytic indicated for stroke
- only start alteplase if still w/in 3-hr window of stroke sx onset (package insert)
* * 4.5 hrs (guidelines)*

[handwritten top margin:] severe h/a / acute HTN / N/V } d/c infusion / obtain ER CT scan

DRUG	DOSING	SAFETY/SIDE EFFECTS/MONITORING
Alteplase (Activase) Must confirm clot on brain imaging (head CT scan) before use	Infuse 0.9 mg/kg (maximum dose 90 mg) IV over 60 minutes with 10% of the dose given as a bolus over 1 minute Dosing is different for MI and pulmonary embolism indications Once reconstituted, use within 8 hours.	**CONTRAINDICATIONS** Active bleed, PLT count < 100,000/mm³, INR > 1.7, ↑ aPTT due to recent heparin use (within previous 48 hours), current use of direct thrombin inhibitors or direct factor Xa inhibitors, previous ICH, severe uncontrolled hypertension (> 185/110 mmHg), recent intracranial or intraspinal surgery, stroke or serious head injury within past 3 months, intracranial neoplasm, and many others. **SIDE EFFECTS** Major bleeding (e.g., ICH), hypotension, angioedema **MONITORING** Neurological assessments every 15 minutes during infusion, then every 30 minutes for next 6 hours, then hourly until 24 hours after treatment. Check BP every 15 minutes for the first 2 hours, then every 30 minutes for 6 hours, then hourly until 24 hours after treatment. Obtain follow-up brain imaging (head CT) at 24 hrs before starting anticoagulants and antiplatelets. **NOTES** Treatment must be initiated within 3 hours of symptom onset (guidelines state benefit in select patients up to 4.5 hours but this is not FDA approved). If severe headache, acute hypertension, nausea, or vomiting occurs, discontinue the infusion and obtain emergency CT scan. If patients are receiving fibrinolytic therapy, the drug should be given ≤ 60 minutes of the patient's arrival in the ED (door to needle time).

[handwritten notes, left margin:]
- *0.9 mg/kg (max 90 mg) IV over 60 min*
  - *10% given as bolus over 1 min*
- *√ neuro q15 min during infusion*
  - *then q30 min x next 6 hrs*
  - *then q hr until 24 hrs post tx*
  - *then q30 min x next 6 hrs*
  - *then q hr until 24 hrs post tx*
- *≤ 60 min door to needle time*

Alteplase Drug Interactions

- Most drug interactions are due to additive effects with other agents that can ↑ bleeding risk. See Drug Interactions chapter for drugs that can increase bleeding risk.

Additional Therapies in the Treatment of Acute Ischemic Stroke

Aspirin Therapy

[handwritten:] if no tPA

Aspirin 325 mg PO within 24 - 48 hours after stroke onset is recommended in most patients to prevent early recurrent stroke. Aspirin should not be given within 24 hours of fibrinolytic therapy.

Hypertension Management

Antihypertensives should be used to lower BP < 185/110 mmHg prior giving alteplase. In patients with malignant hypertension (> 220/120 mmHg), the BP should be ↓ by 15% during the first 24 hours after stroke onset.

Hyperglycemia Management

Maintain BG levels in the range of 140-180 mg/dL and closely monitor to prevent hypoglycemia.

DVT Prevention

SC anticoagulants should be given for DVT prophylaxis in immobilized patients. However, these agents should (not) be used within 24 hours of receiving alteplase therapy.

Arixtra?

Ischemic Stroke Prevention

Modifiable risk factors should be corrected.

- Hypertension – the use of ACE inhibitors and thiazide-type diuretics have shown a reduction in the risk of stroke in addition to lifestyle modifications. This recommendation also holds for patients (without) a history of hypertension as long as they can tolerate the BP reduction. It is reasonable to target SBP level < 140 mmHg and DBP < 90 mmHg. It may be reasonable to target a SBP of < 130 mmHg for patients with a lacunar stroke. *occlusion of penetrating artery that supplies blood to brain's deep structures*

- Dyslipidemia – treat according to the ACC/AHA 2013 lipid guidelines (see Dyslipidemia chapter).

- Diabetes – screening for diabetes should be done in the post stroke period; A1C is the preferred test during this time. Use of existing guidelines for glycemic control and BP targets in patients with diabetes is recommended for patients who have had a stroke or TIA.

- Metabolic syndrome – counsel on lifestyle modification (diet, exercise, and weight loss) for vascular risk reduction.

- Lifestyle changes including smoking cessation, increased physical exercise (at least 30 minutes most days of the week), weight reduction if necessary (maintain a BMI 18.5-24.9 kg/m² and a waist circumference < 35 inches for women and < 40 inches for men) and limit alcohol intake (≤ 2 drinks/day for males, ≤ 1 drink/day for females).

- Nutrition – it is reasonable to recommended sodium restriction to < 2.4 grams/day and further reduction < 1.5 grams/day for greater BP reduction. Follow a Mediterranean-type diet emphasizing vegetables, fruits, whole grains, low-fat dairy products, poultry, legumes and olive oil.

p. 620 (controversial)

Primary Prevention

Primary prevention for ischemic stroke is only recommended for patients with atrial fibrillation. See Anticoagulation chapter for more detail.

3 approved regimens:
① ASA
② ASA/dipyridamole ER
③ clopidogrel

Secondary Prevention

Patients with previous cardioembolic stroke should be placed on anticoagulant therapy for secondary stroke prevention. For patients with noncardioembolic ischemic stroke or TIA, the use of antiplatelet agents rather than oral anticoagulation is recommended to reduce the risk of recurrent stroke and other cardiovascular events. Aspirin, aspirin plus extended-release dipyridamole, or clopidogrel are all acceptable options for initial therapy. For patients allergic to aspirin, clopidogrel should be used. The combination of aspirin and clopidogrel can be considered for initiation within 24 hours of a minor ischemic stroke or TIA and continued for 90 days. When this combination is started days to years after a minor stroke or

2° stroke prevention
• previous cardioembolic stroke → place on anticoag
• previous [non]cardioembolic stroke → place on antiPLT

TIA, it ↑ the risk of hemorrhage and should not be used for routine secondary prevention after ischemic stroke or TIA.

For patients who have an ischemic stroke or TIA while taking aspirin, there is no evidence that ↑ the dose of aspirin provides additional benefit. Although alternative antiplatelet agents are often considered, no single agent or combination has been adequately studied in patients who have had an event while receiving aspirin.

Antiplatelet Therapy

Aspirin binds irreversibly to the cyclooxygenase-1 and 2 (COX-1 and 2) enzymes, resulting in ↓ prostaglandin (PG) and ↓ thromboxane A2 (TxA2) production; TxA2 is a potent vasoconstrictor and facilitates platelet aggregation. Aspirin has anti-platelet, antipyretic, analgesic, and anti-inflammatory properties. Clopidogrel inhibits $P2Y_{12}$ ADP-mediated platelet activation and aggregation. Dipyridamole inhibits the uptake of adenosine into platelets and increases cAMP levels, which indirectly inhibits platelet aggregation.

DRUG	DOSING	SAFETY/SIDE EFFECTS/MONITORING
Aspirin (Ascriptin, Bayer Aspirin, Bufferin, Bufferin Extra Strength, Ecotrin, St. Joseph Adult Aspirin, others)	50-325 mg daily	**CONTRAINDICATIONS** NSAID or salicylate allergy; patients with the syndrome of asthma, rhinitis, and nasal polyps; children < 16 years old with viral infection (due to Reye's syndrome risk) **SIDE EFFECTS** Dyspepsia, heartburn, GI upset, GI bleed/ulceration, bleeding, renal impairment, tinnitus (in toxicity) **MONITORING** Bleeding, bruising See Pain chapter for more information
Dipyridamole ER/Aspirin (Aggrenox)	200 mg/25 mg BID Protect from moisture; keep in original container	**CONTRAINDICATIONS** Allergy to NSAIDs; patients with the syndrome of asthma, rhinitis, and nasal polyps; children < 16 years of age with viral infections **SIDE EFFECTS** Headache (> 10%), dyspepsia, abdominal pain, nausea, diarrhea, and bleeding **MONITORING** Signs of bleeding; Hgb/Hct as necessary **NOTES** Amount of aspirin provided is not adequate for cardiac indications (e.g., MI prophylaxis)

Antiplatelet Therapy Continued

DRUG	DOSING	SAFETY/SIDE EFFECTS/MONITORING
Clopidogrel *(Plavix)* *PRODRUG !*	75 mg daily	**BOXED WARNING** Effectiveness depends on the activation to an active thiol metabolite mainly by CYP 2C19. Poor metabolizers exhibit higher cardiovascular events than patients with normal 2C19 function. Tests to check CYP 2C19 genotype can be used as an aid in determining a therapeutic strategy. Consider alternative treatment strategies in patients identified as 2C19 poor metabolizers. The CYP2C19*1 allele corresponds to fully functional metabolism while the CYP2C19*2 and *3 alleles have reduced function. **CONTRAINDICATIONS** Active pathological bleed (e.g., PUD, ICH) **WARNINGS** Avoid concurrent use of CYP2C19 inhibitors such as omeprazole or esomeprazole. Thrombotic thrombocytopenic purpura (TTP) has been reported; have patients report fever, weakness, extreme skin paleness, purple skin patches, yellowing of the skin or eyes, or neurological changes. **SIDE EFFECTS** Bleeding, bruising, rash, pruritus **MONITORING** Signs of bleeding; Hgb/Hct as necessary **NOTES** Do not start in patients likely to undergo CABG surgery and discontinue 5 days prior to any major surgery MedGuide required
Ticlopidine *Ticlid®* *✓ CBC q 2 wks* *x 1st 3 mo*	250 mg BID with food	**BOXED WARNINGS** May cause life-threatening hematologic reactions, including neutropenia, agranulocytosis, thrombotic thrombocytopenia purpura (TTP), and aplastic anemia. *↓ higher risk than w/ Plavix®* **SIDE EFFECTS** ↑ cholesterol (↑ TGs), N/V/D, rash, neutropenia, bleeding, pruritus **MONITORING** CBC every 2 weeks for first 3 months

(handwritten notes, left margin):
do NOT start in pts likely to undergo CABG

d/c 5 days prior to major surgery

Drug Interactions

- Most drug interactions are due to additive effects with other agents that can ↑ bleeding risk. See Drug Interactions chapter for drugs that can increase bleeding risk.

- Clopidogrel is a prodrug metabolized mainly by CYP 2C19. Avoid concomitant use with strong or moderate 2C19 inhibitors (cimetidine, fluconazole, ketoconazole, voriconazole, fluoxetine, fluvoxamine and others). Avoid concomitant use with omeprazole and esomeprazole as these agents may reduce the effectiveness of clopidogrel due to 2C19 inhibition.

GASTROESOPHAGEAL REFLUX DISEASE (GERD) & PEPTIC ULCER DISEASE (PUD)

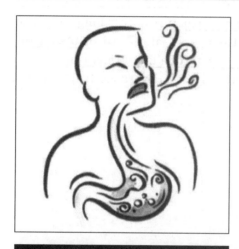

GUIDELINE

Katz PO, Gerson LB, Vela MF. Guidelines for the diagnosis and management of gastroesophageal reflux disease. *Am J Gastroenterol.* 2013; 108:308-28.

GASTROESOPHAGEAL REFLUX DISEASE (GERD)

Background

Gastroesophageal reflux disease (GERD) is a condition in which the stomach contents leak backward into the esophagus. Normally, gastric contents are prevented from backflow into the esophagus by a ring of muscle fibers called the lower esophageal sphincter (LES). In GERD, the LES pressure (muscle tone) is reduced (or transiently relaxes) and allows for backflow of the stomach contents. Typical symptoms of GERD include heartburn, hypersalivation, regurgitation and/or an acid taste in the mouth. Less commonly, symptoms can include recurrent cough, sore throat, hoarseness, and chest pain, which can be difficult to distinguish from cardiac pain. GERD can lead to esophageal erosion, strictures, bleeding and Barrett's esophagus, abnormal cell growth of the esophageal lining due to years of acid reflux which can lead to esophageal cancer.

The stomach epithelial lining contains parietal cells which secrete hydrochloric (HCl) acid and intrinsic factor, G cells which secrete gastrin, mucus-secreting cells, and chief cells which secrete pepsinogen. The parietal cells have receptors for histamine, acetylcholine. These substances stimulate HCl acid secretion by acting on the H^+/K^+ ATPase pumps located on the parietal cell wall.

Treatment Principles

Patient-reported symptoms are used in the initial diagnosis; invasive testing is not required when typical symptoms are present. Patients with alarm symptoms (chest pain, dysphagia, choking, hematemesis, black bloody stools) should be sent for further evaluation. An 8-week course of a proton pump inhibitor (PPI) is the treatment of choice for symptom relief, and is used to heal any erosive esophagitis. There are no major efficacy differences between the various PPIs. If symptoms persist after an 8 week treatment, maintenance PPIs can be used. Histamine-2 receptor antagonists (H$_2$RAs) can be used for maintenance if erosive disease is not present. Metoclopramide and sucralfate are not recommended. Some patients self-treat occasional and less bothersome symptoms with OTC antacids, H$_2$RAs or PPIs. Caution should be used with chronic acid suppression from H$_2$RAs and PPIs because of recent concerns of ↑ risk of GI infections (most commonly caused by *C. difficile)* and ↑ risk of nosocomial pneumonia in hospital-

RECOMMENDED NON-DRUG (LIFESTYLE) TREATMENT

- Weight loss – best evidence in improvement, per guidelines.

- Avoid foods that ↓ LES pressure, these are patient specific and can include: chocolate, caffeine, acidic/spicy food, and carbonated drinks.

- Avoid eating meals with high fat content 2-3 hours before bedtime.

- Elevate the head of the bed 6"-8" (not with pillows, but with a wedge, or by elevating the head-side of the bed under the mattress).

ized patients. In addition, PPIs ↑ risk of osteoporosis and fractures with long-term use. The use of H$_2$RAs in the elderly has risks. According to the Beers Criteria, all H$_2$RAs should be avoided in elderly patients with delirium, dementia or cognitive impairment because of adverse CNS effects that could make these worse. Be careful not to overdose H$_2$RAs. Renal impairment requires lower doses.

Drug Treatment

Antacids

Antacids work by neutralizing gastric acid (producing salt and water) thus increasing gastric pH. This provides relief within minutes since antacids do not require systemic absorption. Antacids work quickly, but the duration of relief is only 30 – 60 minutes. This makes antacids most suitable for mild, infrequent symptoms.

DRUG	DOSING	SAFETY/SIDE EFFECTS/MONITORING
Calcium carbonate *(Tums, others)* **Magnesium [Phillips Milk of Magnesia (MOM),** *others]* **Magnesium + (Aluminum or Calcium) combo** *(Maalox, Mylanta,* Rolaids, *others)* **Mag-Al-Simethicone (anti-gas)** *(Maalox Max, Mylanta Max* **Strength,** *others)* Sodium bicarbonate + aspirin + citric acid (*Alka-Seltzer Original)* Sodium bicarbonate *(Neut)* Antacid + alginic acid *(Gaviscon)* Calcium carbonate, magnesium hydroxide, famotidine *(Pepcid Complete)*	Many formulations including suspensions, chewable tablets, capsules 10-30 mL or 2-4 tablets 4-6x/day	**WARNINGS** Aluminum and magnesium can accumulate with severe renal dysfunction. Use is not recommended in patients with CrCl < 30 mL/min. **SIDE EFFECTS** Calcium may cause constipation or loose stools. Aluminum may cause constipation. Magnesium may cause loose stools (may use together to counter-balance, but still can get loose stools). Unpleasant taste. **NOTES** Onset of relief within minutes; lasts 30-60 minutes. Antacids are the drugs of choice in pregnancy. *Alka Seltzer Original* contains > 500 mg Na+ and 325 mg aspirin per tab. Sodium bicarbonate also used for metabolic acidosis with renal disease. Alginic acid in *Gaviscon* theoretically forms barrier to combat reflux (efficacy?).

Antacid Drug Interactions

- Decreased absorption with concomitant allopurinol, isoniazid, mycophenolate, integrase strand transfer inhibitors (INSTIs), quinolone and tetracycline antibiotics. Doxycycline and minocycline are less likely to be of clinical concern. Separate from these agents (2 hours before or 6 hours after ciprofloxacin, 2 hours before or 2 hours after levofloxacin, 4 hours before or 8 hours after moxifloxacin, 1-2 hours before or 4 hours after tetracycline). Gabapentin should be administered 2 hours after antacids. Thyroid products should be separated from antacids by at least 4 hours.

- Drugs that require an acidic gut for absorption will have ↓ absorption with antacids: Antacids have a short duration of action and can usually be separated from drugs that could interact; use caution with administration of calcium carbonate, iron, itraconazole, ketoconazole, the *Atelvia* formulation of risedronate, dasatinib, bosutinib, erlotinib, nilotinib, pazopanib, rilpivirine, and atazanavir.

Antacid Patient Counseling

- Recommend lifestyle counseling.

- This medicine provides immediate relief, but <u>lasts only about 30 - 60 minutes</u>. If you need a medication that lasts longer, please ask your healthcare provider.
- If you use this product more than 2 times per week, you may have a condition that requires stronger therapy. Discuss the symptoms with your healthcare provider.
- Do not use aluminum or magnesium products if you have advanced kidney disease.
- If you experience constipation, discontinue use of aluminum-containing products.
- If you experience loose stools, discontinue use of magnesium-containing products.
- Do not use antacids that contain sodium if you are on a sodium restricted diet, have heart disease, high blood pressure, heart failure or kidney disease.
- Do not use sugar-containing antacids if you have diabetes.
- Seek urgent care if you have bloody stools or vomit blood or material that looks like coffee grounds.

Histamine-2 Receptor Antagonists (H₂RAs)

H₂RAs <u>reversibly inhibit the H₂ receptors on the gastric parietal cells</u>, which ↓ gastric acid secretion. H₂RAs are used PRN for heartburn and scheduled for GERD. Higher doses are used for ulcer healing and hypersecretory conditions (Zollinger-Ellison syndrome). H₂RAs can be used as maintenance therapy for GERD in patients who experience relief while taking them (patients without erosions) or for patients who complete 8 weeks of PPI therapy (to heal erosions) and are able to remain symptom free on an H₂RA. This could ↓ side effects associated with long-term use of PPIs.

DRUG	DOSING	SAFETY/SIDE EFFECTS/MONITORING
Famotidine *(Pepcid, Pepcid AC, Pepcid AC Max Strength)* Tablet, Oral Suspension, Injection **+ calcium carbonate and magnesium hydroxide** *(Pepcid Complete)* + ibuprofen 800 mg *(Duexis)*	**OTC** 10-20 mg 1-2 times daily PRN **Rx** 20 mg BID	**WARNINGS** Confusion, usually reversible. Risk factors: <u>age > 50, renal or hepatic impairment (see notes)</u>. ECG changes with renal dysfunction (famotidine). Potential for vitamin B12 deficiency with prolonged use (≥ 2 years). **SIDE EFFECTS** Headache, agitation/vomiting in children < 1 year Cimetidine: <u>gynecomastia, impotence</u>
Ranitidine *(Zantac, Zantac Acid Reducer, Deprizine FusePaq Compounding Kit)* Tablet (OTC), Capsule (Rx), Oral Suspension and Syrup, Injection	**OTC** 75-150 mg 1-2 times daily PRN **Rx** 150 mg BID	**NOTES** Onset of relief: 30-45 minutes, duration: 4-10 hours. Generally no benefit to combining with a PPI, except if used at HS for a patient taking a PPI for daytime symptoms.
Nizatidine *(Axid, Axid AR)* Tablet (OTC), Capsule (Rx), Oral Solution	**OTC** 75 mg 1-2 times daily PRN **Rx** 150 mg BID	<u>Decrease dose</u> when CrCl < 50 mL/min (famotidine, ranitidine, nizatidine); CrCl < 30 mL/min (cimetidine). Cimetidine (and to a lesser extent famotidine and ranitidine) can ↑ SCr, without causing renal impairment. Acid suppressive therapy (including H₂RAs and PPIs) ↑ risk of GI <u>infections</u> (including *C. difficile* associated diarrhea) and may ↑ risk of <u>pneumonia</u> in hospitalized patients.
Cimetidine *(Tagamet, Tagamet HB)* Tablet, Injection	**OTC** 200 mg 1-2 times daily PRN **Rx** 400 mg Q6H	<u>Avoid all H₂RAs in elderly with delirium, dementia, cognitive impairment due to risk of adverse CNS effects per Beers Criteria. Avoid cimetidine entirely due to drug interactions and side effects.</u> Take with meals or OTC PRN 30-60 minutes before food causing heartburn.

H₂RA Drug Interactions

- Caution with use of concurrent CNS depressants: risk of additive delirium, dementia, cognitive impairment especially in the elderly. Use lower doses in elderly and renal impairment. <u>Avoid cimetidine entirely in elderly.</u>

- Drugs that require acidic medium for absorption will have reduced or eliminated absorption with antacids, H₂RAs and PPIs: <u>calcium carbonate, iron, itraconazole, ketoconazole, posaconazole, and atazanavir all require an acidic gut for adequate absorption – do not use acid suppressing agents or separate dosing from antacids</u>; dasatinib, pazopanib and risedronate *(Atelvia* formulation only) cannot be used with PPIs and H₂RAs, *Atelvia* can be used with antacids if separated. Rilpivirine and nelfinavir cannot be used with PPIs and requires separation from H₂RAs and antacids.

CIMETIDINE

- <u>Cimetidine is a CYP450 3A4 inhibitor</u> and weak to moderate inhibitor of other CYP450 enzymes. Avoid use with clopidogrel, dofetilide and warfarin. Use caution with many drugs including amiodarone, phenytoin, carbamazepine, quinidine, theophylline, SSRIs, and others.

H₂RA Patient Counseling

- Recommend lifestyle counseling.

- This medicine provides fast relief in about 30 - 45 minutes and it lasts 4 - 10 hours. If your symptoms remain bothersome, discuss with your healthcare provider.

- If you are self-treating for more than 14 days or more than 2 times per week and heartburn persists, discuss your symptoms with a healthcare provider.

- If elderly: This medication could cause you to be confused, dizzy, or have memory problems. If you notice this, discuss the symptoms with your healthcare provider.

WHAT IS ESOMEPRAZOLE STRONTIUM?

Esomeprazole strontium is not generic *Nexium*, but it has the same indications.

- Not approved for infants/children (concerns about bone growth with strontium)

- Pregnancy Category C vs. *Nexium* Category B

- 24.65 mg capsule = 20 mg esomeprazole base

- 49.3 mg = 40 mg esomeprazole base

Proton Pump Inhibitors (PPIs)

PPIs block gastric acid secretion by <u>irreversibly binding to the gastric H⁺/K⁺-adenosine triphosphatase (ATPase) pump in parietal</u> cells. This shuts down the proton pump. An 8-week course of PPI therapy is recommended for relief of GERD symptoms and to heal erosions that may be present. Any PPI can be selected, see table for recommended dosing. After 8 weeks of PPI therapy, symptoms should be reassessed. If symptoms continue, the lowest effective dose of PPI should be used. Intermittent and on-demand PPI therapy are additional options that patients use.

Recommended PPI Dosing for GERD

DRUG	TIMING
Dexlansoprazole (*Dexilant*)	<u>Without regard to meals</u> (pre-meal if needed for symptoms)
Esomeprazole magnesium (*Nexium*)	60 minutes before breakfast
Esomeprazole strontium	60 minutes before breakfast
Lansoprazole (*Prevacid*)	Before breakfast (time not specified)
Omeprazole (*Prilosec*)	Before breakfast (time not specified)
Omeprazole + sodium bicarbonate (*Zegerid*)	60 minutes before breakfast <u>(can also control nighttime symptoms if given at HS)</u>
Pantoprazole (*Protonix*)	30 minutes before breakfast
Rabeprazole (*AcipHex*)	30 minutes before meal (capsules) May take with or without food (tablets)

DRUG	DOSING	SAFETY/SIDE EFFECTS/MONITORING
Omeprazole (*PriLOSEC, PriLOSEC OTC*; *First-Omeprazole, Omeprazole+Syrspend SF Alka* suspension compounding kits) Tablet (OTC), Capsule, Packet, Suspension **+ sodium bicarbonate (*Zegerid, Zegerid OTC*)** Capsule, Packet	*Prilosec*: 20 mg daily *Zegerid* dosing based on omeprazole component: 20 mg daily	**WARNINGS** <u>Can ↑ risk of *C. difficile*-associated diarrhea (CDAD)</u> <u>Can ↑ osteoporosis-related fractures</u>, especially when used long-term <u>Can ↑ risk of pneumonia in hospitalized patients</u> <u>Hypomagnesemia</u> with long-term use; potential for vitamin B12 deficiency with prolonged use (≥ 2 years) **SIDE EFFECTS** Generally mild and infrequent (headache, diarrhea, nausea)
Pantoprazole (*Protonix*) Tablet, Injection, Packet	40 mg daily	**NOTES** PPIs are the most effective agents for severe disease/ symptoms
Lansoprazole (*Prevacid, Prevacid SoluTab, Prevacid 24H-OTC, First-Lansoprazole* suspension compounding kit) Soluble tablet, Capsule, Suspension	15-30 mg daily	All available PPIs have similar efficacy, although an individual patient may respond better to one agent than another
Dexlansoprazole (*Dexilant*) Capsule	30-60 mg daily	Dexlansoprazole, esomeprazole, lansoprazole, omeprazole, and rabeprazole capsules can be opened (not crushed) and mixed in apple sauce or acidic juice if patient cannot swallow pill or for NG tube delivery
Esomeprazole magnesium (*NexIUM, NeXIUM IV*) Capsule, Injection, Packet **+ naproxen 375 or 500 mg (*Vimovo*)** Esomeprazole strontium Capsule	20-40 mg daily (esomeprazole base) Esomeprazole strontium 24.65 mg = 20 mg esomeprazole base and 49.3 mg = 40 mg base	Do not crush, cut, or chew tablets or capsules <u>Pantoprazole and esomeprazole are the only PPIs available IV</u> *Zegerid* 20 mg and 40 mg have same Na$^+$ bicarb content; two 20 mg caps ≠ 40 mg cap; caution in patients on Na$^+$ restricted diet, each cap has 300 mg Na$^+$
RABEprazole (*AcipHex*) Tablet, Capsule Sprinkle	20 mg daily	Suspension kits contain pre-measured powdered drug, suspension liquid (with flavoring) and mixing tools; available in different sizes/strengths

PPI Drug Interactions

- Drugs that require acidic medium for absorption will have reduced or eliminated absorption with antacids, H₂RAs and PPIs: <u>calcium carbonate, iron, itraconazole, ketoconazole, posaconazole, erlotinib, and atazanavir all require an acidic gut for adequate absorption – do not use acid suppressing agents or separate dosing from antacids</u>; dasatinib, pazopanib and risedronate *(Atelvia* formulation only) cannot be used with PPIs and H₂RAs, *Atelvia* can be used with antacids if separated. Rilpivirine and nelfinavir cannot be used with PPIs and requires separation from H₂RAs and antacids. Avoid St. John's wort with PPIs.

- <u>PPIs inhibit CYP450 2C19</u>: Do not use with delavirdine, erlotinib, nelfinavir, and posaconazole. PPIs may ↑ levels of methotrexate, phenytoin, raltegravir, saquinavir, tacrolimus, voriconazole and warfarin.

- <u>PPIs may reduce the effectiveness of clopidogrel via 2C19 inhibition.</u> If using these agents together, <u>avoid omeprazole and esomeprazole.</u>

PPI Patient Counseling

- Recommend lifestyle counseling.
- Refer to chart and counsel accordingly: It is important to take your medicine 30 minutes before breakfast. It will work best to stop acid if taken this way.
- This medicine is not for immediate relief of heartburn and acid symptoms, you need to take it everyday as prescribed to get relief.
- If taking long-term, ensure that calcium and vitamin D intake is optimal. Recommend calcium citrate formulations (improved absorption in basic pH).
- If you are planning to stop this medicine, you should taper the dose to avoid acid rebound. Please discuss with your healthcare provider (recommend decreased dose, then every other day over at least a couple of weeks.)
- Effervescent and orally dissolving formulations *(Prevacid SoluTab)* contain phenylalanine. Do not use in patients with phenylketonuria (PKU).
- If you are self-treating for more than 14 days and heartburn persists, consult your healthcare provider.
- Do not crush or chew any capsules.
- *Prevacid SoluTab*: Do not swallow whole. Place on tongue and allow to dissolve (with or without water), then swallow.

Cytoprotective Agents

Misoprostol is a prostaglandin E_1 analog that replaces the gastro-protective prostaglandins removed by NSAIDs.

Sucralfate is in a sucrose-sulfate-aluminum complex and can interact with albumin and fibrinogen to form a physical barrier over an open ulcer. This protects the ulcer from further insult by HCl acid, pepsin, and bile and allows it to heal.

DRUG	DOSING	SAFETY/SIDE EFFECTS/MONITORING
Misoprostol *(Cytotec)*	Start at 100 mcg right after dinner, increase (if tolerated) to 100 mcg QID or 200 mcg QID. Take right after meals and at bedtime.	**BOXED WARNINGS (2)** Abortifacient – warn patients not to give this drug to others; do not use to ↓ NSAID-induced ulcers in women of childbearing potential unless capable of complying with effective contraceptive measures. **SIDE EFFECTS** Diarrhea, abdominal pain **NOTES** Pregnancy Category X
Sucralfate *(Carafate)*	1 g tablets QID before meals and at bedtime (usual), may be given 1 g Q4H (for treatment of active ulcer)	**WARNINGS** Caution in renal impairment – sucralfate is in an aluminum complex and can accumulate. **SIDE EFFECTS** Constipation **NOTES** Used only as an adjunct for GERD or peptic ulcer disease; no longer recommended by the ACG GERD guidelines.

Sucralfate Drug Interactions

- Avoid taking antacids 30 minutes before or 30 minutes after taking sucralfate.
- Avoid other drugs 2 hours before or 4 hours after administering sucralfate (difficult to use).

Misoprostol Patient Counseling

- Do not use in women of childbearing age unless strict compliance with contraceptive measures.
- Can start with 100 mcg right after dinner (with food in stomach), attempt to increase as-directed. Use of psyllium *(Metamucil)* may help decrease diarrhea.

Sucralfate Patient Counseling

- Major side effect is constipation; drink adequate fluids and use laxatives if directed.
- Discuss other drugs, including OTC products you are using, with your healthcare provider. This drug can decrease the absorption of other medicines.

Metoclopramide

Metoclopramide is a dopamine antagonist. At higher doses, it blocks serotonin receptors in the chemoreceptor zone of the CNS. It also enhances the response to acetylcholine in the upper GI tract causing enhanced motility and accelerated gastric emptying (peristaltic speed) and ↑ LES tone.

DRUG	DOSING	SAFETY/SIDE EFFECTS/MONITORING
Metoclopramide (***Reglan***, *Metozolv ODT*) Tablet, ODT, Oral Solution	5-15 mg QID 30 min before meals and at bedtime	**BOXED WARNING** May cause tardive dyskinesia – increased risk in elderly and with high doses and long-term therapy **CONTRAINDICATIONS** GI obstruction, perforation, hemorrhage; history of seizures; pheochromocytoma; combination with other agents likely to increase extrapyramidal symptoms (EPS) **SIDE EFFECTS** Somnolence, dystonic reactions, restlessness, fatigue, drug-induced Parkinson disease, neuroleptic malignant syndrome (rare) **NOTES** Reduce dose in patients with CrCl < 40 mL/min (use 50% of normal dose) CNS side effects are dose-related and more common in the elderly – use with caution and dose-adjust in renal impairment Avoid use in patients with Parkinson disease Metoclopramide has a short duration of action (must be present in gut when food is present) MedGuide required

Metoclopramide Drug Interactions

- Avoid in patients receiving medications for Parkinson disease (antagonistic effect). Avoid use of antipsychotic agents, promethazine, tetrabenazine, and trimetazidine with metoclopramide due to increase in adverse effects. When used in combination with SSRIs, monitor for possible EPS, NMS, and serotonin syndrome.

- Caution for additive CNS effects, including dizziness, somnolence and fatigue.

Metoclopramide Patient Counseling

- Use caution when driving, operating machinery, or performing other hazardous activities. This drug may cause dizziness or drowsiness.

- Avoid consuming alcohol during treatment with this drug. Alcohol may increase drowsiness and dizziness.

- Contact your healthcare provider right away if you experience any unusual body movements, such as shakiness, stiffness, or uncontrollable movements of the mouth, tongue, cheeks, jaw, arms, or legs.

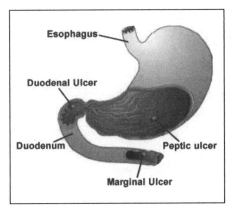

PEPTIC ULCER DISEASE (PUD)

Background

Peptic ulcer disease (PUD) occurs from mucosal erosion within the gastrointestinal tract. Unlike gastritis, the ulcers in PUD extend deeper into the mucosa. Most ulcers occur in the duodenum but a small percent also occur in the stomach. The three most common causes of PUD are *Helicobacter pylori (H. pylori)*-positive ulcers, nonsteroidal anti-inflammatory drug (NSAID)-induced ulcers and

GUIDELINES

Chey WD, Wong BC. American College of Gastroenterology guideline on the management of *Helicobacter pylori* infection. *Am J Gastroenterol.* 2007; 102:1808-25.

Gatta L, Vakil N, Vaira D, Scarpignato C. Global eradication rates for *Helicobacter pylori* infection: systematic review and meta-analysis of sequential therapy. *BMJ.* 2012; 347:4587-99.

stress ulcers in the presence of critical illness and in mechanically-ventilated patients. *H. pylori*, a spiral-shaped, pH sensitive, gram-negative bacterium that lives in the acidic environment of the stomach, is responsible for the majority of peptic ulcers (~70-80%). Other, less common causes of PUD are hypersecretory states, such as Zollinger-Ellison syndrome (causes ↑ gastric acid), G-cell hyperplasia, mastocytosis, and basophilic leukemias.

Under normal conditions, a physiologic balance exists between gastric acid secretion and the gut's repair mechanism. Mucosal defense and repair mechanisms include mucus and bicarbonate secretion, mucosal blood flow, prostaglandin synthesis, cellular regeneration, and epithelial cell renewal. These mechanisms protect the GI mucosa from damage from NSAIDs (including aspirin), *H. pylori*, acid, pepsin, and other GI irritants.

Symptoms

The primary symptom of PUD is gastric pain which can feel like a gnawing or burning pain in the middle or upper stomach. The pain is usually most bothersome between meals or during the night. Other symptoms are bloating, reflux and nausea. If the ulcer is duodenal (usually caused by *H. pylori*), eating generally lessens the pain. With gastric ulcers (primarily from NSAIDs), eating generally worsens the pain. Other symptoms include heartburn, belching, bloating, nausea and anorexia.

H. pylori Diagnostic Tests

H. pylori infection, if left untreated, can lead to cancer. If testing is positive for *H. pylori*, the infection should be treated. Common diagnostic tests for the presence of *H. pylori* include:

- Urea breath test (UBT): Breath test that identifies gas (CO_2) produced by the bacteria. False negatives can be secondary to the recent use of H_2RAs, PPIs, bismuth or antibiotics; discontinue H_2RAs and PPIs 1 to 2 weeks and bismuth and antibiotics 4 weeks prior to the test.

- Fecal antigen test: Detects *H. pylori* in the stool. False negatives can be secondary to the recent use of H_2RAs, PPIs, bismuth, or antibiotics (to a lesser extent than the UBT); discontinue these drugs at least 2-4 weeks prior to test.

H. pylori Treatment

The American College of Gastroenterology guidelines recommend triple therapy with a PPI + 2 antibiotics (clarithromycin and amoxicillin) for 14 days. Metronidazole can be used in place of amoxicillin if the patient has an allergy. Several of the regimens (with various PPIs) are FDA-approved for a 10 day regimen. Due to recent failures with triple therapy (often due to clarithromycin resistance), many patients now receive quadruple therapy. The guidelines do not yet state this recommendation, however many experts discourage the use of triple therapy as first-line due to clarithromycin resistance rates unless local eradication rates are

≥ 90%. Quadruple therapy consists of one of the following regimens: a PPI, clarithromycin, metronidazole/tinidazole and amoxicillin <u>or</u> a PPI, bismuth, tetracycline and metronidazole or the use of <u>sequential therapy</u>, which is now first-line in some countries outside of the U.S. and is used increasingly here. Sequential therapy is a 10-day treatment that switches after 5 days: a PPI plus amoxicillin 1 g BID is taken for 5 days, followed by triple therapy with a PPI, clarithromycin 500 mg BID and tinidazole BID for the remaining 5 days. If the PPI is continued beyond 14 days, this is to help ulcer healing for a short period of time; it should not be continued indefinitely.

<u>Do not make drug substitutions in *H. pylori* eradication regimens</u>. H_2RAs should not be substituted for a PPI, unless the patient cannot tolerate a PPI. Likewise, other antibiotics in the same class should not be substituted in *H. pylori* eradication regimens (for example, do not use ampicillin instead of amoxicillin).

First-Line *H. pylori* Treatment Regimens

DRUG REGIMEN	NOTES

Triple Drug Therapy – Take for 14 days

PPI BID (or esomeprazole 40 mg daily) + **Amoxicillin 1,000 mg BID +** **Clarithromycin 500 mg BID** *(Prevpac* – with lansoprazole as the PPI)	<u>Penicillin or macrolide allergy:</u> replace amoxicillin or clarithromycin with metronidazole 500 mg BID in this regimen OR can use alternative therapy below See GERD section for PPI side effects and Infectious Disease chapter for more on the antibiotics *Prevpac* contains all medications on one blister card. Take entire contents of one card each day for 14 days.

Quadruple Therapy – Take for 10-14 days
(Use if failed above therapy, cannot tolerate above agents, have taken a macrolide or metronidazole in the past, or if high local resistance rates to clarithomycin)

PPI BID (or esomeprazole daily) + **Bismuth subsalicylate 525 mg QID +** **Metronidazole 250-500 mg QID +** **Tetracycline 500 mg QID** Or Regimens Using Combination Products: Bismuth subcitrate potassium 420 mg QID + metronidazole 375 QID + tetracycline 375 mg QID *(Pylera)* + PPI for 10 days Bismuth subsalicylate 525 mg QID + metronidazole 250 mg QID + tetracycline 500 mg QID *(Helidac)* + H_2RA for 28 days	**Alcohol use** Do not use metronidazole **Pregnancy** Do not use tetracycline **Salicylate allergy/children** Do not use bismuth subsalicylate (or tetracycline in children 8 years or less). If patient cannot tolerate a PPI, substitute H_2RA (e.g., ranitidine 150 mg BID, famotidine 40 mg daily, nizatidine 300 mg/d). Swallow all capsules in the *Pylera* regimen; <u>chew the pink bismuth tablets in the *Helidac* regimen</u> and swallow the rest.

Drug Interactions

- Refer to previous sections for drug interactions with antacids, H_2RAs, and PPIs.

- Refer to Infectious Diseases chapter for drug interactions with antibiotics.

H. pylori Patient Counseling

- For all *H. pylori* regimens: These medicines are used for stomach ulcers caused by an infection. It is very important that you take the medicine as prescribed and complete the course of therapy.

- It is common to have some diarrhea while taking these medicines. If it becomes severe or watery, contact your healthcare provider.

- For *Prevpac:* Each card has your dose (4 pills) for the morning and the evening. Take your dose before breakfast and before dinner.

- Other side effects to watch for are bad taste in the mouth, headache, or any sign of allergy like a skin rash.

- For *Helidac:* To treat your stomach ulcers correctly, you will need two prescriptions: *Helidac* and a prescription for an acid reducing medication. You will take the acid reducing medicine for 28 days to help the ulcer heal, but you should not continue taking it after that unless your healthcare provider tells you to.

- This medicine may cause a darkening of your tongue and dark stool. It goes away when you stop the medicine.

- For *Helidac*, you will take 4 pills 4 times per day – breakfast, lunch, dinner and bedtime. It is very important that you chew the round pink tablets and swallow the other three pills. Take with a full glass of water. Take the acid reducing medication as it is prescribed.

- For *Pylera:* To treat your stomach ulcers correctly, you will need two prescriptions: *Pylera* and a prescription for an acid reducing medication. You will take the acid reducing medicine for 10 days to help the ulcer heal, but you should not continue taking it after that unless your healthcare provider tells you to.

- For *Pylera*, you will take 3 capsules 4 times per day – breakfast, lunch, dinner and bedtime with a full glass of water. Swallow the capsules whole. Take the acid reducing medication as it is prescribed.

Non-Steroidal Anti-Inflammatory Drug (NSAID)-Induced Ulcers (Primarily Gastric)

Background

The use of high dose non-steroidal anti-inflammatory drugs (NSAIDs) or chronic NSAID use greatly increases the risk for gastric (GI) ulcers. NSAIDs (including aspirin) can cause gastric mucosal damage by 2 mechanisms: direct irritation of the gastric epithelium and systemic inhibition of prostaglandin synthesis (by inhibiting COX-1).

Prevention and Treatment

Concomitant PPI therapy decreases ulcer risk. High-risk patients using a non-selective NSAID chronically can reduce bleeding risk by using concurrent PPI therapy. The clinician will need to consider long-term risks of acid-suppression therapy. Alternatively, a COX-2 selective agent (e.g., celecoxib) with or without a PPI can be used in high-risk patients if they do not have cardiovascular risk factors. Generic NSAID agents that approach the selectivity of celecoxib are meloxicam, nabumetone and etodolac. Some evidence

RISK FACTORS FOR NSAID-INDUCED ULCERS
Elderly
Previous bleed
Chronic NSAID use or high dose
Concomitant anticoagulant, steroids, SSRIs/SNRIs
Smoking
Poor health

suggests that naproxen may be preferable to other NSAIDs in patients with low-moderate GI risk and high CV risk.

If an ulcer develops, it would be best to discontinue the NSAID, if possible, and treat the ulcer with a PPI for about 8 weeks. Misoprostol is also an option, but diarrhea and cramping along with its four times per day dosing regimen contribute to poor patient compliance. If the NSAID therapy cannot be stopped, then reducing the NSAID dose, switching to acetaminophen or a nonacetylated salicylate or using a more selective COX-2 inhibitor should be considered.

Use caution with NSAIDs in any person with cardiovascular or renal disease since they can elevate blood pressure and decrease renal blood flow. If possible, avoid non-selective NSAIDs and celecoxib in patients with both high GI and CV risk and those at high risk of chronic kidney disease.

Patients who require antiplatelet therapy with a previous history of ulcers should be tested for *H. pylori* and treated, if positive.

PRACTICE CASE

PATIENT PROFILE

Patient Name	Benjamin Specter							
Address	10 Pine Place							
Age	72	**Sex** Male	**Race** White	**Height** 5'6"	**Weight** 160lbs
Allergies	Aspirin (hives)							

DIAGNOSES

GERD	Seasonal allergies, occasional bronchodilator use
Prostate enlargement	Dyslipidemia, CHD, MI x 2 (last ~8 years ago)
Parkinson disease	

MEDICATIONS

Date	No.	Prescriber	Drug & Strength	Quantity	Sig	Refills
6/23/13	35421	Cooper	Clopidogrel 75 mg	#30	1 PO daily	6
6/23/13	35422	Cooper	Protonix 40 mg	#30	1 PO daily	6
6/23/13	35423	Cooper	Pravastatin 20 mg	#30	1 PO BID	6
6/23/13	35424	Cooper	Sinemet 25/250	#90	1 PO tid	6
			Albuterol inhaler	#1	Occasional use	4
			Loratadine 10 mg		1 tablet, as needed	
11/1/13	42877	Kreinfeldt	Metoclopramide 10 mg	#120	1 PO QID	

LAB/DIAGNOSTIC TESTS

Test	Normal Value	Results Date 5/12/13	Date	Date
Protein, T	6.2-8.3 g/dL			
Albumin	3.6-5.1 g/dL			
Alk Phos	33-115 units/L			
AST	10-35 units/L			
ALT	6-40 units/L			
CH, T	125-200 g/dL			
TG	<150 g/dL			
HDL	g/dL			
LDL	g/dL			
GLU	65-99 mg/dL			
Na	135-146 mEq/L			
K	3.5-5.3 mEq/L			
Cl	98-110 mEq/L			
C02	21-33 mmHg			
BUN	7-25 mg/dL	28		
Creatinine	0.6-1.2 mg/dL	1.9		
Calcium	8.6-10.2 mg/dL			
WBC	4-11 cells/mm³			
RBC	3.8-5.1 mL/mm³			
Hemoglobin	Male: 13.8- 17.2 g/dL Female: 12.1-15.1 g/dL			
Hematocrit	Male: 40.7-50.3% Female: 36.1- 44.3%			
MCHC	32-36 g/dL			
MCV	80-100 µm			
Platelet count	140-400 x 10³/mm³			
TSH	0.4-4.0 mIU/L			
FT4	4.5- 11.2 mcg/dL			
Hgb A1c	4-6%			

ADDITIONAL INFORMATION

Date	Notes
11/11/13	PCP (Cooper) on vacation. Reports bothersome heartburn. Reflux after eating dinner and during sleep. Eats dinner 8:30 pm, falls asleep 9:30-10 pm. Enjoys after dinner black tea with honey & pipe. Per discussion, symtpoms appear controlled.

Questions

1. The patient is using *Protonix* once daily. Which of the following is an appropriate substitution?

   a. Omeprazole
   b. Esomeprazole
   c. Pantoprazole
   d. Rabeprazole
   e. Lansoprazole

2. The patient is still experiencing symptoms despite his current therapy. The physician decided to add-on metoclopramide to control the reflux symptoms. Choose the correct statement:

   a. Inappropriate therapy; the physician should increase *Protonix* to 60 mg daily.
   b. Inappropriate therapy; the physician should either increase *Protonix* to BID dosing, or add ranitidine 75 mg at bedtime.
   c. Inappropriate therapy; the physician should add on magnesium citrate prn.
   d. Inappropriate therapy; the physician should start misoprostol 200 mcg QID.
   e. Metoclopramide is appropriate therapy; no change is required.

3. Benjamin can make several lifestyle changes that may help with his evening symptoms. Which of the following are correct counseling points the pharmacist can provide to the patient?

   a. Consider cessation of evening smoke
   b. Eat dinner at an earlier time
   c. Change his evening drink to a non-caffeinated, non-alcoholic option
   d. Elevate the head of his bead 6-8 inches
   e. All of the above

4. The substituting physician prescribed metoclopramide. Which of the following side effects may be present?

   a. Worsening of his Parkinson disease symptoms
   b. Worsening of his prostate disease symptoms
   c. Dizziness, sleepiness
   d. A and B only
   e. A and C only

5. If the metoclopramide was to be used in a different patient with this degree of renal function, what would be the correct dose?

   a. 10 mg four times daily
   b. 10 mg twice daily
   c. 10 mg daily
   d. 2.5-5 mg four times daily
   e. 5 mg once daily

Questions 6-15 are NOT based on the above case.

6. An elderly female presents at the pharmacy. She does not have health insurance coverage. Which of the following PPIs is available over-the-counter?

   a. *Zegerid*
   b. *Prevacid*
   c. *Prilosec*
   d. A and C
   e. All of the above

7. A patient has entered the pharmacy and asked the pharmacy technician to help her locate the store-brand version of *Pepcid*. Which of the following medications should the technician select?

   a. Famotidine
   b. Cimetidine
   c. Ranitidine
   d. Omeprazole
   e. Lansoprazole

8. A physician has written a prescription for *Prevacid*. Which of the following represents an acceptable therapeutic substitution?

   a. Omeprazole
   b. Esomeprazole
   c. Rabeprazole
   d. Pantoprazole
   e. Lansoprazole

9. Which of the following proton pump inhibitors is available in an IV formulation? (Select **ALL** that apply.)

   a. *Dexilant*
   b. *Nexium*
   c. *Protonix*
   d. *AcipHex*
   e. *Prilosec*

10. An elderly female patient has hypertension and heartburn. Her family states she has trouble swallowing large pills. She failed H$_2$RA therapy and has been well-controlled on a PPI. She is currently using *Nexium* 40 mg daily. Which of the following would be a better option?

    a. Gaviscon

    b. Alka Seltzer Original

    c. Zegerid

    d. Prevacid SoluTab

    e. Maalox

11. A 46 year-old man has received a prescription for lansoprazole 15 mg daily, amoxicillin 500 mg BID and clarithromycin 500 mg BID for *H. pylori* treatment. Choose the correct statement:

    a. Contact prescriber to correct dose of lansoprazole.

    b. Contact prescriber to correct doses of lansoprazole and amoxicillin.

    c. Contact prescriber to correct doses of clarithromycin and amoxicillin.

    d. Contact prescriber to correct doses of lansoprazole and clarithromycin.

    e. Fill as written.

12. A female patient presents a prescription to the pharmacy for lansoprazole 30 mg BID, bismuth subsalicylate 525 mg QID, metronidazole 250 mg QID and tetracycline 500 mg QID for 14 days. The patient's other prescriptions include hydrochlorothiazide and the combination oral contraceptive product *Lybrel*. Choose the correct counseling statement:

    a. You will need to use back-up contraception, such as condoms and foam, for the 14 days you are using this antibiotic therapy.

    b. You will need to use back-up contraception, such as condoms and foam, for the 14 days you are using this antibiotic therapy and for 1 week afterwards.

    c. You will need to use back-up contraception, such as condoms and foam, for the 14 days you are using this antibiotic therapy and for 2 weeks afterwards.

    d. You will need to stop the *Lybrel* and use an alternative form of contraception for the 14 days you are using this antibiotic therapy.

    e. It is acceptable to use alcohol in moderation during use of this regimen.

13. A 16 year-old patient has the following allergies noted on her patient profile: ciprofloxacin, aspirin and erythromycin. The allergic reaction is not listed, and the patient is not available by phone. You wish to fill the prescription for *H. pylori* therapy, which includes rabeprazole, amoxicillin and clarithromycin. Choose the correct statement:

    a. It is safe to fill; most allergies to erythromycin are gastrointestinal.

    b. It is safe to fill; there is no cross-reaction with these agents.

    c. It is not safe to fill due to the use of amoxicillin in a patient with ciprofloxacin allergy.

    d. It is not safe to fill due to the patient's age.

    e. It is not safe to fill until the erythromycin "allergy" is clarified.

14. Proton pump inhibitors can increase the risk of: (Select **ALL** that apply.)

    a. Bone fracture

    b. *C. difficile* infection

    c. Stroke

    d. Heart attacks

    e. Pneumonia in hospitalized patients

15. A pharmacist is dispensing tetracycline. Which of the following are correct counseling points? (Select **ALL** that apply.)

    a. Take this medication 1-2 hours before or 4 hours after taking any products containing magnesium, aluminum, or calcium, iron, zinc including vitamins, supplements and dairy products.

    b. Do not use sunlamps while using this therapy.

    c. You should avoid getting pregnant while using this medicine.

    d. You may experience stomach upset, including loose stools and nausea.

    e. Do not take if you are allergic to penicillin.

Answers

1-c, 2-b, 3-e, 4-e, 5-d, 6-e, 7-a, 8-e, 9-b,c, 10-d, 11-b, 12-a, 13-e, 14-a,b,e, 15-a,b,c,d

CONSTIPATION & DIARRHEA

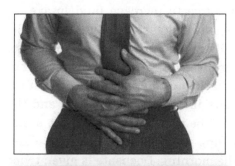

CONSTIPATION

Background
Constipation is defined as infrequent or hard stools, or difficulty passing stools. More specifically, constipation may involve pain during the passage of a bowel movement, the inability to pass a bowel movement after straining or pushing for more than 10 minutes, requiring digital evacuation, or no bowel movements after more than 3 days. The lifestyle measures in the box may help. If not or if inadequate, laxatives are used.

Drug Treatment
The AGA guidelines recommend increasing fiber intake (dietary and as supplements) with the possibility of adding on a relatively inexpensive osmotic agent (milk of magnesia or polyethylene glycol). These are all available OTC. Milk of magnesia contains magnesium and is not used with severe renal impairment. Polyethylene glycol is available OTC as *MiraLax* and in a larger prescription container.

LIFESTYLE MEASURES

These lifestyle modifications may be helpful to reduce constipation:

Look for offending drugs (see chart)

Correct fluid intake (64 oz – caution with CVD)

Limit caffeine and alcohol (to avoid dehydration)

Replace refined foods with whole grain products, bran, fruits & vegetables, beans

Increase physical activity

Do not delay going to the bathroom when the urge to defecate is present; may need to schedule time (important for young children)

If the patient needs to defecate a suppository (bisacodyl or glycerol) will provide fast relief. Preferably, these should be administered 30 minutes after a meal when GI peristalsis has increased, but they can be used at any time of day. Oral stimulants (senna, bisacodyl) can be added on at bedtime as chronic agents. Senna is the usual first-line oral stimulant agent and is given as 2 tablets QHS. These agents take ~10 hours to work and

CONSTIPATION NOTES

Medical conditions where constipation is common

Cerebrovascular events	Multiple sclerosis
Parkinson disease	Irritable Bowel Syndrome (constipation-predominant)
Spinal cord tumors	
Diabetes	Anal disorders (anal fissures, fistulae, rectal prolapse)
Hypothyroidism	

Medications that are constipating

Opioids	Aluminum antacids (magnesium often in combination with aluminum to counteract effect)
Anticholinergic drugs	
Antihistamines, phenothiazines, tricyclic antidepressants, antispasmodics, urge incontinence drugs, especially darifenacin (Enablex)	Aluminum complex in other drugs (sucralfate [Carafate])
	Tramadol, tapentadol
Non-DHP calcium channel blockers, especially verapamil	Colesevelam
	Milnacipran
Clonidine	Ranolazine
Bismuth	Varenicline
Iron (use docusate to avoid hard, compact stools)	5-HT$_3$ receptor antagonists (e.g., ondansetron)
	Phentermine/topiramate
	Aripiprazole

will make it will make it possible to have a bowel movement the following morning, which is when most people defecate. Men most often have a bowel movement most mornings. Women have bowel movements less frequently.

One-third of adults > 60 years have chronic constipation. Prior to recommending fiber consider if the patient will be willing to use an adequate amount of fluids. This is required with fiber. An elderly female with incontinence, for example, would not likely willingly agree to increase fluid intake. In this case, docusate would be reasonable. Patients of any age using iron supplements will generally require docusate. Iron makes the stool hard and compact. It is difficult for fiber to mix in to soften the stool, and the patient will be able to defecate more easily the following morning. Most patients defecate in the morning. Docusate is given twice daily (usually 100 mg BID) to make the stool softer while the food is being processed.

Patients using chronic opioids will often require a stimulant laxative because the opioids reduce the ability to push out the stool. A higher dose (taken ATC) will increase laxative requirement. Certain opioids are more constipating than others (e.g., morphine causes more constipation than fentanyl) but all are constipating, and some patients have more constipation than others. The stool softener docusate is given with the stimulant laxative if the stool is hard. If the stool is not hard but the patient cannot push it out, this is sometimes called "moosh with no push" and is treated with a stimulant alone. There are newer, expensive options for opioid-induced constipation for patients who do not find relief with a stimulant ± stool softener.

Laxative Agents Used for Bowel Prep

A screening colonoscopy is used to detect colorectal cancer, along with fecal occult blood tests. They are also used for other gastrointestinal conditions, such as Crohn's. A successful colonoscopy requires a complete and thorough bowel prep. Several of the agents below (the PEGs, and occasionally sodium phosphate) are used for both bowel prep and as laxatives. Sodium phosphate can cause fluid and electrolyte abnormalities, and is particularly risky in patients with renal or cardiac disease. Some of the PEG formulations are only used for bowel prep, such as Golytely. General counseling for bowel prep agents must include when to take the agent, what the patient can consume during the bowel cleansing process (i.e., after they have started using the bowel prep agent) and what must be avoided. Although usually safe and well-tolerated, in certain patients fluid and electrolyte loss could be critical. For this reason, some of the bowel prep agents require MedGuides. <u>Use extra caution in patients with cardiovascular disease, renal insufficiency, if taking diuretics (loops, due to additional fluid loss) and NSAIDs.</u>

OK to Consume

- "Clear liquid diet," which can include water, clear broth (beef or chicken), fat-free consommé, juices (apple, prune, grape, cranberry, and cider) without pulp, noncarbonated, sodas *(Sprite, 7-Up*, ginger ale, and seltzer), coffee or tea (without milk or cream), clear gelatin (without fruit pieces), popsicles (without fruit pieces or cream), fruit ices (no fruit pieces).

Do not Consume

- <u>Anything with red or blue/purple food coloring</u> (including gelatin and popsicles), milk, cream, tomato, orange or grapefruit juice, cream soups, any soup other than broth. No liquids that they cannot "see through."

- Alcoholic beverages

- No solid or semi-solid foods – liquid only until after the procedure is complete.

Laxatives for Chronic/Maintenance Therapy

Bulk-producing laxatives create a gel-like matrix in the stool, soaking up fluid in loose stool and adding bulk to hard stool. Emollients and lubricants (stool softeners) lubricate and soften fecal mass, making defecation easier. Lubiprostone works by activating chloride channels in the gut, leading to increased fluid in the gut and peristalsis. Linaclotide is an agonist of guanylate cyclase C, which increases chloride and bicarbonate secretion into the intestinal lumen, decreasing GI transit time.

Chronic/Maintenance Therapy

DRUG	DOSING	SAFETY/SIDE EFFECTS/MONITORING

Bulk-producing laxatives

DRUG	DOSING	SAFETY/SIDE EFFECTS/MONITORING
Psyllium (*Metamucil*, others)	2.5-30 g/day in divided doses	**SIDE EFFECTS** Increased gas, bloating, bowel obstruction if strictures present, choking if powder forms are not taken with enough liquid **NOTES** Onset of action – 12 to 24 hours
Calcium polycarbophil (*FiberCon*, others)	1,250 mg 1-4 times/day	<u>Drugs of choice in pregnancy</u> <u>First-line treatment for constipation</u>, +/- an osmotic agent Increase bulk in diet slowly Adequate fluid intake required
Methylcellulose (*Citrucel*)	2 g 1-3 times/day	<u>Take 2 hours before/after drugs</u> (caution with other drugs that stick to fiber) Psyllium: tart-like flavor; sugar-free forms available

Chronic/Maintenance Therapy Continued

DRUG	DOSING	SAFETY/SIDE EFFECTS/MONITORING

Emollients, lubricants (stool softeners)

DRUG	DOSING	SAFETY/SIDE EFFECTS/MONITORING
Docusate Sodium (**Colace**) Docusate Calcium Mineral Oil	Docusate – usually 100 mg BID (max of 500 mg/day)	**NOTES** Onset of action – 24 to 48 hours Bitter taste with liquid only Advise not to use more than 7 days without consulting physician (not that it's harmful, just to rule out more serious problem) Mineral oil – take a multivitamin at a different time due to risk of fat-soluble vitamin depletion (A, D, E & K)

Stimulants and irritants – Use caution when recommending agents by brand name as many brands can refer to multiple products

DRUG	DOSING	SAFETY/SIDE EFFECTS/MONITORING
Senna (**Ex-Lax**, others)	15 mg, usually 2 tabs QHS	**WARNINGS** Avoid use if stomach pain, nausea, vomiting, or a sudden change in bowel movements which lasts > 2 weeks. **SIDE EFFECTS** Stomach upset, cramping, electrolyte imbalance with overdose (e.g., eating disorders)
Bisacodyl (**Dulcolax**, others)	Bisacodyl OTC: 5 mg, take 1-3 tablets once daily	**NOTES** Onset of action – 8-12 hours Do not crush or chew bisacodyl tablets (they are EC), do not take within 1 hr of milk or antacids – may require dose reduction with H_2RAs or PPIs.
Cascara (see Natural Products chapter)		Senna is well-tolerated at the usual dose. Side effects are increased when high doses are used. Caution, brand names can refer to multiple products.

Rx Agents

DRUG	DOSING	SAFETY/SIDE EFFECTS/MONITORING
Lubiprostone (**Amitiza**)	24 mcg capsule twice daily with food IBS dosing: 8 mcg PO once daily to twice daily Decrease dose with severe liver impairment	**SIDE EFFECTS** Nausea, diarrhea, headache, hypokalemia **NOTES** Take with food and water. Swallow whole. Do not break, chew or crush.
Linaclotide (Linzess)	Chronic idiopathic constipation – 145 mcg PO daily IBS with constipation – 290 mcg PO daily	**BOXED WARNING** Do not use in patients less than 18 years of age **SIDE EFFECTS** Diarrhea, abdominal distension, flatulence, headache **NOTES** Must be dispensed with a MedGuide. Keep in tightly closed, original container (contains desiccant). Take at least 30 minutes before breakfast on an empty stomach. Swallow whole; do not break, chew or crush.

Acute (STAT) Treatments and Bowel Preps

Stimulants/irritants work by reducing water and electrolyte absorption by stimulating colonic neurons and irritating the mucosal lining of the colon. Osmotic laxatives cause fluid to be retained in the bowel lumen, with a net increase of fluid secretions in the small intestines. This distends the colon and increases peristalsis.

DRUG	DOSING	SAFETY/SIDE EFFECTS/MONITORING
Bisacodyl Rectal	10 mg PR	**SIDE EFFECTS** Rectal burning **NOTES** Onset of action – 10 minutes If too soft to insert, can cool in refrigerator or cold water first
Osmotics **Magnesium salts (MOM)** Lactulose Sorbitol	30-60 mL 15-30 mL 30-150 mL (as 70% solution)	**SIDE EFFECTS** Electrolyte imbalance, excessive gas, hypermagnesemia, hypocalcemia and hyperphosphatemia in patients with renal dysfunction, dehydration **NOTES** Onset of action – 2 to 48 hours Caution in patients with renal dysfunction (magnesium salts) Lactulose can also be used chronically – titrated to 2-3 soft stools/day
Sodium phosphates *(Fleet enema, OsmoPrep)*	1 enema PR PRN *OsmoPrep*: Evening before colonoscopy: 4 tablets with 8 oz clear liquids Q15 min for a total of 20 tablets Next morning: 4 tablets with 8 oz clear liquids Q15 min for a total of 12 tablets	**WARNINGS** Do not use sodium phosphates in CHF, renal disease, $\downarrow Ca^{2+}$ or $\uparrow PO_4$ **SIDE EFFECTS** Electrolyte imbalance, excessive gas, hypocalcemia and hyperphosphatemia in patients with renal dysfunction, dehydration **NOTES** Onset of action – 1 to 5 minutes Ensure adequate hydration
Nonabsorbable solutions; also used for bowel prep **Polyethylene glycol (Golytely, MiraLax, Carbowax)** *NuLytely, TriLyte* are sulfate free *HalfLytely, HalfLytely +* bisacodyl, *MoviPrep* are less volume (2 L)	PEG – 17 g in 8 oz water (for bowel prep, repeat every 10 minutes until 2 liters are consumed)	**SIDE EFFECTS** Nausea, abdominal fullness, bloating **NOTES** Onset of action – within 4 hours **To ensure adequate bowel prep** Clear liquid diet for one day prior, avoid red or blue/purple drinks If it will help, split the dose of the bowel prep, such as half the night before, and half 4-6 hours before procedure Use flavored agents, or add lemon juice or *Crystal Light* (no sugar-containing products)

Acute (STAT) Treatments and Bowel Preps Continued

DRUG	DOSING	SAFETY/SIDE EFFECTS/MONITORING
Picosulfate, Magnesium Oxide, Anhydrous Citric Acid *(Prepopik)*	150 mL x 2 doses	**SIDE EFFECTS** Hypermagnesemia and reduced GFR Possible headache, hypokalemia, hypochloremia, hyponatremia, nausea, elevated serum creatinine **NOTES** Combination stimulant laxative and osmotic, enables lower fluid intake – used for bowel prep **Directions** If morning procedure, take dose the afternoon before and 6 hours later If later in the day, take first dose night before, 2nd 5 hours prior to procedure Drink 5 glasses of clear liquid after the 1st dose and 3 glasses after the 2nd dose
Glycerin suppository (adult size, peds size) *Babylax* is liquid in rectal applicator (squeeze out liquid around stuck stool into rectum)	Use 1 suppository, can repeat x 1	**SIDE EFFECTS** Anal irritation, stomach cramping **NOTES** Onset of action – 15-30 minutes Insert rectally towards side of rectal wall (at side of stool)

Opioid-Induced Constipation Treatments

Methylnaltrexone and alvimopan block opioid receptors in the gut to reduce the constipating effects of opioids.

DRUG	DOSING	SAFETY/SIDE EFFECTS/MONITORING
Methylnaltrexone *(Relistor)*	8 mg if weight 38-61 kg, 12 mg if 62-114 kg, 0.15 mg/kg if > 114 kg Administer SC every other day (upper arm, abdomen or thigh)	**WARNINGS** Discontinue if severe or persistent diarrhea Gastrointestinal perforation: rare reports; use cautiously if history GI tract lesions, monitor for severe abdominal symptoms **CONTRAINDICATIONS** GI obstruction **SIDE EFFECTS** Abdominal pain, flatulence, nausea **NOTES** Stay close to toilet after injecting Decrease dose if CrCl < 30 mL/min Only for patients on opioids who have failed DSS + laxative (senna, bisacodyl). Do not use routinely; can often increase laxative until the patient can excavate

Opioid-Induced Constipation Treatments Continued

DRUG	DOSING	SAFETY/SIDE EFFECTS/MONITORING
Alvimopan *(Entereg)*	12 mg PO, 30 min-5 hrs prior to surgery, and 12 mg BID for up to 7 days total (15 doses) Must be hospitalized to receive this drug	**BOXED WARNING** Possible MI risk Due to MI risk, drug is available only through the REMS program (EASE) **CONTRAINDICATIONS** Patients who have taken therapeutic doses of opioids for more than 7 consecutive days prior to use **SIDE EFFECTS** Dyspepsia, hypokalemia **NOTES** Use is limited to post-surgical patients to decrease the risk of post-operative ileus
Naloxegol *(Movantik)* C-II Peripherally-acting mu-opioid receptor antagonist (PAMORA) for the treatment of opioid-induced constipation (OIC) in adult patients with chronic, non-cancer pain.	25 mg Q daily in the morning, use 12.5 mg with CrCl < 60 mL/min	**SIDE EFFECTS** Abdominal pain, diarrhea, headache, flatulence **NOTES** Discontinue laxatives prior to use; can reintroduce laxatives as needed if suboptimal response to naloxegol after 3 days. Do not use with strong 3A4 inhibitors. Avoid use or reduce dose to 12.5 mg daily with moderate 3A4 inhibitors. Do not use with grapefruit juice.

DIARRHEA NOTES

Medications that can cause diarrhea

Antacids containing magnesium	Laxatives
Antibiotics, especially broad-spectrum antibiotics and clindamycin, erythromycin (due to prokinetic activity) – rule out *C. difficile* infection	Metoclopramide
	Misoprostol
	Quinidine
	Many drugs include diarrhea as a possible side effect
Colchicine	

DIARRHEA

Background

Diarrhea occurs when there is an increase in the number of bowel movements or bowel movements are more watery and loose than normal. When the intestines push stools through the bowel before the water in the stool can be reabsorbed, diarrhea occurs. Abdominal cramps, nausea, vomiting, or a fever may occur along with the diarrhea. Fluid and electrolyte replacement is essential; review counseling points at end of this section.

Treatment

- Most cases are viral. Diarrhea can be idiopathic, caused by diseases, or can be caused by stomach flu or food poisoning. Drinking untreated water, not washing fruits/vegetables properly, using untreated ice for drinks, or unpasteurized dairy products can cause viral, bacterial, or parasitic infections. *E. coli* is the most common bacterial cause. The treatment of diarrhea caused by a bacterial infection is discussed in the Infectious Disease chapter.

Antidiarrheals

Bismuth subsalicylate exhibits both antisecretory and antimicrobial effects when used as an antidiarrheal. Loperamide acts on intestinal muscles to inhibit peristalsis and to slow intestinal motility. Diphenoxylate works by inhibiting excessive GI motility and GI propulsion. A subtherapeutic amount of atropine is include in the formulation to discourage abuse.

DRUG	DOSING	SAFETY/SIDE EFFECTS/MONITORING
Bismuth subsalicylate (*Pepto-Bismol*, others)	524 mg (30 mL or 2 tablets) every 30-60 minutes as needed up to 8 doses/day; max 2 days	**CONTRAINDICATIONS** Children with viral infections (varicella, influenza) due to risk of Reye's syndrome, patients with a salicylate allergy, history of severe GI bleed or coagulopathy **SIDE EFFECTS** <u>Black tongue/stool</u>, hearing loss/tinnitus (toxicity) **NOTES** Bismuth subsalicylate should be used with caution in patients on aspirin therapy or anticoagulants or those who have renal insufficiency Salicylate toxicity can occur if used excessively
Loperamide (*Imodium, Anti-Diarrheal, Diamode*, others)	2 mg tab/cap; 1 mg liquid 4 mg PO after first loose stool initially; then 2 mg after each subsequent stool; not to exceed 16 mg/d	**CONTRAINDICATIONS** Abdominal pain without diarrhea, children < 2 years of age, acute dysentery (bloody diarrhea and high fever), acute ulcerative colitis, pseudomembranous colitis (*C. difficile*), diarrhea caused by enterotoxin-producing bacteria (*toxigenic E. coli, Salmonella, Shigella*) **SIDE EFFECTS** Abdominal cramping, constipation, nausea **NOTES** <u>Do not self-treat for > 2 days</u>
Diphenoxylate 2.5 mg with atropine 0.025 mg (*Lomotil*) <u>C-V</u>	5 mg up to QID (max 20 mg/day)	**CONTRAINDICATIONS** Children < 2 years of age, pseudomembranous colitis (*C. difficile*), diarrhea caused by enterotoxin-producing bacteria (toxigenic *E. coli, Salmonella, Shigella*) obstructive jaundice **SIDE EFFECTS** Sedation, constipation, urinary retention, tachycardia, blurred vision, dry mouth, depression

Counseling for All Diarrhea Cases

- Do not self-treat if high fever (> 101°F) or blood in stool; see healthcare provider if no improvement in 2 days, if severe abdominal pain, infants (< 6 months), or if patient is pregnant.

- Diarrhea treatment should include <u>fluid and electrolytes</u> – this is important for all but especially so in <u>children</u> or adults with chronic medical illness.

- For moderate-severe fluid loss, replacement is best accomplished with oral rehydration solutions (ORS), which are available at stores and pharmacies (*Pedialyte, Infalyte*, etc) in developed countries. *Gatorade* or similar products are used as alternatives.

- Caution with *Imodium* and *Lomotil* if a decrease in intestinal motility may be due to infection from *Shigella, Salmonella*, and toxigenic strains of *E. coli* – toxic megacolon (usually due to *E. coli* or severe IBS) may occur. <u>These products are also not recommended in *C. difficile*</u> infections – the patient's body must be able to rid itself of the toxin.

- If fever/cold symptoms are present, aspirin rarely causes Reye's Syndrome in children and is avoided except under a healthcare provider's care (it may rarely be used in a child with a heart condition, where benefit may outweigh risk). For fever or mild pain, the parent can treat the child with acetaminophen or ibuprofen but should not exceed recommended daily amounts of acetaminophen or ibuprofen.

- Combination cough and cold products should not be used in children under 2 years old per the FDA (under 6 years old per the American Academy of Pediatrics). Any combination product may contain additional amounts of acetaminophen or ibuprofen – the patient must be counseled to count all sources.

- Rule out lactose intolerance as a cause of the diarrhea by stopping use of dairy products. Physicians can confirm lactose intolerance by tests.

- Bismuth Subsalicylate Counseling

- Do not use if you have an allergy to bismuth, salicylates (including aspirin and NSAIDs, like ibuprofen), or any other part of this drug.

- Tell your healthcare provider prior to starting this medicine if you are also taking a salicylate like aspirin.

- Do not give to children and teenagers who have flu signs, chickenpox, or other viral infections due to the chance of Reye's syndrome.

- Some chewable products have phenylalanine. If you have PKU, do not use this product.

- This medicine may make your tongue and stool dark, this is normal. Contact your healthcare provider right away if you notice tarry or bloody stools or if you are throwing up blood or a substance that looks like coffee grounds.

- If you notice a ringing in the ears or a loss of hearing while taking this medicine, stop taking it and contact your healthcare provider.

- Do not take for longer than 7 days without the approval of your healthcare provider.

66

INFLAMMATORY BOWEL DISEASE (IBD)

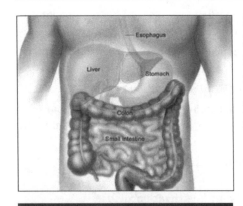

GUIDELINES

Lichtenstein GR, Hanauer SB, Sand-born WJ. Management of crohn's disease in adults. *Am J Gastroenterol.* 2009; 104:465-483.

Kornbluth A, Sachar DB. Ulcerative colitis practice guidelines in adults. *Am J Gastroenterol.* 2010; 105:501-523.

BACKGROUND

Inflammatory Bowel Disease (IBD) is a group of inflammatory conditions of the colon and small intestine. The major types of IBD are ulcerative colitis and Crohn's disease. The hallmark symptom is persistent bloody diarrhea. Other symptoms include rectal urgency and tenesmus (a feeling of having to pass stools, even if the colon is empty). Symptom control (with antidiarrheals or antispasmodics) may be necessary. Symptoms can occur at any time with likely flares when the patient develops an infection, uses NSAIDs, or eats foods that trigger the disease. Food triggers include fatty foods, gas-producing foods (lentils, beans, legumes, cabbage, broccoli, onions) and some others. These are patient-specific. When food triggers are identified they can be avoided or prepared in a way that improves tolerability.

Ulcerative Colitis (UC)

UC is characterized by mucosal inflammation confined to the rectum and colon (often referred to as distal IBD) with superficial ulcerations (in contrast to Crohn's, where the ulcers can be deep). If UC is distal only it will be accessible with topical (rectal) treatment. The larger the affected area, the worse the symptoms. When the disease flares, patients can have numerous stools per day, often with pain, which can significantly decrease quality of life. UC is classified as mild, moderate, severe or fulminant. Moderate disease is characterized by > 4 stools per day with minimal signs of toxicity and patients with severe disease have ≥ 6 bloody stools daily with evidence of toxicity [fever, tachycardia, anemia, or an elevated erythrocyte sedimentation rate (ESR)].

Crohn's Disease (CD)

CD is characterized by deep, transmural (through the tissue) inflammation that can affect any part of the GI tract. The ileum and colon are most commonly affected. Damage to the bowel wall can cause strictures and fistulas (abnormal connections or openings). Symptoms of CD include chronic diarrhea (often nocturnal), abdominal pain, and weight loss. Perianal symptoms (e.g., bleeding, fissures) can be present before bowel symptoms.

CD and UC Symptoms

	CD	UC
Diarrhea	Bloody or non-bloody	Bloody
Smoking	Risk factor	Protective
Location	Entire GI tract (esp. ileum & colon)	Colon (esp. rectum)
Depth	Transmural	Superficial
Pattern	Non-continuous	Continuous
Fistulas/Strictures	Common	Uncommon

Natural Products

For diarrhea in IBD, psyllium (in *Metamucil* and other formulations) or other "bulk-forming" fiber products can be useful.

Peppermint (oil, sometimes teas) can be useful as an antispasmodic. Some use chamomile tea. The probiotic *Lactobacillus* or *bifidobacterium infantis* can reduce abdominal pain, bloating, urgency, constipation or diarrhea in some patients. Antibiotics and probiotics are not taken at the same time; separate the dosing by at least two hours. Fish oils (for the EPA and DHA, the omega fatty acid components) are being used, although the evidence for benefit is contradictory. Indian frankincense gum resin taken TID may be beneficial for UC, based on preliminary studies.

Watch for avoidable problems: Sorbitol is used as a sweetener in some diet foods and is present in various drugs. Sorbitol has laxative properties and can cause considerable GI distress in some patients. Lactose will worsen GI symptoms if lactose-intolerant. Lactose is used in some oral drugs as an excipient. Both sorbitol and lactose are classified as excipients (or binders); they help hold tablets together.

Drug Treatment

Mild cases of UC and CD may only need antidiarrheal medicines, primarily loperamide (*Imodium*). Antispasmodics for UC may be useful. The most common antispasmodic is dicyclomine (*Bentyl*) which is an anticholinergic with a high incidence of side effects (e.g., dizziness, dry mouth, somnolence, urinary retention).

Short courses of oral or IV steroids are used to treat acute exacerbations in both UC and CD. In UC aminosalicylates are used for maintenance therapy to control inflammation and reduce flare-ups. Mesalamine is the primary aminosalicylate used – it is well tolerated and can be taken once daily. The other aminosalicylates (sulfasalazine, basalazide, olsalazine) are converted to mesalamine. Sulfasalazine is used less commonly due to the many side effects associated with the sulfapyridine component. The efficacy of aminosalicylates has been proven in UC; however, guidelines no longer recommend their use in CD (they do not maintain remission). Topical steroids or oral budesonide are first line for mild-moderate CD. In moderate-severe cases, an immunosuppressive agent such as azathioprine, mercaptopurine, or methotrexate are used. Steroids may also be used in moderate-severe cases. Anti-TNF agents (e.g., infliximab) are used in patients with IBD that is refractory to steroids and immunosuppressants. These agents are discussed in the Autoimmune chapter.

Nicotine has been shown to worsen CD but can be protective in UC. In fact, nicotine patches have been used as an adjunct therapy for UC; however, adverse effects (nausea, dizziness) limits the benefit.

Agents Used For Mild Symptom Control: Diarrhea, Cramping/GI Spasms

DRUG	DOSING	SAFETY/SIDE EFFECTS/MONITORING

Antidiarrheals

DRUG	DOSING	SAFETY/SIDE EFFECTS/MONITORING
Loperamide *(Imodium)*	2 mg tab/cap; 1 mg liquid 4 mg PO after first loose stool initially; then 2 mg after each subsequent stool; not to exceed 16 mg/day	**CONTRAINDICATIONS** Abdominal pain without diarrhea, children < 2 years of age, acute dysentery (bloody diarrhea and high fever), acute ulcerative colitis, pseudomembranous colitis *(C. difficile)*, bacterial enterocolitis (caused by *Salmonella, Shigella*, and *Campylobacter*) **SIDE EFFECTS** Abdominal cramping, constipation, nausea **NOTES** Do not self-treat for > 2 days
Bismuth subsalicylate *(Pepto-Bismol,* others)	524 mg (2 tbsp or 2 tablets) every 30-60 min as needed, up to 8 doses/day; max 2 days	**CONTRAINDICATIONS** Children with viral infections (varicella, influenza) due to risk of Reye's syndrome, patients with a salicylate allergy, history of severe GI bleed/ulcer or coagulopathy **SIDE EFFECTS** Black tongue/stool, hearing loss/tinnitus (toxicity) **NOTES** Caution in patients on aspirin therapy, anticoagulants, or those with renal insufficiency Salicylate toxicity can occur if used excessively
Diphenoxylate 2.5 mg with atropine 0.025 mg *(Lomotil)* C-V	5 mg daily-QID (max 20 mg/day)	**CONTRAINDICATIONS** Children < 2 years of age, pseudomembranous colitis *(C. difficile)*, diarrhea caused by enterotoxin-producing bacteria (toxigenic *E. coli, Salmonella, Shigella*), obstructive jaundice **WARNING** Toxic megacolon reported in acute ulcerative colitis patients on agents that inhibit intestinal motility. Observe for abdominal distention and discontinue promptly if noted. **SIDE EFFECTS** Somnolence, urinary retention, tachycardia, dry mouth, dizziness, depression

DRUG	DOSING	SAFETY/SIDE EFFECTS/MONITORING

Antispasmodic

| Dicyclomine *(Bentyl)* | 20 mg QID; max 80 mg/day for > 2 weeks (can use 40 mg QID for < 2 weeks if symptoms respond)

 Take 30-60 minutes before meals | **CONTRAINDICATIONS**
 GI obstruction, severe ulcerative colitis, reflux esophagitis, unstable cardiovascular status in acute hemorrhage, obstructive uropathy, breast feeding, narrow-angle glaucoma, myasthenia gravis, infants < 6 months of age

 WARNINGS
 Anticholinergic – use caution in elderly, per Beer's Criteria; caution in mild-moderate ulcerative colitis (potential for toxic megacolon or paralytic ileus)

 SIDE EFFECTS
 Dizziness, dry mouth, nausea, blurred vision |

Corticosteroids

DRUG	DOSING	SAFETY/SIDE EFFECTS/MONITORING

Oral Steroids

| PredniSONE | 5-60 mg/day | **SIDE EFFECTS**
 Short-term: ↑ appetite/weight gain, fluid retention, emotional instability (euphoria, mood swings, irritability), insomnia, GI upset; higher doses can cause ↑ in BP and blood glucose

 Long-term: Adrenal suppression/Cushing's syndrome, immuno-supression/impaired wound healing, hypertension, hyperglycemia, cataracts, osteoporosis, others. See Asthma chapter.

 NOTES (FOR ALL STEROIDS)
 For acute flare management – steroids should not be used long-term – however, some patients use chronically due to severity of condition.

 If used long-term, assess bone density (consider use of bisphosphonates, optimize calcium and vitamin D intake). |
| **Budesonide** *(Entocort EC, Uceris)*

 Entocort EC – 3 mg extended release capsule

 Uceris – 9 mg extended release tablet | Active disease: 9 mg once daily in the morning for up to 8 weeks

 Maintenance of remission: 6 mg once daily for 3 months

 If changing from prednisone, taper prednisone while starting budesonide | If used longer than 2 weeks, must taper (over 3-4 weeks) to avoid withdrawal symptoms.

 May use alternate day therapy (ADT) to ↓ adrenal suppression and adverse effects.

 For Budesonide
 Undergoes extensive first-pass metabolism; lower systemic exposure than other oral steroids.

 Entocort indicated for mild-moderate Crohn's involving the ileum or ascending colon; *Uceris* indicated in UC only.

 Swallow whole – do not crush, chew or break. |

Corticosteroids Continued

DRUG	DOSING	SAFETY/SIDE EFFECTS/MONITORING
Topical Steroids		
Hydrocortisone (*Cortifoam, Cortenema*)	*Cortenema:* 1 enema (100 mg) QHS for 21 days, then taper *Cortifoam:* 1 applicatorful (80 mg) 1-2 times daily for 2-3 weeks, then taper	**CONTRAINDICATIONS** Enema and foam: obstruction, abscess, perforation, peritonitis, intestinal anastomoses, extensive fistulas Enema only: systemic fungal infections and ileocolostomy in immediate/early post-op period **NOTES** Topical steroids have not been proven effective for maintenance of remission. Advantages of topical therapy include less systemic absorption and less frequent dosing schedule.
Budesonide rectal foam (*Uceris*)	1 metered dose BID x 2 weeks, then 1 metered dose daily x 4 weeks (1 metered dose = 2 mg budesonide)	**NOTES** For mild-moderate distal UC. Propellant is flammable; avoid fire and smoking during and after use.

Budesonide Drug Interactions

- Budesonide is a major CYP450 3A4 substrate; potent inhibitors may require a budesonide dose reduction.

- Avoid the use of grapefruit products when using this medication.

Maintenance Therapy

DRUG	DOSING	SAFETY/SIDE EFFECTS/MONITORING

Aminosalicylates

Mesalamine *(Apriso, Asacol HD, Delzicol, Pentasa* and *Lialda* are all long-acting orals; *Canasa* – suppository; *Rowasa* – enema) 5-ASA (5-aminosalicyclic acid)	Suppository: 1 g rectally QHS Enema: 4 g QHS Oral: *Delzicol*: 800 mg TID or 400 mg QID *Pentasa*: 1 g QID *Lialda*: 2.4-4.8 g once daily *Asacol HD*: 1.6 g TID *Apriso* 1.5 g once daily	**CONTRAINDICATIONS** Hypersensitivity to salicylates or aminosalicylates or any component of the formulation (see notes) **WARNINGS** Caution in patients with renal or hepatic impairment and active peptic ulcer, ↑ blood dyscrasias in elderly, pericarditis/myocarditis, oligospermia (rare) Patients with hypersensitivity to sulfasalazine may have a similar reaction to mesalamine; however, most patients do not. *Apriso* contains pheylalanine – avoid in phenylketonuria (PKU). *Rowasa* enema contains metabisulfite salts – caution in sulfite sensitivity. **SIDE EFFECTS** Abdominal pain, nausea, headache, flatulence, eructation (belching), pharyngitis, acute intolerance syndrome (similar to symptoms of IBD exacerbation) **MONITORING** Renal function, CBC, symptoms of IBD **NOTES** Best to avoid concomitant use of oral formulations with antacids, H₂RAs, or PPIs (interfere with absorption). Mesalamine is better tolerated than other aminosalicylates. Topical mesalamine is more effective than oral mesalamine and steroids for distal disease/proctitis in UC; can use oral and topical together. Topical agents should not be used in proximal disease. Swallow caps/tabs whole; do not crush, chew, or break due to delayed-release coating.
SulfaSALAzine *(Azulfidine, Azulfidine EN-tabs, Sulfazine, Sulfazine EC)* 5-aminosalicylic acid derivative	2-6 g daily divided TID or QID	See Autoimmune chapter.
Balsalazide *(Colazal, Giazo)*	*Colazal*: 2.25 g PO TID *Giazo*: 3.3 g PO BID	**CONTRAINDICATIONS** Salicylate allergy **SIDE EFFECTS** Headache, abdominal pain, diarrhea, vomiting (GI effects more common in children) **MONITORING** Renal function, LFTs, hypersensitivity, symptoms of IBD **NOTES** *Giazo* is only approved in males (failed to show a benefit in females) *Colazal* capsule contents may be sprinkled on applesauce. Beads are not coated, so mixture can be chewed if needed. This may cause staining of teeth/tongue.

Maintenance Therapy Continued

DRUG	DOSING	SAFETY/SIDE EFFECTS/MONITORING
Olsalazine (*Dipentum*)	500 mg PO BID	**CONTRAINDICATIONS** Salicylate allergy **SIDE EFFECTS** Diarrhea, abdominal pain **MONITORING** CBC, LFTs, renal function, symptoms of IBD

Immunosuppressive Agents – these agents can be used if patient fails above therapy or they can be used in combination with above therapies; often called "immunomodulators" or "steroid sparing" therapies

DRUG	DOSING	SAFETY/SIDE EFFECTS/MONITORING
AzaTHIOprine (*Azasan, Imuran*)	2-3 mg/kg/day given IV/PO	**BOXED WARNINGS (2)** Chronic immunosuppression can ↑ risk of neoplasia (esp. lymphomas) Hematologic toxicities (leukopenia, thrombocytopenia) and mutagenic potential **WARNINGS** GI (severe N/V/D), hematologic (leukopenia, thrombocytopenia, anemia), and hepatotoxicity; patients with genetic deficiency of thiopurine methyltransferase (TPMT) are at ↑ risk for myelosuppression and may require lower dose. **SIDE EFFECTS** Severe N/V/D, rash, ↑ LFTs, hematologic toxicities (leukopenia, thrombocytopenia) **MONITORING** LFTs, CBC (weekly for 1st month), renal function **NOTES** Pregnancy Category D Azathioprine is metabolized to mercaptopurine (avoid concurrent use due to myelosuppression) Olsalazine and allopurinol inhibit TPMT – may require ↓ dose of azathioprine
Mercaptopurine (*Purinethol, Purixan*)	1-1.5 mg/kg/day PO	Similar to azathioprine, including TPMT **NOTES** Take on an empty stomach. Avoid old terms "6-Mercaptopurine" and "6-MP" – they caused 6x overdoses.
Methotrexate (*Rheumatrex, Trexall*) *Rasuvo* and *Otrexup* auto-injectors are used for RA	15-25 mg weekly PO	See Autoimmune chapter.

Monoclonal Antibodies to TNF

In patients with moderate-severe disease that has not responded to steroids and/or immunosuppressants or in any patient in which a steroid is contraindicated or not desired, treatment with monoclonal antibodies to TNF is likely to be used next. The drugs used in UC and CD are listed below. These are in the Autoimmune chapter, where they are primarily used. The integrin receptor antagonists are used for both (autoimmune and IBD) and are discussed below.

DRUG	UC	CD
Adalimumab *(Humira)*	FDA approved	FDA approved
InFLIXimab *(Remicade)*	FDA approved	FDA approved
Golimumab *(Simponi)*	FDA approved	
Certolizumab *(Cimzia)*		FDA approved

Monoclonal Antibodies – Integrin Receptor Antagonists

DRUG	DOSING	SAFETY/SIDE EFFECTS/MONITORING
Natalizumab *(Tysabri)* Approved for Crohn's and Multiple Sclerosis	300 mg IV over 1 hour every 4 weeks If taking steroids when initiating *Tysabri*, taper when onset of benefit observed. Stop *Tysabri* if patient cannot taper steroids within 6 months.	**BOXED WARNING** Risk for progressive multifocal leukoencephalopathy (PML) – monitor mental status changes. Risk factors for PML include: anti-JC virus antibodies, ↑ treatment duration and prior immunosuppressant use. **SIDE EFFECTS** Infusion reactions, headache, fatigue, nausea, respiratory infections, rash, hepatotoxicity (rare) **NOTES** Only approved for moderate-severe Crohn's patients who have failed anti-TNF therapy. Discontinue if no response by week 12. REMS: Must be enrolled in manufacturer TOUCH prescribing program. Cannot be used with other immunosuppressants. MedGuide required. Do not shake. Stable in NS only. Requires protection from light during administration.
Vedolizumab *(Entyvio)* Approved for Crohn's and UC	300 mg IV at 0, 2, and 6 weeks, then every 8 weeks. Discontinue if no benefit by week 14	**WARNINGS** Infusion reactions (rare), infections, liver injury, and PML (see monitoring). Patients receiving vedolizumab should not receive live vaccines. **SIDE EFFECTS** Headache, nasopharyngitis, arthralgia, antibody development **MONITORING** LFTs, signs and symptoms of infection, hypersensitivity, neurological symptoms and/or progressive weakness (to monitor for PML – not observed with vedolizumab, but Boxed Warning with natalizumab); routine TB screening **NOTES** Refrigerate and store in original packaging. After reconstitution and dilution, use immediately or refrigerate up to 4 hours. Do not freeze. Infuse over 30 min. All immunizations must be up to date before starting therapy. Cannot be used with other immunosuppressants. MedGuide required.

Mesalamine Patient Counseling

- <u>Do not crush or chew long-acting formulations</u>. You may see a <u>ghost tablet</u> in the feces *(Asacol HD)*; the drug has been absorbed into your body; the tablet is empty.

- *Rowasa* enema: *Rowasa* is an off-white suspension. It can darken over time when removed from the foil pouch. If it has dark brown contents, throw it away. Remove bottle from pouch and shake well. Remove the protective sheath from the applicator tip. Hold the bottle at the neck so as not to cause any of the medicine to be discharged. Best results are obtained by lying on the left side with the left leg extended and the right leg flexed forward for balance. Gently insert the lubricated applicator tip into the rectum to prevent damage to the rectal wall, pointed slightly toward the navel. Grasp the bottle firmly, and then tilt slightly so that the nozzle is aimed toward the back, and squeeze slowly to instill the medication. Steady hand pressure will discharge most of the medicine. After administering, withdraw and discard the bottle. Remain in position for at least 30 minutes, or preferably all night for maximum benefit. *Rowasa* can cause staining of surfaces including, clothing, and other fabrics, flooring, painted surfaces, marble, granite, vinyl and enamel. Take care in choosing a suitable location for administration of this product.

- *Canasa* suppository: For best results, empty your rectum (have a bowel movement) just before using. This medication should be used at bedtime. Detach one suppository from the strip. Remove foil wrapper; avoid excessive handling. Insert the suppository with the pointed end first completely into your rectum, using gentle pressure. For best results, keep the suppository in your rectum for at least 1-3 hours. You may put a little bit of lubricating gel on the suppository. *Canasa* can cause staining of surfaces including, clothing, and other fabrics, flooring, painted surfaces, marble, granite, vinyl and enamel. Keep *Canasa* away from these surfaces to prevent staining.

Hydrocortisone *(Cortifoam)* Patient Counseling

- Preparation: Shake the foam container well for 5 – 10 seconds before using. Hold container upright on a level surface. Place the tip of the applicator onto the nose of the container cap. Pull plunger past the fill line on the applicator barrel. To fill the applicator, press down firmly on the cap flanges, hold for 1 – 2 seconds and release. Wait 5 – 10 seconds for the foam to expand and fill the applicator barrel. Repeat until full and then remove applicator from container.

- Use: hold applicator firmly by the barrel (thumb and middle finger on the barrel "wings") and place index finger on the plunger. Insert tip into anus and push plunger to expel foam. Withdraw applicator. The foam container should never be inserted into the anus – only the applicator.

- After use, take apart and clean all parts with warm water for next use.

- Each aerosol container should deliver 14 doses.

- Store at room temperature.

Budesonide *(Uceris)* Rectal Foam Patient Counseling

- This medicine is for rectal use only.

- The *Uceris* rectal foam kit has 2 aerosol canisters and 28 lubricated applicators. Each canister contains 14 doses of foam. Store at room temperature. Do not puncture or burn the canisters.

- Empty your rectum completely. Warm the canister in your hands and shake well for 10 – 15 seconds before using. Choose a position to administer – standing, lying or sitting on the toilet. Use the evening dose before bedtime and try not to have a bowel movement until morning.

- The aerosol is flammable. Keep it away from fire, flames or smoking during and after use. Do not spray toward a flame.

- Do not use grapefruit or grapefruit juice with this medication. If you have been using grapefruit do not change the amount without discussing this with your healthcare provider.

Budesonide *(Entocort EC* and *Uceris)* Patient Counseling

- Take this medication with a full glass of water before a meal. <u>Do not crush, chew or break open the capsule</u>.

- Tell your healthcare provider if you have changes in the shape or location of body fat (especially in your arms, legs, face, neck, breasts, and waist), high blood pressure, severe headache, fast or uneven heart rate, blurred vision, or a general ill feeling with headache, tiredness, nausea, and vomiting.

- You should have your blood pressure monitored on a regular basis.

- You should have your blood sugar monitored on a regular basis.

- Do not use grapefruit or grapefruit juice products with this medication. If you have been using grapefruit do not change the amount without discussing this with your healthcare provider.

- Avoid being near people who are sick or have infections.

For counseling on the biologic agents, see the Autoimmune chapter.

PRACTICE CASE

Frank Clough: SOAP Note for 09/24/2014
Age on DOS: 75 yrs, DOB: 01/14/1939

San Diego Medical Group
35 La Jolla Drive Suite 100 San Diego, CA 92130
(444) 444-4444

seen by: Alison James
seen on: Wednesday 24 September 2014

VS

Height:	Weight:	BMI:	Blood Pressure:	Temp:	Pulse:	Resp Rate:
65.0 in	148.0 lb	24.6	165 / 92 mmHg	98.9 F	97 bpm	16 rpm

CC | Lots of diarrhea for the past few days and now there's blood in it

S | Mr. Clough presents with a 3 day history of 5-6 diarrhea episodes per day. He describes this as similar to his initial diagnosis of ulcerative colitis in Nevada about 5 months ago. He describes some cramping and bloating in the lower abdomen, but no other associated pain. He doesn't think the pain is worse or better with food, but he hasn't eaten much over the past few days. He has no nausea or vomiting. Today he noticed some streaks of blood in the diarrhea and his wife became concerned and made the appointment at the clinic. He states he is compliant with his mesalamine suppositories and they have worked well in controlling his UC over the past months until now. His usual diarrhea frequency is 1-2 episodes her day. Patient reports an allergy to penicillin. He experiences a severe rash.

O | Past Medical History:
Ulcerative colitis (distal disease) and hypertension

Medications:
Canasa 1 gm suppository daily at HS x 5 months / Tenormin 100 mg daily x "many years"
Both prescribed by MD in Nevada and active. Patient states he is compliant.

Labs (reference range):
Na 139 mEq/L (135 - 145)
K 3.8 mEq/L (3.5 - 5)
Cl 100 mEq/L (95 - 103)
HCO3 26 mEq/L (24 - 30)
BUN 27 mg/dL (7 - 20)
SCr 1.4 mg/dL (0.6 - 1.3)
Glu 109 mg/dL (100 - 125)
WBC 8.6 cells/mm3 (4 - 11 x 10^3)
Hgb 16.8 g/dL (13.5 - 18 male, 12 - 16 female)
Hct 48 % (38 - 50 male, 36 - 46 female)
Plt 250 mm3 (150,000 - 450,000)

A | 75 yo otherwise fairly healthy white gentleman here for an ulcerative colitis exacerbation.
(1) Ulcerative colitis (distal) exacerbation:
Patient has been well-controlled on mesalamine suppositories for his disease and finds this therapy acceptable. He has never required steroids of any kind. He is currently dehydrated as evidenced by objective data (BP, HR and BUN/SCr ratio) and requires therapy to control the acute flare.
(2) Hypertension:
BP is not currently at goal. Since this is a new patient to our clinic, we may need to re-assess once he is more stable and rehydrated. Regardless, need to align therapy with JNC 8 guidelines.

P | Prednisone 10 mg daily for ulcerative colitis flare. Follow-up in clinic in 1 week.

Questions

1. The patient was originally prescribed mesalamine suppositories for distal disease classified as mild-moderate. Which of the following statements are correct? (Select **ALL** that apply.)

   a. Oral therapy is preferred for initial treatment.

   b. Mesalamine is available in oral and rectal (suppositories, enema) formulations.

   c. Sulfasalazine is preferred over mesalamine for distal disease.

   d. Mesalamine cannot be used in a sulfa allergy.

   e. Mesalamine is considered first-line therapy for distal disease.

2. Mesalamine rectal suppository counseling should include the following points: (Select **ALL** that apply.)

   a. Peel open the plastic and remove suppository prior to use.

   b. Handle unwrapped suppository as little as possible.

   c. Should be kept in the rectum for at least 1-3 hours.

   d. Lubricating gel may be used to ease application.

   e. Insert suppository just prior to a bowel movement.

3. The physician prescribed prednisone therapy for the acute flare-up. Which of the following are short-term side effects that may occur and should be conveyed to the patient? (Select **ALL** that apply.)

   a. Elevated blood glucose

   b. Elevated blood pressure

   c. Osteoporosis

   d. Changes in mood

   e. Cataracts

4. ACG guidelines recommend against steroid treatment for long-term control of IBD symptoms; however, many patients use budesonide (or prednisone) daily. Which of the following are long-term side effects that may occur and should be conveyed to the patient? (Select **ALL** that apply.)

   a. Hepatotoxicity

   b. Poor wound healing

   c. Fat redistribution

   d. Adrenal suppression

   e. Peptic ulcers

Questions 5-6 are NOT based on the above case.

5. A female patient has failed her initial therapy for Crohn's disease, which included cyclosporine and methotrexate. Her symptoms are described as severe. She is prescribed infliximab. Which of the following statements is CORRECT?

   a. She can use *Enbrel* instead.

   b. She should have been prescribed *Tysabri* prior to use of infliximab.

   c. Infliximab suppositories are the preferred formulation.

   d. This medication comes in an IV formulation only.

   e. This medication can suppress TB activation.

6. A patient has been prescribed infliximab. Which of the following tests should be ordered prior to the start of therapy? (Select **ALL** that apply.)

   a. Pulmonary function

   b. TSH and FT4

   c. CBC

   d. TB

   e. HBV

Answers

1-b,e, 2-a,b,c,d, 3-a,b,d, 4-b,c,d, e, 5-d, 6-c,d,e

67

ERECTILE DYSFUNCTION

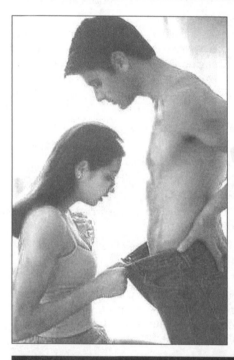

BACKGROUND

The most common direct cause of erectile dysfunction (ED) is reduced blood flow to the penis, which is commonly caused by diseases, including diabetes and metabolic syndrome, obesity, hypertension, heart disease, and nerve damage (commonly due to diabetes). ED is often the "canary in the coal mine" (an early warning) for cardiovascular disease. ED can appear first since the arteries supplying blood to the penis are smaller than those supplying blood to the heart; they can become restricted sooner than the larger vessels. Men with ED should be referred for cardiac evaluation. Hormone imbalances (such as low testosterone), psychological issues (including depression and stress) and neurological illness can also cause ED. Some men will need testosterone replacement therapy in order to sustain an erection. In these cases, they are likely to have other signs of low testosterone. See the Osteoporosis and Hormone

COMMON DRUGS THAT CAN CAUSE SEXUAL DYSFUNCTION

Blood pressure medications – especially beta blockers, clonidine, methyldopa

Antipsychotics – including haloperidol, chlorpromazine, fluphenazine and thioridazine

Antidepressants – particularly SSRIs and SNRIs

Atomoxetine

Proscar® Avodart®

The BPH drugs finasteride, dutasteride (2013-warning of possible persistent sexual dysfunction after discontinuation with the these 2 agents), and silodosin

Chemotherapeutic agents that ↓ sex hormone levels, leuprolide (*Lupron*), etc.

Cimetidine – which blocks androgenic hormones

Opioids, chronic use, including methadone

Nicotine

Therapy chapter for more information on testosterone. Some men have more than one factor contributing to ED. Drugs that can contribute to ED are listed in the table. In some men, lifestyle changes, such as losing weight, quitting tobacco use or reducing alcohol intake can correct the condition.

NON-DRUG TREATMENT

Non-drug options include penile vacuums, implants and surgery.

Natural Products

Yohimbe bark is rated as "possibly effective" by the Natural Medicines Database for impotence and for sexual dysfunction associated with SSRIs. Typical doses can cause a variety of adverse effects, including stomach upset, hypertension and tachycardia. Excessive doses can cause hypotension, seizures and respiratory depression. Concurrent use with MAO inhibitors is contraindicated. Concurrent use with blood pressure agents can be dangerous. Yohimbe can be unsafe and should not be recommended. L-arginine is rated as "possibly effective" for ED – it can cause additive blood-pressure lowering effects with other hypotensive agents – including the PDE-5 inhibitors, nitrates and blood pressure medications. These combinations should be avoided. Some men find panax ginseng helps with ED.

DRUG TREATMENT

The phosphodiesterase 5 (PDE-5) inhibitors are the primary drugs used for ED in males. Men with decreased libido (sexual interest) and ED should have the serum testosterone level tested; if low, hormone replacement may be helpful, alone or with another agent such as a PDE-5 inhibitor. See the Osteoporosis and Hormone Therapy chapter. This chapter does not discuss female sexual dysfunction since there is not, at present, drugs with an indication for this condition. If a patient cannot tolerate PDE-5 inhibitors (or has a contraindication) alprostadil may be used.

Note that the PDE-5 inhibitors are used under different names for pulmonary arterial hypertension (PAH) – do not use same drugs under different names concurrently (duplicate therapy). The PDE-5 inhibitor tadalifil is indicated for Benign Prostatic Hypertrophy (BPH).

Phosphodiesterase 5 (PDE-5) Inhibitors

Following sexual stimulation (which is required), PDE-5 inhibitors increase blood flow to the penis, causing an erection. They are used for problems with impotence. They do not increase desire.

[margin note, left:] do NOT use nitrates until after:

[margin note:] 24 hrs

[margin note:] 48 hrs

[margin note:] 48 hrs

[margin note:] 12 hrs

[margin note:] may be permanent

[margin note:]
• trouble distinguishing blue green
• seeing blue tinge (shade) around objects

DRUG	DOSING	SAFETY/SIDE EFFECTS/MONITORING
Sildenafil (*Viagra*) *Revatio* – for pulmonary arterial hypertension (PAH)	25, 50, 100 mg Start at 50 mg, taken ~1 hr (0.5-4 hr) before intercourse In elderly patients (age > 65) start with 25 mg. Use this lower starting dose for patients with hepatic impairment, CrCl < 30 mL/min or if on strong CYP 3A4 inhibitors.	**CONTRAINDICATIONS** Concurrent use with nitrates If chest pain after taking seek immediate medical help. **WARNINGS** Color discrimination impairment, dose-related, patients with retinitis pigmentosa may have higher risk. Hearing loss, can be sudden, with or without tinnitus/dizziness. Vision loss, rare but may be due to nonarteritic anterior ischemic optic neuropathy (NAION). Risk factors include low cup-to-disc ratio ("crowded disc"), CAD, diabetes, hypertension, hyperlipidemia, smoking, and > 50 years of age. Avoid use with known degenerative retinal disorders (e.g., retinitis pigmentosa).
Vardenafil (*Levitra, Staxyn ODT*) Do not initiate with *Staxyn*; switch over from low-dose regular tablet.	2.5, 5, 10, 20 mg (*Staxyn* only 10 mg ODT, which is equiv to 10 mg *Levitra*) Start at 10 mg, taken ~1 hr before intercourse In elderly patients (age > 65) start with 5 mg. Use this lower starting dose for patients with hepatic impairment, CrCl < 30 mL/min or if on strong CYP 3A4 inhibitors.	Hypotension, due to vasodilation, higher risk if resting BP < 90/50 mmHg, fluid depletion, or autonomic dysfunction. Caution with other agents that cause hypotension, such as alpha blockers and BP drugs. Priapism, instruct to seek emergency medical care if erection lasts > 4 hr.
Tadalafil (*Cialis*) *Adcirca* – for pulmonary arterial hypertension (PAH), *Cialis* – for ED and Benign Prostatic Hypertrophy (BPH) *[margin note:]* w/ or w/o food	2.5, 5, 10, 20 mg Start at 10 mg, with or without food, taken ~ 1 hr before intercourse or 2.5-5 mg daily (for men who use *Cialis* > 2 times per week). ↓ dose to 5-10 mg with renal impairment or moderate liver impairment. Do not use daily dosing and do not exceed 5 mg every 72 hours if CrCl < 30 mL/min, and do not use if severe liver impairment.	**SIDE EFFECTS** Headache, flushing, dyspepsia, color vision changes (blurred vision, increased sensitivity to light) erythema, epistaxis, diarrhea, myalgia **NOTES** Best when taken on an empty stomach, avoid with fatty food (tadalafil is with or without food). For ED, no more than 1 dose/day is recommended. *Stendra* can be taken closest to sexual activity.
Avanafil (*Stendra*) *[margin note:]* max 1 dose/day	50, 100, 200 mg Start at 100 mg, with or without food, as early as 15 minutes prior to intercourse Do not use with severe renal or liver impairment. Do not use with strong CYP 3A4 inhibitors and use lower dose with moderate CYP 3A4 inhibitors.	

Drug Interactions

- PDE-5 inhibitors are contraindicated with nitrates. Concurrent use of nitrate medications [any nitroglycerin-containing drug, including *Nitrostat, Nitrolingual*, isosorbide dinitrate-hydralazine *(BiDil)*, others] increases the potential for excessively low blood pressure. Taking nitrates is an absolute contraindication to the use of these medicines. These include the illicit drugs such as amyl nitrate and butyl nitrate ("poppers").

- If a patient with ED has taken a PDE-5 inhibitor and then develops angina, nitroglycerin should not be used until after 12 hours for avanafil, 24 hours for sildenafil or vardenafil and after 48 hours for tadalafil. (Sometimes nitrates are used in an acute emergency, despite this warning, with careful monitoring.)

- Caution with PDE-5 inhibitor and concurrent alpha-1 blocker therapy: PDE-5 inhibitors may enhance the hypotensive effect of an alpha-1 blocker. The alpha-1 blocker dose should be stable (without excessive dizziness/hypotension) prior to the start of the PDE-5 inhibitor. If *Cialis* is being used for BPH, do not use alpha-1 (non-selective) blockers concurrently.

- CYP450 3A4 inducers (strong) decrease levels; monitor effectiveness. 3A4 inhibitors (moderate) increase the PDE-5 levels (may require lower doses) and 3A4 inhibitors (strong) require lower doses of PDE-5 inhibitors.

Alternative Agents

DRUG	ROUTE	SAFETY/SIDE EFFECTS/MONITORING
Intracavernosal alprostadil *(Caverject Impulse, Edex)* *Prostin VR Pediatric*– patency of ductus arteriosus	Injected via syringe into penis Causes erection 5-10 min after injection, lasts ~1 hr, max 3x/ week and 1x/day	**BOXED WARNING** Risk of apnea when used in neonates. **SIDE EFFECTS** Penile pain, headache, dizziness, hematoma, priapism, scarring at injection site **NOTES** Refrigerate vials, reconstitute prior to use. Syncope can occur within 1 hr of administration, most commonly with concurrent antihypertensives.
Transurethral alprostadil *(MUSE)* Refrigerate	Inserted into urethra (pellets)	**SIDE EFFECTS** Penile pain, headache, dizziness, priapism **NOTES** Alprostadil formulations are Pregnancy Category X/C *(MUSE)*.

[handwritten note:] max 1x/day 3x/wk

PRACTICE CASE

JF is a 60 y/o black male who made an appointment at the Family Medicine clinic to be evaluated for impotence. He cannot sustain an erection. This has caused performance anxiety, which has worsened the situation. His medical conditions include hypertension, anxiety/low mood, obesity and prostate enlargement.

Allergies: NKDA

Medications:
Flomax 0.4 mg daily   *selective*
Inderal LA 160 mg daily
Fosinopril 10 mg daily
Zoloft 100 mg daily
Vitamin D 200 IU daily
Aspirin 325 mg daily
Acetaminophen 325 mg 1-2 tablets PRN headache

Vitals:
Height: 5'9" Weight: 210 pounds
BP: 118/82 mmHg HR: 90 BPM RR: 16 BPM Temp: 98.6°F

Labs: Na (mEq/L) = 140 (135 - 145)
K (mEq/L) = 5.1 (3.5 - 5)
Cl (mEq/L) = 100 (95 - 103)
HCO3 (mEq/L) = 25 (24 - 30)
BUN (mg/dL) = 16 (7 - 20)
SCr (mg/dL) = 1.0 (0.6 - 1.3)
Glucose (mg/dL) = 130 (100 - 125)
Ca (mg/dL) = 10.1 (8.5 - 10.5)
Mg (mEq/L) = 1.9 (1.3 - 2.1)
PO4 (mg/dL) = 4.5 (2.3 - 4.7)

Start sildenafil 50 mg - take 1 hour prior to sexual activity. Schedule follow-up appointment in 2 months. The cardiologist has written a new prescription for amiodarone 200 mg PO daily that AH would like to have filled.

Questions

1. Is sildenafil contraindicated in this patient? (Select **ALL** that apply.)

    a. Yes, the combination of Flomax and sildenafil is contraindicated.

    b. No, but he must be cautioned about dizziness, lightheadedness and fainting.

    c. No, but he has to begin sildenafil at 12.5 mg once daily.

    d. No, but the Flomax should be changed to doxazosin; this is a safer combination.

    e. No, but the dose of the alpha blocker should be stable (well-tolerated) prior to beginning the PDE-5 inhibitor.

2. Which of the following medications could be contributing to Jim's problem with erectile dysfunction? (Select **ALL** that apply.)

    a. Inderal LA

    b. Zoloft

    c. Vitamin D

    d. Aspirin

    e. Acetaminophen

3. If Jim begins sildenafil therapy, he should be counseled concerning the risk of priapism. Select the correct counseling statement:

    a. If you sustain an erection that lasts more than 4 hours, you should stop using the medicine. The erection will go away in about 24 hours.

    b. If you sustain an erection that lasts more than 4 hours, you should stop using the medicine and take 25 mg of over-the-counter diphenhydramine. The erection will go away in about 24 hours.

    c. If you sustain an erection that lasts more than 4 hours, you should stop using the medicine and rest in bed until the erection goes away, which takes about 4-6 hours.

    d. If you sustain an erection that lasts more than 2 hours, you will need to get medical help right away. Priapism must be treated as soon as possible or it can cause lasting damage to the penis.

    e. If you sustain an erection that lasts more than 4 hours, you will need to get medical help right away. Priapism must be treated as soon as possible or it can cause lasting damage to the penis.

4. The pharmacist should call the physician and recommend possible medication changes that could reduce or eliminate the ED problem. Reasonable suggestions could include: (Select **ALL** that apply.)

    a. Change the Zoloft to a medication that is not in the SSRI or SNRI class.

    b. Change the fosinopril to losartan.

    c. Change Inderal LA to a different class of medication, or try a trial with metoprolol.

    d. Change the fosinopril to amlodipine.

    e. Change the Inderal LA to furosemide.

Questions 5-6 do not apply to the above case.

5. A patient is using tadalafil three times weekly. He uses 10 mg, taken 1 hour before sexual intercourse. He has asked the physician to change him to the daily form of the medicine, since he uses it more than twice weekly. Choose the correct dosing range for daily tadalafil when used for ED:

    a. 0.125-2.5 mg daily

    b. 2.5-5 mg daily

    c. 5-10 mg daily

    d. 10-15 mg daily

    e. This medicine cannot be used daily

6. The PDE-5 inhibitors require lower doses, and in some cases avoidance, when a patient is using certain drugs, including saquinavir and clarithromycin. This is due to the following reason: *Invirase*

    a. These are strong CYP 3A4 inducers; they could cause the PDE-5 inhibitor level to decrease to a dangerous level.

    b. These are strong CYP 3A4 inhibitors; they could cause the PDE-5 inhibitor level to increase to a dangerous level.

    c. These are strong CYP 3A4 inducers; they could cause the PDE-5 inhibitor level to increase to a dangerous level.

    d. These are strong CYP 3A4 inhibitors; they could cause the PDE-5 inhibitor level to decrease to a dangerous level.

    e. There is no interaction between PDE-5 inhibitor's and these medications.

Answers

1-b,e, 2-a,b, 3-e, 4-a,c, 5-b, 6-b

68

BENIGN PROSTATIC HYPERPLASIA (BPH)

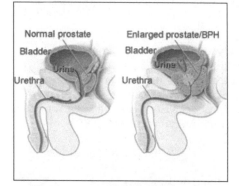

Normal prostate Enlarged prostate/BPH
Bladder Bladder
Urine Urine
Urethra Urethra

GUIDELINES

Update on AUA Guideline on the Management of Benign Prostatic Hyperplasia. *The Journal of Urology.* 2011; 185:1793-1803.

American Urological Association Practice Guidelines Committee. AUA guidelines on management of benign prostatic hyperplasia 2003. Chapter 1: Diagnosis and treatment recommendations. *The Journal of Urology.* 2003; 170:530-547.

BACKGROUND

The prostate is a walnut-sized gland that surrounds the urethra at the base of the bladder. As part of the male reproductive system, the main function of the prostate is to secrete slightly alkaline fluid that becomes part of the seminal fluid carrying sperm.

The prostate is dependent on androgens (mainly testosterone) for development and maintenance of size and function. Testosterone is metabolized to dihydrotestosterone (DHT) by 5 alpha-reductase. DHT is responsible for normal and hyperplastic growth (increase in the number of cells). Benign prostatic hyperplasia (BPH) results from overgrowth of the stromal and epithelial cells of the prostate gland. The enlarged gland contributes to lower urinary tract symptoms (LUTS) via direct bladder outlet obstruction (BOO) and increased smooth muscle tone and resistance. As the prostate enlarges, the layer of tissue surrounding it stops it from expanding, causing the gland to press against the urethra like a clamp on a garden hose. The bladder wall becomes thicker and irritated. The bladder begins to contract even when it contains small amounts of urine, causing more frequent urination. Eventually, the bladder weakens and loses the ability to empty itself. Interestingly, there is not a direct linear correlation between prostate size and symptoms; some men are more bothered even with a smaller prostate size, while others with a larger prostate are not as symptomatic. The enlargement does not usually cause problems until later in life with a peak incidence around 65 years of age. When the prostate becomes larger, prostate specific antigen (PSA) levels can increase; yet, BPH does not increase the risk of prostate cancer.

SYMPTOMS/COMPLICATIONS

The signs and symptoms of BPH are mainly LUTS which include difficulty holding urine (storage) and emptying the bladder (voiding). These disturbances significantly impact the quality of life for the patient. LUTS can include:

- Hesitancy, intermittency, straining or weak stream of urine
- Urinary urgency and leaking or dribbling
- Incomplete emptying of the bladder (bladder always feels full)
- Urinary frequency, especially nocturia (urination at night)
- Bladder outlet obstruction (BOO)

BPH rarely causes more severe symptoms – but, if the blockage is severe, the urine could back up into the kidneys and result in acute renal failure. Urinary tract infections can also be present, but are uncommon in men.

DIAGNOSIS

Prostate cancer symptoms can be similar to the symptoms of BPH. Diagnosis requires a careful patient medical history including surgeries and trauma, current medications including herbal and OTC drugs, focused physical exam including a Digital Rectal Exam (DRE), and urinalysis and serum Prostate Specific Antigen (PSA) to rule out conditions other than BPH (e.g., prostate or bladder cancer, neurogenic bladder, others). Patient may be asked to complete a voiding diary as well to better tailor therapy. PSA, a protein produced by prostate cells, is frequently ↑ in prostate cancer, however, it can also be increased in other conditions including BPH. Note that the recommendations for routine prostate cancer screening have changed (they will be done less frequently than in the past); see Oncology chapter.

DRUGS THAT WORSEN BPH
Decongestants (e.g., pseudoephrine)
Anticholinergics (e.g., benztropine)
Antihistamines (e.g., diphenhydramine, chlorpheniramine)
TCAs, phenothiazines and other drugs with anticholinergic properties
Caffeine (can worsen symptoms)
Diuretics (increase urination–be sure to take early in the day to limit nocturia)
SNRIs (affect urethral resistance)
Testosterone products

DRUG TREATMENT

The patient's perception of the severity of BPH symptoms guides selection of the treatment modality in a patient. Validated questionnaires, such as the AUA Symptom Score, are commonly used to quantify symptoms. The scoring system rates how bothersome the symptoms are to the patient, with higher scores indicating more severe or bothersome symptoms. Treatment options can include watchful waiting, pharmacologic therapy and surgical intervention. Choice of treatment is a shared decision-making process between the patient and the clinician. Mild disease is generally treated with watchful waiting, which entails having the patient return for reassessment yearly. Moderate/severe disease is generally treated with medications, a minimally invasive procedure, or surgery such as transurethral resection of the prostate (TURP). Medications include alpha blockers (selective and non-selective), alone or in combination with a 5 alpha-reductase inhibitor. The 5 alpha-reductase inhibitors should not be used in men with LUTS secondary to BPH without prostatic enlargement (as these medications work by decreasing prostate size). Peripheral-acting anticholinergic agents used for overactive bladder (such as tolterodine) are sometimes a reasonable option for men without an elevated post void residual (PRV) urine and when LUTS are predominately irritative. If anticholinergics are used, PVR should be < 250-300 mL (anticholinergics are discussed in the Overactive Bladder chapter). Another treatment option is using the phosphodiesterase-5 (PDE-5) inhibitor tadalifil. This can be used in men with BPH alone, and can be an attractive option for men with both BPH and erectile dysfunction (ED); the dose is sufficient for both indications. Tadalafil, in combination with an alpha blocker (especially a non-selective agent) would pose risk for additive hypotension and orthostasis in an elderly male.

Historically, alpha blockers have been considered the standard BPH drug treatment. They are used alone in mild symptoms, and often with a 5 alpha-reductase inhibitor with moderate symptoms. Recently, tamsulosin (the most popular alpha-blocker) has been associated with floppy iris syndrome, a condition that makes cataract surgery difficult to complete safely. Cataracts are common in elderly patients, and the use of alpha blockers increases the risk itself. The important thing is to let the ophthalmologist know if a patient has ever taken an alpha-blocker.

Natural Products

Saw palmetto is used for BPH, but it is rated as "possibly ineffective" by The Natural Medicines Database due to contradictory and inconsistent data. Pygeum is another natural product and it is rated as "possibly effective". Do not recommend a pygeum product unless it has been harvested ethically; ripping the bark off the trees to extract pygeum is not sustainable. Other natural products rated as "possibly effective" are beta-sitosterol (which is available as supplements, in margarine substitutes, in African wild potato extract products, in pumpkin seed and in soy and red clover) and rye grass pollen. Lycopene is used for prostate cancer prevention, however, there is no good evidence for taking the supplement for this purpose. Pharmacists should not recommend natural products until the patient has seen a health care provider; it is not prudent to recommend a product that could be masking cancer symptoms. Although the symptoms will primarily be benign, the small risk of prostate cancer must be considered.

Alpha Blockers

These agents inhibit alpha-1 adrenergic receptors and relax the smooth muscle of the bladder neck reducing bladder outlet obstruction and improving urinary flow. There are 3 types of alpha receptors: 1A (prostate primarily has these receptors), 1B, and 1D; terazosin and doxazosin are non-selective and this results in more side effects (orthostasis, dizziness, fatigue, headache) than the selective agents (tamsulosin, alfuzosin, silodosin).

DRUG	DOSING	SAFETY/SIDE EFFECTS/MONITORING

Non-Selective Alpha-1 Blockers

DRUG	DOSING	SAFETY/SIDE EFFECTS/MONITORING
Terazosin	Start at 1 mg at bedtime; titrate slowly to effect – generally 10 mg QHS (may ↑ to 20 mg QHS)	**WARNINGS** Orthostatic hypotension/syncope: typically with first dose, if therapy is interrupted for several days, dosage is increased too rapidly or another antihypertensive agent or PDE-5 inhibitor is started Floppy iris syndrome can occur during cataract surgery Priapism – seek medical attention if lasting > 4 hours Angina – D/C if symptoms of angina begin or worsen **SIDE EFFECTS** Dizziness, fatigue, orthostatic hypotension, headache, muscle weakness **MONITORING** BP, PSA, urinary symptoms
Doxazosin (*Cardura, Cardura XL*)	IR: start at 1 mg; titrate slowly up to 4-8 mg daily, usually given at bedtime XL: Start at 4 mg daily with breakfast; titrate to a max of 8 mg daily	**NOTES** The non-selective agents are often given QHS to help minimize the initial "first dose" effect of orthostasis/dizziness. This requires careful counseling (see below) as the man likely has nocturia, where getting up at night to use the bathroom with dizziness and orthostasis can be dangerous. Alpha blockers work right away, but 4-6 weeks may be required to assess whether beneficial effects have been achieved; they do not shrink the prostate and do not change PSA levels. Take *Cardura XL* with breakfast.

Alpha Blockers Continued

DRUG	DOSING	SAFETY/SIDE EFFECTS/MONITORING

Selective Alpha$_{1A}$ Blockers

DRUG	DOSING	SAFETY/SIDE EFFECTS/MONITORING
Tamsulosin *(Flomax)* + dutasteride *(Jalyn)*	0.4 mg daily, 30 min after the same meal each day; max 0.8 mg daily	**CONTRAINDICATIONS** Concurrent use silodosin or alfuzosin with strong 3A4 inhibitors, hepatic impairment (Child-Pugh class C for silodosin, class B/C for alfuzosin); severe renal impairment (silodosin) **WARNINGS** Orthostatic hypotension/syncope: typically with first dose, if therapy is interrupted for several days, dosage is increased too rapidly or another antihypertensive agent or PDE-5 inhibitor is started Floppy iris syndrome can occur during cataract surgery
Alfuzosin *(Uroxatral)*	10 mg daily, immediately after same meal each day CrCl < 30 mL/min: use with caution	Priapism–seek medical attention if lasting > 4 hours Angina - D/C if symptoms of angina begin or worsen **SIDE EFFECTS** Dizziness, fatigue, hypotension, headache, rhinitis (tamsulosin) Abnormal ejaculation (esp. with tamsulosin and silodosin) **MONITORING** BP, PSA, urinary symptoms **NOTES**
Silodosin *(Rapaflo)*	8 mg daily with a meal CrCl 30-50 mL/min: 4 mg daily CrCl < 30 mL/min: do not use	Do not use alfuzosin in patients at risk for QT prolongation – prolongs QT-interval Silodosin can cause retrograde ejaculation (28%), reversible upon drug discontinuation Alpha blockers – used for bladder outlet obstruction in women (off label)

Alpha Blocker Drug Interactions

■ Caution is advised when PDE-5 inhibitors *(Viagra/Revatio, Cialis/Adcirca, Levitra/Staxyn, Stendra)* are co-administered with alpha blockers. PDE-5 inhibitors and alpha blockers are both vasodilators with BP lowering effects. When they are used in combination, there will be an additive effect on BP. In some patients, concomitant use of these two drug classes can lower BP significantly leading to symptomatic hypotension (dizziness, light headedness, fainting). Patients should be stable on alpha-blocker therapy before PDE-5 inhibition is initiated and the lowest doses of the PDE-5 inhibitor should be used when initiating therapy. Conversely, if a patient is already taking an optimal dose of a PDE-5 inhibitor and an alpha blocker needs to be started, the alpha blocker should be started at the lowest dose, and the selective agents will be preferred (over the non-selective agents).

- Use caution with any hypotensive condition or with other drugs that lower BP.

- Tamsulosin, alfuzosin and silodosin are major CYP 3A4 substrates; avoid use with strong 3A4 inhibitors (ritonavir, itraconazole, ketoconazole, clarithromycin, others).

- Silodosin cannot be used with strong P-gp inhibitors, such as cyclosporine.

- Alfuzosin: can cause QT-prolongation; do not use with other QT-prolongating agents. Use with caution in patients with known QT prolongation (congenital or acquired).

5 Alpha-Reductase Inhibitors

These agents inhibit the 5 alpha-reductase enzyme which blocks the conversion of testosterone to dihydrotestosterone (DHT). This class of medications is indicated for the treatment of symptomatic BPH in men <u>with an enlarged prostate</u> to improve symptoms, decrease the risk of acute urinary retention, and decrease the risk of need for surgery, including TURP or prostatectomy.

DRUG	DOSING	SAFETY/SIDE EFFECTS/MONITORING
Finasteride *(Proscar)* Affects 5α-receptors type 2 For hair loss (*Propecia* 1 mg daily)	5 mg daily	**CONTRAINDICATIONS** Women of child-bearing potential, pregnancy, children **WARNINGS** May ↑ risk of high-grade prostate cancer. **SIDE EFFECTS** Impotence, ↓ libido, ejaculation disturbances, breast enlargement and tenderness, rash – sexual SEs ↓ with time and approach placebo levels at one year of use in some men; in some men sexual issues persist **MONITORING** PSA, urinary symptoms
Dutasteride *(Avodart)* + tamsulosin (*Jalyn*) Affects both types of 5α-receptors (types 1 and 2)	0.5 mg daily	**NOTES** Pregnancy Category X Pregnant women should not handle or take; can be absorbed through skin, can be detrimental to fetus, semen of male taking this drug may present a danger 6 months (or longer) of treatment may be required for maximal efficacy Usually used in men with larger prostate size (40+ grams) or more severe symptoms; due to the slow-onset, often given with α-blocker 5 alpha-reductase inhibitors shrink the prostate and ↓ PSA levels Swallow dutasteride whole. Do not chew or open as contents may cause oropharyngeal irritation. Take *Jalyn* 30 min after same meal each day.

5 Alpha-Reductase Inhibitor Drug Interactions

- Finasteride and dutasteride are minor CYP 3A4 substrates; strong CYP 3A4 inhibitors may increase levels.

- Do not use finasteride in a patient using *Propecia* for hair loss; refer to prescriber.

Phosphodiesterase-5 (PDE-5) Inhibitor

PDE-5 mediated reduction in smooth muscle and endothelial cell proliferation, decreased nerve activity and increased smooth muscle relaxation and tissue perfusion of the prostate and bladder.

DRUG	DOSING	SAFETY/SIDE EFFECTS/MONITORING
Tadalafil *Cialis* – for ED and Benign Prostatic Hypertrophy (BPH) *Adcirca* – for pulmonary arterial hypertension (PAH)	5 mg daily, same time each day CrCl 30-50 mL/min: 2.5 mg CrCl < 30 mL/min: do not use Use 2.5 mg if using strong CYP 3A4 inhibitor	**CONTRAINDICATIONS** Concurrent use of nitrates **WARNINGS** Rare: may cause color discrimination, sudden vision loss in one of both eyes – may be a sign of nonarteritic anterior ischemic optic neuropathy (NAION), decrease or a loss of hearing, priapism, concomitant use with alpha blockers is not recommended–discontinue alpha-blocker at least 1 day before initiating tadalafil. See Erectile Dysfunction chapter for complete review **SIDE EFFECTS** Headache, flushing, nausea, dyspepsia, color vision changes, blurred vision, increased sensitivity to light, epistaxis, erythemia, diarrhea, myalgia, back pain, respiratory tract infection, nasopharyngitis **MONITORING** BP, PSA, urinary symptoms

For drug interactions/counseling for tadalafil, see Erectile Dysfunction chapter.

Alpha Blocker Counseling

- Especially for non-selective agents, such as doxazosin: This medicine can cause a sudden drop in blood pressure. You may feel dizzy, faint or "light-headed," especially after you stand up from a lying or sitting position. This is more likely to occur after you have taken the first few doses or if you increase your dose, but can occur at any time while you are taking the drug. It can also occur if you stop taking the drug and then restart treatment. When you get up from a sitting or lying position, go slowly and hold onto the bed rail or chair until you are steady on your feet.

- Your blood pressure should be checked when you are sitting or lying down and standing.

- If you take the medicine at bedtime, but need to get up from bed to go to the bathroom, get up slowly and cautiously and hold onto the bed rail or chair until you are steady on your feet.

- You should not drive or do any hazardous tasks until you are used to the effects of the medicine. If you begin to feel dizzy, sit or lie down until you feel better.

- This medicine can cause side effects that may impair your thinking or reactions. Be careful if you drive or do anything that requires you to be awake and alert.

- Drinking alcohol can make the dizziness worse, and increase night-time urination if taken close to bedtime.

- Taking cold and allergy medications such as decongestants and antihistamines can make your symptoms worsen. Discuss what to use with your pharmacist if you need assistance.

- Tell your doctor (or ophthalmologist) about the use of this medication before cataract surgery. The doctor will want to know if you have ever taken this medication.

- Rarely, this medication can cause a painful erection which cannot be relieved by having sex. If this happens, get medical help right away. If it is not treated, you may not be able to get an erection in the future.

Tamsulosin

- The dose should be administered approximately half an hour following the same meal each day.

Alfuzosin

- Do not crush, chew, or break the alfuzosin tablets. Swallow them whole.

- Take after same meal each day (food increases absorption).

Silodosin

- The most common side effect seen with this medication is an orgasm with reduced or no semen (dry orgasm). This side effect does not pose a safety concern and is reversible with discontinuation of the drug (lower risk with tamsulosin).

- Take the same time each day with food.

5 Alpha-Reductase Inhibitor Counseling

- This medicine can take several months or longer to help reduce the BPH symptoms. It is effective, it just takes awhile to work because it shrinks the prostate slowly. If your doctor has given you another medicine called an alpha-blocker, that medicine works faster.

- Women who are or may become pregnant should not handle the tablets. (These drugs can cause birth defects to a developing male fetus – Pregnancy Category X). The semen of males using the medicine may also be harmful.

- Your doctor may perform blood tests or other forms of monitoring during treatment with finasteride. One of the tests that may be performed is called PSA (prostate-specific antigen). This drug can reduce the amount of PSA in the blood.

- Tell your doctor if you experience any of these side effects: decreased sex drive, decreased volume of ejaculate, impotence, breast tenderness or enlargement.

- Taking cold and allergy medications such as decongestants and antihistamines can make your symptoms worsen. Discuss what to use with your pharmacist if you need assistance.

69

OVERACTIVE BLADDER (OAB)

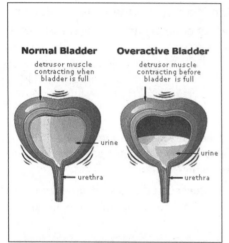

Normal Bladder — detrusor muscle contracting when bladder is full — urine — urethra

Overactive Bladder — detrusor muscle contracting before bladder is full — urine — urethra

GUIDELINE

Diagnosis and Treatment of OverActive Bladder (Non-neurogenic) In Adults: AUA/SUFU Guideline. *J Urol.* 2012 Dec; 188(6 Suppl):2455-63. doi: 10.1016/j. juro.2012.09.079.

BACKGROUND

Overactive bladder (OAB) is a common, disabling urinary disorder that affects many people (1 in 6 people or over 33 million Americans). It is not a normal sign of aging. In overactive bladder, the detrusor muscle contracts frequently and before the bladder is full, leading to the classic symptoms of:

- urinary urgency (a sudden, compelling desire to pass urine which is difficult to defer), and

- urinary frequency (voiding ≥ 8 times in a 24 hour period), and

- nocturia (≥ 2 awakenings to void per night)

Overactive bladder can lead to urinary urge incontinence. About 1/3 of patients have incontinent episodes (OAB wet) and the other 2/3 of patients do not have incontinence (OAB dry).

IMPLICATIONS OF OVERACTIVE BLADDER

Many co-morbidities exist in patients with OAB including falls and fractures, skin breakdown and infections, UTIs, depression, and sexual dysfunction. Due to embarrassment of their condition, there are many social implications of OAB including low self-esteem, lack of sexual intimacy, social and physical isolation, sleep disturbances, limits on travel and dependence on caregivers; all leading to a reduced quality of life. Many patients become dehydrated because they limit their fluid intake. The cost of pads and adult diapers can be a huge financial burden.

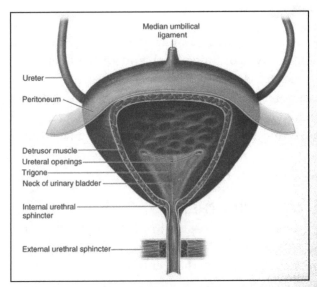

PATHOPHYSIOLOGY

The bladder is commonly referred to as a "balloon" with an outer muscular layer known as the detrusor muscle. The detrusor muscle and the bladder outlet functions are neurologically coordinated to store and expel urine. The detrusor muscle is innervated mainly by the parasympathetic nervous system while the bladder neck is innervated by the sympathetic nervous system. The internal sphincter is also innervated by the sympathetic nervous system and the external sphincter is innervated by the somatic nervous system. Both voluntary and involuntary contractions of the detrusor muscle are mediated by activation of muscarinic receptors via acetylcholine. Of the five known muscarinic receptor subtypes, the human bladder is comprised of M2 and M3 receptors in a 3:1 ratio. It is the M3 receptor that is responsible for both emptying contractions as well as involuntary bladder contractions of incontinence. In overactive bladder, the detrusor muscle is hyperactive (overactive), causing the symptoms of frequent micturitions, urgency, nocturia, and/or incontinence.

Risk Factors for Overactive Bladder

- Age > 40 years
- Diabetes
- Restricted mobility
- Obesity
- Prior vaginal delivery
- Neurologic conditions (e.g., stroke, Parkinson disease, dementia)
- Hysterectomy
- Drugs that can increase incontinence [e.g., ACE inhibitors (due to cough), alcohol, cholinesterase inhibitors, diuretics, sedatives, others]
- Pelvic injury

FORMS OF URINARY INCONTINENCE

Functional
There is no abnormality in the bladder, but the patient may be cognitively, socially, or physically impaired thus hindering him or her from access to a toilet (e.g., patients in wheelchairs).

Overflow
Leakage that occurs when the quantity of urine stored in the bladder exceeds its capacity, often occurring without the urge to urinate (BPH is the most common cause).

Stress
Urine leaks out during any form of exertion (e.g., exercise, coughing, sneezing, laughing, etc.) as a result of pressure on the bladder.

Urge
Patient cannot hold in urine long enough to reach the toilet and is associated with neuropathy; often found in those who have diabetes, strokes, dementia, Parkinson disease, or multiple sclerosis (although people without co-morbidities are affected also).

Mixed
Combination of urge and stress incontinence

Approximately 1/3 of incontinence is stress, 1/3 is urge and 1/3 is mixed.

Diagnosis

Diagnosis requires a careful patient history intake including co-morbid conditions, duration of symptoms, baseline symptoms, fluid intake and type of fluids (with and without caffeine), a physical exam and urinalysis. Validated questionnaires such as the Urinary Distress Inventory (UDI) or the Overactive Bladder Questionnaire (OAB-q) are used to quantify symptoms. Patients may be required to complete a bladder diary to accurately measure intake and voiding information. A urine culture and post-void residual assessment may be performed to rule out other causes.

PELVIC FLOOR MUSCLE EXERCISES

Pelvic Floor Muscle ("Kegel") Exercises
These exercises are done to strengthen the pelvic floor muscles and can diminish OAB symptoms.

Proper technique is key and this means finding the correct muscles. Instruct the patient to imagine that they are trying to stop urination midstream. Squeeze the muscles they would use. If they sense a "pulling" feeling, those are the correct muscles for pelvic exercise.

Pull in the pelvic muscles and hold for a count of 3. Then relax for a count of 3. Work up to 3 sets of 10 kegel exercises per day. Do these exercises 3 times a day to strengthen pelvic floor muscles and reduce wetting episodes.

NON-DRUG THERAPY

Behavioral therapies are considered first-line to improve OAB symptoms by changing patient behavior and/or their environment. Behavioral treatments include bladder training, delayed or scheduled voiding, pelvic floor muscle exercises (Kegel exercises), urge control techniques (distraction, self-assertions), fluid management, dietary changes (avoiding bladder irritants), weight loss and other lifestyle changes. Behavior therapies can be combined with other treatment modalities such as medications. Surgical intervention should be reserved for the rare non-neurogenic patient who has failed all other therapeutic options and whose symptoms are intolerable.

DRUG THERAPY

Behavioral and drug therapies are often used in combination in clinical practice to optimize patient symptom control and quality of life. Anticholinergic drugs are second-line therapy. These agents are antagonists of the muscarinic receptor and block acetylcholine, thus limiting contractions of the detrusor muscle. Patients with a post void residual (PVR) > 250-300 mL should not be started on an anticholinergic agent. Extended-release formulations are preferred over immediate-release formulations due to a lower rate of dry mouth. More selective (for the M3 receptor) anticholinergic agents (solifenacin, darifenacin, fesoterodine) have less CNS side effects over the nonselective, older agents such as oxybutynin. If a patient fails an antimuscarinic agent or develops an adverse effect, it is recommended to try at least one other anticholinergic agent or a dose adjustment before moving on to third-line recommendations, including onabotulinumtoxin A, nerve stimulation or surgical correction. Indwelling catheters are used only as a last resort in select patients. Additive antimuscarinic drugs should be avoided, if possible.

CHOLINERGIC & ANTICHOLINERGIC PHARMACOLOGY

Cholinergic drugs act like acetylcholine at the acetylcholine receptors and cause the "SLUD" symptoms: Salivation, Lacrimation (tearing), Urination and Diarrhea. The classic cholinergic drug bethanechol is used occasionally to <u>treat urinary retention</u> by increasing urination, which occurs with neurogenic bladder. Another cholinergic agent is pilocarpine, which is sometimes used for dry mouth (to increase salivation).*

Anticholinergics have the opposite effect: they block acetylcholine, which is present in the periphery (outside of the CNS) and centrally (inside the CNS) and will cause the anti-SLUD peripheral symptoms of dry mouth, dry/blurry vision, urinary retention and constipation along with the central anticholinergic effects such as sedation, dizziness and cognitive impairment.

This is how diphenhydramine, which blocks acetylcholine in the CNS, works as a sedative. Diphenhydramine has to travel through the periphery (to get to the CNS) and will cause the peripheral side effects as well, including urinary retention. However, it is not an appropriate choice for an elderly patient because of the central effects which can increase fall risk, and the peripheral effects that are not desired.

When incontinence drugs were first developed, the primary goal was to use agents with lower CNS penetration; therefore, exhibiting fewer central side effects. Oxybutynin is an older drug in this class and the prototype peripheral agent. Later on, drugs were designed to be specific for the M3 muscarinic receptor, the subtype present in high density on the bladder wall (the detrusor muscle). When this muscle contracts, there is a sudden urge to urinate; therefore blocking the M3 receptor can reduce the sudden urge to urinate. Darifenacin is an example of an M3-specific drug. Unfortunately, the M3 receptor is also found in high density on the salivary glands, causing dry mouth when this receptor is blocked. The pharmacist must help the patient to manage dry mouth, which is quite uncomfortable and increases the degree of dental decay. It is possible to reduce this side effect with the use of longer-acting agents (instead of IR formulations) and with drugs that bypass first-pass metabolism (patch and gel) since the drug metabolites contribute to the dry mouth. With the long-acting formulations, there are lower "peaks" and, thus, lower side effects. Although there is more drug to hit the "right" receptors (producing the desired effect) during peak concentrations, there will also be more drug to hit the "wrong" receptors (causing side effects).

* Another mechanism to increase acetylcholine is to block the enzyme that breaks it down. These are the acetylcholinesterase inhibitors, which are used for dementia and to reverse neuromuscular blockade.

Anticholinergic Drugs

These agents are competitive antagonists of the muscarinic receptors which inhibit binding of acetylcholine, thus limiting contractions of the detrusor muscle.

DRUG	DOSING	SAFETY/SIDE EFFECTS/MONITORING
Oxybutynin	5 mg PO BID-TID	**CONTRAINDICATIONS** Urinary retention, gastric retention, decreased gastric motility and uncontrolled narrow angle glaucoma
Oxybutynin XL *(Ditropan XL)*	5-30 mg PO daily	
Oxybutynin patch (*Oxytrol*, *Oxytrol for Women – OTC)*	3.9 mg daily (Rx patch is changed every 3-4 days; OTC patch is changed every 4 days)	*Oxytrol for Women* OTC: Pain or burning when urinating, blood in urine, unexplained lower back or side pain, cloudy or foul-smelling urine, males, age < 18 years, urinary or gastric retention, glaucoma, accidental urine loss only due to coughing, sneezing, or laughing
Oxybutynin 10% topical gel *(Gelnique)*	Apply contents of 1 sachet to intact, dry skin daily	
Oxybutynin 3% topical gel *(Gelnique 3%)*	3 pumps daily	**WARNINGS** Anticholinergics may cause agitation, confusion, drowsiness, dizziness, hallucinations, headache, and/or blurred vision, which may impair physical or mental abilities; patients must be cautioned about performing tasks which require mental alertness (e.g., operating machinery or driving).
Tolterodine *(Detrol)*	1-2 mg PO BID	
Tolterodine ER *(Detrol LA)*	2-4 mg PO daily	
Trospium *(Sanctura, Sanctura XR)*	20 mg BID or 60 mg XR daily. Take on empty stomach	**SIDE EFFECTS** Dizziness and drowsiness (greatest with oxybutynin and less with the newer, selective agents), xerostomia (dry mouth), constipation, dry eyes/blurred vision, urinary retention, application site reactions (with topicals and patch)
Solifenacin *(VESIcare)*	5-10 mg PO daily	**NOTES** ↓ dose in renal impairment (CrCl < 30 mL/min) with fesoterodine, solifenacin, tolterodine, and trospium (do not use trospium XR formulation in these patients).
Darifenacin *(Enablex)*	7.5-15 mg PO daily	Extended-release formulations have less incidence of dry mouth than their IR counterparts.
		Oxybutynin patch and gel cause less dry mouth and constipation than oral forms.
Fesoterodine *(Toviaz)*	4-8 mg PO daily	Darifenacin causes more constipation.
		Oxytrol patch should be placed on dry, intact skin on the abdomen, hips or buttocks. Avoid reapplication to the same site within 7 days. Available OTC for women ≥ 18 years. Men who are experiencing OAB symptoms should see their doctors to rule out other conditions.
		Antimuscarinic agents should be used with caution in patients using other medications with anticholinergic properties.

Anticholinergic Drug Interactions

- All of the anticholinergics can have additive effects with other medications that have anticholinergic side effects.

- Acetylcholinesterase inhibitors used for dementia (e.g., donepezil) increase acetylcholine in the CNS, whereas the OAB agents primarily stay in the periphery (outside the CNS). However, some patients may experience some CNS side effects (e.g., memory impairment). The risk vs. benefit must be considered. If little to no improvement in OAB symptoms at 6 weeks, the anticholinergic drug should be discontinued.

- Tolterodine ER – do not exceed 2 mg/day when administered with strong 3A4 inhibitors.

- Solifenacin – do not exceed 5 mg/day when administered with strong 3A4 inhibitors.

- Darifenacin – do not exceed 7.5 mg/day when administered with strong 3A4 inhibitors.

- Fesoterodine – do not exceed 4 mg/day when administered with strong 3A4 inhibitors.

Beta-3 Agonist

Mirabegron relaxes the detrusor muscle during the storage phase of the fill-void cycle by activation of beta-3 receptors which increases bladder capacity.

DRUG	DOSING	SAFETY/SIDE EFFECTS/MONITORING
Mirabegron *(Myrbetriq)*	25-50 mg daily CrCl 15-29 mL/min: 25 mg CrCl < 15 mL/min: not recommended	**SIDE EFFECTS** Hypertension, nasopharyngitis, UTI, headache **MONITORING** BP, HR, urinary symptoms **NOTES** Efficacy seen within 8 weeks

Mirabegron Drug Interactions

- Mirabegron is a moderate CYP2D6 inhibitor. Use caution with co-administration of narrow therapeutic window drugs metabolized by 2D6. Levels of metoprolol and desipramine are increased when co-administered with mirabegron. Use caution when administered concurrently with digoxin (use lowest digoxin dose and monitor levels).

Onabotulinumtoxin A *(Botox)*

Botox is a third-line treatment option for patients who are refractory to first- and second-line treatment options. It affects the efferent pathways of detrusor activity by inhibiting the release of acetylcholine.

DRUG	DOSING	SAFETY/SIDE EFFECTS/MONITORING
Onabotulinumtoxin A *(Botox)*	100 units total dose, as 0.5 mL (5 units) injections, across 20 sites (given intradetrusor) – repeat therapy no sooner than 12 weeks from previous administration In adults treated with *Botox* for more than one indication, do not exceed a total dose of 360 units in a 3 month interval.	**BOXED WARNING** All botulinum toxin products may spread from the area of injection to produce symptoms consistent with botulinum toxin effects. Swallowing and breathing difficulties can be life-threatening. **CONTRAINDICATIONS** Infection at the proposed injection site, urinary tract infection and urinary retention **SIDE EFFECTS** Urinary tract infection, urinary retention, dysuria **MONITORING** Post-void residual volume, symptoms of OAB **NOTES** Potency units of *Botox* are not interchangeable with other preparations of botulinum toxin products. Prophylactic antimicrobial therapy (excluding aminoglycosides) should be administered 1-3 days prior to, on the day of, and for 1-3 days following *Botox* administration. MedGuide required.

Botox Drug Interactions

- Aminoglycosides and other agents affecting neuromuscular transmission can potentiate the effects of *Botox.*

Anticholinergic Patient Counseling

Ditropan XL

- This medication is used to treat symptoms of an over-active bladder.

- Certain medications can interact with this medication. Tell your healthcare provider or pharmacist of the medications you are currently taking including any over the counter products, vitamins and herbal supplements.

- The tablet must be swallowed whole with liquid; do not crush, divide, or chew; take at approximately the same time each day.

- This medication can be taken without regards to meals (unlike trospium which needs to be taken on an empty stomach).

- If you miss a dose, skip it. Take at your next scheduled dose. Do not take 2 doses within the same day.

- This medicine can cause dry mouth. Some formulations cause more dry mouth than others (the longer-lasting forms tend to cause less dry mouth). If dry mouth is bothersome, please discuss with your healthcare provider. Avoiding mouthwashes with alcohol, taking small sips of water, sucking on ice chips or sugar-free candy or chewing sugar-free gum can help with dry mouth symptoms. Take good care of your teeth since dry mouth contributes to tooth decay.

- Another possible side effect of this medicine is constipation. Some formulations cause more constipation than others with darifenacin *(Enablex)* causing the most. Maintain adequate water and dietary fiber, including vegetables and whole-grains. A stool softener, such as docusate, may be helpful. If not, a laxative such as senna may be helpful. You may need to discuss this with your healthcare provider. If you have any type of serious constipation or constipation for ≥ 3 days, or current stomach problems, you should let your healthcare provider know.

- This medication can make you feel dizzy or drowsy. Using alcohol can make this worse. Heat can make this worse. Do not operate any dangerous machinery (such as driving a car) until you know how this medicine affects your concentration and coordination.

- Doing pelvic floor muscle (Kegel) exercises in combination with this medicine will work better than taking the medicine alone. You should get instructions on how to do this correctly, and do them for a few minutes three times daily, so you can slowly build up these muscles.

Oxytrol Patch

- The patch causes less dry mouth than oral formulations.
- Open one pouch and apply immediately. Do not use if pouch is torn or opened.
- Apply one patch to clean, dry, intact skin on the abdomen, hips, or buttocks.
- Apply to an area of skin that is under clothing and protected from sunlight. Avoid applying the patch on your waistline, since tight clothing may rub the patch off.
- The Rx patch is changed every 3 to 4 days; the OTC patch is changed every 4 days.
- Select a new site for each new patch (avoid reapplication to same site within 7 days).
- Do not apply the patch to areas of skin that are irritated, oily, or to where lotions or powders have been applied.
- The patch must be removed prior to having a MRI procedure.
- Contact with water (e.g., swimming, bathing) will not change the way the drug works. Avoid rubbing the patch area during these activities.
- If the area around the patch becomes red, itchy, or irritated, try a new site. If irritation continues or becomes worse, notify your healthcare provider promptly.

Oxybutynin topical *(Gelnique)*

- For topical use only.
- This formulation causes less dry mouth and less constipation than other formulations.
- For *Gelnique* 10%, each packet is for one use only. For *Gelnique* 3%, use 3 pumps (must prime the pump prior to first use with 4 pumps).
- Apply to clean, dry, intact skin on abdomen, upper arm/shoulders, or thighs. Rub into skin until dry. Use a different site each day (cannot use the same site two days in a row).
- Do not apply to recently shaved skin.
- Do not bath, swim or shower for 1 hour after application.
- Wash hands after use.
- Cover treated area with clothing after gel has dried to prevent transfer of medication to others.
- Oxybutynin gel is flammable. Avoid an open flame and do not smoke until the gel has completely dried on the skin.

70

GLAUCOMA, OPHTHALMICS & OTICS

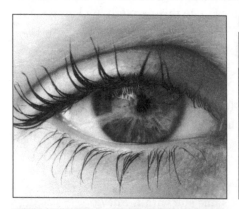

Eye & Ear Rx Interpretation

ABBREVIATION	MEANING	CAUTION
AD, AS, AU	Right Ear, Left Ear, Each Ear	These directions can be mistaken (interchanged) for each other & may mean other things: know how to interpret them but it is safer to write them out: use right eye, left eye, each eye, right ear, left ear, each ear.
OD, OS, OU	Right Eye, Left Eye, Each Eye	
Memory tip: A is from the Latin for ear (auris), O is from eye (oculus), D is from right (dextra) and S is from left (sinistra).		

GUIDELINE

American Academy of Ophthalmology Glaucoma Panel. Preferred Practice Pattern Guidelines. Primary Open-Angle Glaucoma Suspect. 2010. http://one. aao.org/preferred-practice-pattern/ primary-openangle-glaucoma-ppp--october-2010 (accessed 2014 Oct 7).

EYE MEDICATION FORMULATIONS

- Solutions

- Suspensions – shake well or disperse prior to use.

- Ointments – apply to the conjunctival sac or over lid margins (for blepharitis). Ointments will make vision blurry and are not used with contact lenses.

apply to lower lid only

- Gels – with cap on, invert and shake once to get medicine into the tip before instilling into the eye.

GLAUCOMA

Glaucoma is an eye disease caused by an increase in intraocular pressure (IOP). If left untreated, glaucoma can result in damage to the optic nerve and gradual loss of vision. There may be no symptoms felt by the patient, although some may experience eye pain, headache, or decreased vision.

There are two main forms of glaucoma. Angle-closure, or closed-angle glaucoma is treated in the hospital and is a medical emergency. The more common type, open-angle glaucoma, is most commonly treated with eye drops and in some cases, surgery. The decision to treat depends on whether damage to the optic nerve is present, the results from a "visual field" test and the IOP value.

RISK FACTORS

Include family history, increased age, African Americans and nearsightedness (myopia). A history of eye surgeries and diabetes can be contributory.

DRUG TREATMENT

Prostaglandin (PG) analogs and beta-blockers are used most commonly as initial agents. PG analogs are the most effective drugs at ↓ IOP, are safe and are used once daily. If the pressure is high in one eye and not the other a beta blocker would be more likely used as the initial agent because the iris-darkening/eyelash thickening would not be desirable in one eye only. The other classes of glaucoma medications are used as add-ons.

DRUGS THAT CAN INCREASE IOP

Cough/cold/motion sickness medications (antihistamines, including scopolamine)

Anticholinergics (e.g., oxybutynin, tolterodine, benztropine, trihexyphenidyl, tricyclics) *including*

Chronic corticosteroids, especially eye drops such as prednisolone *Pred Forte® ↑ pressure*

Topiramate (Topamax) - *SE (monitor in some pts)*

Adherence & Technique: Improvement Is Needed

There are two likely causes of persistently high IOP: 1) poor eyedrop administration technique and 2) poor adherence. The correct way to administer eye drops is described later in this chapter. The asymptomatic presentation contributes to poor adherence. Counseling is critical for both administration technique and the need for therapy. The patient should understand the consequences of untreated glaucoma (i.e., loss of vision). Yet, even with counseling, the adherence remains poor. For example, in one of the studies referenced in the glaucoma guidelines, less than 45% of the participants took < 75% of the daily doses. The patients had received counseling, and the medication was provided at no charge, and taken once-daily.

DRUG	DOSING	SIDE EFFECTS/CLINICAL CONCERNS
Beta Blockers, Nonselective: reduce aqueous humor production		
Timolol 0.25% and 0.5% (Timoptic, Timoptic-XE, Istalol, Betimol, Timoptic Ocudose)	*Timoptic:* 1 drop Q daily-BID *Timoptic-XE:* 1 drop Q daily (gel)	**CONTRAINDICATIONS** Sinus bradycardia; sinus node dysfunction; heart block > than first degree (except in patients with a pacemaker); cardiogenic shock, uncompensated cardiac failure, bronchospastic disease
+ brominidine (Combigan)		**SIDE EFFECTS** Slight burning, stinging, itching of the eyes or eyelids, changes in vision, increased sensitivity of the eyes to light, bradycardia, bronchospasm with non-selective agents, fatigue
+ dorzolamide (Cosopt, Cosopt PF) *- preservative free*		
Levobunolol (Betagan) بذبذبات		**NOTES** All non-selective beta blockers except for betaxolol.
Carteolol (Ocupress) بأزنق في الكرتونة		Some contain the preservative benzalkonium chloride (BAK) which is absorbed by soft contact lenses. Use eyedrops first, wait 15 minutes before inserting lenses (or remove prior to using eye drops). Occasionally patients have sensitivity to this preservative.
Metipranolol (OptiPranolol)		The PF in *Cosopt PF* stands for "preservative free."
Betaxolol (Betoptic, Betoptic S) *asthma attack → will need taxi*		Some contain sulfites, which can cause allergic reactions.

only selective β-blocker for glaucoma ↑

(different from sulfa allergy)

Timoptic XE® – gel
+ suspension → needs to be mixed ▽
shake contents of tube before use
turn container upside down once

DRUG	DOSING	SIDE EFFECTS/CLINICAL CONCERNS

Prostaglandin Analogs: increase aqueous outflow

[handwritten: no BAK! contains other preservative]

[handwritten left margin: unopened → fridge]
[handwritten left margin: preservative free (PF)]

Travoprost (Travatan Z) **Bimatoprost (Lumigan)** **Latanoprost (Xalatan)** Unoprostone (Rescula) BID Tafluprost (Zioptan) *[handwritten: 10-single use containers in foil pouch * (unopened → fridge) * open pouch is good for 28 days]*	1 drop QHS, except *Rescula* is BID Cannot be administered with contact lenses (preservative BAK will absorb into lenses) – remove and wait 15 min prior to re-insertion (most given QHS- instruct to remove lenses 1st)	**WARNINGS** Ocular effects: darkening of the iris, eyelid skin and eyelashes. Eyelash length and number can increase. Long-term consequences to the eye are not known. Contamination of multiple-dose ophthalmic solutions can cause bacterial keratitis. **SIDE EFFECTS** Blurred vision, stinging, foreign body sensation, increased pigmentation of the iris/eyelashes, eyelash growth/thickening **NOTES** Store unopened bottles of latanoprost in refrigerator. *Zioptan* comes as 10 single-use containers in a foil pouch; store unopened pouches in refrigerator. Once opened the contents are good for 28 days at room temperature. Bimatoprost (*Latisse*) is indicated for eyelash hypotrichosis (to ↑ eyelash growth) – do not use concurrently with same class for glaucoma without MDs approval (using PAs more frequently ↓ effectiveness). *Travatan Z* does not contain BAK, instead has different preservative. This may be helpful to some with reaction to BAK or dry eye, but most are fine with a less expensive generic. *Zioptan:* The single-use containers are (sterile, but no preservative – cannot keep). Discard the container after use, even if medicine is remaining.

[handwritten spanning bottom: apply like gel eyeliner w/ applicator tips provided to upper lash line w/ eyes closed; do not apply to lower lid; blot excess solution w/ tissue]

Cholinergics (Miotics): increase aqueous outflow *[handwritten: stimulates ACh receptors [SLUDGE] lacrimation]*

Carbachol (Isopto Carbachol, Miostat)	1-2 drops up to TID	**SIDE EFFECTS** Corneal clouding, poor vision at night (due to pupil constriction), burning (transient), irritation, hypotension, bronchospasm, abdominal cramps/GI distress
Pilocarpine (Isopto Carpine, Pilopine HS)	Solution: 1-2 drops up to 6x/daily Gel: Instill 0.5" ribbon into lower conjunctival sac once daily, at bedtime	**NOTES** Use with caution with history of retinal detachment or corneal abrasion.

Carbonic Anhydrase Inhibitors: reduce aqueous humor production

[handwritten left margin: TID, BID, TID]

Dorzolamide (Trusopt) **+ timolol (Cosopt, Cosopt PF).** AcetaZOLAMIDE *[handwritten: po!]* (Diamox Sequels) Brinzolamide (Azopt) + brimonidine (Simbrinza) Methazolamide (Neptazane)	Trusopt: 1 drop TID Azopt: 1 drop TID Cosopt: 1 drop BID Acetazolamide 250 mg PO 1-4 x daily, or 500 mg ER PO BID	**WARNINGS** Sulfonamide allergy with the eye drops and the oral acetazolamide: caution with allergy due to risk of systemic exposure **SIDE EFFECTS** Ocular agents: blurred vision, blepharitis, dry eye, discharge Oral agent (acetazolamide): CNS effects (ataxia, confusion), photosensitivity/skin rash (including risk of SJS and TEN), anorexia, nausea, risk of hematological toxicities *[handwritten: bitter taste]* **NOTES** Acetazolamide oral capsules are infrequently used for glaucoma. They are used for prevention and treatment of acute mountain (altitude) sickness. *Cosopt PF* comes in preservative-free (PF), single-use containers.

[handwritten bottom left: SE: CNS (ataxia, confusion) photosensitivity, skin rash (TEN, SJs) anorexia/nausea hematological toxicities]

Glaucoma Medications Continued

DRUG	DOSING	SIDE EFFECTS/CLINICAL CONCERNS
Adrenergic Alpha-2 Agonists: increase aqueous outflow, reduce aqueous humor production		
Brimonidine (Alphagan P) + timolol **(Combigan)** + brinzolamide **(Simbrinza)** Dipivefrin *(Propine, Akpro)* Apraclonidine *(Iopidine)*	*Iopidine, Alphagan* are dosed TID	**WARNINGS** CNS depression: caution with heavy machinery, driving **SIDE EFFECTS** Sedation, burning/stinging/itchy eyes, dry mouth, dry nose

(handwritten margin notes: TID, α₂ agonists, TID)

Patient Counseling (Eye Drops)

- Wash your hands.
- Before you open the bottle, shake it a few times.
- Bend your neck back a little so that you're looking up. Use one finger to pull down your lower eyelid. It is helpful, at least initially, to use a mirror.
- Without letting the tip of the bottle touch your eye or eyelid, squeeze one drop of the medicine into the space between your eye and your lower eyelid. If you squeeze in more than one drop, you are wasting medicine.
- After you squeeze the drop of medicine into your eye, close your eye. Then press a finger between your eye and the top of your nose. Press for at least one full minute. This way, more of the medicine stays in your eye. You will be less likely to have side effects. Blot extra solution from the eyelid with a tissue.
- If you need to take more than one glaucoma medicine:
- Put a drop of the first medicine in your eye. Wait at least 10 minutes to put the second medicine in your eye. If you are taking three eye drops, wait 10 more minutes before putting the third medicine in your eye. If you don't wait 10 minutes between medicines, some of the medicine may run out of your eye. If the medicine runs out of your eye, it does not help.
- If someone else puts your medicines in your eye for you, remind that person to wait 10 minutes between each medicine.

Prostaglandin Analog Counseling Specifics

- Remove contact lenses before using this medication because it contains a preservative that can be absorbed by the lenses, and cause them to become discolored. Wait at least 15 minutes after using this medication before putting your lenses back in.
- You may experience an increase in brown pigment in the iris and gradual changes in eye color (for this reason, they are not usually administered to patients with light eyes who have glaucoma in one eye only). Eyelash growth and pigmentation may increase (which is often pleasing to the patient). The skin on the eyelids and around the eyes may darken.
- This medicine is well-tolerated, but occasionally a patient can experience excessive tearing, eye pain, or lid crusting. If this occurs, please discuss with the optometrist or ophthalmologist..
- Latanoprost *(Xalatan)* unopened bottles should be stored in the refrigerator.
- Tafluprost *(Zioptan)* is kept refrigerated. Once opened the pouch of 10 is good at room temperature for 28 days.

- Do not use this medicine if you are also using Bimatoprost *(Latisse)*, to increase eyelash growth, without the the optometrist's or ophthalmologist's approval. *Latisse* may reduce the effectiveness of the glaucoma medicine.

Timolol *(Timoptic)* Counseling Specifics

- Common side effects from beta blockers include burning/stinging or itching of the eyes, and possible light sensitivity.
- Timolol is a non-selective beta blocker, and although proper application should keep most of the medicine in the eye, it is best to avoid in patients with asthma, COPD, chronic bronchitis, emphysema, or advanced cardiac disease. The medicine might exacerbate the disease symptoms. If you have any of these conditions, please discuss if this medicine is safe to use.
- If dispensing the drops in the *Ocudose* dispenser: To open the bottle, unscrew the cap by turning as indicated by the arrows on the top of the cap. Do not pull the cap directly up and away from the bottle. Pulling the cap directly up will prevent your dispenser from operating properly.
- Invert the bottle, and press lightly with the thumb or index finger over the "Finger Push Area" until a single drop is dispensed into the eye.
- If dispensing the gel *(Timoptic XE)*: Turn the container upside down once and shake the contents prior to use (the gel is a suspension and needs to be mixed). The gel is used once daily.

XE gel

OTHER OCULAR CONDITIONS

Medications can cause ocular adverse effects that disappear once the drug is discontinued (such as blurry vision from an anticholinergic). In other cases the damage can be permanent (such as vision loss with a PDE5-inhibitor). Patients should be instructed to report visual changes immediately; in most cases the damage is reversible if the medication is stopped quickly.

Common Agents Known to Cause Vision Changes/Damage

- Alpha blockers (floppy iris syndrome-causes difficulty in cataract surgery)
- Amiodarone (corneal deposits, optic neuropathy)
- Bisphosphonates (ocular inflammation)
- Digoxin (yellow/green vision, blurriness, halos) *toxicity*
- Chloroquine *(Aralen)* (retinopathy, may cause permanent visual damage)
- Ethambutol *(Myambutol)*, linezolid *(Zyvox)* (optic neuropathy, especially with chronic use) 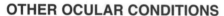 *↑ covers MRSA, VRE faecium*
- Ezogabine *(Potiga)* (retinal changes, vision loss)
- Hydroxychloroquine *(Plaquenil)* (retinopathy)
- Isoniazid (optic neuritis)
- Isotretinoin (↓ night vision which may be permanent, dry eyes/irritation) *WARNING against driving*
- Quinolones (retinal detachment)
- Sildenafil *(Viagra)* and other PDE5-Inhibitors used for ED, PAH, BPH (greenish tinge around objects, possible permanent vision loss in one or both eyes)
- Tamoxifen *(Soltamox)* (corneal changes, decreased color perception)

■ Telithromycin *(Ketek)* (blurry vision, diplopia)

■ Voriconazole *(VFEND)* (abnormal vision, color vision change, photophobia) *in ~ 20% of pts*
    ↳ *WARNING: can cause vision problems; have vision checked if used > 28 days*

Conjunctivitis: Allergic, Bacterial & Viral

Conjunctivitis or "pink eye" occurs in one or both eyes. Symptoms include swelling, itching, burning, and redness of the conjunctiva, the protective membrane that lines the eyelids and covers the white part of the eye (the sclera). Conjunctivitis can be due to a virus, a bacteria, an allergan or from some type of ocular irritant, such as chemicals or contact lenses. In most cases, conjunctivitis causes only mild discomfort, does not harm vision and will clear without medical treatment. Many times, treatment is given even if not clearly indicated. In some cases, treatment is required.

Viral and bacterial conjunctivitis occurs mostly in young children and is highly contagious. Until treatment is initiated, infected children should stay at home and should be allowed to return to school once treatment has begun, unless there are systemic symptoms. Any patient with viral or bacterial conjunctivitis should be instructed to use proper hand hygiene:

■ Don't touch your eyes with your hands.

■ Wash your hands thoroughly and frequently.

■ Change your towel and washcloth daily, and do not share towels with others.

■ Discard eye cosmetics, particularly mascara.

■ Do not use anyone else's eye cosmetics or personal eye-care items.

For any type of conjunctivitis compresses can help alleviate swelling and mild discomfort. To make a compress, soak a clean cloth in warm water (cool water for viral or allergic conjunctivitis), wring it out and apply gently to the closed eyelids. Artificial tears can be used to provide lubrication and help reduce a "gritty" feeling.

Chemical conjunctivitis has no specific drug treatment and is not described in the following table. The irritant should be flushed out of the eyes with saline and inflammation can be reduced with an NSAID or a steroid eye drop. If contact lenses have caused the irritation they should not be used until the condition has cleared. It may be helpful to change the type of contact lens or the brand of disinfectant solution. If the condition is severe, such as a burn, or the chemical is dangerous or unknown, the patient should be referred for emergency care.

Treatment Common to All Conjunctivitis Types

Most cases are mild and will resolve without treatment directed at the cause, such as an antibiotic for suspected bacterial conjunctivitis. However, these are often used and in some cases are helpful in alleviating symptoms more quickly. Inflammation for any type of conjunctivitis can be reduced with NSAID (if mild) or steroid eye drops (if more severe). Artificial tears can help with a "gritty" feeling and will alleviate dryness. Instruct patients to return for follow-up if they do not recover within a few days (or longer with some types). If antibiotics are used the course should be completed.

Conjunctivitis Types

[handwritten: ↗ cold compresses] *[handwritten: cold compresses ↖]*

VIRAL	BACTERIAL	ALLERGIC
Causes: adenovirus (most common), other viruses, most mild but some due to a more severe viral infection (e.g., zoster, HIV)	Causes: *Staph aureus, Strep pneumoniae, H. influenzae, Moraxella catarrhalis* More severe cases can be due to infection with *N. gonorrhoeae* or *Chlamydia*, which will require systemic treatment.	Common allergens include pollen, dust mites, animal dander, molds
No topical treatment for common viral conjunctivitis. The infection will run its course, from several days to 2-3 weeks.	Topical antibiotic eye drops or ointments, selected: *[handwritten: "sight"]* ✱ Azithromycin (*Azasite*) – stored in refrigerator, 14 days at room temp. ✱ Moxifloxacin (*Vigamox*) ✱ Besifloxacin (*Besivance*) Tobramycin/Dexamethasone (*TobraDex, TobraDex ST*) ✱ Ciprofloxacin (*Ciloxan*) ✱ Ofloxacin (*Ocuflox*) Gentamicin (*Garamycin*) Tobramycin (*Tobrex*) Erythromycin ✱ Sulfacetamide (*Bleph-10*) Trimethoprim/Polymyxin B (*Polytrim*) Neomycin/Bacitracin/Polymyxin B (*Neosporin*)	**MAST CELL STABILIZER EYE DROPS** Cromolyn Lodoxamide (*Alomide*) Nedocromil (*Alocril*) Pemirolast (*Alamast*) **ANTIHISTAMINE EYE DROPS** Azelastine (*Optivar*) Epinastine (*Elestat*) Olopatadine (*Patanol*)

Eye Drops to Reduce Inflammation and Add Lubrication (Moisture)

DRUG	USAGE NOTES	EXAMPLES
Eye Drops to ↓ Inflammation	Steroid eye drops should be used short-term due to risk of ↑ IOP. *[handwritten: preferred over PredForte® b/c does not ↑ IOP as much as PredForte® does]*	**STEROIDS** Dexamethasone (*Maxidex, Ozurdex*) Loteprednol (*Alrex, Lotemax* suspension, ointment, gel) Fluorometholone (*Flarex, FML Forte, FML Liquifilm* suspension, ointment) Prednisolone acetate (*Pred Forte*) **NSAIDs** Ketorolac (*Acular, Acular LS, Acuvail*) Flurbiprofen (*Ocufen*) Diclofenac Bromfenac
Artificial Tears to Moisturize Eyes	Common lubricants – mineral oil, glycerin, propylene glycol, dextran, hypromellose Administered multiple times daily, as-needed.	*Systane* *Refresh* *Clear Eyes* *Liquifilm* and others

Blepharitis (Eyelid Inflammation)

Blepharitis most commonly involves the part of the eyelid where the eyelashes come out of the skin. In many patients the condition is chronic and is difficult to treat and in others it is an acute, short-term condition. The primary symptoms are <u>inflamed, irritated and itchy</u>

[handwritten: CsA eye drops (Restasis®) - for dry eyes from autoimmune condition]

eyelids. The preferred treatment is gentle washing and application of compresses: apply a warm compress over the eye for a few minutes to loosen the crusty deposits, then use a warm moist washcloth (water plus a few drops of baby shampoo) to wipe away the debris. In some cases, antibiotic ointments, steroid eye drops and artificial tears are helpful.

OTICS

Background

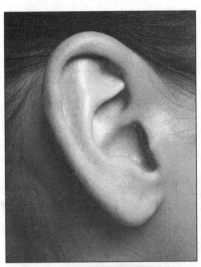

Common conditions treated in the ear include pain (such as from an otitis infection-which may be treated with topical antibiotics, although oral are much more common), inflammation from swimmer's ear (otitis externa) and ear wax (cerumen) impaction. Otitis externa pain can be treated (preferentially) with systemic analgesics (ibuprofen, acetaminophen). During treatment patients should stay out of the water, avoid flying due to the pressure changes, and avoid the use of headphones and ear plugs. Tinnitus (ringing or roaring or buzzing sounds) is caused by drug toxicity (primarily salicylates), noise exposure, or is idiopathic. There is no effective drug treatment for tinnitus. For any condition, eye drops may be used in the ear, but never use ear drops in the eyes; the ear drops may not have an appropriate pH, may not be isotonic and may not be sterile.

Ear drops with antibiotics may also be used for outer ear infections. A few common products:

- Ciprofloxacin and hydrocortisone *(Cipro HC)* — hydrocortisone

- Ciprofloxacin and dexamethasone *(Ciprodex)*

- Neomycin, colistin, hydrocortisone, and thonzonium *(Cortisporin-TC)* — HC, neomycin + colistin thonzonium

Ear Wax (Cerumen) Removal

Earwax blockage occurs when earwax (cerumen) accumulates in the ear or becomes too hard to wash away naturally. It is removed in a medical office. If the condition is chronic, ear-wax removal medication [carbamide peroxide *(Debrox)*, triethanolamine *(Cerumenex)*] is sometimes used every 4 - 8 weeks as a preventive measure. Instruct the patient to tilt the head sideways (see below) and instill 5 - 10 drops twice daily for up to four days.

Otic Medication Application

- If cold, hold the bottle for 1 or 2 minutes to warm the solution. Ear drops that are too cold will be uncomfortable and can cause dizziness.

- Lie down or tilt the head so that the affected ear faces up.

- Gently pull the earlobe up and back for adults (down and back for children) to straighten the ear canal.

- Administer the prescribed number of drops into the ear canal. Keep the ear facing up for about 5 minutes to allow the medicine to coat the ear canal.

- Do not touch the dropper tip to any surface. To clean wipe with a clean tissue.

71

MOTION SICKNESS

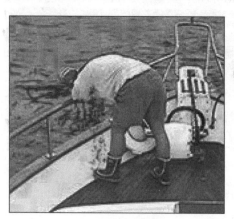

BACKGROUND

Motion sickness (kinetosis) is also called seasickness or airsickness. Symptoms are nausea, dizziness and fatigue. People can get motion sickness on a moving boat, train, airplane, car, or amusement park rides. This is a common condition.

NON-PHARMACOLOGIC TREATMENT

Some patients find benefit with a wrist band that presses on an acupuncture point located on the inside of the wrist, about the length of 2 fingernails up the arm from the center of the wrist crease. One popular brand is *Sea-Band* benefit. The best way to stop motion sickness, if possible, is to stop the motion.

Natural Products

Ginger, in teas or supplements, is used most commonly. Peppermint may be helpful.

PHARMACOLOGIC TREATMENT

Medications for motion sickness are anticholinergics and may cause drowsiness and may impair judgment. Pilots, ship crew members, or anyone operating heavy equipment or driving a car should not take them. The military uses combinations of products (such as oral scopolamine to reduce nausea, taken with a stimulant, such as dextroamphetamine, to counteract the drowsiness from the scopolamine) but these combinations have significant risk and should not be routinely recommended.

Scopolamine *(Transderm-Scop)* is the most commonly prescribed medication for motion sickness. It is not more effective than generically-available OTC agents but is applied topically (behind the ear) and is taken less frequently (apply 4-6 hours prior to need, lasts three days, do not cut patch, alternate ears, do not get into eyes, wash hands afterwards).

<u>Antihistamines</u> used for motion sickness include cyclizine (*Marezine*), diphenhydramine *(Benadryl)*, dimenhydrinate *(Dramamine)* or Meclizine *(Bonine)*. Dimenhydrinate, meclizine and cyclizine are long-acting piperazine antihistamines and are a little less sedating than other antihistamines, but they are still sedating.

Promethazine is used and is prescription only. <u>Do not use promethazine in children</u>. All promethazine products carry a black box warning contraindicating use in children less than 2 years and strongly cautioning use in children age 2 and older. The FDA advises against the use of promethazine with codeine cough syrups in children less than 6 years of age, due to the risk of respiratory depression, cardiac arrest and neurological problems.

<u>All of the antihistamines have anticholinergic effects similar to scopolamine.</u> Make sure the oral agents are taken prior to travel (30-60 minutes prior) and ensure that the patient knows they will get tired. Instruct them not to consume alcohol or other CNS depressants.

DRUG	DOSING	SIDE EFFECTS/FORMULATIONS/CONTRAINDICATIONS
Scopolamine 3-day patch (Transderm-Scop) Applied behind ear Q 72 hrs, rotate ears	1.5 mg, patch placed behind ear (hairless), 4-6 hours before needed (or evening before AM surgery – remove 24 hours after surgery) Primarily for motion sickness and occasionally used inpatient. Do not cut patch, wash hands after application.	**SIDE EFFECTS** Dry mouth, dizziness, stinging eyes (if touch eyes after handling patch), pupil dilation, ↑ risk of intraocular pressure (IOP) Confusion (can be significant in elderly, frail) **RARELY** Hallucinations, tachycardia Remove patch prior to MRI **NOTES** Pregnancy Category C
Meclizine (Dramamine Less Drowsy, Medi-Meclizine, Univert)	12.5-25 mg 30-60 minutes before needed.	**SIDE EFFECTS** Sedation, dry mouth, urinary retention, constipation, dry/blurry vision, tachycardia **NOTES** Pregnancy Category B Worsening of BPH symptoms, can ↑ IOP (glaucoma), and worsen cognition (elderly)

OTHER ANTIHISTAMINES USED
Cyclizine
DiphenhydrAMINE
DimenhyDRINATE

Promethazine [Rx-Do not use in children due to (primarily) risk of respiratory depression.], comes in oral tablets, rectal suppository and injection. Do not administer IV due to risk of severe tissue necrosis; IM route is preferred for injection.

Transderm Scop Counseling
- Wear only one patch at any time.
- <u>No alcohol.</u> Try to avoid other drugs that make you tired – this drug causes significant drowsiness. Do not use in children.
- The most common side effect is dryness of the mouth. Other common side effects are drowsiness, temporary blurring of vision and dilation (widening) of the pupils may occur, especially if the drug is on your hands and comes in contact with the eyes.

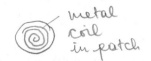

metal coil in patch

- Remover prior to an MRI procedure or the patch will burn your skin.
- Infrequently, some people get disoriented, and others can get confusion, hallucinations or heart palpitations. If any of these occur remove the patch and contact your doctor.

How to use

- Peel off the clear backing from the patch and apply it to a clean, dry, hairless area of the skin behind the ear. Press firmly for at least 30 seconds to make sure the patch sticks well, especially around the edges. The patch will slowly release the medication into your body over 3 days. Do not use the patch if it appears broken, cut, or damaged. Apply at least 4 hours before activity that will cause motion sickness.

- Be sure to wash your hands thoroughly with soap and water immediately after handling the patch, so that any drug that might get on your hands will not come into contact with your eyes.

- Also wash the area behind the ear where the patch was removed.

limit water contact (water sports, etc.)

peripheral antiACh effects
constipation
urinary retention
dry mouth
dry eyes / blurred vision

tolteridine, oxybutinin

* *in order for antiACh drug to help w/ motion sickness it has to be able to cross BBB !! ⇒ CENTRAL AXN RATHER THAN PERIPHERAL!*

* *type of cholinergic receptors in bladder (blocked to tx urinary incontinence = same type of cholinergic receptors in salivary glands ⇒ can't tx overactive bladder w/o getting dry mouth (SE)*

COMMON SKIN CONDITIONS

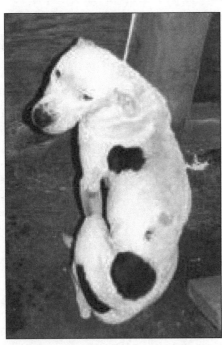

GUIDELINES

There are various conditions presented in this section and treatments for each are presented below. It can be difficult to determine the type of skin condition, which are often presented by the patient to the community pharmacist. *The Handbook of OTC Drugs* has pictures of common conditions, and many more are available at www.dermnet.com. If recommending OTC treatment it is important to tell the patient to be seen by a physician if the condition does not improve or worsens. A pharmacist should be able to recognize a blemish that could be skin cancer; see the pictures and description in the Oncology I chapter.

Natural Products

Aloe is a natural product produced from the aloe vera plant that is used for many skin conditions, including sunburn and psoriasis. It has little proven efficacy but if used as a gel or lotion it may provide a soothing effect. Tea tree oil is used for a variety of skin conditions. It can be useful for treating acne. It may be helpful for onychomycosis symptoms (depending on the dose and application schedule), but is not useful in eradicating the infection in most patients. Lysine is used for cold sore prevention.

DRUGS THAT CAN DISCOLOR SKIN OR SECRETIONS

Brownish
Levodopa, Entacapone
Methyldopa

Brown/Yellowish
Metronidazole, Tinidazole (darkened urine)
Nitrofurantoin
Riboflavin (B2)

Brown/Black/Greenish
Methocarbamol

Purple/Orangeish/Reddish
Chlorzoxazone

Orange/Yellowish
Sulfasalazine

Orange/Reddish/Brownish
Ezogabine

Yellow-Greenish
Propofol
Flutamide

Red-Orangeish
Phenazopyridine
Rifapentine
Rifampin

Reddish
Anthracyclines

Blueish
Mitoxantrone
Methylene blue

Acne, Background & Treatment

- Most people develop acne, including infants, adults (and women, commonly, around the menstrual cycle) and, primarily, adolescents in puberty.

- Androgens (male sex hormones) are the primary determinant of acne (and is why boys often will have worse acne than girls) and the presence of the bacteria *P. acnes* and fatty acids present in oil glands. Where the oil glands are located is where acne occurs: the face, chest, shoulders and back.

- Lesions are classified as whiteheads, blackheads, small bumps, cysts and nodules.

- Treatment is determined by severity: mild (few, occasional pimples), moderate (inflammatory papules), or severe (nodules and cysts).

- Acne is treated with four primary groups of agents: OTC (benzoyl peroxide and salicylic acid), retinoids, systemic isotretinoin and antibiotics.

- Benzoyl peroxide (BPO) is the most effective OTC agent. It comes as Rx, including in combination with hydrocortisone, the retinoid adapalene or with the antibiotics erythromycin or clindamycin. Start with 2.5-5% BPO, which is generally adequate and less irritating than the higher strengths.

- Salicylic acid is a mildly useful OTC agent, and is primarily used in "medicated pads" for facial cleansing.

- Retinoids, primarly topical tretinoin and derivates are the usual Rx drug of choice. [They are also used to reduce fine wrinkles.]

  - Retinoids are vitamin A derivatives. The mechanism is primarily to reduce adherence of the keratinocytes (outer skin cells) in the oil gland.

  - They are well-tolerated when used topically, with mild skin irritation (redness, drying) and photosensitivity possible. Start at night (or every other night) with the correct (pea sized) amount. Use moisturizer each morning, followed by sunscreen.

  - Retinoids take 4-12 weeks to work and acne may worsen initially. An antibiotic (often minocycline) taken concurrently can help.

❏ They are not used in pregnancy or breastfeeding; some are pregnancy category C, others are X. Tazarotene often works better than tretinoin; it is used with difficult cases and is pregnancy category X.

❏ Often a topical antibiotic is used concurrently – the retinoid allows the antibiotic to get into the pores to eradicate the bacteria.

❏ The oral retinoid isotretinoin has many safety considerations, including severe teratogenicity, and is reserved for severe nodular acne only. Cholesterol and pregnancy tests are required, among other monitoring.

■ Some women find benefit with birth control pills, especially if the acne is in combination with irregular periods or symptoms of androgenic excess.

■ Azelaic acid *(Azelex, Finacea)* is a topical dicarboxylic acid cream or gel available OTC and Rx for acne and rosacea. It is well tolerated and can cause mild topical burning or "tingling."

DRUGS	NOTES	SAFETY/COUNSELING
Retinoid topicals are 1st line agents Tretinoin cream *(Atralin, Renova, Retin-A, Retin-A Micro, Avita, Refissa, Tretin-X)* Slower-release, less skin irritation with: ■ Microsphere gel *(Retin-A Micro)* ■ Polymerized cream or gel *(Avita)* **Adapalene *(Differin)*** cream, solution Adapalene + BPO *(Epiduo)* Tazarotene *(Tazorac,* Avage-creams, Fabior-foam) stronger, more irritating Dapsone gel *(Aczone)* Retinoids are popular and there are many other products, such as clindamycin + tretinoin gel *(Ziana)*, others	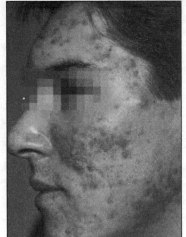 Severe nodular acne – this may be a suitable candidate for istotretinion (oral), but a retinoid with an antibiotic may be tried first.	Apply daily, usually at bedtime, about 20 minutes after washing face. If irritation use lower strength, or every other night. May need to reduce contact initially (wash off every a period of time.) A pea-sized amount is sufficient (for facial application); it should be divided into 4 equal parts and smoothed over the entire surface of the face – not just on acne. Avoid salicylic acid scrubs or astringents while starting a retinoid; this will worsen irritation. Wash only with mild soap twice daily. Takes 4-12 weeks to see response; may worsen acne initially. Limit sun exposure. Do not use dapsone gel if G6PD deficiency.

Acne Background & Treatment Continued

DRUGS	NOTES	SAFETY/COUNSELING
Benzoyl peroxide (most effective OTC agent), salicylic acid is weaker OTC agent OTC (many products) including *Benoxyl, Benzac, Clearasil,* If needed with retinoid. Erythromycin + BPO *(Benzamycin)* Clindamycin + BPO *(Acanya, BenzaClin, Duac, Neuac)* BPO+hydrocortisone *(Vanoxide-HC)* Azelaic acid *(Azelex, Finacea),* OTC, Rx	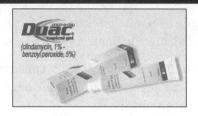 *(clindamycin, 1% - benzoyl peroxide, 5%)* ***Duac*** Dispense with 60 day expiration. Apply QHS to affected areas. Can store at room temp, do not freeze. Limit sun exposure. **Clindamycin Topicals, usual instructions** Clean face, shake (if lotion), apply a thin layer once or twice daily. Avoid contact with eyes; if contact, rinse with cold water. Takes 2-6 weeks for effect and up to 12 weeks for full benefit.	BPO can bleach clothing, hair Limit sun exposure; skin will burn more easily. ***Benzamycin and BenzaClin*** Add indicated amount of purified water to the vial (70% ethyl alcohol for *Benzamycin*) and immediately shake to completely dissolve medication. If needed, add additional purified water to bring level up to the mark. Add the solution in the vial to the gel and stir until homogenous in appearance (1 to 1½ minutes). *Benzamycin* is kept refrigerated. *BenzaClin* is kept at room temp. Place a 3 month expiration date on the label following mixing.
Oral Isotretinoin *(Amnesteem, Claravis, Myorisan, Absorica)* <u>Only for the treatment of severe recalcitrant nodular acne</u> 0.5–1.0 mg/kg/day, divided BID with food (to absorption) for 15-20 weeks. Comes as 10, 20, and 40 mg capsules. Counseling about contraception and behaviors associated with risk of pregnancy must be repeated on a monthly basis. <u>Two forms of birth control</u> are required with taking this medication (not the mini-pill). DRYNESS! Carry bottled water, eye drops and lip balm.	Female patients must sign patient information/informed consent form about birth defects that contains warnings about the risk of potential birth defects if the fetus is exposed to isotretinoin. <u>Must have had 2 negative pregnancy tests prior to starting treatment.</u> Cannot get pregnant for one month before, while taking the drug, or for one month after the drug is stopped. Do not breast feed or donate blood until at least one month has passed after the drug is stopped. <u>Do not use with vitamin A supplements, tetracyclines, steroids, progestin-only contraceptives, or St. John's wort.</u> Must swallow capsule whole, or puncture and sprinkle on applesauce or icecream – this may irritate esophagus	<u>Pregnancy Category X: severe birth defects or miscarriage.</u> <u>Can only be dispensed by a pharmacy registered and activated with the pregnancy risk management iPLEDGE program.</u>1-month Rx at a time, fill within 7 days with yellow sticker attached. Teratogenicity, arthralgias, skeletal hyperostosis, osteoporosis, psychiatric issues (such as depression, psychosis, and risk of suicide), ↓ night vision (may be permanent), difficulty wearing contact lens (<u>dry eyes</u>/irritation), <u>dry skin, chapped lips</u>, elevated cholesterol and blood glucose, transient chest pain and hearing loss, and photosensitivity.
ORAL ANTIBIOTICS USED COMMONLY FOR ACNE **Minocycline ext-rel** *(Solodyn)* 12 years and older, dosed by weight Doxycycline and minocycline are more effective than tetracycline in eradicating *P. acnes* Trimethoprim/Sulfamethoxazole is also used. Erythromycin used to be commonly used but is not currently due to resistance.	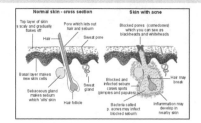	Photosensitivity, rash in susceptible patients, dizziness, diarrhea, somnolence Like other tetracyclines can cause fetal harm if administered during pregnancy. May cause permanent discoloration in teeth if used when teeth are forming (up to 8 years of age).

Cold Sores, Background & Treatment

- Cold sores (Herpes simplex labialis) are ubiquitous and are highly contagious. Children often pick up the infection from family members. Infection is usually due to herpes simplex virus type 1 (HSV-1) in children, but can be caused by HSV-2 when older due to oral/genital sex. Virus can be shed when asymptomatic but is most commonly spread with active lesions; the infectious exudate should not be transmitted (kissing, sharing drinks).

- Sore eruption is preceded by prodromal symptoms (tingling, itching, soreness). In most patients the sore appears in the same location repeatedly. The most common site is the junction between the upper and lower lip. Triggers that instigate sore outbreaks include fatigue/stress, stress to the skin (sun exposure, acid peels) and dental work. Patients should identify their own trigger/s and attempt to avoid them.

- The prodromal period is the optimal time to apply topical or take oral medication to reduce blister duration. If recurrences are frequent (> 4 times/year), chronic suppression, taken daily, can be used. OTC and Rx topicals shorten the duration by up to one day; oral (systemic) antivirals shorten the duration by up to two days.

- The natural product lysine is used commonly for cold sore prevention.

DRUGS	NOTES	SAFETY/COUNSELING
Docosanol *(Abreva)* – OTC **Rx** Acyclovir topical cream *(Zovirax)* Acyclovir buccal tablets *(Sitavig)* Penciclovir topical cream *(Denavir)*	Oral antivirals can be used, are more effective, and are discussed in the ID chapter.	*Abreva* cream: Apply 5x daily at first sign of outbreak, continue until healed. *Zovirax* cream: Apply 5 times daily for 4 days (can be used on genital sores). *Sitavig* tablet: Apply one 50 mg tablet as a single dose to the upper gum region. *Denavir* cream: Apply every 2 hours during waking hours for 4 days.

Dandruff, Background & Treatment

- Dandruff occurs when the scalp is itchy and/or scaling with white oily flakes (dead skin) in the hair and on the shoulders, back or clothing.

- Dandruff can be due to either eczema or fungal (yeast) overgrowth, and worsened by hormones, the weather or shampoo. Seborrheic dermatitis is a common form of eczema that causes flaking, itchy skin on the face, back, chest or head. If it is on the scalp it is commonly referred to as dandruff.

- Patients are not likely to know the cause of the dandruff. A store-brand, inexpensive dandruff shampoo can be tried first, and if this is ineffective, the pricier ketoconazole antifungal shampoo can be used.

DRUGS	NOTES	SAFETY/COUNSELING
Selenium sulfide (*(Dandrex, Selsun, Tersi)*, zinc pyrithone (*Head & Shoulders*), coal tar shampoos, *Suave* or store brands "dandruff" shampoos Ketoconazole shampoo *(Nizoral A-D)* Ketoconazole topical comes in many formulations for dandruff or seborrheic dermatitis (see notes above): cream, foam, gel & shampoo	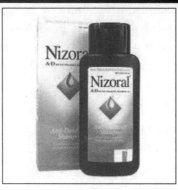 There are many different dandruff shampoos. Shown here is the antifungal shampoo *Nizoral A-D*. It is prudent to have the patient try less expensive formulations first, since these may work as well, including store brands or *Suave* dandruff shampoo.	Rub shampoo in well and leave in for 5 minutes, then rinse out. Shampoo daily. If the shampoo stops working, switch products. *Nizoral A-D* Apply twice weekly, for up to 8 weeks. Do not use if open sores on scalp. Can cause skin irritation.

Skin Fungal Infections, Background & Treatment

Tinea pedis, cruris, corporis, and topical candida infections (vaginal, onychomycosis, diaper rash see separate sections)

Athlete's foot (tinea pedis)

- A fungal infection of the foot caused by various fungi (commonly trichophyton rubrum)

- Symptoms are itching, peeling, redness, mild burning, and sometimes sores. This is a common infection, particularly among those using public pools, showers, and locker rooms. Diagnosis is usually by symptoms, but if unclear (psoriasis and other conditions can cause itchy skin), the skin can be scraped off and viewed under a microscope.

- It is treated topically with antifungals, except in severe cases.

Jock itch (tinea cruris)

- Affects the genitals, inner thighs and buttocks.

- The rash is red, itchy and can be ring-shaped.

- Jock itch is not very contagious, but can be spread person-to-person with close contact.

- Keep the skin dry (use a clean towel after showering) and treat with an antifungal topical. Creams work best.

- Change underwear at least daily.

Ringworm (tinea corporis)

- Not a worm, but a skin fungal infection.

- Ringworm can appear anywhere on the body and typically looks like circular, red, flat sores (one or more, may overlap), usually with dry, scaly skin. Occasionally the ring-like presentation is not present – just itchy red skin.

- The outer part of the sore can be raised while the skin in the middle appears normal. It can spread person-to-person or by contact with infected animals.

- Most cases are treated topically.

- Tinea capitis is "ringworm" on the scalp – this affects primarily young children, mostly in crowded, lower-income situations and requires systemic therapy, with the same drugs used for onychomycosis.

Cutaneous (skin) Candida infections

- Topical candida infections cause red, itchy rashes, most commonly in the groin, armpits or anywhere the skin folds.

- These are more likely in obese persons because they will have more skin with folds; the infection can be in unusual places, such as under the breasts, if the skin is moist. Diabetes is another risk factor.

- Occasionally fungal infections appear in the corner of nails (on the skin, not in the nailbed). If this is a suspected bacterial infection, OTC antibiotic topicals or mupirocin (*Bactroban* – excellent gram positive coverage) can be used.

- Candida can cause diaper rash in infants (discussed under diaper rash.)

DRUGS	NOTES	SAFETY/COUNSELING
Terbinafine and butenafine highly effective: Terbinafine (*Lamisil AT* cream and solution) Butenafine (*Lotrimin Ultra* cream) Clotrimazole (*Lotrimin* cream, lotion, solution, *Desenex*) Miconazole (*Monistat-Derm, Lotrimin* powder and spray) Miconazole+petrolatum (for moisture barrier, used in geriatrics) *(Baza)* *Monistat Derm* cream Tolnaftate (*Tinactin* powder, cream, spray) Undecylenic acid (*Cruex, Desenex*), others **Betamethasone/Clotrimazole (*Lotrisone*)** – popular for tinea with inflammation/itching **Rx** Ketoconazole (cream), ketoconazole foam *(Extina)* Note the same name in OTC products can refer to different active ingredients – do not instruct patient by brand name alone or their could be a product mix-up. The FDA will be attempting to eliminate this confusion by restricting name allocations.	The top picture is tinea corporis (ringworm) – the rings can overlap, or be single) – note the redness. If pictures are not clear please refer to sources at the beginning of the chapter for online images.	Topical antifungals come in creams, ointments, gels, solutions Creams work best and are used in most cases. Solutions can be easier to apply in hairy areas. Powders do not work well for treatment but may be used for prevention, such as in shoes after a gym workout. Use cotton socks. Apply medicine 1-2 inches beyond the rash. Use for at least 2-4 weeks, even if it appears healed. Reduce moisture to the infected area If foot infection, do not walk barefoot (to avoid spreading it) Wear sandals in public showers (to avoid catching it)

Onychomycosis (Tinea Unguium – Toenail or Fingernail Fungal Infections), Background & Treatment

■ Onychomycosis can cause pain, discomfort, and disfigurement and can lead to physical limitations, such as difficulty standing and walking. The discoloration and disfigurement can cause loss of self-esteem and psychological issues.

■ Topical agents are limited to mild cases, patients who cannot tolerate systemic therapies, or are used concurrently with systemic treatment or as prophylaxis. They are <u>not</u> potent enough to cure most infections.

■ Itraconazole and terbinafine are used most commonly and have FDA indications; fluconazole and posaconazole are used off-label. Griseofulvin is rarely used currently.

■ It takes a long time for the nail bed to look better – sometimes up to a year in toenails. Toenails take longer to treat than fingernails, and are more commonly infected.

■ Pulse therapy (intermittent) can be used to reduce costs and possibly toxicity, but may not be as effective.

■ A 20% <u>potassium hydroxide (KOH) smear</u> is essential for diagnosis as other conditions can produce a similar presentation.

DRUGS	NOTES	SAFETY/COUNSELING
Itraconazole *(Sporanox)* Dose 200 mg Q daily x 12 weeks for 12 weeks, or "pulse-dosing" (fingernails only): 200 mg BID x 1 week, repeat 1-week course after 3 weeks off-time Terbinafine *(LamISIL, Terbinex)* – oral (topical is LamISIL AT, and is used for fungal skin infections) 250 mg PO daily for 6 weeks (fingernail) or 12 weeks (toenail) Ciclopirox *(Penlac, Loprox)* Apply evenly over entire nail plate QHS, or 8 hours before washing) to all affected nails with applicator brush Tavabarole *(Kerydin)* Efinaconazole *(Jublia)* *Kerydin* & *Jublia*: apply once daily for 48 weeks, both for toenails	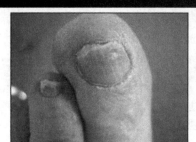 Ciclopirox *(Penlac, Loprox)* – used in combination with orals; poor efficacy when used alone. Occasionally used in patients who cannot tolerate systemic therapy, but generally cannot cure an infection when used alone. Occasionally used as prophylaxis. Tavaborole *(Kerydin)* – oxaborole antifungal, applied topically to toenails Q daily x 48 weeks to entire nail surface and under the nail tip. Efinaconazole *(Jublia)* – azole antifungal, applied topically to toenails Q daily x 48 weeks	For systemic azoles, see ID chapter. Primarily these drugs are hepatotoxic (monitor liver), are QT prolongers (Avoid in QT risk) and are 3A4 substrates & inhibitors (many drug interactions). Nausea and diarrhea are common, monitor LFTs. Itraconazole *(Sporanox)* Black box warning to avoid use in heart failure. Requires gastric acid for absorption; cannot use strong acid suppressing agents concurrently. Terbinafine *(Lamisil, Terbinex)* – oral Primarily headache, rash, nausea, risk of hepatotoxicity. Recurrence is common. Practice proper foot care and keep the nails dry. Keep blood glucose controlled. Do not smoke.

Vaginal Fungal Candida ("Yeast") Infections

This is a common infection; about 75% women will have at least one episode, and half of these women will have recurrence. In a small percentage of women the recurrence is chronic.

- The infection is uncommon before a girl begins menstruating, and occurs most commonly during the week prior to menstruation – this makes treatment decisions around the period important. The woman can begin treatment during menses, or wait until the bleeding stops. Tampons should not be used when medication is applied.

- Vaginal fungal infections are also common during pregnancy. Pregnant patients are hopefully seeing a physician, and require longer (7-10 day treatment).

- Symptoms are primarily itching, with possible soreness and pain (burning) during urination or sex. Some women have a cottage-cheese like discharge (white, thick, clumpy).

- Diagnosis can be confirmed with either a vaginal culture to check for fungal growth or, via a pH test: a pH greater than 4.5 indicates the presence of either a candida or trichomoniasis infection. OTC test kits such as the *Vagisil Screening Kit* test for vaginal pH. Generally, testing is not necessary if the woman has been seen by the physician for the initial infection and is able to recognize the symptoms.

- If the woman has had the infection before and is able to recognize the symptoms, she can self-treat with OTC products. If there are more than four infections in a year, or if symptoms recur within 2 months, refer to the physician to rule-out an underlying condition that could be causative (most likely diabetes, HIV, receiving steroids or other immune-suppressing agents, pregnancy, or irritation from repeated douching or use of lubricants.) Women taking high-dose estrogen in birth control pills or in hormone replacement therapy are at elevated risk. Antibiotic use can be a risk factor; the antibiotic can wipe out the normal flora and lead to fungal overgrowth.

- Lactobacillus or yogurt with active cultures is thought to reduce infection occurrence; however, this is rated as "possibly ineffective" by the *Natural Medicines Database.*

- If self-treating, counsel that condoms and diaphragms may not provide adequate pregnancy protection; the oil in OTC antifungals weakens the latex.

- To avoid future infections, keep the vaginal area clean, wipe from the front to the back, use cotton underwear, avoid tight-fitting clothing, including pantyhose, change pads/tampons often, change out of wet swimsuits or clothing quickly, and recommend against use of vaginal douches, sprays and deodorant tampons; these can alter the vaginal pH and contribute to infection.

DRUGS	NOTES	SAFETY/COUNSELING
Mild-moderate, infrequent infection 1 or 3 day treatment, with vaginal cream, ointment or vaginal suppository/tab **OTC, topical** Butoconazole (*Gynazole-1*, others) Clotrimazole (*Gyne-Lotrimin*, others) Miconazole (*Monistat 3*, others) Terconazole (*Terazol 3*, others) Tioconazole (*Vagistat-1*) **Rx, oral** Fluconazole (*Diflucan*) 150 mg PO x 1 Complicated infections, Pregnancy 7-10 days treatment, or send for referral	The male sexual partner may be tested if the female's infections are recurrent; this is not commonly done. Always counsel on ways to avoid recurrence: avoid douching, wear cotton underwear, avoid tight-fitting pantyhose and pants, change out of wet swimsuits quickly. Some recommend avoiding hot tubs or very hot baths.	Counseling for OTC antifungals: Prior to using the product, wash the vagina with mild soap and water, and pat dry with a towel. Insert applicator, suppository, or vaginal tab at night before bed. Lying down immediately after insertion helps retain the medicine inside the vagina. It may be helpful to use a protective pad. The creams and suppositories are oil-based medications that can weaken latex condoms and diaphragms; avoid sexual intercourse. If you get your menstrual cycle during treatment, continue the treatment, otherwise a woman can wait until her menstrual cycle is over before starting treatment if she desires (this is not necessary.) Do not use tampons during treatment. Complete entire course of treatment. Medical care is warranted if symptoms persist/recur within 2 months after using an OTC product, or if > 4/year.

Eczema (Atopic Dermatitis), Background & Treatment

- Eczema is a general term for many types of skin inflammation, and is used interchangeably with the term atopic dermatitis (which is sometimes used to refer to other conditions – this makes the term "atopic dermatitis" confusing.)

- Eczema is most common in young children and infants, but can occur at any age.

- Eczema presents as skin rashes, which become crusty and scaly; blisters can develop. The rash is very itchy, red, dry and sore.

- Common locations are the insides of elbows, back of knees, face (often on the cheeks), behind the ears, buttocks, hands and feet.

- Outbreak "triggers" can be environmental irritants or allergens, including soaps, perfumes, pollution, stress or weather changes; patients should attempt to avoid triggers.

- Hydration is essential to reduce disease severity. Use moisturizers. Maintain humidity in the home.

- Treatment can include topical corticosteroids (and occasional oral courses, if-needed), antihistamines (for itching), or the immune-suppresant calcineurin inhibitors, if topical steroids with hydration are not adequate.

- In severe, refractive cases oral immune-suppressants (cyclosporine, methotrexate, monoclonal antibody-type drugs such as etanercept and others) can be used. These are described in other chapters.

DRUGS	NOTES	SAFETY/COUNSELING
Tx: topical or oral steroids, antibiotics, antihistamines, keep skin well hydrated (moisturized with petrolatum, lanolin, products such as *Aquaphor, Eucerin, Keri* or store brands) Treat first with topical steroids, only use these agents if failed steroids: **Tacrolimus (Protopic)** **Pimecrolimus (Elidel)** Do not use in children younger than 2 years of age.		Dispense MedGuide for *Elidel* and *Protopic*: Associated with cases of lymphoma and skin cancer; use only as second-line agents for short-term and intermittent treatment of atopic dermatitis (eczema) in patients unresponsive to, or intolerant of other treatments. Apply a thin layer only to the affected skin areas, twice a day. Use the smallest amount needed to control symptoms. Takes weeks to work; continue to apply. Wash your hands after application. Limit sun exposure; photosensitizer. Side effects can include headache, skin burning, itching, cough, flu-like symptoms

Hemorrhoids

- Hemorrhoids are swollen blood vessels in the lower rectum. They are in a sensitive location and have a rich blood vessel supply that can result in engorgement. Common symptoms are pruritus, burning and rectal bleeding. The blood is usually bright red.

- If dietary fiber is not optimum, increasing fiber intake can help reduce straining. Products such as psyllium will mix with the stool to make it spongier and easier to push out. A stool softener (such as docusate) will reduce straining.

- Phenylephrine (*Preparation H*, others) is a vasoconstrictor that shrinks the hemorrhoid and reduces burning and itching.

- Hydrocortisone (*Anusol-HC, Preparation H Hydrocortisone*, others) comes in anal suppositories and various topicals including creams and wipes. These reduce itching and inflammation.

- Witch hazel (*Tucks* pads) is a mild astringent that can relieve mild itching. Barriers (skin protectants) to reduce irritation from stool/urine are helpful in some cases (petrolatum, others – see Diaper Rash section).

- There are many combination products. Example: *Tucks* ointment contains mineral oil (skin protectant), zinc oxide (desiccant) and pramoxine (anesthetic).

DRUGS	NOTES	SAFETY/COUNSELING
Preparation H *Anusol-HC* Many others	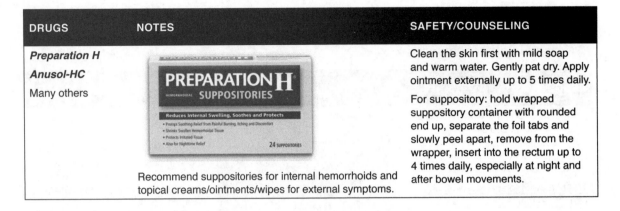 Recommend suppositories for internal hemorrhoids and topical creams/ointments/wipes for external symptoms.	Clean the skin first with mild soap and warm water. Gently pat dry. Apply ointment externally up to 5 times daily. For suppository: hold wrapped suppository container with rounded end up, separate the foil tabs and slowly peel apart, remove from the wrapper, insert into the rectum up to 4 times daily, especially at night and after bowel movements.

Lice, Background & Treatment

NOTE this section discusses lice; SCABIES (mites) are treated with some of the same medications. Scabies are primarily spread through sexual contact. The primary treatment for scabies is permethrin in a cream formulation (*Elimite*) and the prescription drug ivermectin (*Stromectol*), two doses, taken one week apart. Ivermectin, when taken orally, can be difficult to tolerate due to lymph node enlargement, arthralgias, skin tenderness, pruritus and fever. Ivermectin was approved in 2012 in a topical formulation for lice called *Sklice*. Lindane (*Kwell*, others) used to be commonly used for scabies (and lice) but is not used commonly now due to <u>neurotoxicity</u>.

- Lice occurs most commonly in elementary school age children.

- Pyrethrins (permethrin) are the OTC drug of choice; can be used in infants as young as 2 months. Avoid with chrysanthemums or ragweed allergy.

- Malathion lotion 0.5% (*Ovide*) is an organophosphate. Only for use on persons 6 years of age and older. Can irritate the skin and is flammable; do not smoke or use electrical heat sources, including hair dryers, curlers, and curling or flat irons, when applying and while the hair is wet.

- Benzyl alcohol lotion (*Ulesfia* 5% lotion) kills live lice but not nits. Can irritate the skin and eyes; avoid eye contact.

- *Lindane* shampoo 1% is no longer recommended due to neurotoxicity and is reserved for refractive cases, and never in pregnancy, on irritated skin, or in infants, children, persons with small frames and the elderly.

- If the same medication has been used several times it may not be working.

- Repeating the procedure, and removing the nits from hair, bedding, and elsewhere is essential:

  - Wash clothes and bedding in hot water, followed by a hot dryer.

  - If something cannot be washed, seal it in an air-proof bag for 2 weeks or dry clean. Vacuum the carpet well. Soak combs and brushes in hot water for 10 minutes. Make sure to check other children in the household.

❑ Do not use a combination shampoo/conditioner, or conditioner before using lice medicine. Do not re-wash the hair for 1-2 days after treatment.

❑ After each treatment, check the hair and use a nit comb to remove nits and lice every 2-3 days. Continue to check for 2-3 weeks to be sure all lice and nits are gone.

❑ Re-treatment is needed for OTC and prescription products (except *Sklice*) on days 7-10 (they vary; check the product) in order to kill any surviving hatched lice before they produce new eggs.

DRUGS	NOTES	SAFETY/COUNSELING
Permethrin, pyrethrins, OTC DOC for lice *(Nix, RID, Triple X)* 2 months+ Spinosad *(Natroba)* –works well, expensive. 4+ yrs Malathion *(Ovide)* – flammable, do not use near heat source, organophosphate Benzyl Alcohol Lotion *(Ulesfia)* 6+ yrs Ivermectin *(Sklice)* 6+ yrs Lindane *(Kwell*, others) is no longer routinely recommended; high risk neurotoxicity/seizures, requires MedGuide – more commonly used for scabies (mites)	Notice how the nit is cemented to the hair shaft. Egg, Hair, Nit (Louse Egg), Nymph (Juvenile), Adult Louse	In addition to OTC treatment, remove the live lice and nits by inspecting the hair in 1-inch segments and using a lice comb. Without removing live lice and nits, the OTC product will not work. Nits are "cemented" to the hair shaft and do not fall off after treatment. Nit removal requires multiple efforts, which should be continued for two weeks after treatment. See bulleted points above for additional counseling.

Genital Warts, Background & Treatment

■ Genital warts are caused by the human papillomavirus (HPV), a common sexually transmitted disease (STD), spread easily skin-to-skin. Consider recommending HPV vaccine, if series incomplete. *Gardasil* protects against the strains of HPV that cause most genital warts and reduces risk of cervical cancer. *Cervarix* protects against cervical cancer but not genital warts. Condoms reduce risk of STD transmission.

■ Treatment may not be required if no symptoms, but if discomfort or emotional distress treatment can reduce or remove the warts.

■ Imiquimod (*Aldara, Zyclara*) will reduce warts. Avoid sexual contact while the cream is on your skin; weakens condoms, diaphragms and can irritate the partner's skin.

In addition to the treatments below, the warts may be removed by lasers, cryotherapy (with liquid nitrogen to freeze the warts, after which they come off), freezing, electrocautery (electrical current burns off warts) or surgical excision.

DRUGS	NOTES	SAFETY/COUNSELING
Imiquimod cream (*Aldara, Zyclara*) *Aldara* also approved for superficial basal cell carcinoma and actinic keratosis. Podophyllum Resin (*Podocon-25*)	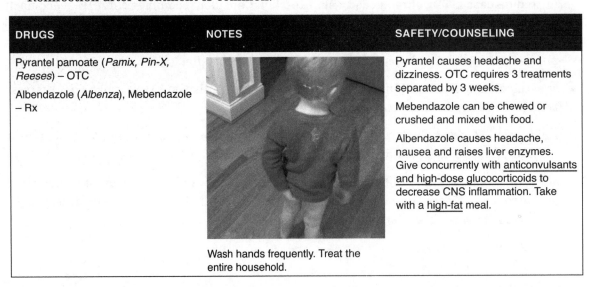 Genital warts: Found on shaft of penis (male), vagina, vulva, cervix (female) and around anus	Imiquimod Apply to entire treatment area before bedtime and rub in until the cream is no longer visible. Use only 1 packet per application. Wash off after 8 hours. Applied 3x/week until clearance or 16 wks duration. Wash hands before and after application. Do not touch eyes, lips or nose. Common skin reactions: burning, edema, erythema, induration, itching, scabbing, crusting, exudate.

Pinworm *(Vermicularis)* Infection

- Anthelmintics, such as mebendazole, pyrantel pamoate, and albendazole, are active against *Enterobius vermicularis.*

- Pinworm infection most commonly occurs in children and presents as anal itching. Pyrantel comes in several OTC products including the popular *Pin-X*. The pinworms can be resistant to treatment. Albendazole and mebendazole are prescription only.

- The "tape" test is used to identify eggs: stick a piece of tape around the anus in the morning prior to voiding/defecating. It can take up to 3 morning tape tests to identify the eggs. Reinfection after treatment is common.

DRUGS	NOTES	SAFETY/COUNSELING
Pyrantel pamoate (*Pamix, Pin-X, Reeses*) – OTC Albendazole (*Albenza*), Mebendazole – Rx	Wash hands frequently. Treat the entire household.	Pyrantel causes headache and dizziness. OTC requires 3 treatments separated by 3 weeks. Mebendazole can be chewed or crushed and mixed with food. Albendazole causes headache, nausea and raises liver enzymes. Give concurrently with anticonvulsants and high-dose glucocorticoids to decrease CNS inflammation. Take with a high-fat meal.

Topical Inflammation (From Various Conditions, Rashes), Background & Treatment

- Primary treatment for skin irritation are topical steroids. Two strengths of hydrocortisone (HC) available OTC, 0.5% and 1%; all other topical steroids are prescription. A chart of Rx topical steroids is at the end of this chapter.

- The steroid vehicle influences the strength of the medication. Usual potency, from highest to weakest: ointment > creams > lotions > solutions > gels > sprays. Ointments have low water content; refer to the Compounding chapter for details.

- Parts of the body with thin skin, such as the face, eyelids and genitals, are highly susceptible to the side effects of topical steroids and low potency products should be used on these areas. Use low potency products on areas of the skin with folds, such as the armpits, groin, and under the breasts, where the absorption is higher.

- Local (skin) steroid side effects, if used long-term include skin thinning, pigment changes (lighter or darker), telangectasia (blood vessel) formation, rosacea, perioral dermatitis and acne, increased risk skin infections, delayed wound healing, irritation/burning/peeling, and possibly contact dermatitis from the steroid itself.

- For urticaria (hives) the second-generation antihistamines can be recommended (OTC) as the initial options due to better tolerability than first-generation antihistamines. Cetirizine is a common choice; see the Allergic Rhinitis, Cough & Cold chapter for a discussion of antihistamines. For hives, higher doses are used. The "non-sedating" antihistamines are more sedating with higher doses. First-generation antihistamines (diphenhydramine, others) can be given at bedtime if the sedative effects are desirable.

- H2-blockers (famotidine, others) are helpful in some patients for hives and urticaria. Hydroxyzine is often prescribed and is in the table below.

DRUGS	NOTES	SAFETY/COUNSELING
OTC steroids are low potency: Hydrocortisone 0.5% (infants) and 1% for mild conditions, thin skin (groin area, elderly) and for children. HC 1% lotion *(Aquanil)* See other steroids in chart at end of this section. Apply high potency Rx steroids once daily – Apply OTC/lower potency 1-2x daily. It is common to see a higher potency product, followed by a lower potency product, to treat acute inflammation. Severe rash likely to require oral steroids for 1-2 weeks.	Ointments often more potent than creams; use ointments for thick or dry skin. Ointments have low water content (reduced absorption) and form a skin barrier. Use lotions, gels and foams for hairy skin. No evidence for use of topical diphenhydramine – can use systemic but caution due to side effects. Skin should be lubricated (hydrated) with moisturizers for most conditions. The steroid vehicle can lubricate. Camphor, menthol, local anesthetics (often in combo creams with HC) can help relieve itching. COMMON STEROIDS, BY POTENCY, AT END OF THIS CHAPTER	 The "finger-tip" unit is used to estimate amount required: the amount that can be squeezed from the fingertip to the 1st joint covers one adult hand (about ½ g) Topical steroid over-use has risks; see top bullet points. Do not apply for longer than 2 weeks. Encourage patient not to use more than directed.
HydrOXYzine *(Vistaril)* 25 mg TID-QID	Used for general urticaria (hives) with severe itching	Anticholinergic; primarily sedation and dry mouth.

Diaper Rash, Background & Treatment

Diaper rash commonly occurs with nearly all babies. The skin is sensitive, and when exposed to the urine and stools, and a diaper moving back and forth, rash appears. Once the skin is damaged it is susceptible to bacteria and yeast overgrowth.

Prevention

- Change diapers frequently, do not cover diapers with plastic, use absorbent diapers.

- Wipe well with unscented wipes or plain water.

- Leave off the diaper, when possible, to let the skin air-dry. The baby can lie on a towel.

- Use a skin protectant:

  - Petrolatum ointment (*A & D* ointment, store brands) – this is a good preventative everyday ointment.

  - Petrolatum with zinc oxide, such as in *Desitin* – is thicker and contains a dessicant (zinc oxide) to dry out the skin; may be preferable for babies more prone to rash.

- "Butt paste" or "Triple paste" – are other alternatives.

- Clotrimazole, miconazole, others – for stubborn rashes, if yeast thought to be involved.

- Hydrocortisone 0.5-1% cream – can be used BID, but not for more than several days at a time.

- Combinations of the above are used.

DRUGS	NOTES	SAFETY/COUNSELING
Desitin (petrolatum + zinc oxide, a dessicant to decrease moisture) *A&D Ointment*, or plain petrolatum, or store-brands. Miconazole+zinc oxide+petrolatum (*Vusion*) Or other products mentioned above.		Review counseling tips above. Infants should be referred to the physician (especially if under 6 months) and older babies if condition appears serious or worsens. Topical antibiotics may be needed if bacterial involvement is suspected. Topical antifungals may be needed if fungal involvement is suspected. Topical steroids, low potency, may be used short-term. Diaper rashes can have more than one contributing organism.

Minor Cuts, Abrasions & Burns, Background & Treatment

- The basic types of minor wounds are lacerations, abrasions, cuts, bites and burns.

- Some can be effectively treated through simple first aid and others, depending on the severity, may need more medical attention than first aid can provide.

- Anything that involves puncture wounds should be referred out.

- Make sure tetanus vaccine is current (Q 10 years, after series has been completed.) If the wound is dirty a repeat tetanus vaccine may be required if it is >5 years since vaccination. The patient should be referred for medical care.

- If wound looks like abuse, contact authorities if able.

- Abrasions are minor injuries to the top layer of skin and are primarily treated with simple first aid.

- Abrasions such as a skinned knee can be cleaned thoroughly, antibiotic ointment applied and allowed to air heal.

- Lacerations are defined as irregular wounds with ragged edges, with the potential for deeper skin damage and bruising under the skin.

- If deep seek medical attention.

- A cut is different than a laceration because the edges will be more uniform or regular.

- After cleaning, if the bleeding does not stop, or it extends far below the surface layers of the skin, seek medical attention because it may require stitching to get the wound to close. If not, regular bandaging should get the edges of the wound to close over time.

- Antibiotic ointment can be applied prior to placing the bandage.

- Tissue adhesives *(Band-Aid Liquid Bandage, Nexcare Skin Crack Care*, others) create a polymer layer, which binds to the skin, keeping the wound clean and keeping moisture out. Some contain topical analgesics. *Seal-On* is a topical sponge (dressing) that can absorb blood and is used for nose-bleeds and other minor bleeds. There are other similar products.

- Bites (except minor insect bites) should never be treated with just simple first aid, because of the high risk of infection, especially with animal or human bites. Certain spider bites in the U.S. can be deadly: the brown recluse, the black widow and the hobo spiders. Spiders tend to stay hidden and are not aggressive. Bites can be generally be avoided by inspecting and shaking out clothing or equipment prior to use, and wearing protective clothing. If bitten, stay calm, identify the type of spider if possible, wash with soap and cold water, apply cold compress with ice, elevate extremity, and get emergency medical care.

- Minor, harmless insect bites can be treated with a topical steroid or systemic antihistamine (such as diphenhydramine) to reduce itching.

- Burns are characterized as first degree (red/painful, minor swelling), second degree (thicker, very painful, produce blisters) and third degree (damage to all layers of skin, skin appears white or charred.) Burns produced by chemical exposure, or in a person with underlying disease that reduces immunity should be referred for emergency medical care.

- If the burn is first or second degree OTC treatment is acceptable if the area is less than 2 inches in diameter and if the burn is not on the face, over a major joint or on the feet or genitals. In diabetes a burn on a foot, even mild, could lead to an amputation. Vigilance is required.

- Minor burns should be treated first by running the burn under cool running water or soaking in cool water for 5-20 minutes.

- Do not apply ice, which can further damage the injured skin. Bandages should be applied if the skin is broken, or if blisters pop. Burns heal best when kept moist (but not wet). Certain bandages designed for burns keep the environment moist, or ointments, such as antibiotic ointment, can be applied.

- Burned skin itches as it heals; the fingernails of children may need to be cut short and filed, or covered. The skin that has been burned will be more sensitive to the sun for up to a year.

- Ointments (80% oil/20% water, such as Aquaphor) should be used for skin protection over a minor burn to hold in moisture and reduce scarring risk.

- Silver sulfadiazene *(Silvadene; SSD; Thermazene)* may be used topically to reduce infection risk and promote healing, although it has not been shown to be very effective. If the skin is broken systemic toxicity could occur. Do not use if sulfa allergy or G6PD deficiency (due to hemolysis risk).

DRUGS	NOTES	SAFETY/COUNSELING
Triple antibiotic ointment (Neosporin, store brands) contains polymyxin, bacitracin & neomycin. If reaction to the neomycin component can use **Polysporin** (bacitracin and polymixin) or **Bacitracin** alone. Either of these is often sufficient. **Mupirocin (Bactroban)** is an Rx antibiotic cream or ointment; very good staph and strep coverage, including MRSA; can be used for nasal MRSA colonization. *(Bactroban nasal is used for MRSA-nasal colonization)* **Bacitracin, Neomycin, Polymyxin B,** and **Hydrocortisone (Cortisporin** ointment) is a popular Rx topical used for superficial skin infections. Tissue adhesives *(Band-Aid Liquid Bandage, Nexcare Skin Crack Care,* others) – "paint on" bandages to protect/keep moisture in skin via polymer layer. *Seal-On,* others (topical dressings for minor bleeds). sponge (dressing) that	The wound may be covered with a sterile bandage if it is in a place that could get dirty. 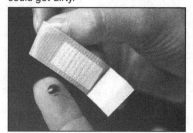 Leaving a wound uncovered helps it stay dry and helps it heal. If the wound is not in an area that will get dirty or be rubbed by clothing, it does not need to be covered.	To apply topical antibiotics: Clean the affected area and apply a small amount of medication (an amount equal to the surface area of the tip of a finger) to the affected area 1 to 3 times daily. If area can get dirty (such as a hand) or be irritated by clothing, cover with an adhesive strip (e.g., *Band-Aid*) or with sterile gauze and adhesive tape +/- antibiotic ointment. Change daily. Certain wounds, like large scrapes, should be kept moist and clean to help reduce scarring and speed healing. Bandages used for this purpose are called occlusive or semi-occlusive bandages. Burns require a moist (but not wet) environment by applying either ointment, or a bandage designed for burns.

Poison Ivy, Oak, Sumac, Background & Treatment

- Poison ivy, oak or sumac poisoning is an allergic reaction that results from touching the sap of these plants, which contain the toxin uroshiol.

- The sap may be on the plant, in the ashes of burned plants, on an animal, or on other objects that came in contact with the plant, such as clothing, garden tools, and sports equipment.

- Small amounts of uroshiol can remain under a person's fingernails for several days unless it is deliberately removed with good cleaning.

- Poison ivy grows around lakes and streams in the midwest and east. Leaves are green in the summer and red in the fall.

- Poison oak grows in the western (along the Pacific coast) and in the east from New Jersey to Texas. The leaves look like oak, usually in clusters of three leaves. The plant has clusters of yellow berries.

- Poison sumac grows in boggy areas, especially in the southeast and west. The leaves have 7-13 smooth-edged leaflets, with pale yellow or cream-colored berries.

DRUGS	NOTES	SAFETY/COUNSELING
Aluminum acetate solution *(Burrow's)* Colloidal oatmeal *(Aveeno)* Calamine lotion – *Caladryl, IvaRest* are calamine + topical analgesics *Zanfel* is supposed to bind urushiol (this is the toxin) – low evidence for efficacy	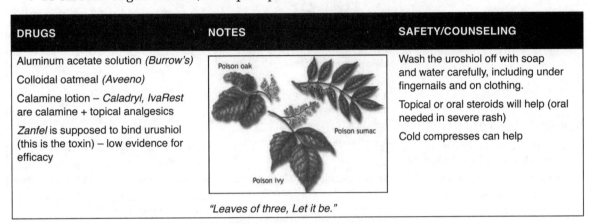 *"Leaves of three, Let it be."*	Wash the uroshiol off with soap and water carefully, including under fingernails and on clothing. Topical or oral steroids will help (oral needed in severe rash) Cold compresses can help

Alopecia (Hair Loss), Background & Treatment

- As people age, hair tends to gradually thin. Other causes of hair loss include hormonal factors, medical conditions and medications.

- The most common cause of hair loss is a hereditary condition called male-pattern baldness, and less commonly, female-pattern baldness.

- Hormonal changes in women that can result in hair loss are usually associated with pregnancy, childbirth or menopause.

- Medical conditions that cause hair loss include hypothyroidism, alopecia areata (an auto-immune condition), scalp infections and some other conditions, including lupus.

- Drugs that can contribute to alopecia include various chemotherapeutics (primarily because hair cells are rapidly dividing and therefore are targeted by the treatment) and infrequently with the following medications: clomiphene, heparin, hydroxychloroquine, interferons, lithium, some types of oral contraceptives, levonorgestrel, procainamide, valproate, spironolactone and warfarin.

- Zinc and vitamin D deficiency is thought to contribute to hair loss.

- Many people will seek surgical intervention for hair loss. The medications work modestly and are presented here. Bimatoprost in the *Latisse* formulation is for thinning eyelashes (hypotrichosis) and should not be used concurrently in patients using a prostaglandin analog for glaucoma (minimally, contact the optometrist or opthamologist to confirm because the IOP may increase if there is excessive use of prostaglandin analogs.)

DRUGS	NOTES	SAFETY/COUNSELING
Finasteride *(Propecia)* 5-alpha reductase type 2 inhibitor <u>Do not dispense with someone on finasteride *(Proscar)* for BPH</u> 1 mg daily, at least 3 months duration to begin to see effect	Male pattern baldness "My Mom always said…god made a few good heads, and put hair on the rest of them."	Preg Categ X: females should not handle – can damage male fetus. Must be used indefinitely or condition reappears. **SIDE EFFECTS** Lower dose than *Proscar*; lower risk of sexual side effects; see overactive bladder chapter for further details
Minoxidil topical OTC 2% and 5% – 5% solution more effective, but more facial hair growth.	Rx tablets indicated for hypertension (very rarely used)	For men and women Must be used indefinitely or condition reappears.
Bimatoprost solution *(Latisse)* For thinning eyelashes (hypotrichosis)	Apply nightly to the skin at the base of the upper eyelashes only (do not apply to the lower lid). Use the applicator brush. Blot any excess. Repeat for other eye. Dispose of the applicator after one use.	May cause itchy eyes and/or eye redness. If discontinued, lashes eventually return to previous appearance. Eyelid skin darkening may occur, which may be reversible. Hair growth may occur in other skin areas that the solution frequently touches. Do not use concurrently with PG analogs used for glaucoma.

Sunscreens, Background & Treatment

- Applying sunscreen is important due to the risk of sun damage and skin cancer. Keep in mind that sunscreen blocks vitamin D production in the skin and many Americans are vitamin-D deficient. This is a difficulty in current practice.

- It is advisable to stay out of the sun when it is strongest (between 10AM-4PM). The sun damaging ultraviolet (UV) rays penetrate clouds; this applies to overcast days as well.

- Another method to avoid the sun is to wear protective clothing.

- Where skin is exposed sunscreen can be applied that provides both UVA (A for aging – causes damage below the skin surface) and UVB (B for burning) protection. Both UVA and UVB contribute to skin cancer. A "broad spectrum" sunscreen should be chosen; it protects against both UVA and UVB. SPF stands for sun protection factor, which is a measure of how well the sunscreen deflects UVB rays.

- Some dermatologists recommend <u>SPF 15</u> and others recommend <u>SPF 30</u>. The key is to apply <u>liberally and at least every two hours</u>. The American Academy of Pediatrics says to keep all babies less than 6 months old out of the sun.

- HOW SPF WORKS: If someone would normally burn in 10 minutes, an SPF of 5 would extend the time they would burn to 50 minutes (5 x 10 = 50.) However, it is not accurate to calculate that if one normally would burn in one hour, then a sunscreen with an SPF of 10 would permit the person to stay in the sun for 10 hours (10 times longer) without burning, since the intensity of the sun varies during the day, and the sunscreen would not last more than a couple of hours.

- Sunscreen labeling is no longer permitted to use "waterproof" or "sweatproof" since they all wash off, at least partially, in the water. They can claim to be "water-resistant" but only for 40-80 minutes. Always reapply after swimming, or sweating.

- The American Academy of Dermatology (AAD) recommends sunscreens with any of the following ingredients: avobenzone, cinoxate, ecamsule, menthyl anthranilate, octyl methoxycinnamate, octyl salicylate, oxybenzone or sulisobenzone.

- Oxybenzone irritates some people's skin; this is not common.

DRUGS	NOTES	SAFETY/COUNSELING
Many products, choose one with UVA and UVB coverage, SPF 15+. UVA: Blocks aging (A for aging – wrinkles). Ingredients that block UVA: ecamsule, avobenzone, oxybenzone, sulisobenzone, titanium dioxide, zinc oxide (zinc and titanium are common barrier agents). UVB: Blocks burning (B for burning). SPF (sun exposure factor) – measures how long it takes to burn versus not using sunscreen (measures UVB only). An SPF of 15 takes 15 times longer for skin to redden than without the sunscreen.	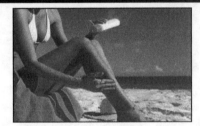 Apply liberally, at least every two hours, prior to sun exposure, and after getting the skin wet from swimming or sweating.	All sunscreens wash off; reapply after going in the water and at least every 2 hours. Avoid peak sun (10AM-4PM), even if overcast. Wear protective clothing. Consider vitamin D deficiency-if avoiding sun or little sun exposure may need supplementation. UVA and UVB exposure increases risk of skin cancer, including most common type (squamous cell). "Broad spectrum" covers both UVA and UVB. Water resistant – means resistant for 40-80 minutes.

Potencies of Topical Steroid Products

TREATMENT	ACTIVE INGREDIENT
Very High Potency	
Clobex Lotion/Spray/Shampoo, 0.05%	Clobetasol propionate
Cormax Cream/Solution, 0.05%	Clobetasol propionate
Diprolene Ointment, 0.05%	**Betamethasone dipropionate**
Olux Foam, 0.05%	**Clobetasol propionate**
Temovate Cream/Ointment/Solution, 0.05%	**Clobetasol propionate**
Ultravate Cream/Ointment, 0.05%	**Halobetasol propionate**
Vanos Cream, 0.1%	**Fluocinonide**
Psorcon Ointment, 0.05%	Diflorasone diacetate
Psorcon E Ointment, 0.05%	Diflorasone diacetate

TREATMENT	ACTIVE INGREDIENT
High Potency	
Diprolene Cream AF, 0.05%	**Betamethasone dipropionate**
Elocon Ointment, 0.1%	**Mometasone furoate**
Florone Ointment, 0.05%	Diflorasone diacetate
Halog Ointment/Cream, 0.1%	Halcinonide
Lidex Cream/Gel/Ointment, 0.05%	**Fluocinonide**
Psorcon Cream, 0.05%	Diflorasone diacetate
Topicort Cream/Ointment, 0.25%	Desoximetasone
Topicort Gel, 0.05%	Desoximetasone

TREATMENT	ACTIVE INGREDIENT
High-Medium Potency	
Cutivate Ointment, 0.005%	Fluticasone propionate
Lidex-E Cream, 0.05%	**Fluocinonide**
Luxiq Foam, 0.12%	Betamethasone valerate
Topicort LP Cream, 0.05%	Desoximetasone

TREATMENT	ACTIVE INGREDIENT
Medium Potency	
Cordran Ointment, 0.05%	Flurandrenolide
Elocon Cream, 0.1%	**Mometasone furoate**
Kenalog Cream/Spray, 0.1%	**Triamcinolone acetonide**
Synalar Ointment, 0.03%	Fluocinolone acetonide
Westcort Ointment, 0.2%	**Hydrocortisone valerate**

Potencies of Topical Steroid Products Continued

TREATMENT	ACTIVE INGREDIENT

Lower Potency

TREATMENT	ACTIVE INGREDIENT
Capex Shampoo, 0.01%	Fluocinolone acetonide
Cordran Cream/Lotion/Tape, 0.05%	Flurandrenolide
Cutivate Cream/Lotion, 0.05%	Fluticasone propionate
DermAtop Cream, 0.1%	Prednicarbate
***DesOwen* Lotion, 0.05%**	**Desonide**
Locoid Cream/Lotion/Ointment/Solution, 0.1%	Hydrocortisone
Pandel Cream, 0.1%	Hydrocortisone
Synalar Cream, 0.03%/0.01%	Fluocinolone acetonide
***Westcort* Cream, 0.2%**	**Hydrocortisone valerate**

Mild Potency

TREATMENT	ACTIVE INGREDIENT
Aclovate Cream/Ointment, 0.05%	Alclometasone dipropionate
***Derma*-Smoothe/FS Oil, 0.01%**	**Fluocinolone acetonide**
Desonate Gel, 0.05%	Desonide
Synalar Cream/Solution, 0.01%	Fluocinolone acetonide
Verdeso Foam, 0.05%	Desonide

Lowest Potency

TREATMENT	ACTIVE INGREDIENT
Cetacort Lotion, 0.5%/1%	Hydrocortisone
Cortaid Cream/Spray/Ointment	**Hydrocortisone**
Hytone Cream/Lotion, 1%/2.5%	Hydrocortisone
Micort-HC Cream, 2%/2.5%	Hydrocortisone
Nutracort Lotion, 1%/2.5%	Hydrocortisone
Synacort Cream, 1%/2.5%	Hydrocortisone

$$BMI = \frac{lbs}{in^2} \cdot 703$$

WEIGHT LOSS

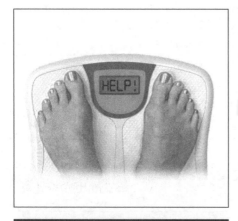

GUIDELINES

2013 AHA/ACC/TOS Guideline for the Management of Overweight and Obesity in Adults: A Report of the American College of Cardiology/American Heart Association Task Force on Practice Guidelines and The Obesity Society. *J Am Coll Cardiol.* 2014; 63(25_PA):2985-3023.

BACKGROUND

Overweight and obesity is a national health threat and a major public health challenge. Data from the CDC (2014) estimates obesity at 35% of U.S. adults and 17% of children and adolescents 2 – 19 years. Obesity is a BMI of ≥ 30, or, for a person 5'9", a weight of ≥ 203 pounds. Overweight puts patients at increased risk for coronary heart disease, hypertension, stroke, type 2 diabetes, certain types of cancer, and premature death. In addition to health risks, overweight reduces quality of life and causes social stigmatization and discrimination. This is sadly true for adults, and for children. Not too long ago it was uncommon to see an overweight child. Today, one-third of children are overweight or obese.

Weight loss is successful only when the patient (and usually the family) is able to make permanent changes in diet and exercise habits. Fad diets may cause an acute weight drop but do not contribute to long-term weight loss and can have harmful health consequences. Many people think they are just "born fat" or have low metabolism. Children become overweight (and grow into overweight adults) primarily due to to poor eating habits in the family and community. If low metabolism is an issue it will show up on lab tests (as hypothyroidism) and will be treated.

fad diet = short-term intense diet

A healthy weight: value and achievement

In 2013 long-awaited obesity guidelines were released as a joint project between the American College of Cardiology, the American Heart Association and the Obesity Society. The guidelines support these actions:

↓ daily caloric intake by 500-750 kcal (↓ ~3500 kcal/wk) = ↓ 1 lb lost /wk

+ physical act. = ↓ up to 2 lbs/wk

Obesity needs to be confronted and addressed – which means it needs to be identified. BMI and waist circumference should be assessed at least annually. Overweight and obese patients should be warned of the health risks.

Counseling should emphasize that lifestyle changes that produce even modest, sustained weight loss of 3%-5% produce clinically meaningful health benefits (decreased triglycerides, A1C, and the risk of developing type 2 diabetes), and greater weight loss produces greater benefits.

Rather than emphasizing one particular type of diet, the guidelines state that "A variety of dietary approaches can produce weight loss in overweight and obese adults." Dietary strategies could consist of any 1 of the following methods:

kcal/day
* 1,200 - 1,500 ♀
* 1,500 - 1,800 ♂

- Reducing food and calorie intake: (1,200–1,500 kcal/day for women and 1,500–1,800 kcal/day for men or using a 500-750 kcal/day energy deficit; (a 500 kcal decrease per day) equals 1 pound weight lost per week (3,500 kcal/pound), or

- Using "one of the diets" that restricts certain food types (such as restricting high-carbohydrate foods, low-fiber foods, or high-fat foods) in order to create an energy deficit by reduced food intake.

- In select patients and only under medical monitoring the use of a very low calorie diet (defined as < 800 kcal/day) can be provided.

In all patients, weight loss support should include regular contact with a trained person, with body weight and diet monitoring and regular physical activity (i.e., 200-300 minutes/week).

bariatric
surgery
- BMI ≥ 40
OR
- BMI ≥ 35
+ comorbidities

The guidelines recommend bariatric surgery for adults with a BMI ≥ 40 or BMI ≥ 35 with an obesity-related comorbid condition. This will involve adjusting medications and nutrient support. Post-bariatric requirements are discussed in more detail later in this chapter.

Drug Treatment: OTC and Rx

produces ephedra
analog

OTC weight loss drugs commonly contain stimulants, such as the ephedra alkaloid bitter orange or related compounds, along with excessive amounts of caffeine. Caffeine is packaged under different names – including as yerba mate, guarana or concentrated green tea powder. Tolerance develops quickly with the use of these agents, requiring higher doses. In patients with cardiovascular (CVD) risk – which is often present in overweight patients – they carry significant risk. A newer OTC product called *Fastin* (the name is taken from the previous Rx drug phentermine) is being marketed as a "thermogenic intensifier." It contains stimulants, including synephrine and caffeine. For CVD-risk patients it should be viewed as a potential heart-attack-in-a-bottle. In February of 2012 Dr. Oz recommended raspberry ketones and sales took off. There is no evidence that this compound works for weight loss, and the structure is similar to synephrine. In the last two years Dr. Oz has promoted garcinia cambogia and green coffee bean extract. None of these products are proven effective. (Thank you Dr. Oz; please stop. These recommendations keep community pharmacists busier than normal, and do not appear to help patients.)

Wow!

Prescription agents are not appropriate for patients with small amounts of weight to lose. Prescription drugs should not be used in patients who are not obese or overweight with at least one weight-related co-morbidity (such as diabetes or hypertension). They are only used in addition to a dietary plan and increased physical activity, per the FDA. However, one may wish to consider what they are eating, as carbohydrates are a culprit to many in obtaining long-term weight loss.

Two new drugs were approved in 2012 for weight loss; both of these drugs were originally rejected by the FDA for psychiatric and cardiovascular effects *(Qsymia)* and for cancer and cardiovascular effects *(Belviq)*. With these two agents, pharmacists should consider the "7 year rule" – which roughly translates to: do not recommend new agents until they have been out for awhile and used in millions – not including your patients, friends and family – in order to get a more complete understanding of the adverse effect profile than might have been evident in clinical trials. Naltrexone/Bupropion *(Contrave)* was approved in 2014. The three newest drugs had variable effects on weight loss in clinical trials (at one year, vs placebo): *Qsymia* (~20 pounds), *Belviq* (~7 pounds) and *Contrave* (~9 pounds). The older stimulant agents are only used short-term to "jump start" a diet. Orlistat is available both OTC *(Alli)* and Rx *(Xenical)*; it is a useful agent to reduce dietary fat absorption, but has GI tolerability issues (flatulence can be embarrassing) and must be taken with a reduced fat diet. The <u>fat</u> contibutes to the <u>flat</u>. Any medication must be taken concurrently with a reasonable dietary plan, and preferably, physical activity that contributes to good health and weight management. *Qysmia, Belviq* and *Contrave,* unlike stimulants, can be continued long-term for maintenance. None of them should continue to be used if the patient did not obtain at least a 5% weight loss in 12 weeks. A 3 mg SC formulation of liraglutide called Saxenda is expected to be approved in 2015 for weight loss. See the diabetes section for detailed drug information; for diabetes the maximum dose is 1.8 mg daily. The primary side effect, even at the lower dose, is nausea.

Handwritten margin note (left): 3-4 wks

Handwritten margin note (right): — sub Q liraglutide · Victoza® max dose for D 1.8 mg/day · Saxenda® wt loss dose 3 mg ✱ main SE: nausea

DRUG	DOSING	SAFETY/SIDE EFFECTS/MONITORING

Phentermine: Sympathomimetic, with effects similar to amphetamines, causing increase in norepinephrine.

Topiramate: Effects due to decreased appetite and satiety, possibly by enhancing GABA, blocking glutamate receptors and/or weak inhibition of carbonic anhydrase.

DRUG	DOSING	SAFETY/SIDE EFFECTS/MONITORING
Phentermine and topiramate extended-release capsules (Qsymia) C-IV REMS drug: only through certified pharmacy network; not all stores will carry. Psychiatric and cardiac monitoring required.	Start at 3.75-23 mg PO Q AM x 14 days, then titrate up based on weight loss.	**CONTRAINDICATIONS** Hyperthyroidism, glaucoma, MAO I use within past 14 days, pregnancy, lactation **SIDE EFFECTS** Dizziness, headache, cognitive impairment, constipation, dry mouth, insomnia, paresthesias, ↓ serum bicarbonate, upper respiratory tract infection, pharyngitis Decrease dose with moderate renal impairment **NOTES** CrCl < 50 mL/min max dose phentermine 7.5 mg/topiramate 46 mg daily. Pregnancy Category X.

Handwritten margin note (left): ↓ ~20 lbs

Handwritten margin note (right of side effects): → from topiramate

Handwritten note (bottom left): REMS - congenital malformations (orofacial clefts) => ♀ w/ reproductive potential

Handwritten note (bottom right): phentermine (topiramate → preg D)

Weight Loss Drugs Continued

DRUG	DOSING	SAFETY/SIDE EFFECTS/MONITORING
Naltrexone/Bupropion *90mg* (Contrave) The naltrexone component ↓ food cravings and the bupropion component ↓ appetite.	ER tab 8 mg/**90** mg Week 1: 1 tab QAM Week 2: 1 tab QAM, 1 tab QPM Week 3: 2 tabs QAM, 1 tab QPM Week 4+: 2 tabs QAM, 2 tabs QPM	**BOXED WARNING** Not approved for treatment of major depressive disorder (MDD) or psychiatric disorders. Antidepressants can increase the risk of suicidal thinking and behavior in children, adolescents, and young adults (18-24 years of age) with MDD and psychiatric disorders; consider risk prior to prescribing. **CONTRAINDICATIONS** Uncontrolled hypertension, seizure disorder, use of other bupropion-containing products, bulimia/anorexia nervosa, chronic opioid or opiate agonist or partial agonist use, or acute opiate withdrawal, abrupt discontinuation of alcohol, benzodiazepines, barbiturates, and antiepileptic drugs, concomitant use of MAO Is, pregnancy **WARNINGS** Use with caution in patients with underlying psychiatric disorders **SIDE EFFECTS** Nausea, constipation, headache, sleep disorder, vomiting (all > 10%) **NOTES** Pregnancy Category X. Do not cut, chew, or crush tablets. 14 days wash-out period between MAO I and *Contrave*. Patients should be off all opioids for minimum of 7-10 days before initiating *Contrave*. Naltrexone will block opioids, which will block analgesia; do not use concurrently.

Handwritten left margin: 8mg; ↓ ~9 lbs; qd then BID

Serotonin 5-HT$_{2c}$ receptor agonist

Lorcaserin *(Belviq)* C-IV	10 mg PO BID Discontinue if 5% weight loss not achieved by week 12	**CONTRAINDICATIONS** Pregnancy **SIDE EFFECTS** Headache, dizziness, fatigue, nausea, dry mouth, constipation, hypoglycemia (in diabetes patients, monitor, ↓ lymphocytes) **NOTES** Per FDA, company required to monitor cardiovascular outcomes after release. Pregnancy Category X. Serotonergic risk with additive agents.

Handwritten left margin: ↓ ~7 lbs; BID dosing

Handwritten note: d/c if ↓ 5% wt not achieved by week 12

Handwritten bottom note:
* use Rx drugs in obese pts (BMI ≥ 30)
 OR overwt pts w/ 1+ wt-related condition
 (BMI = 25 - 29.9)

Weight Loss Drugs Continued

DRUG	DOSING	SAFETY/SIDE EFFECTS/MONITORING

Short term appetite suppressants – sympathomimetics, with effects similar to amphetamines, causing increase in norepinephrine

DRUG	DOSING	SAFETY/SIDE EFFECTS/MONITORING
Phentermine *(Adipex-P, Suprenza-ODT)* C-IV	15-37.5 mg PO, before or after breakfast, or in divided doses	**CONTRAINDICATIONS** MAO Is within past 14 days Avoid use with hypertension, PAH, hyperthyroidism, glaucoma, abuse potential
Diethylpropion *(Tenuate)* C-IV	25 mg PO IR, TID 1 hour before meals and mid-evening 75 mg PO SR, once in midmorning	**SIDE EFFECTS** Dizziness, tremor, agitation, tachycardia, blood pressure elevations, insomnia, cardiovascular complications, dependence, psychotic symptoms possible **NOTES** Used for 3-4 weeks to "jump-start" a diet.

[handwritten: in BMI > 27 w/ health compx OR > 30 ⊖ compx]

Long-term lipase inhibitor

[handwritten left margin: 2 x OTC strength; take w/ fat-containing meals; use w/ low-fat diet plan]

DRUG	DOSING	SAFETY/SIDE EFFECTS/MONITORING
Orlistat Rx *(Xenical)*	120 mg PO w/each meal containing fat Both orlistat formulations must be used with a low-fat diet plan.	**WARNING** (Rare) cases liver damage **SIDE EFFECTS** GI (flatus with discharge, fecal urgency, fatty stool) ~13 lbs in 1 year **NOTES** Increased risk urinary oxalate stones Reduces 1/3 dietary fat Take multivitamin with A, D, E, K and beta carotene at bedtime or separated by 2+ hours from *Xenical*. Do not use with cyclosporine or separate by 3+ hours. Separate levothyroxine by 4 hours. Must stick to dietary plan for both weight improvements and to help moderate side effects.

[handwritten: • ↓ ~ 13 lbs/yr • ↓ 1/3 dietary fat • take w/ multivit (ADEK) + β-carotene 4 hrs or sep. 2+ hrs • separate CsA by 3+ hrs • separate levothyrox by 4 hrs]

OTC

DRUG	DOSING	SAFETY/SIDE EFFECTS/MONITORING
Orlistat OTC *(Alli)*	60 mg PO w/each meal containing fat	Same as *Xenical* (above) for counseling, vitamin and diet/fat intake, and drug interactions. ~5 pounds in 6 months Reduces 1/4 dietary fat

[handwritten: • ↓ ~ 5 lbs/6 mo • ↓ 1/4 dietary fat]

Post-Bariatric Surgery; Pharmacists Role

The guidelines recommend advising adults with a BMI ≥ 40 or BMI ≥ 35 with an obesity-related comorbid conditions who are motivated to lose weight and who have not responded to other options that bariatric surgery may be an appropriate option to improve health, and offer referral to an experienced bariatric surgeon for consultation and evaluation. This

[handwritten: ursodiol (Actigall®, Urso 250®, Urso Forte®)
• dissolves gallstones (do not use if gallbladder removed)
• also for 1° biliary cirrhosis
• give Al-based antacids 2 hrs after ursodiol
• Urso Forte® – may split, ⊖ chew
• Urso® / Urso Forte® } take w/ food]

will correlate with easier payment for these procedures and therefore a higher number of patients receiving them. Bariatric surgery restricts food intake, which leads to weight loss. Patients who have bariatric surgery must commit to a lifetime of healthy eating and regular exercise. These are important to sustain the weight loss.

The procedure may use "open" approaches, which involve cutting the stomach in the standard manner, or by laparoscopy. Most bariatric surgery today is laparoscopic because it requires a smaller cut, creates less tissue damage, leads to earlier hospital discharges, and has fewer problems, especially less hernias occurring after surgery. Not all patients are suitable for laparoscopy. Patients who are extremely obese, who have had previous stomach surgery, or who have complex medical problems may require the open approach.

Weight loss surgery requires changes to the drug regimen, and adjustments in nutrients with decreased absorption, depending on the surgery type. This summary will not distinguish between the needs with various surgeries, but rather provide a short review of common problems.

Micronutrients

- One of the most common problems following bariatric surgery is calcium deficiency. Calcium is mostly absorbed in the duodenum, which may be bypassed. Calcium citrate is preferred as it has non-acid dependent absorption.

- Anemia may result from vitamin B12 and iron deficiency; both may require supplementation. Iron and calcium supplements should be separated. *to prevent chelation*

- Some will require life-long supplementation of the fat-soluble vitamins A, D, E and K due to fat malabsorption.

Medications

- Medications may require dose-reduction, and may need to be crushed or in liquid or transdermal form for up to two-months post-surgery. Pharmacists will need to assess which drugs can be safely crushed.

- Due to the risk of gallstones with rapid weight loss, patients may need ursodiol (Actigall, Urso 250, Urso Forte), which dissolves gallstones, unless the gallbladder has been removed. This drug is also used for primary biliary cirrhosis. It cannot be administered with aluminum-based antacids (if used, give 2 hours after ursodiol). *Urso Forte* can be split into halves for appropriate dosage, not chewed. *Urso* and *Urso Forte* should be taken with food. Ursodiol can be made into a sweetened suspension. The most common side effects are headache, dizziness, constipation or diarrhea (both about 26%) and nausea.

- Avoid drugs that are GI irritants – such as NSAIDs and bisphosphonates.

Dumping Syndrome

Dumping syndrome (rapid gastric emptying) occurs when undigested food moves rapidly into the small intestine, and may occur if the surgery bypasses or removes part or all of the stomach. Dumping syndrome can be separated into early and late forms, depending on the occurrence of symptoms in relation to the time elapsed after a meal. Common symptoms include abdominal cramps, nausea and diarrhea.

Methods to Avoid Dumping Syndrome

- Eat smaller meals, avoid fluids with meals (use only between meals).

- Reduce carbs, especially refined carbs, avoid sugar, including glucose, sucrose, fructose, dextrose, honey and corn syrup. Increase protein. Chew well.

- Increase fiber intake, including psyllium, guar gum and pectin. Avoid alcohol and acidic foods.

- Do not lie down after eating.

The prescription drugs Acarbose *(Precose)* and octreotide *(Sandostatin)* are used in some cases. Acarbose delays carbohydrate absorption (see Diabetes section). Octreotide *(Somatostatin)* and the synthetic analogue *Sandostatin* is rarely used in severe cases. The usual initial dose of octreotide is 50 mcg administered subcutaneously BID/TID 30 minutes prior to each meal. Octreotide can cause bradycardia, chest pain, fatigue, dizziness, gastrointestinal and other adverse effects. It is sometimes (uncommonly) used for diarrhea.

to avoid dumping
- smaller meals
- ↓ fluids w/ meals (use only between meals)
- do not lie down after eating
- chew well

- ↓ carbs (refined)
- Ø sugar (glu, fru, su, dex, honey, corn syrup)
- ↑ protein
- ↑ fiber (psyllium, guar gum, pectin)
- Ø EtOH, acidic foods

APPENDIX

PRESCRIPTION TOP-SELLERS

Brand names are provided as a study aid (generic may be top-seller).

RANK	DRUG	BRAND NAME
1	Hydrocodone/Acetaminophen	*Lortab, Vicodin, Xodol*
2	Lisinopril	*Prinivil, Zestril*
3	Levothyroxine	*Levoxyl, Synthroid*
4	Simvastatin	*Zocor*
5	Amlodipine	*Norvasc*
6	Omeprazole	*Prilosec*
7	Amoxicillin	*Moxatag*
8	Atorvastatin	*Lipitor*
9	Metformin	*Fortamet, Glucophage, Glumetza*
10	Azithromycin	*Zithromax, Z-Pak, Zmax*
11	Alprazolam	*Xanax*
12	Hydrochlorothiazide	*Microzide, Oretic*
13	Tramadol	*Ultram*
14	Gabapentin	*Gralise, Neurontin*
15	Sertraline	*Zoloft*
16	Fluticasone Propionate, nasal inhaler	*Flonase*
17	Zolpidem	*Ambien*
18	Citalopram	*Celexa*
19	Metoprolol Tartrate	*Lopressor*
20	Ibuprofen	

RANK	DRUG	BRAND NAME
21	Prednisone	
22	Furosemide	*Lasix*
23	Metoprolol Succinate	*Toprol XL*
24	Oxycodone/Acetaminophen	*Endocet, Percocet, Roxicet, others*
25	Pravastatin	*Pravachol*
26	Losartan	*Cozaar*
27	Atenolol	*Tenormin*
28	Lisinopril/HCTZ	*Prinzide, Zestoretic*
29	Montelukast	*Singulair*
30	Cyclobenzaprine	*Fexmid*
31	Clonazepam	*Klonopin*
32	Fluoxetine	*Prozac*
33	Albuterol	*ProAir HFA, Proventil HFA, Ventolin HFA*
34	Lorazepam	*Ativan*
35	Amoxicillin/Clavulanate	*Augmentin*
36	Ciprofloxacin oral	*Cipro*
37	Meloxicam	*Mobic*
38	Trazodone	
39	Warfarin	*Coumadin*
40	Sulfamethoxazole/Trimethoprim	*Bactrim, Bactrim DS, Septra DS, Sulfatrim*

Prescription Top-Sellers Continued

RANK	DRUG	BRAND NAME
41	Cephalexin	Keflex
42	Carvedilol	Coreg
43	Clopidogrel	Plavix
44	Pantoprazole	Protonix
45	Escitalopram	Lexapro
46	Rosuvastatin	Crestor
47	Esomeprazole	Nexium
48	Ranitidine	Zantac
49	Tamsulosin	Flomax
50	Naproxen	Anaprox, Naprosyn, others
51	Fluconazole	Diflucan
52	Duloxetine	Cymbalta
53	Oxycodone	OxyContin, Roxicodone
54	Bupropion XL	Wellbutrin XL
55	Potassium Chloride	Klor-Con, Micro-K, others
56	Diazepam	Valium
57	Venlafaxine ER	Effexor XR
58	Allopurinol	Aloprim, Zyloprim
59	Fluticasone/Salmeterol	Advair Diskus
60	Methylprednisolone	Medrol, Medrol Dosepak
61	Triamcinolone	Kenalog, others (topicals)
62	Amitriptyline	
63	Paroxetine	Paxil
64	Amphetamine salts	Adderall
65	Losartan/HCTZ	Hyzaar
66	Clonidine	Catapres, Catapres-TTS
67	Doxycycline	Oracea, Doryx, others
68	Triamterene/HCTZ	Dyazide, Maxzide, Maxzide-25
69	Fenofibrate	Antara, Lofibra, Tricor, Trilipix, others
70	Glimepiride	Amaryl

RANK	DRUG	BRAND NAME
71	Metformin ER	Glucophage XR
72	Lovastatin	Altoprev, Mevacor
73	Vitamin D2, Ergocalciferol	
74	Levofloxacin	Levaquin
75	Acetaminophen/Codeine	Tylenol #2, #3, #4
76	Spironolactone	Aldactone
77	Valacyclovir	Valtrex
78	Promethazine	Phenergan
79	Lamotrigine	Lamictal, Lamictal ODT, Lamictal Starter
80	Topiramate	Topamax
81	Alendronate	Fosamax
82	Valsartan	Diovan
83	Influenza Virus Vaccine	Fluvirin, Fluzone, Afluria, others
84	Quetiapine	Seroquel
85	Metronidazole	Flagyl
86	Lisdexamfetamine	Vyvanse
87	Folic acid	
88	Enalapril	Vasotec
89	Glipizide	Glucotrol
90	Cefdinir	
91	Clindamycin oral	Cleocin
92	Risperidone	Risperdal
93	Methylphenidate ER	Concerta
94	Insulin Glargine	Lantus
95	Carisoprodol	Soma
96	Pregabalin	Lyrica
97	Propranolol	Inderal
98	Latanoprost	Xalatan
99	Ondanestron	Zofran
100	Morphine	MS Contin, Avinza, Kadian, others

Prescription Top-Sellers Continued

RANK	DRUG	BRAND NAME
101	Tiotropium	Spiriva HandiHaler
102	Amphetamine Salts ER	Adderall XR
103	Benazepril	Lotensin
104	Celecoxib	Celebrex
105	Benzonatate	Tessalon Perles, Zonatuss
106	Sumatriptan	Imitrex
107	Isosorbide Mononitrate	Monoket
108	Bactroban	Mupirocin
109	Temazepam	Restoril
110	Bupropion SR	Wellbutrin SR
111	Sildenafil	Viagra
112	Hydroxyzine HCl	
113	Mometasone	Nasonex
114	Amlodipine/Benazepril	Lotrel
115	Diclofenac Gel	Voltaren Gel, Flector
116	Sitagliptan	Januvia
117	Buprenorphine/Naloxone	Suboxone
118	Polyethylene Glycol	Golytely, MoviPrep, Nulytely, TriLyte
119	Tadalafil	Cialis
120	Phentermine	Adipex-P, Suprenza
121	Estradiol patch	Vivelle-Dot
122	Acyclovir	Zovirax
123	Aripiprazole	Abilify
124	Valsartan/HCTZ	Diovan HCT
125	Tizanidine	Zanaflex
126	Mirtazapine	Remeron
127	Buspirone	Buspar
128	Finasteride	Proscar
129	Penicillin VK	Pencillin
130	Nitrofurantoin	Macrobid, Macrodantin, Furadantin

RANK	DRUG	BRAND NAME
131	Donepezil	Aricept
132	Nystatin	Bio-Statin
133	Ramipril	Altace
134	Glipizide ER	Glucotrol XL
135	Famotidine	Pepcid
136	Butalbital/Acetaminophen/ Caffeine	Fioricet
137	Ezetimibe	Zetia
138	Levetiracetam	Keppra
139	Nebivolol	Bystolic
140	Glyburide	Diabeta, Glynase
141	Clobetasol	Clobex, Olux, Temovate, others
142	Ketoconazole	Nizoral
143	Lansoprazole	Prevacid
144	Diltiazem	Cardizem, Tiazac
145	Fluticasone, oral inhaler	Flovent HFA, Flovent Diskus
146	Formoterol/Budesonide	Symbicort
147	Methocarbamol	Robaxin
148	Baclofen	Lioresal
149	Methotrexate	Rheumatrex, Trexall
150	Chlorhexidine	Peridex, others
151	Methylphenidate	Ritalin
152	Oseltamivir	Tamiflu
153	Verapamil SR	Calan SR, Isoptin SR
154	Oxycodone	OxyContin
155	Codeine/Promethazine	
156	Meclizine	UniVert
157	Fentanyl	Duragesic
158	Ethinyl Estradiol/Etonogestrel	NuvaRing
159	Hydralazine	
160	Prednisolone	

Prescription Top-Sellers Continued

RANK	DRUG	BRAND NAME
161	Digoxin	Lanoxin
162	Minocycline	Minocin, Solodyn
163	Doxazosin	Cardura
164	Dexlansoprazole	Dexilant
165	Pioglitazone	Actos
166	Gemfibrozil	Lopid
167	Nifedipine	Adalat CC, Nifediac CC, Procardia
168	Ethinyl Estradiol/Norgestimate	Tri-Sprintec, Sprintec, TriNessa, Ortho Tri-Cyclen Lo
169	Hydroxycholoroquine	Plaquenil
170	Dicyclomine	Bentyl
171	Medroxyprogesterone	Depo-Provera
172	Ropinirole	Requip
173	Clotrimazole/Betamethasone	Lotrisone
174	Thyroid (dessicated)	Armour Thyroid
175	Albuterol	Proventil HFA, Ventolin HFA, others
176	Olmesartan	Benicar
177	Insulin Detemir	Levemir FlexTouch
178	Clindamycin, topical	Cleocin, Clindagel, others
179	Phenazopyridine	Pyridium, Uristat, others
180	Prednisolone	Orapred, Pediapred, Prelone, others
181	Memantine	Namenda
182	Hydroxyzine Pamoate	Vistaril
183	Estrogens (conjugated)	Premarin
184	Omega-3 Fatty Acids	Lovaza
185	Oxybutynin	Gelnique, Oxytrol, Ditropan XL
186	Hydrocortisone	A-Hydrocort, Cortef, Solu-CORTEF

RANK	DRUG	BRAND NAME
187	Nortriptyline	Pamelor
188	Methadone	Dolophine, Methadose
189	Divalproex ER	Depakote ER
190	Nitroglycerin	Nitrostat
191	Dextromethorphan/Promethazine	
192	Lithium	Lithobid
193	Timolol maleate	Timoptic, Istalol, Betimol
194	Cefuroxime	Ceftin
195	Zolpidem ER	Ambien CR
196	Beclomethasone	QVAR
197	Metoclopramide	Reglan, Metozolv ODT
198	Levocetirizine	Xyzal
199	Olmesartan/HCTZ	Benicar HCT
200	Terazosin	
201	Cyanocobalamin	Nascobal
202	Divalproex	Depakote
203	Olanzapine	Zyprexa, Zyprexa Relprevv, Zyprexa Zydis
204	Brompheniramine/Pseudoephedrine/Dextromethorphan	Bromfed DM
205	Fluzone High Dose	Influenza virus vaccine
206	Chlorthalidone	Thalitone
207	Solifenacin	VESIcare
208	Dexmethylphenidate ER	Focalin XR
209	Insulin Aspart	Novolog FlexPen
210	Eszopiclone	Lunesta
211	Hydromorphone	Dilaudid
212	Carbidopa/Levodopa	Sinemet, Sinemet CR

Prescription Top-Sellers Continued

RANK	DRUG	BRAND NAME
213	Erythromycin	E.E.S., Ery-Tab, EryPed, Erythrocin
214	Cetirizine	Zyrtec
215	Ofloxacin	Ocuflox, Floxin Otic
216	Quinapril	Accupril
217	Dextroamphetamine/ Amphetamine ER	Adderall XR
218	Colchicine	Colcrys
219	Oxybutynin ER	Ditropan XL
220	Indomethacin	Indocin
221	Desvenlafaxine	Pristiq
222	Oxcarbazepine	Trileptal
223	Labetalol	Trandate
224	Bisoprolol/HCTZ	Ziac
225	Benztropine	Cogentin
226	Ethinyl Estradiol/ Norethindrone	Loestrin, Loestrin 24 Fe, Microgestin Fe 1/20
227	Rivaroxaban	Xarelto
228	Fluocinonide	Vanos
229	Lidocaine topical	Lidoderm
230	Neomycin/Polymyxin B/ Hydrocortisone	Cortisporin, Cortomycin
231	Ketorolac	Acular, Toradol
232	Sitagliptan/Metformin	Janumet
233	Pramipexole	Mirapex
234	Testosterone gel	AndroGel
235	Lumigan	Bimatoprost
236	Venlafaxine	Effexor

RANK	DRUG	BRAND NAME
237	Insulin Aspart	Novolog
238	Phenytoin	Dilantin, Phenytek
239	Niacin ER	Niaspan
240	Ezetimibe/Simvastatin	Vytorin
241	Terbinafine	Lamisil, Terbinex
242	Insulin lispro	Humalog
243	Nabumetone	Relafen
244	Amiodarone	Cordarone, Pacerone
245	Tretinoin	Atralin, Avita, Refissa, Renova, Renova Pump, Retin-A, Retin-A Micro
246	Guanfacine XR	Intuniv
247	Ethinyl Estradiol/Drospirenone	Yaz, Yasmin, others
248	Olopatadine	Pataday
249	Travoprost	Travatan Z
250	Cyclosporine, eye drops	Restasis
251	Clarithomycin	Biaxin
252	Hydrocodone/ Chlorpheniramine	TussiCaps, Tussionex
253	Glyburide/Metformin	Glucovance
254	Irbesartan	Avapro
255	Medroxyprogesterone	Provera
256	Azelastine	Astelin, Astepro
257	Phenobarbital	Luminal
258	Moxifloxacin	Vigamox
259	Diphenoxylate/Atropine	Lomotil

RxPrep thanks IMS Health and Mr. Robert Hunkler for providing this list to aid the students.

COMMON MEDICAL ABBREVIATIONS

Medical safety warning: Do not use any in the "DO NOT USE" abbreviation list in your institution; the meaning of abbreviations varies.

ABBREVIATION	MEANING
AAA	Abdominal Aortic Aneurysm
A&O	Alert & Oriented
ABG	Arterial Blood Gas
ACOG	American Congress of Obstetricians and Gynecologists
ACTH	Adrenocorticotropic Hormone
ADH	Anti-Diuretic Hormone
ADR	Adverse Drug Reaction
ADT	Alternate Day Therapy
AF	Atrial Fibrillation, or A.Fib
AGEF	Acute Generalized Exanthematous Pustulosis
AIN	Acute Interstitial Nephritis
ALT	Alanine Aminotransferase
ANA	Antinuclear Antibody
ANS	Autonomic Nervous System
APTT	Activated Partial Thromboplastin Time
ARDS	Acute Respiratory Distress Syndrome
ARF	Acute Renal Failure
AST	Aspartate Aminotransferase
ATN	Acute Tubular Necrosis
AVP	Arginine Vasopressin
BEE	Basal Energy Expenditure
BMP	Basic Metabolic Panel
BP	Blood Pressure
BPH	Benign Prostatic Hypertrophy
BPM	Beats Per Minute, Breaths Per Minute
BUN	Blood Urea Nitrogen
C-I, C-II, C-III, C-IV, C-V	Refers to Controlled Drug Categories
C&S	Culture and Sensitivity
C/O	Complaining Of
CA	Cancer
CABG	Coronary Artery Bypass Graft
CAD	Coronary Artery Disease
CAPES	*Citrobacter, Acinetobacter, Providencia, Enterobacter, Serratia*
CBC	Complete Blood Count
CC	Chief Complaint
CCB	Calcium Channel Blocker

ABBREVIATION	MEANING
CD	Crohn's Disease
CF	Cystic Fibrosis
CH	Cholesterol
CHF	Congestive Heart Failure
CI	Cardiac Index, Contraindicated
CMV	*Cytomegalovirus*
CNS	Central Nervous System
CO	Cardiac Output
COPD	Chronic Obstructive Pulmonary Disease
CP	Chest Pain or Cerebral Palsy
CPAP	Continuous Positive Airway Pressure
CPK	Creatine Phosphokinase
CPR	Cardiopulmonary Resuscitation
CrCL	Creatinine Clearance
CRF	Chronic Renal Failure
CRP	C-reactive Protein
CSF	Cerebrospinal Fluid
CT	Computerized Tomography
CV	Cardiovascular
CVA	Cerebrovascular Accident
CVP	Central Venous Pressure
CXR	Chest X-Ray
D1	Dopamine 1 Receptor
D2	Dopamine 2 Receptor
D/C	Discontinue or Discharge
D5W	5% Dextrose in Water
DDIs	Drug-Drug Interactions
DJD	Degenerative Joint Disease (Osteoarthritis)
DKA	Diabetic Ketoacidosis
DM	Diabetes Mellitus
DOC	Drug of Choice
DOE	Dyspnea on Exertion
DRESS Syndrome	Drug Reaction with Eosinophilia and Systemic Symptoms
DVT	Deep Venous Thrombosis
Dx	Diagnosis
EC	Enteric Coated

Common Medical Abbreviations Continued

ABBREVIATION	MEANING
ECG	Electrocardiogram
EIAD	Extended-Interval Aminoglycoside Dosing (PK chapter)
ESBL	Extended Spectrum Beta Lactamases
ESR	Erythrocyte Sedimentation Rate
ETOH	Ethanol
F/U	Follow-Up
FBS	Fasting Blood Sugar
FEV$_1$	Forced Expiratory Volume in 1 second
FT4	Free Thyroxine (T4)
fxn	Function
GFR	Glomerular Filtration Rate
GI	Gastrointestinal
GNR	Gram Negative Rod
GTT	Glucose Tolerance Test
H/O	History Of
HA	Headache
HACEK	*Haemophilus, Actinobacillus, Cardiobacterium, Eikenella, Kingella*
HBV	Hepatitis B Virus
HCG	Human Chorionic Gonadotropin
HCT	Hematocrit
HCTZ, HCT	Hydrochlorothiazide
HCV	Hepatitis C Virus
HDL, HDL-C	High Density Lipoprotein
HF	Heart Failure
Hgb	Hemoglobin
HIV	Human Immunodeficiency Virus
HJR	Hepatojugular Reflex
HNPEK	Haemophilus influenzae, Neisseria spp, Proteus mirabilis, E. coli, Klebsiella pneumonia
HPI	History of Present Illness
HR	Heart Rate
HSV	Herpes Simplex Virus
HTN	Hypertension
HUS/TTP	Hemolytic-Uremic Syndrome and Thrombotic Thrombocytopenic Purpura
Hx	History
I&O	Intake and Output
IBD	Inflammatory Bowel Disease
IBS	Irritable Bowel Syndrome
ICU	Intensive Care Unit

ABBREVIATION	MEANING
IE	Infective Endocarditis
IM	Intramuscular
INR	International Normalized Ratio
IV	Intravenous
IVP	Intravenous Push
LD	Loading Dose
LDH	Lactate Dehydrogenase
LDL, LDL-C	Low-Density Lipoprotein
LFTs	Liver Function Tests
LLSB	Left Lower Sternal Border
LVH	Left Ventricular Hypertrophy
MAO	Monoamine Oxidase
MAO I	Monoamine Oxidase Inhibitor
MAP	Mean Arterial Pressure
MCH	Mean Cell Hemoglobin
MCHC	Mean Cell Hemoglobin Concentration
MCV	Mean Corpuscular Volume
MD	Maintenance Dose
MI	Myocardial Infarction
MRI	Magnetic Resonance Imaging
MRSA	Methicillin-Resistant Staph Aureus
MS	Multiple Sclerosis or Morphine Sulfate (Don't use for Morphine – Dangerous)
MSSA	Methicillin-Sensitive Staph Aureus
MVA	Motor Vehicle Accident
MVI	Multivitamin Injection
N/V	Nausea and Vomiting
N/V/D	Nausea, Vomiting, Diarrhea
NG	Nasogastric
NKA	No Known Allergies
NKDA	No Known Drug Allergies
NOAC	New Oral Anticoagulant
NPO	Nothing By Mouth
NRT	Nicotine Replacement Therapy
NSAIDs	Nonsteroidal Anti-Inflammatory Drugs
NSR	Normal Sinus Rhythm
ODT	Orally Disintegrating Tablet
P-gp	P-glycoprotein
PAP	Pulmonary Artery Pressure

Common Medical Abbreviations Continued

ABBREVIATION	MEANING
PCC	Prothrombin Complex Concentrate
PCI	Percutaneous Coronary Intervention
PCN	Penicillin
PCOS	Polycystic Ovary Syndrome
PCWP	Pulmonary Capillary Wedge Pressure
PE	Pulmonary Embolus, or Physical Exam
PEK	*Proteus mirabilis, E. coli, Klebsiella pneumonia*
PKU	Phenylketonuria
PMH	Past Medical History
PO	Oral
PPD	Purified Protein Derivative
PRBC	Packed Red Blood Cells
PRN	As Needed
PT	Prothrombin Time, or Physical Therapy
Pt	Patient
PTCA	Percutaneous Transluminal Coronary Angioplasty
PTH	Parathyroid Hormone
PUD	Peptic Ulcer Disease
PVC	Polyvinyl Chloride
Q	Every
R/O	Rule Out
RA	Rheumatoid Arthritis
RASS	Richmond Agitation and Sedation Scale
RBC	Red Blood Cell
RML	Right Middle Lobe
ROS	Review of Systems
RSI	Rapid Sequence Intubation
RSV	Respiratory Syncytial Virus
Rx	Treatment, Prescription
rxn	Reaction
S/P	Status Post
SCr	Serum Creatinine
SIADH	Syndrome of Inappropriate Antidiuretic Hormone
SIG	Write on Label
SJS	Stevens Johnson Syndrome
SLE	Systemic Lupus Erythematous

ABBREVIATION	MEANING
SOAP	Subjective, Objective, Assessment, Plan
SOB	Shortness of Breath
SC or SQ	Subcutaneous
STAT	Immediately
S/Sx	Signs and Symptoms
Sx	Symptoms
TB	Tuberculosis
TC	Total Cholesterol
TdP	Torsade de Pointes
TEG	Thromboelastography
TEN	Toxic Epidermal Necrolysis
TG	Triglycerides
TIA	Transient Ischemic Attack
TIBC	Total Iron Binding Capacity
TPN	Total Parenteral Nutrition
TSH	Thyroid Stimulating Hormone
TTP	Thrombotic Thrombocytopenic Purpura
Tx	Treatment
UA	Urinalysis
UC	Ulcerative Colitis
UFH	Unfractionated Heparin
ULN	Upper Limit of Normal
URTI	Upper Respiratory Tract Infection
UTI	Urinary Tract Infection
V1	Vasopressin 1 Receptor
V2	Vasopressin 2 Receptor
VF	Ventricular Fibrillation
VRE	Vancomycin-Resistant Enterococcus
VT	Ventricular Tachycardia
WBC	White Blood Cells
WNL	Within Normal Limits
WPW	Wolff-Parkinson-White Syndrome
y/o	Years Old
yr	Year

INDEX